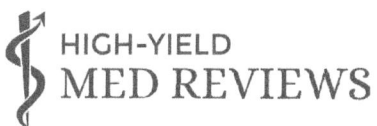

2025

A COMPREHENSIVE *RAPID REVIEW*

NAPLEX

Pharmacology & Drug Classes

Editors

Anthony J. Busti, MD, PharmD, MSc, FNLA, FAHA
Craig Cocchio, PharmD, BCPS, DABAT
Cassie Boland, PharmD, BCACP, CDCES

Contributing Authors

Allison Butts, PharmD, BCOP
Erika Heffner, PharmD, MBA, BCPS
Shawn Riser Taylor, PharmD, CPP, CDCES
Elizabeth Travers, PharmD, BCOP
Christine Vo, PharmD, BCPS

2025 NAPLEX – Pharmacology & Drug Classes: A Comprehensive Rapid Review
Part 2 of the 2025 NAPLEX Comprehensive Rapid Review 3 Book Series

Published in the United States of America by High-Yield Med Reviews
P.O. Box 690044 | San Antonio, TX 78269
www.highyieldmedreviews.com

High-Yield Med Reviews is an official brand of MedEducation, LLC. MedEducation, LLC does business as (dba) High-Yield Med Reviews. High-Yield Med Reviews is a registered trademark of MedEducation, LLC in the United States of America.

Copyright © 2024 by High-Yield Med Reviews

All rights reserved. No part of this publication may be reproduced, stored in a retrieval system, distributed, or transmitted by any means, electronic, mechanical, photocopying, recording and/or otherwise, without the prior written permission of the publishers.

ISBN 979-8-3302-3168-3

Printed and bound in U.S.A by IngramSpark, Lightning Source LLC

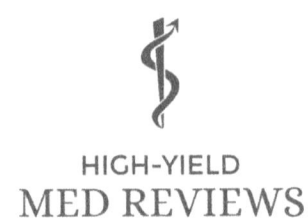

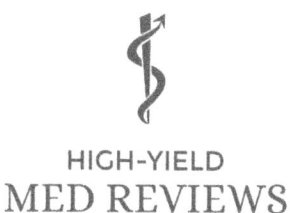

HIGH-YIELD MED REVIEWS

Disclaimer for Educational Material:
All rights reserved. MedEducation LLC, (dba, High-Yield MED Reviews) is a Texas corporation, advised by healthcare providers who provide unbiased education in generally accepted practices. No part of this material may be reproduced, stored, or transmitted in any way whatsoever without written permission from the CEO of MedEducation, LLC. The editors rely primarily on peer-reviewed, published medical information and on the opinions of the editorial staff and independent peer-reviewers. All education and recommendations are considered to be educational and not meant to apply to specific patients. The information provided in our reviews should be used appropriately in the context of the provider's legal role as a healthcare provider in their respective state or country. MedEducation, LLC do not accept responsibility for the application of this information in direct or indirect patient care. It is the responsibility of you, the healthcare provider in training or practice, to ascertain the status of each drug and to check the product information provided by the manufacturer of each drug for any changes. The editors and authors have made every effort to provide accurate and complete information and shall not be held responsible for any damage from any error, possible omission, or inaccuracy.

Disclaimer for Online Material:
The following pertains to any and all online medical or drug information provided online to include, but not limited to, Q-Bank, online lectures, webinars, case-reviews, online drug reference tables, drug reference tables, medical calculators, database material, etc. By your choice to use any of the material available online on the High-Yield MED Reviews website, you agree that your use of this website and its products and services is governed by High-Yield MED Reviews' Terms and Conditions, Individual Customer Agreement, Privacy Policy, and any and all other policies found on websites (regardless of whether you individually registered and paid for access to them).

For additional information, please refer to our policies online.

Table of Contents

Book 2: Pharmacology & Drug Classes

CARDIOLOGY — 1

- Antiarrhythmics
  - Class Ia Agents — 3
  - Class Ib Agents — 8
  - Class Ic Agents — 12
  - Class II Agents — 16
  - Class III Agents — 25
  - Class IV Agents — 31
  - Misc/Unclassified — 36
- Antihypertensives
  - ACE-Inhibitors — 41
  - Alpha-1 Blockers (Non-Selective) — 47
  - Alpha-2 Agonists — 52
  - ARBs — 57
  - Beta-Blockers — 62
  - Calcium Channel Blockers — 70
  - Direct Renin Inhibitor — 77
  - Neprilysin Inhibitors — 79
  - Vasodilators — 82
    - Nitrates — 82
    - Miscellaneous — 87
- Antithrombotic Agents
  - Antiplatelet Agents
    - GPIIbIIIa Receptor Blockers — 94
    - Miscellaneous /Other — 98
    - Thienopyridines (P2Y12 Inhibitors) — 102
  - Anticoagulants — 107
    - Direct Thrombin Inhibitors (DTI) — 107
    - Factor Xa Inhibitors (Oral) — 112
    - Heparin / LMWH — 117
    - Vitamin K Antagonists - Warfarin — 123
  - Thrombolytics — 127
- Antithrombotic Reversal Agents
  - Antidotes — 132
  - Antifibrinolytics — 137
  - Phytonadione and Protamine — 141
- Diuretics
  - Aldosterone Antagonists/Potassium Sparing Diuretics — 145
  - Carbonic Anhydrase Inhibitors & Osmotic Agents — 151
  - Loop Diuretics — 156
  - Thiazide Diuretics — 161

CARDIOLOGY (cont'd)

Hemodynamic Agents
    Inotropes   167
    Vasopressors   171
Lipid Lowering Agents
    Angiopoietin-Like Protein 3 (ANGPTL3) Inhibitor   176
    Bile Acid Binding Sequestrants   178
    Ezetimibe   182
    Fibrates   185
    Niacin   188
    Omega - 3 Fatty Acids   191
    PCSK-9 Inhibitors   194
    Small Interfering Ribonucleic Acid   198
    Statins   200

DERMATOLOGY   207

    Acne Agents   209
    Calcineurin Inhibitors (Topical)   216
    Caustics
        Aluminum chloride, Ferric sulfate, Silver nitrate   219
    Miscellaneous Agents   222
    Non-Steroidal Antiinflammatory Drugs (NSAIDS) - Topical   228

ELECTROLYTES   233

    Magnesium   233
    Potassium   239
    Sodium   244

ENDOCRINOLOGY   251

Androgen Replacement
    Testosterone Replacement   253
Antidiabetic Agents - Non-Insulins
    Alpha Glucosidase Inhibitors   257
    Amylin Analogs   259
    Biguanides (Metformin)   261
    DPP-4 Inhibitors   264
    GIP/GLP-1 Receptor Agonist   267
    GLP-1 Receptor Agonist   270
    Meglitinides   274
    SGLT-2 Inhibitors   276
    Sulfonylureas   283
    Thiazolidinediones (TZDs)   286
Antidiabetic Agents - Insulins
    Insulin (Long Acting or Basal)   289
    Insulin (Rapid & Short Acting)   294

ENDOCRINOLOGY (cont'd)

Antigout Agents	
General Antigout Agents	300
Xanthine Oxidase Inhibitors	305
Corticosteroids	
Long-Acting Corticosteroids	309
Short To Medium Acting Corticosteroids	313
Corticosteroid Summary Table	319
Glucagon	320
Glucagon Receptor Agonist	323
Hormones	
Insulin-Like Growth Factor	341
Nonsteroidal Mineralocorticoid Receptor Antagonist	327
Pancreatic Enzymes	330
Phosphate-Binding Agents	333
Potassium Binding Agents	338
Thyroid Agents	
Iodides	341
Thioamides	344
Thyroid Hormones	348
Vasopressin Receptor Antagonists	352

GASTROENTEROLOGY — 357

5-ASA Derivatives	359
Adsorbents and Antisecretory	362
Antacids	
Histamine H2 Receptor Antagonists	366
Proton Pump Inhibitors (PPIs)	370
Antiemetics	
Dopamine Antagonists	375
Miscellaneous Antiemetics	380

GASTROENTEROLOGY

Serotonin Antagonist Antiemetics	385
Substance P and NK1 Antagonists	389
Antimotility Agents	393
Laxatives	397
Prokinetic Agents	405

GENITOURINARY — 411

5-Alpha Reductase Inhibitors	413
Alpha 1a Blocker (Selective)	416
Antimuscarinics & Beta-3 Receptor Activator	419
Type 5 PDE Inhibitors	425

HEMATOLOGY — 429

- Colony Stimulating Factors (CSA)
  - Erythropoiesis Stimulating Agents — 431
  - Granulocyte colony-stimulating factor — 435
  - Megakaryocyte Growth Factor — 439
- Iron Replacement & Supplements — 442

IMMUNOLOGY — 449

- Antihistamines — 451
- Antirejection Agents
  - Anti-CD52 Monoclonal Antibody — 460
  - Antithymocyte Globulin — 463
  - Calcineurin Inhibitors — 466
  - Interferon — 470
- Immunosuppressant Agent
  - Antimetabolites — 476
  - Antiproliferative Agents (mTOR Inhibitors) — 480
  - DMARDs — 484
  - IL-1 Antagonists — 490
  - IL-2 Antagonists — 494
  - IL-6 Antagonists — 497
  - IL-17 Antagonists — 500
  - IL-23 Antagonists — 503
  - Janus Kinase Inhibitors — 507
  - Selective T-Cell Costimulation Blocker — 511
  - Sphingosine 1-Phosphate (S1P) Receptor Modulator — 514
  - TNF-Alpha Antagonists — 518
- Leukotriene Modifiers — 523
- Vaccines
  - General Concepts and Summary — 527
  - Adult Schedule — 548
  - Infant and Child Schedule — 552
  - Preteen and Teen Schedule — 555
  - SARS-CoV-2 Vaccines — 557

INFECTIOUS DISEASES — 561

- Antibiotics
  - Aminoglycosides — 563
  - Beta-Lactams
    - Aminopenicillins — 568
    - Antistaphylococcal Penicillins — 573
    - Carbapenems — 576
    - Cephalosporins 1st Generation — 580
    - Cephalosporins 2nd Generation — 583
    - Cephalosporins 3rd Generation — 586
    - Cephalosporins 4th-5th Generation — 590
    - Monobactams — 593
    - Natural Penicillin — 596

INFECTIOUS DISEASES (cont'd)	
Chloramphenicol	599
Clindamycin (Lincosamides)	602
Cyclic Lipopeptide	605
Fluoroquinolones	608
Miscellaneous Antibiotics	615
Glycopeptides	618
Macrolides	622
Nitroimidazole (Metronidazole, Tinidazole)	626
Oxazolidinones	629
Polymyxins	632
Quinupristin/dalfopristin	635
Sulfonamide Antibiotics	637
Tetracyclines	642
Antifungals	
Amphotericin	648
Azoles (Systemic Triazoles)	652
Azoles (Topical Imidazoles)	657
Echinocandins	662
Flucytosine	665
Other Antifungals	668
Antimycobacterials	
General Agents	672
Isoniazid	676
Rifamycins	679
Antivirals	
CMV Antivirals	683
COVID Antivirals	688
Hepatitis B Antivirals	694
Hepatitis C Antivirals	698
HSV and VZV Antivirals	703
Influenza Antiviral	708
Palivizumab	713
Ribavirin	715
HIV / Antiretrovirals	
Combination Dosage Forms	718
CYP450 Inhibitors	723
Entry Inhibitors	728
Integrase Inhibitors	732
NNRTIs (Non-Nucleoside Reverse Transcriptase Inhibitors)	737
NRTIs (Nucleotide/Nucleoside Reverse Transcriptase Inhibitors)	742
Protease Inhibitors	749

MUSCULOSKELETAL	755
Anit-FGF23 MABs	757
Bisphosphonates	760
Calcimimetics	765

MUSCULOSKELETAL (cont'd)

Calcitonin	768
Calcium Salts	771
Parathyroid Hormone Analogs	776
RANKL Inhibitor	779
Sclerostin Inhibitor	782
Selective Estrogen Receptor Modulators	785
Vitamin D Analogs	789

NEUROLOGY 795

Alzheimer's Agents	
Acetylcholinesterase Inhibitors	797
Analgesics - Local Anesthetics	801
Analgesics - Non-Opioid	
Acetaminophen	809
NSAIDs	813
Salicylates	823
Skeletal Muscle Relaxants	828
Analgesics - Opioid	
Opioid Analgesics, Long-Acting	837
Opioid Analgesics, Short-Acting	843
Opioid Analgesics, Partial Agonists	851
Opioid Rotation / Conversions	855
Analgesics - Opioid Antagonists	857
Anticonvulsants	
Brain Carbonic Anhydrase Inhibitors	862
GABA Uptake Inhibitors/GABA Transaminase Inhibitors	866
Gabapeninoids	869
NMDA Receptor Antagonist	872
Sodium Channel Modulators	875
SV2A Protein Ligand	881
Voltage Gated Calcium Channel Blockers	884
Antimigraine Agents	
Calcitonin Gene-Related Peptide Receptor Antagonists	889
Serotonin 5-HT1B/d Receptor Agonists	894
Barbiturates	901
Benzodiazepines (Parts 1 & 2)	906
CNS Stimulants	917
Neuromuscular Blockers	
Depolarizing	923
Non-depolarizing	926
Reversal Agents	931
Parkinson's Agents	
Anticholinergics	934
Carbidopa-Levodopa	937
COMT Inhibitors	941
Dopamine Agonists	945

NEUROLOGY (cont'd)

- MAO-B Inhibitors — 949
- Sedative Hypnotics
  - General — 952
  - Etomidate — 957
  - Propofol — 959

OB / GYN — 963

- Contraceptives
  - Non-Oral Contraceptives — 965
  - Oral Contraceptives — 969
- Other Hormones
  - Gonadotropin-Releasing Hormone Agonists and Antagonist — 974

OPHTHALMOLOGY — 979

- Ophthalmic Antiglaucoma Agents
  - Alpha Agonists, Ophthalmic — 981
  - Beta Antagonists, Ophthalmic — 984
  - Carbonic Anhydrase Inhibitors, Ophthalmic — 987
  - Cholinergic Agonists, Ophthalmic — 990
- Ophthalmic/Nasal Antihistamines — 993
- Ophthalmic Anti-inflammatory Agents
  - Glucocorticoids, Ophthalmic — 998
  - Ophthalmic/Nasal Imidazoline — 1003
  - Mast Cell Stabilizer — 1006
  - Non-Steroidal Anti-inflammatory Drugs, Ophthalmic — 1009
- Ophthalmic Prostaglandin Analogs — 1012

OTIC AGENTS — 1017

- Otic Anti-inflammatory and Cerumenolytics — 1019
- Otic Antimicrobials — 1022

PSYCHIATRY / MENTAL HEALTH — 1025

- Allosteric GABA-A Modulator — 1027
- Antidepressants
  - Atypical Antidepressants — 1029
  - MAO-A Inhibitors — 1034
  - SNRI -Serotonin- Norepinephrine Reuptake Inhibitors — 1037
  - SSRI - Selective Serotonin Reuptake Inhibitors — 1041
  - TCA - Tricyclic Antidepressants — 1046
- Antipsychotics
  - Antipsychotics First Generation — 1051
  - Antipsychotics Second Generation — 1057
- Buspirone — 1064
- Lithium — 1066

PSYCHIATRY / MENTAL HEALTH (cont'd)

Insomnia Agents	
Orexin Receptor Antagonists	1070
Non-Benzodiazepines	1074
NMDA Antagonists	1078
Norepinephrine Reuptake Inhibitors	1081
Smoking Cessation Agents	1084
Substance Abuse Deterrents	
Alcohol deterrents	1090

PULMONOLOGY   1095

Bronchodilators, Anticholinergic	
SAMA	1097
LAMA	1100
Bronchodilators, Beta-2 Agonist	
SABA	1104
LABA	1108
CFTR Modulator	1113
Corticosteroids - Inhaled	1117
Inhalers - Combination Products	1121
Methylxanthines	1125
Monoclonal Antibodies (MABs)	
Anti-Asthma	1129
Mucolytics/CF	1133
Phosphodiesterase-4 Inhibitors	1137
Pulmonary Hypertension	
Endothelin-Receptor Antagonists	1141
Guanylate Cyclase Stimulator	1144
Synthetic Prostacyclin & Prostacyclin IP Receptor Agonist	1147

PRACTICE EXAM - DRUG CLASSES   1153

NAPLEX Practice Questions & Answers	1153

Book 1: Foundations of Pharmacy Practice

See Book 1 for full access to the table of contents as part of this book series
- Test Taking Strategies
- Pharmacokinetics & Pharmacodynamics
- Pharmacogenetics
- Herbal Medicines & Nutrition
- Special Topics in Pharmacy
- EBM, Biostastics, & Literature Evaluation

Book 3: Disease States & Pharmacotherapy

See Book 3 for full access to the table of contents as part of this book series
- 370+ Disease State Summaries
- Board Exam Essentials
- Specialized Areas of Pharmacy Practice Reviews
- Practice Questions

COMMON ABBREVIATIONS

A

A1c	Hemoglobin A1c
ABW	Actual body weight
ACE	Angiotensin-converting enzyme
ACS	Acute coronary syndrome
AF	Atrial fibrillation
AID	Automated insulin delivery
AIDS	Acquired Immunodeficiency Syndrome
AKI	Acute kidney injury
AMS	Altered mental status
ANGPTL3	Angiopoietin-like 3
Anti-M	Antimicrosomal antibodies
Anti-Tg	Antithyroglobulin antibodies
AOM	Acute otitis media
Apo B	Apolipoprotein B
AR	Absolute risk
ARB	Angiotensin receptor blocker
ARF	Acute renal failure
ARR	Absolute risk reduction
ASCVD	Atherosclerotic cardiovascular disease

B

BB	Beta-blocker
BBW	Black box warning
bDMARD	Biologic disease modifying antirheumatic drugs
BID	Twice daily
BM	bowel movement
BMD	Bone mineral density
BMI	Body mass index
BMP	Basic metabolic panel
BMS	Bone marrow suppression
BNP	Brain natriuretic peptide
BP	Blood pressure
BPD	Bronchopulmonary dysplasia
BPH	Benign prostatic hypertrophy

C

CABG	Coronary artery bypass graft
CAD	Coronary artery disease
CBC	Complete blood count
CCB	Calcium channel blockers
CGM	Continuous glucose monitoring
CHD	Coronary heart disease or congenital heart disease
CK	Creatine kinase
CMP	Complete metabolic panel
CO	Cardiac output

CPK	Creatine phosphokinase
CrCl	Creatinine clearance
CRP	C-reactive protein
CSII	Continuous subcutaneous insulin infusions
CV	Cardiovascular
CVD	Cardiovascular disease

D

DB	Double-blind
DBP	Diastolic blood pressure
DCT	Distal convoluted tubule
DEXA	Dual-energy x-ray absorptiometry
DKA	Diabetic ketoacidosis
DM	Diabetes mellitus
DOAC	Direct oral anticoagulants
DPP-4	Dipeptidyl-peptidase 4
DTR	Deep tendon reflexes
DVT	Deep vein thrombosis
DXA	Duel-energy x-ray absorptiometry

E

eGFR	Estimated glomerular filtration rate
ECG	Electrocardiogram
ESR	Erythrocyte sedimentation rate
ESRD	End-stage renal disease

F

FPG	Fasting plasma glucose
FXa	Factor Xa

G

GAD	Generalized anxiety disorder
GDM	Gestational diabetes mellitus
GERD	Gastroesophageal reflux disease
GI	Gastrointestinal
GIP	Glucose-dependent insulinotropic polypeptide
GLP-1	Glucagon-like peptide-1
GU	Genitourinary

H

H2RA	Histamine H_2 receptor antagonist
hCG	Human chorionic gonadotropin
Hct	Hematocrit
HCTZ	Hydrochlorothiazide
HCV	Hepatitis C virus
HDL	High density lipoprotein
HF	Heart failure
Hgb	Hemoglobin

HHS	Hyperosmolar hyperglycemic state
HIV	Human immunodeficiency virus
HR	Heart rate
HSV	Herpes simplex virus
HTN	Hypertension

I

IBD	Inflammatory bowel disease
IBS	Irritable bowel syndrome
IBW	Ideal body weight
IL	Interleukin
IM	Intramuscular
IN	Intranasal
INR	International Normalized Ratio
ITT	Intent-to-treat
IV	Intravenous

J

K

K^+	Potassium

L

LD	Loading dose
LDL	Low density lipoprotein
LFT	Liver function test
LVEF	Left ventricular ejection fraction

M

MACE	Major adverse cardiovascular events
MAO	Monoamine oxidase
MD	Maintenance dose
MDD	Major depressive disorder
MEN2	Multiple Endocrine Neoplasia syndrome type 2
MI	Myocardial infarction
MIC	Minimum inhibitory concentration
MRSA	Methicillin resistant staphylococcus aureus
MTC	Medullary thyroid carcinoma

N

Na^+	Sodium
NAFLD	Nonalcoholic fatty liver disease
NASH	Nonalcoholic steatohepatitis
NNH	Number needed to harm
NNT	Number needed to treat
NSTEMI	Non-ST-segment elevation myocardial infarction

O

O₂sats	Oxygen saturation
OA	Osteoarthritis
OCD	Obsessive compulsive disorder
ODT	Orally disintegrating tablet
OGTT	Oral glucose tolerance test
OTC	Over-the-counter

P

PCOS	Polycystic ovarian syndrome
PE	Pulmonary embolism
PO	Oral
PPG	Post-prandial glucose
PPI	Proton-pump inhibitor
PRN	As needed
PTH	Parathyroid hormone

Q

QID	Four times daily

R

R	Randomized
RA	Rheumatoid arthritis
RAAS	Renin-angiotensin-aldosterone system
RBC	Red blood cells
RSV	Respiratory syncytial virus
RR	Relative risk or respiratory rate
RRR	Relative risk reduction

S

SBP	Systolic blood pressure
SC	Subcutaneous
SCD	Sudden cardiac death
SCr	Serum creatinine
SNS	Sympathetic nervous system
STDs	Sexually transmitted diseases
STEMI	ST-segment elevation myocardial infarction
SU	Sulfonylureas
SV	Stroke volume

T

T	Temperature
T1DM	Type 1 diabetes mellitus
T2DM	Type 2 diabetes mellitus
T3	Triiodothyronine
T4	Thyroxine
TAR	Time above range

TBR	Time below range
TC	Total cholesterol
TCA	Tricyclic antidepressant
TFT	Thyroid function test
TG	Triglycerides
TID	Three times daily
TIR	Time in range
TMP/SMX	Trimethoprim/sulfamethoxazole
TSH	Thyroid stimulating hormone
TZD	Thiazolidinediones

U

UA	Urinalysis
UACR	Urine albumin to creatinine ratio
ULN	Upper limit of normal

V

VF	Ventricular fibrillation
VLDL	Very low-density lipoprotein
VRE	Vancomycin resistant enterococci
VTE	Venous thromboembolism
VZV	varicella zoster virus

W

WBC	White blood cells
Wt	Weight

X

Y

YO	Years old

Z

2025

A COMPREHENSIVE *RAPID REVIEW*

NAPLEX

Pharmacology & Drug Classes

Cardiology

CARDIOVASCULAR – VAUGHAN WILLIAMS CLASS 1A

Drug Class
- **Vaughan Williams Class 1a**
  - Disopyramide
  - Procainamide
  - Quinidine

> **Accelerate Your Knowledge**
> ✓ *Procainamide is one of the common drugs of choice for patients needing rate control or pharmacologic cardioversion associated with preexcited a-fib (also known as WPW)..*

Main Indications or Uses

- Supraventricular arrhythmias
- Ventricular arrhythmias

Mechanism of Action
- Slows cardiac conduction decreases cardiac automaticity and increases refractory periods primarily by blocking the opening of sodium channels with intermediate recovery from the blockade during phase 0.
  - Procainamide's active metabolite, N-acetyl procainamide (NAPA), also acts as a sodium channel blocker and blocks the potassium rectifier current.
  - These actions, coupled with their longer duration of action, can produce cardiac arrhythmias.

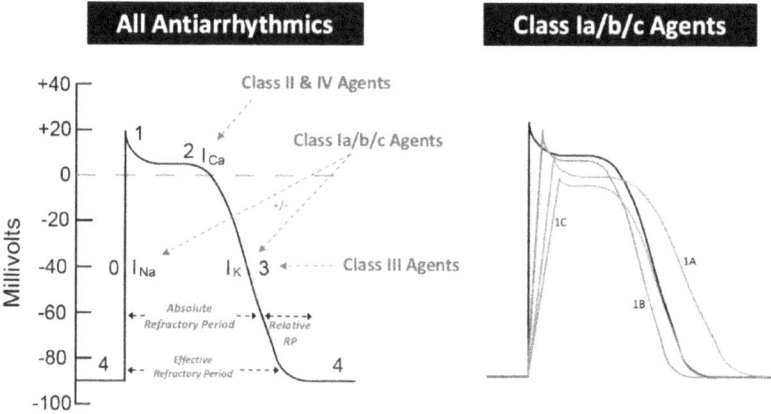

Primary Net Benefit
- Disopyramide and quinidine are rarely used clinically, but procainamide still plays a role in the acute management of supraventricular and ventricular arrhythmias.
- Main Labs to Monitor:
  - ECG, particularly QRS and QT intervals during procainamide infusion.
  - If procainamide continued, CBC, procainamide, and NAPA blood levels.

High-Yield Basic Pharmacology
- **Conduction and Refractoriness**
  - Class 1a agents can convert a reentry arrhythmia to normal conduction by blocking both directions of electrical flow by depressing conduction and prolonging refractoriness.
    - Orthodromic conduction is antegrade conduction through the AV node.
    - Antidromic conduction is retrograde conduction through the AV node.
- **Disopyramide**
  - Due to calcium channel blocking properties, disopyramide produces the most negative inotropic effects among the Class 1a agents.
    - Disopyramide, more specifically its active metabolite, produces the most anticholinergic effects among the Class 1a agents and possesses calcium channel blocking effects.

- Its active metabolite (N-despropyldisopyramide) is produced by hepatic mono-N-dealkylation.
- R-disopyramide possesses a sodium channel blocking effect, whereas S-disopyramide has pharmacologic actions similar to quinidine.
- Should not be used in HFrEF patients
    - Produces more negative inotropy than either procainamide or quinidine
- **Procainamide**
    - Least likely to cause hypotension among the Class 1a agents since procainamide lacks alpha-adrenergic blocking properties.
    - Procainamide therapy can be monitored using serum concentrations, with a normal therapeutic range of 4 to 12 mcg/mL.
        - Additionally, NAPA concentrations (normal range of 10 to 20 mcg/mL) should be followed, particularly in acute overdoses/toxicity and CKD patients
        - NAPA is eliminated renally, with an elimination half-life of 6 to 10 hours, much longer than the parent procainamide half-life of 3 to 4 hours.
- **Quinidine**
    - Anticholinergic adverse events are expected, including dry mucous membranes and flushed skin.
    - Rarely used due to cardiotoxicities, including syncope, QT prolongation, and Torsade de Pointes can occur at normal therapeutic doses.
        - Cinchonism, occurring from acute or chronic quinidine overdose, consists of abdominal pain, diarrhea, tinnitus, and altered mental status

High-Yield Clinical Knowledge
- **Disopyramide and Quinidine Induced Hypoglycemia**
    - Can induce insulin release from pancreatic islet cells via potassium channel blockade.
- **Slow Acetylators and Procainamide**
    - Patients who are "slow acetylators" are at higher risk of the early development of procainamide-induced lupus syndrome.
        - The parent compound, not NAPA, causes this syndrome.
            - Subjects with procainamide-induced lupus exposed to NAPA alone had their lupus-like symptoms resolve.
- **Procainamide Dosing Regimens**
    - Drug references list various loading doses for procainamide and titration parameters.
        - Proper dosing, including infusion loading doses of 10 to 17 mg/kg infusion at 20 to 50 mg/minute, 100 mg IV bolus every 5 minutes.
        - The therapeutic endpoint for these doses includes QRS interval widening by 50% of its original width, a maximum dose of 1 g being reached, or hypotension occurring.

High-Yield Core Evidence
- **PROCAMIO Study**
    - A multicenter randomized, open-labeled study compared procainamide and amiodarone for the acute treatment of stable wide QRS complex tachycardia.
    - Study subjects were randomized to either intravenous procainamide or amiodarone.
    - Compared to amiodarone, significantly fewer subjects who received procainamide had major predefined cardiac adverse events within 40 min after infusion initiation.
    - This result was maintained in a subgroup of patients with structural heart disease.
    - Furthermore, more patients receiving procainamide had their tachycardia terminated within 40 min than subjects receiving amiodarone, with a similar incidence of adverse events.
    - The authors concluded that procainamide therapy was associated with fewer major cardiac adverse events and a higher proportion of tachycardia termination within 40 min. (Eur Heart J. 2017 May 1;38(17):1329-1335.)
- **Procainamide vs Lidocaine**
    - A retrospective study compared procainamide's effect to lidocaine on terminating sustained monomorphic ventricular tachycardia (SMVT).

- Patients receiving procainamide had their SMVT terminated more frequently than patients receiving lidocaine (75.7% vs. 35.0%).
- The mean dose of procainamide used in these patients was relatively low (358 ± 50 mg) compared to patients receiving lidocaine (81 ± 30 mg)
- The study authors concluded that procainamide was more effective than lidocaine in terminating SMVT associated with structural heart diseases. (Circ J. 2010 May;74(5):864-9.)

High-Yield Fast-Facts
- **Amphetamines on UDS**
    - Procainamide shares structural similarities with amphetamine, and some patients may have a false-positive urine screening for amphetamines.
- **Rate Dependent Block**
    - Rate dependence is a term used to describe Class 1 antiarrhythmic effects where the sodium channel blocking effects are lowest at slow heart rates but higher at fast heart rates.
- **Quinidine Salts**
    - The expressed dose of quinidine changes depending on the particular salt form. 267 mg of gluconate salt is equivalent to 200 mg of sulfate salt.
    - The IV formulation of quinidine is no longer available in the US.

HIGH-YIELD BOARD EXAM ESSENTIALS
- **CLASSIC AGENTS:** Disopyramide, procainamide, quinidine
- **DRUG CLASS:** VW Class 1a
- **INDICATIONS:** Supraventricular arrhythmias, ventricular arrhythmias
- **MECHANISM:** Slows cardiac conduction decreases cardiac automaticity and increases refractory periods primarily by blocking the opening of sodium channels with intermediate recovery from the blockade.
- **SIDE EFFECTS:** Negative inotropy (disopyramide), ANA antibody (procainamide), cardiotoxicity (quinidine), QRS widening due to the Na+ channel blockade in phase 0
- **CLINICAL PEARLS:**
    - Disopyramide and quinidine are rarely used clinically, but IV procainamide still has a role in the acute management of supraventricular arrhythmias and ventricular arrhythmias.
    - The QRS widening with procainamide is worsened or magnified in hypokalemia, hypocalcemia, and hypomagnesemia.

Table: Drug Class Summary

Vaughan Williams Class 1a - Drug Class Review			
High-Yield Med Reviews			
Mechanism of Action: *Sodium channel blockers slow cardiac conduction, decrease cardiac automaticity, and increase refractory periods.*			
Class Effects: *Terminates or slows pathologic conduction contributing to arrhythmias*			
Generic Name	**Brand Name**	**Main Indication(s) or Uses**	**Notes**

Disopyramide	Norpace	• Ventricular arrhythmias	• **Dosing (Adult):**
			  − Patients weight less than 50 kg:
			    − Oral loading dose: 200 mg
			    − Maintenance dose: 100 mg q6h (IR), or 200 mg q12h (CR)
			  − Patients weight 50 kg or greater
			    − Oral loading dose: 300 mg
			    − Maintenance dose: 150 to 200 mg q6h (IR), or 300 mg q12h (CR).
			    − Maximum dose: 400 mg q6h)
			• **Dosing (Peds):** Immediate release only
			  − IR: 1.5 to 7.5 mg/kg/dose q6h
			  − Maximum 1,600 mg/day
			• **CYP450 Interactions:** Substrate CYP 3A4
			• **Renal or Hepatic Dose Adjustments:**
			  − Controlled release
			    − Not recommended if GFR is < 40 mL/minute
			  − Immediate release
			    − GFR 10 to 50 mL/minute 100 to 200 mg every 12 to 24 hours
			    − GFR < 10 mL/minute 100 to 200 mg every 24 to 48 hours
			• **Dosage Forms:** Oral (IR capsule, ER capsule)

\multicolumn{4}{c}{**Vaughan Williams Class 1a - Drug Class Review**}

| **Vaughan Williams Class 1a - Drug Class Review** ||||
| **High-Yield Med Reviews** ||||
Generic Name	Brand Name	Main Indication(s) or Uses	Notes
Procainamide	Pronestyl	<ul><li>Supraventricular arrhythmias</li><li>Ventricular arrhythmias</li></ul>	<ul><li>**Dosing (Adult):**<ul><li>IV loading dose: 10 to 17 mg/kg infusion at 20 to 50 mg/minute (maximum 1g)</li><li>IV: 100 mg bolus every 5 minutes (maximum 1g)<ul><li>Administration endpoints<ul><li>QRS interval widening by 50% of its original width</li><li>Maximum dose of 1 g</li><li>Hypotension</li></ul></li></ul></li><li>IV continuous infusion 1 to 4 mg/minute</li></ul></li><li>**Dosing (Peds):**<ul><li>IV loading dose: 10 to 15 mg/kg over 30 to 60 minutes.</li><li>IV infusion: 20 to 80 mcg/kg/minute (maximum 2,000 mg/24 hours)</li></ul></li><li>**CYP450 Interactions:** Substrate of CYP 2D6</li><li>**Renal or Hepatic Dose Adjustments:**</li><li>For continuous infusion only<ul><li>Reduce total dose by 25% to 50%<ul><li>GFR 10 to 50 mL/minute</li><li>Dialysis</li><li>Child-Pugh score of 8-10</li></ul></li><li>Reduce total dose by 50% to 75% and follow NAPA levels.<ul><li>GFR < 10 mL/minutes</li><li>Child-Pugh score greater than 10</li></ul></li></ul></li><li>**Dosage Forms:** IV solution</li></ul>
Quinidine	Quinaglute, Quinidex	<ul><li>Supraventricular arrhythmias</li><li>Ventricular arrhythmias</li></ul>	<ul><li>**Dosing (Adult):**<ul><li>Quinidine sulfate- initial dose 200 to 400 mg/q6h.</li><li>Quinidine gluconate- initial dose 324 to 648 mg q8h</li></ul></li><li>**Dosing (Peds):** Quinidine sulfate- 7.5 mg/kg q6h</li><li>**CYP450 Interactions:** Substrate of CYP 3A4, 2C9, 2E1, P-gp. Inhibits CYP 2D6, 3A4, P-gp.</li><li>**Renal or Hepatic Dose Adjustments:**<ul><li>Reduce to 75% of normal dose if GFR < 10 mL/minute</li></ul></li><li>**Dosage Forms:** Oral tablet (IR and ER)</li></ul>

CARDIOVASCULAR – VAUGHAN WILLIAMS CLASS 1B

Drug Class
- **Vaughan Williams Class 1b**
  - Lidocaine
  - Mexiletine

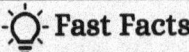

Fast Facts

✓ *Mexiletine is the prodrug of lidocaine and is available as an oral dosage form since lidocaine cannot be absorbed from the GI tract.*

Main Indications or Uses
- Chronic treatment to prevent ventricular tachycardia (VT) and ventricular fibrillation (VF)
- Acute treatment of VF or pulseless VT

Mechanism of Action
- Class 1b antiarrhythmics block inward sodium current by blocking inactivated sodium channels (in Purkinje and ventricular cells) with rapid kinetics during phase 0, preventing myocardial reentry and subsequent dysrhythmias.
  - This action increases the effective refractory period and prolongs the action potential, causing QRS to widen on the ECG.

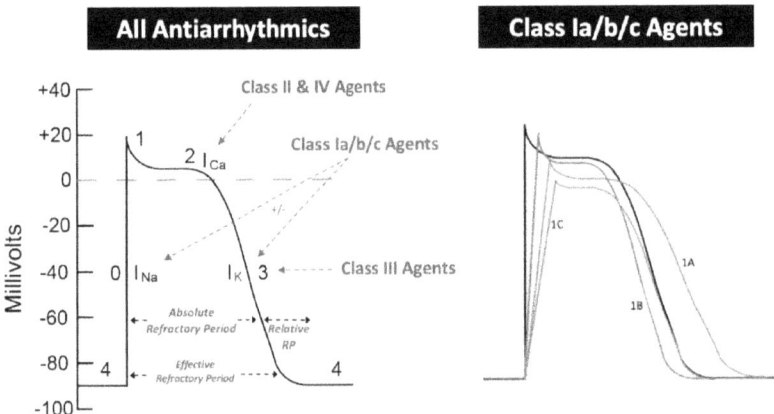

Primary Net Benefit
- Lidocaine may be as effective as amiodarone for shock-refractory ventricular fibrillation or pulseless ventricular tachycardia, avoiding numerous potential drug interactions and adverse events.
- Main Labs to Monitor:
  - Lidocaine concentrations if therapy continues beyond 24 hours.
  - ECG

High-Yield Basic Pharmacology
- **Rapid Kinetics**
  - Rapid kinetics refers to these agents' ability to recover from blockade between action potentials, thus having no effect on conduction. But in depolarized cells, there is a selective depression of conduction because of slower unbinding characteristics.
    - As a result, minimal changes are seen on the ECG after conversion from the pathologic rhythm.
- **Sodium Channel Inhibition**
  - Lidocaine inhibits both the open and inactivated states of cardiac sodium channels.
- **Atrial Arrhythmias**
  - These agents are not effective for managing atrial arrhythmias, potentially due to action potentials in the atrium being too short to permit enhancement of inactivated sodium channels from having any benefit.
- **Phase 4 Action**
  - By decreasing the slope of phase 4 of the myocyte action potential, these agents also decrease automaticity and the threshold for excitability.

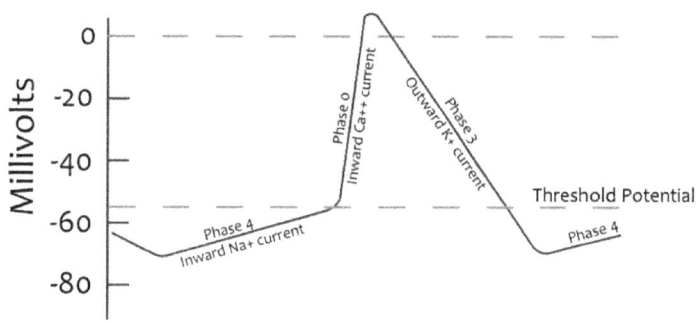

- **Lidocaine**
    - Lidocaine undergoes significant first-pass metabolism, resulting in oral bioavailability of 3%.
        - While this absorption prevents oral use for antiarrhythmic or analgesic effects, it is sufficient to precipitate toxicity, particularly in children.
            - Therapeutic monitoring of lidocaine consists of following the plasma lidocaine concentration and the toxic and active metabolite monoethylglycinexylidide (MEGX).
    - **Mexiletine**
        - It was developed as an analog of lidocaine but desired to permit oral therapy. By specifically reducing first-pass hepatic metabolism, mexiletine can be considered orally available lidocaine.
            - It is used clinically in combination with other antiarrhythmics such as sotalol, which can improve efficacy while limiting dose-related toxicities of either agent.

High-Yield Clinical Knowledge
- **Mexiletine Tremors**
    - A common complaint that may affect compliance is the development of tremors in patients taking mexiletine. However, this effect may be minimized by simply having the patient take mexiletine with food.
- **Neuropathic Pain Management and Opioid-sparing**
    - Numerous agents have been investigated for their potential opioid-sparing effects. For example, mexiletine has been proposed as an agent for chronic neuropathic pain management in patients where opioid-sparing therapies may be helpful.
- **Lidocaine Therapeutic Monitoring**
    - CYP3A4 metabolizes lidocaine into two metabolites, glycinexylidide (GX) and the MEGX, as mentioned above.
    - MEGX is a less potent sodium channel blocker but has a much longer half-life.
        - Target lidocaine levels are 1.5 to 5.0 mcg/mL
            - Heart failure, hepatic impairment, beta-blockers, and patients receiving prolonged infusions of lidocaine should be kept at the lower end of the therapeutic range to prevent toxicity.
- **Conversion to Mexiletine**
    - Patients on IV lidocaine infusions can be transitioned to mexiletine by administering 200 mg of mexiletine when the lidocaine infusion is stopped.
        - Conversion from other Class 1a antiarrhythmics can also be accomplished by administering 200 mg of mexiletine 6 to 12 hours after the last dose of the Class 1a agent.

High-Yield Core Evidence
- **ALPS Trial**
    - A randomized, double-blind trial comparing amiodarone, lidocaine, and placebo in refractory ventricular fibrillation. Adult patients were included if they had a nontraumatic out-of-hospital cardiac arrest with shock-refractory ventricular fibrillation or pulseless ventricular tachycardia after at least one shock and had IV access established.
    - There was a significant improvement in the primary outcome (survival to hospital discharge) in patients receiving amiodarone compared to placebo. But there was no benefit observed in patients receiving lidocaine compared to placebo. Furthermore, when amiodarone and lidocaine were compared, there was no difference in the primary outcome observed.

- However, there was a heterogeneity of treatment effects when the arrest was witnessed.
- Additionally, patients receiving active bystander CPR and active drugs (amiodarone and lidocaine) had a higher survival rate than placebo, but no difference for an unwitnessed arrest.
- The authors concluded that neither amiodarone nor lidocaine resulted in a significantly higher survival rate or favorable neurologic outcome versus placebo in this population. (N Engl J Med. 2016 May 5;374(18):1711-22.)
- **Mexiletine For Myotonic Dystrophy Type 1**
    - This was a publication of two randomized, double-blind, crossover trials evaluating mexiletine or placebo in patients with myotonic dystrophy type 1 with grip or percussion myotonia on examination.
    - Patients receiving mexiletine 150 mg or 200 mg had a significant improvement compared to placebo in the primary outcome of isometric grip force to relax from 90% to 5% of peak force after a 3-second maximum grip contraction.
    - There were no observed treatments associated with severe adverse events, prolonged PR, QRS, or QTc intervals.
    - The authors concluded that mexiletine is effective, safe, and well-tolerated over seven weeks as an anti myotonia treatment in myotonic dystrophy type 1. (Neurology. 2010 May 4; 74(18): 1441–1448.)

High-Yield Fast-Facts
- **Intranasal LEAN**
    - Lidocaine is one of the four "LEAN" drugs that can be administered via an endotracheal tube if IV/IO access is unobtainable.
- **Moricizine and tocainide**
    - Moricizine and tocainide are often mentioned in texts as belonging to the class 1b antiarrhythmic class. Unfortunately, these agents are no longer commercially available in the US.
- **Amphetamines on UDS**
    - Mexiletine has been reported to cause a false-positive urine drug assay for amphetamines.

HIGH-YIELD BOARD EXAM ESSENTIALS
- **CLASSIC AGENTS:** Lidocaine, mexiletine
- **DRUG CLASS:** VW Class 1b
- **INDICATIONS:** Chronic treatment to prevent ventricular tachycardia (VT) and ventricular fibrillation (VF), Acute treatment of VF or pulseless VT
- **MECHANISM:** Block inward sodium current by blocking inactivated sodium channels with rapid kinetics, preventing myocardial reentry and subsequent dysrhythmias.
- **SIDE EFFECTS:** Tremors, headache, seizures (at higher doses), QRS widening
- **CLINICAL PEARLS:**
    - Similar to VW Class 1a agents, due to the sodium channel blockade within the ventricular myocyte there is QRS widening on the ECG with higher doses.
    - Lidocaine is not absorbed when taken by mouth, thus mexiletine is the pro-drug of lidocaine and can be given by mouth.
    - Patients on IV lidocaine infusions can be transitioned to mexiletine by administering 200 mg of mexiletine when the lidocaine infusion is stopped.

Table: Drug Class Summary

\multicolumn{4}{c}{**Vaughan Williams Class 1b - Drug Class Review**}
\multicolumn{4}{c}{High-Yield Med Reviews}
\multicolumn{4}{l}{**Mechanism of Action:** *Block inward sodium current by blocking inactivated sodium channels, preventing myocardial reentry and subsequent dysrhythmias.*}
\multicolumn{4}{l}{**Class Effects:** *Increases the effective refractory period and prolongs the action potential.*}
Generic Name	**Brand Name**	**Main Indication(s) or Uses**	**Notes**

Lidocaine	Xylocaine	• Ventricular arrhythmias	• **Dosing (Adult):**
			— IV or IO (intraosseous): 1 to 1.5 mg/kg bolus.
			  — Maximum 3 mg/kg
			— IV: continuous infusion 1 to 4 mg/minute
			• **Dosing (Peds):**
			— IV or IO (intraosseous): 1 to 1.5 mg/kg bolus.
			  — Maximum 3 mg/kg
			— IV continuous infusion: 20 to 50 mg/kg/minute
			• **CYP450 Interactions:** Substrate of CYP 1A2, 2A6, 2B6, 2C9, 3A4
			• **Renal or Hepatic Dose Adjustments:** No specific dose adjustment, but follow GX/MEGX concentrations.
			• **Dosage Forms:** Solution for injection. Numerous other dosage forms exist, but not for antiarrhythmic indications.

Mexiletine	Mexitil	• Ventricular arrhythmias	• **Dosing (Adult):**
			— Oral: loading dose 400 mg (optional)
			— Oral maintenance dose: 150 to 200 mg q8h to q12h
			  — Maximum dose 1.2 g/day
			• **Dosing (Peds):**
			— Initial oral dose: 6 to 8 mg/kg/day in 2 or 3 divided doses
			  — Maximum dose 15 mg/kg/day or 1.2 g/day, whichever is less
			• **CYP450 Interactions:** Substrate of CYP 1A2, 2D6. Inhibits CYP 1A2
			• **Renal or Hepatic Dose Adjustments:**
			— None recommended, but elimination half-life is doubled in the setting of hepatic failure.
			• **Dosage Forms:** Oral (capsule)

CARDIOVASCULAR – VAUGHAN WILLIAMS CLASS 1C

Drug Class
- **Vaughan Williams Class 1c**
  - Flecainide
  - Propafenone

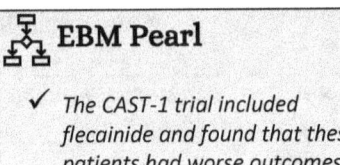

EBM Pearl
- ✓ The CAST-1 trial included flecainide and found that these patients had worse outcomes.

Main Indications or Uses
- **Acute Care:**
  - Pharmacological cardioversion of paroxysmal atrial fibrillation
    - Flecainide
    - Propafenone
- **Chronic Care:**
  - Prevention of paroxysmal atrial fibrillation or flutter and paroxysmal supraventricular tachycardias
    - Flecainide
    - Propafenone
  - Ventricular arrhythmias
    - Flecainide
    - Propafenone

Mechanism of Action
- Prevent reentry pathways by slowing conduction via blocking fast inward sodium current.
  - By slowing the rate of phase 0 depolarization and prolonging refractoriness in all areas of the heart and reducing spontaneous depolarizations.

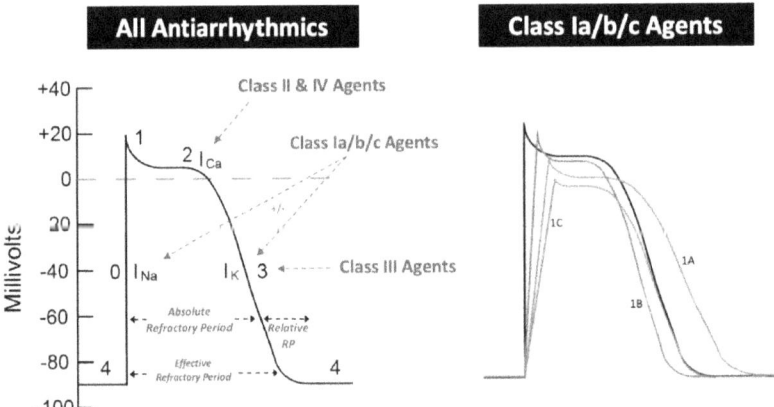

Primary Net Benefit
- Unique role in outpatient oral cardioversion for patients with paroxysmal atrial fibrillation.
- Main Labs to Monitor:
  - ECG at baseline, periodically thereafter
  - Flecainide serum trough concentrations when starting therapy in pediatric patients or adults with renal or hepatic impairment.

High-Yield Basic Pharmacology
- Flecainide and propafenone are inhibitors of the ryanodine receptor 2 (RyR2) calcium channel in cardiac cells. This effect leads to the suppression of delayed afterdepolarizations.
  - This should not be confused with the RyR1 calcium channel, better known for its role in malignant hyperthermia.
- Flecainide, like propafenone, possesses sodium channel blocking properties and potassium rectifier current blocking and calcium channel blocking properties.

- Propafenone is a racemic mixture where only the R-propafenone blocks RyR2 channels. In addition, the S-propafenone possesses beta-blocking properties.
    - Flecainide is also a racemic mixture, but the racemates do not possess different electrophysiologic effects.
- Propafenone undergoes first-pass metabolism to 5-OH-propafenone.
    - This active, equipotent metabolite can be therapeutically relevant in 'extensive metabolizers.'

High-Yield Clinical Knowledge
- **Flecainide**
    - Each of the class 1c agents carries a warning that there is increased mortality in patients with structural heart disease receiving these agents. This warning originated from the results of the CAST trials, described further below.
        - The specific warning pertains to patients receiving these agents for asymptomatic, non-life-threatening ventricular arrhythmias who had a recent myocardial infarction.
            - This stipulation is often omitted, preventing patients without these specific risk factors from potentially receiving these agents for atrial arrhythmias or as a bridge to ablation therapy.
        - Patients with impaired renal function, low urine pH, concomitant CYP2D6 inhibitors, and HFrEF have reduced flecainide clearance
- **Propafenone**
    - In addition to its class 1c sodium channel effects, propafenone acts as a weak beta-adrenergic blocker and is an L-type calcium channel blocker and potassium channel blocker.
        - Propafenone is a structural analog of propranolol. It is hypothesized this similarity gives rise to its beta-blocking properties.
    - The metabolism of propafenone by CYP2D6 is saturable, leading to unpredictable and abrupt increases in plasma levels.
        - In patients with low or absent CYP2D6 (from drug interactions or poor metabolizer patients), the first-pass effect is significantly diminished and will lead to much higher plasma propafenone levels and toxicity
- **Visual Disturbances**
    - Patients taking flecainide commonly complain of visual disturbances and dose-related blurred vision.
- **Anticipated ECG Interval Changes**
    - Flecainide and propafenone are expected to prolong the PR, QRS, and QT intervals.
        - Flecainide toxicity often has prolonged PR and QRS with a normal QT interval.

High-Yield Core Evidence
- **CAST-1 trial**
    - This was a multicenter, double-blind, parallel-group, randomized, placebo-controlled trial examining the effect of a Class 1c antiarrhythmic (encainide, flecainide, or moricizine) or placebo could suppress ventricular ectopy after myocardial infarction, thus reducing the incidence of sudden death.
    - This study was terminated early due to excessive cardiac and non-arrhythmic cardiac causes mortality in patients receiving a class 1c agent.
    - Among the deaths not attributed to an arrhythmia, the causes of death included acute myocardial infarction with shock or chronic congestive heart failure.
    - Furthermore, the active treatments did not lead to a difference between the patients receiving active drug and those receiving placebo in the incidence of nonlethal disqualifying ventricular tachycardia, proarrhythmia, syncope, need for a permanent pacemaker, congestive heart failure, recurrent myocardial infarction, angina, or need for coronary artery bypass grafting or angioplasty.
    - The authors concluded that the active treatment with a class 1c agent leads to excess deaths due to arrhythmia and deaths due to shock after acute recurrent myocardial infarction. (N Engl J Med. 1991 Mar 21;324(12):781-8.)
- **CAST-2 trial**
    - This study involved two blinded, randomized phases. The early phase evaluated moricizine or placebo for 14 days after myocardial infarction. The long-term phase evaluated moricizine in patients with ventricular premature depolarizations adequately suppressed or partially suppressed by moricizine.

- This study was stopped early when it was observed that there was excess mortality among patients receiving early phase moricizine as compared with no treatment or placebo.
- For patients who had completed the long-term phase, there was no difference in deaths or cardiac arrests due to arrhythmias in patients assigned to moricizine or placebo.
- The authors concluded that the use of moricizine to suppress asymptomatic or mildly symptomatic ventricular premature depolarizations to reduce mortality after myocardial infarction is ineffective and harmful. (N Engl J Med. 1992 Jul 23;327(4):227-33.)
- **Pill-In-The-Pocket**
  - This was an open-label, observational study assessing the feasibility and safety of self-administered oral loading of flecainide and propafenone for out-of-hospital treatment of recent-onset atrial fibrillation.
  - Patients were converted to normal sinus from recent-onset atrial fibrillation with either flecainide or propafenone in the emergency department, then discharged with out-of-hospital self-administration of flecainide or propafenone.
  - Patients were followed for a mean follow-up of 15 ± 5 months. Among the patients who had an episode of atrial fibrillation, 92% were rapidly and successfully treated with a resolution of symptoms and was 100% effective in episodes of recurrences.
  - The numbers of monthly visits to the emergency room and hospitalizations were significantly lower during follow-up than during the year before the target episode.
  - The authors concluded that in a selected, risk-stratified population of patients with recurrent atrial fibrillation, pill-in-the-pocket treatment is feasible and safe, with a high rate of compliance by patients, a low rate of adverse events, and a marked reduction in emergency room visits and hospital admissions. (N Engl J Med. 2004 Dec 2;351(23):2384-91.)

High-Yield Fast-Facts
- **Vegetarians and Flecainide**
  - Patients following a strict vegetarian diet may have decreased flecainide clearance if their urine pH is 8 or greater.
- **Propafenone Beta-Blocker**
  - The beta-blocking properties of propafenone are hypothesized to contribute to the increased mortality observed in patients taking propafenone who have a history of HFrEF.
- **Flecainide in Pediatrics**
  - Flecainide can be used in pediatric populations and compounded into an oral suspension.
  - This compound, however, carries a high risk of medication error since the drug may precipitate, leading to dose stacking, or can be confused with other SALAD drugs such as fluoxetine.

HIGH-YIELD BOARD EXAM ESSENTIALS
- **CLASSIC AGENTS:** Flecainide, propafenone
- **DRUG CLASS:** VW Class Ic
- **INDICATIONS:** Pharmacological cardioversion of paroxysmal Afib, Prevention of paroxysmal Afib/flutter and paroxysmal SVT, ventricular arrhythmias
- **MECHANISM:** Prevent reentry pathways by slowing conduction via blocking fast inward sodium current
- **SIDE EFFECTS:** Decreased inotropy, blurry vision, arrhythmias
- **CLINICAL PEARLS:** Each of the class 1c agents carries a warning that there is increased mortality in patients with structural heart disease receiving these agents. This warning originated from the results of the CAST trials.

Table: Drug Class Summary

| \multicolumn{4}{c}{**Vaughan Williams Class 1c - Drug Class Review**} |
|||||

\multicolumn{4}{l}{**Vaughan Williams Class 1c - Drug Class Review** High-Yield Med Reviews}
Mechanism of Action: *Prevent reentry pathways by slowing conduction via blocking fast inward sodium current*			
Class Effects: *Prolonging refractoriness in all areas of the heart and reducing spontaneous depolarizations.*			
Generic Name	**Brand Name**	**Main Indication(s) or Uses**	**Notes**
Flecainide	Tambocor	<ul><li>Pharmacological cardioversion</li><li>Paroxysmal Afib, Aflutter, or PSVT</li></ul>	<ul><li>**Dosing (Adult):**<ul><li>Oral: 50 mg q12h<ul><li>Maximum 300 mg/day</li></ul></li><li>Cardioversion<ul><li>Weight < 70 kg - 200 mg</li><li>Weight 70 kg or greater - 300 mg</li></ul></li></ul></li><li>**Dosing (Peds):**<ul><li>Oral: 50 to 100 mg/m^2/day divided q8 to 12h</li><li>Maximum 200 mg/m^2/day</li></ul></li><li>**CYP450 Interactions:** Substrate CYP2D6, CYP1A2</li><li>**Renal or Hepatic Dose Adjustments:**<ul><li>GFR < or equal to 35 mL/minute: 100 mg q24h</li></ul></li><li>**Dosage Forms:** Oral (tablet)</li></ul>
Propafenone	Rythmol	<ul><li>Pharmacological cardioversion</li><li>Paroxysmal Afib, Aflutter, or PSVT</li></ul>	<ul><li>**Dosing (Adult):**<ul><li>Extended-release - 225 mg q12h<ul><li>Maximum 425 mg q12h</li></ul></li><li>Immediate-release - 150 mg q8h (300 mg every 8 hours)</li><li>Cardioversion (IR tablet)<ul><li>Weight < than 70 kg - 450 mg</li><li>Weight is 70 kg or greater - 600 mg</li></ul></li></ul></li><li>**Dosing (Peds):** Not routinely used</li><li>**CYP450 Interactions:** Substrate CYP3A4, CYP2D6, CYP1A2. Inhibits CYP1A2, CYP2D6, P-gp</li><li>**Renal or Hepatic Dose Adjustments:**<ul><li>No specific recommendations</li></ul></li><li>**Dosage Forms:** Oral (ER capsule, IR tablet)</li></ul>

CARDIOVASCULAR – VAUGHAN WILLIAMS CLASS 2 (BETA-ANTAGONISTS)

Drug Class
- Vaughan Williams Class 2 (Beta-antagonists)
- Acute Care
  - Esmolol
  - Labetalol
  - Metoprolol
- Chronic Care
  - Acebutolol
  - Atenolol
  - Carvedilol
  - Bisoprolol
  - Betaxolol
  - Metoprolol
  - Nadolol
  - Nebivolol
  - Penbutolol
  - Pindolol

Main Indications or Uses
- Acute Care:
  - Atrial fibrillation with rapid ventricular response
  - Hypertensive emergencies
    - Acute aortic syndromes/Acute aortic dissection
    - Acute ischemic stroke
    - Acute hemorrhagic stroke
    - Preeclampsia/eclampsia
- Chronic Care:
  - Angina
  - Atrial fibrillation/flutter, maintenance of ventricular rate control
  - Heart failure with reduced ejection fraction, including left ventricular dysfunction following myocardial infarction
  - Hypertension
  - Myocardial infarction, early treatment, and secondary prevention
  - Variceal hemorrhage prophylaxis

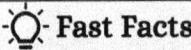

Fast Facts
- All beta-blockers have negative chronotropic and inotropic effects, but carvedilol and labetalol can also reduce afterload through alpha receptor inhibition.

Mechanism of Action
- Beta-antagonists are competitive inhibitors of catecholamines on beta-adrenergic receptors and blunt the chronotropic and inotropic response to catecholamines.
  - This mechanism slows the rate of SA node discharge, prevents ectopic pacemakers, and decreases conduction through the atrial and the AV node.
    - Beta-1 antagonists specifically block Gs proteins and their activation of adenylate cyclase. As a result, decreased cAMP production prevents protein kinase A phosphorylation of L-type calcium channels. This ultimately reduces calcium influx, limiting calcium-dependent calcium release from the sarcoplasmic reticulum and reducing contractility.
    - Beta-2 antagonists in cardiac tissue inhibit primarily block the inhibitory actions of the Gs and Gi protein pathways.
  - They also decrease inotropy by reducing cytosolic calcium levels that allow actin and myosin to interact to facilitate muscle contraction. This component of the mechanism of action is generally not considered a clinical benefit for most patients.
  - They are known to reduce remodeling which has many benefits in those with heart failure. This is likely due to the reduction in RAAS activation where it can reduce angiotensin II mediated effects of remodeling.

Primary Net Benefit
- Beta-blockers exert numerous beneficial effects, including reducing the heart rate and blood pressure, having antiarrhythmic and anti-ischemic properties, and inhibiting ACE release from the juxtaglomerular apparatus.

- In heart failure, beta-blockers confer benefits by inhibiting cardiac remodeling that puts patients at increased risk of sudden cardiac death (i.e., going into pulseless V-tach or V-fib).
- **Main Labs to Monitor:**
  - ECG, heart rate, and blood pressure at baseline and after any change in therapy.

High-Yield Basic Pharmacology
- **Antiarrhythmic Effect**
  - The antiarrhythmic action of beta-blockers is mediated via beta-blockade in the AV node. This is observed on the ECG as PR interval prolongation.
- **Beta-Blocker Effects**
  - Beta-antagonists possess inter-class variations in pharmacologic activity.
    - Aside from the commonly known beta-1 selective and nonselective agents, other classifications include agents with:
      - Intrinsic sympathomimetic activity (ISA; acebutolol, carteolol, pindolol)
      - Mixed alpha- and beta-antagonist activity (carvedilol, labetalol)
      - Increased production of nitric oxide (carteolol, nebivolol)
      - Potassium channel blockade activity (sotalol)
      - Calcium channel blockade (betaxolol, carvedilol)
- **Dose-Dependent Effects**
  - The selective beta-1 antagonists are selective only at normal therapeutic dosing.
    - As doses increase, or exposure increases via drug interactions, selectivity may be lost, and nonselective sequelae can occur.
      - This is where bronchospasms can also occur in asthmatics or those with moderate to severe COPD.

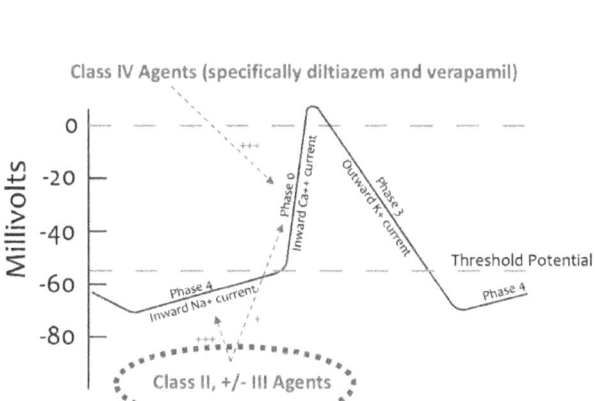
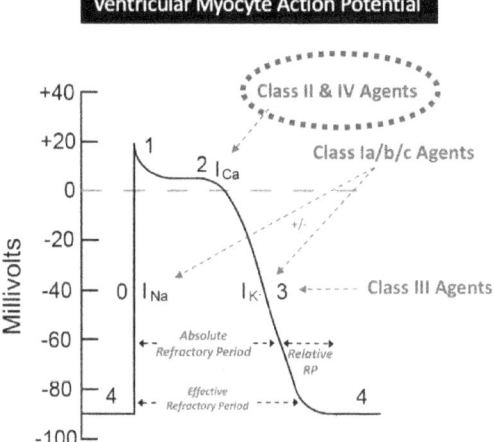

High-Yield Clinical Knowledge
- **Cardiac Effect from Sympathetic Stimuli**
  - Beta receptor antagonists slow the heart rate and decrease myocardial contractility if there are sympathetic stimuli to antagonize.
  - These agents have the most pronounced effect when the sympathetic nervous system stimulates cardiac activity.
    - Acute administration of beta-antagonists may temporarily increase peripheral vascular resistance (PVR) as a response to decreased cardiac output. But over time, PVR returns to baseline values or may even lower in patients with hypertension by inhibiting catecholamine activation of renin in renal juxtaglomerular cells.

- **IV to PO Conversion Errors**
  - When converting propranolol from IV to PO (or vice versa), careful attention must be given to avoid significant drug errors.
  - The oral bioavailability of propranolol is ~25% due to extensive first-pass metabolism. However, there are no empiric dose conversion recommendations because of patient variation, drug interactions, and clinical indication.
    - But considering the use of propranolol in acute indications such as thyroid storms, where both dosage forms are recommended, a general concept of the difference in bioavailability can be inferred: 0.5 to 1 mg IV over 10 minutes versus 60 to 80 mg by mouth.
- **Hypoglycemic Masking**
  - Beta-antagonists diminish sympathetic-mediated responses to hypoglycemia (tachycardia, tremor, and hunger)
  - During the acute hypoglycemic stress response, sweating is not diminished as this response is mediated by nicotinic activation by acetylcholine.
- **Esmolol Loading Dose**
  - In part, the efficacy of esmolol depends on the administration of a loading dose of 0.5 mg/kg.
  - This is a result of esmolol's short elimination half-life of 9 minutes. While the duration of effect is short-lived, this pharmacokinetic parameter is relevant to the importance of administering a bolus before the start of the infusion.
    - Most drug information resources list the bolus dose as 500 mcg/kg. However, it may be relevant to convert the units to 0.5 mg/kg since some clinicians may be hesitant to give a perceived high dose, which would increase the risk of therapeutic failure with esmolol.
- **Rate Control for AF**
  - For acute control rate control in AF, beta-1 selective agents are potentially less effective compared to non-dihydropyridine calcium channel blockers (evidence described below)
    - However, in AF precipitated by increased sympathetic tone such as surgery, or thyrotoxicosis, rapid-acting beta-blockers can be highly effective and should be considered first-line therapy.
- **Paroxysmal Supraventricular Tachycardia (PSVT)**
  - Beta-blockers can be used in the management of acute PSVT. Specifically, beta-1 selective agents act on the AV nodal portion of the reentrant circuit to slow the antegrade electrical flow.
    - Beta-blockers may also benefit PSVT by limiting conduction through slow, calcium-dependent tissues.
- **Bronchoconstriction and Bronchospasm**
  - Nonselective beta-blocking agents and selective beta-1 antagonists used at high doses may cause bronchoconstriction and bronchospasm in some patients.
    - Although selective beta-1 antagonists are less likely to cause these effects, selectivity is lost at doses in the high-end of normal or above, and beta-2 effects can be observed.
    - Agents with ISA activity may be less likely to cause adverse respiratory effects. Still, if the risk of bronchospasm or bronchoconstriction is a concern, alternative rate control agents such as calcium channel blockers should be used.
- **Beta-antagonists And Carbohydrate and Lipid Metabolism**
  - Beta-antagonists prevent catecholamine-mediated glycogenolysis and impair glucose response to hypoglycemia.
    - Nonselective beta-blocking agents can reduce HDL, increase LDL, and increase triglycerides by their action on free fatty acids.
    - These nonselective beta-blockers prevent the release of free fatty acids, reduce their oxidation in muscle tissue, and limit ATP production.
      - As a result, these fatty acids accumulate in adipose tissue and limit lipolysis as a vital source of ATP, particularly under physiologic stress.

High-Yield Core Evidence
- **Diltiazem Vs. Metoprolol for Acute AF-RVR**
  - This was a prospective, observational convenience sample of adult patients presenting with AF-RVR who were randomized to receive diltiazem or metoprolol.

- Significantly more patients receiving diltiazem achieved an HR of fewer than 100 beats per minute within 5 minutes and 30 minutes of drug administration.
- The mean decrease in HR for the diltiazem group was more rapid and substantial than that of the metoprolol group. However, there was no difference between the groups concerning hypotension or bradycardia.
- The authors concluded that diltiazem was more effective in achieving rate control in ED patients with AF-RVR and did so with no increased incidence of adverse effects. (J Emerg Med. 2015 Aug;49(2):175-82.)
- **Rate Control Of Acute AF-RVR With HFrEF**
    - This was a single-center, retrospective cohort study comparing the effect of IV push metoprolol compared to diltiazem in patients with HFrEF in AF with RVR.
    - The primary outcome was successful rate control within 30 min of medication administration, defined as a heart rate (HR) of less than 100 beats per minute or an HR reduction of 20% or greater.
    - There was no difference in the primary outcome of successful rate control within 30 min between the treatment groups and no difference in HR control at predefined time points or adverse events (hypotension, bradycardia, worsening heart failure).
    - The authors concluded that in the acute management of AF with RVR in patients with HFrEF, IVP diltiazem achieved similar rate control with no increase in adverse events compared to IVP metoprolol. (Am J Emerg Med. 2019 Jan;37(1):80-84)
- **OPTIC Trial**
    - In this randomized trial, patients received amiodarone plus beta-blockers, sotalol alone, or beta-blocker within 21 days of placement of an implantable cardioverter-defibrillator (ICD) for inducible or spontaneously occurring ventricular tachycardia or fibrillation.
    - Amiodarone plus beta-blocker significantly reduced the risk of ICD shock compared with beta-blocker alone and sotalol.
    - However, more patients discontinued amiodarone at one year, compared to sotalol and beta-blocker alone, and more patients taking amiodarone experienced adverse events and symptomatic bradycardia.
    - The authors concluded that amiodarone plus beta-blocker effectively prevents these shocks and is more effective than sotalol but has an increased risk of drug-related adverse effects. (JAMA. 2006 Jan 11;295(2):165-71.)
- **POST Trial**
    - This was a multi-center, randomized, placebo-controlled, double-blind trial of metoprolol's effect at the highest tolerated dose in vasovagal syncope over a 1-year treatment period. Patients were followed for a mean of 11 years.
    - There was no significant difference observed between treatment groups regarding the first recurrence of syncope, and there was no difference in the likelihood of recurrent syncope.
    - The authors concluded that metoprolol was ineffective in preventing vasovagal syncope in the study population. (Circulation. 2006 Mar 7;113(9):1164-70.)

High-Yield Fast-Facts
- **Sotalol Beta-Blocker vs Class III**
    - Sotalol has the properties of a beta-blocker; however, it is not classified as a Class 2 antiarrhythmic. Instead, its primary antiarrhythmic action is via potassium channel blocking and is thus a Class 3 agent.
- **Carvedilol and Insulin Sensitivity**
    - Carvedilol is less likely to cause decreased insulin sensitivity and has been associated with increased insulin sensitivity in patients with insulin resistance.
- **Alpha to Beta Ratios**
    - The vasodilatory properties of carvedilol and labetalol are a function of the ratio of alpha to beta antagonist activity. The ratio for carvedilol is 1:10 (alpha: beta), whereas labetalol's ratio changes depending on the route of administration (oral - 1:3; IV - 1:7).

HIGH-YIELD BOARD EXAM ESSENTIALS
- **CLASSIC AGENTS:** Acebutolol, atenolol, carvedilol, bisoprolol, betaxolol, esmolol, metoprolol, nadolol, nebivolol, penbutolol, pindolol
- **DRUG CLASS:** VW Class 2
- **INDICATIONS:** Angina, atrial fibrillation/flutter, HFrEF, hypertension, hypertensive emergency, myocardial infarction, variceal hemorrhage prophylaxis (propranolol).
- **MECHANISM:** Competitive inhibitors of catecholamines on beta-adrenergic receptors and blunt the chronotropic and inotropic response to catecholamines
- **SIDE EFFECTS:** Bradycardia, fatigue, hypotension, poor exercise performance, bronchospasm in asthmatics.
- **CLINICAL PEARLS:**
    - Historically indicated for hypertension but are not the best antihypertensive agents as monotherapy. They can reduce remodeling in heart failure which reduces risk of sudden cardiac death.
    - Beta-antagonists diminish sympathetic-mediated responses to hypoglycemia (tachycardia, tremor, and hunger), during the acute hypoglycemic stress response, sweating is not diminished as this response is mediated by nicotinic activation by acetylcholine.
    - Risk of bronchospasm in asthmatics and some COPD patients.

Table: Drug Class Summary

Vaughn Williams Class 2 (Beta-Antagonists) - Drug Class Review High-Yield Med Reviews			
Mechanism of Action: *Competitive inhibitors of catecholamines on beta-adrenergic receptors blunt the chronotropic and inotropic response to catecholamines*			
Class Effects: *Slows the rate of SA node discharge, prevents ectopic pacemakers, and decreases conduction through the atrial and the AV node*			
Generic Name	**Brand Name**	**Main Indication(s) or Uses**	**Notes**
Acebutolol	Sectral	<ul><li>Hypertension</li><li>Premature ventricular contractions</li></ul>	<ul><li>Dosing (Adult):<ul><li>Oral: 200 to 400 mg once daily</li><li>Maximum 1200 mg daily</li></ul></li><li>Dosing (Peds): Not commonly used</li><li>CYP450 Interactions: none</li><li>Renal or Hepatic Dose Adjustments:<ul><li>GFR 25 to 49 mL/minute: Reduce dose by 50%</li><li>GFR < 25 mL/minute: Reduce dose by 75%</li></ul></li><li>Dosage Forms: Oral (capsule, tablet)</li></ul>
Atenolol	Tenormin	<ul><li>Hypertension</li><li>Premature ventricular contractions</li></ul>	<ul><li>Dosing (Adult):<ul><li>Oral: 25 to 100 mg once daily</li><li>Maximum 100 mg daily</li></ul></li><li>Dosing (Peds):<ul><li>Oral: 0.3 to 1 mcg/kg/day once daily or in divided doses q12h</li></ul></li><li>CYP450 Interactions: none</li><li>Renal or Hepatic Dose Adjustments:<ul><li>GFR 15 to 35 mL/minute: Maximum daily dose of 50 mg</li><li>GFR < 15: Maximum daily dose of 25 mg</li><li>Hemodialysis: Administer after dialysis</li></ul></li><li>Dosage Forms: Oral (tablet)</li></ul>
Carvedilol	Coreg	<ul><li>HFrEF</li><li>Hypertension</li></ul>	<ul><li>Dosing (Adult):<ul><li>IR: 3.125 mg to 25 mg BID</li><li>If over 85 kg, maximum 50 mg BID</li><li>ER 20 mg daily</li><li>Maximum 80 mg/day</li></ul></li><li>Dosing (Peds):<ul><li>Oral: 0.075-0.08 mg/kg/dose BID</li><li>Maximum 50 mg BID.</li></ul></li><li>CYP450 Interactions: Inhibits P-gp. Substrate of P-gp, CYP 2C9, 2D6, 3A4, 1A2</li><li>Renal or Hepatic Dose Adjustments: None</li><li>Dosage Forms: Oral (tablet, capsule)</li></ul>

Vaughn Williams Class 2 (Beta-Antagonists) - Drug Class Review High-Yield Med Reviews			
Generic Name	**Brand Name**	**Main Indication(s) or Uses**	**Notes**
Betaxolol	Kerlone	• Hypertension	• **Dosing (Adult):** − Oral: 5 to 20 mg once daily • **Dosing (Peds):** Not used • **CYP450 Interactions:** Minor substrate of CYP1A2, 2D6 • **Renal or Hepatic Dose Adjustments:** None • **Dosage Forms:** Oral (tablet)

Bisoprolol	Zebeta	• Hypertension	• **Dosing (Adult):**
			  − Oral: 1.25 to 10 mg daily
			    − Maximum 10 mg/day
			• **Dosing (Peds):** None
			• **CYP450 Interactions:** Substrate of CYP2D6, and CYP3A4
			• **Renal or Hepatic Dose Adjustments:**
			  − GFR less than 40 mL/minute, initial dose no more than 2.5 mg daily
			• **Dosage Forms:** Oral (tablet)

Esmolol	Brevibloc	• Atrial fibrillation/flutter
		• Intraoperative and/or postoperative tachycardia and/or hypertension
		• Sinus tachycardia
		• Supraventricular tachycardia
			• **Dosing (Adult):**
			  − IV bolus: 500 to 1000 mcg/kg over 30 to 60 seconds
			  − IV infusion: 50 to 300 mcg/kg/min
			• **Dosing (Peds):**
			  − IV bolus: 100 to 500 mcg/kg over 30 to 60 seconds
			  − IV infusion: 50 to 300 mcg/kg/min
			• **CYP450 Interactions:** None
			• **Renal or Hepatic Dose Adjustments:** None
			• **Dosage Forms:** IV solution

Labetalol	Trandate	• Acute aortic dissection
		• Acute ischemic stroke
		• Acute hemorrhagic stroke
		• Hypertension
		• Preeclampsia/eclampsia
			• **Dosing (Adult):**
			  − Oral: 100 mg twice daily up to
			    − Maximum 400 mg twice daily
			  − IV: 10-20 mg IV push every 10 minutes
			• **Dosing (Peds):**
			  − Oral: 1 to 3 mg/kg/day in 2 divided doses
			    − Maximum 10 to 12 mg/kg/day, or 1,200 mg/day
			  − IV: 0.2 to 1 mg/kg/dose
			    − Maximum 40 mg/dose
			• **CYP450 Interactions:** Extensive first pass, hepatic glucuronidation
			• **Renal or Hepatic Dose Adjustments:** None
			• **Dosage Forms:** Oral (tablet), IV solution

Vaughn Williams Class 2 (Beta-Antagonists) - Drug Class Review
High-Yield Med Reviews

Generic Name	Brand Name	Main Indication(s) or Uses	Notes

Metoprolol	Lopressor Toprol	<ul><li>Angina</li><li>HFrEF</li><li>Hypertension</li><li>Myocardial infarction</li></ul>	<ul><li>**Dosing (Adult):**
			− Oral: IR 12.5 to 200 mg BID
			   − Maximum 400 mg daily
			− Oral: ER 50 to 200 mg
			   − Maximum 400 mg daily
			− IV: 2.5 to 5 mg IV push q5minutes as needed
			   − Maximum total dose 15 mg</li><li>**Dosing (Peds):**
			− Oral: 0.1 to 0.2 mg/kg/dose BID
			   − Maximum 2 mg/kg/day, or 200 mg/day
			− IV: 0.1 to 0.2 mg/kg
			   − Maximum 10 mg/dose</li><li>**CYP450 Interactions:** Substrate CYP 2D6, and CYP 2C19</li><li>**Renal or Hepatic Dose Adjustments:** None</li><li>**Dosage Forms:** Oral (tablet [IR and ER], capsule [IR and ER]), IV solution</li></ul>

Nebivolol	Bystolic	<ul><li>Hypertension</li></ul>	<ul><li>**Dosing (Adult):** − Oral: 5 mg once daily − Maximum 40 mg daily</li><li>**Dosing (Peds):** Not used</li><li>**CYP450 Interactions:** Extensive first pass, hepatic glucuronidation</li><li>**Renal or Hepatic Dose Adjustments:** − GFR < 30 mL/minute: Initial dose of 2.5 mg once daily</li><li>**Dosage Forms:** Oral (tablet)</li></ul>
Nadolol	Corgard	<ul><li>Angina</li><li>Hypertension</li></ul>	<ul><li>**Dosing (Adult):** − Oral: 10 to 240 mg once daily</li><li>**Dosing (Peds):** − Oral: for SVT - Initial dose of 0.5 to 1 mg/kg/day − Maximum 2.5 mg/kg/day</li><li>**CYP450 Interactions:** None, but major P-gp substrate</li><li>**Renal or Hepatic Dose Adjustments:** − GFR > 50 mL/minute, every 24 hours. − GFR 31 to 50 mL/minute, every 24 to 36 hours − GFR 10 to 30 mL/minute, every 24 to 48 hours − GFR <10 mL/minute, every 40 to 60 hours − HD - administer post-dialysis</li><li>**Dosage Forms:** Oral (tablet)</li></ul>

\multicolumn{4}{c}{**Vaughn Williams Class 2 (Beta-Antagonists) - Drug Class Review**}
\multicolumn{4}{c}{High-Yield Med Reviews}
Generic Name	Brand Name	Main Indication(s) or Uses	Notes

Pindolol	Visken	- Hypertension	- **Dosing (Adult):**
			  – Oral: 2.5 to 30 mg BID
			    – Maximum 60 mg daily
			- **Dosing (Peds):** Not routinely used
			- **CYP450 Interactions:** Substrate of CYP2D6
			- **Renal or Hepatic Dose Adjustments:** No specific recommendations.
			- **Dosage Forms:** Oral (tablet)

Propranolol	Inderal	- Angina
		- Cardiac arrhythmias
		- Essential tremor
		- Hypertension
		- Migraine prophylaxis
		- MI
		- Obstructive hypertrophic cardiomyopathy
		- Pheochromocytoma
		- Proliferating infantile hemangioma
			- **Dosing (Adult):**
			  – Oral: IR 10 to 320 mg once to four times daily
			    – Maximum 320 mg daily
			  – Oral: ER 80 to 320 mg daily
			    – Maximum 320 mg daily
			  – IV: solution 1 mg IV q2minutes
			    – Maximum 3 doses
			- **Dosing (Peds):**
			  – Oral: IR 0.5 to 1 mg/kg/day in 3 divided doses
			    – Maximum 4 mg/kg/day
			  – IV 0.01 to 0.15 mg/kg/dose q6 to 8 hours
			  – Age-dependent maximum of 1 mg/dose for infants, and 3 mg/dose for children and adolescents
			- **CYP450 Interactions:** Extensive first pass, oxidation via CYP1A2, CYP2C19, CYP2D6, and CYP3A4. Inhibits CYP 1A2
			- **Renal or Hepatic Dose Adjustments:** None
			- **Dosage Forms:** Oral (tablet, capsule [ER], solution), IV solution

CARDIOVASCULAR – VAUGHAN WILLIAMS CLASS 3 - POTASSIUM CHANNEL BLOCKER

Drug Class
- Vaughan Williams Class 3 - Potassium Channel Blocker
- Acute Care
  - Amiodarone
  - Bretylium
  - Dofetilide
  - Ibutilide
  - Sotalol
- Chronic Care
  - Amiodarone
  - Dronedarone
  - Sotalol

Fast Facts
- The oral and IV forms of amiodarone contain high concentrations of iodine which can contribution to thyroid dysfunction overtime.

Main Indications or Uses
- Acute/Chronic Care:
  - Atrial fibrillation/atrial flutter
  - Ventricular arrhythmias

Drug Interaction Pearl
- Amiodarone is a potent inhibitor of CYP450 2C9, 3A4 and P-gp resulting in clinically relevant drug interactions. Watch out for warfarin and digoxin in particular.

Mechanism of Action
- Potassium channel antagonists in cardiac tissues block the rapidly activating component of the delayed rectifier potassium current during phase 3 of the action potential, thereby prolonging refractoriness in atrial and ventricular tissues and delaying repolarization.
  - Class III agents prevent and terminate reentry dysrhythmias by prolonging the action potential and refractoriness.

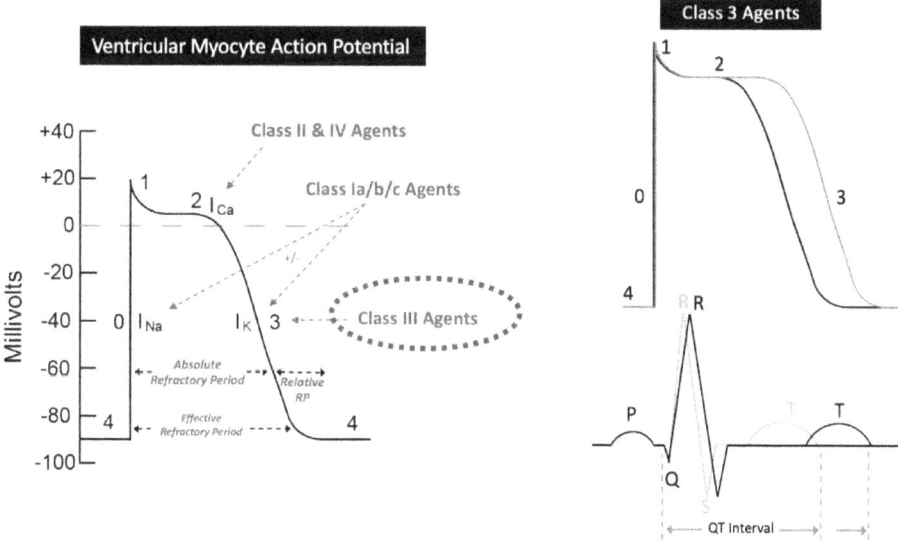

Primary Net Benefit
- Acute and chronic management of atrial and ventricular arrhythmias. Several agents have significant toxicities and may only be initiated in acute care settings.
- Main Labs to Monitor:
  - ECG, blood pressure at baseline and with therapeutic changes.
  - Amiodarone requires extensive baseline and routine laboratory measures for nearly every organ system.

High-Yield Basic Pharmacology
- **Reverse Use-Dependence**
  - Reverse use-dependence describes the class effect of preferentially prolonging the cardiac action potential at slow heart rates and a diminished impact at fast heart rates.
    - This causes both decreased efficacy at controlling tachyarrhythmias and increases the risk of torsades de pointes at slow heart rates.
- **Amiodarone Analog**
  - Dronedarone is an analog of amiodarone that has been de-iodinated but with the addition of a methylsulfonyl group.
    - Developed to decrease the toxicities associated with chronic amiodarone use, dronedarone failed to demonstrate the same effectiveness for broad cardiac indications. As a result, it carried specific warnings for NYHA Class III and IV heart failure patients.
- **Racemic Mixture**
  - Sotalol is a racemic mixture of d- and l-isomers which are both class III potassium channel blockers, with the l-isomer possessing beta-blocking properties.
  - There is some evidence to suggest that d-sotalol may be proarrhythmic.

High-Yield Clinical Knowledge
- **Amiodarone pharmacokinetics, toxicities, drug interactions**
  - Amiodarone possesses antiarrhythmic properties of each Vaughn Williams class: Sodium channel antagonist, beta-antagonist, potassium channel antagonist, and calcium channel antagonist.
    - Amiodarone is known to cause dose-limiting toxicities in all tissues except for the kidneys.
    - However, acute renal failure can indirectly result from cardiovascular, hepatic, hematologic, or endocrine-related toxicities.
  - The hepatic metabolism and impact on hepatic oxidation by amiodarone are extensive. Amiodarone is a substrate of CYP1A2, CYP2C19, CYP2C8, CYP2D6, CYP3A4, and P-gp. It also inhibits CYP2C9, CYP2D6, CYP3A4, and P-gp.
    - Although amiodarone prolongs the PR, QRS, and QT interval, the incidence of torsades de pointes associated with amiodarone is infrequent.
- **Dronedarone warnings**
  - Specific patient populations are uniquely unable to receive dronedarone due to an increased risk of morbidity or mortality.
    - The use of dronedarone is contraindicated in patients with permanent atrial fibrillation, those with symptomatic heart failure and/or a recent decompensation requiring hospitalization or NYHA Class III or IV symptoms, and liver or lung toxicity related to previous amiodarone use.
      - Other contraindications include patients with pre-existing second-degree or third-degree AV block or sick sinus syndrome without a functioning pacemaker, concomitant use of potent CYP3A4 inhibitors, other QT-interval prolonging drugs, and severe hepatic impairment, or if the patient is pregnant or breastfeeding.
- **Dofetilide FDA warning**
  - Dofetilide initiation is associated with a relatively high risk of Torsade De Pointes of approximately 3%. Therefore, initiation or dose adjustments must be in an acute care setting where the patient can be observed for a minimum of 3 days.
    - Facilities must have the capacity to conduct continuous cardiac monitoring, renal function assessments, and the ability to perform cardiac resuscitation.
- **Sotalol**
  - Sotalol is fundamentally a beta-blocker but possesses potassium channel blocking properties. Therefore, the class III action (potassium channel antagonist activity) is the desired clinical effect.
    - Similar to other beta-antagonists, sotalol can precipitate acute decompensation of HFrEF.

- **Benzyl Alcohol and Polysorbate 80**
  - Amiodarone is poorly soluble in water; therefore, it is commercially available as an IV solution in benzyl alcohol and polysorbate 80. As a result, when further diluted with D5W, there is a high risk of precipitation, requiring administration with a 5-micron in-line filter.

- Rapid administration of amiodarone is associated with hypotension. However, this effect is hypothesized to be due to polysorbate 80-induced vasodilation.
    - Polysorbate and benzyl alcohol-free "aqueous" amiodarone preparation was commercially available and did reduce the incidence of hypotension. However, due to the increased cost, and lack of patient-oriented benefit of this agent, it is not commonly available.
- **Weight-based Vs. Fixed Amiodarone Doses**
  - The commonly used IV doses of amiodarone (300mg or 150 mg IV bolus followed by 1mg/min for 6 hours, then 0.5 mg/min for 16 hours) is not appropriate for all indications.
    - For pharmacologic cardioversion of adult patients with atrial tachyarrhythmias, the appropriate dose is 5 mg/kg IV over 30 minutes, followed by an infusion of 10 mg/kg over 20 hours.
      - Due to hypotension, many patients do not tolerate this 5 mg/kg loading dose and fail this pharmacologic strategy.
- **Pharmacologic Cardioversion**
  - Bretylium, dofetilide, and ibutilide are used primarily for acute pharmacologic cardioversion. Therefore, these agents must be initiated in a critical care setting capable of continuous cardiac monitoring and cardiac resuscitation.
- **Dronedarone**
  - The role of dronedarone in practice is narrow due to the risks of worsening heart failure.
    - When combined with either a beta-blocker or calcium channel blocker, it may be an alternative to amiodarone to treat atrial fibrillation in patients with hypertrophic cardiomyopathy with an implantable cardioverter-defibrillator.
- **Sotalol Metabolism**
  - Sotalol does not undergo metabolism and is almost eliminated in the urine. Thus, it may be an ideal agent in patients with a high risk of drug interactions with amiodarone or dronedarone.
    - Pharmacodynamic interactions may still occur with relevant agents, including other beta-blockers, calcium channel blockers, and antiarrhythmics.
      - Sotalol should not be administered with antacids due to a significant reduction in bioavailability.
      - The concomitant use of sotalol and citalopram, clarithromycin, fluoroquinolones, or quetiapine is contraindicated due to excessive QT prolongation risk.

High-Yield Core Evidence
- **DIAMOND**
  - This was a multicenter, randomized, placebo-controlled, double-blind study of dofetilide or placebo in patients undergoing cardioversion in a hospital setting.
  - Dofetilide was not significantly different compared to placebo regarding the primary endpoint of death from any cause.
  - Dofetilide did improve secondary endpoints, including the risk of hospitalization for worsening congestive heart failure, converting atrial fibrillation to sinus rhythm, and maintaining sinus rhythm.
  - Significantly more patients receiving dofetilide experienced torsade de pointes than the placebo group.
  - The authors concluded that dofetilide effectively converted atrial fibrillation, prevented its recurrence, and reduced the risk of hospitalization for worsening heart failure, but dofetilide had no effect on mortality. (N Engl J Med. 1999 Sep 16;341(12):857-65.)
- **SAFIRE-D**
  - This was a multicenter, randomized, placebo-controlled, double-blind study of dofetilide or placebo that evaluated the incidence of converting atrial fibrillation or atrial flutter to sinus rhythm.
  - Dofetilide at any dose studied was significantly better than the placebo at converting study subjects to sinus rhythm and maintaining sinus rhythm assessed one year later.
  - The majority of pharmacological cardioversions with dofetilide occurred within 24 hours and nearly all within 36 hours.
  - The authors concluded that dofetilide is moderately effective in cardioverting atrial fibrillation or atrial flutter to sinus rhythm and significantly effectively maintains sinus rhythm for one year. (Circulation. 2000;102:2385 –2390.)

- **Sotalol Amiodarone Atrial Fibrillation Efficacy Trial**
  - This was a multicenter, randomized, placebo-controlled, double-blind of patients with persistent atrial fibrillation on anticoagulation comparing amiodarone, sotalol, or placebo.
  - Amiodarone was superior to sotalol and placebo in the primary endpoint of time to recurrence of atrial fibrillation beginning on day 28. Sotalol was superior to the placebo. Amiodarone also had a significantly longer time to recurrent atrial fibrillation than either sotalol or placebo.
  - The incidence of major adverse events was similar between the three groups.
  - The authors concluded that amiodarone and sotalol are equally efficacious in converting atrial fibrillation to sinus rhythm, but amiodarone is superior for maintaining sinus rhythm. (N Engl J Med. 2005;352:1861.)
- **ATHENA**
  - This was a multicenter, randomized trial of patients with atrial fibrillation who had additional risk factors for death, comparing dronedarone to placebo.
  - Dronedarone significantly reduced the risk of the primary outcome, which was the first hospitalization due to cardiovascular events or death.
  - Secondary outcomes were death from any cause, death from cardiovascular causes, and hospitalization due to cardiovascular events.
  - There was also a significant reduction in the risk of cardiovascular deaths in patients receiving dronedarone compared to placebo.
  - More patients receiving dronedarone experienced bradycardia, QT-interval prolongation, nausea, diarrhea, rash, and an increased serum creatinine level than the placebo group.
  - The authors concluded that dronedarone reduced the incidence of hospitalization due to cardiovascular events or death in patients with atrial fibrillation. (N Engl J Med. 2009 Feb 12;360(7):668-78.)

High-Yield Fast-Facts
- **Iodine and Amiodarone**
  - Amiodarone is 40% by weight iodine.
- **Iodine Allergy**
  - Iodine allergy is incompatible with life. If patients report iodine allergy to amiodarone, there is likely another mechanism underlying that effect, and other iodine-containing medications (thyroid hormones) can be safely continued.
- **Amiodarone Half-Life**
  - After a single dose of amiodarone, its elimination half-life is approximately 58 days. With chronic use, the elimination half-life is up to 142 days.

HIGH-YIELD BOARD EXAM ESSENTIALS
- **CLASSIC AGENTS:** Amiodarone, bretylium, dronedarone, dofetilide, ibutilide, sotalol
- **DRUG CLASS:** VW Class III
- **INDICATIONS:** Atrial fibrillation/atrial flutter, ventricular arrhythmias
- **MECHANISM:** Potassium channel antagonists block the delayed rectifier potassium current and prolong refractoriness in atrial and ventricular tissues. The QRS can widen and QT interval can be prolonged. It also has a half-life of about 58 days.
- **SIDE EFFECTS:** Arrhythmias, amiodarone (hyper/hypothyroid, hepatotoxicity, pulmonary toxicity, skin discoloration)
- **CLINICAL PEARLS:**
  - Amiodarone is a well-known inhibitor of CYP2C9, 3A4 and P-gp and causes a lot of drug interactions (warfarin, diltiazem, verapamil, simvastatin, and many other drugs). Amiodarone possesses antiarrhythmic properties of each Vaughn Williams class. Amiodarone also has a long half-life
  - Sotalol is renally eliminated and thus requires dose adjustments to avoid bradycardia or heart block.

Table: Drug Class Summary

Vaughan Williams Class 3 - Drug Class Review			
High-Yield Med Reviews			
Mechanism of Action: *Potassium channel antagonists block the delayed rectifier potassium current and prolong refractoriness in atrial and ventricular tissues.*			
Class Effects: *Prevent and terminate reentry dysrhythmias.*			
Generic Name	**Brand Name**	**Main Indication(s) or Uses**	**Notes**

Amiodarone	Nexterone, Pacerone	• Ventricular arrhythmia	• **Dosing (Adult):**
			   − IV: (with pulses) 150 mg over 10 minutes, then 1 mg/minute for 6 hours, then 0.5 mg/minute for 18 hours.
			   − IV: (pulseless) 300 mg bolus, may be followed by an additional 150 mg
			   − Oral: 400 to 600 mg daily in divided doses for 2 to 4 weeks, adjusting to doses range from 100 to 400 mg once daily.
			• **Dosing (Peds):**
			   − IV: 5 mg/kg
			• Maximum 3 doses or 15 mg/kg
			   − Oral: 10 to 15 mg/kg/day in 1 to 2 divided doses, adjusting to 2.5 to 5 mg/kg/day
			• **CYP450 Interactions:** Substrate of CYP1A2, CYP2C19, CYP2C8, CYP2D6, CYP3A4, P-gp. Inhibits CYP2C9, CYP2D6, CYP3A4, P-gp
			• **Renal or Hepatic Dose Adjustments:**
			   − No specific recommendations, but reduced doses in hepatic failure should be considered.
			• **Dosage Forms:** IV solution, oral (tablet)

Bretylium	Bretylol	• Ventricular arrhythmia	• **Dosing (Adult):** − IV: bolus 5 mg/kg • Repeat 10 mg/kg q15 to 30 minutes, as necessary • **Dosing (Peds):** Not routinely used • **CYP450 Interactions:** None known • **Renal or Hepatic Dose Adjustments:** No specific adjustments • **Dosage Forms:** IV (solution)

Dofetilide	Tikosyn	• Atrial fibrillation/atrial flutter	• **Dosing (Adult):**
			   − Oral: 500 mcg BID
			• **Dosing (Peds):** Not routinely used
			• **CYP450 Interactions:** Substrate of CYP3A4
			• **Renal or Hepatic Dose Adjustments:**
			   − GFR between 40 to 60 mL/minute reduce initial dose to 250 mcg twice daily
			   − GFR between 20 to 39 mL/minute reduce initial dose to 125 mcg twice daily
			   − Do not use if GFR is < 20 mL/minute
			   − Child-Pugh class C - use caution
			• **Dosage Forms:** Oral (capsule)

\multicolumn{4}{c}{**Vaughan Williams Class 3 - Drug Class Review**}
\multicolumn{4}{c}{High-Yield Med Reviews}
Generic Name	**Brand Name**	**Main Indication(s) or Uses**	**Notes**
Dronedarone	Multaq	<ul><li>Paroxysmal or persistent atrial fibrillation</li></ul>	<ul><li>**Dosing (Adult):**<ul><li>Oral: 400 mg BID with meals.</li></ul></li><li>**Dosing (Peds):** Not routinely used</li><li>**CYP450 Interactions:** Substrate of CYP3A4. Inhibits CYP2D6, CYP3A4, P-gp</li><li>**Renal or Hepatic Dose Adjustments:**<ul><li>Contraindicated in severe hepatic impairment</li></ul></li><li>**Dosage Forms:** Oral (tablet)</li></ul>
Ibutilide	Corvert	<ul><li>Atrial fibrillation/flutter</li></ul>	<ul><li>**Dosing (Adult):**<ul><li>Patients < 60 kg - IV 0.01 mg/kg over 10 minutes</li><li>Patients 60 kg or greater - IV 1 mg over 10 minutes</li></ul></li><li>**Dosing (Peds):** Not routinely used</li><li>**CYP450 Interactions:** None known</li><li>**Renal or Hepatic Dose Adjustments:** No specific adjustments</li><li>**Dosage Forms:** IV (solution)</li></ul>
Sotalol	Betapace, Sorine, Sotylize	<ul><li>Atrial fibrillation/flutter, symptomatic</li><li>Ventricular arrhythmias</li></ul>	<ul><li>**Dosing (Adult):**<ul><li>Oral: 40 to 160 mg BID</li></ul></li><li>Maximum 480 mg/day<ul><li>IV: 75 mg over 5 hours q12h</li></ul></li><li>**Dosing (Peds):**<ul><li>30 mg/m^2/dose q8h</li></ul></li><li>Dose adjustment based on age-related factor graph</li><li>**CYP450 Interactions:** None known</li><li>**Renal or Hepatic Dose Adjustments:**<ul><li>GFR 30 to 60 mL/minute reduce frequency to every 24 hours.</li><li>GFR 10 to 29 mL/minute reduce frequency to every 36 to 48 hours.</li><li>GFR < 10 mL/minute use not recommended</li></ul></li><li>**Dosage Forms:** IV (solution), Oral (solution, tablet)</li></ul>

CARDIOVASCULAR – VAUGHAN WILLIAMS CLASS 4

Drug Class
- **Vaughan Williams Class 4**
  - Diltiazem
  - Verapamil

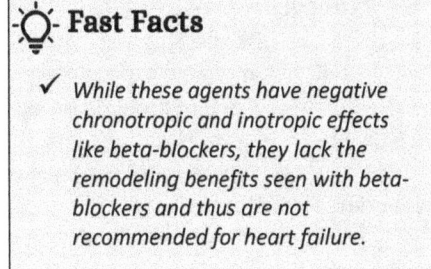

Fast Facts
✓ *While these agents have negative chronotropic and inotropic effects like beta-blockers, they lack the remodeling benefits seen with beta-blockers and thus are not recommended for heart failure.*

Main Indications or Uses
- **Acute Care:**
  - Atrial fibrillation or atrial flutter rate control
  - Supraventricular tachycardia
- **Chronic Care:**
  - Chronic stable angina
  - Hypertension
  - Vasospastic angina

Mechanism of Action
- Slows rate of phase 0 recovery of nodal tissue by decreasing calcium flow into cardiac nodal cells. In nodal tissue, calcium influx initiates depolarization instead of sodium which initiates depolarization in other cardiac tissues.
  - This results in the slowing the pulse (i.e., a negative chronotropic effect)
- They also impair phase 2 mediated calcium influx into the ventricular myocyte where calcium is then used to aid the binding of actin and myosin to facilitate the contraction of the ventricular myocardium.
  - By inhibition this calcium into the ventricular myocyte reduces the force of contraction (i.e., a negative inotropic effect)

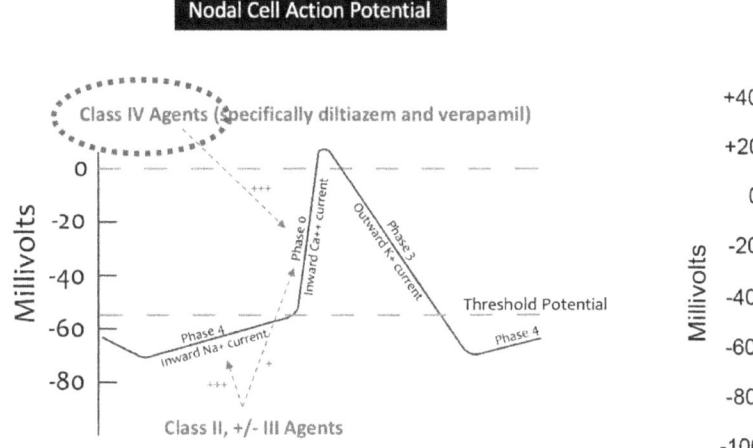
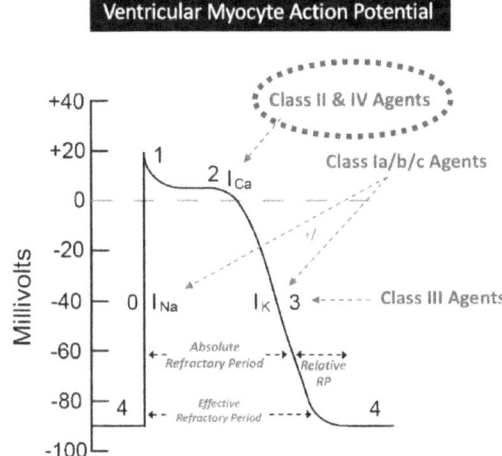

Primary Net Benefit
- Routinely used for acute ventricular rate control in patients with atrial fibrillation with a rapid ventricular response.
- Main Labs to Monitor:
  - ECG and blood pressure at baseline and periodically thereafter.
  - Periodic liver function tests

High-Yield Basic Pharmacology
- **Calcium Channels**
  - The L-type calcium channel is not the only clinically relevant voltage-gated calcium channel. These less commonly known channels include P, N, R, T, and Q -type channels.
    - These channels are located in the heart, nervous system, pancreas, and skeletal muscles.

- Ligand-gated calcium channels include the inositol-trisphosphate receptors and the ryanodine receptor (RyR) family.
- **Non-DHP**
  - Diltiazem and verapamil proportionally increase the degree of calcium channels when there is a high frequency of opening, as in fast heart rates.
    - While this partially explains the non-dihydropyridine selectivity for cardiac effects, resting membrane potential plays a larger role.
    - For dihydropyridine agents, due to the more negative resting potential for cardiac muscle, agents such as amlodipine, clevidipine, or nicardipine preferentially bind to vascular smooth muscle, where there is a less negative resting potential.
- **Ryanodine Receptor**
  - In cardiac tissue, the inhibition of calcium entry into cells limits the activation of the ryanodine receptor on the sarcoplasmic reticulum and limits calcium-dependent calcium release.
    - Without this massive efflux of calcium from the sarcoplasmic reticulum, there will be insufficient calcium to bind with troponin C, which is essential for displacing troponin and tropomyosin from actin and freeing actin to bind with myosin.

High-Yield Clinical Knowledge
- **Myocardial Muscle and Smooth Muscle Calcium Channel Block**
  - Binds to prevent calcium entry through "long-type" or L-type calcium channels on myocardial and smooth muscle.
    - The reduction in calcium influx intracellularly prevents the calcium-calmodulin complex from stimulating myosin light chain kinase phosphorylation and ultimately activating actin-myosin interaction and a resulting contraction.
- **Verapamil Racemate**
  - Knowledge of verapamil being a racemic mixture is clinically relevant. This is because of L-verapamil's significant first-pass metabolism, which is the more potent calcium channel blocker.
  - Therefore, when administered intravenously, verapamil has a more pronounced effect on the PR interval than when taken orally.
    - Since this first-pass effect results from several CYP450 isoenzymes, this effect can also be observed if drug interactions inhibit the first-pass metabolism.
    - Diltiazem also undergoes first-pass metabolism but does not appear to have appreciable differences in action between ingestion routes.
- **Atrial Fibrillation with Rapid Ventricular Response**
  - Diltiazem or verapamil can rapidly control ventricular rates in patients with atrial fibrillation. In these patients, diltiazem is commonly used in a fixed-dose (10 mg IV) or weight-based dose regimen (0.25 mg/kg IV followed by 0.35 mg/kg if inadequate response). An infusion of diltiazem can follow successful rate control at 5 to 15 mg/hr.
    - Avoid in patients who also have Wolff-Parkinson-White (WPW) syndrome, which can worsen the tachycardia.
- **Supraventricular Tachycardia**
  - Verapamil can be used as an alternative to adenosine. As a result of the significant first-pass metabolism of oral verapamil, the intravenous dose is 5 to 10 mg. In contrast, the oral dose for atrial fibrillation rate control is up to 480 mg/day.
- **Atrial Fibrillation Rate Control**
  - Non-dihydropyridine calcium channel blockers can be used for rate control of patients with atrial fibrillation.
  - However, these agents should be avoided in patients with HFrEF and atrial fibrillation.
- **Constipation**
  - Non-dihydropyridine calcium channel blockers are associated with constipation.
    - This is no trivial adverse event leading to GI obstruction and potentially perforation.

High-Yield Core Evidence
- **Diltiazem Fix or Variable Weight-based Dosing**
    - This was a retrospective review of patients with atrial fibrillation and rapid ventricular response, comparing a fixed dose of diltiazem to the variable weight-based dose.
    - The investigators observed that the fixed dose of 10 mg diltiazem was non-inferior to weight-based dosing in regards to the primary outcome of successful treatment of atrial fibrillation (a composite of the heart rate less than 100 beats/min, reduction of HR at least 20%, or conversion to normal sinus rhythm.)
    - The authors concluded that the standard diltiazem dose was non-inferior to weight-based dosing in the initial treatment of atrial fibrillation and rapid ventricular response. (J Emerg Med. 2016 Oct;51(4):440-446.)
- **Diltiazem vs Verapamil for SVT**
    - Single-center, randomized study comparing the effect of verapamil or diltiazem as slow infusions in terminating spontaneous supraventricular tachycardia in the emergency department.
    - There was no difference between verapamil and diltiazem in converting patients to sinus rhythm, and the incidence of adverse events was similar between groups.
    - The authors concluded that calcium channel blocker infusions were safe and efficacious in terminating spontaneous SVT. (Resuscitation. 2002 Feb;52(2):167-74.)
- **AFFIRM**
    - This was a landmark multicenter, parallel-group, randomized, controlled trial that compared a rate-control strategy to a rhythm-control strategy to manage atrial fibrillation.
    - The primary outcome of this study (5-year mortality) was not significantly different between groups.
    - However, more patients in the rhythm-control group were hospitalized more frequently, had a PEA or bradycardic event, and more patients crossed over from the rhythm control to rate control arms rather than vice versa.
    - A subgroup analysis associated the rhythm-control strategy with a higher risk of death than the rate-control strategy among older patients, patients with CAD, and patients without HF.
    - The authors concluded that the rhythm-control strategy offers no survival advantage over the rate-control strategy. However, the rate-control strategy has potential benefits, such as a lower risk of adverse drug effects. (N Engl J Med. 2002 Dec 5;347(23):1825-33.)
- **AF-CHF**
    - This was a multicenter, randomized trial comparing the rhythm control with rate control in patients with HFrEF and a history of atrial fibrillation.
    - There was no significant difference in the primary outcome of time to death from cardiovascular causes.
    - There were also no differences in the secondary outcomes of death from any cause, stroke, worsening heart failure, and the composite of death from cardiovascular causes, stroke, or worsening heart failure.
    - The authors concluded that patients with atrial fibrillation and HFrEF, a systematic strategy of rhythm control, do not reduce the rate of death from cardiovascular causes compared with a rate-control strategy. (N Engl J Med. 2008 Jun 19;358(25):2667-77.)

High-Yield Fast-Facts
- **Not Just L-Type**
    - Cardiac calcium channels are predominantly L-type; however, T-type calcium channels are also present. Mibefradil was a T-type cardiac calcium channel blocker but was withdrawn from the market.
- **Non-Cardiac Indications**
    - Verapamil can be used for numerous non-cardiac indications, including cluster headaches, migraines, and cocaine-induced chest pain.
- **Overdose**
    - Non-dihydropyridine calcium channel blocker overdose can be treated with high-dose insulin therapy (insulin regular 1 unit/kg).

> **HIGH-YIELD BOARD EXAM ESSENTIALS**
> - **CLASSIC AGENTS:** Diltiazem, verapamil
> - **DRUG CLASS:** VW Class IV
> - **INDICATIONS:** Atrial fibrillation or atrial flutter rate control, SVT, chronic stable angina, hypertension, vasospastic angina
> - **MECHANISM:** L-type calcium channels inhibition, ultimately leading to vasodilation, negative inotropy (myocardial muscle and smooth muscle); slows heart rate and rate of recovery in nodal tissue by decreasing calcium flow into cardiac nodal cells (SA and AV nodal tissue)
> - **SIDE EFFECTS:** Bradycardia, hypotension, constipation, worsening of GERD
> - **CLINICAL PEARLS:**
>   - Avoid both agents in patients with WPW along with AFib with RVR.
>   - Verapamil can be used as an alternative to adenosine for SVT.
>   - As a result of the significant first-pass metabolism of oral verapamil, the intravenous dose is 5 to 10 mg. Whereas the oral dose for atrial fibrillation rate control is up to 480 mg/day.

Table: Drug Class Summary

Vaughan Williams Class 4 - Drug Class Review High-Yield Med Reviews			
Mechanism of Action: *Myocardial muscle and smooth muscle* *-L-type calcium channel inhibition, ultimately leading to vasodilation and negative inotropy.* *SA and AV nodal tissue* *-Slows heart rate and the recovery rate in nodal tissue by decreasing calcium flow into cardiac nodal cells.*			
Class Effects: *Vasodilation decreased chronotropic and inotropic effect*			
Generic Name	**Brand Name**	**Main Indication(s) or Uses**	**Notes**
Diltiazem	Cardizem, Cartia, Matzim, Taztia, Tiadylt, Tiazac	<ul><li>Angina</li><li>Atrial fibrillation or atrial flutter</li><li>Hypertension</li><li>Ventricular tachycardia</li><li>SVT</li></ul>	<ul><li>**Dosing (Adult):**<ul><li>IR: 30 mg 4 times daily<ul><li>Maximum 240 to 360 mg/day</li></ul></li><li>12-hour (twice-daily) formulations: 60 mg twice daily; Max: 240 to 360 mg/day</li><li>24-hour (once-daily) formulations: 120 to 180 mg once daily<ul><li>Maximum 240 to 360 mg/day</li></ul></li><li>IV: 0.25 or 0.35 mg IV push<ul><li>Alternatively 10 mg IV push</li></ul></li><li>IV: infusion 5 to 15 mg/hour</li></ul></li><li>**Dosing (Peds):**<ul><li>IR: 1.5 to 2 mg/kg/day in 3 to 4 divided doses<ul><li>Maximum 6 mg/kg/day or 360 mg/day, whichever is less</li></ul></li><li>IV 0.25 or 0.35 mg IV push</li></ul></li><li>**CYP450 Interactions:** Major substrate of CYP3A4, P-gp</li><li>**Renal or Hepatic Dose Adjustments:** None</li><li>**Dosage Forms:** Oral (solution, capsule or tablet), IV solution</li></ul>
Verapamil	Calan, Verelan	<ul><li>Angina</li><li>Atrial fibrillation or atrial flutter</li><li>Hypertension</li><li>Ventricular tachycardia</li><li>SVT</li></ul>	<ul><li>**Dosing (Adult):**<ul><li>IR: 80 to 120 mg 3 times daily.</li><li>ER: 180 mg once daily</li></ul></li><li>Maximum 480 mg/day<ul><li>IV: bolus 2.5 to 10 mg IV push</li></ul></li><li>**Dosing (Peds):**<ul><li>IR: 2 to 8 mg/kg/day in 3 divided doses</li></ul></li><li>Maximum 480 mg/day<ul><li>IV: 0.1 to 0.3 mg/kg/dose; Maximum 5 mg/dose</li></ul></li><li>**CYP450 Interactions:** Major substrate of CYP3A4</li><li>**Renal or Hepatic Dose Adjustments:**<ul><li>Cirrhosis, reduce oral dose to 20-30% of normal, IV dose 50% reduction</li></ul></li><li>**Dosage Forms:** Oral (capsule or tablet), IV solution</li></ul>

CARDIOVASCULAR – VAUGHAN WILLIAMS UNCLASSIFIED

Drug Class
- Vaughan Williams Unclassified
- Acute Care
    - Adenosine
    - Digoxin
    - Magnesium sulfate
- Chronic Care
    - Digoxin

Main Indications or Uses
- Acute Care:
    - Paroxysmal supraventricular tachycardia
        - Adenosine
    - Ventricular fibrillation or ventricular tachycardia
        - Magnesium
- Chronic Care:
    - Atrial fibrillation or atrial flutter, rate control
        - Digoxin
    - Heart failure with reduced ejection fraction (HFrEF)
        - Digoxin
    - Seizures in severe eclampsia
        - Magnesium sulfate

> **Fast Facts**
> - Digoxin is one of the few drugs that is dosed on lean body mass due to its high penetration into the cardiac muscle.
> - Digoxin is a substrate of P-gp, not CYP450 3A4.
> - Magnesium sulfate is sometimes used for COPD exacerbations for bronchodilation. This is due to its ability to compete with calcium mediated interaction with actin and myosin.

Mechanism of Action
- Adenosine
    - Activates inward rectifier potassium current and inhibition of calcium current in the SA and AV nodes.
        - This shortens the action potential duration, hyperpolarization, and slowing of normal automaticity
- Digoxin
    - Antiarrhythmic properties from increasing parasympathetic tone, thereby decreasing the rate of depolarization of the SA node and decreasing the rate of conduction through the AV node
        - It also inhibits the sodium-potassium ATPase pump resulting in increased myocardial cell calcium concentration and causing a positive inotropic effect.
            - Inhibition of this pump causes increased sodium within the cell, permitting exchange for calcium via calcium-sodium antiporter. This enhances the calcium release from the sarcoplasmic reticulum during systole, which increases the cardiac muscle contraction force.
- Magnesium sulfate
    - May cause a decrease in the rate of calcium entry, thereby limiting the rate of initial depolarizations of early afterdepolarizations associated with torsade de pointes.
        - Magnesium is also a cofactor of the Na+,-K+-ATPase exchange, with enhanced function associated with magnesium administration, decreasing calcium entry to cardiac cells.

Primary Net Benefit
- Adenosine has a crucial role in the acute management of supraventricular arrhythmias, and magnesium sulfate is a safe and effective adjunct to therapy in ventricular arrhythmias. However, the role of digoxin continues to become limited due to the safety of the drug and more advanced electrophysiologic cardiac interventions.
- Main Labs to Monitor:
    - ECG continuously during treatment (Adenosine)
    - Digoxin serum concentrations, potassium, and magnesium serum concentrations (at baseline and periodically throughout therapy)

High-Yield Basic Pharmacology
- **Digoxin ECG Changes**
  - Digoxin can have numerous effects on the ECG, including QT interval shortening, and characteristic scooping of the ST segments, mainly seen with toxicity.
- **Calcium, Potassium, and Digoxin**
  - While hyperkalemia may represent severe digoxin toxicity, hypocalcemia and hypokalemia may increase the risk of digoxin toxicity when initiating digoxin.
    - Hyperkalemia occurs due to the relatively higher degree of sodium-potassium ATPase pump inhibition, which causes relative increases in extracellular potassium.
      - There is a hypothetical risk of administration of calcium to treat hyperkalemia due to digoxin toxicity. However, the risk of causing cardiac tetany, otherwise known as "stone heart," appears to be minimal based on observational literature.
- **Cardiac Stress Testing**
  - Adenosine can be used for thallium cardiac stress testing due to adenosine's ability to cause coronary vasodilation and increases blood flow in normal coronary arteries with little to no increase in stenotic coronary arteries.
    - The dose is much lower (140 mcg/kg/min) and administered via IV infusion for 6 minutes.

High-Yield Clinical Knowledge
- **Rapid administration of adenosine**
  - The conventional method of rapidly pushing adenosine through a proximal Y-site on IV tubing, followed by a fluid bolus from a more distal Y-site, may not be the most effective method of administration.
    - Adenosine can be administered through the same IV Y-site as the subsequent fluid bolus using a device known as a 3-way stopcock.
    - Adenosine may also be diluted into the 20 mL sodium chloride 0.9% flush without compromising activity.
- **Digoxin for atrial fibrillation rate control**
  - Digoxin is widely used in patients with atrial fibrillation; however, intravenous diltiazem is safe and more effective in achieving ventricular rate control and leads to a shorter hospital stay in patients with acute atrial fibrillation. (Crit Care Med. 2009 Jul;37(7):2174-9)
- **Magnesium sulfate rate of administration**
  - For use as an antiarrhythmic, magnesium sulfate 1 to 4.5g must be administered rapidly to achieve the rate and rhythm control effects.
    - Many hospitals' computerized order entry systems default magnesium sulfate infusions to run over 1 hour. However, for use as an antiarrhythmic, 4.5g must be administered over approximately 10 minutes or faster if hemodynamically unstable.
- **Digoxin Loading Doses Onset**
  - Digoxin has a relatively slow onset of action in its ability to control the ventricular rate.
    - Initial rate control can be achieved within 1 hour of the first component of a loading dose; the maximum benefit isn't achieved for 24 to 48 hours.
- **Adenosine Alternative Administration**
  - Adenosine may be administered via a central intravenous catheter; however, the dose must be lowered to 3 mg followed by 6 mg twice if the desired response is not achieved.
- **Digifab**
  - Digifab is the digoxin immune antigen-binding fragment that binds to and eliminates digoxin renally.
    - It can be used for other non-digoxin cardiac glycosides.
- **Digoxin Drug Interactions - Amiodarone Or Dronedarone**
  - By inhibiting P-gp, amiodarone can potentially double digoxin concentrations; therefore, the digoxin dose should be empirically lowered by 50% when amiodarone is started.
    - Like amiodarone, dronedarone also inhibits P-gp and can increase digoxin concentrations by about 2.5-fold. The same empiric digoxin dose reduction of 50%.

High-Yield Core Evidence
- **Adenosine Vs. Diltiazem or Verapamil For SVT**
  - This was a prospective, randomized controlled trial comparing adenosine to verapamil or diltiazem in the emergency treatment of spontaneous supraventricular tachycardia (SVT).
  - Significantly more patients receiving calcium-channel blockers converted to sinus rhythm than the adenosine group.
  - There was one event of hypotension in the calcium channel group and none in the adenosine group.
  - The authors concluded that calcium channel blockers are an alternative to adenosine in the emergency treatment of stable patients with SVT. (Resuscitation. 2009 May;80(5):523-8.)
- **LOMAGHI Trial**
  - This was a multicenter, randomized, controlled, double-blind clinical trial comparing magnesium sulfate to placebo in rate control of rapid atrial fibrillation in the emergency department.
  - Magnesium sulfate was superior to placebo concerning the primary outcome of reducing baseline ventricular rate to 90 beats/min or less or reducing the ventricular rate by 20% or greater from baseline.
  - This effect was sustained at both high (9g) and low dose (4.5g) magnesium sulfate compared to placebo at 24 hours.
  - The authors concluded that intravenous magnesium sulfate appears to have a synergistic effect when combined with other AV nodal blockers resulting in improved rate control. (Acad Emerg Med. 2019 Feb;26(2):183-191.)
- **A subgroup of the TREAT-AF Study**
  - This was a subgroup analysis from the TREAT-AF study to assess the association of digoxin with mortality in atrial fibrillation.
  - A retrospective study of Veterans Affairs patients with newly diagnosed, nonvalvular atrial fibrillation was seen in an outpatient setting.
  - Patients treated with digoxin had significantly higher cumulative mortality rates than untreated patients.
  - Furthermore, digoxin use was independently associated with mortality after multivariate adjustment and propensity matching, even after adjustment for drug adherence.
  - The authors concluded that digoxin was associated with an increased risk of death in patients with newly diagnosed atrial fibrillation, independent of drug adherence, kidney function, cardiovascular comorbidities, and concomitant therapies. (J Am Coll Cardiol. 2014;64:660 –668.)
- **Digoxin And Mortality In Atrial Fibrillation**
  - This was a subgroup analysis of the ARISTOTLE study using a propensity score-adjusted analysis in new digoxin users compared to a propensity score-matched control group.
  - Digoxin was associated with a significantly higher risk of death and sudden death in the propensity score-matched analysis.
  - If serum digoxin concentration was above the normal therapeutic limit, patients had a 56% increased mortality hazard compared with those not on digoxin.
  - When analyzed as a continuous variable, serum digoxin concentration was associated with a significantly higher adjusted hazard of death for each 0.5-ng/ml increase in patients with and without heart failure.
  - The authors concluded that in patients with atrial fibrillation taking digoxin, the risk of death was independently related to serum digoxin concentration and highest in patients with concentrations above normal therapeutic ranges, and initiating digoxin was independently associated with higher risk mortality in patients with AF, regardless of heart failure. (J Am Coll Cardiol. 2018 Mar 13;71(10):1063-1074.)

High-Yield Fast-Facts
- **Adenosine and P2Y12 Inhibitors**
  - The bradycardic effects of cangrelor and ticagrelor are mediated by a relative increase in adenosine interaction with cardiac tissue.
- **Chronic Theophylline and Adenosine**
  - Patients chronically taking theophylline or high dose caffeine may require higher than normal doses of adenosine due to increased adenosine metabolism.

- **Vagal Maneuvers**
    - Vagal maneuvers are non-pharmacologic interventions used for SVT before pharmacologic therapy. While these methods are of questionable efficacy, provided they do not delay definitive care, these procedures have minimal risk.

HIGH-YIELD BOARD EXAM ESSENTIALS
- **CLASSIC AGENTS:** Adenosine, digoxin, magnesium sulfate
- **DRUG CLASS:** VW unclassified
- **INDICATIONS:** Paroxysmal SVT (adenosine), Vfib/Vtach (magnesium), Afib/flutter, HFrEF (digoxin), seizures in severe eclampsia (magnesium)
- **MECHANISM:** Activates inward rectifier potassium current and inhibition of calcium current in the SA and AV nodes (adenosine); increases parasympathetic tone, decreases rate of depolarization of the SA node and decreasing the rate of conduction through the AV node (digoxin); may decrease in the rate of calcium entry, thereby limiting the rate of initial depolarizations of early after depolarizations associated with torsade de pointes (magnesium).
- **SIDE EFFECTS:** Bradycardia, hyperkalemia, paralysis (magnesium)
- **CLINICAL PEARLS:**
    - Digoxin is widely used in patients with atrial fibrillation, however, intravenous diltiazem is safe and more effective in achieving ventricular rate control and leads to a shorter hospital stay in patients with acute atrial fibrillation.
    - Digoxin is a major substrate of P-gp and thus is prone to drug interactions.
    - Adenosine is the drug of choice for SVT but must be given by rapid IV push due to its very short half-life.

Table: Drug Class Summary

Vaughan Williams Unclassified - Drug Class Review High-Yield Med Reviews			
Mechanism of Action: Adenosine - Activates inward rectifier potassium current and inhibition of calcium current in the SA and AV nodes. Digoxin - increases parasympathetic tone, decreases the rate of depolarization of the SA node, and decreases the rate of conduction through the AV node. Magnesium sulfate - May decrease the calcium entry rate, thereby limiting the rate of initial depolarizations early afterdepolarizations associated with torsade de pointes.			
Class Effects: Slows conduction through cardiac tissue.			
Generic Name	**Brand Name**	**Main Indication(s) or Uses**	**Notes**
Adenosine	Adenocard	• Paroxysmal SVT	• **Dosing (Adult):** — IV: bolus 6 mg; May repeat 12 mg twice • **Dosing (Peds):** — IV: bolus of 0.1 mg/kg (max: 6 mg) — May repeat 0.2 mg/kg (max: 12 mg) twice • **CYP450 Interactions:** None known • **Renal or Hepatic Dose Adjustments:** None • **Dosage Forms:** IV: (solution)
Digoxin	Digitek, Digox, Lanoxin	• Atrial fibrillation or atrial flutter • HFrEF	• **Dosing (Adult):** — IV: LD 0.25 to 0.5 mg, followed by 0.25 mg IV q6h — Maximum 1 to 1.5 mg/24 hours — Oral: LD 0.5 mg, followed by 0.125 to 0.25 mg q6h — Maintenance 0.125 to 0.25 mg daily • **Dosing (Peds):** — Complex dosing exists for pediatrics. — Best to look it up or consult with expert • **CYP450 Interactions:** Substrate of CYP3A4, P-gp • **Renal or Hepatic Dose Adjustments:** — LD: GFR 15 mL/min or less = 50% of normal dose. — Maintenance dose: GFR 45 to 60 mL/min, reduce to 0.0625 to 0.125 mg once daily. — GFR 30 to < 45 mL/min 0.0625 mg once daily. — GFR < 30 mL/min 0.0625 mg every 48 • **Dosage Forms:** IV (solution), Oral (tablet)
Magnesium sulfate	N/A	• Torsades de Pointes: • Polymorphic VT with QT prolongation, with pulse • Ventricular fibrillation/ Pulseless VT	• **Dosing (Adult):** — IV: bolus 1 to 4.5 g over 1 to 5 minutes. — IV: infusion 0.5 to 1g hour (initial rate). • **Dosing (Peds):** — IV: bolus 25 to 50 mg/kg/dose — Maximum 2g/dose • **CYP450 Interactions:** None • **Renal or Hepatic Dose Adjustments:** None • **Dosage Forms:** IV (solution)

CARDIOVASCULAR – ACE-INHIBITORS

Drug Class
- Angiotensin-converting Enzyme Inhibitors (ACEi)
  - Acute Care
    - Captopril
    - Enalaprilat
  - Chronic Care
    - Benazepril
    - Captopril
    - Enalapril
    - Fosinopril
    - Lisinopril
    - Moexipril
    - Perindopril
    - Quinapril
    - Ramipril
    - Trandolapril

Main Indications or Uses
- Acute Care:
  - Acute HTN
  - Acute myocardial infarction (MI)
  - Acute decompensated HF
  - Scleroderma renal crisis
- Chronic Care:
  - HTN
  - Heart failure
  - Acute coronary syndromes
  - Chronic kidney disease (CKD, +/- diabetes)

> **Fast Facts**
> - ACEi are first line in patients with HTN and HFrEF especially if the patient has diabetes.
> - ACEi are considered to be renal protective due to reductions in glomerular filtration pressures and reduced remodeling.
> - ACEi are contraindicated in pregnancy, in patients with AKI or ARF, and those with hyperkalemia.

Mechanism of Action
- ACE-inhibitors ultimately reduce angiotensin II (Ang II, vasoconstrictor) and lower blood pressure (BP).
  - ACE inhibitors block angiotensin-converting enzyme from converting angiotensin I to Ang II, thus preventing activation of Ang II receptors and vasoconstriction as well as other effects.
  - Ang II has mitogenic effects that result in remodeling of the vasculature and heart leading to worsening heart disease over time. Note: this is one of the main benefits of ACE inhibitors in the treatment of heart failure.

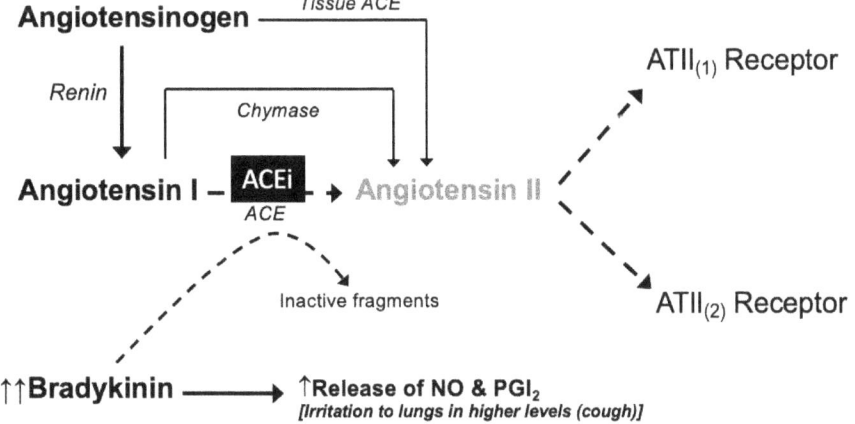

Primary Net Benefit
- ACE inhibitors are first-line disease-modifying agents for HTN that vasodilate and reduce BP.
- Main Labs to Monitor:
  - Basic metabolic panel (potassium, creatinine [SCr])

High-Yield Basic Pharmacology
- **Clinical Pharmacology**
  - ACE inhibitors have other clinically beneficial effects, including cardiac remodeling prevention, renal perfusion improvements, renal complications reduction, and improved mortality with left ventricular systolic dysfunction.
- **ACE "Escape"**
  - ACE levels do not decrease with chronic ACE inhibitor therapy. ACE levels become normal after 1-3 months of ACE inhibitor therapy, called "ACE escape," which is a result of other Ang I metabolism pathways, including chymase, neutral endopeptidase (aka neprilysin), and cathepsin.
- **Prodrugs**
  - Enalapril and ramipril are pro-drugs that require activation via hepatic metabolism (active metabolites enalaprilat and ramiprilat).

High-Yield Clinical Knowledge
- **Inpatient Setting**
  - Due to delayed vasodilatory effects, use in acute HTN is limited, even with IV forms (up to 15 min).
  - Enalaprilat IV has an onset of 15 min but a potential 6-hour duration of action. Use caution with boluses.
  - Captopril can be used as an oral agent for acute HTN to avoid IV administration if not required.
- **Hypertension**
  - ACE inhibitors are a potential first-line agent for HTN but are not as effective at preventing HF or stroke as thiazide diuretics or CCBs. This is especially true in African American patients.
  - Compelling indications for ACE-inhibitor therapy include post-myocardial infarction, HF, CKD Stage 3-5 or with albuminuria, or diabetes with albuminuria.
- **Heart Failure**
  - ACE inhibitor starting doses should be low. Caution in patients with a history or increased risk of orthostatic hypotension, the elderly, CKD, sodium or volume depletion, acute HF exacerbation, or taking concomitant vasodilators/thiazide diuretics.
  - Titration to the maximum tolerated dose and specific hemodynamic targets should still be the goal.
- **CKD**
  - ACE inhibitors or ARBs should be used in patients with Stage 3 CKD or higher or any stage with albuminuria and patients with diabetes and albuminuria to reduce the progression of nephropathy.
- **Monitoring Considerations**
  - ACE inhibitors can cause hyperkalemia, especially in combination with other agents that can cause hyperkalemia.
  - ACE inhibitors can cause an increase in baseline SCr due to changes in renal perfusion. If an increase in SCr is >35% or > 1 mg/dL, then dosage reduction or discontinuation may be required.
- **Acute Kidney Injury**
  - May cause hyperkalemia and AKI, especially with unilateral/bilateral renal artery stenosis.
  - Consider other agents that can cause AKI, such as NSAIDs and others.
- **Combination Therapy**
  - ACE inhibitors are not recommended in combination with ARBs.
  - Avoid ACE inhibitors in combination with or within 36 hours of switching from or to neprilysin inhibitors.
  - SGLT-2 inhibitors can be used in combination to further improve renal and CV outcomes in patients with CKD +/- diabetes, HF +/- diabetes, or for secondary prevention of CV events with diabetes.

High-Yield Core Evidence
- **TRANSCEND**
  - ACE inhibitor-induced angioedema eliminates the potential use of the ACE inhibitor class.
  - ARBs have been investigated for safety in patients with ACE inhibitor-induced angioedema due to RAAS inhibition benefits.
  - 75 patients were enrolled with a history of ACE inhibitor-induced angioedema and randomized to placebo or ARB therapy. No events of angioedema were reported.

- Angioedema can occur any time during RAAS agent therapy, but this study supports a potential role for ARBs in selected patients. (Lancet 2008;372(9644):1174–1183.)
- **SOLVD 1 and SOLVD 2**
  - Examined the effects of enalapril on mortality and hospitalizations in patients with HF.
  - SOLVD 1 demonstrated that enalapril added to conventional therapy significantly reduced mortality and hospitalizations for HF in patients with HF and reduced ejection fraction.
  - SOLVD2 added to this data by further examining subsets of patients and describing improvements in progressive LV dilatation and systolic dysfunction in response to randomization to enalapril. (N Engl J Med 1991 Aug 1;325(5):293-302.; Circulation 86;431–438.)

High-Yield Fast-Facts
- ACE inhibitors, ARBs, and DRIs are contraindicated in pregnancy as they are teratogens.
- ACE inhibitors block the breakdown of the vasodilatory peptide bradykinin, which likely causes the ACE inhibitor-induced cough and impaired endothelial function that leads to angioedema.
- While most ACE inhibitors are eliminated exclusively by the kidneys, fosinopril, trandolapril, and quinapril are eliminated by the liver and kidneys.
- ACE inhibitors are well-known for increasing the risk of angioedema, but ARBs, direct renin inhibitors, DPP-4 inhibitors, and neprilysin inhibitors also carry an increased risk, especially in combination. The highest risk is with sacubitril in combination with ACE inhibitors.

HIGH-YIELD BOARD EXAM ESSENTIALS
- **CLASSIC AGENTS:** Benazepril, captopril, enalapril, fosinopril, lisinopril, moexipril, ramipril
- **DRUG CLASS:** ACE inhibitors
- **INDICATIONS:** Acute HTN, acute myocardial infarction, acute decompensated HF (captopril, enalaprilat), HTN, HF, CKD, post-MI
- **MECHANISM:** Decrease Ang II and lower BP. Also, inhibit Ang II-mediated vascular remodeling.
- **SIDE EFFECTS:** Dry cough, hyperkalemia, transient SCr bump, AKI, angioedema
- **CLINICAL PEARLS:**
  - A potential first-line monotherapy agent for HTN. Consider comorbidities when choosing as a first-line agent (HF, post-MI, or Stage 3-5 CKD or w/ albuminuria or DM with albuminuria).
  - African American patients may not benefit from ACE inhibitor monotherapy as much as combination therapy.
  - ACE inhibitors can cause hyperkalemia and AKI, especially with "bilateral" renal artery stenosis.
  - Choose an ARB in patients with a history of ACE inhibitor-induced angioedema for RAAS inhibition.
  - Counsel to avoid the use of potassium-containing salt substitutes to avoid hyperkalemia.
  - All ACE inhibitors are contraindicated in pregnancy.

Table: Drug Class Summary

ACE-Inhibitors - Drug Class Review High-Yield Med Reviews			
Mechanism of Action: *ACE-inhibitors reduce the actions of Ang II via ACE inhibition and lower BP.*			
Class Effects: *BP lowering, decreased cardiac remodeling, improved renal perfusion, and improvements in other microvascular complications*			
Generic Name	**Brand Name**	**Main Indication(s) or Uses**	**Notes**

Benazepril	Lotensin	- Hypertension	- **Dosing (Adult):**
			  – Oral: 5 to 10 mg once daily, maximum 40 mg daily in 1-2 divided doses
			- **Dosing (Peds):**
			  – 6 years or older: oral initial dose 0.2 mg/kg/dose once daily and titrate to 0.1 to 0.6 mg/kg/dose, max daily dose = 40 mg
			- **CYP450 Interactions:** No CYP interactions
			- **Renal or Hepatic Dose Adjustments:**
			  – GFR < 30 mL/min or hemodialysis: initial dose 5 mg then titrate to maximum tolerated dose
			- **Dosage Forms:** Oral (tablet)

Captopril	Capoten	- Diabetic nephropathy
		- HF with reduced ejection fraction
		- Hypertension
		- Myocardial infarction with left ventricular dysfunction
			- **Dosing (Adult):**
			  – Oral: 6.25 mg 3 times daily, titrate to 50 mg 3 times daily as tolerated
			- **Dosing (Peds):**
			  – Starting dose 0.1 to 0.3 mg/kg/dose every 6 to 24 hours, titrate to target dose of 0.3 to 3.5 mg/kg/day divided every 6-12 hours, maximum 6 mg/kg/day
			- **CYP450 Interactions:** None
			- **Renal or Hepatic Dose Adjustments:**
			  – GFR 10 to 50 mL/min: initial dose 75% of normal dose every 12 hours
			  – GFR < 10 mL/min: 50% of normal dose every 24 hours
			- **Dosage Forms:** Oral (tablet)

Enalapril	Vasotec	- Heart failure
		- Hypertension
			- **Dosing (Adult):**
			  – Oral starting dose 2.5 mg twice daily, target dose of 10 to 20 mg twice daily, maximum 40 mg/day
			  – IV (enalaprilat) 0.625 to 1.25 mg IV every 6 hours
			- **Dosing (Peds):**
			  – Oral initial dose 0.1 mg/kg/day in 1-2 divided doses, maximum = 0.5 mg/kg/day
			  – IV (enalaprilat) 5-10 mcg/kg/dose every 8 to 24
			- **CYP450 Interactions:** None

			- **Renal or Hepatic Dose Adjustments:**
			  − GFR < 30 mL/min, or in heart failure patients with serum creatinine >1.6 mg/dL: start with 2.5 mg daily
			  − Hemodialysis: administer 50% of normal dose after dialysis
			- **Dosage Forms:** Oral (solution, tablet), IV (enalaprilat)

Fosinopril	Monopril	- Heart failure
		- Hypertension
			- **Dosing (Adult):**
			  − Initial dose 10 mg once daily, increasing dose as tolerated to target range 20-40 mg daily, maximum dose of 40 mg/day
			- **Dosing (Peds):**
			  − Initial dose 0.1 mg/kg/dose daily, titrate to maximum daily dose 0.6 mg/kg/day, or 40 mg/day, whichever is less
			- **CYP450 Interactions:** None
			- **Renal or Hepatic Dose Adjustments:**
			  − GFR < 30 mL/min initial dose 5 mg then titrate to maximum tolerated dose
			- **Dosage Forms:** Oral (tablet)

Lisinopril	Zestril	- Heart failure
		- Hypertension
		- ST-elevation myocardial infarction
			- **Dosing (Adult):**
			  − Initial dose 2.5-10 mg daily, increasing dose as tolerated to target range 40 mg daily
			- **Dosing (Peds):**
			  − Initial dose 0.07 mg/kg/dose once daily, titrate to maximum daily dose 0.6 mg/kg/day, or 40 mg/day, whichever is less
			- **CYP450 Interactions:** None
			- **Renal or Hepatic Dose Adjustments:**
			  − GFR < 30 mL/min: initial dose 2.5 mg daily then titrate to maximum tolerated dose.
			- **Dosage Forms:** Oral (solution or tablet)

Perindopril	Aceon	- Heart failure
		- Stable coronary artery disease
			- **Dosing (Adult):**
			  − Initial dose 2 mg daily, target dose 8-16 mg daily
			- **Dosing (Peds):** None
			- **CYP450 Interactions:** None
			- **Renal or Hepatic Dose Adjustments:**
			  − GFR 30-80 mL/min: maximum dose 8 mg/day
			  − GFR < 30 mL/min: initial 2.5 mg every other day
			  − HD: administer on dialysis days
			- **Dosage Forms:** Oral (tablet)

ACE-Inhibitors - Drug Class Review High-Yield Med Reviews			
Generic Name	**Brand Name**	**Main Indication(s) or Uses**	**Notes**

Moexipril	Univasc	• Hypertension	• **Dosing (Adult):**
			  – Initial dose 3.75 to 7.5 mg daily, target maximum dose 30 mg/day in 1-2 divided doses
			• **Dosing (Peds):** None
			• **CYP450 Interactions:** None
			• **Renal or Hepatic Dose Adjustments:**
			  – GFR < 40 mL/min: 2.5 mg daily, maximum 15 mg/day.
			• **Dosage Forms:** Oral (tablet)

Quinapril	Accupril	• Heart failure
		• Hypertension
			• **Dosing (Adult):**
			  – Initial dose 5 mg twice daily, target maximum tolerated dose 80 mg/day divided
			• **Dosing (Peds):**
			  – Initial dose 0.2 mg/kg
			• **CYP450 Interactions:** None
			• **Renal or Hepatic Dose Adjustments:**
			  – GFR < 30 mL/min: start with 2.5 mg daily
			• **Dosage Forms:** Oral (tablet)

Ramipril	Altace	• Heart failure
		• Hypertension
			• **Dosing (Adult):**
			  – Initial dose 1.25 to 2.5 mg daily, titrate to a target maximum 10 mg daily
			• **Dosing (Peds):** None
			• **CYP450 Interactions:** None
			• **Renal or Hepatic Dose Adjustments:**
			  – GFR < 40 mL/min: initial 25% of normal dose, titrate to maximum tolerated dose or 10 mg daily, whichever is less.
			• **Dosage Forms:** Oral (capsule or tablet)

Trandolapril	Mavik	• Hypertension
		• Post-myocardial infarction heart failure or left-ventricular dysfunction
			• **Dosing (Adult):**
			  – Initial dose 1 mg daily, maximum dose 4 mg daily
			• **Dosing (Peds):** None
			• **CYP450 Interactions:** None
			• **Renal or Hepatic Dose Adjustments:**
			  – GFR < 30 mL/min: initial dose 0.5 mg daily, titrate to maximum tolerated dose or 4 mg, whichever is less.
			• **Dosage Forms:** Oral (capsule or tablet)

CARDIOVASCULAR – ALPHA 1 BLOCKERS (NON-SELECTIVE)

Drug Class
- Alpha 1 Blockers (Nonselective)
  - For selective alpha 1a blockers, see the Genitourinary section
- Agents
  - **Acute Care**
    - Phentolamine
  - **Chronic Care**
    - Doxazosin
    - Phenoxybenzamine
    - Prazosin
    - Terazosin

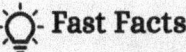

Fast Facts
- ✓ Alpha-1 blockers are NOT first line or preferred treatments for the chronic management of hypertension.
- ✓ Prazosin is one of the few drugs indicated for PTSD. This is a common question on exams.

Main Indications or Uses
- **Acute Care:**
  - Extravasation of sympathomimetic vasopressors (phentolamine only)
  - Pheochromocytoma (any of the agents)
- **Chronic Care:**
  - Phenoxybenzamine
    - Pheochromocytoma treatment
  - Doxazosin, terazosin
    - Benign prostatic hyperplasia
    - Hypertension
    - Ureteral calculi expulsion (off-label)
  - Prazosin
    - Hypertension
    - PTSD-related nightmares and sleep disruption (off-label)
    - Raynaud syndrome (off-label)

Mechanism of Action
- Nonselective alpha-1 antagonism leads to vasodilation via inhibition of Gq-protein coupled receptors in the systemic vasculature.
  - Inhibition of these Gq receptors inhibits the IP3 pathway and ultimately inhibits SR calcium release.
- Additional Consideration:
  - Phenoxybenzamine is unique among alpha-1 antagonists in that it causes an irreversible blockade.
    - This is due to a reactive ethylenediammonium intermediate which covalently binds to these receptors and causes an irreversible blockade.

Primary Net Benefit
- Potent vasodilation in many patients that results in reflex tachycardia and risk of orthostasis in older patients.
- Main Labs to Monitor:
  - No routine monitoring

High-Yield Basic Pharmacology
- **Arterial and Venous Dilation**
  - Contrary to nitrates, nonselective alpha-1 blockers may cause vasodilation in arteriolar resistance vessels and veins at normal therapeutic dosing.
    - These potent vasodilatory effects elicit the classic reflex tachycardia and orthostatic hypotension as adverse events.
- **CNS Penetration**
  - Due to its lipophilicity, prazosin can penetrate the CNS to suppress sympathetic outflow.

- While this may further improve blood pressure lowering, it can also increase the risk of falls in patients by causing dizziness, drowsiness, confusion, and vertigo.
    - Furthermore, since prazosin may depress the baroreflex function in hypertensive patients, rapid changes from seated or supine to a standing position may pose a risk of falls to patients taking prazosin.
- This is the primary reason the first dose of prazosin should be directly observed. In addition, the patient should be monitored in a medical office or facility for up to 90 minutes after the first dose of prazosin and 6 hours for the first dose of doxazosin.
- **Phentolamine**
    - Although phentolamine is typically classified as an alpha-1 antagonist, it has numerous other receptor activities, inducing postsynaptic alpha-2 antagonist properties on vascular smooth muscle and presynaptic alpha-2 antagonism (which would cause an increase in norepinephrine release).
    - Furthermore, phentolamine is also a minor inhibitor of serotonin, antihistaminic, and antimuscarinic effects.

High-Yield Clinical Knowledge
- **Extravasation of a Sympathomimetic Vasopressor:**
    - Phentolamine (when available) should be considered as an agent to prevent tissue necrosis of the affected tissue.
        - The administration of phentolamine should be a subcutaneous injection of phentolamine using 25 gauge or smaller needles.
    - Phentolamine should be prepared as a 5 mg in NS to a final total volume of 10 mL.
    - Then, incremental doses of up to 10 mg should be injected through the catheter and subcutaneously around the site.
    - There should be an immediate response to the tissue, and if not, consider additional dose(s).
    - However, additional doses should be used with caution since phentolamine may cause systemic hypotension, and given the patient was already on a vasopressor, this may be clinically relevant.
- **Ureteral Calculi Expulsion:**
    - Tamsulosin is commonly used to enhance the passage of ureteral stones in both male and female patients.
    - However, the efficacy of this treatment is questionable.
- **Hypertension and Dyslipidemia:**
    - In patients with uncontrolled hypertension and uncontrolled lipids, alpha-1 antagonists exert a pleiotropic effect on lipids.
    - Alpha-1 antagonists can help lower LDL and triglycerides and increase concentrations of HDL.
- **Urethral Underactivity:**
    - Alpha-1 antagonists may be useful in patients with urethral underactivity since they can relax the internal bladder sphincter.
- **Adverse Effects (Floppy Iris Syndrome):**
    - Tamsulosin is associated with floppy iris syndrome. Although it has been reported with doxazosin and silodosin, it is more prevalent with tamsulosin.
    - This adverse effect occurs due to the alpha-1a antagonist effects in iris dilator muscles, increasing the likelihood of post-ophthalmologic operative complications, including posterior capsular rupture, retinal detachment, residual retained lens material, or endophthalmitis. In addition, permanent loss of vision can result.
- **Erectile Dysfunction:**
    - Since phentolamine can reduce peripheral adrenergic tone and enhance cholinergic tone, it can be used to improve cavernosal filling. This use as an erectogenic agent has fallen out of favor given the availability of PDE-5 inhibitors but can still be occasionally seen in practice. To avoid excessive hypotension, phentolamine is combined with papaverine.

High-Yield Core Evidence
- **Terbutaline for Extravasation Study**
  - Phentolamine has been intermittently available, making it difficult to rely upon.
  - Terbutaline, a beta-2 selective agonist, has been proposed as an alternative to phentolamine for the extravasation of specific cytotoxic agents.
  - A case series of 4 patients suffering extravasations from dopamine and dobutamine and three patients having epinephrine injected into the thumb (from inadvertent epinephrine auto-injector deployment).
  - These cases highlighted the potential use of terbutaline as a reasonable alternative.
  - This literature recommended using terbutaline locally and infiltrating the extravasation area using a solution of 1 mg diluted in 10 mL of 0.9% sodium chloride.
  - The necessary volume of terbutaline solution administered varied from 3 to 10 mL. (Am J Emerg Med. 1999 Jan;17(1):91-4.)
- **ALLHAT**
  - The ALLHAT study was a multicenter, double-blinded, parallel-group, randomized controlled trial of patients randomized to base therapy of doxazosin, lisinopril, amlodipine, or chlorthalidone.
  - The primary objective was to compare the combined endpoint of fatal CHD and nonfatal MI.
  - A total of 42,418 patients aged 55 and older with hypertension and one additional CV risk factor were randomized to one of these four treatment groups and were followed for a mean of 4.9 years.
  - This study was stopped early when more secondary endpoints of stroke, HF, and CV events were seen with doxazosin than chlorthalidone.
  - There was no difference in the primary endpoint of fatal coronary heart disease and nonfatal MI but demonstrated that chlorthalidone is superior to doxazosin in preventing CV events in patients with hypertension. (JAMA. 2002;288(23):2981–2997.)
- **PATHWAY-2**
  - The PATHWAY-2 study was a multicenter, double-blind, crossover, controlled trial of patients with resistant hypertension randomized to one of four treatment groups: spironolactone, doxazosin modified release, bisoprolol, or placebo.
  - Specifically, regarding the a priori comparison of spironolactone to doxazosin, patients randomized to spironolactone had a statistically significant improvement in mean SBP reduction. Still, the clinical relevance of this 4 mm Hg reduction has been debated. (Lancet. 2015;386(10008):2059–2068.)

High-Yield Fast-Facts
- **Epinephrine as a vasodilator**
  - As a result of the selective alpha-1 antagonism, an effect of "epinephrine reversal" may occur. In addition, since there would be an alpha-1 blockade but beta-2 activation, vasodilation could occur.
- **Reflex tachycardia**
  - Alpha-1 antagonists as individual agents like prazosin will cause vasodilation but a reflex tachycardia. Therefore, a medication such as carvedilol or labetalol possesses nonselective beta-blocking properties and alpha-1 antagonism. Thus, any reflex tachycardia would be blunted.

HIGH-YIELD BOARD EXAM ESSENTIALS
- **CLASSIC AGENTS:** Doxazosin, phenoxybenzamine, phentolamine, prazosin, terazosin
- **DRUG CLASS:** Alpha-1 blockers (nonselective)
- **INDICATIONS:** Extravasation of sympathomimetic vasopressors (phentolamine); pheochromocytoma treatment (phenoxybenzamine); Benign prostatic hyperplasia, ureteral calculi expulsion (doxazosin, terazosin)
- Hypertension (doxazosin, prazosin, terazosin), PTSD-related nightmares and sleep disruption, Raynaud syndrome (prazosin).
- **MECHANISM:** Vasodilation via inhibition of Gq-protein coupled receptors in the systemic vasculature.
- **SIDE EFFECTS:** Hypotension, reflex tachycardia, headache
- **CLINICAL PEARLS:** Contrary to nitrates, nonselective alpha-1 blockers may cause vasodilation in arteriolar resistance vessels and veins at normal therapeutic dosing. Nitrates need larger doses to achieve both. None of these agents are recommended as monotherapy for the treatment of hypertension. They are most commonly used for secondary causes of elevated BP and/or as adjunct to other treatments. Use with caution if the patient is also taking type 5 PDE inhibitors for erectile dysfunction due to the risk of hypotension.

Table: Drug Class Summary

Alpha-1 Antagonists (Nonselective) - Drug Class Review High-Yield Med Reviews			
Mechanism of Action: *Vasodilation systemic vasculature to result in a lowering of the blood pressure.*			
Class Effects: *Vasodilation, reflex tachycardia, risk of orthostasis in older patients.*			
Generic Name	**Brand Name**	**Main Indication(s) or Uses**	**Notes**
Doxazosin	Cardura, Cardura XL	<ul><li>Benign prostatic hyperplasia</li><li>Hypertension</li><li>Ureteral calculi expulsion</li></ul>	<ul><li>**Dosing (Adult):**<ul><li>IR: 1 mg once daily, maximum 16 mg/day.</li><li>Extended-release: 4 mg once daily, maximum 16 mg/day</li></ul></li><li>**Dosing (Peds):**<ul><li>IR: 0.5 mg once daily at bedtime, maximum 2 mg/day</li></ul></li><li>**CYP450 Interactions:** Substrate of CYP3A4, 2C19, 2D6</li><li>**Renal or Hepatic Dose Adjustments:**<ul><li>Contraindicated for patients with moderate or severe hepatic impairment (Child-Pugh class B/C)</li></ul></li><li>**Dosage Forms:** Oral tablet (immediate-release and extended-release)</li></ul>
Phenoxybenzamine	Dibenzyline	<ul><li>Pheochromocytoma treatment</li></ul>	<ul><li>**Dosing (Adult):**<ul><li>Oral: 10 mg twice daily, maximum 240 mg/day</li></ul></li><li>**Dosing (Peds):**<ul><li>Oral: 0.2 to 0.25 mg/kg/dose once or twice daily; maximum dose: 40 mg/dose</li></ul></li><li>**CYP450 Interactions:** None</li><li>**Renal or Hepatic Dose Adjustments:** None</li><li>**Dosage Forms:** Oral (capsule)</li></ul>
Phentolamine	OraVerse, Rogitine	<ul><li>Extravasation of sympathomimetic vasopressors</li><li>Pheochromocytoma diagnosis</li></ul>	<ul><li>**Dosing (Adult):**<ul><li>Local infiltration: Inject 5 to 10 mg (diluted in 10 mL 0.9% sodium chloride) into extravasation area.</li></ul></li><li>**Dosing (Peds):**<ul><li>Infiltrate the area of extravasation with a small amount of 0.5 to 1 mg/mL.</li></ul></li><li>**CYP450 Interactions:** None</li><li>**Renal or Hepatic Dose Adjustments:** None</li><li>**Dosage Forms:** IV solution</li></ul>

\multicolumn{4}{c}{**Alpha-1 Antagonists (Nonselective) - Drug Class Review**}
\multicolumn{4}{c}{High-Yield Med Reviews}
Generic Name	**Brand Name**	**Main Indication(s) or Uses**	**Notes**
Prazosin	Minipress	<ul><li>Hypertension</li><li>PTSD-related nightmares and sleep disruption</li><li>Raynaud syndrome (off-label)</li></ul>	<ul><li>**Dosing (Adult):**<ul><li>Oral: 1 mg 2 to 3 times daily, maximum 40 mg/day.</li></ul></li><li>**Dosing (Peds):**<ul><li>Oral: 0.05 to 0.1 mg/kg/day in divided doses every 8 hours, maximum 20 mg/day</li></ul></li><li>**CYP450 Interactions:** None</li><li>**Renal or Hepatic Dose Adjustments:** None</li><li>**Dosage Forms:** Oral (capsule)</li></ul>
Terazosin	Hytrin	<ul><li>Benign prostatic hyperplasia</li><li>Hypertension</li><li>Ureteral calculi expulsion</li></ul>	<ul><li>**Dosing (Adult):**<ul><li>Oral: 1 mg at bedtime, maximum 20 mg/day.</li></ul></li><li>**Dosing (Peds):**<ul><li>Oral: 1 mg at bedtime, maximum 20 mg/day.</li></ul></li><li>**CYP450 Interactions:** None</li><li>**Renal or Hepatic Dose Adjustments:** None</li><li>**Dosage Forms:** Oral (capsule)</li></ul>

CARDIOVASCULAR – ALPHA-2 AGONISTS

Drug Class
- Alpha-2 Agonists
  - Clonidine and dexmedetomidine are also commonly pharmacologically classified as imidazoline agonists.
  - Dexmedetomidine is also classified as a sedative
- Agents:
  - **Acute Care**
    - Clonidine
    - Dexmedetomidine
    - Methyldopa
  - **Chronic Care**
    - Clonidine
    - Guanfacine
    - Tizanidine

> **Fast Facts**
> ✓ The extended-release formulations of clonidine and guanfacine are indicated for the management of ADHD and are one of the "non-stimulant" options.

Main Indications or Uses
- **Acute Care:**
  - Hypertension
  - ICU Sedation
    - Mainly only dexmedetomidine, but sometimes clonidine is initiated in transition from dexmedetomidine.
  - Opioid Withdrawal Syndrome (off-label)
    - Mainly clonidine
- **Chronic Care:**
  - Attention-Deficit/Hyperactivity Disorder (ADHD)
    - Only extended-release formulations of clonidine and guanfacine
  - Hypertension
  - Muscle spasm and/or musculoskeletal pain
  - Spasticity

Mechanism(s) of Action
- Centrally acting alpha-2 agonist
  - These agents exert an agonist effect on the presynaptic alpha-2 receptors in the central nervous system (CNS), thereby enhancing the activity of inhibitory neurons in the vasoregulatory regions of the CNS.
  - This ultimately leads to a *decrease* in the release of norepinephrine.
- Imidazoline receptor agonism
  - The antihypertensive effects of clonidine and dexmedetomidine are also facilitated via imidazoline-1 receptor activation.
    - This activation mediates the hypotensive effect observed with these agents due to a reduction in the sympathetic outflow from the intermediolateral cell columns of the thoracolumbar spinal tracts into the periphery. This also lowers the heart rate, reduces vascular tone, and lowers arterial blood pressure.

Primary Net Benefit
- Potent vasodilators with a wide range of indications, including hypertension, Attention-Deficit/Hyperactivity Disorder, muscle spasms, and spasticity.
- Main Labs to Monitor:
  - No routine monitoring

High-Yield Basic Pharmacology
- **Transient Vasoconstriction:**
  - Although oral clonidine's ultimate effect is vasodilation, transient vasoconstriction occurs due to peripheral alpha-2 agonist effects, followed by more prolonged hypotension from central alpha-2 agonist effects.
- **Methyldopa is Unique:**
  - Methyldopa is a prodrug converted to α-methylnorepinephrine in the brain, which ultimately activates central alpha-2 receptors similar to clonidine.
    - However, chronic use can result in sodium and water retention, complicating comorbidities such as heart failure.
- **Ophthalmic Agents:**
  - Apraclonidine and brimonidine are topical ophthalmic agents that are also alpha-2 agonists. These agents lower intraocular pressure in patients with ocular hypertension or open-angle glaucoma. Brimonidine should be used with caution in patients already on clonidine or another systemic alpha-2 agonist since it is systemically absorbed.

> **Counseling Points**
> ✓ Counsel patients on immediate release clonidine for the treatment of hypertension to NOT abruptly stop it as it is well known to result in rebound tachycardia and worsening BP.

High-Yield Clinical Knowledge
- **Hypertension**
  - Clonidine is an oral agent with a rapid onset that can facilitate blood pressure lowering in patients with hypertensive urgency. In these patients, where oral antihypertensive agent interventions are appropriate, clonidine can be titrated and reduced as blood pressure goals are assessed.
- **Pre-eclampsia/Eclampsia**
  - Many drug references and textbooks continue to list methyldopa as a potential first-line agent for pre-eclampsia. However, since safer and agents with more predictable pharmacokinetics and clinical effects are available (i.e., labetalol), methyldopa is seldom used for this indication any longer.
- **Opioid Withdrawal**
  - Clonidine has been used as an adjunct agent in the management of opioid withdrawal.
    - However, it is essential to note that despite its I2 agonist properties, clonidine primarily acts via its central alpha-2 agonist effects and masks the sympathetic effects of opioid withdrawal.
- **Attention-Deficit/Hyperactivity Disorder (ADHD)**
  - Only the extended-release dosage formulations are indicated for this indication in pediatric patients.
    - Those formulations include extended-release clonidine (Kapvay) and extended-release guanfacine (Intuniv).
- **Hypertension**
  - If one of these agents is to be discontinued, abrupt cessation must be avoided.
    - This is because of rebound hypertension and a withdrawal-like syndrome.
    - This effect is thought to be a result of a compensatory increase in norepinephrine release, as well as CNS manifestations of nervousness, agitation, headache, and tremor.
  - Although methyldopa is seldom used anymore, it can also cause hepatitis or hemolytic anemia, which should prompt rapid discontinuation.
- **Muscle spasm and/or musculoskeletal pain**
  - Although tizanidine shares similar pharmacology with clonidine, in that they are both central alpha-2 agonists.
  - Tizanidine largely lacks any antihypertensive effects at normal therapeutic dosing and is primarily used as a skeletal muscle relaxant.
  - However, if combined with clonidine, there could be additional antihypertensive responses observed.

High-Yield Core Evidence
- **Acute Care**
  - To examine the difference between clonidine and labetalol for treating severe hypertension in an emergency department setting, 36 patients were randomized to one of these treatments in a blinded fashion.
  - The study investigators observed similar blood pressure lowering effects between the two treatments with a similar safety profile, and no statistically significant differences were noted.
  - The authors concluded that labetalol was comparable to clonidine for treating severe hypertension in an emergency department setting. (Am J Med Sci. 1992 Jan;303(1):9-15.)
- **ReHOT**
  - The ReHOT study was a randomized, multicenter trial that compared spironolactone to clonidine as the fourth drug in patients with resistant hypertension.
  - Resistant hypertension was defined as patients with poor blood pressure control despite treatment with three drugs, including a diuretic, for 12 weeks.
  - There was no difference between each treatment in blood pressure control during office visits and 24-h ambulatory blood pressure monitoring (RR, 1.01 [0.55-1.88]; P=1.00).
  - The authors concluded that clonidine was not superior to spironolactone in true resistant hypertensive patients. (Hypertension. 2018;71:681–690.)

High-Yield Fast-Facts
- **ADHD Use**
  - Use guanfacine with extreme caution if the patient lives with children younger than two since guanfacine can potentially cause fatal toxicity from a single tablet/capsule ingestion in children.
- **Imidazoline Agonists**
  - The imidazoline compounds oxymetazoline and tetrahydrozoline, normally administered as ophthalmic agents, can have effects similar to clonidine toxicity.
- **COMT Metabolism**
  - Methyldopa is metabolized by COMT, and thus competitive inhibitors of COMT or inhibitors of MAO may increase the risk of toxicity of methyldopa.

HIGH-YIELD BOARD EXAM ESSENTIALS
- **CLASSIC AGENTS:** Clonidine, dexmedetomidine, guanfacine, methyldopa, tizanidine
- **DRUG CLASS:** Alpha-2 agonists
- **INDICATIONS:** Hypertension, ICU Sedation (dexmedetomidine), ADHD (extended-release formulations of clonidine and guanfacine)
- **MECHANISM:** Central alpha-2 agonist, enhancing the activity of inhibitory neurons in the vasoregulatory regions of the central nervous system. Imidazoline receptor agonism (clonidine).
- **SIDE EFFECTS:** Hypotension, reflex tachycardia
- **CLINICAL PEARLS:**
  - Clonidine should not be used as monotherapy for the treatment of chronic HTN but can be used as monotherapy for ADHD. It is used as an adjunct or for short-term use in acute hypertension. Abrupt discontinuation of chronic clonidine will result in tachycardia and elevated BP.
  - Dexmedetomidine can be used to aid in weaning patients off the vent in ICU (does not suppress respiratory drive).
  - Guanfacine is available in a sustained-release form that is FDA approved for treating ADHD in children aged 6–17 years. Use extreme caution if the patient lives with children younger than two since guanfacine can potentially cause fatal toxicity from a single tablet/capsule ingestion in children.

Table: Drug Class Summary

Alpha-2 Agonists - Drug Class Review High-Yield Med Reviews			
Mechanism of Action: *Central alpha-2 agonist, enhancing the activity of inhibitory neurons in the vasoregulatory regions of the central nervous system. Imidazoline receptor agonism (clonidine).*			
Class Effects: *Vasodilation, potential sedating effects*			
Generic Name	**Brand Name**	**Main Indication(s) or Uses**	**Notes**

Clonidine	Catapres
	Kapvay
		• Hypertension	• **Dosing (Adult):**
			  – Oral: Initial: 0.1 mg twice daily, > 0.6 mg/day not recommended.
			  – TD Patch: 0.1 mg/24-hour patch once every 7 days
			• **Dosing (Peds):**
			  – Weight 45 kg or less: Initial: 0.05 mg at bedtime
			  – Weight more than 45 kg: Initial: 0.1 mg at bedtime.
			    – Max is based on patient weight: 27 to 40.5 kg: 0.2 mg/day; 40.5 to 45 kg: 0.3 mg/day; > 45 kg: 0.4 mg/day
			• **CYP450 Interactions:** No CYP interactions
			• **Renal or Hepatic Dose Adjustments:** None
			• **Dosage Forms:** Topical (transdermal patch), Oral (tablet, IR and ER (Kapvay))

Dexmedetomidine	Precedex	• ICU Sedation	• **Dosing (Adult):**
			  – D: 1 mcg/kg x 10 min IV, then 0.2-0.7 mcg/kg/hr.
			• **Dosing (Peds):**
			  – LD: 0.5-1 mcg/kg x 10 min IV, then 0.2-0.5 mcg/kg/hr.
			• **CYP450 Interactions:** Substrate of CYP2A6
			• **Renal or Hepatic Dose Adjustments:** None
			• **Dosage Forms:** Solution for IV injection

Guanfacine	Intuniv	• Hypertension
		• Attention-deficit/hyperactivity disorder
			• **Dosing (Adult):**
			  – Oral: 0.5 to 1 mg once daily at bedtime, maximum 3 mg.
			• **Dosing (Peds):**
			  – Oral: 0.5 to 1 mg once daily at bedtime, maximum is based on patient weight: 27 to 40.5 kg: 2 mg/day; 40.5 to 45 kg: 3 mg/day; > 45 kg: 4 mg/day.
			• **CYP450 Interactions:** Major substrate of CYP3A4
			• **Renal or Hepatic Dose Adjustments:** None
			• **Dosage Forms:** Oral (tablet IR and ER (Intuniv))

Alpha-2 Agonists - Drug Class Review
High-Yield Med Reviews

Generic Name	Brand Name	Main Indication(s) or Uses	Notes

Methyldopa	Aldomet	- Hypertension	- **Dosing (Adult):**
			  - Oral: 250 mg 2 to 3 times daily, maximum 3000 mg/day.
			
			- **Dosing (Peds):**
			  - Oral: 10 mg/kg/day in 2 to 4 divided doses, max 65 mg/kg/day or 3000 mg
			- **CYP450 Interactions:** Major substrate of COMT
			- **Renal or Hepatic Dose Adjustments:** Every 12 or 24 hours if CrCl <10 mL/minute. Give after HD
			- **Dosage Forms:** Oral (tablet)

Tizanidine	Zanaflex	- Muscle spasm and/or musculoskeletal pain
		- Spasticity
			- **Dosing (Adult):**
			  - Oral: 2 to 4 mg every 6 to 12 hours as needed and/or at bedtime, maximum 24 mg/day
			- **Dosing (Peds):**
			  - Oral: 1 mg at bedtime, titrate as needed
			- **CYP450 Interactions:** Major substrate of CYP1A2
			- **Renal or Hepatic Dose Adjustments:**
			  - Use with caution in patients with CrCl <25 mL/minute
			- **Dosage Forms:** Oral (capsule or tablet)

CARDIOVASCULAR – ANGIOTENSIN RECEPTOR BLOCKER

Drug Class
- **Angiotensin Receptor Blocker**
- **Chronic Care**
    - Azilsartan
    - Candesartan
    - Irbesartan
    - Losartan
    - Olmesartan
    - Telmisartan
    - Valsartan

Main Indications or Uses
- **Chronic Care:**
    - HTN
    - Heart failure
    - Acute coronary syndromes (ACS)
    - Chronic kidney disease (CKD, +/- diabetes)

> **Fast Facts**
> ✓ ARBs don't cause the dry cough seen with ACEi and thus are generally used after failing a trial with an ACEi for the treatment of hypertension and/or heart failure.

Mechanism of Action
- ARBs ultimately reduce the actions of angiotensin II (Ang II) and lower blood pressure (BP) via vasodilation.
    - ARBs block Ang II preferentially at the Ang II type 1 (AT1) receptors, which causes vasodilation and reduces aldosterone, catecholamine, and arginine vasopressin release. Remodeling is also reduced.

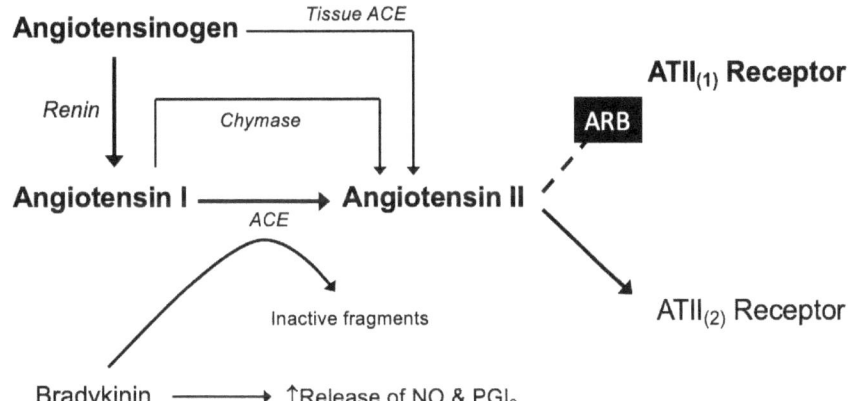

Primary Net Benefit
- ARBs are alternatives to ACE inhibitors to decrease BP by vasodilation.
- Main Labs to Monitor:
    - Basic metabolic panel (potassium, creatinine [SCr])

High-Yield Basic Pharmacology
- **Clinical Pharmacology**
    - ARBs have clinically beneficial effects like ACE inhibitors, including preventing cardiac remodeling, slowing the progression of renal disease, and improving mortality.
- **Serum Creatinine Changes**
    - ARBs are associated with an increase in serum creatinine (SCr) caused by the inhibition of Ang II vasoconstriction on the efferent arteriole.
    - Modest elevations of < 35% increase from baseline or absolute increases SCr < 1 mg/dL should be followed closely. If larger changes occur, ARB therapy should be stopped, or the dose reduced.
- **Hyperkalemia**

- Hyperkalemia is more likely with ARBs when combined with potassium-sparing diuretics, potassium supplements, mineralocorticoid receptor antagonists, ACE inhibitors, or direct renin inhibitors.

High-Yield Clinical Knowledge
- **Hypertension**
  - ARBs are alternatives to ACE inhibitors for post-ACS, HF, CKD, or diabetes with albuminuria.
- **Heart Failure (HF)**
  - ARBs can prevent HF hospitalizations with reduced EF. Titrate to maximum tolerated dose.
- **Post-Ischemic Stroke**
  - Patients receiving ARBs for secondary stroke prevention have a lower risk of recurrent stroke than patients receiving a calcium channel blocker.
- **CKD**
  - ARBs are alternatives to ACE inhibitors for reducing the progression of nephropathy in patients with Stage 3-5 CKD or CKD with albuminuria.
- **Acute Kidney Injury (AKI)**
  - May cause hyperkalemia and AKI, especially with unilateral/bilateral renal artery stenosis.
  - Consider other agents that can cause AKI, such as NSAIDs, vancomycin, and others.
- **Combination Therapy**
  - ACE inhibitors are not recommended in combination with ARBs.
  - SGLT-2 inhibitors can be used in combination to improve renal and CV outcomes in patients with CKD +/- diabetes, HF +/- diabetes, or for secondary prevention of CV events with diabetes.

High-Yield Core Evidence
- **VALLIANT**
  - Patients were randomized to therapy with valsartan, valsartan plus captopril, or captopril alone post-MI to compare cardiac remodeling and hypertrophy effects.
  - There was no difference between treatment groups for the primary endpoint of death from any cause.
  - More adverse events were reported in the combination group compared to other groups.
  - Valsartan is as effective as captopril in patients at high risk for CV events post-MI (N Engl J Med 349: 1893–1906).
- **ON-TARGET**
  - ON-TARGET was a double-blind, randomized trial comparing ramipril, telmisartan, or both to assess a composite outcome of CV death, MI, stroke, or hospitalization for HF.
  - There was no difference between treatment groups for the primary outcome.
  - Telmisartan use was associated with lower rates of cough and angioedema but more hypotension.
  - The combination therapy group had no benefit but an increased risk of hypotension, syncope, and renal dysfunction.
  - Telmisartan causes less cough than ramipril, but otherwise, they are clinically interchangeable (N Engl J Med. 2008 Apr 10;358(15):1547-59).

High-Yield Fast-Facts
- ARBs are teratogens and contraindicated in pregnancy.
- ARBs do not affect bradykinin breakdown, so ACE inhibitor-induced cough can be eliminated. Bradykinin offers benefits for vasodilation, cardiac remodeling, and increased tissue plasminogen activator levels that may be lost.
- ARBs may be less effective at lowering BP in African Americans due to HTN with low-renin patterns. This effect will also reduce the response to beta-blockers and ACE-inhibitors. ARBs may be preferred over ACE inhibitors.
- African Americans have a higher risk of angioedema from ACE-inhibitors or ARBs compared with Caucasians.
- ARBs were developed to overcome deficiencies in ACE inhibitors' mechanism of action, but evidence has not solidified this benefit of antagonizing AT1 receptors versus blocking the primary ACE pathway.

HIGH-YIELD BOARD EXAM ESSENTIALS
- **CLASSIC AGENTS:** Azilsartan, candesartan, irbesartan, losartan, olmesartan, telmisartan, valsartan
- **DRUG CLASS:** ARB
- **INDICATIONS:** Hypertension, HF, CKD, ACS
- **MECHANISM:** Reduce the actions of Ang II and lower BP by antagonizing AT1 receptors
- **SIDE EFFECTS:** Hyperkalemia, transient SCr bump; cough and angioedema (both less than ACE inhibitors)
- **CLINICAL PEARLS:**
    - ARBs are alternatives to ACE inhibitors for HTN, HF, CKD, and post-ACS to provide BP and other benefits.
    - ARBs may be less effective in African American patients but may reduce the risk of angioedema.
    - Counsel to avoid the use of potassium-containing salt substitutes to prevent hyperkalemia.
    - All ARBs are contraindicated in pregnancy.

Table: Drug Class Summary

\multicolumn{4}{c}{**Angiotensin II Receptor Blocker - Drug Class Review**}
\multicolumn{4}{c}{High-Yield Med Reviews}
\multicolumn{4}{l}{**Mechanism of Action:** ARBs block the actions of Ang II preferentially at AT1 receptors and lower BP}
\multicolumn{4}{l}{**Class Effects:** Vasodilation, BP reduction, decreased cardiac remodeling, and improved renal perfusion. Associated with hyperkalemia. Avoid in pregnancy.}
Generic Name	**Brand Name**	**Main Indication(s) or Uses**	**Notes**
Azilsartan	Edarbi	- Hypertension	- **Dosing (Adult):** − Oral: 40 mg daily, maximum 80 mg daily - **Dosing (Peds):** None - **CYP450 Interactions:** CYP2C9 substrate - **Renal or Hepatic Dose Adjustments:** None - **Dosage Forms:** Oral (tablet)

Candesartan	Atacand	- HF with reduced ejection fraction
		- Hypertension
			- **Dosing (Adult):**
			  − Initial starting dose 4-8 mg daily, titrated to maximum dose 32 mg daily
			- **Dosing (Peds):**
			  − Initial dose 0.2 mg/kg/day, adjusted to target range 0.05 to 0.4 mg/kg/day in 1-2 divided doses, maximum 0.4 mg/kg/day, or 32 mg, whichever is less.
			- **CYP450 Interactions:** CYP2C9 substrate
			- **Renal or Hepatic Dose Adjustments:** Child-Pugh class C, reduce starting dose
			- **Dosage Forms:** Oral (tablet)

Irbesartan	Avapro	- Diabetic nephropathy
		- Hypertension
			- **Dosing (Adult):**
			  − Initial dose 150 mg daily, maximum 300 mg once daily
			- **Dosing (Peds):**
			  − Fixed weight-based dosing: 10-20 kg: initial 37.5 mg daily; 21-40 kg: initial 75 mg daily; >40 kg: initial 150 mg daily
			- **CYP450 Interactions:** CYP2C9 substrate
			- **Renal or Hepatic Dose Adjustments:** None
			- **Dosage Forms:** Oral (tablet)

Telmisartan	Micardis	- Cardiovascular risk reduction - Hypertension	- **Dosing (Adult):** − Initial dose 20-40 mg daily, maximum 80 mg daily - **Dosing (Peds):** Not used. - **CYP450 Interactions:** None - **Renal or Hepatic Dose Adjustments:** None - **Dosage Forms:** Oral (tablet)

\multicolumn{4}{c}{**Angiotensin II Receptor Blocker - Drug Class Review**}

Generic Name	Brand Name	Main Indication(s) or Uses	Notes

Olmesartan	Benicar	- Hypertension	- **Dosing (Adult):**
			  – Initial dose 20 mg daily, maximum 40 mg daily
			- **Dosing (Peds):**
			  – 5-20 kg: Initial dose 0.3 mg/kg/dose daily, maximum dose 0.6 mg/kg/dose
			  – 20-35 kg: Initial dose 10 mg daily, maximum dose 20 mg/day
			  – > 35 kg: see adult dosing
			- **CYP450 Interactions:** None, OATP1B1/1B3 substrate
			- **Renal or Hepatic Dose Adjustments:**
			  – GFR < 20 mL/min, maximum dose 20 mg
			- **Dosage Forms:** Oral (tablet)

Losartan	Cozaar	- Hypertension
		- Proteinuric chronic kidney disease
			- **Dosing (Adult):**
			  – Initial 25- 50 mg daily, maximum 100 mg/day
			- **Dosing (Peds):**
			  – Children > 6 years: 0.7 mg/kg daily, maximum initial dose 50 mg/dose, titrated to a maximum daily dose of 1.4 mg/kg/day or 100 mg/day.
			- **CYP450 Interactions:** Substrate of CYP2C9, CYP3A4
			- **Renal or Hepatic Dose Adjustments:**
			  – Mild to moderate hepatic impairment, initial dose of 25 mg once daily
			- **Dosage Forms:** Oral (tablet)

Valsartan	Diovan	- Hypertension	- **Dosing (Adult):**
			  – Initial 20 mg twice daily, maximum dose 160 mg twice daily
			- **Dosing (Peds):**
			  – Initial 0.25-4 mg/kg/dose daily, maximum 1.35 mg/kg/dose twice daily, or 160 mg/day, whichever is less.
			- **CYP450 Interactions:** OATP1B1/1B3 substrate
			- **Renal or Hepatic Dose Adjustments:** none
			- **Dosage Forms:** Oral (tablet)

CARDIOVASCULAR – BETA-BLOCKERS

Drug Class
- Beta-blockers
  - Acute Care
    - Esmolol
    - Labetalol
    - Metoprolol
    - Propranolol
  - Chronic Care
    - Atenolol
    - Carvedilol
    - Betaxolol
    - Bisoprolol
    - Labetalol
    - Propranolol
    - Metoprolol
    - Nadolol
    - Nebivolol

Main Indications or Uses
- Acute Care:
  - Hypertensive emergency
    - Acute aortic syndromes/Acute aortic dissection
    - Acute ischemic stroke
    - Acute hemorrhagic stroke
    - Preeclampsia/eclampsia
- Chronic Care:
  - Angina
  - Atrial fibrillation/flutter, maintenance of ventricular rate control
  - Heart failure with reduced ejection fraction, including left ventricular dysfunction following myocardial infarction
  - Hypertension
  - Myocardial infarction, early treatment, and secondary prevention
  - Variceal hemorrhage prophylaxis

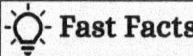

Fast Facts

✓ While most beta-blockers are not the best antihypertensive medications and thus no longer recommended first line in most patients, bisoprolol, carvedilol, and metoprolol succinate are very beneficial in heart failure despite their negative inotropic properties.

Mechanism of Action
- Beta-1 antagonist
  - Antagonists of beta-1 decrease calcium-dependent calcium release from the sarcoplasmic reticulum and limit the actin-myosin interaction in cardiac tissue.
    - This is done by antagonism of the beta-1 receptor, a Gs-protein coupled receptor that prevents adenylate cyclase activation.
    - This prevents the increased intracellular production of cAMP and prevents the activation of protein kinase A (PKA).
    - Without activated PK), there is no phosphorylation of voltage-sensitive calcium channels and the ryanodine receptor calcium release (RyR) channels on the sarcoplasmic reticulum.
- Beta-2 antagonist
  - Beta-2 receptors exist primarily in bronchioles, skeletal muscle, and arteries.
  - Activation or stimulation of these Gs- or Gi-protein coupled receptors leads to increased actin-myosin activity and muscle contraction.
  - Thus, antagonist activity on these receptors causes bronchoconstriction, skeletal muscle vasculature contraction, and arterial contraction.
- Alpha-1 antagonist
  - Alpha-1 antagonists lead to vasodilation via inhibition of Gq-protein coupled receptors. Inhibition of these Gq receptors inhibits the IP3 pathway and ultimately inhibits SR calcium release.
- Antiarrhythmic properties
  - Beta-blockers are known to slow phase 4 within the action potential of nodal cells thereby resulting in a negative chronotropic effect (i.e., reduction in the pulse).

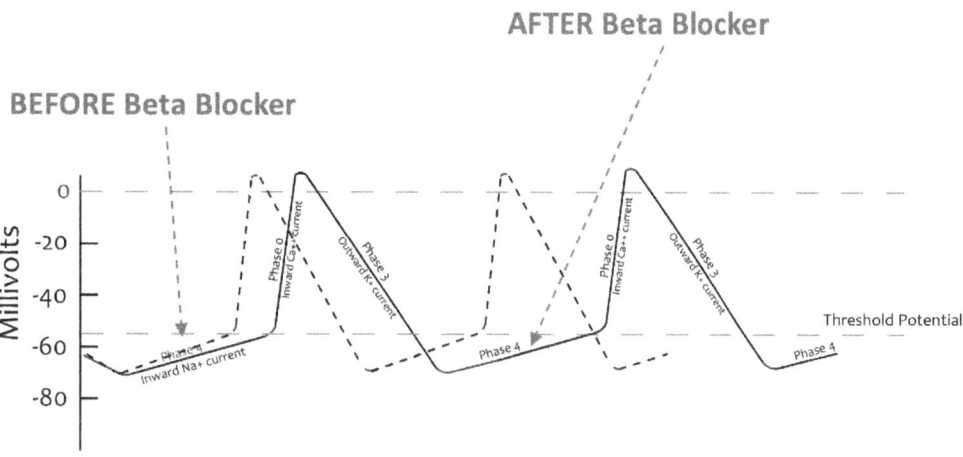

Primary Net Benefit
- Lowers blood pressure with minimal or no change in heart rate also contributes to the prevention of cardiac remodeling post-myocardial infarction.
- Main Labs to Monitor:
    - No routine laboratory monitoring in general but serum Cr if on atenolol or nadolol due to renal elimination

High-Yield Basic Pharmacology
- **Clinical Classifications**
    - Beta-blockers are also commonly pharmacologically categorized as:
        - Selective (i.e., beta-1 selective antagonists)
        - Non-selective (beta-1 and beta-2 nonselective antagonists)
        - Non-selective beta and alpha-1 antagonists (beta-1, beta-2, and alpha-1 antagonists)
        - Intrinsic sympathomimetic activity (Can have beta-agonist or antagonist properties)
        - Membrane stabilizing activity (Sodium channel blocking properties)
        - Class II antiarrhythmics (Vaughan Williams Classification)
- **Ophthalmic Agents**
    - Vasodilation from specific beta-1 selective agents like carteolol (ophthalmic) and nebivolol can occur through increased nitric oxide production, whereas others possess calcium channel blocking properties such as carvedilol and betaxolol.
- **Alpha Antagonist Properties**
    - Alpha-1 antagonists as individual agents like prazosin will cause vasodilation but a reflex tachycardia.
    - Therefore, a medication such as carvedilol or labetalol possesses non-selective beta-blocking properties and alpha-1 antagonism.
    - Thus, any reflex tachycardia would be blunted.

High-Yield Clinical Knowledge
- **Vasodilatory Properties**
    - Most beta-blockers do not possess vasodilatory properties at normal therapeutic dosing.
    - Beta-1 selective agents work primarily in the heart, where approximately 80% of beta receptors are beta-1.
    - Beta-2 antagonist activity in the vasculature leads to vasoconstriction (consider beta-2 agonists like albuterol cause bronchodilation and how non-selective beta-blockers precipitate bronchospasm).
    - Only beta-blockers with alpha-1 antagonist effects and some with intrinsic sympathomimetic activity can cause vasodilation.
        - The former was used for this action; the latter was not used as vasodilators.
    - The vasodilatory properties of carvedilol and labetalol are a function of the ratio of alpha to beta antagonist activity. The ratio for carvedilol is 1:10 (alpha: beta), whereas labetalol's ratio changes depending on the route of administration (oral - 1:3; IV - 1:7).

- **Antihypertensive Actions**
  - Beta-1 antagonists exert their antihypertensive effect mainly through the RAAS system (beta-1 inhibition of renin release from the juxtaglomerular cells), not through decreased cardiac output (which would cause a reflex increase in MAP).
- **Acute Blood Pressure Lowering**
  - In patients with acute ischemic stroke who are eligible for fibrinolysis with rt-PA, their blood pressure must be less than 185 mmHg systolic and less than 110 mmHg diastolic.
  - Labetalol is a first-line agent to manage blood pressure in this scenario and should be given as an IV bolus at a dose of 20 mg.
  - While patients are receiving rt-PA and for the next 24 hours, blood pressure should be maintained less than 180/105 mmHg.
  - These patients can be managed with labetalol as an IV agent or transitioned to oral dosage forms.
- **Esophageal Varices**
  - Carvedilol's mixed beta-blocking and alpha-1 antagonist activity benefit patients with esophageal varices and primary variceal bleeding prophylaxis.
  - These benefits from carvedilol result from downregulation of intrahepatic resistance and an additional decrease in hepatic venous pressure gradient.
- **Non-Selective Beta Effects**
  - Non-selective inhibits vasodilation and can increase vascular tone.
  - This action is why in patients with pheochromocytoma, non-selective beta-blockers are contraindicated.
  - If these patients receive a beta-blocker, there would be an uncompensated alpha receptor-mediated vasoconstriction caused by epinephrine secreted from the tumor.

High-Yield Core Evidence
- **INTERACT-2**
  - The INTERACT-2 trial was a multicenter, prospective, randomized, open-treatment, blinded trial comparing intensive blood pressure-lowering treatment (target systolic BP <140 mm Hg within 1 hour) or guideline-recommended treatment (target systolic BP <180 mm Hg) in patients with acute hemorrhagic stroke.
  - Labetalol and nicardipine, hydralazine, metoprolol, and urapidil were used in each group to achieve their respective target pressures.
  - However, intensive blood pressure lowering did not reduce the risk of death or severe disability, but there was no increase in adverse safety events. (N Engl J Med. 2013 Jun 20;368(25):2355-65.)
- **CLUE**
  - The CLUE study was a multicenter clinical trial of 226 patients with hypertension in the ED (2 systolic blood pressure ≥180 mmHg) randomized to either nicardipine or labetalol.
  - More patients in the nicardipine arm achieved an adequate blood pressure target (SBP decrease of at least 20 mmHg) within 30 minutes compared to patients receiving labetalol (91.7 vs. 82.5%, P = 0.039). (Crit Care. 2011; 15(3): R157.)
- **CAPRICORN**
  - The CAPRICORN study was a landmark paper demonstrating the mortality benefit of carvedilol in patients with acute MI and evidence of LV systolic dysfunction when compared to placebo.
  - This study was a multicenter, randomized, placebo-controlled study of 1,959 patients with hemodynamically stable myocardial infarction (within 3-21 days before randomization and with reduced LVEF of 40% or less and on an ACE inhibitor) were randomized to receive carvedilol or placebo.
  - There was no difference in the primary endpoint of all-cause mortality or hospital admission for CV problems. Still, all-cause mortality alone was significantly lower in the carvedilol group than placebo (12% vs. 15%, HR 0.77, CI 0.60-0.98, P=0.031). (Lancet. 2001. 357(9266):1385-1390.)

- **COMET**
  - The COMET study built upon the results of the CAPRICORN study and extended the observed benefits of carvedilol to patients with HFrEF (EF ≤35%) and NYHA II-IV symptoms.
  - In this multicenter, randomized 3,029 patients with HFrEF and class II-IV heart failure to carvedilol or metoprolol twice daily and other medical therapies, patients who received carvedilol had lower all-cause mortality compared to the patients receiving metoprolol tartrate (34% vs. 40%; P=0.0017). (Lancet. 2003. 362(9377):7-13.)

High-Yield Fast-Facts
- Beta-blockers can mask important signs of hypoglycemia; however, they do not mask all crucial signs. For example, beta-blockers may inhibit the tachycardic response to hypoglycemia and tremors, although sweating as a warning sign of hypoglycemia is preserved. This is because tachycardia and tremors are sympathetic responses, whereas sweating is parasympathetic and not blunted by beta-blockers.
- Beta-3 receptors exist in the heart, adipose tissue, and bladder. However, their only current therapeutic role is with mirabegron, a beta-3 agonist used for overactive bladder with symptoms of urge urinary incontinence, urgency, and urinary frequency.
- Esmolol is an ultrashort-acting beta-1 selective antagonist. While its use is in the hyperacute setting, it has more of a cardiac effect (negative inotropy and chronotropy) and minimal vasodilation at normal therapeutic dosing.

HIGH-YIELD BOARD EXAM ESSENTIALS
- **CLASSIC AGENTS:** Atenolol, carvedilol, betaxolol, bisoprolol, labetalol, propranolol, metoprolol, nebivolol
- **DRUG CLASS:** Beta-blockers
- **INDICATIONS:** Angina, atrial fibrillation/flutter, HFrEF, hypertension, hypertensive emergency, myocardial infarction, variceal hemorrhage prophylaxis (propranolol).
- **MECHANISM:** Reduces pulse (negative chronotropy), decreases cardiac output (due to negative inotropy), reduces renin release to lower BP via indirect inhibition of ATII levels. Improves remodeling in HF.
- **SIDE EFFECTS:** Bradycardia, fatigue, hypotension, poor exercise performance.
- **CLINICAL PEARLS:**
  - Beta-1 antagonists exert their antihypertensive effect mainly through the RAAS system (beta-1 inhibition of renin release from the juxtaglomerular cells), not through decreased cardiac output (which would cause a reflex increase in MAP).
  - Beta-blockers can reduce remodeling seen in HF which can reduce the risk of sudden cardiac death. Only metoprolol succinate and carvedilol are approved for HF.
  - In most cases can be safely used in pregnancy (e.g., labetalol).
  - This class may mask the effects of hypoglycemia in diabetics (though they can still sweat).
  - Use in patients with moderate to severe asthma or COPD can experience SOB due to bronchospasm.

Table: Drug Class Summary

Beta-Blockers - Drug Class Review High-Yield Med Reviews			
Mechanism of Action: *Beta-1 antagonist, beta-2 antagonist, alpha-1 antagonist (Carvedilol, Labetalol)* *Beta-1 antagonist, beta-2 antagonist (Nadolol, Propranolol)* *Beta-1 antagonist with increased NO production (Nebivolol)* *Beta-1 antagonist with L-type calcium channel blocking properties (Betaxolol)* *Beta-1 antagonists, selective (Atenolol, Betaxolol, Bisoprolol, Metoprolol, Nebivolol, Esmolol)*			
Class Effects: *Lowers blood pressure with minimal or no change in heart rate*			
Generic Name	**Brand Name**	**Main Indication(s) or Uses**	**Notes**

Atenolol	Tenormin	- Acute MI
		- Angina pectoris
		- Hypertension
			- **Dosing (Adult):**
			  – Oral: 25 to 100 mg once daily, maximum 100 mg daily
			- **Dosing (Peds):**
			  – Oral: 0.3 to 1 mcg/kg/day once daily or in divided doses q12h.
			- **CYP450 Interactions:** none
			- **Renal or Hepatic Dose Adjustments:**
			  – GFR 15 to 35 mL/minute - Maximum daily dose of 50 mg
			  – GFR less than 15 - Maximum daily dose of 25 mg
			  – Hemodialysis: moderately dialyzable, normal dosing range 25 to 50 mg/day administered after dialysis.
			- **Dosage Forms:** Oral (tablet)

Carvedilol	Coreg	- Heart failure with reduced ejection fraction, including left ventricular dysfunction following myocardial infarction
		- Hypertension
			- **Dosing (Adult):**
			  – IR: 3.125 mg twice daily up to 25 mg twice daily (≤ 85 kg) or 50 mg (> 85 kg); ER 20 mg daily up to maximum 80 mg/day.
			- **Dosing (Peds):**
			  – 0.075-0.08 mg/kg/dose twice daily. Maximum dose of 50 mg twice daily.
			- **CYP450 Interactions:** Inhibits P-gp; substrate of P-gp, CYP 2C9, 2D6, 3A4, 1A2
			- **Renal or Hepatic Dose Adjustments:** None
			- **Dosage Forms:** Oral (tablet, capsule)

Betaxolol	Kerlone	- Hypertension	- **Dosing (Adult):**
			  – Oral: 5 to 20 mg once daily
			- **Dosing (Peds):**
			  – Not routinely used
			- **CYP450 Interactions:** Minor substrate of CYP1A2, 2D6
			- **Renal or Hepatic Dose Adjustments:** None
			- **Dosage Forms:** Oral (tablet)

Cardiology

Beta-Blockers - Drug Class Review
High-Yield Med Reviews

Generic Name	Brand Name	Main Indication(s) or Uses	Notes

Bisoprolol	Zebeta	- Hypertension	- **Dosing (Adult):**
			  - Oral: 1.25 to 10 mg once daily up to a maximum 10 mg/day.
			- **Dosing (Peds):**
			  - Not routinely used
			- **CYP450 Interactions:** Substrate of CYP2D6 and CYP3A4
			- **Renal or Hepatic Dose Adjustments:**
			  - GFR < 40 mL/minute use initial dose of 2.5 mg daily with very slow titration
			- **Dosage Forms:** Oral (tablet)

Esmolol	Brevibloc	- Intraoperative and postoperative tachycardia and/or hypertension
		- Sinus tachycardia
		- Supraventricular tachycardia and atrial fibrillation/flutter
			- **Dosing (Adult):**
			  - IV: bolus 500 to 1000 mcg/kg over 30 to 60 seconds followed by 50 to 300 mcg/kg/min
			- **Dosing (Peds):**
			  - IV: bolus 100 to 500 mcg/kg over 30 to 60 seconds followed by 50 to 300 mcg/kg/min
			- **CYP450 Interactions:** None
			- **Renal or Hepatic Dose Adjustments:** None
			- **Dosage Forms:** IV solution

Labetalol	Trandate	- Hypertension
		- Acute aortic syndromes/Acute aortic dissection
		- Acute ischemic stroke
		- Acute hemorrhagic stroke
		- Preeclampsia/eclampsia
			- **Dosing (Adult):**
			  - Oral: 100 mg twice daily up to maximum 400 mg twice daily
			  - IV: 10-20 mg IV push every 10 minutes
			- **Dosing (Peds):**
			  - Oral: 1 to 3 mg/kg/day in 2 divided doses, maximum daily dose of 10 to 12 mg/kg/day, or 1,200 mg/day
			  - IV: 0.2 to 1 mg/kg/dose, maximum dose: 40 mg/dose
			- **CYP450 Interactions:** Extensive first pass, hepatic glucuronidation
			- **Renal or Hepatic Dose Adjustments:** None
			- **Dosage Forms:** Oral (tablet), IV solution

Beta-Blockers - Drug Class Review
High-Yield Med Reviews

Generic Name	Brand Name	Main Indication(s) or Uses	Notes

Metoprolol	Lopressor
	Toprol
		- Angina
		- Heart failure with reduced ejection fraction (ER oral formulation)
		- Hypertension
		- Myocardial infarction
			- **Dosing (Adult):**
			  - Oral: IR 12.5 to 200 mg twice daily up to maximum 400 mg daily; Oral ER 50 to 200 mg, up to maximum 400 mg daily;
			  - IV: 2.5 to 5 mg IV push over 2 minutes and repeat every 5 minutes as needed. Maximum total dose of 15 mg.
			- **Dosing (Peds):**
			  - Oral: initial dose of 0.1 to 0.2 mg/kg/dose twice daily, titrating up to 1 to 2 mg/kg/day. Maximum daily dose of 2 mg/kg/day or 200 mg/day
			  - IV: 0.1 to 0.2 mg/kg; maximum dose: 10 mg/dose
			- **CYP450 Interactions:** Substrate CYP 2D6, and CYP 2C19
			- **Renal or Hepatic Dose Adjustments:** None
			- **Dosage Forms:** Oral (tablet [IR and ER], capsule [IR and ER]), IV solution

Nebivolol	Bystolic	- Hypertension	- **Dosing (Adult):**
			  - Oral: 5 mg once daily, maximum 40 mg daily
			- **Dosing (Peds):**
			  - Not routinely used
			- **CYP450 Interactions:** Extensive first pass, hepatic glucuronidation
			- **Renal or Hepatic Dose Adjustments:**
			  - GFR <30 mL/minute: Initial dose of 2.5 mg once daily
			- **Dosage Forms:** Oral (tablet)

Nadolol	Corgard	- Angina
		- Hypertension
			- **Dosing (Adult):**
			  - Oral: 10 to 240 mg once daily
			- **Dosing (Peds):**
			  - Oral: for SVT - Initial dose of 0.5 to 1 mg/kg/day once daily or in 2 divided doses. Maximum 2.5 mg/kg/day
			- **CYP450 Interactions:** None, but major P-gp substrate
			- **Renal or Hepatic Dose Adjustments:**
			  - GFR > 50 mL/minute, every 24 hours.
			  - GFR 31 to 50 mL/minute, every 24 to 36 hours
			  - GFR 10 to 30 mL/minute, every 24 to 48 hours
			  - GFR <10 mL/minute, every 40 to 60 hours
			  - HD - administer post-dialysis
			- **Dosage Forms:** Oral (tablet)

		Beta-Blockers - Drug Class Review High-Yield Med Reviews	
Generic Name	**Brand Name**	**Main Indication(s) or Uses**	**Notes**
Propranolol	Inderal	<ul><li>Angina, chronic stable</li><li>Cardiac arrhythmias</li><li>Essential tremor</li><li>Hypertension</li><li>Migraine headache prophylaxis</li><li>Myocardial infarction, early treatment and secondary prevention</li><li>Obstructive hypertrophic cardiomyopathy</li><li>Pheochromocytoma</li><li>Proliferating infantile hemangioma</li></ul>	<ul><li>**Dosing (Adult):**<ul><li>Oral: immediate release 10 to 320 mg once to four times daily, maximum 320 mg daily</li><li>Oral: extended-release 80 to 320 mg daily, maximum 320 mg daily</li><li>IV: solution 1 mg IV every 2 minutes as needed, maximum 3 doses.</li></ul></li><li>**Dosing (Peds):**<ul><li>Oral: immediate release initial dose of 0.5 to 1 mg/kg/day in 3 divided doses. Maximum daily dose of 4 mg/kg/day</li><li>IV: solution 0.01 to 0.15 mg/kg/dose slow IV over 10 minutes every 6 to 8 hours as needed. The max dose is age-dependent with maximum of 1 mg/dose for infants, and 3 mg/dose for children and adolescents</li></ul></li><li>**CYP450 Interactions:** Extensive first pass, oxidation via CYP1A2, CYP2C19, CYP2D6, and CYP3A4. Inhibits CYP 1A2</li><li>**Renal or Hepatic Dose Adjustments:** None</li><li>**Dosage Forms:** Oral (tablet, capsule [ER], solution), IV solution</li></ul>

CARDIOVASCULAR – CALCIUM CHANNEL BLOCKERS

Drug Class
- **Calcium Channel Blockers**
    - Acute Care
        - Clevidipine
        - Diltiazem
        - Nicardipine
        - Nifedipine
        - Nimodipine
        - Verapamil
    - Chronic Care
        - Amlodipine
        - Diltiazem
        - Felodipine
        - Isradipine
        - Nicardipine
        - Nifedipine
        - Nisoldipine
        - Verapamil

Main Indications or Uses
- **Acute Care**
    - Acute Ischemic Stroke with Hypertensive Crisis
    - Angina / Acute Coronary Syndrome
    - Atrial fibrillation with rapid ventricular response
    - Cocaine-induced chest pain
    - Supraventricular tachycardia (verapamil)
    - Preeclampsia/Eclampsia
    - Subarachnoid hemorrhage
    - Ventricular arrhythmias
- **Chronic Care**
    - Angina pectoris
    - Atrial fibrillation rate control
    - Migraine/Cluster headache (verapamil)
    - Hypertension
    - Pulmonary artery hypertension
    - Raynaud phenomenon

> **Fast Facts**
> ✓ Nimodipine is not used for the treatment of hypertension but is instead only used for the prevention of neurological complications associated from subarachnoid hemorrhage.

Mechanism of Action
- **Myocardial muscle and smooth muscle**
    - Bind to and prevent calcium entry through "long-type" or L-type calcium channels on myocardial and smooth muscle. The reduction in calcium influx intracellularly prevents the calcium-calmodulin complex from stimulating myosin light chain kinase phosphorylation and ultimately activating actin-myosin interaction and a resulting contraction.
- **SA and AV nodal tissue**
    - Slows rate of phase 4 recovery of nodal tissue by decreasing calcium flow into cardiac nodal cells. In nodal tissue, calcium influx initiates depolarization instead of sodium which initiates depolarization in other cardiac tissues.

Primary Net Benefit
- Calcium channel blockers provide a wide range of cardiovascular and neurologic benefits and, depending on the agent, provide vasodilation, decreased chronotropy, and inotropy.
- Main Labs to Monitor:
    - Liver function (INR/PT, albumin, protein, bilirubin)
    - Liver enzymes (AST/ALT, alk phos)
    - Serum creatinine

Cardiology

High-Yield Basic Pharmacology
- **Classification**
  - Calcium channel blockers are also commonly pharmacologically categorized as dihydropyridine vs. non-dihydropyridine
- **Nitric-Oxide and Amlodipine**
  - Amlodipine can cause vasodilation through another mechanism - nitric oxide release.
- **Cardiac Calcium Channels**
  - In cardiac tissue, the inhibition of calcium entry into cells limits the activation of the ryanodine receptor on the sarcoplasmic reticulum, limiting calcium-dependent calcium release.
  - Without this massive efflux of calcium from the sarcoplasmic reticulum, there will be insufficient quantities of calcium to bind with troponin C, which is essential for displacing troponin and tropomyosin from actin, freeing actin to bind with myosin.

High-Yield Clinical Knowledge
- **Dihydropyridines**
  - Dihydropyridine calcium channel blockers are more selective for smooth muscle calcium channels at normal therapeutic doses.
    - This specificity yields vasodilation and little to no effect on heart rate or contractility.
  - The specificity of dihydropyridines is owed to their preference for less negative resting potentials of calcium-binding site tissues. For example, since the typical resting potential of smooth muscle is -70mV, dihydropyridines preferentially bind there and not to the more negative myocardial tissue (-90mV).
  - At normal therapeutic dosing, dihydropyridines do not have a measurable effect on the SA node. However, isradipine is the exception to this rule as it has a significant depressant effect on the SA node at therapeutic dosing sufficient to blunt any reflex tachycardia from its vasodilation.
- **Hypertension**
  - The JNC 8 guidelines include dihydropyridine and non-dihydropyridine calcium channel blockers as first-line options for managing hypertension.
- **High-Risk Drug-Interactions:**
  - All undergo the first-pass metabolism
  - Diltiazem/Verapamil inhibits 2C9, 2D6, 3A4 and P-glycoprotein; 3A4 substrates
  - Dihydropyridines substrates of 3A4, 2D6, and 2C9 inhibit 3A4
    - Clevidipine - red blood cell hydrolysis (no known pharmacokinetic interactions)
- **Acute Ischemic Stroke with Hypertensive Crisis**
  - Clevidipine or nicardipine are options to lower blood pressure in ischemic stroke patients who are potential candidates for fibrinolysis. These agents would be used if fibrinolytic candidates' systolic blood pressure is greater than 185 mmHg and/or diastolic greater than 110 mmHg.
- **Angina**
  - Immediate-release nifedipine must be avoided for this indication as sharp reductions in blood pressure have occurred.
- **Atrial Fibrillation with Rapid Ventricular Response**
  - Diltiazem or verapamil can rapidly control ventricular rates in patients with atrial fibrillation. In these patients, diltiazem is commonly used in a fixed-dose (10 mg IV) or weight-based dose regimen (0.25 mg/kg IV followed by 0.35 mg/kg if inadequate response). An infusion of diltiazem can follow successful rate control at 5 to 15 mg/hr.
- **Cocaine Induced Chest Pain (Non-Dihydropyridines)**
  - Diltiazem or verapamil can be used for this indication, as beta-blockers should be avoided. However, sinus tachycardia from cocaine is best managed with crystalloid volume and short-acting benzodiazepines.
- **Supraventricular Tachycardia**
  - Verapamil can be used as an alternative to adenosine. As a result of the significant first-pass metabolism of oral verapamil, the intravenous dose is 5 to 10 mg. Simultaneously, the oral dose for atrial fibrillation rate control is up to 480 mg/day.

- **Preeclampsia/Eclampsia**
  - Although labetalol is preferred, clevidipine or nicardipine are options for managing hypertension related to preeclampsia or eclampsia. Nifedipine is an oral option for this off-label indication.
- **Subarachnoid hemorrhage**
  - Nimodipine is used almost exclusively for this indication and only exists as an oral dosage form.
- **Angina pectoris**
  - Although beta-blockers are preferred, dihydropyridine (or rarely diltiazem) can be used in addition. These agents can assist in the re-establishment of the myocardial oxygen supply-demand relationship.
- **Atrial fibrillation rate control**
  - Non-dihydropyridine calcium channel blockers can be used for rate control of patients with atrial fibrillation. However, these agents should be avoided in patients with HFrEF and atrial fibrillation.
- **Migraine/Cluster headache (verapamil)**
  - As a prophylaxis agent, verapamil may be used to prevent migraines or cluster headaches. However, it's important to note that this is not meant as an abortive agent but a preventative maintenance intervention.
- **Pulmonary Arterial Hypertension**
  - Patients with group-1 pulmonary hypertension may receive nifedipine, diltiazem, or verapamil can be used in a small select group of patients. This small group of patients, otherwise known as "responders," are those who demonstrate a significant acute response to calcium channel blockers.
- **Raynaud Phenomenon**
  - Nifedipine is the drug of choice for patients with recurrent vasospasm of the fingers and toes, otherwise known as the Raynaud phenomenon.

High-Yield Core Evidence
- **Fixed or Weight-Based Diltiazem Dosing**
  - The practice of a progressive weight-based diltiazem dose for managing atrial fibrillation with rapid ventricular response has been questioned in emergency medicine practice, but little evidence has guided therapy.
  - This study was the first to compare the higher weight-based dose of 0.2 to 0.3 mg/kg if inadequate response was compared retrospectively to a fixed dose of 10 mg IV in patients with Afib with RVR.
  - The investigators observed that the fixed dose of 10 mg diltiazem was non-inferior to weight-based dosing in the initial treatment of AF with RVR. (J Emerg Med. 2016 Oct;51(4):440-446.)
- **British Aneurysm Nimodipine Trial**
  - This was a randomized, double-blind placebo-controlled trial of patients with acute subarachnoid hemorrhage admitted to a neurosurgical center within 96 hours of the onset of signs/symptoms.
  - Patients were randomized to nimodipine 60mg q4h orally x 21 days or a placebo.
  - The primary outcome of incidence of cerebral infarction occurred less in the nimodipine group than placebo, with an absolute risk reduction of 11%, translated to an NNT of 9.
  - This persisted after adjusting for the potential imbalance of independent poor prognostic factors between groups. (BMJ, 298(6674), 636–642.)
- **AFFIRM**
  - The AFFIRM trial was a landmark multicenter, parallel-group, randomized, controlled trial that compared a rate-control strategy to a rhythm-control strategy to manage atrial fibrillation.
  - Contrary to popular opinion, there was no difference between groups concerning the primary outcome of this study (5-year mortality, 25.9% vs. 26.7% (HR 1.15; 95% CI 0.99-1.34; P=0.08))
  - However, more patients in the rhythm-control group were hospitalized more frequently, had a PEA or bradycardic event, and more patients crossed over from the rhythm control to rate control arms rather than vice versa.
  - A subgroup analysis associated the rhythm-control strategy with a higher risk of death than the rate-control strategy among older patients, patients with CAD, and patients without HF.
  - The authors concluded that the rhythm-control strategy offers no survival advantage over the rate-control strategy, and there are potential advantages, such as a lower risk of adverse drug effects, with the rate-control strategy. (N Engl J Med. 2002. 347(23):1825-1833.)

- **ACCOMPLISH**
  - The ACCOMPLISH trial was a randomized, double-blind trial that compared benazepril-amlodipine to benazepril-hydrochlorothiazide in patients with hypertension at high risk of cardiovascular complications and death and a primary outcome of time to the first event of the composite of a cardiovascular event and death from cardiovascular causes.
  - Fewer patients in the benazepril–amlodipine group met the primary outcome than in the benazepril–hydrochlorothiazide group (relative risk reduction of 19.6%).
  - The authors concluded that the benazepril-amlodipine combination was superior in reducing cardiovascular events in high-risk hypertensive patients. (N Engl J Med. 2008;359(23):2417-2428.)

High-Yield Fast-Facts
- In calcium channel blocker overdose, the 'selectivity' of dihydropyridines for smooth muscle can become lost, and negative inotropic and negative chronotropic effects can occur. Although calcium (chloride or gluconate, the provided dose is adjusted accordingly) can help overcome this blockade, high dose insulin (aka hyperinsulinemia-euglycemia therapy) can be used early on in the resuscitation of these patients)
- Diltiazem has numerous oral dosage forms that can increase the risk of drug errors. Immediate release, extended-release 12-hour, and extended-release 24-hour dosage forms exist. To make things more confusing, each of the 12 or 24-hour release forms uses interchangeable terms, including "extended-release" or "long-acting" and "controlled release."

HIGH-YIELD BOARD EXAM ESSENTIALS
- **CLASSIC AGENTS:** Amlodipine, clevidipine, diltiazem, nicardipine, nifedipine, verapamil.
- **DRUG CLASS:** Calcium channel blockers
- **INDICATIONS:** Acute ischemic stroke, angina / ACS, AFib +/- RVR, SVT, preeclampsia/eclampsia, subarachnoid hemorrhage, ventricular arrhythmias, migraine/cluster headache (verapamil), hypertension, pulmonary artery hypertension, Raynaud phenomenon
- **MECHANISM:** L-type calcium channels inhibition, ultimately leading to vasodilation. Diltiazem and verapamil exhibit additional negative inotropy (myocardial muscle and smooth muscle) which slows heart rate and rate of recovery in nodal tissue by decreasing calcium flow into cardiac nodal cells (SA and AV nodal tissue).
- **SIDE EFFECTS:** Bradycardia, hypotension, constipation; case reports of gingival hyperplasia
- **CLINICAL PEARLS:**
  - The non-DHP CCB (diltiazem & verapamil) can be useful when rate control needed in AFib with RVR, but they do prevent cardiac remodeling or protect patients from sudden cardiac death (like beta-blockers). These two agents are also known to inhibit CYP3A4 and P-gp causing drug-interactions.
  - Nimodipine is used almost exclusively for subarachnoid hemorrhage indication and only exists as an oral dosage form.
  - CCB can be used in pregnancy for treatment of hypertension.

Table: Drug Class Summary

Calcium Channel Blockers - Drug Class Review High-Yield Med Reviews			
Mechanism of Action: *Myocardial muscle and smooth muscle* *-L-type calcium channels inhibition, ultimately leading to vasodilation and negative inotropy.* *SA and AV nodal tissue* *-Slows heart rate and rate of recovery in nodal tissue by decreasing calcium flow into cardiac nodal cells.*			
Class Effects: *Vasodilation, decreased chronotropy, and inotropy*			
Generic Name	**Brand Name**	**Main Indication(s) or Uses**	**Notes**

Amlodipine	Katerzia, Norliqva, Norvasc	• Angina
		• Hypertension
		• Raynaud phenomenon
			• **Dosing (Adult):**
			  – Oral: 2.5 to 5 mg once daily, maximum 10 mg/day
			• **Dosing (Peds):**
			  – Oral: 0.1 mg/kg/dose once daily up to 5 mg for < 6 yrs and up to 10 mg for ≥ 6 yrs old
			• **CYP450 Interactions:** Major CYP 3A4 substrate
			• **Renal or Hepatic Dose Adjustments:** None
			• **Dosage Forms:** Oral tablet, oral suspension (Katerzia), oral solution (Norliqva)

Clevidipine	Cleviprex	• Hypertension	• **Dosing (Adult):**
			  – IV: Initial: 1 to 2 mg/hour, doubled every 5 to 10 min to a maximum of 21 mg/hour
			• **Dosing (Peds):**
			  – Not routinely used
			• **CYP450 Interactions:** No CYP interactions
			• **Renal or Hepatic Dose Adjustments:** None
			• **Dosage Forms:** IV solution (20% emulsion)

Diltiazem	Cardizem, Cartia, Maztim, Taztia, Tiadilt, Tiazac	• Angina
		• Atrial fibrillation or atrial flutter, rate control
		• Hypertension
		• Nonsustained ventricular tachycardia or ventricular premature beats, symptomatic
		• Supraventricular tachycardia
			• **Dosing (Adult):**
			  – IR: 30 mg 4 times daily (maximum 240 to 360 mg/day);
			  – 12-hour (twice-daily) formulations: 60 mg twice daily (maximum 240 to 360 mg/day,
			  – 24-hour (once-daily) formulations: 120 to 180 mg once daily (maximum 240 to 360 mg/day)
			  – IV: 0.25 or 0.35 mg IV push, alternatively 10 mg IV push. Continuous infusion 5 to 15 mg/hour.
			• **Dosing (Peds):**
			  – IR: initial 1.5 to 2 mg/kg/day in 3 to 4 divided doses to maximum 6 mg/kg/day or to 360 mg/day whichever is less
			  – IV: 0.25 or 0.35 mg IV push
			• **CYP450 Interactions:** Major substrate of CYP3A4, P-gp
			• **Renal or Hepatic Dose Adjustments:** None
			• **Dosage Forms:** Oral (solution, capsule or tablet), IV solution

Calcium Channel Blockers - Drug Class Review
High-Yield Med Reviews

Generic Name	Brand Name	Main Indication(s) or Uses	Notes

Isradipine	DynaCirc	- Hypertension	- **Dosing (Adult):**
			  – Oral: 2.5 mg twice daily, maximum 5 mg twice daily.
			- **Dosing (Peds):**
			  – Oral: 0.05 to 0.1 mg/kg/dose 2 to 3 times daily, up to 0.6 mg/kg/dose or 10 mg/day (lesser of the two)
			- **CYP450 Interactions:** Major substrate of CYP3A4
			- **Renal or Hepatic Dose Adjustments:** None
			- **Dosage Forms:** Oral (capsule)

Nicardipine	Cardene	- Angina
		- Hypertension
			- **Dosing (Adult):**
			  – Oral: 20 to 40 mg 3 times daily
			  – IV: 5 mg/hour titrate by 2.5 mg/hour every 5-10 minutes, maximum dose 15 mg/hour
			- **Dosing (Peds):**
			  – Oral: 0.5 to 1 mcg/kg/minute, maximum dose 4 to 5 mcg/kg/minute
			- **CYP450 Interactions:** Major substrate of CYP3A4, inhibits 2D6
			- **Renal or Hepatic Dose Adjustments:**
			  – Oral: Initial: 20 mg 3 times daily
			- **Dosage Forms:** Oral (capsule), IV solution

Nifedipine	Procardia; Procardia XL	- Angina, Hypertension, Pre-eclampsia, Pulmonary arterial hypertension (group 1)	- **Dosing (Adult):**
			  – ER: 30 to 90 mg once daily; maximum: 120 mg/day
			- **Dosing (Peds):**
			  – ER: 0.25 to 0.5 mg/kg/day once daily or divided in 2 doses; maximum daily dose of 3 mg/kg/day (or 120 mg/day)
			- **CYP450 Interactions:** Major substrate of CYP3A4
			- **Renal or Hepatic Dose Adjustments:** None
			- **Dosage Forms:** Oral immediate or extended-release (capsule or tablet)

Nimodipine	Nimotop, Nymalize	- Subarachnoid hemorrhage	- **Dosing (Adult):**
			  – Oral: 60 mg every 4 hours for 21 consecutive days
			- **Dosing (Peds):**
			  – Not routinely used
			- **CYP450 Interactions:** Major substrate of CYP3A4
			- **Renal or Hepatic Dose Adjustments:**
			  – Cirrhosis - 30 mg every 4 hours
			- **Dosage Forms:** Oral (capsule), oral solution

Calcium Channel Blockers - Drug Class Review
High-Yield Med Reviews

Generic Name	Brand Name	Main Indication(s) or Uses	Notes
Nisoldipine	Sular	• Hypertension	• **Dosing (Adult):** — Geomatrix delivery system (brand name Sular) Initial: 17 mg once daily, maximum 34 mg per day; ER oral tablet 20 mg once daily, maximum 60 mg/day • **Dosing (Peds):** — Not routinely used • **CYP450 Interactions:** Major substrate of CYP3A4 • **Renal or Hepatic Dose Adjustments:** — Hepatic impairment, no more than 8.5 mg/day (Sular), or no more than 10 mg/day ER dosage form • **Dosage Forms:** Oral (tablet)
Verapamil	Calan, Verelan	• Angina pectoris (IR form only)	• **Dosing (Adult):** — IR form: 80 to 120 mg 3 times daily. — Extended-release: Initial: 180 mg once daily. Maximum 480 mg/day — IV: bolus 2.5 to 10 mg IV push (2 minutes) • **Dosing (Peds):** — IR: 2 to 8 mg/kg/day in 3 divided doses; maximum daily dose: 480 mg/day — IV: 0.1 to 0.3 mg/kg/dose, maximum 5 mg/dose • **CYP450 Interactions:** Major substrate of CYP3A4 • **Renal or Hepatic Dose Adjustments:** — Cirrhosis, reduce oral dose to 20-30% of normal, IV: dose 50% reduction. • **Dosage Forms:** Oral (capsule or tablet), IV solution

CARDIOVASCULAR – DIRECT RENIN INHIBITOR

Drug Class
- Direct Renin Inhibitor
- Agents:
  - Chronic Care
    - Aliskiren

Main Indications or Uses
- Chronic Care:
  - Hypertension

Mechanism of Action
- Direct renin inhibitors reduce the actions of angiotensin II (Ang II) and lower blood pressure (BP).
  - Aliskiren inhibits renin that mediates the conversion of angiotensinogen to angiotensin I (Ang I), which reduces Ang II and causes vasodilation.

Primary Net Benefit
- Aliskiren results in vasodilation and BP reduction.
- Main Labs to Monitor:
  - Potassium
  - Serum creatinine (SCr)
  - Liver enzymes (AST/ALT, Alk Phos)
  - Creatine kinase (CK)

High-Yield Basic Pharmacology
- Oral Absorption
  - The oral absorption of aliskiren can be substantially decreased (71%) if taken with a high-fat meal.
- Drug Interactions
  - Aliskiren is a CYP 3A4 substrate as well as a P-glycoprotein substrate.
  - Combination therapy with aliskiren and ACE inhibitors or ARBs should be avoided, especially in patients with diabetes or CrCl < 60 mL/min.
    - Combination therapy increases risk of hyperkalemia and CV and renal adverse effects.
    - Eur Heart J, 2013, 34:2159–2219.
  - Cyclosporine and itraconazole should be avoided.

High-Yield Clinical Knowledge
- Clinical Effects
  - In addition to BP-reducing effects, aliskiren down-regulates sympathetic discharge, promotes natriuresis and diuresis, and inhibits cardiac and vascular remodeling.
- CK Elevations
  - Aliskiren has been associated with 300% increases in CK and angioedema in ≤ 1% of patients.
- Combination Therapy
  - Caution when combined with other drugs that can increase potassium or reduce renal function, such as potassium supplements, potassium-sparing diuretics, potassium-containing salts, NSAIDs, and others.
  - Combination with other RAS modulating agents should be avoided.

High-Yield Core Evidence
- ALTITUDE
  - ALTITUDE was a double-blind, randomized, placebo-controlled study investigating the role of aliskiren plus an ACE-inhibitor or ARB versus placebo plus either an ACE-inhibitor or ARB in reducing cardiovascular and renal sequelae among patients with CVD, type 2 diabetes and CKD, or both.

- The study was stopped early due to increased adverse effects and lack of benefit for the primary endpoint (composite of time to CV death or first occurrence of cardiac arrest with resuscitation, nonfatal myocardial infarction, nonfatal stroke, unplanned hospitalization for HF, end-stage renal disease, death attributable to kidney failure, or the need for renal-replacement therapy with no dialysis or transplantation, or doubling of the baseline SCr).
- Due to the absence of clinical benefit and increased risk of renal failure, hyperkalemia, and hypotension, aliskiren added to ACE-inhibitors or ARBs has no role in HTN. (N Engl J Med. 2012;367(23):2204–2213.)

High-Yield Fast-Facts
- Aliskiren is not typically utilized as monotherapy in clinical practice.
- **Lithium and Aliskiren**
    - Lithium is known to cause nephrogenic diabetes insipidus (NDI). Lithium does so via numerous mechanisms, but one immediate action is decreased cAMP, leading to reduced vasopressin-regulated water channel aquaporin-2 (AQP2).
    - Aliskiren can upregulate AQP2 protein expression in inner medullary collecting duct principal cells and is a possible agent to manage lithium-induced NDI.

HIGH-YIELD BOARD EXAM ESSENTIALS
- **CLASSIC AGENTS:** Aliskiren
- **DRUG CLASS:** Direct renin inhibitor
- **INDICATIONS:** Hypertension
- **MECHANISM:** Directly inhibits renin which mediates the conversion of angiotensinogen to angiotensin I.
- **SIDE EFFECTS:** Hyperkalemia and SCr elevation; CK elevation and angioedema (rare)
- **CLINICAL PEARLS:**
    - Aliskiren is less utilized in clinical practice due to better alternatives.
    - Do not use in combination with ACE inhibitors or ARBs in patients with diabetes or CrCl < 60 mL/min.
    - Aliskiren is a CYP 3A4 and P-glycoprotein substrate. Do not use in pregnancy.

Table: Drug Class Summary

Direct Renin Inhibitor - Drug Class Review			
High-Yield Med Reviews			
Generic Name	**Brand Name**	**Indication(s) or Uses**	**Notes**

Aliskiren	Tekturna	• Hypertension	• **Dosing (Adult):**
			  – Initial 150 mg daily, maximum 300 mg daily
			• **Dosing (Peds):**
			  – For children > 6 with weight 20-50 kg: initial 75 mg daily, maximum 150 mg/day
			• **CYP450 Interactions:** CYP3A4 and P-gp substrate
			• **Renal or Hepatic Dose Adjustments:** None
			• **Dosage Forms:** Oral (tablet)

Cardiology

CARDIOVASCULAR – NEPRILYSIN INHIBITOR

Drug Class
- Neprilysin Inhibitor
- Agents:
  - Chronic Care
    - Sacubitril (co-formulated with valsartan in US)

Main Indications or Uses
- Chronic Care
  - Heart failure with reduced ejection fraction (HFrEF)
    - Sacubitril and Valsartan

> **EBM Pearl**
> ✓ The PARADIGM HF study was huge because sacubitril + valsartan went head-to-head with an active comparator and beat it in a well-designed clinical trial.

Mechanism of Action
- Sacubitril
  - Inhibits neprilysin (aka neutral endopeptidase), preventing the breakdown of natriuretic peptides, bradykinin, and other vasodilators.
- Valsartan (ARB)
  - Inhibits angiotensin II (Ang II) type 1 receptors (AT1), reducing the actions of Ang II and lowering BP.

Primary Net Benefit
- In HFrEF, the combination of sacubitril-valsartan significantly improves cardiovascular morbidity and mortality compared to ACE inhibitor therapy alone.
- Main Labs to Monitor:
  - Serum potassium & renal function (baseline and periodically)

High-Yield Basic Pharmacology
- ARB Component Effects
  - Most monitoring and safety concerns are related to valsartan, like hyperkalemia and increased SCr.
- Bradykinin Effect
  - Sacubitril prevents bradykinin breakdown and allows for the beneficial effects of bradykinin, including vasodilation, modulating cardiac remodeling, and increased levels of tissue plasminogen activator.
- Prodrug
  - Sacubitril is a prodrug metabolized by esterases to its active metabolite.

High-Yield Clinical Knowledge
- Heart Failure
  - HFrEF and NYHA Class II-III
    - AHA currently recommends replacing an ACE inhibitor or ARB with sacubitril-valsartan in patients with HFrEF and NYHA class II-III symptoms to reduce morbidity and mortality.
    - Consider in patients with SBP ≥ 100 mmHg, no increase in IV diuretic in ≤ 6 hours, no IV inotrope in ≤ 24 hours, and K^+ < 5 mEq/L.
    - May need to decrease the dose of loop diuretic.
  - HF with Preserved Ejection Fraction (HFpEF)
    - Sacubitril-valsartan in HFpEF patients with EF ≥ 45% did not demonstrate reductions in CV outcomes, but in HFpEF patients with EF < 45%, HF hospitalizations were reduced.
    - Consider after optimizing mineralocorticoid receptor antagonist or SGLT2 inhibitor therapy in patients with HFpEF.
- Sacubitril and ACE-Inhibitors
  - When switching from an ACE-inhibitor to sacubitril-valsartan, the ACE-inhibitor must be discontinued 36 hours before initiating sacubitril.
  - The risk of angioedema is very high with the combination of sacubitril and an ACE inhibitor.

- The initial clinical investigation of omapatrilat (neprilysin inhibitor) combined with ACE-inhibitors demonstrated a 3.2-fold increase in the risk of angioedema. (Am J Hypertens 2004 Feb;17(2):103-11.)
- **Use in Pregnancy**
  - Sacubitril should not be used in pregnancy due to the risk of fetal toxicity.

High-Yield Core Evidence
- **PARADIGM-HF**
  - A multicenter, prospective, randomized, comparative trial was studied in patients with HFrEF (EF < 40%) randomized to either sacubitril-valsartan or enalapril plus standard therapy.
  - Sacubitril-valsartan significantly improved the primary outcome of the composite of death from CV causes or hospitalization for HF and was stopped early because of this benefit.
  - There was also a significant reduction in the rate of HF symptoms, hospitalization for HF, CV mortality, and all-cause mortality among patients receiving sacubitril-valsartan compared to enalapril.
  - Patients receiving sacubitril-valsartan had a higher incidence of hypotension and nonserious angioedema but a lower incidence of renal impairment, hyperkalemia, and cough than the enalapril group.
  - Sacubitril-valsartan was superior to enalapril in reducing the risks of death and hospitalization for HF. (NEJM 2014 Sep 11;371(11):993-1004.)
- **PARAGON-HF**
  - A multinational, double-blind, randomized, parallel-group, active-controlled trial of patients with NYHA class II-IV HF, an EF of 45% or higher, an elevated level of natriuretic peptides, and structural heart disease with patients randomized to receive sacubitril-valsartan or valsartan.
  - There was no difference between groups in the primary outcome (composite of total hospitalizations for HF and death from CV causes).
  - Patients in the sacubitril-valsartan group had a higher incidence of hypotension and angioedema and a lower incidence of hyperkalemia.
  - Sacubitril-valsartan did not significantly decrease total hospitalizations for HF and death from CV causes among patients with HF and an EF of 45% or higher, but it did demonstrate a benefit driven by a reduction in HF hospitalizations in HFpEF with lower EFs in a prespecified analysis.
    - NEJM 2019 Oct 24;381(17):1609-1620.

High-Yield Fast-Facts
- No washout period is required when patients were previously on an ARB.
- Valsartan in sacubitril/valsartan is more bioavailable, so valsartan 26, 51, and 103 mg are equivalent to valsartan 40, 80, and 160 mg, respectively.
- African Americans have a higher risk of angioedema from ACE-inhibitors or ARBs compared with Caucasians, but the risk of angioedema is even higher (4-fold) with sacubitril.

HIGH-YIELD BOARD EXAM ESSENTIALS
- **CLASSIC AGENTS:** Sacubitril
- **DRUG CLASS:** Neprilysin inhibitor
- **INDICATIONS:** HFrEF and HFpEF with low EF
- **MECHANISM:** Inhibits neprilysin, preventing the breakdown of natriuretic peptides, bradykinin, and other vasodilators to reduce BP.
- **SIDE EFFECTS:** Cough, hyperkalemia and SCr increase (due to valsartan) and/or AKI, angioedema
- **CLINICAL PEARLS:** When switching therapy from ACE inhibitors to sacubitril-valsartan, the ACE-inhibitor must be discontinued 36 hours before initiating sacubitril. No washout period for ARBs.

Table: Drug Class Summary

	Neprilysin Inhibitor - Drug Class Review High-Yield Med Reviews
	**Mechanism of Action:** Inhibits neprilysin and prevents the breakdown of natriuretic peptides, bradykinin, and other vasodilators Valsartan reduces the actions of Ang II and lowers BP by inhibiting Ang II AT1 receptors.
	**Class Effects:** *Vasodilation, BP-lowering, decreased cardiac remodeling.*
Generic Name	Brand Name	Main Indication(s) or Uses	Notes
Sacubitril-valsartan	Entresto	• Heart failure	• **Dosing (Adult):** — Sacubitril-valsartan: 24mg/26mg BID — May start 49mg/51 mg BID if previously taking a moderate-high dose of ACE inhibitor or ARB (> 10 mg enalapril or > 160 mg valsartan or equivalent) — Titrate: every two weeks to target sacubitril-valsartan 97mg/103mg BID • **Dosing (Peds):** — 1.6 mg/kg/dose BID (based on the combined dose of sacubitril-valsartan) — Target dose of 2.3 mg/kg/dose BID • **CYP450 Interactions:** None known • **Renal or Hepatic Dose Adjustments:** — GFR < 30 mL/minute: initial 24mg/26mg BID — Severe hepatic impairment (Child-Pugh C) - not recommended • **Dosage Forms:** Oral (tablet)

CARDIOVASCULAR – ANTIHYPERTENSIVES – NITRATES

Drug Class
- **Drug Class: Nitrates**
  - Nitrates are also commonly pharmacologically categorized as:
    - Antianginal agent
    - Antidote, extravasation
    - Vasodilator
- **Agents:**
  - **Acute Care**
    - Nitroglycerin
    - Nitroprusside
  - **Chronic Care**
    - Isosorbide dinitrate (Dilatrate SR; Isordil)
    - Isosorbide mononitrate (Imdur)
    - Nitroglycerin

> **Fast Facts**
> ✓ Nitroglycerin comes in a large number of different dosage formulations from sublingual tablets and sprays to transdermal ointment, to solutions for injection thereby allowing it to be used for a wide variety of clinical scenarios.

Main Indications or Uses
- **Acute Care:**
  - Hypertensive emergencies (ex., myocardial infarction, acute pulmonary edema)
  - Cardiac Angina (including Prinzmetal angina)
  - Extravasation of Vasopressors (when applied topically)
- **Chronic Care:**
  - Chronic stable angina
  - Heart failure with reduced ejection fraction (HFrEF) (Isosorbide dinitrate with hydralazine)
  - Prevent of Esophageal spasms
  - Anal Fissures (when used topically)

Mechanism of Action
- Acts as a nitric oxide (NO) donor, replacing NO that would normally be produced by endothelial cells, leading to vasodilation.
  - Vasodilation occurs in the peripheral veins to reduce preload (i.e., the volume of blood returning to the heart or left ventricular end-diastolic dysfunction) and in arteries to reduce afterload to improve forward flow.
    - Vasodilation of the coronary arteries can also improve collateral flow to the myocardium, thereby reducing cardiac ischemia.

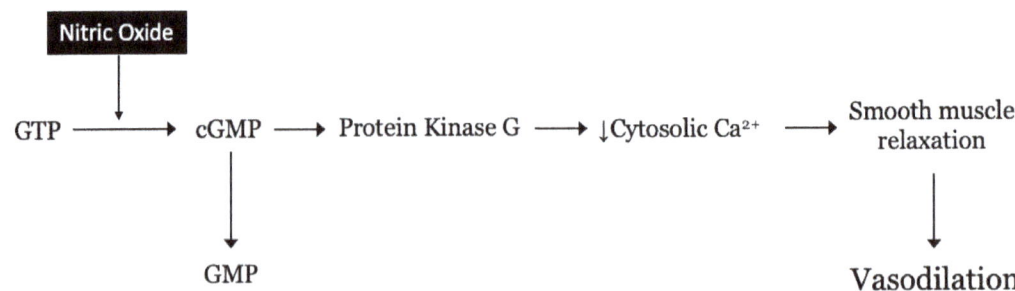

- **Clinical Considerations:** Vasodilators aren't necessarily dilators of veins. Many are arterial dilators, but their action can be dose-dependent.
  - E.g., at low doses (10 to 50 mcg/min), nitroglycerin is primarily a venodilator. However, arterial dilation occurs at higher doses (200-400 mcg/min).
    - Clinical scenarios and disease-specific therapeutic goals can determine the appropriate drug and dose strategy.

Primary Net Benefit
- At standard doses reduces preload and offers a reduction in preload and vasodilation of coronary vasculature. Higher doses can also reduce afterload. It also comes in different dosage forms allowing for broad use.

High-Yield Basic Pharmacology
- Isosorbide dinitrate can be thought of as a prodrug from isosorbide mononitrate.
  - After absorption, isosorbide dinitrate is hepatically (or in smooth muscle) denitration to isosorbide mononitrate.
- Nitroprusside is metabolized to ONE molecule of Nitric Oxide and FIVE molecules of CN, or cyanide.
  - These CNs are rapidly metabolized to less toxic thiocyanate. Still, if nitroprusside is administered at a high rate (2 mcg/kg/minute), exposure of the drug to UV light, or in the setting of renal impairment, toxicity can occur.
- Nitroglycerin tachyphylaxis can occur with uninterrupted or chronic use.

High-Yield Clinical Knowledge
- **Acute Care**
  - **Acute Ischemic Stroke with Hypertensive Crisis:**
    - In patients with acute ischemic stroke, the use of nitroprusside to control blood pressure (i.e., > 185 mm Hg systolic or > 110 mm Hg diastolic) is a relative contraindication for fibrinolysis with acute ischemic stroke rt-PA.
      - Since it is the last line agent, other therapies such as labetalol and nicardipine should have been attempted and optimized but failed.
    - Such a degree of hypertension that is difficult to control could increase the risk of hemorrhagic conversion to the ischemic stroke, which would be made worse in the presence of rt-PA.
  - **Acute Pulmonary Edema in Heart Failure:**
    - Consider using sublingual nitroglycerin with a short course (~20 min) of BiPap to reduce reload and reduce afterload to encourage forward flow that will relieve vascular congestion.
    - Given 0.4 mg or 400 mcg sublingually every 5 minutes until desired effect can offer an estimated equivalent of about 80 mcg/min (400 mcg / 5 minutes = ~80 mcg/min). While an SL tab does not function as a controlled release drug, this convenient and readily available treatment can be simllar to the IV doses up to 200 mcg/min.
  - **Angina / Acute Coronary Syndrome:**
    - Although nitroglycerin is a common component in the acute management of myocardial infarction, its clinical impact is minimal, if any is present. While using a nitroglycerin dosage form in this scenario may relieve chest pain or discomfort, it has not demonstrated a patient-oriented clinical benefit with no change in morbidity or mortality.
  - **Cyanide Toxicity from Nitroprusside Infusions:**
    - To reduce the risk of cyanide toxicity from nitroprusside infusions, it can be formulated with sodium thiosulfate, one of the antidotes of cyanide.
    - Also, preventing exposure to UV light (not fluorescent lighting in most pharmacy departments) can limit the risk of cyanide toxicity.

- **Extravasation of a Vasopressor:**
  - In the event of the extravasation of a vasopressor, phentolamine is often cited as the ideal agent to treat the surrounding tissue. However, it is rarely available, often on shortage.
  - An acceptable alternative can be nitroglycerin in its topical ointment dosage form. Although, patients may have systemic hypotensive effects due to the absorption of the topical nitroglycerin.
- **High-Risk Drug-Interactions:**
  - It is critically important to avoid nitrates in patients taking type 5 phosphodiesterase inhibitors within 24 hours or up to 48 hours if tadalafil due to the risk of severe hypotension.
- **Chronic Care**
  - With long-term use of nitrates, tolerance or tachyphylaxis can occur.
    - This diminishing effect is due to counterregulatory neurohumoral mechanisms opposing nitric oxide.
    - This is thought to occur because of an impairment in the bioconversion of nitrates, thus limiting NO release or an increase in NO clearance due to the generation of superoxide.

- Nitroglycerin exists in numerous dosage forms: sublingual tablet, sublingual packet, translingual aerosol, extended-release capsule, transdermal ointment, transrectal ointment, transdermal patch, and an intravenous solution.

High-Yield Core Evidence
- **Acute Care**
  - **The ECLIPSE Study:**
    - An analysis of three prospective, randomized, open-label, parallel comparison studies compared clevidipine to nitroglycerin, nitroprusside, or nicardipine for asymptomatic hypertension in perioperative patients. There was no difference in the incidence of myocardial infarction, stroke, or renal dysfunction between the therapies. -- *Anesth Analg. 2008;107(4):1110-1121.*
  - **Nitroglycerin Use for Acute Pulmonary Edema:**
    - High-dose nitroglycerin bolus dosing for acute pulmonary edema has been suggested as a possible therapeutic strategy to reduce ICU admissions in this population. A retrospective study evaluated the incidence of ICU admission and hospital LOS in acute pulmonary edema patients who received intermittent high-dose nitroglycerin bolus (2 mg IV every 3-5 minutes) vs. standard nitroglycerin infusion (10-50 mcg/min) vs. bolus and infusion. Patients receiving the combination bolus and infusion had a significantly lower incidence of ICU admission and hospital LOS with a low incidence of hypotension. -- *Am J Emerg Med. 2017;35(1):126-31.*
- **Chronic Care**
  - **The A-HeFT Trial (African-American Heart Failure Trial):**
    - Evaluated the use of hydralazine-isosorbide dinitrate compared to standard therapy plus placebo in patients who were self-identified African Americans with NYHA class III or IV HFrEF. Unfortunately, this trial was terminated early because of a significant 43% reduction in all-cause mortality in patients receiving hydralazine/isosorbide compared with placebo. Thus earning the branded combination product known as BiDil FDA approval to treat HFrEF in African Americans. -- *N Engl J Med 2004; 351:2049-2057.*
  - **Isosorbide mononitrate in patients with HFpEF.**
    - A multicenter, double-blind crossover study in 110 patients with HFpEF was randomized to escalating doses of isosorbide mononitrate or placebo, subsequent crossover to the other group for six weeks. The primary endpoint in this study was the daily activity level. Isosorbide did not improve activity levels compared to the placebo. In addition, isosorbide mononitrate was associated with a dose-dependent reduction in activity levels, did not improve the quality of life, or plasma NT-proBNP concentrations with more frequent adverse events, which included worsening HF and syncope. -- *N Engl J Med 2015; 373:2314-2324.*

High-Yield Fast-Facts
- **Nitroglycerin Exploding:**
  - While it can spontaneously explode in its commonly available dosage forms, the concentration of nitroglycerin is well below the threshold for this risk.
- **NitRITE vs. Nitrate:**
  - Amyl nitrite is a nitRITE, not a nitRATE. It was once used as an inhaled vasodilator but is no longer used for this indication. Instead, its role is as a cauterizing agent for certain types of hemorrhages.
- **Anesthesia:**
  - Nitric oxide used as an anesthetic gas can induce methemoglobin.

HIGH-YIELD BOARD EXAM ESSENTIALS
- **CLASSIC AGENTS:** Isosorbide dinitrate, Isosorbide mononitrate, Nitroglycerin, Nitroprusside
- **DRUG CLASS:** Nitrates, Vasodilators
- **INDICATIONS:** Hypertensive emergency, Angina, Esophageal Spasms, Extravasation of Vasopressors (Topical), Anal Fissures (topical use)
- **MECHANISM:** Acts as a nitric oxide (NO) donor, replacing NO that would normally be produced by endothelial cells that leads to vasodilation.
- **SIDE EFFECTS:** Hypotension, reflex tachycardia, headache
- **CLINICAL PEARLS:**
  - At standard doses reduces preload and offers a reduction in preload and vasodilation of coronary vasculature. At higher doses can also reduce afterload. It also comes in different dosage forms allowing for broad use.
  - Avoid with the co-administration of type 5 PDE inhibitors (i.e., sildenafil) due to risk of hypotension.
  - Nitroprusside is formulated with cyanide (CN) and prolonged infusions can result in accumulation with toxicity. It also must be protected from the light.
  - With chronic use, tachyphylaxis can occur which may warrant a "nitrate free interval".

Table: Drug Class Summary

	Nitrates - Drug Class Review High-Yield Med Reviews		
Mechanism of Action: Act as a nitric oxide donor, replacing NO that would normally be produced by endothelial cells.			
Class Effects: Vasodilation, lowering of blood pressure with potential reflex tachycardia depending on route of admin.			
Generic Name	Brand Name	Main Indication(s) or Uses	Notes
Nitroglycerin	Nitro-Bid Nitro-Dur NitroMist Nitrostat Tridil	• Acute decompensated heart failure • Angina • Acute coronary syndrome • Anal fissures, chronic (topical) • Esophageal spasm • Extravasation of vasopressors	• **Dosing (Adult): IV:** – Initial: 10 to 20 mcg/minute, with subsequent titration (eg, 10 to 20 mcg/minute every 5 to 15 minutes) up to 200 mcg/minute • **Dosing (Peds):** – 0.25 to 0.5 mcg/kg/minute; titrate by 1 mcg/kg/minute every 15 to 20 minutes • **CYP450 Interactions:** – No CYP interactions but important interactions with PDE5 inhibitors • **Renal or Hepatic Dose Adjustments:** None • **Dosage Forms:** IV solution, Oral (sublingual, capsule, translingual), topical (patch, ointment)
Nitroprusside	Nipride RTU Nitropress	• Acute decompensated heart failure • Acute hypertension • Aortic dissection (in combination with esmolol most cases)	• **Dosing (Adult):** – 0.3 to 0.5 mcg/kg/minute; may be titrated by 0.5 mcg/kg/minute every few minutes (max 2 mcg/kg/min) • **Dosing (Peds):** – Initial: 0.3 to 0.5 mcg/kg/minute, titrate every 5 minutes to desired effect; usual dose: 3 to 4 mcg/kg/minute; maximum dose: 10 mcg/kg/minute • **CYP450 Interactions:** – No CYP interactions, but contraindicated with PDE5 inhibitors. • **Renal or Hepatic Dose Adjustments:** – GFR < 30 ml/min increases the risk of cyanide toxicity. Limit mean infusion rate to <3 mcg/kg/minute. • **Dosage Forms:** IV solution
Isosorbide dinitrate	Dilatrate-SR Isordil, Titradose, BiDil (with hydralazine)	• Angina pectoris, prevention	• **Dosing (Adult):** – IR form: 5 to 80 mg BID or TID, SR form: 40 to 160 mg/day • **Dosing (Peds):** not used • **CYP450 Interactions:** Major substrate of CYP3A4 • **Renal or Hepatic Dose Adjustments:** None • **Dosage Forms:** Oral (capsule or tablet)
Isosorbide mononitrate	Imdur	• Angina pectoris (IR form only)	• **Dosing (Adult):** – IR: 5 to 20 mg BID. ER 30 to 60 mg QD, max 240 mg. • **Dosing (Peds):** not used • **CYP450 Interactions:** Major substrate of CYP3A4 • **Renal or Hepatic Dose Adjustments:** None • **Dosage Forms:** Oral (capsule or tablet)

CARDIOVASCULAR – VASODILATORS - MISC

Drug Class
- **Miscellaneous Cardiovascular Agents and Vasodilators**
    - Fenoldopam
    - Hydralazine
    - Ivabradine
    - Phenoxybenzamine
    - Phentolamine
    - Minoxidil
    - Ranolazine

Main Indications or Uses
- **Acute Care:**
    - Acute hypertension
        - Fenoldopam
        - Hydralazine
    - Pheochromocytoma (treatment)
        - Phenoxybenzamine
    - Pheochromocytoma (Diagnosis, prevention, treatment)
        - Phentolamine
    - Extravasation management
        - Phentolamine
- **Chronic Care:**
    - Chronic angina
        - Ranolazine
    - Management of hypertension
        - Minoxidil
    - Risk reduction of hospitalization for worsening heart failure
        - Ivabradine

Mechanism of Action
- **Fenoldopam**
    - Selective dopamine-1 receptor agonist, causing arterial dilation.
        - D1 agonist effects can also enhance renal perfusion, diuresis, and natriuresis.
        - Does possess some moderate affinity to alpha-2 adrenergic receptors.
- **Hydralazine**
    - Smooth muscle relaxation/vasodilation
        - Stimulation of nitric oxide is the release from vascular endothelial cells, causing stimulation of guanylate cyclase to produce cyclic guanosine monophosphate.
        - Also, by reducing intracellular calcium concentrations by inhibiting inositol trisphosphate–induced release of calcium from storage sites.
- **Ivabradine**
    - Decreases spontaneous depolarization of the SA node resulting in a dose-dependent lowering of the heart rate.
        - Selective inhibition of hyperpolarization-activated cyclic nucleotide-gated channels and ion current flow reduces the SA node's spontaneous depolarization rate and prolongs diastolic depolarization.
- **Minoxidil**
    - Produces vasodilation from the opening of vessel wall potassium channels, hyperpolarizing and relaxing vascular smooth muscle.
- **Phenoxybenzamine**
    - Nonselective, irreversible alpha-1 receptor antagonists.

- **Phentolamine**
  - Competitive, reversible alpha-1 and alpha-2 receptor antagonist.
- **Ranolazine**
  - Decreases inward sodium current during repolarization, ultimately decreasing cardiac cell calcium, specifically in ischemic myocytes.
    - As a result, ranolazine enhances the relaxation of ventricular tension and decreases myocardial oxygen consumption.

Primary Net Benefit
- Vasodilation, but the degree of vasodilation and arterial dilation differ by agent and dose used.
- Main Labs to Monitor:
  - No routine lab monitoring

High-Yield Basic Pharmacology
- **Hydralazine**
  - The vasodilation caused by hydralazine often leads to baroreceptor reflex activation.
    - This results in tachycardia due to increased sympathetic outflow to the heart, increasing rate, and contractility.
- **Ivabradine**
  - Ivabradine's actions are specific to the SA node.
    - As a result, there are no direct actions affecting blood pressure, cardiac contractility, or AV nodal conduction.
- **Phenoxybenzamine**
  - In addition to its unique, irreversible alpha-1 blocking properties, phenoxybenzamine has also been described as a serotonin receptor antagonist with H1 antagonist effects.
- **Fenoldopam**
  - It is primarily a D1 receptor agonist but has also been described as possessing antagonist effects on prejunctional alpha-2 autoreceptors at postganglionic sympathetic axons.

High-Yield Clinical Knowledge
- **Fenoldopam**
  - Limited use in clinical practice but may be a reasonable alternative to nitroprusside in patients with a high risk of cyanide/thiocyanate toxicity (high dose, prolonged use, renal impairment).
- **Hydralazine**
  - Despite being frequently used for acute hypertension, it has an unpredictable clinical response, onset, and duration of action. Therefore, alternative agents should be recommended.
- **Ivabradine**
  - Narrow spectrum of HFrEF patients due to FDA-approved indication. With greater clinical experience, these indications may change over time.
- **Phenoxybenzamine**
  - Uniquely used for the management of the sequelae of pheochromocytoma.
- **Phentolamine**
  - Use is limited to the management of extravasation or pheochromocytoma.
- **Minoxidil**
  - Not used clinically for acute hypertension but used during other indications that may affect blood pressure.
- **Ranolazine**
  - Despite numerous drug interactions (CYP3A4, P-gp, and metformin) and a lack of established benefits, it is still commonly used.
- **Hydralazine and NSAIDs**
  - Hydralazine should not be used concomitantly with NSAIDs.
    - Hydralazine is thought to augment the arachidonic acid, COX, and prostacyclin pathways.
      - The administration of NSAIDs could blunt these vasodilatory effects of hydralazine.
- **Acute Care Use of Phentolamine**

- Limited to the management of extravasation of norepinephrine and other sympathomimetic vasopressors.
  - Administered directly into the extravasation area.
    - The dose is typically between 5 and 10 mg but first diluted to a final volume of 10 mL with normal saline.
- **Pheochromocytoma Diagnosis Vs. Management**
  - Both phentolamine and phenoxybenzamine are used for pheochromocytoma.
    - Phentolamine is used primarily in the diagnosis of pheochromocytoma via the phentolamine-blocking test.
    - Phenoxybenzamine is used in the treatment, or more specifically, managing the sequelae of pheochromocytoma such as hypertension and sweating.
- **Fenoldopam And Hypokalemia Risk**
  - Fenoldopam can cause hypokalemia and typically occurs within 6 hours from the start of the infusion.
- **Hydralazine Combination in HFrEF**
  - Hydralazine/isosorbide dinitrate should be used in patients who can't tolerate an ACE inhibitor, ARB, or angiotensin II-neprilysin inhibitor.
- **Visual Disturbances with Ivabradine**
  - Ivabradine may cause unique visual disturbances in patients.
    - Due to the blockade of the hyperpolarization-activated cyclic nucleotide-gated channels, ivabradine induces phosphenes which can cause partial inhibition of the retinal ion current.
      - The visual manifestations have been described as transient enhanced brightness limited to a specific visual field area, halos, image decomposition, colored bright lights, or multiple images.
- **Minoxidil Prodrug and Beta-Blocker Use**
  - The active metabolite of minoxidil, minoxidil sulfate produced via hepatic sulfation, ultimately acts as a potassium channel opener.
  - Because of the vasodilation that accompanies minoxidil use, concomitant beta-blockers are often required to control reflex tachycardia.
- **Ranolazine Drug-Interactions**
  - Ranolazine is a p-glycoprotein substrate, and significant accumulation can occur with PGP inhibitors' concomitant use, including digoxin and cyclosporine.
  - Ranolazine is also a substrate of CYP3A4 and 2D6 with a high potential for drug interactions since many other potential concomitant cardiovascular agents are either substrates or inhibitors of one or both of these enzymes (ex, verapamil, diltiazem, simvastatin, TCAs, tramadol).

High-Yield Core Evidence
- **The INTERACT-2 trial**
  - This was a multicenter, prospective, randomized, open-treatment, blinded trial of patients with spontaneous intracerebral hemorrhage within the previous 6 hours and who had elevated systolic blood pressure to receive intensive treatment to lower their blood pressure or guideline-recommended treatment.
  - Among the possible antihypertensive agents locally available include urapidil, labetalol, hydralazine, metoprolol, and nicardipine.
  - There was no statistically significant difference in the primary outcome of death or major disability between the two treatment strategies; however, a secondary ordinal analysis showed significantly lower modified Rankin scores with intensive treatment.
  - The incidence of nonfatal serious adverse events was similar between the groups.
  - The authors concluded that in patients with intracerebral hemorrhage, intensive lowering of blood pressure did not significantly reduce the rate of the primary outcome of death or severe disability. (N Engl J Med. 2013 Jun 20;368(25):2355-65.)
- **Fenoldopam Phase 3 Trial**
  - Fenoldopam was evaluated in phase 3, a prospective, randomized, open-label, multicenter international trial in adult patients with supine diastolic blood pressures greater than or equal to 120 mm Hg.

- Eligible patients were randomized to receive fenoldopam or nitroprusside to a target diastolic blood pressure of 95 to 110 mm Hg, or a maximum reduction of 40 mm Hg, followed by an infusion for at least six hours, then the patients were weaned off the IV therapy, and oral medication was started.
       - There was no difference between the two antihypertensives in controlling and maintaining diastolic blood pressure and no difference in time to achieve target pressure. In addition, there was no difference in the incidence of adverse effects.
       - The authors concluded that fenoldopam was equivalent to nitroprusside in efficacy and acute adverse events. (Acad Emerg Med. 1995 Nov;2(11):959-65.)
   - **The SHIFT Trial**
       - This was a randomized, double-blind, placebo-controlled, parallel-group study to determine the effect of heart-rate reduction with ivabradine on heart failure outcomes in patients with symptomatic heart failure.
       - Patients receiving ivabradine had a significantly lower incidence in the primary endpoint (composite of cardiovascular death or hospital admission for worsening heart failure), driven by reduced hospital admissions for worsening heart failure and deaths due to heart failure.
       - Patients receiving ivabradine had fewer serious adverse events in the ivabradine group than in the placebo group; however, more patients receiving ivabradine had symptomatic bradycardia and visual side effects.
       - The authors concluded that ivabradine might assist in improving clinical outcomes in heart failure. (Lancet 2010;376:875–885.)
   - **RIVER-PCI Trial**
       - The effect of ranolazine on the improvement in the prognosis of patients with incomplete revascularization after the percutaneous coronary intervention was evaluated in a multicenter, randomized, parallel-group, double-blind, placebo-controlled, event-driven trial.
       - Patients with a history of chronic angina with incomplete revascularization after percutaneous coronary intervention received either ranolazine or a matching placebo.
       - There was no difference in the primary endpoint of time to the first occurrence of ischemia-driven revascularization or ischemia-driven hospitalization without revascularization. Additionally, more patients receiving ranolazine had discontinued study drugs because of an adverse event than placebo.
       - The authors concluded that ranolazine did not reduce the composite rate of ischemia-driven revascularization or hospitalization without revascularization in patients with a history of chronic angina who had incomplete revascularization after percutaneous coronary intervention. (Lancet. 2016 Jan 9;387(10014):136-45.)

High-Yield Fast-Facts
   - **Ranolazine And Metformin Dose Limits**
       - There is yet another unique interaction between ranolazine and metformin among the many drug interactions with ranolazine. Specifically, when ranolazine 1g BID is used with metformin 1g BID, these agents compete for the organic cation transporter 2, affecting their renal clearances.
           - As a result, the risk of metformin accumulation and an increased risk of lactic acidosis.
   - **Cocaine Induced Hypertension Management**
       - Phentolamine has been used for the management of cocaine-induced hypertension.
           - While this may be a reasonable option, the first-line management of cocaine-induced chest pain and hypertension should be benzodiazepines.
   - **Drug Shortage and Alternatives**
       - Phentolamine has been intermittently unavailable due to drug shortages.
           - As an alternative for managing extravasation, terbutaline may be considered in specific circumstances such as norepinephrine extravasation.

   - **Specific Population for Ivabradine**
       - Ivabradine is indicated explicitly in adult patients with NYHA class II to III chronic heart failure with left ventricular ejection fraction less than or equal to 35%, who are in sinus rhythm with a resting heart rate

of at least 70 beats per minute and either is on maximally tolerated doses of beta-blockers or have a contraindication to beta-blocker use.

HIGH-YIELD BOARD EXAM ESSENTIALS
- **CLASSIC AGENTS:** Fenoldopam, hydralazine, ivabradine, phenoxybenzamine, phentolamine, minoxidil, ranolazine
- **DRUG CLASS:** CV agents and vasodilators
- **INDICATIONS:** Acute hypertension (fenoldopam, hydralazine), pheochromocytoma treatment (phenoxybenzamine), pheochromocytoma diagnosis, prevention (phentolamine), extravasation management (phentolamine), chronic angina (ranolazine), hypertension (minoxidil), risk reduction of hospitalization for worsening heart failure (ivabradine)
- **MECHANISM:**
    - Fenoldopam: D1 receptor agonist, causing arterial dilation
    - Ivabradine: Vasodilation from stimulation of nitric oxide release and reduction of intracellular calcium concentrations (hydralazine), decreases spontaneous depolarization of the SA node
    - Minoxidil: Opening of potassium channels, hyperpolarizing, and relaxing vascular smooth muscle
    - Phenoxybenzamine: Nonselective, irreversible alpha-1 receptor antagonists
    - Phentolamine: Competitive, reversible alpha-1 and alpha-2 receptor antagonist
    - Ranolazine: Decreases inward sodium current during repolarization, enhancing relaxation of ventricular tension and decreases myocardial oxygen consumption
- **SIDE EFFECTS:** Hypotension, reflex tachycardia, headache
- **CLINICAL PEARLS:** Hydralazine/isosorbide dinitrate should be used in patients who can't tolerate an ACE inhibitor, ARB, or angiotensin II-neprilysin inhibitor.

Table: Drug Class Summary

Miscellaneous Vasodilators - Drug Class Review High-Yield Med Reviews			
Mechanism of Action: *Fenoldopam - D1 receptor agonist, causing arterial dilation.* *Hydralazine - Vasodilation from stimulation of nitric oxide release and reduction of intracellular calcium concentrations.* *Ivabradine - Decreases spontaneous depolarization of the SA node* *Minoxidil - Opening of potassium channels, hyperpolarizing, and relaxing vascular smooth muscle.* *Phenoxybenzamine - Nonselective, irreversible alpha-1 receptor antagonists.* *Phentolamine - Competitive, reversible alpha-1 and alpha-2 receptor antagonist.* *Ranolazine - Decreases inward sodium current during repolarization, enhancing ventricular tension relaxation and decreasing myocardial oxygen consumption.*			
Class Effects: *Vasodilation, but the degree of vasodilation and arterial dilation differ by agent and dose used.*			
Generic Name	**Brand Name**	**Main Indication(s) or Uses**	**Notes**

Fenoldopam	Corlopam	• Short-term treatment of severe hypertension	• **Dosing (Adult):**
			  − IV: infusion 0.01 to 0.3 mcg/kg/minute, titrate by 0.05 to 0.1 mcg/kg/minute q15min to target blood pressure
			    − Maximum 1.6 mcg/kg/minute for 48 hours.
			• **Dosing (Peds):**
			  − IV: infusion 0.2 mcg/kg/minute, titrate by 0.3 to 0.5 mcg/kg/minute q20 to 30min
			    − Maximum 0.8 mcg/kg/minute
			• **CYP450 Interactions:** None
			• **Renal or Hepatic Dose Adjustments:** None
			• **Dosage Forms:** IV solution

Hydralazine	Apresoline	• Hypertension
		• Hypertensive emergency in pregnancy or postpartum
			• **Dosing (Adult):**
			  − Oral: initial dose 10 to 25 mg q6h
			    − Maximum 100 to 200 mg/day
			  − IM or IV: 5 to 20 mg q4-6hours
			    − Maximum 20-40 mg/dose
			• **Dosing (Peds):**
			  − Oral: initial dose 0.75 to 3 mg/kg/day divided q6-12h
			    − Maximum 7 mg/kg/day or 200 mg/day, whichever is less
			• **CYP450 Interactions:** None
			• **Renal or Hepatic Dose Adjustments:**
			  − CrCl > or equal to 10 mL/minute- frequency of q8h
			  − CrCl <10 mL/minute- frequency of q8-16h.
			  − Intermittent hemodialysis: Dose after dialysis
			• **Dosage Forms:** IV solution, Oral (tablet)

Miscellaneous Vasodilators - Drug Class Review
High-Yield Med Reviews

Generic Name	Brand Name	Main Indication(s) or Uses	Notes
Ivabradine	Corlanor	• Hospitalization risk reduction in patients with symptomatic heart failure and an ejection fraction of 35% or less.	• **Dosing (Adult):** — Oral: initial dose of 2.5 to 5 mg twice daily • **Dosing (Peds):** — < 40 kg- initial dose of 0.05 mg/kg/dose twice daily; Max: 7.5 mg twice daily — > or equal to 40 kg, see adult dosing • **CYP450 Interactions:** Major substrate of CYP3A4 • **Renal or Hepatic Dose Adjustments:** — Child-Pugh class C, contraindicated • **Dosage Forms:** Oral (capsule or tablet)
Minoxidil	Loniten	• Management of hypertension • Hair growth (topical only)	• **Dosing (Adult):** — Oral: initial dose of 5 mg daily — Maximum dose of 100 mg/day • **Dosing (Peds):** — Oral: initial dose 0.2 mg/kg/dose once — Maximum dose 5 mg/dose • **CYP450 Interactions:** None known • **Renal or Hepatic Dose Adjustments:** None • **Dosage Forms:** Oral (tablet)
Phenoxybenzamine	Dibenzyline	• Management of pheochromocytoma • Hair growth (topical only)	• **Dosing (Adult):** — Oral initial 10 mg twice daily — Maximum dose of 240 mg daily • **Dosing (Peds):** — Oral initial 0.2 to 0.25 mg/kg/dose once or twice daily; Maximum 10 mg/dose • **CYP450 Interactions:** None • **Renal or Hepatic Dose Adjustments:** None • **Dosage Forms:** Oral (capsule)
Phentolamine	Rogitine OraVerse	• Diagnosis & management of pheochromocytoma • Extravasation management	• **Dosing (Adult):** — IV or IM: 5 mg once — Local infiltration of 5 to 10 mg • **Dosing (Peds):** — IV: 1 mg bolus or IM 3 mg once — Local infiltration of 0.5 to 1 mg/mL • **CYP450 Interactions:** None • **Renal or Hepatic Dose Adjustments:** None • **Dosage Forms:** IV (solution)
Ranolazine	Ranexa	• Chronic angina	• **Dosing (Adult):** — Oral: initial dose of 500 mg twice daily — Maximum 1,000 mg twice daily • **Dosing (Peds):** Not used • **CYP450 Interactions:** Substrate and inhibitor of CYP3A4, CPY2D6, and P-gp • **Renal or Hepatic Dose Adjustments:** None • **Dosage Forms:** Oral (tablet)

CARDIOVASCULAR – GLYCOPROTEIN IIB/IIIA INHIBITOR

Drug Class
- **Acute Care**
    - Abciximab
    - Eptifibatide
    - Tirofiban

Main Indications or Uses
- **Acute Care:**
    - Acute myocardial infarction, adjunct to percutaneous coronary intervention

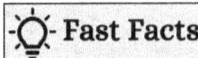 **Fast Facts**

✓ Out of the agents in this class, only abciximab is a monoclonal antibody with irreversible inhibition of the GPIIb/IIIa receptor on the platelet surface.

Mechanism of Action
- These agents block fibrinogen from binding to the platelet glycoprotein IIb/IIIa receptors.
    - The GPIIb/IIIa receptor is the final step in platelet aggregation, which anchors platelets to one another via fibrinogen and prevents further platelet activation by inhibiting the von Willebrand factor.

Primary Net Benefit
- These agents are potent inhibitors of platelet aggregation at the final point of platelet-to-platelet adherence.
    - However, despite this, all of the agents require the coadministration of anticoagulation with heparin or low molecular weight heparins.
- Main Labs to Monitor:
    - CBC
    - INR/PT, PTT, ACT
    - Fibrinogen
    - Fibrin split products

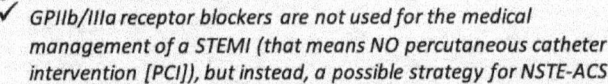 **Knowledge Integration**

✓ GPIIb/IIIa receptor blockers are not used for the medical management of a STEMI (that means NO percutaneous catheter intervention [PCI]), but instead, a possible strategy for NSTE-ACS.
✓ If a patient then undergoes delayed catheter intervention after medical management of NSTE-ACS, the use of GPIIb/IIIa agents may be considered.

High-Yield Basic Pharmacology
- **Drug Production**
    Each agent is produced differently, communicating unique pharmacologic and pharmacokinetic properties.
    - Abciximab is a humanized mouse monoclonal Fab fragment antibody with irreversible binding to the GPIIb/IIIa receptor.
    - Whereas eptifibatide is a peptide inhibitor of GPIIb/IIIa, tirofiban is a non-peptide inhibitor. Each of these agents demonstrates reversible inhibition of GPIIb/IIIa.
- **Reversibility and Receptor Affinity**
    - Abciximab is a relatively nonspecific chimeric monoclonal antibody (MAB) that irreversibly inhibits platelet aggregation with a receptor binding ratio of approximately 2:1.
    - Conversely, both eptifibatide and tirofiban are highly specific, reversible platelet aggregation inhibitors. In therapeutic terms, the latter agents are associated with a higher degree of acute inhibition of platelet activity in a ratio of approximately 1000:1.
    - Should hemorrhage occur with either eptifibatide or tirofiban, it is unlikely that platelet transfusions would be of any benefit not be able to absorb the excess drug and would not be helpful in the management of bleeding with eptifibatide or tirofiban.
- **Snake Venom**
    - Eptifibatide is derived from the disintegrin proteins found in the venom of the Southeastern Pygmy Rattlesnake (Sistrurus miliarius).

Cardiology

High-Yield Clinical Knowledge
- **Abciximab Antibodies**
  - Abciximab use can induce the formation of human antichimeric antibodies, leading to acute hypersensitivity reactions.
  - Patients receiving abciximab for the first time have a risk of reaction of approximately 6%, but with repeated exposure after the second administration increases to 27%.
  - If patients receive abciximab four or more times, their risk of acute hypersensitivity is as high as 44%.
- **Contraindications**
  - The contraindications to using a GPIIb/IIIa inhibitor are analogous to the contraindications to fibrinolytics (i.e., alteplase).
  - These contraindications include any patient with a history of hypersensitivity to any product component, active internal bleeding or a history of bleeding diathesis, major surgical procedure, or severe physical trauma within the previous 4 to 6 weeks.
  - There are additional agent-specific contraindications, including the presence of abciximab antibodies or previous exposure.
- **Acute Myocardial Infarction**
  - Thrombocytopenia due to GPIIb/IIIa inhibitors may be difficult to distinguish from heparin-induced thrombocytopenia since these agents are given concomitantly.
    - However, thrombocytopenia due to GPIIb/IIIa inhibitors is more likely to cause rapid thrombocytopenia within hours of administration and a more significant absolute reduction in platelet level.
- **Antithrombotic Strategy**
  - There is clinical equipoise with regards to adjunct antithrombotic strategy during PCI.
  - Depending on clinical practice, either a GPIIb/IIIa receptor antagonist plus anticoagulation (heparin or LMWH) or bivalirudin alone are acceptable practices.
  - While head-to-head clinical trials have suggested these strategies are interchangeable in preventing secondary major cardiac events, there is significantly less bleeding observed in patients receiving bivalirudin.
  - Patients receiving fibrinolytic therapy for STEMI should not receive a GPIIb/IIIa receptor antagonist due to the significantly higher risk of hemorrhage.
- **Acute Stroke**
  - Eptifibatide was investigated as an adjunct to alteplase for acute ischemic stroke. However, the results of the CLEAR-ER study did not demonstrate a therapeutic benefit.

High-Yield Core Evidence
- **ISAR-REACT 2**
  - The ISAR-REACT 2 trial was a randomized, double-blind trial that examined the role of abciximab plus heparin with NSTEMI ACS undergoing PCI after pretreatment with aspirin and clopidogrel, compared to placebo plus heparin and aspirin plus clopidogrel.
  - The use of abciximab was associated with a 25% reduction in the risk of death, myocardial infarction, or urgent target vessel revascularization occurring within 30 days compared to placebo.
  - Additionally, the use of abciximab did not increase the risk of major and minor bleeding and the need for transfusion.
  - However, there was no difference in the primary efficacy outcome of the composite of death, myocardial infarction, or urgent target vessel revascularization occurring within 30 days after randomization in patients without an elevated troponin. (JAMA. 2006 Apr 5;295(13):1531-8.)

- **PRISM-PLUS**
    - The PRISM-PLUS study evaluated the GPIIb/IIIa inhibitor's use, tirofiban, in unstable angina and NSTEMI population.
    - This study randomized patients who met inclusion criteria to either blinded tirofiban alone, heparin alone, or tirofiban plus heparin.
    - Since these patients were not undergoing immediate PCI but rather within 48 hours, the study drugs were infused for a mean of approximately 72 hours before PCI.
    - However, this study was prematurely stopped because of excess 7-day mortality in the group receiving tirofiban alone. But for the available data, patients receiving tirofiban plus heparin had a significantly lower risk of 7-day, 30-day, and 6-month mortality, significantly lower compared to patients receiving heparin alone.
    - In terms of safety, major bleeding occurred similarly across patient groups. (N Engl J Med. 1998 May 21;338(21):1488-97.)

High-Yield Fast-Facts
- **PCI Techniques**
    - GPIIb/IIIa receptor antagonist's role continues to decline due to advances in PCI procedure techniques and bivalirudin use.
        - However, patients suffering an NSTEMI undergoing PCI and receiving clopidogrel may still represent an existing population where GPIIb/IIIa receptor antagonist plus heparin/LMWH may be reasonable.

HIGH-YIELD BOARD EXAM ESSENTIALS
- **CLASSIC AGENTS:** Abciximab, eptifibatide, tirofiban
- **DRUG CLASS:** GP IIb/IIIa inhibitors
- **INDICATIONS:** Acute myocardial infarction, adjunct to percutaneous coronary intervention
- **MECHANISM:** Inhibit fibrinogen from binding to the platelet glycoprotein IIb/IIIa receptors.
- **SIDE EFFECTS:** Acute hypersensitivity (abciximab), hemorrhage
- **CLINICAL PEARLS:**
    - These agents are potent inhibitors of platelet aggregation, but all require the coadministration of anticoagulation with heparin or low molecular weight heparins.
    - Abciximab is the only agent that is a monoclonal antibody (MAB) that irreversibly inhibits platelet aggregation whereas the agents are not MABs and are reversible.

Table: Drug Class Summary

Glycoprotein IIb/IIIa inhibitor - Drug Class Review High-Yield Med Reviews			
Mechanism of Action: *Reversibly inhibits platelet aggregation by binding to the GPIIb/IIIa receptor on the platelet surface and prevents fibrin binding.*			
Class Effects: *Prevents early thrombosis of coronary artery and stenting devices. Increases risk of hemorrhage.*			
Generic Name	**Brand Name**	**Main Indication(s) or Uses**	**Notes**
Abciximab	ReoPro	<ul><li>Percutaneous coronary intervention</li><li>Unstable angina/non-ST-elevation myocardial infarction</li></ul>	<ul><li>**Dosing (Adult):** − IV: bolus of 0.25 mg/kg 10 to 60 minutes prior PCI. Can continue 0.125 mcg/kg/minute (maximum: 10 mcg/minute) for 12 hours. − For NSTEMI, use an initial bolus of 0.25 mg/kg followed by infusion at 10 mcg/minute until 1 hour after PCI.</li><li>**Dosing (Peds):** Not used</li><li>**CYP450 Interactions:** No CYP interactions</li><li>**Renal or Hepatic Dose Adjustments:** None</li><li>**Dosage Forms:** IV: solution</li></ul>
Eptifibatide	Integrilin	<ul><li>Percutaneous coronary intervention with or without coronary stenting</li></ul>	<ul><li>**Dosing (Adult):** − IV: bolus of 180 mcg/kg q10minutes for 2 doses. − Start a continuous infusion of 2 mcg/kg/minute after the first bolus. (Maximum bolus: 22.6 mg; maximum infusion: 15 mg/hr)</li><li>**Dosing (Peds):** Not used</li><li>**CYP450 Interactions:** No CYP interactions</li><li>**Renal or Hepatic Dose Adjustments:** − CrCl less than 50 mL/minute lower continuous infusion starting dose of 1 mcg/kg/minute (maximum 7.5 mg/hour). − Should not be used in ESRD patients on HD.</li><li>**Dosage Forms:** IV solution</li></ul>
Tirofiban	Aggrastat	<ul><li>Unstable angina/non-ST-elevation myocardial infarction</li></ul>	<ul><li>**Dosing (Adult):** − IV: bolus 25 mcg/kg over 5 minutes followed by 0.15 mcg/kg/minute continued for up to 18 hours.</li><li>**Dosing (Peds):** Not used</li><li>**CYP450 Interactions:** None</li><li>**Renal or Hepatic Dose Adjustments:** − CrCl less than or equal to 60 mL/minute, no change in bolus, but a lower infusion of 0.075 mcg/kg/minute continued for up to 18 hours.</li><li>**Dosage Forms:** IV solution</li></ul>

CARDIOVASCULAR – OTHER ANTIPLATELET (DIPYRIDAMOLE, CILOSTAZOL, VORAPAXAR)

Drug Class
- Acute Care
  - Dipyridamole
- Chronic Care
  - Dipyridamole
  - Cilostazol
  - Vorapaxar

Main Indications or Uses
- Acute Care:
  - Diagnostic agent in coronary artery disease
- Chronic Care:
  - Stroke prevention
  - Thrombotic risk reduction (post-MI or PAD)

Mechanism of Action
- Dipyridamole
  - Causes inhibition of platelet aggregation by inhibiting adenosine deaminase and phosphodiesterase, thus preventing the degradation of cyclic AMP to 5'-AMP, leading to intraplatelet accumulation of cyclic AMP.
  - It can also cause an increase in the release of prostacyclin or prostaglandin D2 and causes coronary vasodilation.
- Cilostazol
  - Inhibits phosphodiesterase III, thus preventing the degradation of cyclic AMP, causing a reversible inhibition of platelet aggregation, vasodilation, and inhibition of vascular smooth muscle cell proliferation.
- Vorapaxar
  - Leads to inhibition of platelet aggregation by inhibiting protease-activated receptor-1 (PAR-1), thrombin-induced, and thrombin receptor agonist peptide (TRAP)-induced platelet aggregation.

Primary Net Benefit
- Antiplatelet agents have fallen out of favor for the thienopyridine antiplatelet agents but remain used for unique indications, including diagnostic aids in CAD.
- Main Labs to Monitor:
  - CBC

High-Yield Basic Pharmacology
- Irreversible Inhibition
  - Vorapaxar results in prolonged, irreversible inhibition of platelet activity within one week and persists for up to 4 weeks.
    - Consequently, vorapaxar is contraindicated in patients with active bleeding and patients with a history of stroke, transient ischemic attacks, or intracranial hemorrhage.
- Half-Life
  - The half-life of vorapaxar is very long compared to other agents in this class.
    - Its half-life ranges between 3 to 5 days.
- Classification
  - These antiplatelet agents do not fall within other identifiable classes of similarly acting agents, including the thienopyridines, salicylates, or GPIIb/IIIa agents.
- The Lesser-Known CYP450 Isoenzyme
  - Vorapaxar is a substrate of CYP2J2.
  - This CYP enzyme is a major cardiac CYP450 and primarily metabolizes arachidonic acid to cardioactive epoxyeicosatrienoic acids.

- Inhibition of CYP2J2 has been associated with cardiotoxicity but tumor regression. Conversely, the overexpression of CYP2J2 results in tumor proliferation and cardioprotection.
- The clinical effect of vorapaxar in these scenarios is not known.

High-Yield Clinical Knowledge

- **Dipyridamole and Cardiac Stress Testing**
  - Although used orally as an antiplatelet agent, dipyridamole also is used parenterally in pharmacologically-based cardiac nuclear stress tests.
    - This diagnostic procedure involves the injection of radioactive tracer, administered in conjunction with dipyridamole (or adenosine, or regadenoson), utilizing its coronary vasodilation properties.
- **Cilostazol, Milrinone, and FDA Warnings**
  - As a phosphodiesterase III inhibitor, cilostazol exists in the same medication class as milrinone.
    - In the past, milrinone was used orally to improve cardiac output in heart failure patients.
    - Still, it was found to increase mortality and subsequently removed from the market (oral dosage form only).
    - As a result of being in the same class, cilostazol also now carries an FDA warning stating its use is contraindicated with patients with heart failure of any severity.
- **Symptomatic Bradycardia And Exacerbation Of Angina**
  - Dipyridamole, as described previously, can increase adenosine concentration through its actions on adenosine deaminase.
    - As a result, although platelet function is affected, the risk of adenosine exerting an effect on cardiac conduction increases.
    - Thus, the high incidence of chest pain and bradycardia can be linked to this known effect. Its use should be limited in patients taking agents or food that can further prevent adenosine metabolism, including methylxanthines (caffeine, theobromine, or theophylline).
- **Secondary Stroke Prevention**
  - The American Stroke Association guidelines for secondary stroke prevention recommend either clopidogrel or the combination of aspirin-dipyridamole as antiplatelet therapy.
    - Many patients cannot tolerate the bradycardic and or angina-related adverse events accompanying dipyridamole therapy; thus, clopidogrel is often the primary agent.
      - Clopidogrel has strong evidence supporting its role in secondary stroke prevention from several landmark trials, including the CAPRIE and CHANCE studies.
- **Doctor Who? Double Vs. Triple Antiplatelet Therapy**
  - The TARDIS study analyzed aspirin plus dipyridamole plus clopidogrel compared to aspirin and either clopidogrel or dipyridamole in a search for additional secondary stroke prevention.
    - Despite the additional antiplatelet actions, there was no improvement in recurrent stroke between groups, but unsurprisingly, there was an increased risk of major bleeding in the triple therapy group.

High-Yield Core Evidence

- **Dipyridamole vs Regadenoson**
  - Dipyridamole was compared to regadenoson in patients undergoing single-photon emission tomography myocardial perfusion imaging (MPI) in a single-center, retrospective cohort study.
  - Patients receiving regadenoson had a significantly higher incidence in the primary endpoint of the composite occurrence of any documented adverse event compared to patients receiving dipyridamole.
  - There were no differences between treatment groups concerning required early MPI study termination and no difference in the use of aminophylline or other interventions to treat adverse events.
  - The authors concluded that dipyridamole offers a safe and cost-effective alternative to regadenoson for cardiac imaging studies. (Pharmacotherapy. 2017 Jun;37(6):657-661.)
- **PRoFESS**
  - The PRoFESS trial compared extended-release dipyridamole plus aspirin with clopidogrel and assessed the risk of recurrent stroke between the two antiplatelet agents.

- Study investigators randomized patients with ischemic stroke to receive either aspirin and extended-release dipyridamole, as Aggrenox, clopidogrel, and either telmisartan or placebo once per day.
- There was no difference in the primary outcome of recurrent strokes in patients randomized to Aggrenox or patients randomly assigned to telmisartan or placebo.
- Furthermore, there was no difference in any secondary efficacy outcomes; however, clopidogrel was better tolerated with less bleeding and headache.
- The authors concluded that no therapy investigated had a significantly different effect on recurrent stroke and cognitive decline in patients with ischemic stroke. (Lancet Neurol. 2008 Oct;7(10):875-84.)
- **Cilostazol vs Pentoxifylline**
    - Cilostazol was compared to pentoxifylline or placebo in patients with moderate-to-severe claudication.
    - This study was a randomized, double-blind, placebo-controlled, multicenter trial with a primary outcome of mean maximal walking distance.
    - Patients receiving cilostazol had a significantly greater improvement in maximal walking distance compared to pentoxifylline.
    - This benefit continued for 24 weeks, whereas pentoxifylline was no better than the placebo.
    - Deaths and serious adverse event rates were similar in each group, but more patients receiving cilostazol complained of adverse effects, including headache, palpitations, and diarrhea. However, withdrawal rates were similar in the cilostazol and pentoxifylline groups.
    - The authors concluded that cilostazol was significantly better than pentoxifylline or placebo for increasing walking distances in patients with intermittent claudication but was associated with a greater frequency of minor side effects. (Am J Med. 2000 Nov;109(7):523-30.)

High-Yield Fast-Facts
- **Newer, safer agents**
    - Cilostazol and aspirin-dipyridamole are no longer used routinely due to newer agents, including the thienopyridines.
- **Cilostazol and Vasodilation**
    - In addition to antiplatelet effects, cilostazol can contribute to vasodilation. As a result, patients are at risk of orthostatic hypotension, compounded by the antiplatelet effects, could develop intracranial bleeding with a head injury.

HIGH-YIELD BOARD EXAM ESSENTIALS
- **CLASSIC AGENTS:** Cilostazol, dipyridamole, vorapaxar
- **DRUG CLASS:** Antiplatelet
- **INDICATIONS:** Stroke prevention, thrombotic risk reduction (post-MI or PAD)
- **MECHANISM:** Cilostazol inhibits phosphodiesterase III, thus preventing the degradation of cyclic AMP, causing a reversible inhibition of platelet aggregation, vasodilation, and inhibition of vascular smooth muscle cell proliferation. Dipyridamole inhibits adenosine deaminase and phosphodiesterase, preventing the degradation of cyclic AMP to 5'-AMP, which leads to intraplatelet accumulation of cyclic AMP. Vorapaxar leads to inhibition of platelet aggregation by inhibiting protease-activated receptor-1 (PAR-1), thrombin-induced, and thrombin receptor agonist peptide (TRAP)-induced platelet aggregation.
- **SIDE EFFECTS:** Bleeding, bradycardia (dipyridamole), angina (dipyridamole)
- **CLINICAL PEARLS:** Dipyridamole, through its actions on adenosine deaminase as described previously, can increase the concentration of adenosine.

Table: Drug Class Summary

Other Antiplatelet - Drug Class Review High-Yield Med Reviews			
Mechanism of Action: *Dipyridamole* - inhibits adenosine deaminase and phosphodiesterase, preventing the degradation of cyclic AMP to 5'-AMP, which leads to intraplatelet accumulation of cyclic AMP. *Cilostazol* - inhibits phosphodiesterase III, thus preventing the degradation of cyclic AMP, causing a reversible inhibition of platelet aggregation, vasodilation, and inhibition of vascular smooth muscle cell proliferation. *Vorapaxar* - leads to inhibition of platelet aggregation by inhibiting protease-activated receptor-1 (PAR-1), thrombin-induced, and thrombin receptor agonist peptide (TRAP)-induced platelet aggregation.			
Class Effects: Antithrombotic, antiplatelet effect			
Generic Name	Brand Name	Main Indication(s) or Uses	Notes

Cilostazol	Pletal	• Intermittent claudication	• **Dosing (Adult):**
			   – Oral: 100 mg twice daily
			 • **Dosing (Peds):** Not used
			 • **CYP450 Interactions:**
			   – Inhibitor of CYP3A4.
			   – Substrate of CYP 3A4, 2CYP C19, CYP 2D6, and CYP1A2
			 • **Renal or Hepatic Dose Adjustments:** None
			 • **Dosage Forms:** Oral (tablet, capsule)

Dipyridamole	Persantine
	 Aggrenox
		• Secondary stroke and CV prevention
		 • Diagnostic agent in CAD
			• **Dosing (Adult):**
			   – IV: bolus of 0.56 mg/kg over 4 minutes (maximum dose 70 mg)
			   – Oral: aspirin 25 mg/dipyridamole ER 200 mg twice daily
			 • **Dosing (Peds):**
			   – IV: bolus of 0.56 mg/kg over 4 minutes (maximum dose 70 mg)
			   – Oral: 2 to 5 mg/kg/day in divided doses
			 • **CYP450 Interactions:** None
			 • **Renal or Hepatic Dose Adjustments:** None
			 • **Dosage Forms:** IV solution, Oral (tablet, capsule)

Vorapaxar	Zontivity	• Thrombotic risk reduction with a history of MI or PAD	• **Dosing (Adult):** – Oral: 2.08 mg once daily in combination with aspirin and/or clopidogrel • **Dosing (Peds):** Not used • **CYP450 Interactions:** Substrate of CYP3A4, CYP2J2 • **Renal or Hepatic Dose Adjustments:** None • **Dosage Forms:** Oral (tablet)

CARDIOVASCULAR – THIENOPYRIDINES (AKA P2Y12 INHIBITORS)

Drug Class
- Acute Care
    - Cangrelor
    - Clopidogrel
    - Prasugrel
    - Ticagrelor
- Chronic Care
    - Clopidogrel
    - Prasugrel
    - Ticagrelor

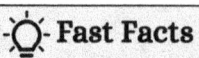

Fast Facts

✓ *The irreversible inhibition of the platelet P2Y12 receptor by clopidogrel allows for once-a-day dosing and is more forgiving if a patient were to miss a dose but results in a pharmacologic that can last for several days which could be harmful if the patient is bleeding or needs surgery.*

Main Indications or Uses
- Acute Care:
    - Acute coronary syndrome
- Chronic Care:
    - Primary and secondary prevention of MI, stroke, or PAD

Mechanism of Action
- Irreversible (clopidogrel, prasugrel) or reversible (cangrelor, and ticagrelor) inhibitor of platelet P2Y12 receptor, preventing ADP from binding and activating the glycoprotein GPIIb/IIIa complex, thereby inhibiting platelet aggregation.

Primary Net Benefit
- First-line antiplatelet agents for post-myocardial infarction, stroke, or peripheral arterial disease patients.
    - Can also serve as a alternative treatment option in patients with an aspirin sensitivity but need antiplatelet effects.
- Main Labs to Monitor:
    - CBC

High-Yield Basic Pharmacology
- Reversibility
    - The reversible inhibitors of P2Y12 are reversible because they disassociate from their binding site, which permits restoration of normal platelet aggregation.
        - This is one of the reasons that ticagrelor must be dosed twice daily.
- Bradycardia
    - Ticagrelor's unique mechanism increases the risk of symptomatic bradycardia and shortness of breath in some patients.
        - This results from ticagrelor's effect on the inhibition of adenosine degradation and inhibition of adenosine uptake by erythrocytes.
        - This interaction increases adenosine exposure which likely explains these unique adverse effects.
- Cangrelor and Loading Doses
    - If patients receive cangrelor, their loading dose of clopidogrel or prasugrel must be delayed.
        - This is due to cangrelor's ability to interfere with the action of clopidogrel or prasugrel to irreversibly inhibit platelet function by directly preventing the binding of their active metabolites.
            - However, when cangrelor infusion is stopped, this effect stops.
            - Thus, if cangrelor is used, clopidogrel or prasugrel loading doses should be delayed until the infusion is stopped.
    - This interaction does not exist with ticagrelor.

High-Yield Clinical Knowledge
- **Clopidogrel 300 mg vs 600 mg**
  - Clopidogrel loading doses of 600 mg should be administered to patients with STEMI undergoing emergent PCI, PCI at least 24 hours after fibrinolytic therapy, and NSTEMI patients undergoing an early invasive approach.
    - The lower 300 mg loading dose should be used in STEMI if PCI occurs after a fibrinolytic strategy is chosen.
    - NSTEMI patients can receive either 300 mg or 600 mg loading dose if using an ischemia-guided approach.
- **Continuing Beyond 12 Months**
  - The AHA guidelines recommend dual antiplatelet therapy (DAPT) for at least 12 months in patients after PCI with drug-eluting stents.
    - However, continuing DAPT beyond 12 months is an area of uncertainty regarding the ideal duration and patient characteristics where the benefit outweighs the risk.
      - The DAPT, DES-LATE, PEGASUS, and OPTIDUAL trials evaluated the role of DATP beyond 12 months.
      - In these studies, there were mixed results regarding the added benefit of continuing DAPT up to 36 months. Any added benefit was often matched with an increased offsetting risk of bleeding.
- **P2Y12 Prodrugs**
  - Clopidogrel and prasugrel are prodrugs that require CYP2C19 (clopidogrel) or CYP3A4 and CYP2B6 (prasugrel) for activation.
    - However, ticagrelor and its metabolite are active. Therefore, the risk of decreased absorption from PPI agents, strong CYP2B6 or 2C19 inhibitors does not exist with ticagrelor.
      - But since CYP3A4 metabolizes ticagrelor, inhibitors of CYP3A4 would increase the exposure and risk of bleeding.
- **Parenteral Agent**
  - Cangrelor is the only thienopyridine available in the US as a parenteral dosage form.
  - After the loading dose, it can achieve platelet inhibition within 2 minutes, and once the infusion is stopped, restoration of normal platelet reactivity occurs within 1 to 2 hours.
    - In the CHAMPION trials, cangrelor may be as effective as a GP IIb/IIIa-based strategy but is associated with less bleeding risk.
    - However, it is still yet to be determined whether cangrelor maintains similar efficacy and benefits compared to a bivalirudin-based PCI strategy since only 19% of the population of the CHAMPION-PHOENIX received this PCI strategy.
- **Aspirin and Ticagrelor**
  - In the PLATO study, there seemed to be an increased risk of stent thrombosis in patients receiving aspirin plus ticagrelor.
  - While this contradictory finding led to an FDA warning and limiting aspirin's dose in patients receiving ticagrelor, this finding was later linked to a small subgroup of patients in the United States (it was a multinational study) with other significant differences in baseline characteristics and clinical outcomes.
    - Therefore, the warning not to exceed 100mg of aspirin daily with ticagrelor, analysis, and evaluation in additional patients established no clinically relevant interaction, causing the combination to increase the risk of thrombosis.
- **Prasugrel Lower Dose 5 Mg Vs 10 Mg**
  - The TRITON-TIMI 38 study described below established the role of prasugrel in managing acute coronary syndromes where PCI is planned.
    - In this study, patients who are elderly (75 years or older) with low body weight (less than 60 kg) had a higher risk of bleeding.
    - But in a follow-up trial (TRILOGY ACS), these at-risk patients were given a lower dose of 5 mg, which mitigated the bleeding risk and preserved the efficacy.

High-Yield Core Evidence
- **CURRENT-OASIS-7**
    - The CURRENT-OASIS-7 trial was a major clinical trial evaluating the use of different clopidogrel dosing strategies in patients with acute coronary syndrome undergoing an invasive strategy (i.e., PCI).
    - Patients were randomized to either double-dose clopidogrel (LD: 600-mg loading x 1, then 150 mg daily x6 days, 75 mg daily after that) or standard-dose clopidogrel (300-mg, then 75 mg daily) and either aspirin 300 to 325 mg daily or aspirin 75 to 100 mg daily.
    - The primary outcome (cardiovascular death, myocardial infarction, or stroke at 30 days) did not differ between the high versus standard clopidogrel dose or the higher dose of aspirin.
    - However, more patients in the high-dose clopidogrel group suffered major bleeding.
    - The authors concluded no significant difference between a double-dose clopidogrel regimen and the standard-dose regimen in patients with ACS undergoing an invasive strategy, or between higher-dose aspirin and lower-dose aspirin, concerning the primary outcome of cardiovascular death, myocardial infarction, or stroke. (N Engl J Med. 2010 Sep 2;363(10):930-42.)
- **CHAMPION PHOENIX**
    - Cangrelor's role as an adjunct to PCI was assessed in a double-blind, placebo-controlled trial that randomized patients undergoing either urgent or elective PCI to receive cangrelor or a loading dose of clopidogrel (300mg or 600mg).
    - The primary endpoint (composite of death, myocardial infarction, ischemia-driven revascularization, or stent thrombosis at 48 hours after randomization) occurred significantly less often in the cangrelor group than in the clopidogrel group, and no difference in the safety endpoints.
    - The authors concluded that cangrelor significantly reduced the rate of ischemic events, including stent thrombosis, with no significant increase in severe bleeding during PCI. (N Engl J Med. 2013 Apr 4;368(14):1303-13.)
- **TRITON-TIMI 38**
    - The TRITON-TIMI 38 trial compared prasugrel with clopidogrel in patients with acute coronary syndromes with planned PCI.
    - Prasugrel was associated with a significant reduction in the primary efficacy endpoint (death from cardiovascular causes, nonfatal myocardial infarction, or nonfatal stroke) compared to clopidogrel and a significant improvement in the incidence of MI urgent-revascularization and stent thrombosis.
    - However, there was no difference in mortality and a significantly higher incidence of major bleeding, life-threatening bleeding, and nonfatal bleeding in patients receiving prasugrel.
    - The authors concluded that in patients with ACS undergoing PCI, prasugrel therapy was associated with significantly reduced rates of ischemic events, including stent thrombosis, but with an increased risk of major bleeding, including fatal bleeding. (N Engl J Med. 2007 Nov 15;357(20):2001-15.)
- **PLATO**
    - The PLATO compared was a multicenter, double-blind, randomized trial that compared ticagrelor to clopidogrel in patients with the acute coronary syndrome, with or without ST-segment elevation.
    - Ticagrelor use was associated with a significantly lower incidence of the primary composite endpoint (death from vascular causes, myocardial infarction, or stroke) than patients receiving clopidogrel.
    - Ticagrelor also reduced the risk of all-cause mortality and death from vascular causes. There was no significant difference in major bleeding, but ticagrelor was associated with a higher rate of major bleeding not related to coronary-artery bypass grafting.
    - The authors concluded that in patients with ACS, ticagrelor significantly reduced the rate of death from vascular causes, myocardial infarction, or stroke without an increase in the overall major bleeding rate but with an increase in the rate of non-procedure-related bleeding. (N Engl J Med. 2009 Sep 10;361(11):1045-57.)

Cardiology

High-Yield Fast-Facts
- **Crushed or Not Crushed**
  - In patients with an acute STEMI who undergo PCI, if they are intubated, each oral agent (clopidogrel, prasugrel, and ticagrelor) may be crushed and administered via a nasogastric or orogastric tube.
- **Ticlopidine Removed from Market**
  - Ticlopidine is a thienopyridine antiplatelet agent but is no longer available in the United States due to the increased risk of neutropenia/agranulocytosis, thrombotic thrombocytopenic purpura, and aplastic anemia.
- **Clopidogrel and TTP**
  - Although ticlopidine was removed from the market, clopidogrel also carries a risk, albeit much lower, of thrombotic thrombocytopenic purpura.

HIGH-YIELD BOARD EXAM ESSENTIALS
- **CLASSIC AGENTS:** Cangrelor, clopidogrel, prasugrel, ticagrelor
- **DRUG CLASS:** P2Y12 inhibitors
- **INDICATIONS:** Acute coronary syndrome, primary and secondary prevention of MI, stroke, or PAD
- **MECHANISM:** Irreversible (clopidogrel, prasugrel) or reversible (cangrelor, and ticagrelor) inhibitor of platelet P2Y12 receptor, preventing ADP from binding and activating the glycoprotein GPIIb/IIIa complex, thereby inhibiting platelet aggregation.
- **SIDE EFFECTS:** Bleeding, bradycardia (ticagrelor)
- **CLINICAL PEARLS:**
  - The reversible inhibitors of P2Y12 are reversible in the sense that they disassociate from their binding site, which permits restoration of normal platelet aggregation.
  - Traditionally, clopidogrel and prasugrel are considered to be irreversible inhibitors of platelet activation.
  - Cangrelor is a parenterally administered option for those going to the cath lab.

Table: Drug Class Summary

Thienopyridines - Drug Class Review
High-Yield Med Reviews

Mechanism of Action:
Irreversible (clopidogrel, prasugrel) or reversible (cangrelor, and ticagrelor) inhibitor of platelet P2Y12 receptor, preventing ADP from binding and activating the glycoprotein GPIIb/IIIa complex, thereby inhibiting platelet aggregation

Class Effects: *First-line antiplatelet agents for patients post-myocardial infarction, stroke, or peripheral arterial disease.*

Generic Name	Brand Name	Main Indication(s) or Uses	Notes
Cangrelor	Kengreal	- Adjunct to PCI	- **Dosing (Adult):** – IV: bolus 30 mcg/kg before PCI, 4 mcg/kg/minute for at least 2 hours or for the duration of the PCI. - **Dosing (Peds):** Not used - **CYP450 Interactions:** None - **Renal or Hepatic Dose Adjustments:** None - **Dosage Forms:** IV solution

Clopidogrel	Plavix	- Acute coronary syndrome
		- Secondary prevention of MI, stroke, or PAD
			- **Dosing (Adult):**
			   – Oral: LD 300 to 600 mg, then 75 mg daily
			- **Dosing (Peds):**
			   – Oral: 0.2 to 1 mg/kg once daily
			- **CYP450 Interactions:** Inhibits CYP2B6, CYP2C8, a substrate of CYP3A4, and CYP2C19
			- **Renal or Hepatic Dose Adjustments:** None
			- **Dosage Forms:** Oral (tablet)

Prasugrel	Effient	- Acute coronary syndrome	- **Dosing (Adult):**
			   – Oral: LD 60 mg before PCI, followed by 5 to 10 mg daily
			      – Over 60 kg, 10 mg once daily
			      – < 60 kg, 5 mg once daily
			- **Dosing (Peds):** Not used
			- **CYP450 Interactions:** Substrate of CYP2B6, CYP3A4
			- **Renal or Hepatic Dose Adjustments:** None
			- **Dosage Forms:** Oral (tablet)

Ticagrelor	Brilinta	- Acute coronary syndrome - CAD primary prevention	- **Dosing (Adult):** – Oral: LD 180 mg once, followed by 90 mg BID for 12 months. After 12 months, reduce dose to 60 mg BID. - **Dosing (Peds):** Not used - **CYP450 Interactions:** Substrate of CYP3A4 - **Renal or Hepatic Dose Adjustments:** None - **Dosage Forms:** Oral (tablet)
Ticlopidine	Ticlid (Not available in the USA)	- Stroke primary and secondary prevention	- **Dosing (Adult):** Oral: 250 mg twice daily - **Dosing (Peds):** Not used - **CYP450 Interactions:** Substrate of CYP3A4, CYP1A2, CYP2B6, CYP2C19, CYP2D6 - **Renal or Hepatic Dose Adjustments:** None - **Dosage Forms:** Oral (tablet)

CARDIOVASCULAR – DIRECT THROMBIN INHIBITORS

Drug Class
- **Acute Care**
  - Argatroban
  - Bivalirudin
- **Chronic Care**
  - Dabigatran

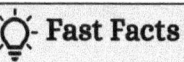

Fast Facts
- ✓ Dabigatran is the only oral dosage formulation option of the DTI's whereas the other options are all given parenterally.
- ✓ Dabigatran is also a pro-drug and must be functionally activated.
- ✓ Dabigatran is reversed by idarucizumab.

Main Indications or Uses
- **Acute Care:**
  - Heparin-induced thrombocytopenia (HIT)
  - STEMI/Percutaneous coronary intervention
- **Chronic Care:**
  - Deep venous thrombosis and pulmonary embolism treatment and prophylaxis
  - Nonvalvular atrial fibrillation
  - Venous thromboembolism prophylaxis in total hip arthroplasty

Mechanism of Action
- Direct thrombin inhibitors (DTI), as their name suggests, inhibit thrombin (factor II) by directly binding to its active site.
  - In other words, unlike heparin, these agents do not require antithrombin (AT) to exert this action.

Primary Net Benefit
- DTIs play an essential role in managing thromboembolic disease states where heparin or other anticoagulants cannot be used or preferred in some circumstances.
- Main Labs to Monitor:
  - CBC (trending of Hgb/HCT for bleeding)
  - INR/PT, PTT, ACT

High-Yield Basic Pharmacology
- **Thrombin Binding Sites**
  - DTIs bind to one or two binding sites on thrombin, relevant to DTIs as there are two subcategories.
  - The bivalent DTI (bivalirudin) binds to the thrombin's active site and at the substrate recognition site.
  - Conversely, the monovalent DTIs (argatroban and dabigatran) are smaller molecules and bind exclusively to the thrombin's active site.
- **Clot-Bound Thrombin**
  - DTIs can penetrate clots and inhibit clot-bound thrombin because of the drugs' small size, which is an advantage of restricting further thrombus formation compared to heparins.

High-Yield Clinical Knowledge
- **DTI for HIT With Renal Impairment**
  - In patients with heparin-induced thrombocytopenia, there is a delicate balance between ongoing antithrombotic therapy and hemorrhage risk.
  - Therefore, careful selection of the appropriate DTI or fondaparinux is essential.
  - Argatroban is preferred for renal insufficiency, although bivalirudin can be used if an appropriate dosage adjustment is considered.
- **Argatroban Conversion to Warfarin**
  - Argatroban prolongs the INR. Therefore, when transitioning to warfarin, bridging requires considering the argatroban dose and a longer INR than typically encountered in practice.
    - For patients on argatroban at more than 2 mcg/kg/minute, argatroban should be lowered to 2 mcg/kg/minute with a repeated measure INR 4 to 6 hours after the dose.

- For patients on argatroban at 2 mcg/kg/minute or less, it can be stopped when the INR is greater than 4 on combined warfarin and argatroban therapy. If argatroban is stopped, remeasure the INR 4 to 6 hours after, and restart argatroban if the INR is below 2.
- **Dabigatran Dyspepsia**
  - Many patients who begin dabigatran therapy cannot tolerate the associated dyspepsia and require conversion to an alternative antithrombotic strategy. If patients experience dyspepsia, suggest taking it with meals, but remind patients that the capsules cannot be opened. Other interventions such as PPIs, H2RA, or antacids may play a role but require consideration for drug-drug or drug-disease interactions.
- **STEMI DTI Strategy**
  - Only bivalirudin currently has a role in the management of STEMI.
  - Depending on clinical practice, either a GPIIb/IIIa receptor antagonist plus anticoagulation (heparin or LMWH) or bivalirudin alone are acceptable strategies for adjuncts to primary PCI.
  - However, while head-to-head clinical trials have suggested these strategies are interchangeable in preventing secondary major cardiac events, there is significantly less bleeding observed in patients receiving bivalirudin.
- **Therapeutic Monitoring**
  - While either argatroban or bivalirudin can be therapeutically monitored using the aPTT, dabigatran does not reliably prolong this test and should not be used clinically for this purpose.
  - For dabigatran, less commonly available coagulation assays, including the dilute thrombin time (dTT), thrombin time (TT), and the ecarin clotting time (ECT), are hypothetically more accurate reflections of the anticoagulation effect.
  - However, these tests are neither commonly available nor are they FDA approved.
- **Prodrug**
  - Dabigatran etexilate is a prodrug that is converted by serum esterase to active dabigatran.
  - Similar to other DOACs, peak concentrations occur 2 hours after an appropriate therapeutic dose.
  - But despite being 85% eliminated renally (85%), dose adjustments are not generally recommended except for patients receiving dabigatran for non-valvular atrial fibrillation and a CrCl less between 15 - 30 mL/minute.

High-Yield Core Evidence
- **HORIZONS-AMI**
  - The HORIZONS AMI was a landmark clinical trial that randomized patients to either bivalirudin or heparin plus glycoprotein IIb/IIIa inhibitors in patients with UA or NSTEMI undergoing primary PCI.
  - Patients receiving bivalirudin-based therapy had a significantly lower incidence in 30-day net adverse clinical events, a lower rate of significant bleeding, but a higher rate of acute stent thrombosis within 24 hours.
  - But since bivalirudin was still superior to heparin plus glycoprotein IIb/IIIa inhibitors in terms of the secondary efficacy outcomes of 30-day cardiac and all-cause mortality, the authors concluded that anticoagulation with bivalirudin alone, as compared with heparin plus glycoprotein IIb/IIIa inhibitors, results in significantly reduced 30-day rates of major bleeding and net adverse clinical events. (N Engl J Med. 2008 May 22;358(21):2218-30.)
- **ISAR-REACT 3**
  - The ISAR-REACT 3 trial was a randomized, double-blinded trial that evaluated patients with stable or unstable angina undergoing PCI to either bivalirudin or unfractionated heparin after pretreatment with clopidogrel.
  - There was no difference between groups regarding the primary outcome of the composite of death, myocardial infarction, urgent target-vessel revascularization due to myocardial ischemia within 30 days after randomization, or major bleeding during the index hospitalization.
  - However, there was a significantly lower incidence of major bleeding with bivalirudin.
  - The authors concluded that although there was no net clinical benefit in patients receiving bivalirudin, they did have less major bleeding, thus making bivalirudin the preferred agent in this patient population. (N Engl J Med. 2008 Aug 14;359(7):688-96.)

- **RELY**
  - The RELY trial was a noninferiority trial that randomized with atrial fibrillation and a stroke risk to receive blinded fashion dabigatran (110 mg or 150 mg twice daily) or unblinded warfarin adjusted to target INR.
  - Dabigatran at a dose of 110 mg compared to warfarin demonstrated noninferiority to warfarin regarding the primary outcome of stroke or systemic embolism.
  - However, the patients who received dabigatran 150 mg twice daily met the criteria for superiority compared to warfarin and had a significantly lower incidence of hemorrhagic stroke. Still, the incidence of major bleeding was similar.
  - The authors concluded that dabigatran 150 mg twice daily was associated with a lower incidence of stroke and systemic embolism with similar major bleeding rates to warfarin. (N Engl J Med. 2009 Sep 17;361(12):1139-51.)

High-Yield Fast-Facts
- Although no longer used in the USA, hirudin, and lepirudin were derived from the saliva of leeches (Hirudo medicinalis). Leeches have been used medicinally for hundreds of years to prevent thrombosis in the fine vessels of reattached digits. Hirudin was derived directly from leech saliva, whereas lepirudin was a recombinant form.
- Patients on in-hospital left ventricular assist devices (LVAD) who have or are suspected of having HIT may receive argatroban or bivalirudin as a substitute. While systemic DTI may be reasonable, the heparin in the LVAD purge solution can be replaced with argatroban to limit heparin exposure in these patients.
- DTIs are also used as primary antithrombotics during extracorporeal membrane oxygenation (ECMO). However, there is a lack of evidence to support the use of DTIs compared to heparin in the setting of ECMO.
- Dabigatran is the only DTI with a specific reversal agent, idarucizumab (Praxbind).

HIGH-YIELD BOARD EXAM ESSENTIALS
- **CLASSIC AGENTS:** Argatroban, bivalirudin, dabigatran
- **DRUG CLASS:** Direct thrombin inhibitors
- **INDICATIONS:** HIT, STEMI, DVT/PE, Afib
- **MECHANISM:** Inhibit thrombin by directly binding to its active site. In other words, these agents do not require antithrombin to exert this action.
- **SIDE EFFECTS:** Hemorrhage, dyspepsia (dabigatran)
- **CLINICAL PEARLS:**
  - Dabigatran is the only oral DTI and is used for the prevention of cardioembolic stroke on-valvular atrial fibrillation. It can be reversed with idarucizumab.
  - Argatroban and bivalirudin are commonly the drugs of choice for HIT on board exams.
  - Argatroban prolongs the INR. Therefore, when transitioning to warfarin, bridging requires consideration of both the dose of argatroban and a longer INR than typically encountered in practice.

Table: Drug Class Summary

Direct Thrombin Inhibitors - Drug Class Review High-Yield Med Reviews			
Mechanism of Action: Direct thrombin inhibitors (DTI), as their name suggests, inhibit thrombin by directly binding to its active site. In other words, these agents do not require antithrombin to exert this action.			
Class Effects: Decreased thrombin generation and increased risk of bleeding.			
Generic Name	**Brand Name**	**Main Indication(s) or Uses**	**Notes**
Argatroban	Acova	<ul><li>Heparin-induced thrombocytopenia (HIT)</li><li>Percutaneous coronary intervention</li></ul>	<ul><li>**Dosing (Adult):**<ul><li>STEMI: Initial dose of 2 mcg/kg/minute IV infusion then adjusted until the steady-state aPTT is 1.5 to 3 times</li><li>HIT: IV infusion of 0.1 to 1.5 mcg/kg/minute</li></ul></li><li>**Dosing (Peds):**<ul><li>HIT: IV infusion initial rate of 0.75 mcg/kg/minute</li></ul></li><li>**CYP450 Interactions:** No CYP interactions</li><li>**Renal or Hepatic Dose Adjustments:**<ul><li>Child-Pugh B or C - start continuous IV infusion at 0.5 mcg/kg/minute and adjust to target aPTT.</li></ul></li><li>**Dosage Forms:** IV solution</li></ul>
Bivalirudin	Angiomax	<ul><li>Percutaneous coronary intervention</li></ul>	<ul><li>**Dosing (Adult):**<ul><li>During PCI: IV 0.75 mg/kg bolus immediately before the procedure, then 1.75 mg/kg/hour for the remainder of the procedure adjusted to ACT target.<ul><li>Can continue at 1.75 mg/kg/hour for up to 4 hours post-procedure.</li></ul></li><li>Prior to PCI: 0.1 mg/kg bolus, then 0.25 mg/kg/hour continued until PCI.</li></ul></li><li>**CYP450 Interactions:** None</li><li>**Renal or Hepatic Dose Adjustments:**<ul><li>PCI: CrCl < 30 mL/minute, no bolus adjustment, but start infusion at 1 mg/kg/hour. If on hemodialysis, the initial rate should be 0.25 mg/kg/hour.</li><li>PCI: CrCl < 30 mL/min or on HD initial infusion rate of 0.04 to 0.07 mg/kg/hour.</li></ul></li><li>**Dosage Forms:** IV solution</li></ul>

| Direct Thrombin Inhibitors - Drug Class Review ||||
| High-Yield Med Reviews ||||
Generic Name	Brand Name	Main Indication(s) or Uses	Notes
Dabigatran	Pradaxa	<ul><li>Deep venous thrombosis and pulmonary embolism treatment and prophylaxis</li><li>Nonvalvular atrial fibrillation</li><li>Venous thromboembolism prophylaxis in total hip arthroplasty</li></ul>	<ul><li>**Dosing (Adult):**<ul><li>Oral: 150 mg twice daily</li></ul></li><li>**Dosing (Peds):**<ul><li>Dosage forms not interchangeable mg:mg</li><li>Oral pellets: base on weight AND age (3 months – 12 years)</li><li>Capsules: base on weight AND age (8 – 12 years)</li></ul></li><li>**CYP450 Interactions:**<ul><li>None, P-glycoprotein substrate</li></ul></li><li>**Renal or Hepatic Dose Adjustments:**<ul><li>CrCl between 30 and 50 mL/minute AND receiving concomitant dronedarone or ketoconazole, 75 mg twice daily.</li><li>CrCl between 15 and 30 mL/min adjust to 75 mg twice daily. CrCl less than 15 mL/min do not use.</li><li>Pediatrics: avoid eGFR < 50 mL/min/1.73m^2</li></ul></li><li>**Dosage Forms:** Oral (capsule)</li></ul>

CARDIOVASCULAR – FACTOR Xa INHIBITORS - ORAL

Drug Class
- Oral Factor Xa Inhibitors, or Direct Oral Anticoagulants (DOACs)
- Agents:
    - Apixaban
    - Edoxaban
    - Rivaroxaban

> **Fast Facts**
> ✓ These anticoagulants can be reversed by andexanet alfa and aPCC.
> ✓ Unlike heparin or fondaparinux, none of these agents require antithrombin to work.

Main Indications or Uses
- Acute/Chronic Care:
    - Venous Thromboembolism (deep vein thrombosis, DVT or pulmonary embolism, PE)
        - Treatment and prophylaxis
    - Nonvalvular Atrial Fibrillation (AF)

Mechanism of Action
- Oral FXa inhibitors prevent the conversion of prothrombin to thrombin by direct, selective, and reversible inhibition of free and clot-bound FXa.
    - FXa is part of the prothrombinase complex that catalyzes the conversion of prothrombin to thrombin.
    - Thrombin promotes platelet activation and fibrin clot formation; therefore, preventing the conversion of prothrombin to thrombin affects both.

Primary Net Benefit
- Oral Factor Xa inhibitors have antithrombotic therapeutic benefits as good as warfarin (rivaroxaban) and superior to warfarin (apixaban) with less routine monitoring and drug interactions.
- Main Labs to Monitor:
    - Prior to initiation
        - CBC
        - Serum creatinine (SCr)
        - Liver function tests (albumin, total protein, bili, aPTT, and PT)
        - Liver enzyme tests (AST, ALT, AlkPhos)

High-Yield Basic Pharmacology
- Basic Pharmacokinetics:
    - Peak plasma levels of apixaban and rivaroxaban are achieved within 2 hours, which is comparable to the initiation of parenteral heparin.
        - This rapid and reliable onset of action permits patients to be discharged from emergency departments on apixaban or rivaroxaban for the treatment of VTE to follow up in an outpatient setting.
    - FXa half-lives are shorter than warfarin (average 40 hours); therefore, their therapeutic effects will decrease faster, which increases the risk of stroke or VTE.
        - Rivaroxaban: 5-9 hours
        - Apixaban and edoxaban: approximately 12 hours
    - Administer rivaroxaban 15-20 mg with food to increase bioavailability.
- Drug Interactions
    - Apixaban: Avoid with strong CYP3A4 inducers
    - Rivaroxaban: Avoid with strong CYP3A4 and P-glycoprotein inducers and inhibitors
    - The most significant drug interactions include those including CYP3A4 and P-glycoprotein involvement.
- Renal Function Considerations
    - Edoxaban
        - CrCl > 95 mL/min or < 15 mL/min: Avoid
    - Rivaroxaban for AF:

- CrCl 15-50 mL/min: 15 mg daily
- CrCl < 15 mL/min: Avoid
- Rivaroxaban for VTE
  - CrCl < 30 mL/min: Avoid
- **Hepatic Function Considerations**
  - Apixaban: Avoid with Child-Pugh Class C
  - Rivaroxaban or edoxaban: Avoid with Child-Pugh Class B or C

> **Knowledge Integration**
> ✓ While these agents are increasing in their clinical use in some special populations their preference is limited until more evidence emerges. For example, LMWHs are preferred in oncology patients with VTE.

High-Yield Clinical Knowledge

- **Apixaban Dose Adjustments**
  - Patients receiving apixaban for nonvalvular AF should receive a reduced dose of 2.5 mg twice daily if they have at least two of the following:
    - Age 80 years or older, Wt 60 kg or less, or SCr 1.5 mg/dL or higher.
  - Current prescribing information does not provide support for using apixaban in patients on hemodialysis.
    - Emerging data exists to suggest its use in this population is at least as effective and safe compared to warfarin.
      - An observational study supported the use of apixaban by demonstrating a reduced incidence of stroke but had a relatively high rate of major and intracerebral bleeding as well as drug discontinuation (Circulation. 2018; 138:1519–1529).
- **Reversal of Oral Factor Xa Inhibitors**
  - Prothrombin complex concentrate (PCC) can be used to reverse the antithrombotic effects of FXa inhibitors in patients with acute major hemorrhage, those who require emergent surgical intervention, and/or have supratherapeutic INRs.
    - Kcentra (PCC) dosing utilizes a low fixed-dose regimen, which reduces thrombosis risk.
  - Andexanet alfa
    - Directly binds and sequesters apixaban and rivaroxaban, halting their antithrombotic actions, in addition to inhibition of tissue factor pathway inhibitors.
    - Edoxaban can be utilized off-label.
- **Obesity and Oral FXa Inhibitors**
  - Patients who weigh more than 120 kg have not been adequately prospectively studied to develop strong recommendations regarding the use of oral FXa inhibitors.
    - Subgroup analyses of ARISTOTLE, ROCKET-AF, and EINSTEIN have suggested apixaban and rivaroxaban maintain clinical efficacy and safety compared to warfarin in patients up to 150 kg.
      - Properly calibrated anti-Xa monitoring can help guide oral FXa inhibitor therapy in obese patients.
- **Edoxaban Special Considerations**
  - Unlike the other available oral FXa inhibitors and warfarin, the use of edoxaban for VTE and AF is limited to specific populations.
    - VTE treatment with edoxaban is permitted after 5-10 days of initial therapy with a parenteral anticoagulant.
    - For edoxaban use in patients with nonvalvular AF, patients must have a CrCl ≤ 95 mL/min.
- **Pediatric Use**
  - Rivaroxaban may be used in infants (after oral feeding for 10 days) through 12 years for thromboprophylaxis after the Fontan procedure for congenital heart disease, VTE, and risk reduction of recurrent VTE.
- **Mechanical Valves**
  - Avoid oral FXa inhibitors for patients with mechanical valves.
- **Monitoring Considerations**
  - Reduced clinical monitoring is mostly an advantage of oral FXa inhibitors over warfarin; however, when patient-specific factors contribute to increased concentrations (i.e., renal or hepatic impairment), clinically relevant bleeding can occur and may be difficult to monitor.

High-Yield Core Evidence

- **AMPLIFY**
  - This was a randomized, double-blind study comparing apixaban with the combination of subcutaneous enoxaparin followed by warfarin for acute venous thromboembolism.
  - There was no difference in the primary efficacy outcome (recurrent symptomatic venous thromboembolism or death related to venous thromboembolism) between the apixaban group and the conventional-therapy group.
  - Fewer patients on apixaban experienced the composite safety endpoint (major bleeding and clinically relevant nonmajor bleeding) and major bleeding (treated as an independent outcome) when compared with conventional therapy.
  - The authors concluded that a fixed-dose regimen of apixaban alone was non-inferior to conventional therapy for the treatment of acute venous thromboembolism and was associated with significantly less bleeding. (NEJM 2013 Aug 29;369(9):799-808.)
- **ROCKET-AF**
  - ROCKET-AF was a landmark, multicenter, prospective, randomized, double-blind trial of patients with nonvalvular AF that compared the effect of rivaroxaban or warfarin in preventing the primary endpoint of stroke or systemic embolism.
  - At a mean follow-up of 2 years, rivaroxaban was non-inferior to warfarin for the composite endpoint of stroke or systemic embolism without increasing bleeding rates.
  - In the ITT analysis, rivaroxaban maintained a non-inferior effect but did not meet statistical significance for superiority.
  - There was no difference in the incidence of major and nonmajor clinically relevant bleeding between the rivaroxaban and warfarin groups.
  - The authors concluded that in patients with AF, rivaroxaban was non-inferior to warfarin for the prevention of stroke or systemic embolism. (NEJM 2011 Sep 8;365(10):883-91.)
- **ARISTOTLE**
  - This was a landmark multicenter, double-blind, randomized trial that compared apixaban to warfarin in patients with AF and at least one additional risk factor for stroke with a primary outcome of ischemic or hemorrhagic stroke or systemic embolism.
  - Patients receiving apixaban had a significantly lower incidence of ischemic or hemorrhagic stroke compared to the warfarin group and met both pre-defined criteria for noninferiority and superiority.
  - Significantly fewer patients who received apixaban experienced major bleeding and death from any cause compared with patients receiving warfarin.
  - The authors concluded that apixaban was superior to warfarin in patients with AF for preventing stroke or systemic embolism, caused less bleeding, and resulted in lower mortality. (NEJM 2011 Sep 15;365(11):981-92.)
- **ENGAGE AF-TIMI**
  - This was a randomized, double-blind, double-dummy trial comparing two once-daily regimens of edoxaban with warfarin in patients with moderate-to-high-risk AF.
  - Edoxaban 30 mg was shown to be noninferior to warfarin regarding the primary endpoint (stroke or systemic embolism), and edoxaban 60 mg was shown to be superior to warfarin.
  - Major bleeding was more frequent with warfarin compared with both doses of edoxaban.
  - The authors concluded that both once-daily regimens of edoxaban were noninferior to warfarin with respect to the prevention of stroke or systemic embolism and were associated with significantly lower rates of bleeding and death from cardiovascular causes. (NEJM 2013 Nov 28;369(22):2093-104.)

High-Yield Fast-Facts

- **Risk Scoring System for AF**
  - The CHA_2DS_2-VASc risk scoring system has been recommended for stroke risk stratification in patients with AF to assist in determining anticoagulation needs.

- **TEG The New(ish) Coagulation Test**
  - Thromboelastography (TEG) is a novel method to acutely determine coagulopathy in the acute care setting. This test is primarily used when hemorrhage is observed or suspected, not for therapeutic monitoring.
- **Antithrombin**
  - Unlike fondaparinux, these agents are all oral and do not require the presence of antithrombin to work.

HIGH-YIELD BOARD EXAM ESSENTIALS
- **CLASSIC AGENTS:** Apixaban, edoxaban, rivaroxaban
- **DRUG CLASS:** Oral FXa inhibitors
- **INDICATIONS:** Nonvalvular AF, VTE (treatment and prophylaxis)
- **MECHANISM:** Prevent the conversion of prothrombin to thrombin by direct, selective, and reversible inhibition of free and clot bound FXa.
- **SIDE EFFECTS:** Bleeding
- **CLINICAL PEARLS:**
  - Oral FXa inhibitors have shorter onset than warfarin, which allows earlier discharge depending on the drug and indication. Oral FXa inhibitor half-lives are also shorter, which can result in decreased efficacy more quickly than with warfarin.
  - Edoxaban should not be used in patients that have either normal renal function (CrCl above 95 mL/min) or severely impaired renal function (CrCl less than 15 mL/min).
  - Andexanet alfa can reverse these agents.

Table: Drug Class Summary

Oral Factor Xa Inhibitors - Drug Class Review High-Yield Med Reviews			
Mechanism of Action: *Oral FXa Inhibitors (apixaban, edoxaban, rivaroxaban) – direct, reversible, and selective FXa inhibition, preventing the conversion of prothrombin to thrombin.*			
Class Effects: *Increases clotting time, decreasing the risk of thrombosis. Associated with drug interactions via P-gp & CYP3A4. Also require renal dose adjustments.*			
Generic Name	**Brand Name**	**Main Indication(s) or Uses**	**Notes**

Apixaban	Eliquis	- Atrial fibrillation
		- Treatment of VTE
			- **Dosing (Adult):**
			   – AF: 5 mg twice daily
			   – DVT/PE - 10 mg twice daily for 7 days, then 5 mg twice daily
			- **Dosing (Peds):** No specific recommendations
			- **CYP450 Interactions:** Substrate of CYP1A2, CYP2C19, CYP2C8, CYP2C9, CYP3A4, and P-gp
			- **Renal or Hepatic Dose Adjustments:**
			   – AF: Reduce to 2.5 mg twice daily if:
			   – Age 80 years or older
			   – Wt 60 kg or less
			   – SCr 1.5 mg/dL or higher
			   – Child-Pugh C - Not recommended
			- **Dosage Forms:** Oral (tablet)

Edoxaban	Savaysa	- Atrial fibrillation
		- Treatment of VTE
			- **Dosing (Adult):**
			   – AF: 60 mg daily
			   – DVT/PE
			      – Wt greater than 60 kg: 60 mg daily
			      – Wt 60 kg or less: 30 mg daily
			- **Dosing (Peds):** No specific recommendations
			- **CYP450 Interactions:** Substrate P-gp
			- **Renal or Hepatic Dose Adjustments:**
			   – CrCl > 95 mL/minute OR less than 15 mL/minute: not recommended
			   – CrCl 15 to 50 mL/minute: 30 mg daily
			   – Child-Pugh B or C: not recommended
			- **Dosage Forms:** Oral (tablet)

Rivaroxaban	Xarelto	- Atrial fibrillation
		- Treatment of VTE
			- **Dosing (Adult):**
			   – AF: 20 mg daily with food
			   – DVT/PE - 15 mg twice daily w/ food for 21 days followed by 20 mg daily w/ food
			- **Dosing (Peds):** Administer after oral feeding for at least 10 days.
			   – Dose and frequency based on weight
			- **CYP450 Interactions:** Substrate of CYP2J2, CYP3A4, P-gp
			- **Renal or Hepatic Dose Adjustments:**
			   – AF: 15 mg daily with food if CrCl between 15 to 50 mL/minute
			   – Avoid use if CrCl is < 15 mL/minute
			- **Dosage Forms:** Oral (tablet), suspension

CARDIOVASCULAR – HEPARIN AND LOW MOLECULAR WEIGHT HEPARINS

Drug Class
- Acute Care
  - Dalteparin
  - Enoxaparin
  - Fondaparinux
  - Heparin
- Chronic Care
  - Dalteparin
  - Enoxaparin
  - Fondaparinux

> **Fast Facts**
> - ✓ All of these agents require antithrombin to be present to exert their pharmacologic effect.
> - ✓ All are administered parenterally. There are no oral options.

Main Indications or Uses
- Acute Care:
  - ST-elevation acute coronary syndromes
  - Non-ST elevation acute coronary syndromes
  - Venous thromboembolism treatment
- Chronic Care:
  - Venous thromboembolism prophylaxis

> **Accelerate Your Knowledge**
> - ✓ While LMWH are most commonly given by subcutaneous (SC) administration, enoxaparin has FDA approved dosing in STEMI where patients can be given 30 mg IV push before the first SC dose.

Mechanism of Action
- Heparin and low molecular weight heparins (LMWH) have no intrinsic anticoagulant properties but activate antithrombin and enhance its ability to inactivate coagulation factors along the coagulation pathway through a confirmation change that improves its binding to factors II and Xa.

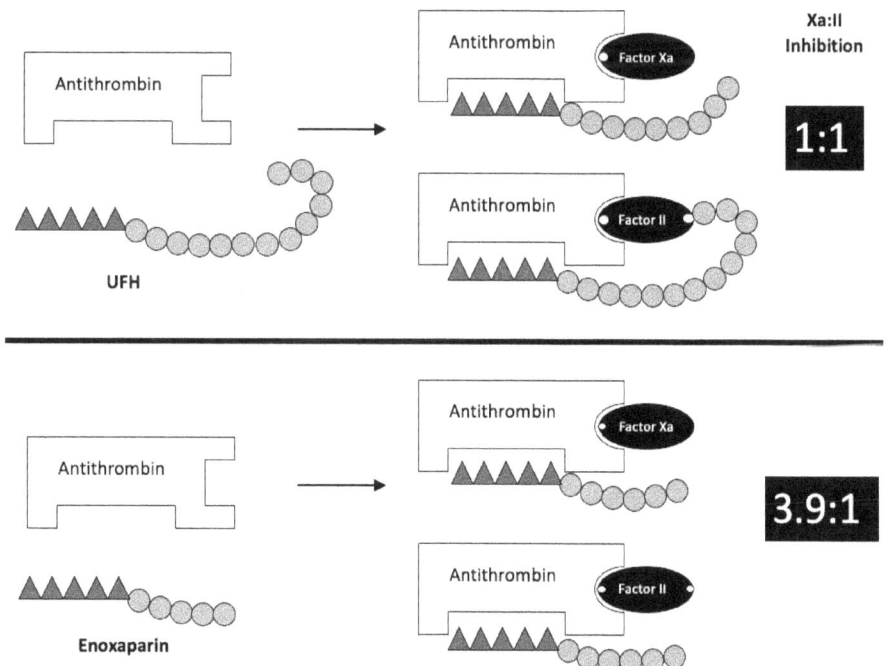

Primary Net Benefit
- Heparin, LMWH, and fondaparinux are used extensively for anticoagulant indications, and each possesses unique pharmacokinetics that can be used to help guide the selection of the appropriate therapy.

- Main Labs to Monitor:
  - CBC (to evaluate platelets due to risk of HIT and trends in Hgb/HCT due to risk of bleeding)
  - INR/PT, PTT, ACT

High-Yield Basic Pharmacology
- **Unfractionated vs. Fractionated**
  - As the name suggests, unfractionated heparin is a long polysaccharide chain with a therapeutically active pentasaccharide component.
  - The larger amount of sufficiently sized polysaccharide chains of heparin gives it a ratio of its anti-factor-Xa capacity to the anti-factor-IIa capacity of 1:1.
  - Conversely, the ratio anti-factor-Xa capacity to anti-factor-IIa for LMWHs is approximately 3 to 4:1.
  - With fondaparinux, it does not possess long pentasaccharide chains to bridge antithrombin to thrombin.
- **Bovine or Porcine**
  - Heparin is produced from cell lines of either bovine origin or porcine.
  - While the majority of the commercially available heparin HIT may be higher in individuals treated with UFH of bovine origin compared with porcine heparin and is lower in those treated exclusively with LMW heparin.
- **Indirect Anticoagulants**
  - These agents are considered "indirect" anticoagulants since they require antithrombin (also known as antithrombin III) to exert any anticoagulant activity. In patients with antithrombin deficiency, these agents would have an insufficient clinical response and warrant alternative therapy with a direct anticoagulant.

High-Yield Clinical Knowledge
- **Antithrombin**
  - Heparin, LWMH, and fondaparinux bind to antithrombin, creating a conformational change that exposes the active site more readily to target coagulation factors (in addition to other proteases).
  - Antithrombin bound to heparin, LWMH, and fondaparinux accelerates the factor Xa inhibition.
  - For factor IIa (thrombin) inhibition, only heparin and LMWHs (but not fondaparinux) with sufficient polysaccharide chains (ones longer than 18 saccharide units) to bridge both antithrombin and thrombin.
  - After antithrombin binds to either factor, the anticoagulant dissociates from the complex and catalyzes other antithrombin molecules.
- **Body Weight Dosing**
  - Weight-based doses of 1 mg/kg of enoxaparin subcutaneously every 12 hours have been reliably used in patients up to 150 kg.
  - In morbidly obese patients weighing more than 150 mg/kg, there is observational literature to guide dosing, but in general, dosing enoxaparin on actual body weight in morbidly obese patients over-exposes patients to enoxaparin and should be dosed on ideal or adjusted body weight and titrated to target anti-Xa level.
- **LMWH Bridge And Once-daily Dosing**
  - LMWH may be continued for a short period of outpatient as a form of the antithrombotic bridge for patients beginning warfarin therapy.
  - In some patients, a 1.5 mg/kg once daily dose may be an acceptable alternative with the hopes of increasing compliance.
  - However, this is limited to patients receiving up to 150 mg per day since that is the largest commercially available enoxaparin dosage form.
  - Furthermore, patients should be counseled on the safety sheath component on almost all enoxaparin syringes.
  - This can be activated by depressing the plunger until a spring-loaded sheath extends, locks, and covers the needle. These devices should still be disposed of in safety sharps containers.

- **Reversal Of Anticoagulation**
  - The anticoagulant effects of heparin, LMWH, and (potentially) fondaparinux may be reversed with protamine sulfate.
  - Protamine sulfate rapidly reverses heparin's anticoagulant effect by binding directly to heparin, thereby reversing its anticoagulant effect.
  - Protamine should be dosed as a function of the remaining therapeutic heparin, with an empiric dose of 1 mg of protamine for every 100 units of heparin remaining in the patient.
  - However, caution should be taken to estimate the remaining heparin (based on t1/2 of 1.5 hours) since excessive protamine sulfate can exert an anticoagulant effect.
  - It's also important to note that protamine only partially reverses the anticoagulant activity of LMWH and has no effect on that fondaparinux.
- **ACT vs. aPTT**
  - In patients undergoing percutaneous coronary intervention (PCI), or cardiac bypass, large doses of heparin are generally used to prevent early clotting.
  - However, the doses used in this scenario are often much higher than those used elsewhere clinically.
  - These doses are sufficiently high to prolong the aPTT.
  - Therefore, an alternative, less-sensitive coagulation test, the ACT, is utilized to monitor therapy in this situation.
- **Clotting Initiation**
  - Numerous elements can initiate the clotting process, but negatively charged phospholipids and particulate substances are essential factors.
    - The aPTT monitors heparin measured by adding particulate substances (commonly kaolin) to the blood sample, which activates factor XII.
    - The presence and concentration of heparin (and antithrombin) will impair activation of factor XII, thus prolonging the aPTT.
- **Pregnant Patients With VTE**
  - Pregnancy increases the risk of thromboembolic disease.
  - Should a pregnant patient be diagnosed with a VTE, the preferred outpatient therapy is an LMWH since warfarin is contraindicated and the DOAC agents have insufficient data (at this time).
- **HIT**
  - Platelet factor 4 (PF4) is a protein released during platelet activation and binds to heparin, preventing it from activating antithrombin.
  - In patients with heparin-induced thrombocytopenia, the PF4 assay can be used to identify these patients.

High-Yield Core Evidence
- **EXTRACT-TIMI 25**
  - The EXTRACT-TIMI 25 trial was a landmark randomized, blinded clinical trial of over twenty-thousand patients with STEMI who were scheduled to undergo fibrinolysis and were randomized to receive weight-based enoxaparin or weight-based unfractionated heparin for at least 48 hours in patients.
  - The primary efficacy endpoint was death or nonfatal recurrent myocardial infarction through 30 days was significantly lower in patients receiving enoxaparin therapy.
  - Enoxaparin therapy was also associated with favorable outcomes, including nonfatal reinfarction and the composite outcome of death, nonfatal reinfarction, or urgent revascularization. Furthermore, enoxaparin caused less major bleeding. (N Engl J Med. 2006 Apr 6;354(14):1477-88.)
- **ACUITY**
  - The ACUITY trial was another landmark trial that randomized patients with acute coronary syndromes to either unfractionated heparin (UH) or enoxaparin plus a glycoprotein IIb/IIIa inhibitor (GPIIb/IIIa), bivalirudin plus a GPIIb/IIIa, or bivalirudin alone.
  - In the two planned comparisons between patients receiving UH/enoxaparin plus GPIIb/IIIa compared to bivalirudin plus GPIIb/IIIa, and UH/enoxaparin plus GPIIb/IIIa compared to bivalirudin alone was noninferiority was met for the primary outcome of the composite endpoint of death, myocardial infarction, or unplanned revascularization for ischemia.

- However, patients receiving bivalirudin alone had less major bleeding than UH/enoxaparin plus GPIIb/IIIa compared to bivalirudin alone. (N Engl J Med. 2006 Nov 23;355(21):2203-16.)
- **MENDOX**
  - The MEDENOX trial established the role of enoxaparin for VTE prophylaxis in hospitalized patients.
  - The study investigators conducted a randomized, double-blind trial of hospitalized patients receiving enoxaparin at a dose of 40 mg once daily, 20 mg once daily, or placebo subcutaneously once daily for 6 to 14 days.
  - Patients receiving enoxaparin 40 mg had a significantly lower risk of in-hospital VTE compared to placebo, and there was no difference between patients who received enoxaparin 20 mg compared to placebo.
  - Furthermore, there were no significant adverse events, namely bleeding, in either treatment group compared to placebo. (N Engl J Med. 1999 Sep 9;341(11):793-800.)
- **ARTEMIS**
  - The ARTEMIS study examined the role of fondaparinux in hospitalized patients over 60 and at moderate to high risk of venous thromboembolism.
  - This study randomized hospitalized patients to either fondaparinux 2.5 subcutaneously daily or placebo and examined VTE incidence during hospitalization.
  - Patients randomized to fondaparinux had a significantly lower VTE incidence, translating to an absolute risk reduction of 46.7% and no significant difference in bleeding risk or mortality. (BMJ. 2006 Feb 11;332(7537):325-9.)

High-Yield Fast-Facts
- **Unit of Heparin**
  - One "unit" of heparin reflects the quantity of heparin that prevents the clotting of 1 mL of citrated sheep plasma 1 hour after calcium addition.

HIGH-YIELD BOARD EXAM ESSENTIALS
- **CLASSIC AGENTS:** Dalteparin, enoxaparin, fondaparinux, heparin
- **DRUG CLASS:** Heparin and LMWH
- **INDICATIONS:** Acute MI, DVT/PE treatment and prophylaxis
- **MECHANISM:** Activate antithrombin and enhance its ability to inactivate coagulation factors along the coagulation pathway.
- **SIDE EFFECTS:** Bleeding or hemorrhage, HIT
- **CLINICAL PEARLS:**
  - All agents require antithrombin to be present to provide anticoagulation. Thus, patients with AT deficiency may not receive a therapeutics effect.
  - Only unfractionated heparin can be monitored with aPTT or ACT.
  - The risk of HIT is greatest with heparin > LMWH > fondaparinux.
  - Heparin, LMWH, and (potentially) fondaparinux may be reversed with protamine sulfate, which rapidly reverses heparin's anticoagulant effect by binding directly to heparin, thereby reversing its anticoagulant effect.

Table: Drug Class Summary

Heparin and Low Molecular Weight Heparins - Drug Class Review High-Yield Med Reviews			
Mechanism of Action: *Indirect anticoagulants that activate antithrombin, which then exerts an antithrombotic effect by inhibiting coagulation factors.*			
Class Effects: *Heparin, LMWH, and fondaparinux are used extensively for anticoagulant indications, and each possesses unique pharmacokinetics that can help guide the selection of the appropriate therapy. Risk of HIT is greatest with heparin and then LMWH.*			
Generic Name	**Brand Name**	**Main Indication(s) or Uses**	**Notes**
Dalteparin	Fragmin	<ul><li>Non-ST elevation acute coronary syndromes</li><li>Venous thromboembolism prophylaxis</li><li>Venous thromboembolism treatment in patients with active cancer</li><li>Venous thromboembolism treatment in pediatric patients</li></ul>	<ul><li>**Dosing (Adult):**<ul><li>NSTEMI with non-invasive intervention: 120 units/kg sq every 12 hours for 5 to 8 days (maximum 10,000 units).</li><li>VTE prophylaxis: 5,000 units sq daily</li></ul></li><li>**Dosing (Peds):**<ul><li>VTE prophylaxis: <50 kg, 100 units/kg/dose sq q24h (target anti-Xa 0.2 to 0.4 units/mL) (maximum 5,000 units)</li><li>VTE treatment: Age under 2 years 150 units/kg/dose sq q12h.</li><li>2 years to 8 years, 125 units/kg/dose sq q12h.</li><li>8 years or older 100 units/kg/dose sq q12h.</li></ul></li><li>**CYP450 Interactions:** No CYP interactions</li><li>**Renal or Hepatic Dose Adjustments:**<ul><li>CrCl < 30 mL/minute is not recommended, although this is controversial.</li></ul></li><li>**Dosage Forms:** Subcutaneous solution</li></ul>
Enoxaparin	Lovenox	<ul><li>Acute coronary syndromes</li><li>Deep vein thrombosis treatment (acute)</li><li>Venous thromboembolism prophylaxis</li></ul>	<ul><li>**Dosing (Adult):**<ul><li>ACS or VTE treatment: 1 mg/kg SQ q12h.</li><li>STEMI with PCI: Younger than 75 years: IV bolus of 30 mg plus 1 mg/kg SQ q12h (maximum of 100 mg). No IV bolus for patients 75 years or older.</li><li>VTE prophylaxis: 40 mg SQ daily, or 30 mg SQ q12h.</li></ul></li><li>**Dosing (Peds):**<ul><li>VTE Prophylaxis: 1 to 2 months, 0.75 mg/kg/dose SQ q12h. Two months or older, 0.5 mg/kg/dose SQ q12h.</li><li>Therapeutic dosing: 1 to 2 months, 1.5 mg/kg/dose SQ q12h</li></ul></li><li>**CYP450 Interactions:** No CYP interactions</li><li>**Renal or Hepatic Dose Adjustments:**<ul><li>VTE prophylaxis- 30 mg SQ daily</li><li>ACS or VTE treatment: 1 mg/kg SQ daily</li></ul></li><li>**Dosage Forms:** Injection solution, subcutaneous solution</li></ul>

Heparin and Low Molecular Weight Heparins - Drug Class Review
High-Yield Med Reviews

Generic Name	Brand Name	Main Indication(s) or Uses	Notes
Fondaparinux	Arixtra	<ul><li>Deep vein thrombosis</li><li>Pulmonary embolism</li><li>Venous thromboembolism prophylaxis in surgical patients</li></ul>	<ul><li>**Dosing (Adult):**<ul><li>VTE treatment for patients < 50 kg: 5 mg SQ daily; patients between 50 to 100 kg: 7.5 mg SQ daily; > 100 kg: 10 mg SQ daily.</li><li>VTE prophylaxis: 2.5 mg SQ daily</li></ul></li><li>**Dosing (Peds):**<ul><li>VTE treatment: 0.1 mg/kg/dose SQ daily</li></ul></li><li>**CYP450 Interactions:** None</li><li>**Renal or Hepatic Dose Adjustments:**<ul><li>Contraindicated in patients with CrCl less than 30 mL/minute</li></ul></li><li>**Dosage Forms:** Subcutaneous solution</li></ul>
Heparin	N/A	<ul><li>Anticoagulation</li></ul>	<ul><li>**Dosing (Adult):**<ul><li>ACS: 60 units/kg IV bolus followed by 12 units/kg/hour IV infusion. If using a fibrinolytic strategy, the maximum bolus dose of 4000 units, and the maximum infusion rate of 1000 units/hour.</li><li>VTE treatment: 80 units/kg IV bolus followed by 18 units/kg/hour IV infusion.</li><li>VTE prophylaxis: 5000 units SQ q8h.</li></ul></li><li>**Dosing (Peds):**<ul><li>Systemic heparinization:<ul><li>Age 0 to 1 year: 75 units/kg IV bolus (over 10 minutes) followed by 28 units/kg/hour</li><li>Age over 1 year: 75 units/kg IV bolus (over 10 minutes) followed by 20 units/kg/hour</li></ul></li></ul></li><li>**CYP450 Interactions:** None</li><li>**Renal or Hepatic Dose Adjustments:**<ul><li>None, adjust doses to target aPTT or anti-Xa</li></ul></li><li>**Dosage Forms:** Injection solution</li></ul>

CARDIOVASCULAR – VITAMIN K ANTAGONIST

Drug Class
- **Vitamin K Antagonist**
- **Agent**
  - Warfarin

Main Indications or Uses
- **Acute/Chronic Care:**
  - Atrial fibrillation
  - Myocardial infarction, secondary prevention
  - Venous Thromboembolism (deep vein thrombosis, DVT; pulmonary embolism, PE)
    - Treatment and prophylaxis

> **Fast Facts**
> ✓ Warfarin has a delayed onset of action and thus requires bridge therapy when an active VTE is present.
> ✓ Warfarin is metabolized by both CYP2C9 and 3A4 and is associated with a high risk for drug interactions.

Mechanism of Action
- Warfarin
  - Warfarin inhibits the reduction of oxidized vitamin K to vitamin K hydroquinone, which prevents the carboxylation (activation) of the coagulation factors II, VII, IX, and X and proteins C and S.
    - Warfarin specifically prevents the reactivation of the clotting factors by inhibiting vitamin K epoxide reductase complex 1 (VKORC1).

Primary Net Benefit
- Warfarin is an anticoagulant with an extensive history of preventing thromboembolism (stroke and VTE) but higher risk of clinically relevant bleeding than oral Factor-Xa inhibitors.
- Main Labs to Monitor:
  - Before initiation
    - CBC
    - Serum creatinine (SCr)
    - Liver function tests (albumin, total protein, bilirubin, aPTT, and PT)
    - Liver enzyme tests (AST, ALT, Alk Phos)
    - May consider genotyping of CYP2C9 and VKORC1 before initiation of therapy.
  - After initiation
    - PT/INR at a patient-specific interval (once per week to every 12 weeks)

High-Yield Basic Pharmacology
- **Racemic Mixture**
  - Warfarin is a racemic mixture of R- and S-warfarin. S-warfarin is the more active component and is metabolized by CYP2C9.
    - R-warfarin is metabolized specifically by CYP1A2 and CYP3A4.
- **Pharmacokinetics**
  - Onset can be within 24-72 hours, but steady state is typically achieved in 5-7 days.
    - The delayed effect is because the existing stores of vitamin K must be depleted, and the active coagulation factors must be eliminated from circulation according to their half-lives.
      - Factor VII: 5 hours
      - Factor IX: 24 hours
      - Factor X: 48 hours
      - Factor II: 60 hours
      - Protein C/S: 7 hours
  - Warfarin's half-life is approximately 35 hours, causing continued drug activity days after discontinuation.
    - While the half-lives of the coagulation factors are often associated with the onset of therapy, the half-life of warfarin itself is also relevant to its duration of action.
  - Warfarin is extensively bound to plasma albumin (90%).

- Patients will be exposed to more active (free) drug with drug interactions that displace or compete with warfarin for albumin, or disease states causing hypoalbuminemia.
- **Drug Interactions**
    - Four drugs can result in major interactions with warfarin and increase the risk of bleeding (increase INR): amiodarone, trimethoprim/sulfamethoxazole, fluconazole, and metronidazole.
        - Others may include fluoroquinolones, doxycycline, steroids, or statins.
    - Rifampin may decrease warfarin's therapeutic effect (decrease INR).
    - Drugs that increase bleeding include aspirin, NSAIDs, antiplatelet agents, SSRIs, SNRIs, or fish oil.
- **Food Interactions**
    - Foods high in vitamin K can reduce the INR, including green, leafy vegetables.
    - Counsel patients to consistently eat high vitamin K-containing foods, not to avoid them.
- **Polymorphisms**
    - Patients with polymorphisms in CYP2C9 and/or in VKORC1 gene expression can have substantially different responses to warfarin.
    - In poor metabolizer CYP2C9 subtypes (increased risk of bleeding), there is no evidence suggesting measurable differences in clinically relevant bleeding or thromboembolic outcomes.
- **Clotting Factor Concentration**
    - A typical therapeutic INR of 2 to 3 for warfarin therapy requires vitamin K-dependent factor concentrations to decline to approximately 25% to 30% of normal values.
    - Elderly, Asian, and patients with decreased CrCl may demonstrate an increased response to warfarin.

High-Yield Clinical Knowledge
- **Dosing and Monitoring**
    - Warfarin therapy is adjusted to target INR, typically 2 to 3, but varies depending on the indication.
        - Atrial fibrillation and VTE: INR 2-3
        - Mechanical valves: INR 2.5-3.5
        - INR target may change if patients experience a thrombotic event at a therapeutic INR.
    - Make 5-25% dose adjustments (up or down) based on the average weekly dose.
    - Once target INR is achieved, the monitoring interval can increase (up to 12 weeks), with acute adjustments for surgical procedures, new or discontinued drugs, or changes in clinical status.
- **Vitamin K Reversal**
    - When vitamin K is required for warfarin reversal, the thrombotic risk increases.
        - The most cautious method to correct hemorrhaging should be considered in patients with a high thromboembolism risk. Use appropriately dosed vitamin K (phytonadione) to avoid INR overcorrection.
    - Asymptomatic INR elevations (i.e., no acute bleeding) can be managed by holding warfarin alone.
- **INR Ranges and Interventions**
    - INR 4.5-10 without bleeding
        - Hold warfarin or consider oral vitamin K 1-2.5 mg once
    - INRs > 10 without bleeding
        - Oral vitamin K 2.5 mg once
    - Serious bleeding at any INR
        - IV Vitamin K 5-10 mg IVPB over at least 30 minutes PLUS either fresh frozen plasma (FFP) or prothrombin complex concentrate
- **Vitamin K SQ vs IV vs PO**
    - Oral vitamin K is the preferred route of administration in patients without severe bleeding.
    - Subcutaneous vitamin K has a slower time of onset than IV administration.
    - Vitamin K IM should be avoided with elevated INR due to increased risk of bleeding and hematoma formation in the muscle.
- **Prothrombin Complex Concentrate**
    - As an alternative to FFP, prothrombin complex concentrates (PCC) can be used to rapidly replace factors II, VII, IX, and X.
        - There exist two different subtypes of PCC: four-factor PCC and activated PCC.

- Four-factor PCC (Kcentra) contains factors II, VII, IX, and X.
- Activated PCC (FEIBA) contains the same factors, but factor VII is activated (Factors II, VIIa, IX, and X).
- **Effect on Existing Thrombi**
  - At therapeutic INRs, warfarin may prevent existing thrombi from expanding but has no direct effect on previously circulating clotting factors or previously formed thrombi.
- **Warfarin and Pregnancy**
  - Warfarin is contraindicated in pregnancy since it can cross the placenta, causing hemorrhagic disorders in the fetus and interfering with fetal proteins in bone and blood, leading to abnormal bone formation.

High-Yield Core Evidence
- **Emergency Department (ED) Discharge of Pulmonary Embolism Patients**
  - A multicenter, open-label randomized trial in a low-risk PE population that compared discharging ED patients on either rivaroxaban or enoxaparin followed by warfarin to determine if there was a difference between these therapies in the hospital length of stay.
  - Treatment with rivaroxaban significantly improved the primary outcome of the total number of initial hospital hours, plus hours of hospitalization for bleeding or venous thromboembolism (VTE), x 30 days.
  - Patients receiving rivaroxaban had a significantly better 90-day composite safety endpoint of major bleeding, clinically relevant nonmajor bleeding, and mortality.
  - Low-risk ED PE patients receiving rivaroxaban on early discharge have similar outcomes to standard of care but fewer total hospital days and lower costs over 30 days. (Acad Emerg Med. 2018;25(9):995-1003.
- **European Atrial Fibrillation Trial (EAFT)**
  - A randomized trial compared open-label warfarin therapy or double-blinded treatment with aspirin or placebo in patients with non-rheumatic atrial fibrillation (NRAF) with a recent transient ischemic attack (TIA) or minor ischemic stroke.
  - Patients with contraindications to warfarin were randomized to receive aspirin or placebo.
  - Patients receiving warfarin had a significantly lower incidence of death from vascular disease, any stroke, myocardial infarction (MI), or systemic embolism compared to placebo.
  - However, there was no difference in the annual incidence of outcome events compared to placebo for patients receiving aspirin alone.
  - The incidence of major bleeding events was similar between warfarin and aspirin therapy.
  - Warfarin effectively reduces the risk of recurrent vascular events in NRAF patients with a recent TIA or minor ischemic stroke. (Lancet. 1993;342: 1255 –1262.)
- **ACTIVE W**
  - A randomized, open treatment, controlled trial comparing clopidogrel plus aspirin to warfarin to prevent vascular events in patients with atrial fibrillation (AF) plus one or more risk factors for stroke.
  - Trial was stopped early as warfarin was superior to clopidogrel plus aspirin in reducing the incidence of the primary outcome of the first occurrence of stroke, non-CNS systemic embolism, MI, or vascular death.
  - Patients receiving warfarin pre-enrollment and during the trial trended towards a greater reduction in vascular events and a significantly lower risk of major bleeding.
  - Oral warfarin therapy is superior to clopidogrel plus aspirin to prevent vascular events in patients with AF at high risk of stroke, especially in those already taking oral anticoagulation therapy. (Lancet. 2006 Jun 10;367(9526):1903-12.)
- **Bridging for Invasive Procedures**
  - A large, retrospective cohort study of warfarin with and without bridge therapy for patients undergoing invasive diagnostic or surgical procedures was conducted to describe the rates of clinically relevant bleeding and recurrent VTE among these patients.
  - There was significantly more clinically relevant bleeding within 30 days after the procedure in the patients receiving bridge therapy than patients who did not.
  - There was no significant difference in thirty-day clinically relevant bleeding, recurrent VTE, and all-cause mortality. No deaths occurred in either group.
  - Bridge therapy was associated with an increased risk of bleeding during warfarin therapy interruption for invasive procedures in patients receiving treatment for a history of VTE and is likely unnecessary for most of these patients. (JAMA Intern Med. 2015;175:1163–1168.)

High-Yield Fast-Facts
- **Interaction with Bactrim (Trimethoprim/Sulfamethoxazole, TMP/SMX)**
  - TMP/SMX interacts with warfarin via two different synergistic mechanisms. Trimethoprim and sulfamethoxazole inhibit CYP2C9, and sulfamethoxazole also displaces warfarin from albumin.
- **TEG vs. INR**
  - Thromboelastography (TEG) is a novel method in acute settings to determine coagulopathy. This test is primarily used when bleeding is observed or suspected, not for therapeutic monitoring.
- Warfarin tablets have different colors to avoid dosing or filling errors.

HIGH-YIELD BOARD EXAM ESSENTIALS
- **CLASSIC AGENTS:** Warfarin
- **DRUG CLASS:** Vitamin K antagonist
- **INDICATIONS:** AF, secondary CV prevention, VTE (treatment and prophylaxis)
- **MECHANISM:** Inhibits the activation of coagulation factors II, VII, IX, and X as well as proteins C and S.
- **SIDE EFFECTS:** Bleeding
- **CLINICAL PEARLS:**
  - Dosing is patient-specific. Duration of therapy is indication-specific.
  - Although warfarin rapidly achieves peak concentrations and inhibits vitamin K regeneration, its therapeutic onset is 5-7 days. Existing vitamin K stores must be depleted and the active coagulation factors removed from circulation in accordance with the duration of their half-life to attain effect.
  - Contraindicated in pregnancy.
  - Reversal agent is vitamin K.

Table: Drug Class Summary

Vitamin K Antagonist - Drug Class Review High-Yield Med Reviews			
Generic Name	**Brand Name**	**Main Indication(s) or Uses**	**Notes**

Warfarin	Coumadin
	Jantoven
		- Treatment of VTE
		- Atrial fibrillation
		- Stroke
		- Post-myocardial infarction
			- **Dosing (Adult):** Dosing depends on target INR based on indication and patient-specific comorbidities/factors
			  - Initial 2.5-10 mg daily
			- **Dosing (Peds):** Dosing depends on target INR
			  - Initial 0.2 mg/kg daily, maximum 10 mg
			- **CYP450 Interactions:** CYP2C19, CYP2C9, CYP3A4, and CYP1A2 substrate
			- **Renal or Hepatic Dose Adjustments:**
			  - No empiric adjustments; with hepatic failure, may increase sensitivity to warfarin
			- **Dosage Forms:** Oral (tablet)

CARDIOVASCULAR – THROMBOLYTICS

Drug Class
- Acute Care
  - Alteplase
  - Reteplase
  - Tenecteplase
- Chronic Care
  - Defibrotide

> **Fast Facts**
> ✓ Alteplase is not only used for acute ischemic stroke, but also for submassive/massive PE, and STEMI within 12 hours of onset.
> ✓ In the context of myocardial infarction, the use of thrombolytics is only indicated for STEMI, not NSTEMI.

Main Indications or Uses
- Acute Care:
  - Acute ischemic stroke
  - Acute myocardial infarction (STEMI)
  - Acute pulmonary embolism (PE)
- Chronic Care:
  - Hepatic sinusoidal obstruction syndrome

Mechanism of Action
- Fibrinolytics break susceptible fibrin via activation of plasmin from plasminogen. Specifically, these agents promote the initiation of fibrinolysis by producing plasmin from fibrin-bound plasminogen.

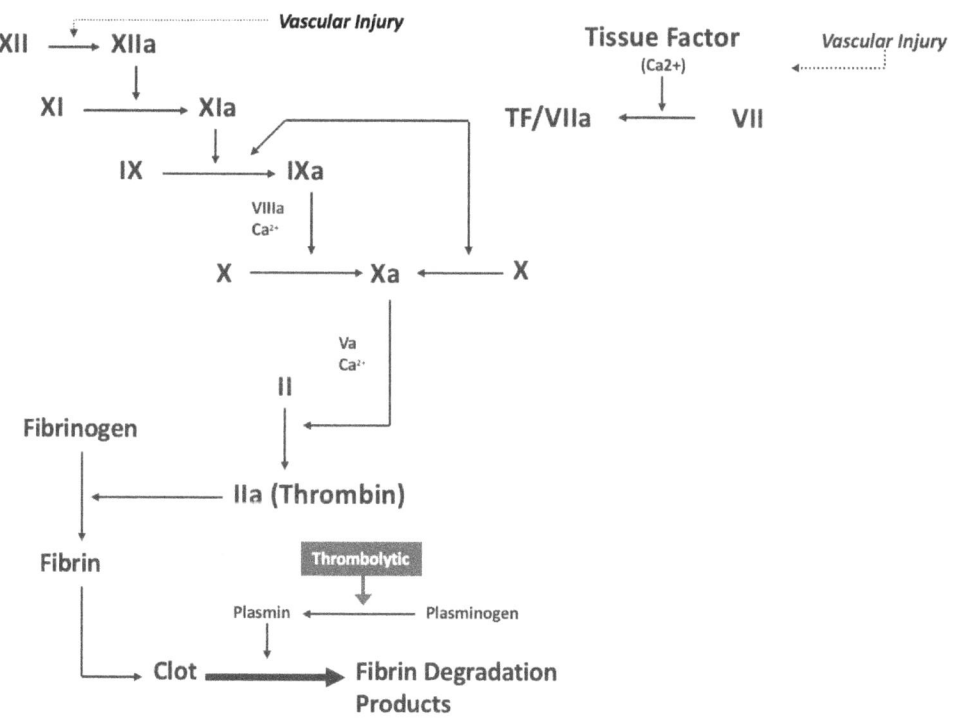

Primary Net Benefit
- Fibrinolytics are often referred to as thrombolytics. While these drugs work to dissolve a thrombus (a clot), they do so by ultimately breaking down fibrin.
  - To prevent confusion and an erroneous assumption that they have a direct effect on thrombin, these drugs will be referred to hereafter as fibrinolytics.
- Main Labs to Monitor:
  - CBC (Hgb/HCT due to the risk of bleeding)
  - INR/PT, PTT, ACT

High-Yield Basic Pharmacology
- **Other Fibrinolytics**
    - Streptokinase and urokinase are no longer used clinically in the United States.
    - In patients with antistreptococcal antibodies receiving streptokinase, they are at risk of fever, allergic reactions, and therapeutic resistance.
- **Alteplase Half-Life**
    - Alteplase has a short pharmacologic half-life of approximately 5 minutes.
        - This results from alteplase being rapidly inactivated by plasminogen activator inhibitor 1 (PAI-1) and PAI-2.
        - But since alteplase promotes the activation of plasminogen to plasmin, the duration of effect is up to 2 hours; then, plasmin is ultimately inactivated by alpha-2 antiplasmin.
- **Von Willebrand Factor**
    - Defibrotide is also classified as an antiplatelet agent through its actions of decreasing von Willebrand factor.

High-Yield Clinical Knowledge
- **Contraindications to Fibrinolysis**
    - Absolute Contraindications
        - Prior intracranial hemorrhage
        - Known structural cerebral vascular lesion
        - Known malignant intracranial neoplasm
        - Ischemic stroke within three months
        - Suspected aortic dissection
        - Active bleeding or bleeding diathesis (excluding menses)
        - Significant closed-head trauma or facial trauma within three months
    - Relative contraindications
        - Uncontrolled hypertension (systolic blood pressure > 180 mm Hg or diastolic blood pressure > 110 mm Hg)
        - Traumatic or prolonged CPR or major surgery within three weeks
        - Recent (within 2–4 weeks) internal bleeding
        - Noncompressible vascular punctures
        - Current use of warfarin and INR > 1.7
- **Acute Ischemic Stroke Caveats to Contraindications**
    - Recent changes in recommendations have relaxed contraindications to alteplase for acute ischemic stroke. The specific contraindications that have been revised include:
        - Patients may receive alteplase in the setting of a historic intracranial hemorrhage, but not an acute hemorrhage.
        - Patients currently taking a DOAC and have taken a dose within 48 hours should not receive alteplase.
- **Hemorrhage and Angioedema**
    - Complications of fibrinolytics include bleeding, which is intuitive.
    - However, angioedema is a relatively prevalent adverse event occurring in 1% of patients.
        - To put this in context, angioedema occurs in approximately 0.8% of patients on ACE-inhibitors.
- **Fibrin Specific**
    - Tenecteplase and reteplase are often referred to as fibrin specific, meaning their activation of plasminogen is more specific to plasminogen bound to fibrin even though alteplase has a 100-fold preference for fibrin (clot) bound plasminogen compared to plasminogen in the circulation.
    - In other words, they are more likely to promote fibrinolysis in relatively new thrombi.
    - These agents are also more resistant to PAI-1 and have a longer duration of effect.
    - However, there is still a risk of plasmin generation that can dissolve fibrin in nonpathological hemostatic plugs as well as that in pathological thrombi.
- **Agent Selection**

- Although alteplase and tenecteplase may be interchangeable for myocardial infarction and PE, alteplase is still preferred in acute ischemic stroke.
- **Hepatic Sinusoidal Obstruction Syndrome (SOS)**
    - Fibrinolytics such as alteplase have been used for SOS; however, they have been associated with a high incidence of hemorrhage, overshadowing any potential benefit.
    - The use of defibrotide, however, is a reasonable option.
    - Although it functions differently to achieve fibrinolysis by increasing endogenous t-PA, increasing thrombomodulin expression, decreasing von Willebrand factor, and plasminogen activator inhibitor-1.
    - Furthermore, if defibrotide is initiated early after identifying SOS, its use was associated with a significantly higher 100-day post-transplant survival.

High-Yield Core Evidence
- **NINDS**
    - The NINDS trial was a randomized, double-blinded, placebo-controlled, multicenter trial in acute ischemic stroke patients.
    - Patients who met extensive inclusion and exclusion criteria were randomized to receive alteplase or placebo and were followed to two primary outcomes.
    - For the first primary outcome of early effect (within 24 hrs), there was no significance between the treatment groups; however, patients who received alteplase demonstrated an improvement in neurologic outcome at 90 days.
    - The incidence of symptomatic intracranial hemorrhage occurred significantly more frequently in the alteplase group, but there was no significant difference in mortality at three months.
    - As a result of the net clinical benefit of improved neurologic functioning at 90 days, the authors supported the positive outcomes at three months despite a higher risk of intracranial bleeding. (N Engl J Med. 1995 Dec 14;333(24):1581-7.)
- **TROICA**
    - The TROICA trial was a double-blind, multicenter trial of adult patients with witnessed out-of-hospital cardiac arrest randomized to receive either tenecteplase or placebo during CPR.
    - There was no difference in the primary end-point of 30-day survival but a significantly higher incidence of intracranial hemorrhages in the tenecteplase group. As a result of an interim analysis, the study was stopped prematurely for futility. (N Engl J Med. 2008 Dec 18;359(25):2651-62.)
- **ASSENT-2**
    - The ASSENT-2 trial was a double-blind, randomized trial to evaluate the use of tenecteplase compared to alteplase for patients with acute myocardial infarction of less than six hour duration.
    - All patients received aspirin and heparin.
    - There was no difference in the primary outcome of all-cause mortality at 30 days, as well as the incidence of ICH or non-fatal stroke at 30 days.
    - Tenecteplase was associated with a lower incidence of non-cerebral bleeding and a lower incidence of blood transfusion. (Lancet. 1999;354:716–722.)
- **Defibrotide**
    - The use of defibrotide in SOS was assessed in an open-label, historically controlled, phase 3 study, which investigated the safety and efficacy of defibrotide in patients with established SOS.
    - Defibrotide was associated with a significant improvement in survival at day +100 post-hematopoietic stem cell transplantation (HSCT) and improved complete response rates.
    - Patients receiving defibrotide reported pulmonary alveolar hemorrhage and GI bleeding rates similar between it and the control groups. (Int J Hematol Oncol. 2017;6:75–93.)

High-Yield Fast-Facts
- Some agents like tenecteplase are referred to as more 'fibrin specific.' This translates to less likely to activate counterregulatory enzymes such as PAI-1 (plasminogen activator inhibitor 1). However, the clinical benefit of this action has not always translated into patient-oriented benefits.
- Low doses of alteplase can be used to assist catheter clearance from thrombosed access sites. Under the brand name Cathflo, alteplase given at a dose of 2 mg can assist in catheter recanalization.

Table: Drug Class Summary

Thrombolytics - Drug Class Review High-Yield Med Reviews			
Mechanism of Action: *Fibrinolytics break susceptible fibrin via activation of plasmin from plasminogen. Defibrotide achieves fibrinolysis via increases in endogenous t-PA, increasing thrombomodulin expression, decreasing von Willebrand factor, and plasminogen activator inhibitor-1.*			
Class Effects: *Fibrin cross-link degradation and dissolution of a fibrin-based thrombus.*			
Generic Name	**Brand Name**	**Main Indication(s) or Uses**	**Notes**
Alteplase	Activase Cathflo Activase	• Acute ischemic stroke (AIS) • Pulmonary embolism (PE) • ST-elevation myocardial infarction (STEMI)	• **Dosing (Adult):** – AIS: 0.9 mg/kg with 10% (0.09 mg/kg) as IV bolus over 1 minute, followed immediately by 90% (0.81 mg/kg) over 1 hour. Maximum 90 mg total dose. – PE: 100mg IV over 2 hours; 50 mg IV over OR 50 mg IV bolus repeated 15 minutes later by another 50 mg IV bolus (for massive PE cardiac arrest) – STEMI: Patients over 67 kg receive 100 mg over 1.5 hours; administered as a 15 mg IV bolus over 1 to 2 minutes followed by infusions of 50 mg over 30 minutes, then 35 mg over 1 hour. Patients < or equal to 67 kg receive 15 mg IV bolus over 1 to 2 minutes followed by infusions of 0.75 mg/kg (maximum of 50 mg) over 30 minutes, then 0.5 mg/kg (maximum 35 mg) over 1 hour. Maximum total dose of 100 mg • **Dosing (Peds):** – Same weight-based dose as adults. Additional off-label uses exist with varied specific doses. • **CYP450 Interactions:** No CYP interactions • **Renal or Hepatic Dose Adjustments:** None • **Dosage Forms:** IV solution
Defibrotide	Defitelio	• Sinusoidal obstruction syndrome (SOS)	• **Dosing (Adult):** – IV: solution 6.25 mg/kg over 2 hours, q6h for at least 21 days (maximum of 60 days). Must be infused with a 0.2-micron in-line filter. • **Dosing (Peds):** – IV: solution 6.25 mg/kg over 2 hours, q6h for at least 21 days (maximum of 60 days). Must be infused with a 0.2-micron in-line filter. • **CYP450 Interactions:** No CYP interactions • **Renal or Hepatic Dose Adjustments:** None • **Dosage Forms:** IV solution

Thrombolytics - Drug Class Review
High-Yield Med Reviews

Generic Name	Brand Name	Main Indication(s) or Uses	Notes
Reteplase	Retavase	- ST-elevation myocardial infarction (STEMI)	- **Dosing (Adult):** - Initial dose of 10 mg once daily, increasing dose as tolerated to target range 20 to 40 mg once daily with maximum dose of 40 mg/day. - **Dosing (Peds):** Not used - **CYP450 Interactions:** None - **Renal or Hepatic Dose Adjustments:** None - **Dosage Forms:** IV solution
Tenecteplase	TNKase	- ST-elevation myocardial infarction (STEMI)	- **Dosing (Adult):** - Scaled weight based dosing. < 60 kg: 30 mg; ≥60 to <70 kg: 35 mg, ≥70 to <80 kg: 40 mg; ≥80 to <90 kg: 45 mg; ≥90 kg: 50 mg. Maximum dose of 50 mg - **Dosing (Peds):** Not used - **CYP450 Interactions:** None - **Renal or Hepatic Dose Adjustments:** None - **Dosage Forms:** IV solution

HIGH-YIELD BOARD EXAM ESSENTIALS
- **CLASSIC AGENTS:** Alteplase, reteplase, tenecteplase, defibrotide
- **DRUG CLASS:** Thrombolytics
- **INDICATIONS:** Acute ischemic stroke, acute myocardial infarction, acute pulmonary embolism, hepatic sinusoidal obstruction syndrome
- **MECHANISM:** Break susceptible fibrin via activation of plasmin from plasminogen. Specifically, these agents promote the initiation of fibrinolysis by producing plasmin from fibrin-bound plasminogen.
- **SIDE EFFECTS:** Hemorrhage, angioedema
- **CLINICAL PEARLS:**
  - Fibrinolytics are often referred to as thrombolytics. While these drugs work to dissolve a thrombus (a clot), they do so by ultimately breaking down fibrin.
  - Alteplase is indicated for acute ischemic stroke within 3 hrs of onset, submassive & massive PE, and STEMI within 12 hrs of onset.
  - Tenecteplase has the longest half-life and thus can be given as a single IVP dose for STEMI.

CARDIOVASCULAR – ANTIDOTES & REVERSAL AGENTS

Drug Class
- Acute Care
  - Activated prothrombin complex concentrate (aPCC)
  - Andexanet Alfa / coagulation factor Xa - (recombinant) inactivated-zhzo
  - Four-factor prothrombin complex concentrate (PCC)
  - Idarucizumab

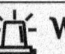

Warnings or Alerts

✓ *While activated prothrombin complex concentrate (aPCC) can reverse bleeding from apixaban, edoxaban, rivaroxaban, and warfarin, it can also cause an over-correction leading to clotting.*

Main Indications or Uses
- Acute Care:
  - Life-threatening bleeding associated with:
    - Apixaban or rivaroxaban (andexanet alfa)
    - Apixaban, rivaroxaban, edoxaban, warfarin (aPCC, PCC)
    - Dabigatran (idarucizumab)
  - Urgent reversal warfarin therapy in patients with acute major bleeding or a need for an urgent surgery/invasive procedure (PCC)
  - Hemorrhage in patients with hemophilia (aPCC)
- Chronic Care:
  - Routine prophylaxis of bleeding events in patients with hemophilia (aPCC)

Primary Net Benefit
- PCC products provide a concentrated, rapid means of replacing vitamin K-dependent clotting factors (clotting factors that are functionally activated), where andexanet alfa presents an inactive factor Xa to bind circulating oral FXa inhibitors, and idarucizumab is a specific monoclonal antibody directed against dabigatran.
- Main Labs to Monitor:
  - INR/PT, PTT
  - CBC
  - Thromboelastography/Thromboelastronomy (if available)

Mechanism of Action
- Activated prothrombin complex concentrate
  - Replaces factors II, IX, and X, as well as activated factor VII (VIIa)
- Andexanet Alfa
  - Directly binds and sequestered apixaban and rivaroxaban, halting their antithrombotic actions, in addition to inhibition of tissue factor pathway inhibitor (TFPI)
- Four-factor prothrombin complex concentrate
  - Replaces the vitamin K-dependent coagulation factors II, VII, IX, and X in addition to protein C and protein S.
- Idarucizumab
  - Humanized monoclonal antibody fragment specific to free and thrombin bound dabigatran, neutralizing its anticoagulant.

High-Yield Basic Pharmacology
- **Reversal, Not Procoagulant**
  - Idarucizumab does not intrinsically possess procoagulant activity, which differs from andexanet alfa, aPCC, and PCC.

- **Procoagulants**
  - Andexanet alfa is thought to exert a procoagulant effect by inhibiting TFPI (a double-negative statement, and inhibitor of tissue factor, thus allowing tissue factor activity) and activating the extrinsic coagulation pathway.
    - Since there is no more anti-Xa activity, the initial thrombin burst from extrinsic pathway activation allows for intrinsic pathway activation and clot formation.
  - Both aPCC and PCC contribute to supraphysiologic concentrations of vitamin-K-dependent clotting factors and promote coagulation.
- **Heparin Content**
  - PCC contains approximately 40 units of heparin for every 500 FIX units.
    - Therefore, a patient could receive anywhere from 200 to 400 units of heparin per dose of PCC.
    - Because of this, there is a risk of exacerbation/reactivation of HIT.
- **Activated PCC**
  - aPCC contains activated factor VII (VIIa) and can rapidly reverse prolonged INRs due to warfarin.
    - There is disagreement among clinicians about the safety of VIIa, given the history of NovoSeven (activated factor VIIa) for the reversal of warfarin.
    - This agent was found to have an unacceptable increase in the incidence of arterial thrombi.
- **Fixed-dose vs. variable weight-based dosing PCC**
  - Upon initial FDA approval, PCC was dosed in a variable dose based on the INR and the patient's weight.
  - This dosing was based on presumed factor deficiencies and was tested in a small group of patients in the study described below.
  - However, when clinicians gained experience with the drug, fixed dosing schedules of 1000 to 2000 units were widely adopted.
  - After the publication of numerous single centers and some multicentered studies, fixed-dose PCC was suggested to effectively achieve target INRs and reduce the risk of thrombosis and overall drug cost.
    - With more advanced coagulation assays such as thromboelastography, these doses may change further and become more patient-specific.
- **Andexanet vs PCC or Andexanet plus PCC for DOAC**
  - The initial phase 3 and phase 4 evidence with andexanet alfa was not compared to any other therapy.
  - This made a comparison between the currently used interventions of DOAC reversal (PCC and aPCC) difficult to assess.
  - However, there is a rationale that andexanet alfa may not replace the need for PCC or aPCC but rather act as an adjunct.
  - Since andexanet alfa does not have strong intrinsic procoagulant activity (other than inhibition of TFPI), it primarily sequesters the DOAC molecule preventing further anticoagulant effect.
  - While this is undoubtedly a desirable clinical outcome, in acute major hemorrhage in the setting of a DOAC, there may also be an acute need for procoagulant activity.
  - It's currently unknown what dose of aPCC or PCC is relevant to andexanet alfa function and whether the increased risk of thrombosis would offset any potential benefit.

High-Yield Clinical Knowledge
- **Clinical Considerations**
  - Kcentra (PCC) also contains heparin and carries a small but present risk of thrombocytopenia in patients with heparin-induced thrombocytopenia.
  - Andexanet alfa has been recommended in guideline statements as the suggested reversal agent for patients with major bleeding at a critical site and patients with major life-threatening bleeding associated with a DOAC. However, if andexanet alfa is not available in these scenarios, PCC is recommended as the alternative.

- **Dental Procedure or Other Minor Medical/Surgical Procedures**
  - The aPCC product (FEIBA) has been used in hemophilia before its use as an emergent anticoagulation reversal agent.
  - In some hemophilia patients with factor VIII inhibitors who have planned dental procedures, or other minor medical or surgical procedures can receive prophylactic factor replacement.
  - Some patients who require routine prophylaxis can receive 85 units/kg every other day, whereas other patient undergoing dental and minor surgical procedures may need up to 50 to 100 units/kg every 6 hours for at least one day or until bleeding is resolved up to a maximum of 100 units/kg/dose or 200 units/kg/day.

High-Yield Core Evidence
- **RE-VERSE AD**
  - This was a multicenter, prospective, open-label study examining the safety of idarucizumab and its potential to reverse the anticoagulant effects of dabigatran in patients who had serious bleeding or required an urgent procedure.
  - Idarucizumab achieved a near-complete median maximum percentage reversal of dabigatran based on the diluted thrombin time or the ecarin clotting time.
  - Among the patients with gastrointestinal bleeding or intracranial hemorrhage, the median time to the cessation of bleeding was 2.5 hours.
  - For patients undergoing an urgent procedure, the median time to initiate that procedure was 1.6 hours, with normal periprocedural hemostasis for almost all patients.
  - At 90 days, thrombotic events occurred in 6.3% of the patients in group A and 7.4% in group B, and the mortality rate was 18.8% and 18.9%, respectively.
  - There were no serious adverse safety signals.
  - The authors concluded that idarucizumab rapidly, durably, and safely reversed the anticoagulant effect of dabigatran. (N Engl J Med. 2017 Aug 3;377(5):431-441.)
- **ANNEXA-4**
  - A single-arm trial evaluated the use of andexanet alfa in patients who had acute major bleeding within 18 hours after administering a factor Xa inhibitor.
  - Andexanet alfa effectively decreased the median anti-factor Xa activity in patients taking apixaban or rivaroxaban and achieved excellent or good hemostasis in most patients.
  - However, despite the achievement of hemostasis in a majority of patients, andexanet was associated with a high rate of thrombosis and death.
  - The authors concluded that in patients with acute major bleeding associated with the use of a factor Xa inhibitor, treatment with andexanet markedly reduced anti-factor Xa activity. (N Engl J Med. 2019 Apr 4;380(14):1326-1335.)
- **Kcentra**
  - A phase 3b, multicenter, open-label study compared PCC to plasma in warfarin-treated patients needing urgent surgical or invasive procedures.
  - Significantly more patients receiving PCC achieved the primary endpoint of effective hemostasis and the co-primary endpoint of rapid INR reduction to less than or equal to 1.3, 30 minutes after the end of the infusion.
  - These outcomes achieved both non-inferiority and superiority of PCC over plasma with similar safety in the incidence of thromboembolic adverse events, fluid overload, or similar cardiac events and late bleeding events.
  - The authors concluded that PCC is non-inferior and superior to plasma for rapid INR reversal and effective hemostasis in patients needing VKA reversal for urgent surgical or invasive procedures. (Lancet. 2015 May 23;385(9982):2077-87.)

High-Yield Fast-Facts
- Fresh frozen plasma replaces a relatively fixed percentage of coagulation factors with an intrinsic INR of 1.6 to 1.8. For many clinicians, FFP is not regarded as an effective method to correct the INR below 1.6 to 1.8 since the volume of FFP required to do so is functionally not possible to administer safely. Therefore, when PCC was compared to FFP with a co-primary outcome of achieving an INR of 1.3, there was a very low likelihood that FFP had a chance to accomplish this endpoint and may not have been an appropriate endpoint for comparison. Furthermore, INR reduction is a surrogate marker for hemostasis, a surrogate marker for mortality.
- The administration of idarucizumab has been associated with numerous drug errors. This results from the total 5 g dose being commercially available exclusively as two 2.5 g vials. Methods to reduce the risk of error include combining each dose into a single container or using programmable IV infusion pumps.
- Andexanet alfa is very expensive, even compared to aPCC and PCC. The AWP of andexanet alfa is up to $58,080 for the high dose regimen.

HIGH-YIELD BOARD EXAM ESSENTIALS
- **CLASSIC AGENTS:** aPCC, andexanet alfa, PCC, idarucizumab
- **DRUG CLASS:** Reversal agents
- **INDICATIONS:** Life-threatening bleeding associated with: apixaban or rivaroxaban (andexanet alfa), apixaban, rivaroxaban, edoxaban, warfarin (aPCC, PCC), dabigatran (idarucizumab), urgent reversal warfarin therapy in patients with acute major bleeding or a need for an urgent surgery/invasive procedure (PCC), hemorrhage in patients with hemophilia (aPCC).
- **MECHANISM:**
    - aPCC: Replaces factors II, IX, and X, as well as VIIa.
    - PCC: Replaces the vitamin K-dependent coagulation factors II, VII, IX, and X in addition to protein C and protein S (PCC).
    - Andexanet alfa: Directly binds and sequestered apixaban and rivaroxaban, halting their antithrombotic actions, in addition to inhibition of TFPI.
    - PCC: Replaces the vitamin K-dependent coagulation factors II, VII, IX, and X in addition to protein C and protein S (PCC).
    - Idarucizumab: Humanized monoclonal antibody fragment specific to free and thrombin bound dabigatran, neutralizing its anticoagulant.
- **SIDE EFFECTS:** Thrombosis, HIT (Kcentra)
- **CLINICAL PEARLS:** PCC and aPCC use has departed from the prescribing information recommended dosing, and commonly use fixed dosing schedules of 1000 to 2000 units are widely accepted.

Table: Drug Class Summary

Reversal Agents - Drug Class Review High-Yield Med Reviews			
Mechanism of Action: ***Andexanet Alfa*** - *directly binds and sequestered apixaban and rivaroxaban, halting their antithrombotic actions, in addition to inhibition of tissue factor pathway inhibitor (TFPI)* ***Idarucizumab*** - *binds to free and thrombin-bound dabigatran, neutralizing its anticoagulant effect.* ***Activated prothrombin complex concentrate*** - *replaces factors II, IX, and X, as well as activated factor VII (VIIa)* *Four-factor prothrombin complex concentrate replaces the vitamin K-dependent coagulation factors II, VII, IX, and X and protein C and S.*			
Class Effects: *Reversal of therapeutic anticoagulation*			
Generic Name	**Brand Name**	**Main Indication(s) or Uses**	**Notes**

Andexanet Alfa	Andexxa	• Life-threatening bleeding associated with apixaban or rivaroxaban	• **Dosing (Adult):**
			   – Dose-dependent on dose and time since the last dose.
			   – IV: 400 mg (low dose) bolus, followed immediately by 4 mg/minute IV infusion for up to 120 minutes.
			   – High dose: 800 mg (low dose) bolus, followed immediately by 8 mg/minute IV infusion for up to 120 minutes.
			• **Dosing (Peds):** Not used
			• **CYP450 Interactions:** None
			• **Renal or Hepatic Dose Adjustments:** None
			• **Dosage Forms:** IV solution

Activated prothrombin complex concentrate	FEIBA	• Control and prevention of bleeding episodes in patients with hemophilia • Life-threatening bleeding associated with oral anticoagulants	• **Dosing (Adult):** IV: 50 to 100 units/kg/dose • **Dosing (Peds):** IV: 50 to 100 units/kg/dose • **CYP450 Interactions:** None • **Renal or Hepatic Dose Adjustments:** None • **Dosage Forms:** IV lyophilized powder for reconstitution. Also known as Anti-inhibitor Coagulant Complex

Four-factor prothrombin complex concentrate	Kcentra	• Control and prevention of bleeding episodes in patients with hemophilia
		• Life-threatening bleeding associated with oral anticoagulants
			• **Dosing (Adult):**
			   – For warfarin-associated hemorrhage - INR 2 to <4: 25 units/kg (max 2,500 units); INR 4 to 6: 35 units/kg (max 3,500 units), INR >6: 50 units/kg (max 5,000 units).
			   – DOAC associated hemorrhage- IV 2,000 units once or 25-50 units/kg once
			• **Dosing (Peds):** use adult dosing
			• **CYP450 Interactions:** None
			• **Renal or Hepatic Dose Adjustments:** None
			• **Dosage Forms:** IV lyophilized powder for reconstitution

Idarucizumab	Praxbind	• Life-threatening hemorrhage due to dabigatran	• **Dosing (Adult):** IV: infusion of 5 g • **Dosing (Peds):** Not routinely used • **CYP450 Interactions:** None • **Renal or Hepatic Dose Adjustments:** None • **Dosage Forms:** IV solution

CARDIOVASCULAR – ANTIFIBRINOLYTICS

Drug Class
- **Acute Care**
  - Epsilon-aminocaproic acid (aminocaproic acid)
  - Tranexamic acid (TXA)
- **Chronic Care**
  - Tranexamic acid

Main Indications or Uses
- **Acute Care:**
  - Adjunct to cardiac surgery
  - Acute major hemorrhage
  - Acute trauma
  - Postpartum hemorrhage
- **Chronic Care:**
  - Menstrual bleeding, heavy
  - Tooth extraction in patients with hemostatic defects

> **Fast Facts**
> ✓ Tranexamic acid (TXA) is most commonly used in current clinical practice during traumatic injury with acute hemorrhage.

Mechanism of Action
- Fibrinolysis occurs due to plasminogen activation and its binding to fibrin's lysine residues.
  - The process of antifibrinolysis from the lysine analogs (aminocaproic acid and TXA) occurs due to their occupation of these lysing binding sites in plasminogen.

Primary Overall Net Benefit
- Analogs of lysine occupy lysing binding sites in plasminogen, thus interfering with the fibrinolysis process and promoting hemostasis.
- Main Labs to Monitor:
  - CBC
  - INR/PT, PTT

High-Yield Basic Pharmacology
- The pharmacologic effects of aminocaproic acid and TXA are similar to the plasmin activator inhibitor-1 (PAI-1) (which inhibits tissue plasminogen activator), PAI-2 (which inhibits urokinase plasminogen activator), and thrombin activatable fibrinolysis inhibitor (TAFI).
- Alpha-2-antiplasmin has a similar role; however, it prevents prothrombin activation to thrombin by inhibiting plasmin.
- Inhibition of plasmin generation can have numerous other benefits, including anti-inflammation, reduced cytokine production, and reduced proteolytic activation of matrix-metalloproteinases.

High-Yield Clinical Knowledge
- **Hyperfibrinolysis Vs. Fibrinolytic Shutdown**
  - The role of antifibrinolytics in acute care medicine was postulated based on the predicted physiology that accompanies massive trauma, surgery, or extracorporeal circulation.
    - In these scenarios, the normal physiologic capacity to regulate fibrinolysis is overwhelmed, coagulopathy ensues and results in a scenario referred to as hyperfibrinolysis.
      - Hyperfibrinolysis exists on a spectrum where, depending on the pathologic state, a patient can exist in hyperfibrinolysis, the opposing polar end of fibrinolysis shutdown, or somewhere in between.
      - It's unclear which antifibrinolytics may benefit as we are still developing our clinical understanding of fibrinolytic shutdown and hyperfibrinolysis.

- **Stabilization of Fibrin**
  - These agents promote the stabilization of fibrin already existing in clots, not an actual procoagulant effect.
    - This occurs from the preservation of the lysine residues on fibrin and can promote clot maturity via the actions of factor XIIIa and TAFI.
      - After fibrin polymerizes to form protofibrils and is subsequently stabilized by XIIIa, these fibrin protofibrils create a mesh linking platelets via the GPIIb/IIIa receptor (which was mobilized to the surface via P2Y12 receptor activation).
      - TAFI, activated by the thrombin-thrombomodulin complex, removes the C-terminal lysine residues from fibrin, thus slowing the rate of fibrin degradation and ultimately yielding fibrin resistant to lysis.
- **TXA For Angioedema**
  - TXA may play a role in managing angioedema, either from a RAAS agent (ACE-inhibitor, ARB, DRI) or hereditary angioedema.
    - TXA can prevent the consumption of C1-esterase and reduce the activation of the complement pathway by limiting the production of plasmin.
      - C1-esterase inhibition limits the production of kallikrein and bradykinin and thus the generation of angioedema.
- **Hereditary Angioedema**
  - TXA is a reasonable, third-line option for long-term *prophylaxis* in patients with hereditary angioedema (HAE), according to the International World Allergy Organization/European Academy of Allergy and Clinical Immunology guidelines. Its role in acute attacks of HAE is controversial.
    - TXA is not recommended for the treatment of acute HAE attacks.
    - TXA may not be harmful, but the magnitude of the clinical effect may include no effect. In other words, the drug is not specifically harmful in this indication but is not expected to independently change the course of treatment.
- **Dose-dependent Risk of Seizures**
  - Aminocaproic acid and TXA have been associated with generalized tonic-clonic seizures in up to 7.6% of patients.
    - This data is based on the historical application of these agents in cardiac surgery where doses greater than 50 mg/kg (i.e., 4000mg in an 80 kg patient).
      - In the CRASH-2 trial, CRASH-3, and the WOMAN trial, there was no increase in the risk of seizures in patients receiving TXA compared to those who received a placebo.
- **Adult Women with Heavy Menstrual Bleeding**
  - The specific branded product of TXA, Lysteda, is approved for use in adult women with heavy menstrual bleeding. It should be reserved for patients who decline or should not use hormonal therapy. The specific branded product allows for the evidence-supported dosing of 1.3 g three times daily for up to 5 days during monthly menstruation (see evidence summary below).

High-Yield Core Evidence
- **CRASH-2**
  - The CRASH-2 was a large, pragmatic landmark clinical trial of TXA in trauma patients.
  - This study was a multicenter, double-blind, placebo-controlled trial that randomized acute trauma patients with, or at risk of, significant bleeding to either TXA 1g IV over 10 minutes followed by 1g IV over 8 hours or placebo within 8 h of injury.
  - Patients receiving TXA had a significantly lower all-cause mortality and lower risk of death due to bleeding than patients receiving placebo.
  - The authors concluded that TXA safely reduced the risk of death in bleeding trauma patients in this study. (Lancet. 2010 Jul 3;376(9734):23-32.)
- **WOMAN**
  - The WOMAN Trial was a landmark clinical trial investigating the effects of early administration of TXA on death, hysterectomy, and other relevant outcomes in women with postpartum hemorrhage.
  - The study investigators conducted a randomized, double-blind, placebo-controlled trial of women aged 16 years and older with a clinical diagnosis of postpartum hemorrhage after vaginal birth or cesarean

section who were subsequently randomized to TXA 1 g IV or placebo with the option of another dose of TXA 1 g IV or placebo if bleeding continued after 30 min, or stopped and restarted within 24 h.
- There was no difference in the composite primary endpoint of death from all causes or hysterectomy in patients receiving TXA or placebo.
- However, patients receiving TXA had a significantly lower risk of death due to bleeding, with those receiving treatment within 3 hours of giving birth having the greatest benefit.
- All other causes of death did not differ significantly by the group, and there was no decrease in the incidence of hysterectomy with TXA.
- There was no difference in the incidence of adverse events in the TXA versus the placebo group.
- The authors concluded that in the treatment for postpartum hemorrhage, TXA should be given as soon as possible after bleeding onset. (Lancet. 2017 May 27;389(10084):2105-2116.)
- **TXA and Heavy Menstrual Bleeding**
  - The role of TXA in adult women with heavy menstrual bleeding was assessed in a double-blind, placebo-controlled study.
  - Study subjects underwent randomization to receive either TXA 1300 mg PO TID for up to 5 days per menstrual cycle through six cycles or placebo.
  - Patients who received TXA had a significantly greater reduction in menstrual blood loss, reduction of menstrual blood loss, and reduction of menstrual blood loss considered meaningful to women.
  - Patients tolerated TXA with similar adverse events reported between active treatment & placebo groups.
  - The authors concluded that TXA significantly improved menstrual blood loss and health-related quality of life in women with heavy menstrual bleeding. (Obstet Gynecol. 2010 Oct;116(4):865-75)

High-Yield Fast-Facts
- **Topical TXA**
  - Topical or oral use of TXA is a valuable adjunct for dental procedures in patients at a high risk of bleeding or on oral anticoagulants.
- **Nebulized TXA**
  - Nebulized TXA can play a role in managing hemoptysis or nasopharyngeal bleeding. In addition, as a topical agent, it can avoid the need for a systemic reversal of oral anticoagulants, preserving thrombotic risk prevention in select patients.
- **TEG Monitoring of TXA**
  - Viscoelastic monitoring with rotational thromboelastometry or thromboelastography should be used as a guide for using TXA for hyperfibrinolysis.
- **Alternative Antifibrinolytic**
  - Aprotinin is a protease inhibitor isolated from bovine lung, often grouped with aminocaproic acid and TXA. However, aprotinin is not available in the United States, nor has it been available.

HIGH-YIELD BOARD EXAM ESSENTIALS
- **CLASSIC AGENTS:** Epsilon-aminocaproic acid (aminocaproic acid), tranexamic acid (TXA)
- **DRUG CLASS:** Antifibrinolytics
- **INDICATIONS:** Adjunct to cardiac surgery, acute major hemorrhage, acute trauma, postpartum hemorrhage, menstrual bleeding, tooth extraction in patients with hemostatic defects.
- **MECHANISM:** Analogs of lysine analogs occupy lysing binding sites in plasminogen, thus interfering with the fibrinolysis process.
- **SIDE EFFECTS:** Thrombosis, seizures
- **CLINICAL PEARLS:** TXA may help reduce the risk of death in major trauma with high risk or already with severe bleeding. In addition, TXA may play a role in the management of angioedema, by preventing the consumption of C1-esterase and reduce the activation of the complement pathway by limiting the production of plasmin.

Table: Drug Class Summary

	Antifibrinolytics - Drug Class Review High-Yield Med Reviews		
Mechanism of Action: *Analogs of lysine analogs occupy lysing binding sites in plasminogen, thus interfering with the fibrinolysis process.*			
Class Effects: *Hemostasis, hemorrhage control.*			
Generic Name	**Brand Name**	**Indication(s) or Uses**	**Notes**
Epsilon-aminocaproic acid	Amicar	<ul><li>Acute hemorrhage from surgery</li><li>Postpartum hemorrhage</li></ul>	<ul><li>**Dosing (Adult):**<ul><li>Loading dose oral or IV: 4 to 5 g<ul><li>IV: infusion 1 g IV per hour</li></ul></li><li>Oral: 1.25 g q1h for 8 hours or until bleeding controlled<ul><li>Maximum daily dose of 30 g</li></ul></li></ul></li><li>**Dosing (Peds):**<ul><li>Loading dose (oral or IV): 50-100 mg/kg/dose every 6 hours<ul><li>Maximum daily dose 24 g/day</li></ul></li></ul></li><li>**CYP450 Interactions:** None</li><li>**Renal or Hepatic Dose Adjustments:**<ul><li>Cardiac surgery in anephric patients, reduce infusion to 5 mg/kg/hour</li></ul></li><li>**Dosage Forms:** IV: solution, oral (tablet)</li></ul>
Tranexamic acid	Cyklokapron Lysteda	<ul><li>Acute hemorrhage from surgery</li><li>Acute trauma</li><li>Postpartum hemorrhage</li><li>Menstrual bleeding, heavy</li><li>Tooth extraction</li></ul>	<ul><li>**Dosing (Adult):**<ul><li>Loading dose oral or IV: 4 to 5 g<ul><li>IV: infusion 1 g IV per hour</li></ul></li><li>Oral: 1.25 g q1h for 8 hours or until bleeding controlled<ul><li>Maximum daily dose of 30 g</li></ul></li></ul></li><li>**Dosing (Peds):**<ul><li>Loading dose (oral or IV) 50-100 mg/kg/dose every 6 hours<ul><li>Maximum daily dose 24 g/day</li></ul></li></ul></li><li>**CYP450 Interactions:** None</li><li>**Renal or Hepatic Dose Adjustments:**<ul><li>Cardiac surgery in anephric patients, reduce infusion to 5 mg/kg/hour</li></ul></li><li>**Dosage Forms:** IV solution, oral (tablet)</li></ul>

CARDIOVASCULAR – PHYTONADIONE AND PROTAMINE

Drug Class
- Anticoagulant Reversal
- Agents:
  - Acute Care
    - Phytonadione
    - Protamine

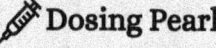

Dosing Pearl

✓ Protamine 1 mg will reverse 100 units of available unfractionated heparin in the body. However, as the dose of protamine exceeds 50 mg, there is a risk that it can function as an anticoagulant and thereby causing bleeding.

Main Indications or Uses
- Acute Care
  - Protamine:
    - Reversal of heparin or low molecular weight heparin
  - Phytonadione:
    - Warfarin-associated INR elevation or hemorrhage

Mechanism of Action
- Phytonadione
  - Provides exogenous vitamin K to allow gamma-carboxylation (activation) of coagulation factors (II, VII, IX, X).
- Protamine Sulfate
  - Rapidly reverses the anticoagulant effect of heparin by binding directly to heparin, thereby reversing its anticoagulant effect.

Primary Net Benefit
- Protamine rapidly reverses the antithrombotic effects of heparin and may partially reverse low-molecular-weight heparins. Phytonadione is a crucial component to warfarin reversal, regardless of acute strategies, including FFP or PCC.
- Main Labs to Monitor:
  - CBC; INR/PT, PTT

High-Yield Basic Pharmacology
- Protamine
  - Patients with prior exposure to protamine in insulin, vasectomy, or fish allergy are at higher risk for protamine-induced adverse reactions.
- IV Suspension
  - Parenteral phytonadione is an aqueous colloidal suspension of a castor oil derivative, dextrose, and benzyl alcohol.
  - These excipients have been attributed to the risk of anaphylactoid reactions associated with phytonadione use.

High-Yield Clinical Knowledge
- Warfarin Reversal
  - Phytonadione reverses INR to normal values between 8 to 24 hours, depending on the dosage form.
  - For patients with no acute hemorrhage, there is no difference in efficacy between oral and IV.
  - In settings of acute hemorrhage, IV phytonadione is more appropriate than oral, as the onset of action is significantly faster (1-2 hours vs. 6 hours).
- Phytonadione IV Administration
  - Phytonadione must be diluted and administered slowly over 1 hour.
  - Slow IV infusion is required to reduce the risk of an anaphylactoid reaction.
  - Subcutaneous administration should be limited when IV administration is unnecessary, but patients cannot tolerate oral phytonadione.
  - IM should be avoided in patients with coagulopathies due to the risk of hematoma and bleeding.

- **Protamine Reversal of Anticoagulation**
  - The anticoagulant effects of heparin, LMWH, and (potentially) fondaparinux may be reversed with protamine sulfate.
  - It's also important to note that protamine only partially reverses the anticoagulant activity of LMWH and has no effect on that fondaparinux.
- **Protamine Dosing**
  - Protamine should be dosed as a function of the remaining therapeutic heparin, with an empiric dose of 1 mg of protamine for every 100 units of heparin remaining in the patient.
  - However, caution should be taken to estimate the remaining heparin (based on t1/2 of 1.5 hours) since excessive protamine sulfate can exert an anticoagulant effect.
- **Protamine Maximum Dose**
  - The maximum single dose of protamine is 50 mg.
  - Higher doses can cause paradoxical anticoagulant effects.
- **Other Anticoagulants**
  - Protamine sulfate is not effective for reversing fondaparinux, direct thrombin inhibitors, or any direct oral anticoagulant.
- **Thrombosis Risk**
  - Whenever vitamin K is used to reverse the antithrombotic effect of warfarin, the underlying thrombotic risk returns.
  - In patients with a high thromboembolism risk, the most cautious method to correct hemorrhaging should be considered and use appropriately dosed vitamin K (phytonadione) of INR overcorrection.

High-Yield Core Evidence
- **Oral Vs. IV Phytonadione**
  - This was a prospective, controlled trial of consecutive patients presenting with excessive anticoagulation without major bleeding who were randomized to receive oral phytonadione 2.5 mg or IV phytonadione 0.5 mg for INRs between 6 to 10, or oral phytonadione 5 mg or phytonadione IV 1 mg for INR greater than 10.
  - Among patients with baseline INR between 6 to 10, the response to IV phytonadione was more rapid than in the oral group.
  - The proportion of patients reaching the therapeutic range INR at 6 and 12 hours was significantly higher.
  - At 24 hours, the mean INR was similar between groups.
  - In patients with baseline, INR values greater than 10, efficacy and safety were comparable for both routes of administration.
  - The authors concluded that oral administration of phytonadione had similar efficacy and safety as IV administered phytonadione and may be suitable for treating patients with excessive anticoagulation. (Arch Intern Med. 2003 Nov 10;163(20):2469-73.)
- **IV or SQ Phytonadione**
  - This was a prospective, controlled trial of consecutive patients presenting with excessive anticoagulation without major bleeding who were randomized to receive either IV phytonadione 1 mg or SQ phytonadione 1 mg.
  - Patients randomized to IV phytonadione had a significantly lower INR at 8 and 24 hours than SQ phytonadione.
  - The mean decrease in INR 8 hours after administration of phytonadione was 3.4 in the IV group and 0.4 in the SQ group, and the mean reduction in INR after 24 hours was 4.9 in the IV group and 3.4 in the SC group.
  - The authors concluded that for excessively anticoagulated patients with warfarin, small doses of SC phytonadione might not correct the INR as rapidly or as effectively as when administered IV. (Arch Intern Med. 1999 Dec 13-27;159(22):2721-4.)

High-Yield Fast-Fact
- **Rat poison**
  - Ingestion of a long-acting anticoagulant rodenticide such as brodifacoum may require high doses of phytonadione (50 mg daily) for days to weeks.
  - Contamination of "k2" in the Chicago area led to numerous patients being exposed to brodifacoum, causing fatal hemorrhages in some and long-term treatment with phytonadione.

HIGH-YIELD BOARD EXAM ESSENTIALS
- **CLASSIC AGENTS:** Phytonadione, protamine
- **DRUG CLASS:** Anticoagulant reversal
- **INDICATIONS:** Reversal of heparin or low molecular weight heparin (protamine), warfarin-associated INR elevation or hemorrhage (phytonadione)
- **MECHANISM:**
  - Phytonadione (vitamin K) provides exogenous vitamin K to allow gamma-carboxylation (activation) of coagulation factors.
  - Protamine rapidly reverses heparin's anticoagulant effect by binding directly to heparin, thereby reversing its anticoagulant effect.
- **SIDE EFFECTS:** Anaphylaxis, infusion reaction (phytonadione), thrombosis, hemorrhage (protamine).
- **CLINICAL PEARLS:**
  - Phytonadione (vitamin K) reverse warfarin but its onset is delayed.
  - Protamine should be dosed as a function of the remaining therapeutic heparin, with an empiric dose of 1 mg of protamine for every 100 units of heparin remaining in the patient (max dose is considered 50 mg because it can start act like an anticoagulant in higher doses).

Table: Drug Class Summary

Anticoagulant Reversal - Drug Class Review **High-Yield Med Reviews**			
Mechanism of Action: *Phytonadione - Provides exogenous vitamin K to allow gamma-carboxylation (activation) of coagulation factors (II, VII, IX, X).* *Protamine Sulfate - Rapidly reverses heparin's anticoagulant effect by binding directly to heparin, thereby reversing its anticoagulant effect.*			
Class Effects: Protamine rapidly reverses the antithrombotic effects of heparin and may partially reverse low-molecular-weight heparins. Phytonadione is a key component to warfarin reversal, regardless of acute strategies, including FFP or PCC.			
Generic Name	**Brand Name**	**Main Indication(s) or Uses**	**Notes**

Phytonadione	Mephyton	• Warfarin-associated INR elevation or hemorrhage (phytonadione)	• **Dosing (Adult):**
			  − IV/Oral/SQ/IM: 1 to 10 mg once
			• **Dosing (Peds):**
			  − IV/Oral/SQ/IM: 0.5 to 10 mg once
			• **CYP450 Interactions:** None
			• **Renal or Hepatic Dose Adjustments:** None
			• **Dosage Forms:** Injection (aqueous colloidal), Oral (tablet)

Protamine	Prosulf	• Reversal of heparin or low molecular weight heparin (protamine)	• **Dosing (Adult):**
			  − IV: dose determined based on heparin administration where 1 mg of protamine neutralizes approximately 100 units of heparin.
			  − Enoxaparin within 8 hours - dosed 1mg to 1 mg of protamine, maximum 50 mg/dose
			  − Enoxaparin 8 to 12 hours ago - 0.5 mg protamine for every 1 mg enoxaparin
			  − Dalteparin, nadroparin, tinzaparin - 1 mg for every 100 anti-factor Xa units
			• **Dosing (Peds):**
			  − IV: dose determined based on heparin administration where 1 mg of protamine neutralizes approximately 100 units of heparin.
			• **CYP450 Interactions:** None
			• **Renal or Hepatic Dose Adjustments:** None
			• **Dosage Forms:** IV (solution)

CARDIOVASCULAR – POTASSIUM-SPARING DIURETICS

Drug Class
- **Potassium-sparing Diuretics**
- **Agents:**
  - Amiloride
  - Eplerenone
  - Finerenone
  - Spironolactone
  - Triamterene

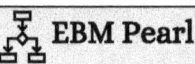 **EBM Pearl**
- ✓ Both eplerenone and spironolactone have been shown to improve mortality in those with heart failure.

Main Indications or Uses
- **Chronic Care:**
  - Ascites
    - Spironolactone
  - CKD in Type 2 DM
    - Finerenone
  - Heart failure
    - Eplerenone, spironolactone
  - Hypertension
    - Amiloride, eplerenone, spironolactone, triamterene
  - Primary hyperaldosteronism
    - Spironolactone

Counseling Point
- ✓ Warn patients about the use of salt substitutes as this can increase the risk of hyperkalemia since the replace the Na+ with K+.

Mechanism of Action
- Eplerenone and Spironolactone (aldosterone receptor antagonists)
  - Competitively inhibit aldosterone from binding to the mineralocorticoid receptor, preventing aldosterone-induced protein production and increasing potassium secretion into the renal tubular lumen.
- Amiloride and Triamterene
  - Inhibit transepithelial sodium transport in the late distal convoluted tubule and collecting duct, decreasing intracellular sodium and impaired function of the sodium-potassium-ATPase pump, causing potassium retention.

Primary Net Benefit
- Potassium-sparing diuretics are weak diuretics on their own but can be added to loop diuretic therapy with synergistic effects. Aldosterone antagonists provide secondary benefits in HF.
- Main Labs to Monitor:
  - Serum potassium at baseline, 3, and 7 days of initiation or dose titration and regularly thereafter

High-Yield Basic Pharmacology
- **Aldosterone Antagonists**
  - These agents could be thought of as aldosterone antagonists rather than diuretics since the latter effect is weak.
    - Diuresis from aldosterone antagonists is a function of aldosterone concentrations, with elevated levels producing greater diuresis and urinary excretion.
- **Steroid Effect**
  - Spironolactone contains a key structural group that confers its affinity to progesterone and androgen receptors and classic adverse events of gynecomastia, impotence, and menstrual irregularities.
    - Eplerenone lacks this epoxide group and does not produce the same degree of affinity for progesterone and androgen receptors, so these adverse effects are less.
- **Acidemia**

- Aldosterone antagonists can elicit acidemia because the same process that prevents potassium elimination also prevents the elimination of hydrogen in the collecting tubule's intercalated cells, similar to a type IV renal tubular acidosis.

High-Yield Clinical Knowledge
- **Hyperkalemia Risk**
  - These agents demonstrate an increased risk of hyperkalemia, especially in some populations.
    - Aldosterone antagonists should be avoided in patients with:
      - SCr concentration above 2.0 mg/dL in women or above 2.5 mg/dL in men or a CrCl of less than 30 mL/minute
      - Serum potassium concentration is greater than 5.0 mEq/L
      - Taking potassium supplements
      - Concomitant NSAIDs or COX-2 inhibitors
      - Concomitant high-dose ACE inhibitors or ARBs
  - When starting eplerenone or spironolactone, potassium concentrations, and kidney function should be checked 3 and 7 days after the initial dose.
- **Cardiac Remodeling**
  - Spironolactone or eplerenone should be used in HFrEF, specifically in patients with NYHA class II to IV HF, in patients with acute HF, or in diabetes early after MI.
    - Eplerenone and spironolactone exert a specific aldosterone antagonist effect in cardiac tissue that ultimately inhibits collagen deposition in the cardiac extracellular matrix and reduces cardiac fibrosis and ventricular remodeling.
- **Ascites**
  - Spironolactone and furosemide are used in combination in patients with ascites.
    - This combination has a specific ratio of spironolactone to furosemide of 100:40 (spironolactone 100 mg and furosemide 40 mg).
    - Maximum combination dose is spironolactone 400 mg and furosemide 160.
- **Heart Failure**
  - According to the current AHA guidelines, low-dose aldosterone antagonists should be added to standard therapy to improve HF symptoms, reduce the risk of HF hospitalizations, and increase survival in select patients.
  - As described above, spironolactone or eplerenone should be used in HFrEF, specifically in patients with NYHA class II to IV HF, in patients with acute HF, or in diabetes early after MI.
    - Among patients with NYHA class II HF, spironolactone or eplerenone are recommended in patients with a prior hospitalization for CV reasons or an elevated plasma BNP.
    - Either agent should also be added to decrease hospitalization risk for HF in patients with HFpEF and elevated BNP.
- **Resistant Hypertension**
  - In patients with treatment-resistant HTN (on ACE inhibitor or ARB, CCB, and diuretic), spironolactone significantly improved the likelihood of achieving BP targets more than bisoprolol, doxazosin, or placebo.
  - In this study, the BP reduction with spironolactone was approximately double that of doxazosin and bisoprolol. (PATHWAY-2. Lancet. 2015 Nov 21;386(10008):2059-2068.)
- **Drug-Interactions**
  - Eplerenone and finerenone are major substrates of CYP3A4 with a high risk for drug interactions that can result in a dose- or concentration-dependent risks of hyperkalemia.

High-Yield Core Evidence
- **RALES Trial**
  - This was a multicenter, prospective, double-blind study that randomized HF patients with LVEF of no more than 35% treated with an ACE-inhibitor, a loop diuretic, or digoxin to either spironolactone or placebo.
  - There was a statistically significant reduction in death (30%) in patients receiving spironolactone, and the study was discontinued early.

- Patients receiving spironolactone were also significantly less likely to be hospitalized for worsening HF and had a significant improvement in HF symptoms.
- More patients receiving spironolactone had serious hyperkalemia compared to placebo.
- The authors concluded that blockade of aldosterone receptors by spironolactone, in addition to standard therapy, substantially reduces the risk of both morbidity and death among patients with severe HF. (N Engl J Med. 1999 Sep 2;341(10):709-17.)

- **EPHESUS Trial**
    - This was a double-blind, placebo-controlled study designed to examine morbidity and mortality in patients with acute MI complicated by left ventricular dysfunction and HF that were randomized to eplerenone or placebo in addition to optimal medical therapy.
    - Patients randomized to eplerenone had a statistically significant improvement in the primary endpoints of death from any cause and death from CV causes or hospitalization for HF, acute MI, stroke, or ventricular arrhythmia.
    - Eplerenone also significantly reduced the incidence of death from any cause or any hospitalization compared to placebo.
    - More patients receiving eplerenone had serious hyperkalemia compared to placebo.
    - The authors concluded that the addition of eplerenone to optimal medical therapy reduces morbidity and mortality among patients with acute MI complicated by left ventricular dysfunction and HF. (N Engl J Med. 2003 Apr 3;348(14):1309-21.)
- **EMPHASIS-HF Trial**
    - This was a randomized, double-blind trial comparing eplerenone to placebo, in addition to recommended therapy, with a primary outcome of the composite of death from CV causes or hospitalization for HF.
    - Eplerenone significantly reduced the primary outcome risk (composite of death from CV causes or hospitalization for HF), causing the study to be stopped early.
    - Patients receiving eplerenone were also less likely to be hospitalized for HF and any cause.
    - More patients receiving eplerenone had serious hyperkalemia compared to placebo.
    - The authors concluded that eplerenone reduced both the risk of death and the risk of hospitalization among patients with systolic HF and mild symptoms compared to placebo. (N Engl J Med. 2011 Jan 6;364(1):11-21.)
- **TOPCAT Trial**
    - This was a multicenter, double-blind trial that randomized patients with HFpEF to receive either spironolactone or placebo to assess the primary outcome of death from CV causes, aborted cardiac arrest, or hospitalization for HF.
    - There was no significant difference between the groups concerning the primary outcome.
    - Spironolactone significantly reduced hospitalization risk for HF but did not significantly decrease death from cardiac arrest or death from CV causes.
    - Treatment with spironolactone was associated with increased SCr levels and a doubling of hyperkalemia rate compared to placebo.
    - The authors concluded that in patients with HFpEF, treatment with spironolactone did not significantly reduce the incidence of the primary composite outcome of death from CV causes, aborted cardiac arrest, or hospitalization to manage HF. (N Engl J Med. 2014 Apr 10;370(15):1383-92.)

High-Yield Fast-Facts
- **Active Metabolites**
    - Spironolactone has two active metabolites with prolonged half-lives. These agents are canrenone (half-life 12-20 hours) and 7-alpha-spironolactone (half-life 14 hours).
- **Triamterene and Folic Acid**
    - In patients with hepatic cirrhosis taking triamterene, folic acid supplementation should be considered since triamterene is a weak folic acid antagonist and may increase the risk of megaloblastic anemia.
- **Amiloride Alternative Uses**
    - Amiloride may improve mucociliary clearance in patients with cystic fibrosis and may be useful for lithium-induced nephrogenic DI.

HIGH-YIELD BOARD EXAM ESSENTIALS
- **CLASSIC AGENTS:** Amiloride, eplerenone, finerenone, spironolactone, triamterene
- **DRUG CLASS:** Potassium sparing diuretics
- **INDICATIONS:** Ascites (spironolactone), CKD in DM2 (finerenone), HF (eplerenone, spironolactone), HTN (amiloride, eplerenone, spironolactone, triamterene), primary hyperaldosteronism (spironolactone)
- **MECHANISM:** Amiloride, triamterene: inhibits sodium reabsorption by blocking sodium channels in the late DCT; eplerenone, spironolactone: inhibition of aldosterone on mineralocorticoid receptors in collecting tubules.
- **SIDE EFFECTS:** Gynecomastia (mainly spironolactone), impotence, and menstrual irregularities (spironolactone), dose-dependent hyperkalemia, renal insufficiency.
- **CLINICAL PEARLS:**
    - Aldosterone antagonists can prevent remodeling in patients with HF and are recommended by the guidelines (supported by RALES and EPHESUS).
    - They can elicit acidemia because the same process that prevents potassium elimination also prevents the elimination of hydrogen in the collecting tubule's intercalated cells, like a type IV renal tubular acidosis.
    - Spironolactone is commonly used in the chronic management of ascites from cirrhosis in high doses with a lower dose of furosemide (dose ratio is 100:40) to prevent hyperkalemia.
    - Finerenone use is mainly as an adjunct to other standard treatments in patients with Type 2 DM + CKD and albumin-to-creatinine ratio > 30 mg/g despite other treatments.
    - Eplerenone and finerenone are major substrates of CYP3A4 and prone to interactions that can cause concentration dependent risk for hyperkalemia.

Table: Drug Class Summary

\multicolumn{4}{c}{**Potassium-Sparing Diuretics - Drug Class Review**}
\multicolumn{4}{c}{High-Yield Med Reviews}
\multicolumn{4}{l}{**Mechanism of Action:** *Amiloride, triamterene: inhibits sodium reabsorption by blocking sodium channels in the late DCT; eplerenone, spironolactone: inhibition of aldosterone on mineralocorticoid receptors in collecting tubules.*}
\multicolumn{4}{l}{**Class Effects:** *Weak diuresis, aldosterone antagonism reducing cardiac remodeling (eplerenone, spironolactone), resistant HTN management (spironolactone), hyperkalemia*}
Generic Name	**Brand Name**	**Main Indication(s) or Uses**	**Notes**

Amiloride	Midamor	• Heart failure
		• Hypertension
			• **Dosing (Adult):**
			   – Oral: 5 mg daily; Max 40 mg/day
			• **Dosing (Peds):**
			   – Oral: 0.3 to 0.625 mg/kg/day; Max 20 mg/day
			• **CYP450 Interactions:** None
			• **Renal or Hepatic Dose Adjustments:**
			   – CrCl 10-50 mL/min: Reduce dose by 50%
			   – CrCl < 10 mL/minute: Avoid use
			• **Dosage Forms:** Oral (tablet)

Eplerenone	Inspra	• Heart failure, post-MI
		• Hypertension
			• **Dosing (Adult):**
			   – Oral: 25 mg daily; Max 50 mg/day
			• **Dosing (Peds):** Not routinely used
			• **CYP450 Interactions:** CYP 3A4 substrate
			• **Renal or Hepatic Dose Adjustments:**
			   – eGFR 31-49: Initial: 25 mg every other day, max 25 mg/day
			   – eGFR 30 or less: Not recommended
			• **Dosage Forms:** Oral (tablet)

Finerenone	Kerendia	• CKD on Type 2 DM	• **Dosing (Adult):**
			   – Oral (only if K+ is < 5 mEq/L and GFR > 25 mL/min): 10-20 mg daily; Max 20 mg/day
			• **Dosing (Peds):** Not routinely used
			• **CYP450 Interactions:** CYP 3A4 substrate (major)
			• **Renal or Hepatic Dose Adjustments:**
			   – eGFR >25 to < 60 mL/min: Initial: 10 mg daily
			   – eGFR 25 or less: Not recommended
			• **Dosage Forms:** Oral (tablet)

Spironolactone	Aldactone	• Ascites
		• Heart failure
		• Hypertension
		• Primary hyperaldosteronism
			• **Dosing (Adult):**
			   – Oral: 12.5 mg daily
			     – Max 200 mg/day
			• **Dosing (Peds):**
			   – Oral: 1-3 mg/kg/day
			     – Max 3 mg/kg/day or 100 mg/day
			• **CYP450 Interactions:** None
			• **Renal or Hepatic Dose Adjustments:**
			   – eGFR 30-50: Initial: 12.5 mg every other day, max 25 mg/day
			   – eGFR < 30: Not recommended
			• **Dosage Forms:** Oral (solution, tablet)

Potassium-Sparing Diuretics - Drug Class Review				
High-Yield Med Reviews				
Mechanism of Action: *Amiloride, triamterene: inhibits sodium reabsorption by blocking sodium channels in the late DCT; eplerenone, spironolactone: inhibition of aldosterone on mineralocorticoid receptors in collecting tubules.*				
Class Effects: *Weak diuresis, aldosterone antagonism reducing cardiac remodeling (eplerenone, spironolactone), resistant HTN management (spironolactone), hyperkalemia*				
Generic Name	**Brand Name**	**Main Indication(s) or Uses**	**Notes**	

Triamterene	Dyrenium	• Edema
		• Hypertension
			• **Dosing (Adult):**
			  – Oral: 50 mg daily
			    – Max 300 mg/day
			• **Dosing (Peds):**
			  – Oral: 1-4 mg/kg/day divided into 1 to 2 doses
			    – Max 6 mg/kg/day or 300 mg/day
			• **CYP450 Interactions:** None
			• **Renal or Hepatic Dose Adjustments:**
			  – CrCl 50 mL/min or less: avoid
			  – Severe hepatic impairment: Contraindicated
			• **Dosage Forms:** Oral (capsule)	

CARDIOVASCULAR – DIURETICS - CARBONIC ANHYDRASE INHIBITORS & OSMOTIC AGENTS

Drug Class
- **Carbonic Anhydrase Inhibitors**
    - Acetazolamide
    - Methazolamide
- **Osmotic Diuretics**
    - Mannitol

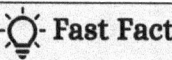 **Fast Facts**

✓ *The three most common uses of acetazolamide in current clinical practice are for prevention of mountain sickness, patients with acute glaucoma with sudden worsening of intraocular pressure (IOP) that can lead to blindness, and in patients with pseudotumor cerebri.*

Main Indications or Uses
- **Acute Care:**
    - Acute altitude/mountain sickness
        - Acetazolamide
    - Elevated intraocular or intracranial pressure
        - Mannitol
- **Chronic Care:**
    - Edema
        - Acetazolamide
    - Epilepsy
        - Acetazolamide

Mechanism of Action
- **Carbonic anhydrase inhibitor**
    - Inhibition of carbonic anhydrase blunts sodium bicarbonate reabsorption, promoting diuresis.
        - Carbonic anhydrase is responsible for converting carbonic acid to carbon dioxide at the renal luminal membrane and rehydration of carbon dioxide to the carbonic acid in the cytoplasm.
        - By blocking these processes, carbonic anhydrase inhibitors promote a reduction of hydrogen secretion and increased renal excretion of sodium, potassium, bicarbonate, and water.
- **Osmotic diuretic**
    - Mannitol is a solute that cannot be reabsorbed and increases the glomerulus' osmotic pressure, causing inhibition of tubular reabsorption of water and nearly all electrolytes.

Primary Net Benefit
- **Carbonic Anhydrase Inhibitors**
    - The limited diuretic effect and clinically used for other indications where carbonic anhydrase inhibitors may be beneficial.
- **Osmotic Diuretics**
    - Used to decrease elevated intracranial pressure, a notable sequela for this agent, with osmotic diuresis. As a result, hypertonic saline is preferred since it maintains hemodynamic effects but does not induce osmotic diuresis.
- **Main Labs to Monitor:**
    - **Acetazolamide**
        - Urine output, urine osmolarity daily
        - Serum electrolytes daily
        - Intraocular pressure every 30 to 60 minutes for acute angle-closure glaucoma
    - **Mannitol**
        - Intracranial pressure
            - Serum osmolality maintained less than 320 mOsm/kg.
                - Osmole gap less than 20
            - Urine output, urine osmolarity daily
            - Serum electrolytes daily

High-Yield Basic Pharmacology
- Carbonic anhydrase inhibitors are sulfonamide derivatives.
  - There is a theoretical risk of cross-reactivity in patients with a history of sulfonamide hypersensitivity.
    - As a result of its sulfonamide structure, carbonic anhydrase inhibitors carry a risk of bone marrow depression, Stevens-Johnson Syndrome, and sulfonamide-like kidney injury.
- Acetazolamide and methazolamide may cause a diversion of ammonia from urine into the systemic circulation, which can worsen existing hepatic encephalopathy.

High-Yield Clinical Knowledge
- **Hyperchloremic Metabolic Acidosis**
  - Carbonic anhydrase inhibitors block the excretion of hydrogen ions accumulating in the plasma.
    - In normal healthy kidneys, reabsorb bicarbonate and offsets the accumulation of hydrogen and ensuing acidosis.
    - With impaired renal function, high doses, or otherwise altered metabolic function, renal tubules' capacity to reabsorb bicarbonate is impaired, increasing acidosis.
      - The acidosis typically resolves upon discontinuation of the carbonic anhydrase inhibitor.
- **Reflection coefficient**
  - The reflection coefficient is the relative impermeability of a given agent concerning the blood-brain barrier, where a reflection coefficient of zero suggests a free permeability molecule. At the same time, a value of 1 represents an entirely impermeable molecule.
    - The reflection coefficient for mannitol is 0.9, and with a high dose and prolonged use, it can cross the blood-brain barrier.
    - With repeated dosing, mannitol crosses the blood-brain barrier, diminishing the osmotic gradient and the response to elevated intracranial.
- **Mannitol Administration**
  - Mannitol must be administered with a 5-micron in-line filter.
    - Mannitol is poorly soluble in water, frequently precipitates, and could cause vascular trauma and decreased therapeutic response to mannitol.
      - Mannitol may be stored in a warm environment to reduce the risk of crystallization. However, even after visual inspection, it is still required to be administered with an in-line filter.
- **Mannitol and Hypernatremia**
  - Although mannitol promotes water and sodium elimination, the proportion of natriuresis is relatively lower than free water diuresis.
  - With prolonged use, this effect can produce hypernatremia.
- **Starling Forces and Intracranial Pressure**
  - In addition to diuresis, mannitol promotes a shift in Starling forces and promotes water movement out of cells, reducing intracellular volume.
    - This effect is used to reduce intracranial pressure or intraocular pressure.
    - However, the effect is not sustained with continued use as mannitol can cross the blood-brain barrier in small quantities and reduce free water movement.
      - Hyponatremia can occur in patients with severe renal impairment because of the relative increase in free water movement into the extracellular space without a corresponding free water elimination in the kidney.
- **Limited Carbonic Anhydrase Inhibitor Use as a Diuretic**
  - The use of carbonic anhydrase inhibitors as diuretics is rare, given the likelihood of developing metabolic acidosis with long-term use.
  - Carbonic anhydrase inhibitors are primarily used for open-angle glaucoma (brinzolamide and dorzolamide).
  - Oral acetazolamide can treat glaucoma but is more commonly used in patients with absence seizures.
  - Although acetazolamide is often referenced to be useful in patients with high-altitude illness or mountain sickness, an inspection of the wilderness medicine literature reveals that this effect is small and similar to that of ibuprofen.

High-Yield Core Evidence
- **HEAT Trial**
  - This prospective, double-blind, randomized, placebo-controlled trial compared ibuprofen, acetazolamide, or placebo to prevent high-altitude headaches and acute mountain sickness in healthy western trekkers in Nepal Himalaya.
  - There was no difference between ibuprofen and acetazolamide concerning the primary outcome of the incidence of high-altitude headaches and acute mountain sickness. Still, both agents were significantly more effective than the placebo.
  - The authors concluded that ibuprofen and acetazolamide were similarly effective in preventing high-altitude headaches and acute mountain sickness. (Wilderness Environ Med. 2010 Sep;21(3):236-43.)
- **Mannitol Vs. HTS**
  - This study was a prospective, parallel-group, randomized, controlled trial designed to compare the effects of equimolar doses of 20% mannitol solution and 7.45% hypertonic saline solution in treating patients with sustained elevated intracranial pressure (ICP).
  - There was no difference between treatments in the reduction of ICP during the experiment.
  - Cerebral perfusion pressure and diastolic and mean blood flow velocities were increased in the mannitol group compared to hypertonic saline, but this did not lead to any major changes in brain tissue oxygen tension.
  - Mannitol caused a significantly greater increase in urine output than hypertonic saline.
  - The authors concluded that a single equimolar infusion of 20% mannitol is as effective as 7.45% sodium chloride in decreasing ICP in patients with brain injury. (Crit Care Med. 2008 Mar;36(3):795-800.)
- **Acetazolamide for Nephrotic Edema**
  - This randomized, double-blind, parallel-arm trial was designed to assess acetazolamide plus hydrochlorothiazide followed by furosemide compared to furosemide plus hydrochlorothiazide by furosemide for the treatment of refractory nephrotic edema.
  - Patients randomized to the acetazolamide regimen had a significantly larger absolute change in weight before and after each treatment phase.
  - The increase in 24-hour urine volume was also significantly higher in group 1 at the end of phase 2.
  - The authors concluded that acetazolamide and hydrochlorothiazide followed by furosemide are more effective than furosemide and hydrochlorothiazide, followed by furosemide to treat refractory nephrotic edema. (Am J Kidney Dis. 2017 Mar;69(3):420-427.)
- **Acetazolamide Plus Loop Diuretic vs Loop Diuretic Alone**
  - This was a multicenter, prospective study designed to determine acetazolamide's effect on natriuresis, decongestion, kidney function, and neurohumoral activation in acute heart failure patients randomized to either acetazolamide plus bumetanide or high-dose bumetanide alone.
  - There was no difference in the primary outcome of natriuresis after 24 h.
  - Acetazolamide improved loop diuretic efficiency assessed by natriuresis corrected for loop diuretic dose.
  - There was a non-significant trend towards lower all-cause mortality or heart failure readmissions in the group receiving acetazolamide. More patients in the combinational treatment arm increased serum creatinine levels of more than 0.3 mg/dL from baseline.
  - The authors concluded that acetazolamide's addition increases the natriuretic response to loop diuretics compared to an increase in loop diuretic dose in AHF at high risk for diuretic resistance. (Eur J Heart Fail. 2019 Nov;21(11):1415-1422.)

High-Yield Fast-Facts
- **Slow Administration**
  - Mannitol should be administered slowly over at least 30 minutes to reduce the risk of hypotension.
- **Topical Carbonic Anhydrase Inhibition**
  - The ophthalmologic carbonic anhydrase inhibitors (brinzolamide and dorzolamide) are critical components of glaucoma management.
- **Mannitol Crystallization**
  - If mannitol crystallizes, it can be placed into the pharmacy's specific mannitol warming storage area to allow for re-solubilization.

HIGH-YIELD BOARD EXAM ESSENTIALS
- **CLASSIC AGENTS:** Acetazolamide, mannitol, methazolamide
- **DRUG CLASS:** Osmotic diuretics (mannitol), carbonic anhydrase inhibitors (acetazolamide, methazolamide)
- **INDICATIONS:** Acute altitude/mountain sickness, edema, epilepsy (acetazolamide), elevated intraocular or intracranial pressure (mannitol),
- **MECHANISM:** Inhibits the reabsorption of sodium bicarbonate, promoting diuresis (carbonic anhydrase inhibitor). Increases osmotic pressure of the glomerulus and inhibition of tubular reabsorption of water and electrolytes (osmotic diuretic).
- **SIDE EFFECTS:** Hyperkalemic metabolic acidosis, hypernatremia, acute kidney injury.
- **CLINICAL PEARLS:** The use of carbonic anhydrase inhibitors as diuretics is rare, given the likelihood of developing metabolic acidosis with long-term use; carbonic anhydrase inhibitors are primarily used for open-angle glaucoma (brinzolamide and dorzolamide). However, acetazolamide is probably most commonly used in pseudotumor cerebri.

Table: Drug Class Summary

| \multicolumn{4}{c}{**Osmotic Diuretics - Drug Class Review**} |
| \multicolumn{4}{c}{High-Yield Med Reviews} |

Mechanism of Action:
Carbonic anhydrase inhibitor - *inhibits the reabsorption of sodium bicarbonate, promoting diuresis.*
Osmotic diuretic - *Increases osmotic pressure of the glomerulus and inhibition of tubular reabsorption of water and electrolytes thereby promoting some degree of diuresis.*

Class Effects: *Diuresis, intravascular volume decreases, electrolyte abnormalities.*

Generic Name	Brand Name	Main Indication(s) or Uses	Notes
Acetazolamide	Diamox	<ul><li>Acute altitude/mountain sickness</li><li>Glaucoma/Elevated intraocular pressure</li><li>Edema</li><li>Epilepsy</li></ul>	<ul><li>**Dosing (Adult):**<ul><li>Oral: 125 to 500 mg once to four times per day</li><li>Maximum 30 mg/kg/day</li><li>IV: 500 mg once</li></ul></li><li>**Dosing (Peds):**<ul><li>Oral: 2.5 to 30 mg/kg/dose q12h</li><li>Maximum 1000 mg/day</li></ul></li><li>**CYP450 Interactions:** None</li><li>**Renal or Hepatic Dose Adjustments:**<ul><li>Contraindicated in severe renal impairment</li><li>Contraindicated in patients with cirrhosis or marked liver disease</li></ul></li><li>**Dosage Forms:** IV solution, oral (extended-release capsule, immediate-release tablet)</li></ul>
Mannitol	Osmitrol	<ul><li>Elevated intracranial pressure</li><li>Elevated intraocular pressure</li></ul>	<ul><li>**Dosing (Adult):**<ul><li>IV: 0.25 to 2 g/kg/dose</li><li>May repeat every 6 to 8 hours</li></ul></li><li>**Dosing (Peds):**<ul><li>IV: 0.25 to 2 g/kg/dose</li><li>May repeat every 6 to 8 hours</li></ul></li><li>**CYP450 Interactions:** None</li><li>**Renal or Hepatic Dose Adjustments:**<ul><li>PI states contraindicated in severe renal impairment, but this may not be observed clinically for these indications.</li></ul></li><li>**Dosage Forms:** IV solution</li></ul>
Methazolamide	Neptazane	<ul><li>Glaucoma/Elevated intraocular pressure</li></ul>	<ul><li>**Dosing (Adult):**<ul><li>Oral: 50 to 100 mg 2 to 3 times/day</li></ul></li><li>**Dosing (Peds):**<ul><li>Not routinely used</li></ul></li><li>**CYP450 Interactions:** None</li><li>**Renal or Hepatic Dose Adjustments:**<ul><li>Contraindicated in severe renal impairment</li><li>Contraindicated in patients with cirrhosis or marked liver disease</li></ul></li><li>**Dosage Forms:** Oral (tablet)</li></ul>

CARDIOVASCULAR – LOOP DIURETICS

Drug Class
- **Loop Diuretics**
  - Bumetanide
  - Ethacrynic acid
  - Furosemide
  - Torsemide

Main Indications or Uses
- **Acute & Chronic Care:**
  - Edema
  - Hypertension
  - Heart failure

> 💡 **Fast Facts**
>
> ✓ Ethacrynic acid is not hard to find but clinically almost never used. However, it is a common teaching point that it is the only loop diuretic without a sulfa moiety though the clinical relevance of the sulfa moiety in the other agents is very questionable.

Mechanism of Action
- Prevent the kidney's ability to concentrate urine by inhibiting the activity of the sodium-potassium-2-chloride symporter in the thick ascending limb of the loop of Henle.
  - The primary effect is the increased urinary elimination of sodium and chloride; however, numerous other solutes are also eliminated (bicarbonate, hydrogen, magnesium, phosphate, potassium, and uric acid).

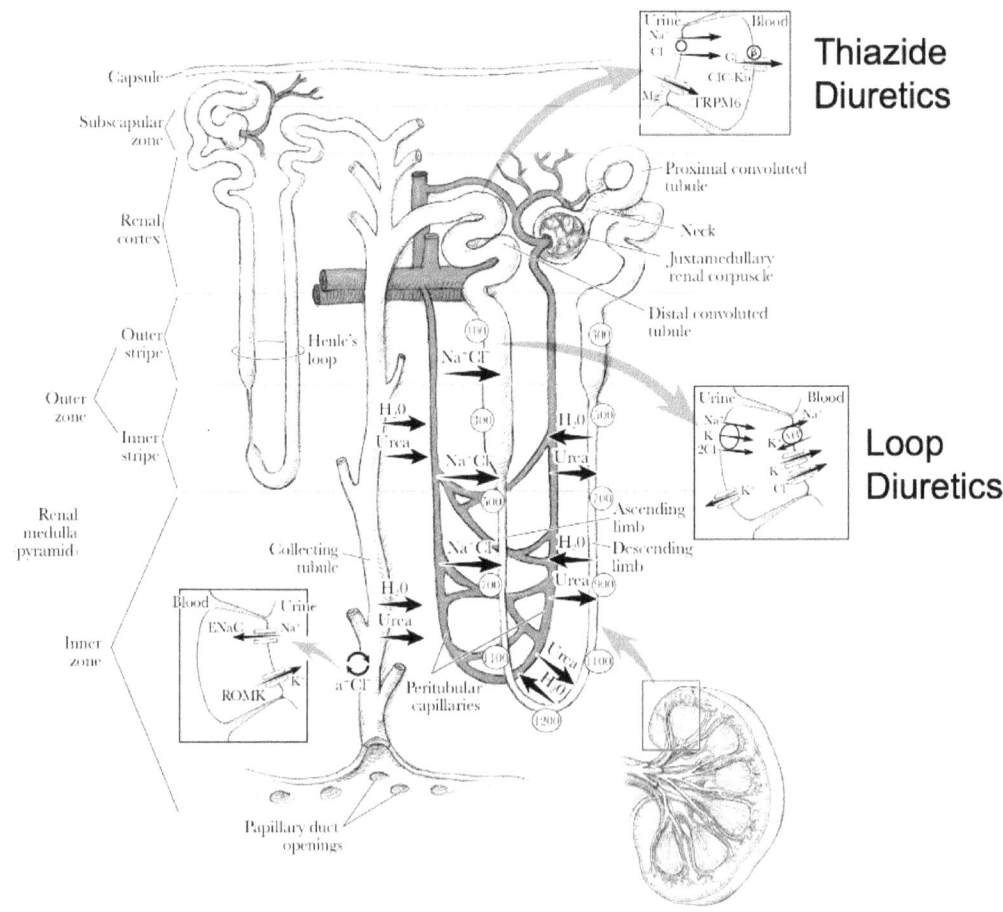

Primary Net Benefit
- Loop diuretics produce acute and sustained diuresis more than most available diuretics on the market. As such, they are most useful for fluid overload or edema.
    - However, long-term effects may be net-negative to therapeutic outcomes if the counterregulatory neurohormonal response is not accounted for.
- Main Labs to Monitor:
    - Blood pressure, particularly orthostatic pressures initially.
    - Serum electrolytes (Na, K, Mg, Ca since they all can be lost in the urine)
    - Renal function (baseline, after one week, then periodically) due to risk of over diuresis leading to pre-renal azotemia

High-Yield Basic Pharmacology
- Acute administration of loop diuretics increases uric acid excretion, but with chronic administration, uric acid excretion is inhibited.
    - This effect may result from enhanced proximal tubule transport or competition between uric acid and the loop diuretic for organic acid secretion in the proximal tubule.
- Loop diuretics can enhance renal blood flow by increasing prostaglandin synthesis and prostaglandin-induced vasodilation.
- Diuretic braking is a counterregulatory process of balancing sodium excretion with sodium intake and occurs in response to the short-lived natriuretic effect of diuretics.
    - This finite course natriuresis results from renal compensatory mechanisms that bring sodium excretion in line with sodium intake, including the sympathetic nervous system activation, RAAS activation, decreased MAP, renal epithelial cell hypertrophy, and increased renal epithelial transporter expression.

High-Yield Clinical Knowledge
- Not For All Heart Failure Patients
    - In patients with AHA Stage C or higher HFrEF or HFpEF, loop diuretics may be added for patients with persistent peripheral or pulmonary edema.
        - Early use of loop diuretics without appropriate RAAS inhibition (ACE-inhibitor/ARB/neprilysin-ARB, and beta-blocker) and sympathetic nervous system inhibition (beta-blocker) can potentially worsen heart failure due to activation of these neurohormonal responses.
- Acute Decompensated Heart Failure
    - The benefit of loop diuretics in acute decompensated heart failure is more relevant to their vasodilatory effects than diuretic effects.
        - Loop diuretics can acutely increase systemic venous capacitance and decrease left ventricular filling pressure via prostaglandin production and thus vasodilation.
    - Some ADHF patients may be depleted intravascularly, and loop diuretic administration alone can worsen their clinical condition.
        - In patients with ADHF from a myocardial infarction or rapid vascular resistance increases or afterload, plasma volume may be contracted.
            - In this setting attempts to reduce volume with diuresis or even vasodilation would be met with worsening ADHF. These patients often require IV fluid bolus administered in delicate aliquots to maintain cardiac output.
- Dose equivalents
    - Changing between loop diuretic agents can be accomplished using accepted approximate oral dose equivalencies.
    - These should only be used in patients with normal renal function.
        - Furosemide 40 mg = bumetanide 1 mg = torsemide 20 mg
- Non-CYP450 Drug Interactions
    - Aminoglycosides
        - Loop diuretic-associated ototoxicity manifests as tinnitus, hearing impairment, deafness, vertigo, and a sense of fullness in the ears.
        - Different from aminoglycoside ototoxicity, loop diuretic hearing impairment is usually reversible upon discontinuation or dose adjustment.

- Ototoxicity can also occur with concomitant amphotericin B, carboplatin, and paclitaxel.
- Digoxin
    - Loop diuretics promote potassium and magnesium clearance, which may predispose patients to digoxin toxicity, even if there are therapeutic levels before initiation.
        - Hypokalemia reduces the sodium-potassium-ATPase pump activity and enhances pump inhibition induced by digoxin, increasing dysrhythmias risk.
        - Hypomagnesemia increases the risk of dysrhythmias from digoxin toxicity due to decreased sodium-potassium-ATPase pump exchange activity.
- Lithium
    - Loop diuretics increase urinary sodium loss and decrease lithium excretion.
- Insulin & Sulfonylureas
    - Loop diuretics may increase insulin resistance and decrease insulin release.
- NSAIDs
    - Blunted diuretic effect by preventing prostaglandin-mediated increases in renal blood flow and risk of nephrotoxicity.
    - Increase RAAS activation, blunting diuretic response, and increased risk of hyperkalemia.
- Probenecid
    - Increases serum concentrations but blunt therapeutic effects of loop diuretic by competing for active tubular secretion.
- **Sulfa Allergy**
    - The loop diuretics bumetanide and furosemide contain a sulfonamide moiety, and torsemide is a sulfonylurea. This often raises the concern of sulfonamide allergy and cross-sensitivity to other "sulfa" containing drugs.
        - A retrospective study found that despite an association between hypersensitivity after receiving sulfonamide antibiotics and a subsequent allergic reaction after receiving a sulfonamide nonantibiotic, this association appears to be due to a predisposition to allergic reactions rather than to cross-reactivity with sulfonamide-based drugs. (N Engl J Med. 2003 Oct 23;349(17):1628-35.)
- **Clinical Difference Between Agents**
    - While furosemide is the most commonly used agent in this class, there is no proven benefit over bumetanide or torsemide.

High-Yield Core Evidence
- **DOSE Study**
    - This prospective, double-blind, randomized trial of patients with acute decompensated heart failure comparing a continuous infusion or intermittent bolus strategy AND a high or low dose furosemide regimen.
    - There was no difference between any treatment comparison (continuous infusion or intermittent bolus AND high or low dose strategy) in the primary outcome of global assessment of symptoms or the mean change in the creatinine level.
    - Patients randomized to high-dose saw a nonsignificant trend toward greater improvement in patients' global assessment of symptoms.
    - This benefit and the observed greater diuresis in the high-dose strategy group were offset by the transient renal function's transient worsening.
    - The authors conclude that among patients with acute decompensated heart failure, there were no significant differences in patient's global assessment of symptoms or in the change in renal function when diuretic therapy was administered by bolus as compared with a continuous infusion or at a high dose as compared with a low dose. (N Engl J Med. 2011 Mar 3;364(9):797-805.)

- **ADHERE Registry Data**
  - This is a subgroup analysis of the ADHERE registry to examine the impact of diuretic dosing.
  - This analysis's primary outcome was to describe the baseline demographic and clinical characteristics of patients hospitalized for ADHF and to examine associations between in-hospital management and clinical outcomes.
  - In this analysis, 62,866 patients receiving less than 160 mg and 19,674 patients with at least 160 mg of furosemide were analyzed.
  - The patients receiving the lower doses had a lower risk for in-hospital mortality, ICU stay, prolonged hospitalization, or adverse renal effects.
  - These findings suggest that future studies should evaluate strategies for minimizing exposure to high doses of diuretics. (Cardiology. 2009;113(1):12-9.)
- **ESCAPE trial**
  - This was a subgroup analysis of the ESCAPE trial, which was a randomized trial of pulmonary artery catheter-guided therapy versus standard therapy in patients hospitalized with decompensated heart failure with a primary endpoint of the number of days since randomization; the patient was neither dead nor hospitalized within 180 days after randomization.
  - In this subgroup, there was no statistically significant difference between patients receiving diuretics compared to those not receiving diuretics in hospital in relation to maximal in-hospital diuretic dose to weight loss, changes in renal function, and mortality in hospitalized heart failure (HF) patients.
  - The authors noted a strong relationship between diuretic doses and mortality was seen notably when doses exceeded 300 mg/day.
  - Dose remained a significant predictor of mortality after adjusting for baseline variables that significantly predicted mortality.
  - The authors concluded that high diuretic doses during heart failure hospitalization are associated with increased mortality and poor 6-month outcome. (Eur J Heart Fail. 2007 Oct;9(10):1064-9.)

High-Yield Fast-Facts
- **Oral Diuretic and Food**
  - When bumetanide or furosemide are administered with food, bioavailability can significantly decrease. There is no effect from food on the bioavailability of torsemide.
- **Oral or IV for ADHF**
  - While oral loop diuretic dosing regimens exist, the true bioavailability in this scenario may be lower or unpredictable due to decreased gut perfusion.
- **Limited primary literature**
  - Despite loop diuretics being a component of cardiovascular and renal therapeutics for decades, there is limited high-quality prospective evidence to support their use in this setting.

HIGH-YIELD BOARD EXAM ESSENTIALS
- **CLASSIC AGENTS:** Bumetanide, ethacrynic acid, furosemide, torsemide
- **DRUG CLASS:** Loop diuretics
- **INDICATIONS:** Edema, hypertension, heart failure
- **MECHANISM:** Prevent the kidney's ability to concentrate urine by inhibiting the activity of the sodium-potassium-2-chloride symporter in the thick ascending limb of the loop of Henle.
- **SIDE EFFECTS:** Volume depletion, hypokalemia, hyponatremia, ototoxicity
- **CLINICAL PEARLS:**
  - In patients with AHA Stage C or higher HFrEF or HFpEF, loop diuretics may be added for patients with persistent peripheral or pulmonary edema, but early use of loop diuretics without appropriate RAAS inhibition and sympathetic nervous system inhibition can potentially worsen heart failure due to activation of these neurohormonal responses.
  - Low dose loops are usually added to high dose spironolactone for the management of ascites.
  - Loop diuretics are commonly associated with causing hypokalemia and hypomagnesemia.

Table: Drug Class Summary

Loop Diuretics - Drug Class Review High-Yield Med Reviews			
Mechanism of Action: *Inhibits the sodium-potassium-2-chloride symporter in the thick ascending limb of the loop of Henle.*			
Class Effects: *Cause relevant diuresis in those with fluid overload and edema. However, can cause loss of Na+, K+, Mg++, and Calcium. Over diuresis can also result in pre-renal azotemia. They cause dose-dependent ototoxicity.*			
Generic Name	**Brand Name**	**Main Indication(s) or Uses**	**Notes**
Bumetanide	Bumex	• Edema • Heart failure • Hypertension	• **Dosing (Adult):** – Oral: 0.5 to 2 mg divided once to TID – IV: bolus 0.5 to 1 mg, or 1 to 2.5 times the total daily dose – IV: infusion 0.5 to 2 mg/hour • **Dosing (Peds):** – All routes (oral, IM, IV) 0.01 to 0.1 mg/kg/dose every 6 to 24 hours. – Maximum 10 mg/day – IV: infusion 1 to 10 mcg/kg/hour • **CYP450 Interactions:** None • **Renal or Hepatic Dose Adjustments:** None • **Dosage Forms:** IV solution, oral (tablet)
Ethacrynic acid	Edecrin	• Edema • Heart failure	• **Dosing (Adult):** – Oral: 50 mg daily; Maximum 400 mg daily – IV: 0.5 to 1 mg/kg/dose or fixed 50 mg • **Dosing (Peds):** – Oral: 1 mg/kg/dose Q24H – IV: 0.5 mg/kg/dose q8 to 24h or IV: infusion of 0.1 mg/kg/hour • **CYP450 Interactions:** None • **Renal or Hepatic Dose Adjustments:** None • **Dosage Forms:** IV solution, oral (tablet)
Furosemide	Lasix	• Edema • Heart failure • Hypertension	• **Dosing (Adult):** – Oral: 20 to 40 mg daily; Max: 160 mg daily – IV: 20 to 40 mg or 1 to 2.5 times the total daily dose; Max: 100 mg/dose – IV: 5 to 20 mg/hour; Max: 600 mg/day • **Dosing (Peds):** – IM or IV: 0.5 to 2 mg/kg/dose q6 to 12h – Maximum 6 mg/kg/day • **CYP450 Interactions:** None • **Renal or Hepatic Dose Adjustments:** – Acute renal failure - may need to increase the dose to a total daily dose of 1 to 3 g • **Dosage Forms:** IV solution, oral (tablet)
Torsemide	Demadex	• Edema • Heart failure • Hypertension	• **Dosing (Adult):** – Oral: 10 to 20 mg once daily; Max: 200 mg/day • **Dosing (Peds):** Not routinely used • **CYP450 Interactions:** Substrate of CYP2C8, CYP2C9 • **Renal or Hepatic Dose Adjustments:** None • **Dosage Forms:** Oral (tablet)

CARDIOVASCULAR – THIAZIDE DIURETICS

Drug Class
- **Thiazide Diuretics**
- **Agents:**
  - Chronic Care
    - Chlorthalidone
    - Chlorothiazide
    - Hydrochlorothiazide
    - Indapamide
    - Metolazone

> **Warnings or Alerts**
>
> ✓ The chronic use of any thiazide diuretic can commonly cause moderate to severe hyponatremia, especially in elderly patients due to the inability of the nephron to reabsorb Na+ being blocked at the DCT and thus eliminated from the body in urine slowly over time.

Main Indications or Uses
- **Chronic Care:**
  - Edema
  - Hypertension

Mechanism of Action
- Inhibit sodium and chloride transport in the early segment of the distal convoluted tubule (DCT) to promote the excretion of primarily sodium and water.

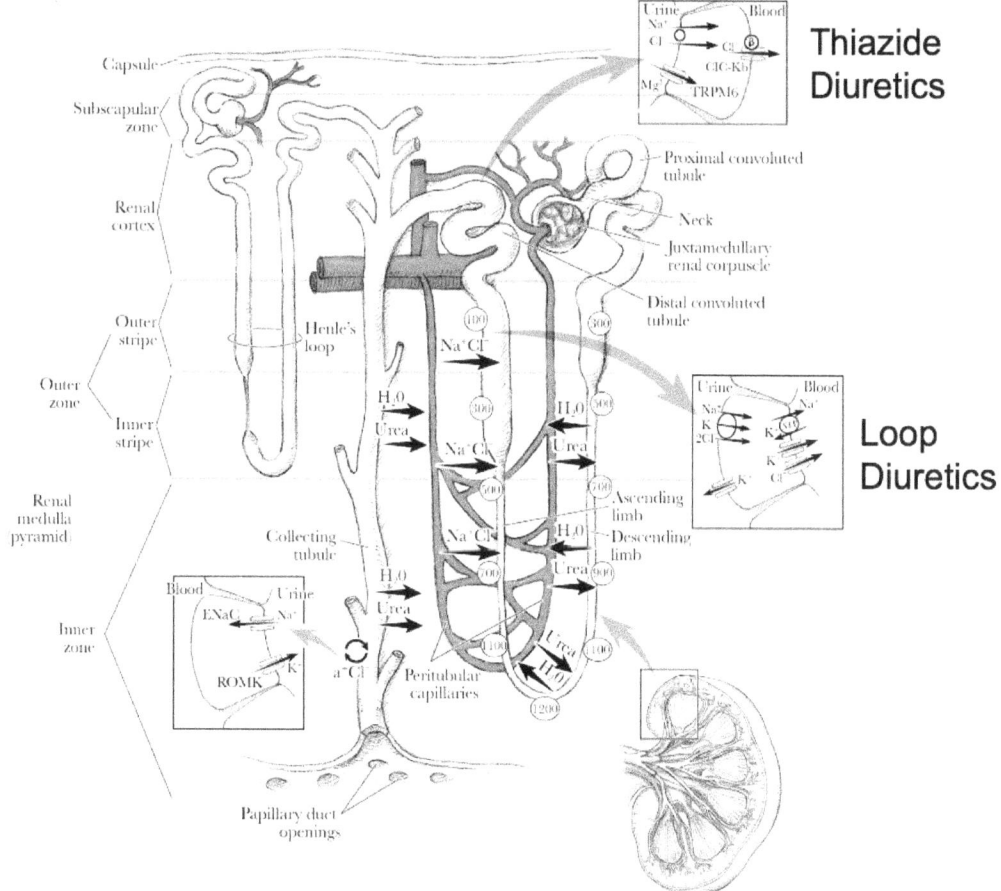

Primary Overall Benefit
- Long-standing history of clinical benefit in patients with HTN from a mechanism other than diuresis.
- Main Labs to Monitor:
  - BP, serum electrolytes, renal function at baseline then intermittently
  - Monitor glucose more frequently when starting in patients with diabetes to note any increase

High-Yield Basic Pharmacology
- **Chlorthalidone CV Benefits**
  - Chlorthalidone may possess greater CV benefits owing to its ability to inhibit carbonic anhydrase relative to other thiazide agents.
    - Carbonic anhydrase inhibition may affect CV (fluid volume balance, remodeling, vasodilation) and platelet functions. (Hypertension 2010;56:463-470.)
    - Hydrochlorothiazide and chlorthalidone both contain a sulfonamide moiety, which has been proposed to exert this carbonic anhydrase activity, but chlorthalidone possesses additional carbonic anhydrase properties.
- **Duration of Action**
  - Thiazides have a much longer duration and half-life, allowing daily dosing in most scenarios, compared to loop diuretics that have short half-lives (generally < 2 hours) and require multiple daily doses.
- **Calcium Reabsorption**
  - Thiazides increase renal tubular reabsorption of calcium and may be beneficial in patients with nephrolithiasis, osteopenia, or osteoporosis.

High-Yield Clinical Knowledge
- **Mechanism of Antihypertensive Effect**
  - Thiazide diuretics do not appear to exert their antihypertensive effect from their diuretic action as plasma and extracellular volumes return to baseline values within 4–6 weeks of initiation.
    - Thiazide-induced volume loss leads to decreased venous return, RAAS activation, sympathetic nervous system activation, reduced cardiac output, and decreased BP.
      - The leading theory describes the inhibition of norepinephrine-induced calcium influx in arteries and unidentified indirect vasodilatory actions.
  - Expert Rev Cardiovasc Ther 2010;8(6):793-802.
- **Lipids and Glucose**
  - Thiazide diuretics may increase total cholesterol, LDL, and triglycerides, as well as cause hyperglycemia via three proposed mechanisms (insulin resistance, decreased insulin release, and inhibition of glucose uptake).
    - There is speculation that thiazide-induced hyperglycemia may result from the effect of these agents on potassium.
      - Additional theories of thiazide-induced hyperglycemia involve hyperuricemia, changes in fat distribution, and PPAR-gamma downregulation.
    - Thiazide diuretics may also increase serum calcium by increasing calcium reabsorption in the distal convoluted tubule.
    - Similar to loop diuretics, thiazide agents may cause hyperuricemia.
- **Nephrogenic Diabetes Insipidus (DI)**
  - Thiazide diuretics are a key component in treating nephrogenic DI since they can reduce urine volume by half.
    - This action is mediated by thiazide-induced increased proximal tubular water reabsorption and the prevention of the distal convoluted tubule's ability to form dilute urine and increases urine osmolality.
- **Dosing Target**
  - Unlike other antihypertensive agents, thiazide diuretics do not need to be titrated to the maximum tolerated dose. HCTZ 50 mg does not typically confer additional benefits.
  - Most patients respond with a clinically relevant effect at initial doses and do not benefit from aggressive titration.
    - This effect may worsen HTN due to the unopposed activation of RAAS and the sympathetic nervous system.

- **Hydrochlorothiazide Versus Chlorthalidone**
    - Chlorthalidone and indapamide may reduce BP to a greater degree and further reduce CV events in hypertensive patients compared to hydrochlorothiazide (Hypertension. 2015, 65:1033–1040. Hypertension. 2015 May;65(5):1041-6.).
        - Despite a lack of head-to-head data, this effect is supported by their longer half-life relative to hydrochlorothiazide and better control of arterial BP.
    - In contrast, a large database comparative cohort study of 730,255 patients determined there was no difference in efficacy between chlorthalidone and HCTZ, but worse safety outcomes were observed with chlorthalidone.
        - JAMA Intern Med. 2020;180(4):542-551.

High-Yield Core Evidence
- **ALLHAT**
    - This was a landmark randomized, double-blind, active-controlled trial that randomly assigned patients to receive chlorthalidone, amlodipine, or lisinopril for planned follow-up of approximately 4-8 years.
    - There was no significant difference between any treatment regarding the primary outcome of combined fatal CHD or nonfatal MI.
    - When all-cause mortality was independently examined, there was no difference between groups.
    - The authors concluded that thiazide-type diuretics are superior in preventing 1 or more major forms of CVD and are less expensive. They should be preferred for first-step antihypertensive therapy. (JAMA. 2002 Dec 18;288(23):2981-97.)
- **CONVINCE**
    - This was a multicenter, double-blind, randomized trial of patients with HTN who had 1 or more additional risk factors for CVD randomized to receive verapamil and either atenolol or hydrochlorothiazide.
    - There was no significant difference between treatment groups regarding the primary outcome of the first occurrence of stroke, MI, or CVD-related death.
    - No significant difference was noted with stroke, MI, or CVD-related death treated as individual outcomes.
    - However, non-stroke hemorrhage was more common in patients receiving verapamil compared with atenolol or hydrochlorothiazide.
    - The authors concluded that calcium-channel therapy's effectiveness in reducing CVD is similar but not better than diuretic or beta-blocker treatment. (JAMA. 2003;289(16):2073–2082.)
- **ACE-inhibitor or Thiazide in the Elderly**
    - This study was a randomized, open-label study of patients with HTN who were 65-84 years old and randomized to either ACE inhibitors or thiazide diuretics.
    - There was a statistically significant difference in the primary outcome of CV events or deaths from any cause, which favored treatment with an ACE inhibitor. Benefits were larger in male than female patients.
    - The authors concluded that initiation of ACE inhibitors in older subjects, particularly men, appears to lead to better outcomes than treatment with diuretics, despite similar BP reductions. (N Engl J Med. 2003;348(7):583–592.)
- **ASCOT-BPLA**
    - This trial was a multicenter, prospective, randomized controlled trial that compared combinations of atenolol with a thiazide versus amlodipine with perindopril on nonfatal MI and fatal CHD.
    - There was no statistically significant difference in the primary endpoint of nonfatal MI and fatal CHD between groups.
    - However, fewer patients in the amlodipine-based arm had fatal and nonfatal strokes, total CV events and procedures, and all-cause mortality.
    - The authors concluded that amlodipine-based regimens prevented more major CV events and induced less diabetes than the atenolol-based regimen. (Lancet. 2005;366(9489):895–906.)

High-Yield Fast-Facts
- **Thiazide vs Thiazide-Like**
  - The true thiazide agents (chlorothiazide, hydrochlorothiazide) are benzothiadiazide derivatives, whereas the thiazide-like agents (chlorthalidone, indapamide, metolazone) are pharmacologically similar to thiazide diuretics but differ structurally.
- **Impaired Renal Function**
  - Thiazide diuretics should not be used in patients with impaired renal function (GFR < 30 mL/min) since their effects may be diminished or eliminated.
- **Diuretic Resistance**
  - Metolazone may be combined with a loop diuretic to overcome 'diuretic resistance' where a synergistic effect occurs with significantly improved diuresis.

HIGH-YIELD BOARD EXAM ESSENTIALS
- **CLASSIC AGENTS:** Chlorthalidone, chlorothiazide, hydrochlorothiazide, indapamide, metolazone
- **DRUG CLASS:** Thiazide diuretics
- **INDICATIONS:** Edema, hypertension
- **MECHANISM:** Inhibit sodium and chloride transport in the early segment of the distal convoluted tubule.
- **SIDE EFFECTS:** Volume depletion, electrolyte abnormalities (low Na, elevated Ca), increased total cholesterol, triglycerides, glucose elevations, hyperuricemia.
- **CLINICAL PEARLS:**
  - Thiazide diuretics do not appear to exert their antihypertensive effect from their diuretic action, as plasma and extracellular volumes return to baseline values within 4–6 weeks of initiation.

Cardiology

Table: Drug Class Summary

	Thiazide Diuretics - Drug Class Review High-Yield Med Reviews		
Mechanism of Action: *Inhibit sodium and chloride transport in the early segment of the distal convoluted tubule.*			
Class Effects: *Moderate sodium and chloride diuresis.*			
Generic Name	**Brand Name**	**Main Indication(s) or Uses**	**Notes**

Chlorthalidone	Thalitone	• Edema
		• Hypertension
			• **Dosing (Adult):**
			  – Oral: 12.5-25 mg once daily
			    – Max 100 mg/day
			• **Dosing (Peds):**
			  – Oral: 0.3 mg/kg/dose daily
			    – Max 2 mg/kg/day or 50 mg/day
			• **CYP450 Interactions:** None
			• **Renal or Hepatic Dose Adjustments:**
			  – CrCl < 30 mL/min: Use with loop
			  – CrCl < 10 mL/min: Avoid use
			• **Dosage Forms:** Oral (tablet)

Chlorothiazide	Diuril	• Edema
		• Hypertension
			• **Dosing (Adult):**
			  – Oral: 250-2,000 mg daily divided into 1-2 doses
			  – IV: 500-1000 mg daily
			• **Dosing (Peds):**
			  – Oral: 10-40 mg/kg/day in 1-2 divided doses
			    – Max 375 mg/day (children under 2).
			  – IV: 5-10 mg/kg/day in divided doses
			    – Max 20 mg/kg/day
			• **CYP450 Interactions:** None
			• **Renal or Hepatic Dose Adjustments:**
			  – CrCl 10-30 mL/min: Diuretic response significantly diminished but no specific dose adjustment
			  – CrCl < 10 mL/min: Avoid use
			• **Dosage Forms:** IV solution, oral (tablet)

Hydrochloro-thiazide	Microzide	• Edema
		• Hypertension
			• **Dosing (Adult):**
			  – Oral: 12.5-25 mg once daily
			    – Max 50 mg/day
			• **Dosing (Peds):**
			  – Oral: 1-2 mg/kg/day in 1-2 divided doses
			    – Max 37.5 mg/day
			• **CYP450 Interactions:** None
			• **Renal or Hepatic Dose Adjustments:**
			  – CrCl 10-30 mL/min: Diuretic response significantly diminished
			  – CrCl < 10 mL/min: Avoid use
			• **Dosage Forms:** Oral (capsule, tablet)

Thiazide Diuretics - Drug Class Review			
High-Yield Med Reviews			
Generic Name	**Brand Name**	**Main Indication(s) or Uses**	**Notes**

Indapamide	Indipam	- Heart Failure
		- Hypertension
			- **Dosing (Adult):**
			  - Oral: 1.25 mg daily
			    - Max 5 mg/day
			- **Dosing (Peds):**
			  - Not routinely used
			- **CYP450 Interactions:** None
			- **Renal or Hepatic Dose Adjustments:**
			  - GFR < 50: 1.25-2.5 mg/day
			- **Dosage Forms:** IV solution, oral (tablet)

Metolazone	Zaroxolyn	- Edema
		- Hypertension
			- **Dosing (Adult):**
			  - Oral: 2.5 mg
			    - Max 20 mg/day
			- **Dosing (Peds):**
			  - Oral: 0.2-0.4 mg/kg/day
			    - Usually in combination with furosemide
			    - Max 20 mg/day
			- **CYP450 Interactions:** None
			- **Renal or Hepatic Dose Adjustments:**
			  - Diuretic response significantly diminished, but no specific dose adjustment
			- **Dosage Forms:** Oral (tablet)

CARDIOVASCULAR – INOTROPES

Drug Class
- **Inotropes**
- **Agents:**
  - **Acute Care**
    - Dobutamine
    - Isoproterenol
    - Milrinone

> **Knowledge Integration**
> ✓ Dobutamine's beta-2 agonist activity can cause vasodilation in the vasculature thereby leading to a reduction in blood pressure despite the increase in cardiac output. This is why some patients require the addition of a vasopressor.

Main Indications or Uses
- **Acute Care**
  - Cardiac decompensation (dobutamine)
  - Heart failure with a reduced ejection fraction (milrinone)
  - Mild or transient episodes of heart block (Isoproterenol)

Mechanism of Action
- Dobutamine, isoproterenol, and milrinone share a common pathway in their action: increasing the heart's contractility by increasing cAMP, which allows for increased phospholipase activity, and enhanced calcium influx to cardiac cells during systole.
  - Dobutamine is a beta-1 and beta-2 agonist and alpha-1 agonist (dose-dependent).
  - Isoproterenol is a beta-1 and beta-2 agonist.
  - Milrinone is a phosphodiesterase-3 (PDE3) inhibitor.

Primary Net Benefit
- Inotropes increase the heart rate and force contraction to increase the stroke volume (SV) which all leads to the improvement in cardiac output but often are accompanied by vasodilation with escalating doses.
- Main Labs to Monitor:
  - No routine labs

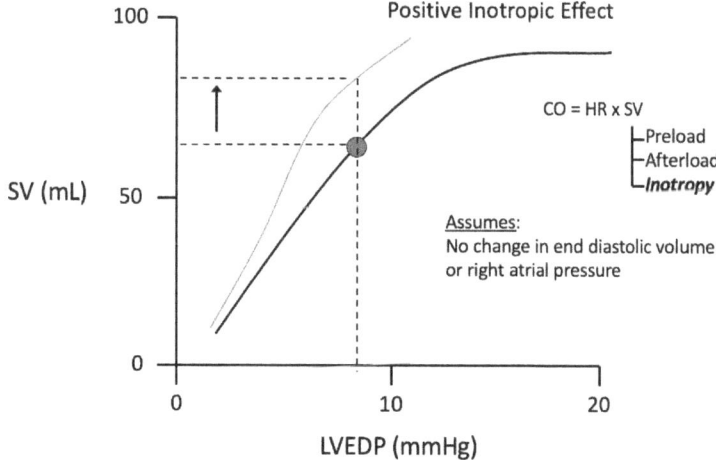

High-Yield Basic Pharmacology
- **Catecholamines Vs. Pressor/Inotropes**
  - The clinical classification of agents as vasopressors and inotropes describes the physiologic action of these drugs.
  - However, it is worth noting that these agents also differ in chemical classification.
    - The common term "catecholamine" refers to the drugs that share a beta-phenylethylamine core structure with hydroxyl groups substituted at positions 3 and 4 of the benzene ring.

- **Beta-Agonists**
  - Beta-1 agonists exert their effects through interaction with Gs protein receptors.
  - Secondary messaging promotes calcium uptake into the sarcoplasmic reticulum through activation of calcium-ATPase channels.
  - A similar interaction occurs via beta-2 agonist effects; however, the physiologic result is relaxation (vasodilation and bronchodilation).
- **Milrinone**
  - Phosphodiesterase inhibitors (PDEs) such as milrinone or amrinone increase cAMP, similar to beta-agonists; however, they do so by preventing its metabolism (through PDE-3 inhibition)

High-Yield Clinical Knowledge
- **Dobutamine Dose Response**
  - When the dose of dobutamine exceeds 20 mcg/kg/min, the proportional selectivity of beta-1 is lost, and beta-2 effects increase.
  - This change's net effect will likely lead to vasodilation and decreases in mean arterial pressure; this may be detrimental to cardiac perfusion and venous return.
  - Alternative agents and re-evaluation of the clinical strategy are needed if doses reach this threshold.
- **Ino-DILATORS**
  - While dobutamine, isoproterenol, and milrinone can increase cardiac output, they can also decrease peripheral vascular resistance.
  - In some scenarios, this can be beneficial by reducing preload and improving venous return but can lead to hypotension and hypoperfusion if not closely titrated.
- **Milrinone Warning**
  - Milrinone carries a black boxed warning that it should not be used for long-term management of heart failure.
  - However, many patients with end-stage heart failure or awaiting heart transplant may be on continuous/chronic outpatient infusions of milrinone.
  - This use is intended to prolong life until definitive care (i.e., a heart transplant or perhaps an LVAD) can be arranged.
- **Dobutamine/Isoproterenol Use**
  - Dobutamine may be used in clinical scenarios with preserved mean arterial pressure but a decreased cardiac output.
    - The use of isoproterenol is narrower, as it is used in patients with decreased cardiac output who are hypertensive.
  - As dopamine levels extend towards and beyond its upper limit of 20 mcg/kg/minute, heart rate will continue to increase, systemic vascular resistance will decrease, and stroke volume will decline due to impaired diastole leading to decreases in cardiac output.
- **Milrinone Use**
  - Milrinone is not often considered first-line due to a higher propensity to decrease vascular resistance and cause hypotension.
  - This decrease in vascular resistance extends to the pulmonary vasculature, making milrinone preferable in specific patient populations, such as pulmonary hypertension.
  - Since milrinone can bypass beta-blockade to exert its inodilatory effects compared to dobutamine, milrinone may be beneficial in supporting cardiac output in patients exposed to beta-blockers.
  - However, due to the prolonged onset of action (as a result of foregoing the bolus dose to avoid excessive hypotension), a four to six-hour half-life, and medication accumulation in renal failure patients, the clinical use of this drug is limited.

High-Yield Core Evidence
- **ADHERE**
  - This was a retrospective analysis of observational patient data from the Acute Decompensated Heart Failure National Registry (ADHERE), a multicenter registry designed to prospectively collect data on each episode of hospitalization for ADHF and its clinical outcomes.
  - Specific cases in which patients received nitroglycerin, nesiritide, milrinone, or dobutamine were identified and reviewed in this analysis.
  - The authors observed that patients who received intravenous nitroglycerin or nesiritide had lower in-hospital mortality than those treated with dobutamine or milrinone.
  - The authors concluded that therapy with either a natriuretic peptide or vasodilator was associated with significantly lower in-hospital mortality than positive inotropic treatment in patients hospitalized with ADHF. The risk of in-hospital mortality was similar for nesiritide and nitroglycerin. (J Am Coll Cardiol. 2005 Jul 5;46(1):57-64.)
- **Milrinone-Dobutamine Study Group**
  - This was a multicenter, open-label clinical trial designed to compare milrinone's hemodynamic and clinical effects with dobutamine in patients with congestive heart failure following acute myocardial infarction.
  - Dobutamine and milrinone were titrated to achieve a 30% increase in the cardiac index from the mean baseline or at least a 25% decrease in mean pulmonary capillary wedge pressure from baseline.
  - Both drugs improved cardiac index and mean pulmonary capillary wedge pressure.
  - Maximal reduction in mean pulmonary capillary wedge pressure over 0-3 hours was more significant in the milrinone group than in the dobutamine group, and reductions were sustained over 24 h.
  - Both drugs improved echocardiographic global ejection fraction and were generally well tolerated.
  - The authors concluded that the short-term infusion of milrinone might have a role in CHF management following AMI, especially when the aim is to reduce pulmonary congestion rapidly. (Clin Cardiol. 1996 Jan;19(1):21-30.)

High-Yield Fast-Fact
- **Digoxin**
  - Digoxin could also be considered an inotrope, as it increases the force of contraction of the heart.

HIGH-YIELD BOARD EXAM ESSENTIALS
- **CLASSIC AGENTS:** Dobutamine, isoproterenol, milrinone
- **DRUG CLASS:** Inotropes
- **INDICATIONS:** Cardiac decompensation (dobutamine), heart failure with a reduced ejection fraction (milrinone), mild or transient episodes of heart block (Isoproterenol)
- **MECHANISM:** Increasing the heart's contractility by increasing cAMP, which allows for increased phospholipase activity, and enhanced calcium influx to cardiac cells during systole.
- **SIDE EFFECTS:** Tachycardia, vasodilation
- **CLINICAL PEARLS:** Dobutamine can also stimulate the beta-2 receptor. When the dose of dobutamine exceeds 20 mcg/kg/min, the proportional selectivity of beta-1 is lost, and beta-2 effects increase; this change's net effect will likely lead to vasodilation and decreases in mean arterial pressure; this may be detrimental to cardiac perfusion and venous return. Due to this effect, sometimes a vasopressor may need to be added.

Table: Drug Class Summary

Inotropes - Drug Class Review			
High-Yield Med Reviews			
Mechanism of Action: Dobutamine is a beta-1 and beta-2 agonist and alpha-1 agonist (dose-dependent). Isoproterenol is a beta-1 and beta-2 agonist. Milrinone is a phosphodiesterase-3 (PDE3) inhibitor.			
Class Effects: Inotropes increase contractility and heart rate to improve cardiac output but often are accompanied by vasodilation with escalating doses.			
Generic Name	**Brand Name**	**Main Indication(s) or Uses**	**Notes**

Dobutamine	Dobutrex	• Cardiac decompensation	• **Dosing (Adult):**
			  – 2 to 20 mcg/kg/minute IV infusion
			• **Dosing (Peds):**
			  – 2 to 20 mcg/kg/minute IV infusion
			• **CYP450 Interactions:** Non-CYP (Linezolid- may enhance the hypertensive effect)
			• **Renal or Hepatic Dose Adjustments:** None
			• **Dosage Forms:** IV (solution)

Isoproterenol	Isuprel	Mild or transient episodes of heart block	• **Dosing (Adult):**
			  – 2 to 20 mcg/minute IV infusion
			• **Dosing (Peds):**
			  – 0.05 to 0.5 mcg/kg/minute IV
			• **CYP450 Interactions:** Non-CYP (Riociguat coadministration contraindicated)
			• **Renal or Hepatic Dose Adjustments:** None
			• **Dosage Forms:** IV (solution)

Milrinone	Primacor	• Heart failure with a reduced ejection fraction	• **Dosing (Adult):**
			  – Initial dose 0.375 mcg/kg/min (0.125 to 0.75 mcg/kg/minute) IV infusion
			• **Dosing (Peds):**
			  – 0.25 to 0.75 mcg/kg/minute IV infusion
			• **CYP450 Interactions:** Non-CYP (Linezolid- may enhance the hypertensive effect)
			• **Renal or Hepatic Dose Adjustments:**
			  – GFR 41-50 mL/minute: Initial dose 0.25 mcg/kg/min
			  – GFR 31-40 mL/minute: 0.125 mcg/kg/min
			  – GFR 21-30 mL/minute: 0.0625 mcg/kg/min
			  – GFR < 20 mL/minute: avoid use.
			• **Dosage Forms:** IV (solution)

CARDIOVASCULAR – VASOPRESSORS

Drug Class
- Vasopressors
- Agents:
  - Epinephrine
  - Norepinephrine
  - Phenylephrine
  - Dopamine
  - Vasopressin
  - Angiotensin II

> **Fast Facts**
> - Norepinephrine is the drug of choice in patients with septic shock still not achieving MAPs of 65 mm Hg or more with appropriate IV fluids and antibiotics.
> - Epinephrine is the drug of choice for the treatment of anaphylaxis or Type 1 hypersensitivity reaction.

Main Indications or Uses
- Hypotension, Septic Shock

Mechanism of Action
- **Dopamine, Epinephrine, Norepinephrine, Phenylephrine**
  - Activation of G protein-coupled receptors, causing activation, leads to numerous intracellular secondary signaling activation that ultimately drives a muscle contraction (in the case of alpha-1, beta-1) or relaxation (alpha-2, beta-2).
- **Vasopressin**
  - Vasopressin stimulates V1 by activating PLC-beta producing IP3 and DAG and ultimately calcium-dependent calcium release.
- **Angiotensin II**
  - Angiotensin II causes a rapid increase in peripheral resistance through the stimulation of AT1 receptors.

Primary Net Benefit
- Essential medications for hemodynamic support in emergency medicine and critical care. Vasopressors generally increase mean arterial pressure, improving perfusion to essential organs during resuscitation.
- Main Labs to Monitor:
  - No routine lab monitoring

High-Yield Basic Pharmacology
- **Vasopressin V1 Receptors**
  - V1 agonism causes vasoconstriction by inhibiting vascular potassium-sensitive ATP channels and inhibiting IL-1beta.
- **Angiotensin II**
  - Angiotensin II has numerous other effects contributing to changes in hemodynamics, including an increase in blood pressure set point for baroreceptor reflex through actions in the CNS, inhibition of norepinephrine reuptake, and enhancing the vascular response to norepinephrine, and depolarization of adrenal chromaffin cells leading to release of catecholamines.

High-Yield Clinical Knowledge
- **Inopressors Vs. Pure Vasopressors**
  - Although commonly referred to as vasopressors or inotropes, reclassifying these drugs differently better matches their clinical effects.
  - The *"inopressors"* (norepinephrine, epinephrine) deliver both increases in vascular resistance and provide inotropic effects.
  - Whereas the "pure vasopressors" (vasopressin, phenylephrine, angiotensin II) provide almost exclusively vasoconstriction without effect on inotropic or chronotropic effects.
    - There also exist "inodilators" such as dobutamine or milrinone, which cause increases in cardiac output but can cause vasodilation.

- **Catecholamine Resistance**
  - In critically ill patients, evidence suggests resistance to exogenous catecholamine via receptor desensitization, downregulation of receptors from exogenous catecholamine infusions, overproduction of NO via iNOS, and promotion of inflammatory cytokines IL-1 and TNF-alpha.
  - These patients may require higher dosing, non-catecholamine pressors (vasopressin or angiotensin II), corticosteroids, or a combination of these therapies.
- **Dopamine Dose**
  - Dopamine is often quoted in pharmacology teaching as having discrete receptor activity at specific doses: D1 agonism 0-3 mcg/kg/min, beta agonism 3-10mcg/kg/min and alpha agonist activity > 10 mcg/kg/min.
  - However, these effects have significant (10 to 75-fold) interpatient variability, meaning each patient may respond differently to different doses.
- **Epinephrine Lab Changes**
  - Epinephrine can potentially produce numerous laboratory changes relevant to patient care.
  - Hyperlactatemia secondary to epinephrine is caused by the inhibition of pyruvate dehydrogenase, causing a pyruvate shunt towards lactate production.
    - Thus, while not a result of tissue hypoperfusion and has no impact on clinical outcome, it may limit the usefulness of tracking lactate clearance as a marker of resuscitation.
  - Hyperglycemia is another common effect caused by increased liver glycogenolysis, reduced tissue uptake of glucose, and inhibition of pancreatic secretion of insulin.
  - Finally, hypokalemia results from an intracellular shift of potassium due to epinephrine.
- **IV Push**
  - Vasopressors can be used in an IV push format and the conventional IV infusion.
  - "Push-dose pressors" using phenylephrine or epinephrine are temporary measures to maintain perfusion in critically ill patient care scenarios.
  - Temporary measures such as push doses rather than continuous IV infusions could augment perfusion while other definitive therapies are prepared (i.e., pressor drips, central lines, various procedures).
- **Drug of Choice**
  - The vast majority of clinical scenarios where a vasopressor is indicated, norepinephrine will be the drug of choice.
  - While the initial dosing should be weight-based and adjusted body weight used for morbidly obese patients, guideline statements do not provide any recommendations on which dosing strategy is preferred.

High-Yield Core Evidence
- **SOAP II**
  - The SOAP II trial was a multicenter, randomized trial of 1679 patients with septic shock was conducted to compare dopamine to norepinephrine as first-line vasopressor therapy.
  - There was no difference in all-cause mortality at 28 days. However, there was a significantly almost double the incidence of arrhythmias in the dopamine group (24.1% vs. 12.4%).
  - Many experts use this landmark trial as a rationale for the first-line use of norepinephrine. (De Backer D, et al. Comparison of Dopamine and Norepinephrine in the Treatment of Shock. N Engl J Med 2010; 362:779-789)
- **Low Dose Dopamine**
  - The use of low-dose dopamine to increase urine output, while it temporarily does improve urine output, is associated with significant adverse events, including death. The risk of low-dose dopamine outweighs any benefit of this therapy. (Ann Intern Med. 2005 Apr 5;142(7):510-24).

- **VASST**
  - Prior iterations of the Surviving Sepsis guidelines recommended the initiation of vasopressin if the patient was not appropriately responding to fluid boluses and required at least 5 mcg/min norepinephrine (or equivalent) for at least 6 hours.
  - The VASST trial failed to observe a mortality benefit from adding vasopressin but did not demonstrate an overabundance of harm.
  - While this was a negative trial and caused vasopressin to fall off of standard sepsis care, it can still be used as a secondary or tertiary vasopressor in sepsis. (N Engl J Med 2008;358:877-87)

High-Yield Fast-Facts
- The common adverse events of tachycardia and arrhythmia from vasopressor beta stimulation can be managed with esmolol.
- Extravasation of vasopressors can cause severe tissue injury. The management of extravasation should include phentolamine, an alpha-adrenergic antagonist to promote vasodilation, 5-10mg in 10-20ml NS, injected into multiple sites of the symptomatic area.
- In rare situations where IV pumps may not be available (such as high patient volumes due to a pandemic), epinephrine can be given without a pump using the so-called "dirty epi drip." Using 1mg of epinephrine in 1 L of NS is made for a 1 mcg/mL concentration. Utilizing a drip chamber or another in-line rate adjustment device, patients could be started on a vasopressor without a pump.

HIGH-YIELD BOARD EXAM ESSENTIALS
- **CLASSIC AGENTS:** Angiotensin II, dopamine, epinephrine, norepinephrine, phenylephrine, vasopressin
- **DRUG CLASS:** Vasopressors
- **INDICATIONS:** Hypotension, septic shock
- **MECHANISM:** Increases vascular resistance and perfusion via alpha and/or beta-agonist activity, V1 agonist activity or AT1 agonist activity.
- **SIDE EFFECTS:** Arrythmias (tachycardia), decreased lactate clearance, extravasation
- **CLINICAL PEARLS:**
  - Dopamine is often quoted in pharmacology teaching as having discrete receptor activity at specific doses: D1 agonism 0-3 mcg/kg/min, beta agonism 3-10mcg/kg/min and alpha agonist activity > 10 mcg/kg/min. However, these effects have significant (10 to 75-fold) interpatient variability, meaning each patient may respond differently to different doses.
  - Dopamine is known to be associated with tachydysrhythmias when compared to norepinephrine and thus is not the vasopressor of choice in septic shock.

Table: Drug Class Summary

	VASOPRESSOR - Drug Class Review High-Yield Med Reviews		
Mechanism of Action: *Increases vascular resistance and perfusion via alpha and/or beta-agonist activity, V1 agonist activity, or AT1 agonist activity.*			
Class Effects: *Vasoconstriction, increase in mean arterial pressure*			
Generic Name	**Brand Name**	**Main Indication(s) or Uses**	**Notes**

Epinephrine	Adrenalin	• Hypotension/shock	• **Dosing (Adult):**
			  − IV: 0.1 to 3 mcg/kg/min continuous
			  − IV: push 1 mg (cardiac arrest)
			  − IV: push 10 to 100 mcg (push-dose)
			• **Dosing (Peds):**
			  − IV: 0.1 to 3 mcg/kg/min continuous
			• **CYP450 Interactions:** None, but metabolized by COMT and MAO
			• **Renal or Hepatic Dose Adjustments:** None
			• **Dosage Forms:** IV solution

Norepinephrine	Levophed	• Hypotension/shock	• **Dosing (Adult):**
			  − IV: 0.1 to 3 mcg/kg/min continuous IV
			• **Dosing (Peds):**
			  − IV: 0.1 to 3 mcg/kg/min continuous IV
			• **CYP450 Interactions:** None, but metabolized by COMT and MAO
			• **Renal or Hepatic Dose Adjustments:** None
			• **Dosage Forms:** IV solution

Phenylephrine	Neosynephrine	• Hypotension/shock	• **Dosing (Adult):**
			  − IV: 0.5 to 10 mcg/kg/min continuous
			  − IV: 40 to 250 mcg bolus q1-2minutes
			  − Intercavernous 100 to 500 mcg
			• **Dosing (Peds):**
			  − IV: 0.5 to 10 mcg/kg/min continuous
			  − IV: 40 to 250 mcg bolus q1-2minutes
			• **CYP450 Interactions:** None, but metabolized by COMT and MAO
			• **Renal or Hepatic Dose Adjustments:** None
			• **Dosage Forms:** IV solution

Dopamine	None	• Hypotension/shock	• **Dosing (Adult):**
			  − IV: 1 to 20 mcg/kg/min continuous
			• **Dosing (Peds):**
			  − IV: 1 to 20 mcg/kg/min continuous
			• **CYP450 Interactions:** None, but metabolized by COMT and MAO
			• **Renal or Hepatic Dose Adjustments:** None
			• **Dosage Forms:** IV solution

VASOPRESSOR - Drug Class Review High-Yield Med Reviews			
Generic Name	Brand Name	Main Indication(s) or Uses	Notes

Vasopressin	Vasostrict	• Hypotension/shock	• **Dosing (Adult):**
			   – IV: 0.03 or 0.04 units/minute continuous
			   – IV: 40 units push
			• **Dosing (Peds):**
			   – IV: 0.5 to 10 milliunits/kg/hour
			• **CYP450 Interactions:** None
			• **Renal or Hepatic Dose Adjustments:** None
			• **Dosage Forms:** IV solution

Angiotensin II	Giapreza	• Hypotension/shock	• **Dosing (Adult):**
			   – IV: 10 to 20 nanogram/kg/min continuous
			• **Dosing (Peds):**
			   – Not routinely used
			• **CYP450 Interactions:** None
			• **Renal or Hepatic Dose Adjustments:** None
			• **Dosage Forms:** IV solution

CARDIOVASCULAR – ANGPTL3 INHIBITOR

Drug Class
- Angiopoietin-like 3 (ANGPTL3) Inhibitor
- Agents:
  - Chronic Care
    - Evinacumab

Main Indications or Uses
- Chronic Care
  - Homozygous familial hypercholesterolemia (HoFH) as an adjunct to other LDL-lowering therapies

Mechanism of Action
- A recombinant human monoclonal antibody that inhibits ANGPTL3, which is an angiopoietin-like protein mainly in the liver that inhibits lipoprotein lipase and endothelial lipase to prevent VLDL catabolism to LDL.

Primary Net Benefit
- Reduces LDL independently of LDL receptor function, which is often significantly reduced in HoFH.
- Main Labs to Monitor:
  - LDL, HDL, TG, TC (baseline, as early as 2 weeks, and periodically)
  - Pregnancy test

High-Yield Basic Pharmacology
- Half-life
  - Long half-life allows for less frequent administration.
    - Note: As with all monoclonal antibodies (MABs) they have a long half-life.
- Drug Interactions
  - Statin concentrations are not altered by evinacumab.

High-Yield Clinical Knowledge
- Evinacumab Administration
  - Do not shake. Utilize a maximum volume of 250 mL of NS or D5W for the solution
  - IV infusion administered over 60 minutes. Do not infuse concomitantly with other medications.
  - Slow rate if signs of infusion or hypersensitivity reactions occur.
  - Schedule every 4 weeks from the date of last dose.
- Adverse Events
  - The most common adverse events were nasopharyngitis, influenza-like illness, dizziness, rhinorrhea, and nausea.
  - Hypersensitivity reactions can occur.
- Pregnancy Considerations
  - May cause fetal harm based on animal studies.
  - Obtain a pregnancy test prior to initiation and use contraception during treatment and for at least 5 months following the last dose.

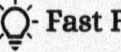
Fast Facts

- If you divide the triglycerides by 5, you get the estimated VLDL.

- The long half-life of evinacumab is like all monoclonal antibodies (MABs). This is helpful to reduce the frequency of administration.

Cardiology

High-Yield Core Evidence
- ELIPSE-HoFH
    - This was a double-blind, randomized, placebo-controlled trial that evaluated evinacumab versus placebo in patients with homozygous familial hypercholesterolemia for 24 weeks with the potential for an open-label 24-week extension.
    - 65 patients were evaluated who were on other lipid-lowering therapies (statins, ezetimibe, PCSK9 inhibitors, lomitapide, and lipoprotein apheresis.
    - The primary endpoint was change in LDL, with a mean change from baseline of 49% compared to placebo.
    - TG and TC were also similarly reduced. HDL was reduced 30%.
    - Similar results were seen in patients 12 years or older (n=14 patients).

High-Yield Fast-Facts
- Cost
    - The annual cost is estimated at $450,000.

HIGH-YIELD BOARD EXAM ESSENTIALS
- **CLASSIC AGENTS:** Evinacumab
- **DRUG CLASS:** ANGPTL3 inhibitor
- **INDICATIONS:** Homozygous familial hypercholesterolemia as an adjunct to other LDL-lowering therapies
- **MECHANISM:** A recombinant human monoclonal antibody that inhibits ANGPTL3, which is an angiopoietin-like protein mainly in the liver that inhibits lipoprotein lipase and endothelial lipase to prevent VLDL catabolism leading to LDL formation.
- **SIDE EFFECTS:** nasopharyngitis, influenza-like illness, dizziness, rhinorrhea, nausea
- **CLINICAL PEARLS:**
    - Administered as IV infusion.
    - Lowers HDL in addition to reducing LDL and TG.
    - May cause fetal harm. Administer pregnancy test before starting and use contraception up to 5 months after discontinuation.

Table: Drug Class Summary

ANGPTL 3 Inhibitor - Drug Class Review			
High-Yield Med Reviews			
Mechanism of Action: A recombinant human monoclonal antibody that inhibits ANGPTL3, which is an angiopoietin-like protein mainly in the liver that inhibits lipoprotein lipase and endothelial lipase.			
Class Effects: Reduces LDL, TG, HDL, TC, and apo B; It is also teratogenic			
Generic Name	Brand Name	Main Indication(s) or Uses	Notes

Evinacumab	Evkeeza	- Homozygous familial hypercholesterolemia	- **Dosing (Adult):**
			  - 15 mg/kg IV every 4 weeks
			- **Dosing (Peds):**
			  - 15 mg/kg IV every 4 weeks
			- **CYP450 Interactions:** None
			- **Renal or Hepatic Dose Adjustments:** None
			- **Dosage Forms:**
			  - Solution for IV infusion

CARDIOVASCULAR – BILE ACID SEQUESTRANTS

Drug Class
- **Bile Acid Sequestrants**
- **Agents:**
    - Chronic Care
        - Cholestyramine resin
        - Colesevelam
        - Colestipol

Main Indications or Uses
- **Chronic Care**
    - Dyslipidemia
        - Cholestyramine resin
        - Colesevelam
        - Colestipol
    - Pruritus associated with cholestasis
        - Cholestyramine resin
    - Type 2 Diabetes
        - Colesevelam

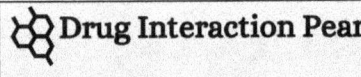

> **Knowledge Integration**
> ✓ These agents only work if they are taken at the same time as when bile acids are present in the GI tract. This means they must be taken with meals which lead to problems with compliance.

> **Drug Interaction Pearl**
> ✓ Counsel to separate the administration of cholestyramine with other medications due to risk of drug interactions.

Mechanism of Action
- Cholesterol is a major precursor of bile acid. When bile acid sequestrants bind bile acids in the intestine and produce an insoluble complex that is eliminated in the feces, the concentration of bile acids decreases so that more cholesterol is oxidized to bile acids, which lowers cholesterol.
    - Reduced hepatocyte cholesterol causes an increase in LDL receptor expression and reductions in LDL.

Primary Net Benefit
- Modest LDL reduction of up to 20%, which generally limits clinical use except in pregnancy.
- Main Labs to Monitor:
    - HDL, LDL, TG, TC (baseline, 4 to 12 weeks after starting, then periodically).
    - Note: Can worsen the TG levels.

High-Yield Basic Pharmacology
- **Pregnancy and Lack of Absorption**
    - Their lack of systemic absorption makes them an appropriate choice for LDL reduction in pregnancy.
- **Increased Triglycerides**
    - The decreased hepatic concentration of cholesterol from bile acid sequestrant therapy causes a subsequent increase in hepatic cholesterol and triglyceride synthesis.
    - These agents should not be used in patients with triglyceride levels above 300 mg/dL.
- **Dosage Form Differences**
    - Cholestyramine and colestipol have poor palatability, so colesevelam was created as a tablet dosage form.
    - Colesevelam tablet dosage forms are associated with a lower incidence of patient discontinuation.

High-Yield Clinical Knowledge
- **Oral Administration and Adverse Effects**
    - Cholestyramine and colestipol are available in powdered resin dosage forms that require mixing with water or juice for oral administration with meals so that it can bind the bile acids.
        - These are notoriously poor-tasting and are accompanied by dose-dependent GI adverse events, including constipation, bloating, epigastric fullness, nausea, and flatulence.
    - Colesevelam and colestipol are available as tablets, which eliminates poor palatability, but GI adverse effects still occur.

- Patients rarely tolerate titration to target doses to achieve maximum LDL reduction because of GI adverse events.
- **Fat-soluble Vitamin Depletion**
  - Decreased GI absorption of bile acids also has the deleterious effect of decreasing fat-soluble vitamin absorption.
    - Appropriate spacing of cholestyramine and colestipol can permit sufficient absorption of necessary fat-soluble vitamins.
    - Colesevelam does not appear to affect fat-soluble vitamin absorption.
- **Drug-Interactions**
  - Cholestyramine and colestipol may also decrease the absorption of many orally administered drugs, including aspirin, ascorbic acid, digoxin, diuretics (thiazides and loops), iron, levothyroxine, propranolol, phenytoin, tetracycline, and warfarin.
    - Other medications should be spaced by 1 hour before or 4 hours after bile acid sequestrants.
  - Fluvastatin, ezetimibe, and pravastatin absorption may also be decreased; therefore, if combination therapy is needed, use an alternative statin.
  - Colesevelam does not appear to interfere with the absorption of digoxin, lovastatin, metoprolol, valproic acid, and warfarin.
- **Pediatric Use**
  - Cholestyramine and colestipol have significant clinical data in pediatric patients (older than 10 years) compared to statins, ezetimibe, and PCSK9 inhibitors.
- **Combination with Statins**
  - As described above, the action of bile acid sequestrants causes an increase in hepatic cholesterol synthesis by upregulating HMG-CoA reductase.
    - The combination of statin therapy can substantially increase the effectiveness of bile acid sequestrants.
- **Diverticulitis**
  - In patients diagnosed with diverticulitis, bile acid sequestrants should be avoided.

High-Yield Core Evidence
- **The Lipid Research Clinics Coronary Primary Prevention Trial**
  - Multicenter, randomized, double-blind study that evaluated the impact of cholestyramine compared to placebo in reducing the risk of CHD.
  - Patients randomized to cholestyramine experienced a significantly lower incidence of the primary endpoint of definite CHD death and/or definite nonfatal MI compared to placebo.
  - Cholestyramine use was also associated with a lower incidence of new positive exercise tests, angina, and coronary bypass surgery.
  - However, there was no significant change in the risk of death from all causes.
  - The authors concluded that reducing total cholesterol by lowering LDL-C levels can diminish the incidence of CHD morbidity and mortality in men at high risk for CHD because of raised LDL-C levels. (JAMA. 1984 Jan 20;251(3):351-64.)

High-Yield Fast-Fact
- **GI Upset Hack**
  - For patients that must take a bile acid sequestrant, the GI intolerances may be reduced by allowing the drug (cholestyramine or colestipol) to be completely suspended in liquid for several hours before the scheduled dose.
- **Type 2 Diabetes Indication**
  - Colesevelam is indicated to improve glucose control in patients with T2DM but is rarely used due to modest efficacy and availability of better alternatives.
- **Use in Diaper Dermatitis**
  - Cholestyramine resin can be compounded with Aquaphor and used TOPICALLY for diaper dermatitis in infants and children.

HIGH-YIELD BOARD EXAM ESSENTIALS
- **CLASSIC AGENTS:** Cholestyramine resin, colesevelam, colestipol
- **DRUG CLASS:** Bile acid sequestrants
- **INDICATIONS:** Dyslipidemia (cholestyramine resin, colesevelam, colestipol), pruritus associated with cholestasis (cholestyramine resin), T2DM (colesevelam)
- **MECHANISM:** Cholesterol is a major precursor of bile acid. When bile acid sequestrants bind bile acids in the intestine and produce an insoluble complex that is eliminated in the feces, the concentration of bile acids decreases so that more cholesterol is oxidized to bile acids, which lowers cholesterol.
- **SIDE EFFECTS:** GI intolerance, decreased absorption of fat-soluble vitamins, elevated TG
- **CLINICAL PEARLS:**
  - Can reduce LDL but must be taken with each meal to capture the bile.
  - Avoid using these agents if the patient has elevated TG at baseline as they can worsen the risk of developing TG-induced pancreatitis.
  - Cholestyramine and colestipol may also decrease the absorption of many orally administered drugs including aspirin, ascorbic acid, digoxin, diuretics (thiazides, loop diuretics), iron, levothyroxine, propranolol, phenytoin, tetracycline, and warfarin.
  - May be used in pregnancy if needed due to lack of systemic absorption.

Table: Drug Class Summary

| \multicolumn{4}{c}{**Bile Acid Sequestrants - Drug Class Review**} |
|||||
| \multicolumn{4}{l}{**Mechanism of Action:** *Bind to bile acids in the intestinal lumen, increasing hepatic consumption of cholesterol to increase bile acid production*} |
| \multicolumn{4}{l}{**Class Effects:** *LDL reduction, small ASCVD risk improvement compared to alternatives, elevated TG, GI intolerance, decrease in fat-soluble vitamin absorption*} |

Generic Name	Brand Name	Main Indication(s) or Uses	Notes

Cholestyramine resin	Prevalite
	Questran
	Questran Light
		• Dyslipidemia
		• Pruritus associated with cholestasis
			• **Dosing (Adult):**
			  – Oral: 4 g once to twice daily, increase to target 8-16 g/day
			    – Max 24 g/day
			• **Dosing (Peds):**
			  – Oral: 2-4 g per day in divided doses (or 240 mg/kg/day), increase to target 8 g/day
			• **CYP450 Interactions:** None, but other clinically relevant interactions (absorption) exist.
			• **Renal or Hepatic Dose Adjustments:** None
			• **Dosage Forms:** Oral (packet, powder)

Colesevelam	Welchol	• Dyslipidemia
		• T2DM
			• **Dosing (Adult):**
			  – Oral: 3.75 g/day in 1-2 divided doses
			• **Dosing (Peds):**
			  – Oral: 3.75 g/day in 1-2 divided doses
			• **CYP450 Interactions:** None, but other clinically relevant interactions (absorption) exist.
			• **Renal or Hepatic Dose Adjustments:** None
			• **Dosage Forms:** Oral (packet, tablet)

Colestipol	Colestid	• Dyslipidemia	• **Dosing (Adult):**
			  – Oral: granules 5 g once to twice daily, increase to target 30 g/day
			  – Oral: tablets 2 g once to twice daily, increase to target 16 g/day
			• **Dosing (Peds):**
			  – Oral: 2-12 g daily in divided doses (or 125-250 mg/kg/day), increase to target 10 g/day
			• **CYP450 Interactions:** None, but other clinically relevant interactions (absorption) exist.
			• **Renal or Hepatic Dose Adjustments:** None
			• **Dosage Forms:** Oral (granules, packet, tablet)

CARDIOVASCULAR – EZETIMIBE

Drug Class
- Antilipemic
- Agents:
  - Chronic Care
    - Ezetimibe

Dosing Pearl
✓ The high degree of enterohepatic recirculation of ezetimibe allows it to be dosed once-a-day and continue to work.

Main Indications or Uses
- Chronic Care
  - Homozygous familial hypercholesterolemia
  - Homozygous sitosterolemia
  - Primary hyperlipidemia

Mechanism of Action
- Inhibits Niemann-Pick C1-Like-1, a sterol transport protein in the brush border of the small intestine, ultimately decreasing hepatic cholesterol delivery, hepatic cholesterol storage, and increased clearance from the blood.
  - Effects on lipids include decreasing total cholesterol, LDL, apolipoprotein-B, and TG and increasing HDL.

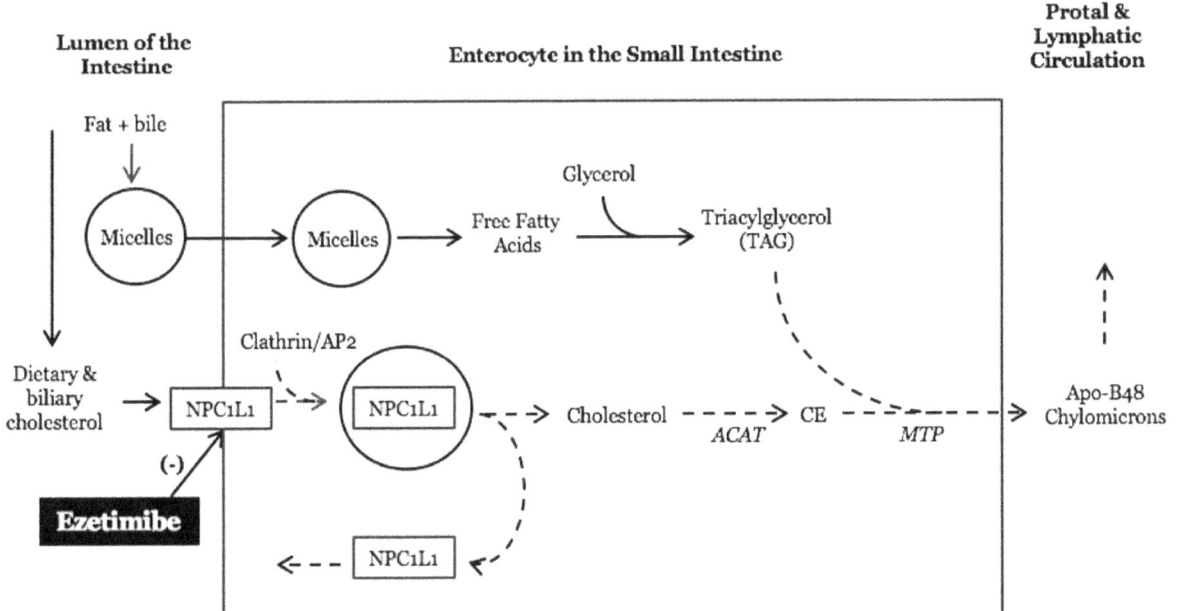

Primary Net Benefit
- Ezetimibe is a moderately potent LDL-lowering agent but has controversial evidence that supports this translation to patient-oriented outcomes (i.e., improved CV mortality).
- Ezetimibe is mostly utilized in combination with statins for patients requiring additional LDL reductions who cannot tolerate maximum statin dosing or who need additional LDL reduction in addition to maximum statin therapy.
- Main Labs to Monitor:
  - HDL, LDL, TG, Total Cholesterol (baseline, 4 to 12 weeks after starting, then periodically)
  - Liver function (albumin, bilirubin, total protein, PT/INR), liver enzymes (AST, ALT, Alk Phos)

High-Yield Basic Pharmacology
- **Prodrug Metabolism**
  - Ezetimibe undergoes glucuronide conjugation in the small intestine and liver to an active metabolite.
- **Duration of Action**
  - The long duration of action of ezetimibe is related to its enterohepatic recirculation.
    - Once ezetimibe is metabolized (via glucuronide conjugation) in the small intestine and liver, it's excreted in the bile back into the intestinal lumen (a primary site of action).
    - This pathway also partially accounts for the risk of cholelithiasis.

High-Yield Clinical Knowledge
- **Adverse Effects**
  - Ezetimibe is generally well-tolerated, but sinusitis, arthralgias, LFT elevations, and myopathy may occur. Statins result in a greater incidence of myopathy compared to ezetimibe.
- **Severe Primary Hypercholesterolemia**
  - In patients with severe primary hypercholesterolemia, if high dose statin is started and LDL is still above 100 mg/dL or does not achieve a 50% reduction, ezetimibe may be added to further target LDL.
- **Very High-Risk Patients**
  - Ezetimibe may be used in combination with a statin in very high-risk ASCVD patients to target an LDL < 70 mg/dL.
    - After the addition of ezetimibe to high-dose statin therapy, if LDL is still > 70 mg/dL, a PCSK9 inhibitor is a reasonable addition.
- **Drug interactions**
  - Ezetimibe has few drug interactions relative to other lipid-lowering drug classes; however, there is a clinically relevant interaction with cyclosporine and fibrates.
    - Coadministration of cyclosporine and ezetimibe increases ezetimibe AUC 2.5 times and nearly triples peak concentration.
    - Cyclosporine peak concentrations are also increased by 15%, and AUC increased by 10%.
    - Fibrates in combination with ezetimibe may increase the risk of myopathy and cholelithiasis.
- **Use Without A Statin**
  - In patients whose statin therapy is contraindicated, ezetimibe may be used in combination with other lipid-lowering interventions.
- **Add-On Therapy**
  - Ezetimibe can be a key add-on therapy to statins that provides additional LDL lowering and a potential 2% absolute risk reduction in CV morbidity and mortality (NNT = 50).
    - It is not only safe but significantly less costly than the newer PCSK-9 inhibitors and provides a similar add-on benefit to statin therapy (ezetimibe NNT = 50; PCSK-9 inhibitor NNT = 67).

High-Yield Core Evidence
- **IMPROVE-IT**
  - This was a multicenter, double-blind, randomized controlled trial of patients who had been hospitalized for ACS within the preceding ten days and elevated LDL to assess the combination of simvastatin plus ezetimibe compared with simvastatin plus placebo.
  - The combination of simvastatin plus ezetimibe significantly improved the primary endpoint of the composite of CV death, nonfatal MI, unstable angina requiring rehospitalization, coronary revascularization, or nonfatal stroke.
  - The rates of prespecified muscle, gallbladder, and hepatic adverse effects and cancer were similar in the two groups.
  - The authors concluded that ezetimibe added to statin therapy resulted in an incremental lowering of LDL levels and improved CV outcomes. (N Engl J Med. 2015 Jun 18;372(25):2387-97.)

- **ENHANCE**
  - This was a multicenter, double-blind, randomized, active comparator trial in patients with familial hypercholesterolemia designed to assess the efficacy of simvastatin-ezetimibe compared to simvastatin alone on the progression of atherosclerosis.
  - There was no significant difference between groups concerning the primary outcome of the change in the mean carotid artery intima-media thickness.
  - Furthermore, secondary outcomes assessing the intima-media thickness of the carotid and femoral arteries did not differ significantly between the two groups.
  - These outcomes occurred despite a significant improvement in the mean LDL cholesterol level (as well as TG and C-reactive protein) with the combination of simvastatin-ezetimibe compared to simvastatin alone.
  - The authors concluded that simvastatin-ezetimibe did not result in a significant difference in changes in intima-media thickness in patients with familial hypercholesterolemia, as compared with simvastatin alone, despite decreases in levels of LDL cholesterol and C-reactive protein. (N Engl J Med. 2008 Apr 3;358(14):1431-43.)

High-Yield Fast-Facts
- **NPC1L1 Polymorphisms**
  - Individuals with polymorphisms of Niemann-Pick C1-Like1 generally have lower LDL-C levels and decreased ASCVD risk than individuals without these polymorphisms.
- **No Increased Risk of Cancer**
  - In preliminary clinical evidence, a small increased risk of cancer seemed to occur with ezetimibe. However, this increased risk of cancer was not seen in the IMPROVE-IT study.

HIGH-YIELD BOARD EXAM ESSENTIALS
- **CLASSIC AGENTS:** Ezetimibe
- **DRUG CLASS:** Antilipemic
- **INDICATIONS:** Homozygous familial hypercholesterolemia, homozygous sitosterolemia, primary hyperlipidemia
- **MECHANISM:** Inhibits Niemann-Pick C1-Like-1, a sterol transport protein in the brush border of the small intestine, ultimately decreasing hepatic cholesterol delivery, hepatic cholesterol storage, and increased clearance from the blood.
- **SIDE EFFECTS:** Well-tolerated, but may see sinusitis, increased LFTs, arthralgias, myopathy (less than statins)
- **CLINICAL PEARLS:** Dosed once-a-day due to enterohepatic recirculation. Very well tolerated and no major drug interactions. In patients with severe primary hypercholesterolemia, if high dose statin is started and LDL is still above 100 mg/dL or does not achieve a 50% reduction, ezetimibe may be added to target LDL below this threshold.

Table: Drug Class Summary

Ezetimibe - Drug Class Review			
High-Yield Med Reviews			
Generic Name	Brand Name	Indication(s) or Uses	Notes
Ezetimibe	Zetia	• Homozygous familial hypercholesterolemia • Homozygous sitosterolemia • Primary hyperlipidemia	• **Dosing (Adult):** Oral: 10 mg once daily • **Dosing (Peds):** Oral: 10 mg once daily • **CYP450 Interactions:** None • **Renal or Hepatic Dose Adjustments:** – Child-Pugh class B or C: Not recommended • **Dosage Forms:** Oral (tablet)

CARDIOVASCULAR – FIBRATES

Drug Class
- Fibrates
- Agents:
  - Fenofibrate
  - Gemfibrozil

Main Indications or Uses
- Chronic Care
  - Hyperlipidemia
  - Hypertriglyceridemia

Mechanism of Action
- Fibrates activate peroxisome proliferator-activated receptor type alpha (PPAR-alpha), facilitating PPAR-alpha mediated stimulation of fatty acid oxidation, increasing lipoprotein lipase synthesis, and decreasing apolipoprotein C-III production.
  - Enhances the clearance of triglyceride-rich lipoproteins, VLDLs, and LDL.
  - PPAR-alpha stimulation increases HDL from activation of apolipoprotein A-I and A-II.

Primary Overall Net Benefit
- Fibrate therapy has fallen out of favor, with the guidelines preferring initiating statin therapy or intensifying statin therapy in patients with severe hypertriglyceridemia and ASCVD risk of 7.5% or higher.
  - If triglycerides are greater than 1000 mg/dL, fibrate therapy could be considered to avoid pancreatitis AFTER addressing the following: a very low-fat diet, avoidance of refined carbohydrates and alcohol, and consumption of omega-3 fatty acids.
- Main Labs to Monitor:
  - HDL, LDL, TG, Total Cholesterol (baseline, three months, then periodically)
  - Liver function (albumin, bilirubin, total protein, PT/INR), liver enzymes (AST, ALT, Alk Phos)
  - Hgb and Hct (may decrease)
  - SCr (may increase)

High-Yield Basic Pharmacology
- Fenofibrate and Coagulation
  - Fenofibrate possesses antithrombotic effects via inhibition of tissue factor, a critical cofactor in initiating the extrinsic clotting pathway.
    - In addition to inhibiting the metabolism of warfarin (CYP2C9 inhibition), fenofibrate may also increase hemorrhage risk due to tissue factor inhibition.
      - Therefore, an increased risk of bleeding could still occur if the patient is converted to dabigatran or an oral factor Xa inhibitor.
- Fenofibrate Dosage Forms
  - Fenofibrate is commercially available in numerous dosage forms (capsules and tablets), as well as fenofibric acid (choline salt).

High-Yield Clinical Knowledge
- Renal Dose Adjustment
  - Fibrates should be used with caution in renal impairment. Avoid with CrCl < 30 mL/min.
  - With gemfibrozil, dose adjustments should begin when the patient's CrCl < 50 mL/min.
- LDL Increase
  - When used for hypertriglyceridemia, fibrates may lead to modest reciprocal rises in LDL, mainly when baseline triglycerides > 1000 mg/dL.
    - Although the LDL concentration increases, this effect is still considered to be beneficial as the morphology of the LDL changes, preserving a potential CV benefit.

- **Drug Interactions**
    - Gemfibrozil should not be combined with statins due to the significant risk of enhanced toxicity (myopathy or rhabdomyolysis) and limited clinical benefit.
        - Specifically, gemfibrozil should not be used with lovastatin, pravastatin, and simvastatin.
        - However, experts suggest use can be considered in combination with atorvastatin, pitavastatin, and rosuvastatin, provided that lower doses are used and the patient is followed closely.
        - Fluvastatin may be used in combination with gemfibrozil without any specific dose adjustments.
- **Place in Therapy**
    - According to the ACC/AHA guidelines, due to the lack of patient-oriented clinical benefit and statin efficacy for TG reduction, fibrates are considered last-line for hypertriglyceridemia.
- **Fibrates and Protease Inhibitors**
    - Protease inhibitors (used for HIV) are known to cause metabolic abnormalities, including hypercholesterolemia and hypertriglyceridemia.
        - Fenofibrate can be used to manage this effect, but ensure the patient is not taking raltegravir (an integrase inhibitor) since the risk of myopathy is increased.
- **Hypersensitivity and Photosensitivity**
    - Can result in mild or severe rashes or other cutaneous eruptions.

High-Yield Core Evidence
- **ACCORD LIPID**
    - Multicenter, placebo-controlled, randomized trial that compared a statin plus a fibrate with statin monotherapy on the risk of CVD in patients with T2DM who were at high risk for CVD.
    - There was no significant difference between groups concerning the primary outcome of the first occurrence of nonfatal MI, nonfatal stroke, or CV death.
    - Furthermore, there was no difference in any secondary outcome or the annual rates of death.
    - In a preplanned subgroup analysis, the authors noted a benefit for men, possible harm for women, and a possible benefit for patients with a high baseline TG and a low baseline HDL.
    - The authors concluded that the combination of fenofibrate and simvastatin did not reduce the rate of fatal CV events, nonfatal MI, or nonfatal stroke compared with simvastatin alone. (N Engl J Med. 2010 Apr 29;362(17):1563-74.)
- **FIELD**
    - Multicenter, placebo-controlled, randomized trial to assess the effect of fenofibrate on CVD events in adults with T2DM not taking a statin.
    - There was no difference in the primary outcome of coronary events defined as CHD death or nonfatal MI.
    - When considered as individual outcomes, fenofibrate was associated with a significant reduction in nonfatal MI, but there was no significant difference in CHD mortality.
    - Fenofibrate was associated with an increase in pancreatitis and pulmonary embolism but no other significant adverse effects.
    - The authors concluded that fenofibrate did not significantly reduce the risk of the primary outcome of coronary events. (Lancet. 2005 Nov 26;366(9500):1849-61.)

High-Yield Fast-Fact
- **Gallstone Risk**
    - Fibrates lower cholesterol, in part by enhancing its elimination in bile and thus increasing the cholesterol content of bile. In some patients, this can increase the risk of cholesterol-based gallstones.
- **FDA Indication Update**
    - The FDA has withdrawn the approval of fenofibrate for use in combination with a statin for ASCVD risk reduction.
- **Pseudo-Cushing Syndrome**
    - Fenofibrate administration may cause a false elevation of urinary-free cortisol values in patients evaluated for Cushing Syndrome.
    - If Cushing Syndrome is suspected in a patient taking fenofibrate, an HPLC-mass spectrometry method should be used to assess urinary-free cortisol.

HIGH-YIELD BOARD EXAM ESSENTIALS
- **CLASSIC AGENTS:** Fenofibrate, gemfibrozil
- **DRUG CLASS:** Fibrates
- **INDICATIONS:** Hyperlipidemia, hypertriglyceridemia
- **MECHANISM:** Activate PPAR-alpha, facilitating PPAR-alpha mediated stimulation of fatty acid oxidation, increasing lipoprotein lipase synthesis, and decreasing apolipoprotein C-III production.
- **SIDE EFFECTS:** LDL increase, gallstones, dyspepsia, diarrhea, photosensitivity, hypersensitivity (rash), hepatotoxicity, myopathy, SCr increase (especially fenofibrate), Hgb/Hct decrease
- **CLINICAL PEARLS:**
  - According to the guidelines, due to the lack of patient-oriented clinical benefit, and the effectiveness of statins at lowering TG, fibrates are considered last-line for hypertriglyceridemia.
  - Fenofibrate may increase risk of bleeding.
  - Gemfibrozil interacts with some statins in combination. Avoid in ESRD.

Table: Drug Class Summary

Fibrates - Drug Class Review High-Yield Med Reviews			
Mechanism of Action: *Activate PPAR-alpha causing fatty acid oxidation, increased lipoprotein lipase synthesis, decreased apolipoprotein C-III production, and activation of apolipoprotein A-I and A-II.*			
Class Effects: *Decreasing TG, VLDL, LDL, increasing HDL. Avoid in ESRD, myopathy, hepatotoxicity, gallstones, delayed hypersensitivity reactions, photosensitivity*			
Generic Name	**Brand Name**	**Indication(s) or Uses**	**Notes**

Fenofibrate	Antara
	Fenoglide
	Fibricor
	Lipofen
	Tricor
	Trilipix
		▪ Hypertriglyceridemia	▪ **Dosing (Adult):** Various, depending on dosage form:
			  – Tablets of 48 and 145 mg
			  – Capsules of 67, 134, and 200 mg
			▪ **Dosing (Peds):** Not routinely used
			▪ **CYP450 Interactions:** Inhibits CYP2C9
			▪ **Renal or Hepatic Dose Adjustments:**
			  – GFR < 30 mL/minute: contraindicated
			  – Hepatic impairment: contraindicated
			▪ **Dosage Forms:** Oral (capsule, tablet)

Gemfibrozil	Lopid	▪ Hypertriglyceridemia	▪ **Dosing (Adult):**
			  – Oral: 600 mg BID, 30 minutes before food
			▪ **Dosing (Peds):** Not routinely used
			▪ **CYP450 Interactions:** CYP3A4 substrate, inhibits CYP2C8
			▪ **Renal or Hepatic Dose Adjustments:**
			  – GFR 10 to 50 mL/minute: reduce dose by 25%
			  – GFR < 10 mL/minute: reduce dose by 50%
			  – Hepatic impairment: contraindicated
			▪ **Dosage Forms:** Oral (tablet)

CARDIOVASCULAR – NIACIN

Drug Class
- Other Lipid-Lowering Agents
- Agents:
  - **Chronic Care**
    - Niacin

Main Indications or Uses
- **Chronic Care**
  - Dyslipidemia

> **Fast Facts**
> ✓ The dose of OTC immediate release niacin is not interchangeable with the prescription formulation, Niaspan. If a switch occurs between formulations, the dosing and titration should start over.

Mechanism of Action
- This is not fully understood, but niacin may inhibit free fatty acid release from adipose tissue, increase lipolysis of triglycerides, and promote chylomicron triglyceride removal from plasma.
- Increases HDL by reversing cholesterol transport in hepatocytes by apolipoprotein A1.

Primary Overall Net Benefit
- Reduction in LDL, TG, and TC, as well as increase in HDL. Also, reduces VLDL, apolipoprotein B, and lipoprotein (a)
- Main Labs to Monitor:
  - Blood glucose (if diabetic)
  - HDL, LDL, TG, TC (baseline, 4-12 weeks, then periodically)
  - Liver function (albumin, bilirubin, total protein, PT/INR), liver enzymes (AST, ALT, Alk Phos), Uric acid

High-Yield Basic Pharmacology
- **Hyperuricemia**
  - In patients with pre-existing gout, initiating niacin may acutely worsen gout and cause flares.
    - Niacin inhibits uricase, decreasing oxidation of uric acid, or it may decrease uric acid excretion.

High-Yield Clinical Knowledge
- **Place in Therapy**
  - Niacin combination therapy with statins is not recommended by the guidelines because clinical evidence has not demonstrated additional clinical benefit or ASCVD risk reduction
  - May be used in special patient scenarios, such as TG > 500 mg/dL or statin intolerance.
  - May consider for augmentation to increase HDL, but patient outcomes are lacking in clinical data.
- **Niacin Vs Niacinamide**
  - Niacinamide is the amide derivative of niacin.
  - At appropriate therapeutic doses, niacin is capable of lowering LDL; however, niacinamide has no lipid-lowering effect.
- **Flushing**
  - Niacin is notorious for causing flushing or the sensation of warmth after each dose.
    - This effect is dose-dependent, with lipid-lowering doses promoting flushing.
    - Taking niacin with warm beverages (i.e., coffee or tea), hot or spicy foods, or alcohol can increase the likelihood and severity of flushing.
  - Tachyphylaxis may occur within 3 consecutive days of therapy, but aspirin can be added to blunt this prostaglandin-mediated response. Take 30 min before niacin.
  - Use extended-release formulations, take with food, and titrate slowly, in addition to aspirin.
- **GI Adverse Effects**
  - Avoid in patients with active peptic ulcer disease.
  - May cause GI distress, vomiting, or diarrhea. Manage with titration and administration with food.
- **Dose-Dependent Hepatic Risk**
  - Niacin use in patients with acute hepatic failure is contraindicated, and there is a dose-dependent risk of hepatotoxicity.

- However, doses less than 3 g per day are generally well-tolerated and not associated with sustained changes in liver enzymes or liver function.
- **Insulin Resistance**
  - Patients with diabetes should not take niacin because of an association with increased insulin resistance.
    - Diabetes medications could be adjusted to manage this effect, but since there is a lack of patient-oriented benefits for ASCVD, this may not be preferable.
    - This insulin resistance is also linked to acanthosis nigricans, another adverse event linked to niacin use.
- **Administration and Dosage Forms**
  - Take with food to reduce flushing.
  - Titration reduces flushing. Titrate Niaspan by 500 mg every 4 weeks. Regular release niacin can be titrated faster.
  - If therapy is stopped for an extended period, retitration is necessary.
  - Dosage forms are not all interchangeable.

High-Yield Core Evidence
- **AIM-HIGH**
  - Multicenter, randomized, placebo-controlled trial that randomized patients to receive extended-release niacin plus simvastatin-ezetimibe or matching placebo plus simvastatin-ezetimibe to increase low HDL levels. Patients had low LDL levels (<70 mg/dL)
  - The study was stopped early when an interim analysis demonstrated no difference in the primary endpoint of the first event of the composite of death from coronary heart disease, nonfatal myocardial infarction, ischemic stroke, hospitalization for acute coronary syndromes, or symptom-driven coronary or cerebral revascularization.
  - Despite no difference in the primary outcome, niacin therapy had significantly increased the median HDL level, lowered the triglyceride level, and lowered the LDL level.
  - Ischemic strokes occurred at low rates but were higher in the niacin group.
  - The authors concluded that among patients with ASCVD and LDL cholesterol levels of < 70 mg/dL, there was no incremental clinical benefit from the addition of niacin to statin therapy during a 36-month follow-up period, despite significant improvements in HDL and TG. (N Engl J Med. 2011 Dec 15;365(24):2255-67.)
- **HPS2-THRIVE**
  - Multicenter, randomized, placebo-controlled trial of patients with CVD on a statin randomized to extended-release niacin plus laropiprant or placebo.
  - There was no difference in the primary outcome of the first major vascular event, including nonfatal myocardial infarction, death from coronary causes, stroke, or arterial revascularization.
  - This observation occurred despite niacin plus laropiprant being associated with a lower LDL and higher HDL level compared to placebo.
  - But the niacin plus laropiprant combination was associated with an increased incidence of disturbances in diabetes control that were considered serious and an increased incidence of diabetes diagnosis, as well as increases in serious adverse events.
  - The authors concluded that among participants with ASCVD, the addition of extended-release niacin-laropiprant to statin-based LDL cholesterol-lowering therapy did not significantly reduce the risk of major vascular events but did increase the risk of serious adverse events. (N Engl J Med. 2014 Jul 17;371(3):203-12.)

High-Yield Fast-Fact
- **Fibrinogen and tPA**
  - Niacin may also play a physiologic role in coagulation since it has been associated with decreased levels of fibrinogen and increased levels of tissue plasminogen activator.
- **Pellagra**
  - Niacin can be used to cure primary pellagra, as the cause of this disease is insufficient dietary intake of niacin.

- **Other Proposed Uses**
  - Niacin has numerous other proposed clinical uses, including acute MI, cancer, migraines, and psychiatric disorders (anxiety, depression, schizophrenia).

HIGH-YIELD BOARD EXAM ESSENTIALS
- **CLASSIC AGENTS:** Niacin
- **DRUG CLASS:** Lipid-Lowering Agents
- **INDICATIONS:** Dyslipidemia
- **MECHANISM:** inhibits release of free fatty acids from adipose tissue, increases lipolysis of triglycerides, and promotes chylomicron triglyceride removal from plasma.
- **SIDE EFFECTS:** Flushing, GI effects, hepatotoxicity, hyperuricemia, increases in glucose
- **CLINICAL PEARLS:**
  - At appropriate therapeutic doses, niacin is capable of lowering LDL, however, niacinamide has no lipid-lowering effect.
  - Patients must be titrated to appropriate doses over time to avoid worsening side effects and risk of liver toxicity.
  - Flushing can be attenuated with aspirin premedication, extended-release formulations, taking with food, and titration.

Table: Drug Class Summary

Niacin - Drug Class Review			
High-Yield Med Reviews			
Mechanism of Action: *Decreases free fatty acids, increases lipolysis of triglycerides, and promotes chylomicron triglyceride removal from plasma.*			
Class Effects: Can improve LDL, TG, and HDL; no ASCVD benefit, flushing, GI effects, increase in uric acid or glucose			
Generic Name	**Brand Name**	**Main Indication(s) or Uses**	**Notes**

Niacin	Niacor
	Niaspan
	Slo-Niacin
		• Dyslipidemia	• **Dosing (Adult):**
			  – Oral: (regular release) 250 mg daily. Titrate weekly up to 2 gm daily divided, then every 2-4 weeks up to 3 gm daily divided
			    – Max 6 g total daily
			  – Oral: (sustained or controlled release) 250-750 mg daily.
			  – Oral: (extended-release) 500 mg at bedtime. Titrate every 4 weeks by 500 mg.
			    – Max 2 g daily
			• **Dosing (Peds):** Age over 10 years
			  – Oral: (regular release) 100-250 mg daily
			    – Max 10 mg/kg/day
			  – Oral: (sustained or controlled release) 500-1500 mg daily
			    – Max 10 mg/kg/day
			• **CYP450 Interactions:** None
			• **Renal or Hepatic Dose Adjustments:** None
			• **Dosage Forms:** Oral (ER capsule, powder, IR tablet, SR tablet, ER tablet)

CARDIOVASCULAR – OMEGA-3 POLYUNSATURATED FATTY ACID

Drug Class
- Omega-3 Polyunsaturated Fatty Acid
- Agents:
    - Chronic Care
        - Omega-3-acid ethyl ester of EPA/DHA (Lovaza)
        - Icosapent ethyl (Omega-3-acid ethyl ester of EPA [Vascepa])

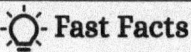 **Fast Facts**

✓ OTC forms of "fish oil" may not contain only omega-3 fatty acids. They may be mixed with other agents like cholesterol, vitamins, or other fats. Read the label on back of the product for the actual amount of omega-3 fatty acids (EPA + DHA) the product offers per dose.

Main Indications or Uses
- Chronic Care
    - Hypertriglyceridemia

Mechanism of Action
- Reduce the hepatic synthesis of triglyceride-rich VLDL. Mechanisms that reduce CV events are not fully known but may include increased EPA composition from carotid plaques, increased circulating EPA/arachidonic acid ration, or inhibition of platelet aggregation.

Primary Overall Net Benefit
- Omega-3 fatty acids containing only EPA (icosapent) are associated with a significant reduction in the rate of ischemic cardiac events, an effect that the former omega-3 fatty acids with EPA/DHA did not demonstrate.
- Main Labs to Monitor:
    - TG, HDL, LDL, TC (baseline, three months, then periodically).
    - Signs/symptoms of bleeding (only at very high doses or if taking anticoagulants/antiplatelet drug).

High-Yield Basic Pharmacology
- Absorption
    - De-esterified to EPA, which is the active metabolite and is absorbed in the small intestine.
- EPA/DHA vs. EPA
    - EPA-only icosapent may hypothetically derive its benefit from a lack of DHA, preventing its effect on increasing LDL in patients with severe hypertriglyceridemia.
- Cardiovascular Benefit
    - The proposed mechanism for reduced cardiovascular disease events is inhibiting platelet aggregation due to an increase in EPA/arachidonic acid ratio.

High-Yield Clinical Knowledge
- Bleeding Risk
    - Omega-3 agents independently may prolong bleeding time by impairing platelet function and reducing several coagulation factors (antithrombin, thrombin, fibrinogen, factor V, factor VII, and von Willebrand factor).
    - Use with warfarin may increase INR in patients with an otherwise stable INR.
    - Although more challenging to quantify clinically, omega-3 agents may also increase the risk of bleeding from dabigatran, oral factor Xa inhibitors (apixaban, edoxaban, rivaroxaban), salicylates, thienopyridines (clopidogrel, cangrelor, prasugrel, ticagrelor), SSRIs, ibrutinib, and NSAIDs.
- Fishy Burps
    - A common complaint of omega-3 products (OTC and the EPA/DHA combination) is abdominal bloating, dyspepsia, and "fishy burps."
        - Minimize these effects by keeping the capsules refrigerated.
- Fish or Shellfish Allergies
    - Patients with known hypersensitivity to fish or shellfish should not take omega-3 products, including icosapent.

- Fish or shellfish allergies should not preclude patients from receiving iodinated contrast agents, as shellfish allergies are not a result of iodine (true iodine allergies are incompatible with life).
- **OTC vs. Rx**
    - As opposed to niacin products, the various omega-3 EPA/DHA OTC products are generally similar to the prescription version (Lovaza).
    - The main difference is that the relative dose of omega-3 EPA/DHA is much higher than available OTC formulations.
        - A 4 g dose of Lovaza (4 capsules) is roughly equivalent to 6 to 8 capsules of OTC omega-3.

High-Yield Core Evidence
- **ORIGIN**
    - Multicenter, double-blind, 2-by-2 factorial randomized controlled trial of patients with recent myocardial infarction or heart failure randomized to omega-3 ethyl esters or placebo to assess the risk of CV mortality.
    - Despite a significant reduction in triglyceride levels associated with omega-3 treatment, there was no significant difference between groups in the primary outcome of death from CV causes.
    - There was also no significant effect of the omega-3 ethyl esters on the rates of major vascular events, death from any cause, or death from arrhythmia.
    - The authors concluded that daily supplementation with omega-3 fatty acids did not reduce the rate of CV events in patients at high risk for CV events. (N Engl J Med. 2012 Jul 26;367(4):309-18.)
- **REDUCE-IT**
    - Multicenter, randomized, double-blind, placebo-controlled trial of patients with ACSVD on a statin but who had a fasting triglyceride level of 135-499 mg/dL and an LDL of 41-100 mg/dL to assess the incidence of CV events in patients taking icosapent compared to placebo.
    - Icosapent was associated with a significant reduction in the primary endpoint of the composite of CV death, nonfatal myocardial infarction, nonfatal stroke, coronary revascularization, or unstable angina, as well as in the key secondary endpoint of the composite of CV death, nonfatal myocardial infarction, or nonfatal stroke.
    - A significantly larger proportion of patients were admitted for atrial fibrillation compared to placebo, but other serious adverse events were similar between groups.
    - The authors concluded that among patients with elevated triglyceride levels despite statins, the risk of ischemic events, including CV death, was significantly lower among those who received 2 g of icosapent ethyl twice daily than among those who received placebo. (N Engl J Med. 2019 Jan 3;380(1):11-22.)

High-Yield Fast-Fact
- **Dietary Omega-3**
    - The AHA recommends eating various fish at least twice per week to maintain healthy omega-3 acquisition from dietary sources. Omega-3 supplementation should be reserved for those with CVD or high TG.

HIGH-YIELD BOARD EXAM ESSENTIALS
- **CLASSIC AGENTS:** Omega-3-acid ethyl ester of EPA/DHA, icosapent ethyl (Omega-3-acid ethyl ester of EPA)
- **DRUG CLASS:** Omega-3 polyunsaturated fatty acid
- **INDICATIONS:** Hypertriglyceridemia
- **MECHANISM:** Reduce the hepatic synthesis of triglyceride-rich VLDL.
- **SIDE EFFECTS:** Increased risk of bleeding (very small risk), fishy breath/burps
- **CLINICAL PEARLS:**
    - These agents are effective at decreasing triglycerides especially in doses of 2,000 mg or more per day and are overall well-tolerated.
    - The risk of drug interactions is very low.
    - Omega-3 agents independently may prolong bleeding time by impairing platelet function and reducing several coagulation factors. The clinical relevance of this is unknown but appears to be minimal.

Table: Drug Class Summary

Omega-3 Polyunsaturated Fatty Acid - Drug Class Review			
High-Yield Med Reviews			
Mechanism of Action: *Reduce the hepatic synthesis of triglyceride-rich VLDL.*			
Class Effects: *Decrease TG, increase HDL, possible increase in LDL; Side effects: fishy burps, potential bleeding risk*			
Generic Name	**Brand Name**	**Indication(s) or Uses**	**Notes**
Icosapent ethyl (Omega-3-acid ethyl ester of EPA)	Vascepa	• Hypertriglyceridemia	• **Dosing (Adult):** − Oral: 2 g BID with meals • **Dosing (Peds):** Not routinely used • **CYP450 Interactions:** None • **Renal or Hepatic Dose Adjustments:** None • **Dosage Forms:** Oral (capsule)
Omega-3-acid ethyl ester of EPA/DHA	Lovaza	• Hypertriglyceridemia	• **Dosing (Adult):** − Oral: 2 g BID or 4 g daily • **Dosing (Peds):** Not routinely used • **CYP450 Interactions:** None • **Renal or Hepatic Dose Adjustments:** None • **Dosage Forms:** Oral (capsule)

CARDIOVASCULAR – PCSK-9 INHIBITORS

Drug Class
- Proprotein Convertase Subtilisin/Kexin Type 9 (PCSK-9) Inhibitors
- Agents:
  - Chronic Care
    - Alirocumab
    - Evolocumab

> **Dosing Pearl**
> ✓ As with other MABs (monoclonal antibodies), these agents have to be administered parenterally as the drug can be damaged by the gastric acid if taken by mouth and is also too large of a molecule to usually be absorbed.

Main Indications or Uses
- Chronic Care
  - Hyperlipidemia, including HoFH
  - Secondary prevention of cardiovascular events

Mechanism of Action
- Inhibition of proprotein convertase subtilisin/kexin type 9 (PCSK-9) permits the recycling of the LDL receptor on hepatocytes and lowers plasma LDL by enhancing the hepatic clearance of LDL.

Primary Net Benefit
- PCSK9 inhibitors are potent reducers of LDL (up to 60%) in patients already taking maximally tolerated statin therapy and other lipid-lowering therapies (ezetimibe) who are not at goal.
  - Provide secondary prevention of ASCVD.
- Main Labs to Monitor:
  - LDL, TG, HDL, TC (baseline, 4 to 12 weeks after starting, then periodically)

High-Yield Basic Pharmacology
- Half-life
  - Long half-life of agents allows for less frequent administration.
- Parenteral Administration
  - Must be administered parenterally to avoid GI degradation since they are monoclonal antibodies. These are also large molecules that tend to be hydrophilic.
- Statins and PCSK9 Expression
  - Although statins are a cornerstone of lipid pharmacotherapy, their inhibition of HMG-CoA reductase activates sterol regulatory element-binding protein (SREBP), which increases the expression of genes promoting the production of PCSK9 and LDL receptors.
  - Therefore, while LDL receptor density increases with statins, these receptors are not recycled because of the increased expression of PCSK9 and its digestion of the LDL receptor.
- Consequences of Significant LDL Reduction
  - PCSK9 inhibitors have been demonstrated to lower LDL levels to less than 20 mg/dL, which led to speculation as to whether such significant absolute reductions are beneficial or safe.
  - Follow-up evaluations from a pre-planned secondary analysis of the FOURIER trial supported the safety of such a significant reduction in LDL with a median follow-up of 2.2 years; however, the long-term effects have not been described. (Lancet. 2017 Oct 28;390(10106):1962-1971.)

High-Yield Clinical Knowledge
- Alirocumab Administration
  - Alirocumab has specific administration requirements that must be followed to ensure full clinical benefit.
  - The solution for injection must stand at room temperature (not aided by heat or hot water) for at least 30-45 minutes prior to use. Do not shake.
  - Appropriate administration sites include the abdomen (>2 inches from the navel), thigh, or upper arm.
  - The administration itself may take up to 20 seconds
  - If the patient is prescribed 300 mg, administer two 150 mg injections consecutively at two different injection sites (i.e., two 20-second injections).

- **Evolocumab Administration**
  - Similar to alirocumab, evolocumab has specific administration requirements that must be followed to ensure full clinical benefit.
  - The solution for injection must stand at room temperature (not aided by heat or hot water) for at least 30 (prefilled autoinjector or prefilled syringe) to 45 (on-body infusor with prefilled cartridge) minutes prior to use.
  - Appropriate administration sites include the abdomen (>2 inches from the navel), thigh, or upper arm.
  - If patients are taking a once-monthly dose, the subcutaneous injection is over 5 minutes with a single-dose on-body infusor!
    - If the patient doesn't use the single-use infusor, they can take three consecutive, individual, subcutaneous 140 mg injections within a 30-minute period.
- **Adverse Events**
  - Hypersensitivity reactions can occur.
  - Aside from a 15% incidence of injection site reactions, the PCSK9 inhibitors are associated with a relatively high incidence of bacterial infections (UTI and respiratory from 5-6%) and influenza (up to 9%).
- **Dose Adjustments**
  - For dose changes (i.e., changing from every two weeks to every four weeks, or vice versa), the first dose of the new regimen should be administered at the time of the next scheduled day of the prior regimen.
- **Missed Doses**
  - Missed doses for every 2-week regimens: if the dose is not administered within 7 days of the missed dose, skip the missed dose and resume the normal dosing schedule.
  - Missed doses for monthly regimens: if the dose is not administered within 7 days of the missed dose, start a new schedule based on this date.
- **PCSK9 Inhibitor or Ezetimibe?**
  - Although the addition of a PCSK9 inhibitor to statin therapy is associated with a 60% further reduction in LDL, the evidence supporting their effect on mortality is lacking.
    - Clinical experts encourage weighing the cost-effectiveness difference between PCSK9 inhibitors and ezetimibe until head-to-head data is available.

High-Yield Core Evidence
- **FOURIER**
  - Multicenter, randomized, double-blind, placebo-controlled trial of patients with ASCVD and LDL levels of 70 mg/dL or higher who were receiving statin therapy and randomized to evolocumab or placebo.
  - Evolocumab significantly reduced the primary endpoint of the composite of CV death, myocardial infarction, stroke, hospitalization for unstable angina, or coronary revascularization compared to placebo.
  - This translates to an absolute 1.5% reduction in major CV events, which was driven primarily by reductions in nonfatal MI, stroke, and revascularization.
  - There was no overall CV mortality benefit observed with evolocumab.
  - There were more injection site reactions with evolocumab, but other adverse events were similar between groups, including new-onset diabetes and neurocognitive events.
  - The authors concluded that evolocumab reduced the risk of CV events. (N Engl J Med. 2017 May 4;376(18):1713-1722.)
- **ODYSSEY OUTCOMES**
  - Multicenter, randomized, double-blind, placebo-controlled trial in patients with ASCVD and dyslipidemia already receiving a high-intensity statin who were given alirocumab or placebo.
  - Alirocumab was associated with a significant reduction in the primary endpoint of the composite of death from coronary heart disease, nonfatal myocardial infarction, fatal or nonfatal ischemic stroke, or unstable angina requiring hospitalization compared to placebo.
  - Similar to FOURIER, there was no difference in mortality.
  - There were more injection site reactions with alirocumab, but other adverse events were similar between groups, including new-onset diabetes and neurocognitive events.
  - The authors concluded that among patients who had a previous acute coronary syndrome and who were receiving high-intensity statin therapy, the risk of recurrent ischemic CV events was lower among those

who received alirocumab than among those who received placebo. (N Engl J Med. 2018 Nov 29;379(22):2097-2107.)

High-Yield Fast-Facts
- **No Neurocognitive Adverse Effects**
  - In the initial preclinical data, there was an observation of potential increased risk for neurocognitive adverse effects. These effects were not associated with either of the PCSK9 inhibitor agents when investigated further in randomized trials.
- **Cost**
  - PCSK9 inhibitors are currently expensive, and their long-term benefit is uncertain, so the value of the agents is difficult to assess. With additional agents and increased clinical use, the cost generally decreases.
- **Other Use Considerations**
  - PCSK9 inhibitors are also associated with reductions in apolipoprotein B-100, lipoprotein A, and triglycerides.
  - Consider for patients who are statin intolerant and uncontrolled on other agents.

HIGH-YIELD BOARD EXAM ESSENTIALS
- **CLASSIC AGENTS:** Alirocumab, evolocumab
- **DRUG CLASS:** PCSK9 inhibitors
- **INDICATIONS:** Hyperlipidemia (mainly heterozygous and homozygous familial), secondary prevention of CV events
- **MECHANISM:** Inhibition of PCSK-9 permits the recycling of the LDL receptor on hepatocytes and lowers plasma LDL by enhancing the hepatic clearance of LDL
- **SIDE EFFECTS:** Injection site reactions, increased risk of infection (UTI, respiratory, influenza)
- **CLINICAL PEARLS:**
  - Consider as add-on to statin if goals are unachieved (typically after also adding ezetimibe).
  - Must be given parenterally every 2-4 weeks since they are monoclonal antibodies and have long half-lives.
  - If the dose is not administered within seven days of the missed date, skip the missed dose and resume the normal dosing schedule, or if dosage is monthly, start a new schedule based on this date.

Table: Drug Class Summary

PCSK-9 Inhibitors - Drug Class Review High-Yield Med Reviews			
Mechanism of Action: *Inhibits PCSK-9, promoting LDL receptor recycling and lowering plasma LDL.*			
Class Effects: *Potent LDL reduction, ASCVD morbidity reduction, hypersensitivity, injection-site reactions, specific administration requirements, increased infection risk*			
Generic Name	**Brand Name**	**Main Indication(s) or Uses**	**Notes**

Alirocumab	Praluent	• Hyperlipidemia (primary and secondary prevention)	• **Dosing (Adult):**
			  – SubQ: 75 mg q2weeks
			  – SubQ: 300 mg q4weeks
			    – Max 150 mg q2weeks
			• **Dosing (Peds):** Not routinely used
			• **CYP450 Interactions:** None
			• **Renal or Hepatic Dose Adjustments:** None
			• **Dosage Forms**: Solution for subcutaneous injection

Evolocumab	Repatha	• Hyperlipidemia (primary and secondary prevention)
		• Homozygous familial hypercholesterolemia
			• **Dosing (Adult):**
			  – SubQ: 140 mg q2weeks
			  – SubQ: 420 mg q4weeks
			    – Max 420 mg q2weeks
			• **Dosing (Peds):**
			  – Children 10 years and older - SubQ 420 mg q4weeks
			    – Max 420 mg q2weeks
			• **CYP450 Interactions:** None
			• **Renal or Hepatic Dose Adjustments:** None
			• **Dosage Forms**: Auto-injector, prefilled syringe, solution cartridge for on-body infusor

CARDIOVASCULAR – SMALL INTERFERING RNA AGENT

Drug Class
- Small Interfering RNA Agent
- Agents:
    - Chronic Care
        - Inclisiran

Main Indications or Uses
- Chronic Care
    - Heterozygous familial hypercholesterolemia
    - Secondary prevention of CV events

Mechanism of Action
- Prevents formation of PCSK9 proteins that degrade LDL receptors, which increases LDL uptake into hepatocytes, resulting in LDL clearance.
    - Inclisiran is a small interfering RNA that is selectively taken up by hepatocytes and put into their endosome and released into the cytoplasm to create a complex with the body's RNA-induced silencing complex (RISC). This complex cleaves multiple copies of PCSK9 mRNA to prevent its formation, which allows for an increase in LDL receptors.

Primary Net Benefit
- Provides LDL-lowering of approximately 50% by increasing LDL receptors and complements statin therapy.
- Main Labs to Monitor:
    - Lipid profile (baseline, 4-12 weeks, then every 3-12 months)
        - May evaluate LDL as early as 30 days after initial dose.

High-Yield Basic Pharmacology
- Absorption
    - Concentrations are undetectable 24-48 hours after administration.
- Distribution
    - Selectively targets hepatocytes for uptake and action.

High-Yield Clinical Knowledge

- Inclisiran Administration
    - Dosing frequency is as follows: initial dose, then again in 3 months, then every 6 months.
    - Must be administered by a healthcare provider.
- Adverse Events
    - Injection site reactions, arthralgias, pain in lower extremities, UTIs, bronchitis, dyspnea, and diarrhea were common adverse events.
- Missed Doses
    - If a dose is missed by more than 3 months, start a new dosing schedule (initial dose, then at 3 months, then every 6 months).
- Place in Therapy
    - May use as an adjunct to maximum statin therapy and lifestyle management.
    - CV outcomes on CV morbidity and mortality have not been determined.
    - After initial dosing, the twice-yearly dosing may be beneficial for compliance.

High-Yield Core Evidence
- **ORION-9**
  - This was a multicenter, double-blind, randomized, placebo-controlled trial in patients (n=482) with HeFH on maximum tolerated statins (74% on high-intensity) who received inclisiran or placebo.
  - The primary endpoint was LDL change from baseline, which demonstrated a 48% reduction.
    - NEJM 2020;382:1520-1530.
- **ORION-10-11**
  - These were multicenter, double-blind, randomized, placebo-controlled trials in approx. 1400-1600 patients with ASCVD taking maximum tolerated statins in each trial who were evaluated for 18 months while taking inclisiran or placebo.
  - The primary endpoint was LDL change from baseline, which demonstrated approx. 51-52% reductions.
  - More injection site reactions were reported with inclisiran than placebo.
    - NEJM 2020;382:1507-1519.

High-Yield Fast-Facts
- **Cost**
  - Inclisiran costs approximately $5,200 annually after the first year. Consider cost-effectiveness.

HIGH-YIELD BOARD EXAM ESSENTIALS
- **CLASSIC AGENTS:** Inclisiran
- **DRUG CLASS:** Small interfering RNA agent
- **INDICATIONS:** Hyperlipidemia (heterozygous familial), secondary prevention of CV events
- **MECHANISM:** Prevents formation of PCSK9 proteins by forming a complex with RISC to cleave PCSK9 mRNA, which prevents PCSK9 from removing LDL receptors, allowing LDL uptake into hepatocytes.
- **SIDE EFFECTS:** Injection site reactions, arthralgias, UTIs, bronchitis, diarrhea, pain in lower extremities, dyspnea
- **CLINICAL PEARLS:**
  - Administration by a healthcare professional every 6 months after initial dosing schedule.

Table: Drug Class Summary

Small Interfering RNA Agent - Drug Class Review			
High-Yield Med Reviews			
Mechanism of Action: *Prevents formation of PCSK9 proteins by forming a complex with RISC to cleave PCSK9 mRNA, which prevents PCSK9 from removing LDL receptors, allowing LDL uptake into hepatocytes.*			
Class Effects: *Reduces LDL (approx. 50%)*			
Generic Name	**Brand Name**	**Main Indication(s) or Uses**	**Notes**
Inclisiran	Leqvio	<ul><li>Heterozygous familial hypercholesterolemia</li><li>Secondary ASCVD prevention</li></ul>	<ul><li>**Dosing (Adult):** 284 mg SC initially, at 3 months, then every 6 months</li><li>**Dosing (Peds):** N/A</li><li>**CYP450 Interactions:** None</li><li>**Renal or Hepatic Dose Adjustments:** None</li><li>**Dosage Forms:** Single-dose prefilled syringe</li></ul>

CARDIOVASCULAR – STATINS (HMG-COA REDUCTASE INHIBITORS)

Drug Class
- Statins (HMG-CoA Reductase Inhibitor)
- Agents:
    - Chronic Care
        - Atorvastatin
        - Fluvastatin
        - Lovastatin
        - Pitavastatin
        - Pravastatin
        - Rosuvastatin
        - Simvastatin

> **Fast Facts**
> ✓ Statins can lower LDL-c by up to 60% from baseline, which is relevant.
> ✓ Statins have been studied in both primary and secondary prevention of CVD and shown to reduce mortality.
> ✓ The risk of liver and muscle toxicity is a dose or concentration dependent effect. At standard recommended doses this risk is very low.

Main Indications or Uses
- Chronic Care
    - Hypercholesterolemia
    - Atherosclerotic cardiovascular disease (primary and secondary prevention)

Mechanism of Action
- Inhibit HMG-CoA reductase, reducing the conversion of HMG-CoA to mevalonic acid, the rate-limiting enzyme in cholesterol synthesis.

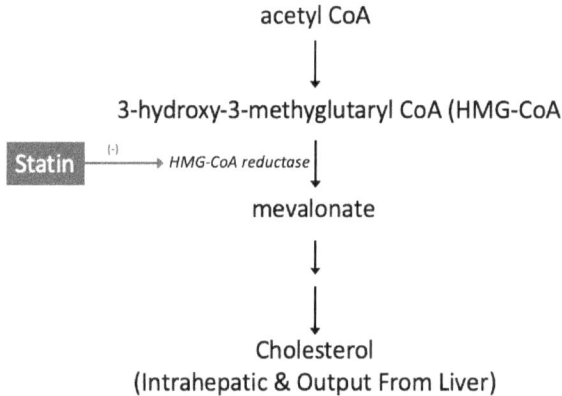

Primary Net Benefit
- Statins reduce LDL and the incidence of CV events, CV mortality, and all-cause mortality.
- Main Labs to Monitor:
    - Lipid profile (baseline, 4-12 weeks after initiation, then periodically)
    - Liver enzymes (AST, ALT; baseline, with suspected hepatic injury, and consider periodically)

High-Yield Basic Pharmacology
- **Statin Half-Life and Time of Administration**
    - Most statins should be administered at bedtime to have the largest lipid-lowering effect, which takes advantage of cholesterol biosynthesis occurring at night (between midnight and 2 am).
        - As a result of their longer half-life, atorvastatin and rosuvastatin may be administered at any point throughout the day if needed to improve compliance.
- **Hepatic Cholesterol Synthesis**
    - In response to the inhibition of HMG-CoA reductase by statins, hepatic cholesterol synthesis is decreased, which induces upregulation of surface LDL receptors, and decreased breakdown of LDL receptors, which results in LDL being increasingly removed from the plasma.
        - Triglycerides are also removed from the plasma by this mechanism.

- **Drug Interactions**
  - Gemfibrozil is contraindicated with statins due to increased risk of rhabdomyolysis.
  - Statins are substrates of the CYP450 enzyme system, although most are minor substrates.
    - Simvastatin, atorvastatin, and lovastatin are major substrates of CYP3A4; fluvastatin is a major substrate of CYP2C9.
    - Consider drug interactions for each agent.

High-Yield Clinical Knowledge
- **Statin Intensity**
  - Statins are subdivided into high-intensity, moderate-intensity, and low-intensity agents and dosed based on their LDL-lowering potential.
    - High-intensity (> 50%): Atorvastatin 40-80 mg, rosuvastatin 20-40mg
    - Moderate-intensity (30-49%): Atorvastatin 10-20 mg, fluvastatin 40 mg BID (or XL 80 mg), lovastatin 40 mg, pitavastatin 1-4 mg, pravastatin 40-80 mg, rosuvastatin 5-10 mg, simvastatin 20-40 mg
    - Low-intensity (< 30%): Fluvastatin 20-40 mg BID, lovastatin 20 mg, pravastatin 10-20 mg, simvastatin 10 mg
  - Once established on therapy, the doubling of the statin dose further decreases LDL by 6%.
- **Pleiotropic Effects**
  - Statins are also used for pleiotropic effects that are not specific to HMG-CoA reductase inhibition.
  - These include anti-inflammatory effects, stabilization of coronary plaques, prevention of endothelial dysfunction, activation of nitric oxide synthase, and reduction of blood viscosity, fibrinogen levels, platelet aggregation, and tissue factor release.
- **Hepatotoxicity**
  - All statins are associated with a dose or concentration dependent risk of causing liver damage.
  - According to updated FDA guidance, statin therapy no longer requires routine hepatic monitoring.
    - This is based on observations that suggest traditional routine monitoring does not appear to be effective in either detecting or preventing serious liver injury.
    - Hepatic enzymes should be measured only if there is clinical suspicion suggestive of liver injury following initiation or changes in statin treatment.
- **Myopathy and Management**
  - Routine screening for myopathy (CPK) is not recommended unless there is clinical suspicion of statin-induced myopathy.
    - Patients at higher risk of myopathies from statins are characterized by those who are over 80 years, have pre-existing hepatic or renal dysfunction, post-surgical or perioperative use of statins, low BMI, and untreated or undiagnosed hypothyroidism.
    - Drug interactions that increase the risk of statin-induced myopathy include fibrates (particularly gemfibrozil), niacin, protease inhibitors, amiodarone, digoxin, cyclosporine, warfarin, macrolide antibiotics, and azole antifungals.
  - Statins may be dosed every other day or weekly to manage myalgias and improve tolerance while providing ASCVD benefit.
  - Co-enzyme Q10 supplementation and vitamin D replacement can also improve myalgias and statin tolerance.
- **Diabetes**
  - Statin therapy is associated with a slightly increased risk of diabetes primarily from decreased insulin release from pancreatic beta-cells.
  - The reduction in the risk of major adverse coronary events greatly outweighs this small increased risk of developing diabetes.
    - Potential alternative mechanisms include inhibition of glucose uptake by pancreatic beta cells, beta-cell apoptosis from nitric oxide production, and glucokinase inhibition due to increased hepatic LDL uptake.

High-Yield Core Evidence
- **PROVE IT - TIMI22**
    - This was a landmark multicenter, double-blind, randomized, comparative, non-inferiority study of patients who were hospitalized for an acute coronary syndrome and compared pravastatin 40 mg daily with atorvastatin 80 mg daily.
    - Patients receiving atorvastatin had a significantly lower incidence in the primary endpoint (death from any cause, MI, documented unstable angina requiring rehospitalization, revascularization, and stroke).
    - The authors concluded that among patients who have recently had an acute coronary syndrome, an intensive lipid-lowering statin regimen provides greater protection against death or major CV events than does a standard regimen. (N Engl J Med. 2004 Apr 8;350(15):1495-504).
- **SPARCL**
    - This was a multicenter, double-blind, parallel group, randomized, placebo-controlled trial of patients who had had a stroke or TIA within one to six months before study entry, had LDL levels of 100-190 mg/dL, and had no known coronary heart disease randomized to atorvastatin 80 mg daily or placebo.
    - Patients randomized to atorvastatin had a significantly lower incidence of the primary endpoint of first nonfatal or fatal stroke.
    - Atorvastatin was also associated with a five-year absolute reduction in the risk of major CV events.
    - The authors concluded that in patients with recent stroke or TIA and without known coronary heart disease, atorvastatin 80 mg reduced the overall incidence of strokes and CV events, despite a small increase in the incidence of hemorrhagic stroke. (N Engl J Med. 2006 Aug 10;355(6):549-59.)
- **JUPITER**
    - This was a multicenter, double-blind, parallel group, placebo-controlled trial that randomized patients with LDL < 130 mg/dL and high-sensitivity C-reactive protein levels of 2.0 mg/L or higher to rosuvastatin 20 mg daily or placebo.
    - Rosuvastatin significantly lowered the occurrence of the combined primary endpoint of MI, stroke, arterial revascularization, hospitalization for unstable angina, or death from CV causes.
    - The reduction in the composite endpoint was driven by rosuvastatin associated improvements in the incidence of MI, stroke, revascularization, or unstable angina.
    - The rosuvastatin group did not have a significant increase in myopathy or cancer but did have a higher incidence of physician-reported diabetes.
    - The authors concluded that rosuvastatin significantly reduced the incidence of major CV events in healthy persons without hyperlipidemia but with elevated high-sensitivity C-reactive protein levels. (N Engl J Med. 2008 Nov 20;359(21):2195-207.)

High-Yield Fast-Facts
- **Use in Pregnancy and Breastfeeding**
    - Statins have been contraindicated in pregnancy. The FDA has recommended that statin contraindications be removed to allow patient-specific use during pregnancy.
    - Statin discontinuation is still recommended in most cases.
    - Patients at very high-risk of CV events, such as those with established CVD or homozygous familial hypercholesterolemia, may continue statin therapy.
    - Breastfeeding is still not recommended. Statins should be discontinued, or infant formula should be used.
- **Great Grapefruit Misunderstanding**
    - Grapefruit inhibits intestinal (not hepatic) CYP3A4 and has the potential to increase absorption of statins, leading to potential adverse events. However, the amount of grapefruit required is generally more than an individual can reasonably consume in a meal. Therefore, if patients desire to eat grapefruit, it is possible with close monitoring and titration of statin therapy.
- **Acute Statin for Acute MI**
    - Patients with an acute STEMI may receive high-intensity statin therapy prior to PCI, with the goal of achieving stabilization of existing (non-ruptured) plaques.

- **Protein Prenylation**
  - Statin therapy may also impair prenylation of certain proteins, with specific benefits in Alzheimer's disease pathophysiology.
    - The proposed mechanism involves statin-mediated prevention of the prenylation of Rab proteins relevant to neuronal protein synthesis.
- **Red Yeast Rice**
  - Red yeast rice should be avoided with statins due to increased risk for toxicity; it is structurally similar to lovastatin.

HIGH-YIELD BOARD EXAM ESSENTIALS
- **CLASSIC AGENTS:** Atorvastatin, fluvastatin, lovastatin, pitavastatin, pravastatin, rosuvastatin, simvastatin
- **DRUG CLASS:** Statins; HMG-CoA reductase Inhibitors
- **INDICATIONS:** ASCVD, hypercholesterolemia
- **MECHANISM:** Inhibit HMG-CoA reductase, reducing the conversion of HMG-CoA to mevalonic acid, the rate-limiting enzyme in cholesterol synthesis, which also results in LDL receptor upregulation.
- **SIDE EFFECTS:** Myalgia, rhabdomyolysis (rare), hepatic enzyme elevation and/or liver failure
- **CLINICAL PEARLS:** Statins have good evidence in both primary and secondary prevention of CVD. Statins are also used for their pleiotropic effects not specific to the HMG-CoA reductase inhibition. Muscle and liver toxicity is a dose or concentration dependent problem. May use alternative dosing to manage myalgias. Statin use should be avoided in most during pregnancy. Statins are not recommended in breastfeeding.

Table: Drug Class Summary

| Statins (HMG-CoA Reductase Inhibitors) - Drug Class Review ||||
High-Yield Med Reviews			
Mechanism of Action: *Inhibit HMG-CoA reductase, reducing the conversion of HMG-CoA to mevalonic acid, the rate-limiting enzyme in cholesterol synthesis.*			
Class Effects: *Decreases LDL, VLDL, TG, TC, increase HDL; Dose or concentrated risk of liver and muscle toxicity.*			
Generic Name	**Brand Name**	**Main Indication(s) or Uses**	**Notes**
Atorvastatin	Lipitor	<ul><li>Atherosclerotic cardiovascular disease</li><li>Heterozygous familial hypercholesterolemia</li><li>Homozygous familial hypercholesterolemia</li></ul>	<ul><li>**Dosing (Adult):** − Oral: 10-80 mg daily</li><li>**Dosing (Peds):** − Oral: 2.5-80 mg daily</li><li>**CYP450 Interactions:** CYP3A4, Pgp substrate</li><li>**Renal or Hepatic Dose Adjustments:** − Active liver disease: contraindicated</li><li>**Dosage Forms:** Oral (tablet)</li></ul>
Fluvastatin	Lescol	<ul><li>Atherosclerotic cardiovascular disease</li><li>Heterozygous familial hypercholesterolemia</li><li>Homozygous familial hypercholesterolemia</li></ul>	<ul><li>**Dosing (Adult):** − Oral: 40-80 mg twice daily</li><li>**Dosing (Peds):** − Oral: 20 mg daily − Max 40 mg BID</li><li>**CYP450 Interactions:** CYP2C8, CYP2C9, CYP2D6, and CYP3A4 substrate</li><li>**Renal or Hepatic Dose Adjustments:** − Active liver disease: contraindicated − Severe renal impairment: max 40 mg/day</li><li>**Dosage Forms:** Oral (tablet)</li></ul>
Lovastatin	Altoprev	<ul><li>Atherosclerotic cardiovascular disease</li><li>Heterozygous familial hypercholesterolemia</li><li>Homozygous familial hypercholesterolemia</li></ul>	<ul><li>**Dosing (Adult):** − Oral: 20-60 mg daily</li><li>**Dosing (Peds):** − Oral: 20-60 mg daily</li><li>**CYP450 Interactions:** CYP3A4 substrate</li><li>**Renal or Hepatic Dose Adjustments:** − GFR < 30 mL/min: Max 20 mg/day</li><li>**Dosage Forms:** Oral (tablet)</li></ul>
Pitavastatin	Livalo Zypitamag	<ul><li>Atherosclerotic cardiovascular disease</li><li>Heterozygous familial hypercholesterolemia</li></ul>	<ul><li>**Dosing (Adult):** − Oral: 1-4 mg daily</li><li>**Dosing (Peds):** − Oral: 1-4 mg daily</li><li>**CYP450 Interactions:** CYP2C8, CYP2C9 substrate</li><li>**Renal or Hepatic Dose Adjustments:** − GFR 15 to 59 mL/min: Max 2 mg/day − Active liver disease: contraindicated</li><li>**Dosage Forms:** Oral (tablet)</li></ul>

| Statins (HMG-CoA Reductase Inhibitors) - Drug Class Review ||||
| High-Yield Med Reviews ||||
Generic Name	Brand Name	Main Indication(s) or Uses	Notes
Pravastatin	Pravachol	<ul><li>Atherosclerotic cardiovascular disease</li><li>Heterozygous familial hypercholesterolemia</li><li>Homozygous familial hypercholesterolemia</li></ul>	<ul><li>**Dosing (Adult):** – Oral: 20-80 mg daily</li><li>**Dosing (Peds):** – Oral: 5-80 mg daily</li><li>**CYP450 Interactions:** CYP3A4, Pgp substrate</li><li>**Renal or Hepatic Dose Adjustments:** – Active liver disease: contraindicated – Severe renal impairment: max 10 mg daily</li><li>**Dosage Forms:** Oral (tablet)</li></ul>
Rosuvastatin	Crestor	<ul><li>Atherosclerotic cardiovascular disease</li><li>Familial hypercholesterolemia</li></ul>	<ul><li>**Dosing (Adult):** – Oral: 5-40 mg daily</li><li>**Dosing (Peds):** – Oral: 5-40 mg daily</li><li>**CYP450 Interactions:** CYP2C9, CYP3A4 substrate</li><li>**Renal or Hepatic Dose Adjustments:** – GFR < 30 mL/min: max 10 mg daily</li><li>**Dosage Forms:** Oral (table)</li></ul>
Simvastatin	Zocor	<ul><li>Atherosclerotic cardiovascular disease</li><li>Heterozygous familial hypercholesterolemia</li><li>Homozygous familial hypercholesterolemia</li></ul>	<ul><li>**Dosing (Adult):** – Oral: 20-40 mg daily</li><li>**Dosing (Peds):** – Oral: 10-40 mg daily</li><li>**CYP450 Interactions:** CYP3A4 substrate</li><li>**Renal or Hepatic Dose Adjustments:** – Active liver disease: contraindicated – Severe renal impairment: initial 5 mg</li><li>**Dosage Forms:** Oral (tablet)</li></ul>

2025

A COMPREHENSIVE *RAPID REVIEW*

NAPLEX
Pharmacology & Drug Classes

Dermatology

DERMATOLOGY – ACNE

Drug Class
- Acne
- Agents:
  - Chronic Care
    - Azelaic Acid
    - Adapalene
    - Benzoyl peroxide
      - Adapalene, benzoyl peroxide
      - Benzoyl peroxide, hydrocortisone
      - Benzoyl peroxide, clindamycin
      - Benzoyl peroxide, erythromycin
    - Erythromycin
    - Isotretinoin
    - Minocycline
    - Salicylic acid
    - Sarecycline
    - Sulfacetamide
      - Sulfacetamide and sulfur
    - Tazarotene
    - Tretinoin
      - Clindamycin, tretinoin
    - Trifarotene

Main Indications or Uses
- Chronic Care
  - Acne

Mechanism of Action
- **Benzoyl Peroxide**
  - Converts to benzoic acid and releases free-radical oxygen to oxidize bacterial proteins in sebaceous follicles, which provides antimicrobial activity against anaerobic bacteria and reduces free fatty acids.
- **Retinoic Acid Derivatives**
  - Expulsion of open comedones and transformation of closed to open comedones by decreasing cohesion between epidermal cells and increased epidermal cell turnover.
- **Azelaic Acid, Clindamycin, Erythromycin, Minocycline, Sarecycline**
  - Antimicrobial action against Cutibacterium acnes and Staphylococcus epidermidis.

Primary Net Benefit
- Topical and systemic interventions for the treatment of acne. Serious teratogenic effects due to retinoids and isotretinoin are core knowledge for health care providers.
- Main Labs to Monitor:
  - Isotretinoin: CBC with differential; Glucose, CPK; Liver function (INR/PT, albumin, bilirubin, protein); Lipid panel
    - Pregnancy test (two negative tests prior to beginning therapy, monthly negative tests during and one month after discontinuation)

High-Yield Basic Pharmacology
- **Retinoic Acid Derivatives**
  - The effect of retinoic acid and derivatives on epithelial tissue is varied, including stabilizing lysosomes, increasing RNA polymerase activity, and increasing PGE2, cAMP, and cGMP.
  - The acid form of vitamin A, tretinoin, is an effective topical treatment for acne.

- Isotretinoin is the 13-cis-retinoic acid analog of vitamin A.
- Tazarotene is an acetylenic retinoid derivative.
- **Retinoid Alternatives**
    - Adapalene is structurally similar to retinoic acid but is a derivative of naphthoic acid.
        - The advantages of adapalene compared to tretinoin include co-formulation with benzyl peroxide and a less irritating effect.

High-Yield Clinical Knowledge
- **Isotretinoin**
    - The use of isotretinoin in women of childbearing potential must utilize the iPLEDGE registration and follow-up system to ensure the risk of teratogenic effects is eliminated.
    - Before initiation of isotretinoin, women must have a negative serum pregnancy test within two weeks of starting isotretinoin.
    - Women who will begin isotretinoin must use an effective means of contraception for at least one month before isotretinoin therapy and continuously throughout isotretinoin therapy.
        - Effective birth control must also be continued for two menstrual cycles following discontinuation of isotretinoin.
    - Isotretinoin therapy must be started on the second or third day of the next normal menstrual period cycle.
    - Patients may experience an acne flair shortly after starting oral isotretinoin therapy, an effect similar to topical retinoid therapy.
- **Acne Management Approach**
    - Retinoids are considered the first-line treatment of inflammatory acne and should be used in combination with benzoyl peroxide.
    - Isotretinoin can be used as a first-line agent for cystic and conglobate acne and continued until complete clearance of acne is achieved.
    - Topical or systemic antibiotics must not be used empirically as monotherapy to treat acne.
    - For pregnant women, azelaic acid topical therapy can be used as retinoids are contraindicated.
- **Application of Retinoic Acids**
    - For the topical application of retinoic acids, the initial concentration should be sufficient to induce mild erythema and peeling.
        - Dose titration is required if too much irritation or too little irritation occurs.
- **Onset of Retinoic Acid Effect**
    - The full onset of the effect of retinoic acid on acne lesions takes approximately 8 to 12 weeks.
    - Patients may be discouraged by the appearance of worsening acne lesions during the first 4 to 6 weeks of treatment, but these lesions will clear with continued therapy.
- **Photosensitivity**
    - Patients using topical tretinoin are at increased susceptibility to UV light and sunburns.
    - Use a daily sunscreen and other protective measures while applying topical tretinoin agents.
    - Caution is also warranted in patients with a personal or family history of skin cancer, as UV exposure with retinoid therapy may increase cancer risk.
- **Benzoyl Acid Combinations**
    - Benzoyl acid has a concentration-dependent irritant effect on the skin and is often co-formulated with other anti-acne antibiotics or retinoids to reduce irritation while maintaining efficacy.
- **Antimicrobial Agents**
    - Moderate to severe acne and resistant inflammatory acne may require systemic antimicrobial therapy.
    - Systemic erythromycin is rarely tolerated due to dose-dependent nausea and vomiting, but minocycline, doxycycline, and sarecycline are routinely used.
    - Tooth discoloration that may be associated with tetracycline use is largely reversible with or without cosmetic dentist interventions. Alternative therapies are recommended for children ≤8 years old.
- **Benzoyl Alternatives**
    - Other topical exfoliating agents, including salicylic acid and sulfacetamide, may be used in patients intolerant to benzoyl acid products.

High-Yield Core Evidence
- **Oral Isotretinoin Meta-Analysis**
    - This was a meta-analysis to assess the efficacy and safety of oral isotretinoin for acne vulgaris.
    - Selected studies included all randomized clinical trials (RCTs) of oral isotretinoin in participants with clinically diagnosed acne compared against placebo, any other systemic or topical active therapy, and itself in a different formulation, dose, regimen, or course duration.
    - From a total of thirty-one RCTs, a total of 3836 participants were included in this meta-analysis.
    - There was significant heterogeneity among included studies and low quality of evidence for most outcomes assessed.
    - Isotretinoin may slightly improve acne severity, assessed by physician's global evaluation, but resulted in more adverse effects including dry lips/skin, cheilitis, vomiting, and nausea; however, there was no difference in decreasing investigator-assessed inflammatory lesions in three studies.
    - Studies using a wide range of dosing supported isotretinoin's efficacy in decreasing total inflammatory lesion count after 20 weeks.
    - There was no report of serious adverse events observed among fourteen RCTs when comparing different doses/therapeutic regimens of oral isotretinoin during treatment or follow-up after the end of treatment (up to 48 weeks). There were reported congenital disabilities.
    - The authors concluded that although the evidence was low-quality for most assessed outcomes, they were unsure if isotretinoin improved acne severity compared with a standard oral antibiotic and topical treatment when assessed by a decrease in total inflammatory lesion count, but it may slightly improve physician-assessed acne severity. (Cochrane Database Syst Rev. 2018 Nov 24;11(11):CD009435.)

High-Yield Fast-Facts
- **Oral Contraceptives**
    - Estrogen-containing oral contraceptives can also help treat acne in some women.
- **Spironolactone**
    - Although there is insufficient data to support its use routinely, some dermatologists reserve spironolactone for acne treatment in some women.

> ## HIGH-YIELD BOARD EXAM ESSENTIALS
> - **CLASSIC AGENTS:** Azelaic acid, adapalene, benzoyl peroxide, erythromycin, isotretinoin, minocycline, salicylic acid, sarecycline, sulfacetamide, tazarotene, tretinoin, trifarotene
> - **DRUG CLASS:** Anti-acne
> - **INDICATIONS:** Acne
> - **MECHANISM:**
>   - Benzoyl peroxide: converts to benzoic acid and releases free-radical oxygen to oxidize bacterial proteins in sebaceous follicles, which provides antimicrobial activity against anaerobic bacteria and reduces free fatty acids.
>   - Retinoic acid derivatives: expulsion of open comedones and transformation of closed to open comedones by decreasing cohesion between epidermal cells and increased epidermal cell turnover
>   - Azelaic acid, clindamycin, erythromycin, minocycline, sarecycline: antimicrobial action against Cutibacterium acnes and Staphylococcus epidermidis.
> - **SIDE EFFECTS:** Dry skin, erythema, teratogen (isotretinoin)
> - **CLINICAL PEARLS:** Retinoids are considered the first-line treatment of inflammatory acne and should be used in combination with benzoyl peroxide. Isotretinoin must be utilized through the iPLEDGE program. Pregnancy must be prevented with contraception and negative pregnancy tests verified before treatment.

Table: Drug Class Summary

Acne - Drug Class Review High-Yield Med Reviews			
Mechanism of Action: *Benzoyl Peroxide* – Converts to benzoic acid and releases free-radical oxygen to oxidize bacterial proteins in sebaceous follicles, which provides antimicrobial activity against anaerobic bacteria and reduces free fatty acids. *Retinoic Acid Derivatives* - Expulsion of open comedones and transformation of closed to open comedones by decreasing cohesion between epidermal cells and increased epidermal cell turnover. *Azelaic Acid, Clindamycin, Erythromycin, Minocycline, Sarecycline* - Antimicrobial action against Cutibacterium acne and Staphylococcus epidermidis			
Class Effects: Topical and systemic interventions for the treatment of acne, serious teratogenic effects due to retinoids and isotretinoin			
Generic Name	**Brand Name**	**Main Indication(s) or Uses**	**Notes**

Azelaic Acid	Azelex, Finacea	▪ Acne vulgaris
		▪ Acne rosacea
			▪ **Dosing (Adult):**
			   – Topical: twice daily
			▪ **Dosing (Peds):**
			   – Topical: twice daily
			▪ **CYP450 Interactions:** None
			▪ **Renal or Hepatic Dose Adjustments:** None
			▪ **Dosage Forms:** Topical (cream, foam, gel)

Adapalene	Differin	▪ Acne vulgaris	▪ **Dosing (Adult):**
			   – Topical: once daily before bedtime
			▪ **Dosing (Peds):**
			   – Topical: once daily before bedtime
			▪ **CYP450 Interactions:** None
			▪ **Renal or Hepatic Dose Adjustments:** None
			▪ **Dosage Forms:** Topical (cream, gel, lotion, pad)

Adapalene, benzoyl peroxide	Epiduo, Epiduo Forte	▪ Acne vulgaris	▪ **Dosing (Adult):**
			   – Topical: once daily before bedtime
			▪ **Dosing (Peds):**
			   – Topical: once daily before bedtime
			▪ **CYP450 Interactions:** None
			▪ **Renal or Hepatic Dose Adjustments:** None
			▪ **Dosage Forms:** Topical (gel, pad)

Benzoyl peroxide	Numerous names including: Acne Medication, Benzac, BenzePrO, Benzoyl Peroxide, BP Gel, Clearskin, Inova, PanOxyl, and others	▪ Acne vulgaris	▪ **Dosing (Adult):**
			   – Topical: once daily in the evening before bedtime
			      – Up to 2-3 times daily
			▪ **Dosing (Peds):**
			   – Topical: once daily in the evening before bedtime
			      – Up to 2-3 times daily
			▪ **CYP450 Interactions:** None
			▪ **Renal or Hepatic Dose Adjustments:** None
			▪ **Dosage Forms:** Topical (cream, foam, gel, kit, liquid, lotion, pad, solution)

Acne - Drug Class Review
High-Yield Med Reviews

Generic Name	Brand Name	Main Indication(s) or Uses	Notes

Benzoyl peroxide, hydrocortisone	Vanoxide-HC	- Acne vulgaris	- **Dosing (Adult):**
			  - Topical: 1-3 times daily
			- **Dosing (Peds):**
			  - Topical: 1-3 times daily
			- **CYP450 Interactions:** None
			- **Renal or Hepatic Dose Adjustments:** None
			- **Dosage Forms:** Topical (lotion)

Benzoyl peroxide, clindamycin	Acanya, Neuac, Onexton	- Acne vulgaris	- **Dosing (Adult):**
			  - Topical: 1-2 times daily
			- **Dosing (Peds):**
			  - Topical: 1-2 times daily
			- **CYP450 Interactions:** None
			- **Renal or Hepatic Dose Adjustments:** None
			- **Dosage Forms:** Topical (gel, kit)

Benzoyl peroxide, erythromycin	Benzamycin	- Acne vulgaris	- **Dosing (Adult):**
			  - Topical: 1-2 times daily
			- **Dosing (Peds):**
			  - Topical: 1-2 times daily
			- **CYP450 Interactions:** None
			- **Renal or Hepatic Dose Adjustments:** None
			- **Dosage Forms:** Topical (gel)

Clindamycin, tretinoin	Veltin, Ziana	- Acne vulgaris	- **Dosing (Adult):**
			  - Topical: once daily before bedtime
			- **Dosing (Peds):**
			  - Topical: once daily before bedtime
			- **CYP450 Interactions:** None
			- **Renal or Hepatic Dose Adjustments:** None
			- **Dosage Forms:** Topical (gel)

Erythromycin	Ery, Erygel	- Acne vulgaris	- **Dosing (Adult):**
			  - Topical: 1-2 times daily
			- **Dosing (Peds):**
			  - Topical: 1-2 times daily
			- **CYP450 Interactions:** None
			- **Renal or Hepatic Dose Adjustments:** None
			- **Dosage Forms:** Topical (gel, pad, solution)

Isotretinoin	Absorica, Accutane, Amnesteem, Claravis, Myorisan, Zenatane	- Acne vulgaris	- **Dosing (Adult):**
			  - Oral: 0.5 mg/kg/day x 1 month, then 1 mg/kg/day in 2 divided doses
			  - Oral: (micronized) 0.4 to 0.8 mg/kg/day in 2 divided doses
			- **Dosing (Peds):**
			  - Children over 12 years, use adult dosing
			- **CYP450 Interactions:** None
			- **Renal or Hepatic Dose Adjustments:** None
			- **Dosage Forms:** Oral (capsule)

Acne - Drug Class Review
High-Yield Med Reviews

Generic Name	Brand Name	Main Indication(s) or Uses	Notes

Minocycline	Amzeeq, Zilxi	- Acne vulgaris	- **Dosing (Adult):**
			   − Topical: once daily before bedtime
			- **Dosing (Peds):**
			   − Topical: once daily before bedtime
			- **CYP450 Interactions:** None
			- **Renal or Hepatic Dose Adjustments:** None
			- **Dosage Forms:** Topical (Foam)

Salicylic acid	AcNesic, Atrix, Exuviance, Neutrogena, SalAc	- Acne vulgaris	- **Dosing (Adult):**
			   − Topical: 1-3 times daily
			- **Dosing (Peds):**
			   − Topical: 1-3 times daily
			- **CYP450 Interactions:** None
			- **Renal or Hepatic Dose Adjustments:** None
			- **Dosage Forms:** Topical (cream, foam, gel, kit, liquid)

Sarecycline	Seysara	- Acne vulgaris	- **Dosing (Adult):**
			   − Oral: 60-150 mg daily
			- **Dosing (Peds):**
			   − Oral: 60-150 mg daily
			- **CYP450 Interactions:** None
			- **Renal or Hepatic Dose Adjustments:** None
			- **Dosage Forms:** Oral (tablet)

Sulfacetamide	Klaron, Ovace Plus, Plexion NS, Seb-Prev	- Acne vulgaris	- **Dosing (Adult):**
			   − Topical: 1-3 times daily
			- **Dosing (Peds):**
			   − Topical: 1-3 times daily
			- **CYP450 Interactions:** None
			- **Renal or Hepatic Dose Adjustments:** None
			- **Dosage Forms:** Topical (cream, gel, liquid, shampoo)

Sulfacetamide and sulfur	AVAR, Clarifoam, Clenia, Plexion, SulfaCleanse, Sumadan, SSS, Sumaxin	- Acne vulgaris	- **Dosing (Adult):**
			   − Topical: 1-3 times daily
			- **Dosing (Peds):**
			   − Topical: 1-3 times daily
			- **CYP450 Interactions:** None
			- **Renal or Hepatic Dose Adjustments:**
			   − Renal impairment - contraindicated
			- **Dosage Forms:** Topical (cleanser, cream, foam, lotion, pad, suspension, wash)

Tazarotene	Arazlo, Fabior, Tazorac	- Acne vulgaris	- **Dosing (Adult):**
			   − Topical: once daily before bedtime
			- **Dosing (Peds):**
			   − Topical: once daily before bedtime
			- **CYP450 Interactions:** None
			- **Renal or Hepatic Dose Adjustments:** None
			- **Dosage Forms:** Topical (cream, foam, gel, lotion)

Acne - Drug Class Review
High-Yield Med Reviews

Generic Name	Brand Name	Main Indication(s) or Uses	Notes

Tretinoin	Altreno, Atralin, Avita, Refissa, Renova, Retin-A, Retin-A Micro	- Acne vulgaris	- **Dosing (Adult):**
			  - Topical: once daily before bedtime
			- **Dosing (Peds):**
			  - Topical: once daily before bedtime
			- **CYP450 Interactions:** None
			- **Renal or Hepatic Dose Adjustments:** None
			- **Dosage Forms:** Topical (cream, gel, lotion)

Trifarotene	Aklief	- Acne vulgaris	- **Dosing (Adult):**
			  - Topical: once daily before bedtime
			- **Dosing (Peds):**
			  - Topical: once daily before bedtime
			- **CYP450 Interactions:** None
			- **Renal or Hepatic Dose Adjustments:** None
			- **Dosage Forms:** Topical (cream)

DERMATOLOGY – CALCINEURIN INHIBITORS (TOPICAL)

Drug Class
- Calcineurin Inhibitors
- Agents:
  - Acute & Chronic Care
    - Pimecrolimus
    - Tacrolimus

Main Indications or Uses
- Acute & Chronic Care
  - Atopic dermatitis

Mechanism of Action
- Bind to cyclophilin (cyclosporine) or FKBP12 (tacrolimus), which inhibits calcineurin, halting the transcription of numerous key cytokines (specifically IL-2) necessary for T-cell activation.

Primary Net Benefit
- Topical calcineurin inhibitors are second-line agents for the temporary and intermittent treatment of atopic dermatitis.
- Main Labs to Monitor:
  - No routine monitoring

High-Yield Basic Pharmacology
- Calcineurin Inhibition
  - Calcineurin usually is responsible for the dephosphorylation and then the movement of a component of the nuclear factor of activated T lymphocytes, which induces cytokine genes for IL-2.
    - Thus, blocking calcineurin activity (calcineurin inhibitor) or its secondary downstream effects (everolimus, sirolimus) prevents the activation of IL-2.

High-Yield Clinical Knowledge
- Malignancy Warning
  - Tacrolimus and pimecrolimus are associated with the rare development of lymphoma or skin malignancies and should be avoided in patients with premalignant dermatologic disorders.
  - The FDA issued a black-boxed warning specific to this effect for topical tacrolimus and pimecrolimus.
- Warts
  - New skin papillomas, otherwise known as warts, are associated with topical tacrolimus and pimecrolimus therapy.
  - Treatment with tacrolimus or pimecrolimus may continue if warts occur; however, it's recommended to discontinue calcineurin inhibitor therapy if warts do not respond to conventional therapies.
- Alcohol Consumption
  - Systemic calcineurin inhibitors inhibit aldehyde dehydrogenase and prevent ethanol metabolism, producing a disulfiram-like effect.
  - Topical tacrolimus or pimecrolimus are minimally absorbed and will not likely cause this effect; however, the warning exists in the prescribing information.

- Netherton Syndrome
  - Topical calcineurin inhibitors should not be used in patients with Netherton syndrome where systemic absorption of tacrolimus or pimecrolimus occurs.
  - Netherton syndrome is an autosomal recessive genetic disorder characterized by an increased incidence of atopic eczema, scaling skin, and hair abnormalities.

High-Yield Core Evidence
- **Pimecrolimus In Atopic Dermatitis**
  - This was a randomized, open-label study of infants with mild-to-moderate atopic dermatitis that compared pimecrolimus 1% cream with topical corticosteroids.
  - Both interventions with pimecrolimus or topical corticosteroids achieved rapid onset and success within three weeks.
  - After five years, pimecrolimus achieved an 85% success rate compared to topical corticosteroids, which reached a 95% success rate.
  - However, the pimecrolimus group required significantly fewer steroid days than the topical corticosteroid group.
  - The profile and frequency of adverse events were similar in the two groups; there was no evidence for both groups' impairment of humoral or cellular immunity.
  - The authors concluded that long-term management of mild-to-moderate atopic dermatitis in infants with either agent was safe without any effect on the immune system, and pimecrolimus may have a steroid-sparing effect. (Pediatrics. 2015 Apr;135(4):597-606.)

High-Yield Fast-Fact
- **Cyclosporine and Eye Color**
  - Ophthalmic cyclosporine administration has been associated with eyelash growth and iris color change.
  - This adverse event has been used for cosmetic purposes.

HIGH-YIELD BOARD EXAM ESSENTIALS
- **CLASSIC AGENTS:** Pimecrolimus, tacrolimus
- **DRUG CLASS:** Topical calcineurin Inhibitors
- **INDICATIONS:** Atopic dermatitis
- **MECHANISM:** Bind to FKBP12, which inhibits calcineurin, halting the transcription of numerous key cytokines (specifically IL-2) necessary for T-cell activation.
- **SIDE EFFECTS:** New skin papillomas
- **CLINICAL PEARLS:** Tacrolimus and pimecrolimus are associated with the rare development of lymphoma or skin malignancies and should be avoided in patients with premalignant dermatologic disorders.

Table: Drug Class Summary

Calcineurin Inhibitors - Drug Class Review			
High-Yield Med Reviews			
Mechanism of Action: *Bind to cyclophilin (cyclosporine) or FKBP12 (tacrolimus), which inhibits calcineurin, halting the transcription of numerous key cytokines (specifically IL-2) necessary for T-cell activation.*			
Class Effects: *Topical calcineurin inhibitors are second-line agents for the temporary and intermittent treatment of atopic dermatitis.*			
Generic Name	**Brand Name**	**Indication(s) or Uses**	**Notes**

Pimecrolimus	Elidel	▪ Atopic dermatitis	▪ **Dosing (Adult):**
			  − Topical: application twice daily
			▪ **Dosing (Peds):**
			  − Topical: application twice daily
			▪ **CYP450 Interactions:** Substrate CYP3A4
			▪ **Renal or Hepatic Dose Adjustments:** None
			▪ **Dosage Forms:** Topical (cream)

Tacrolimus	Protopic	▪ Atopic dermatitis	▪ **Dosing (Adult):**
			  − Topical: application twice daily
			▪ **Dosing (Peds):**
			  − Topical: application twice daily
			▪ **CYP450 Interactions:** Substrate CYP3A4
			▪ **Renal or Hepatic Dose Adjustments:** None
			▪ **Dosage Forms:** Topical (ointment)

DERMATOLOGY – CAUSTICS

Drug Class
- Caustics
  - Aluminum chloride
  - Ferric subsulfate
  - Silver nitrate

Main Indications or Uses
- Acute care
  - Hemostasis (including nosebleeds)
- Chronic care
  - Wart and granulated tissue removal

> **Knowledge Integration**
> ✓ Sliver nitrate is commonly used for nose bleeds where a bleeding lesion can be easily visualized, butt the key determinant is being "clearly visualized" so that the tip of the silver nitrate can only touch that part to stop the bleed.

Mechanism of Action
- **Aluminum chloride**
  - Results in mechanical hemorrhage obstruction from precipitation in tissue and blood proteins.
- **Ferric sulfate**
  - Permits thrombosis from the replacement of iron found in hemoglobin and myoglobin.
- **Silver nitrate**
  - Induced coagulation inhibits fungal DNAse from interchelation with DNA without damaging double helix, binds to electron donor groups inhibiting enzymatic activity, and promotes protein denaturation and precipitation.

Primary Net Benefit
- Topical prothrombotic agents that result in local hemostasis in acute care and surgical care areas.
- Main Labs to Monitor:
  - No routine monitoring parameters.

High-Yield Basic Pharmacology
- **Bactericidal Activity**
  - Silver salts possess strong bactericidal properties and have been implemented as an additive on Foley catheters, endotracheal tubes, and surgically implanted devices, establishing antimicrobial properties.
- **Chemical Cautery**
  - Silver nitrate possesses the ability to produce chemical cautery of nasal mucosa resulting in hemostasis from nasal hemorrhage.
  - Chemical cautery may also benefit exuberant granulations in other scenarios, including bleeding at the site of corns, calluses, plantar warts, or impetigo vulgaris.

High-Yield Clinical Knowledge
- **Silver Dressings**
  - The role of silver in burn patients is its topical application with burn wound dressings, resulting in improved tissue healing and reduced tissue scarring, enhancing the rate of reepithelialization in partial-thickness wounds.
- **Ophthalmic Silver**
  - Although rarely used, silver nitrate has a role in newborns as it prevents gonorrheal ophthalmia neonatorum.
    - Note: applicator sticks of silver nitrate should NOT be used for ophthalmic use.
  - However, erythromycin has largely replaced silver for this use.
- **Monsel's Use**
  - Monsel's solution (ferric subsulfate) is used in surgical departments to control post-procedural hemorrhage.

- **Epistaxsis (Nose Bleeds)**
  - Only use if the bleeding site is clearly visible and then roll the tip over the bleeding site for 4 to 5 seconds until an eschar forms. N Engl J Med 2021;384:e101.

High-Yield Core Evidence
- **Monsel's Solution In Severe Hemorrhage**
  - Case report of the use of Monsel's solution (ferric subsulfate) to arrest excessive uterine bleeding after the evacuation of retained products of conception after a miscarriage.
  - Monsel's solution impregnated into a uterine pack was used to secure hemostasis.
    - Am J Obstet Gynecol. 2007 Feb;196(2):e6-7.

High-Yield Fast-Facts
- **Silver Expansion**
  - The use of silver in numerous surgical devices has been expanding, including its use as a biofilm on titanium orthopedic implants and silver nanoparticles in oral/dental procedures to reduce infection.

HIGH-YIELD BOARD EXAM ESSENTIALS
- **CLASSIC AGENTS:** Aluminum chloride, ferric subsulfate, silver nitrate
- **DRUG CLASS:** Caustics
- **INDICATIONS:** Topical hemostasis (including nose bleeds or epistaxsis)
- **MECHANISM:** Direct coagulant effects unique to each agent.
- **SIDE EFFECTS:** Silver toxicity (argyria)
- **CLINICAL PEARLS:** Silver has an expanding clinical role as an additive to surgically implanted devices to reduce risk of infection.

Table: Drug Class Summary

\multicolumn{4}{c}{**Caustics - Drug Class Review**}
\multicolumn{4}{c}{High-Yield Med Reviews}
Class Effects: *Topical prothrombotic agents that result in local hemostasis in acute care and surgical care areas.*			
Generic Name	**Brand Name**	**Main Indication(s) or Uses**	**Notes**
Aluminum chloride	Hemoban Hemodent ViscoStart Clear	▪ Hemostasis	▪ **Mechanisms of Action:** − Results in mechanical hemorrhage obstruction from precipitation in tissue and blood proteins ▪ **Dosing (Adult):** − Topical application of soaked cotton pellet or retraction cord ▪ **Dosing (Peds):** − No routinely used ▪ **CYP450 Interactions:** None ▪ **Renal or Hepatic Dose Adjustments:** None ▪ **Dosage Forms:** Solution (topical)
Ferric subsulfate	Astringyn, Monsels Ferric Subsulfate	▪ Hemostasis	▪ **Mechanism of Action:** − Permits thrombosis from the replacement of iron found in hemoglobin and myoglobin ▪ **Dosing (Adult):** − Topical application to wound ▪ **Dosing (Peds):** − No routinely used ▪ **CYP450 Interactions:** None ▪ **Renal or Hepatic Dose Adjustments:** None ▪ **Dosage Forms:** Solution (topical)
Silver nitrate	N/A	▪ Antiseptic wound cauterization ▪ Hemostasis (including nose bleeds)	▪ **Mechanism of Action:** − Induced coagulation inhibits fungal DNAse from interchelation with DNA without damaging double helix, binds to electron donor groups inhibiting enzymatic activity, and promotes protein denaturation and precipitation. ▪ **Dosing (Adult):** − Topical application to the wound ▪ **Dosing (Peds):** − Topical application to the wound ▪ **CYP450 Interactions:** None ▪ **Renal or Hepatic Dose Adjustments:** None ▪ **Dosage Forms:** Solution (topical)

DERMATOLOGY – Miscellaneous Agents

Drug Class
- Miscellaneous Agents
- Agents:
    - Acute & Chronic Care
        - Aluminum acetate (Burow Solution)
        - Calamine
        - Capsaicin
        - Coal Tar
        - Lanolin
        - Odevixibat
        - Selenium sulfide
        - Silver sulfadiazine
        - Urea
        - Zinc oxide

Main Indications or Uses
- Acute & Chronic Care
    - Analgesia (capsaicin)
    - Dandruff (coal tar, selenium sulfide)
    - Seborrhea (coal tar)
    - Skin irritation (aluminum acetate, calamine)
    - Protective coating for skin irritations (zinc oxide)
    - Pruritus due to progressive familial intrahepatic cholestasis
    - Psoriasis (coal tar)

Mechanism of Action
- Aluminum Acetate, Calamine, Lanolin
    - Topical soothing effect on the skin.
- Capsaicin
    - Agonist of the transient receptor potential vanilloid (TRPV1) receptor modulating noxious stimulation and the sensation of heat.
- Coal Tar
    - Anti-inflammatory, antimicrobial, and antipruritic activity results from suppressing DNA synthesis.
- Odevixibat
    - Odevixibat is a reversible ileal bile acid transporter inhibitor (IBAT) inhibitor.
- Selenium sulfide
    - Slows the production of corneocytes and skin flaking on the epidermis and epithelium through cytostatic activity.
- Silver sulfadiazine
    - Silver ions complex with chloride in tissues to form silver chloride, causing cellular protein coagulation and the formation of an eschar.
- Urea
    - Dissolves intracellular matrix, disrupting the horny layer of skin or debriding of the nail plate.
- Zinc oxide
    - Mild astringent and antiseptic activity.

Primary Net Benefit
- Commonly available over-the-counter topical skin products that can be used with or without concomitant topical corticosteroids.
- Main Labs to Monitor:
    - Nor routine monitoring.

High-Yield Basic Pharmacology
- **Capsaicin Analgesia**
  - After applying capsaicin, the sensation of heat represents the initial stimulation of TRPV1 receptors, followed by local depletion of substance P, leading to analgesia.
  - Capsaicin is responsible for the sensation of heat from spicy foods.
- **Prolonged Onset**
  - Capsaicin must be regularly applied for up to two weeks before the full effect.
  - This is a result of the time for the depletion of substance P.
- **Coal Tar**
  - Occupational exposure to coal tar has been associated with scrotal cancer; however, the therapeutic use of coal tar for atopic dermatitis has not been associated with an increased risk of cancer.
- **IBAT Inhibition**
  - Odevixibat acts by causing decreased reabsorption of salt-formed bile acids at the terminal ileum.

High-Yield Clinical Knowledge
- **Butt Paste**
  - Diaper dermatitis is a common skin irritation due to infrequent diaper changes and poor cleansing techniques, among other causes.
  - Barriers such as zinc oxide 40% ointment (commercially available under the brand name Butt Paste, among others) can be used to manage diaper dermatitis.
  - Once diaper dermatitis is resolved, a lower concentration of zinc oxide can be used with each diaper change to prevent a recurrence.
- **Washing Hands**
  - Patients must be instructed to wash their hands before and after applying topical skin products to avoid oral ingestion.
  - This is particularly important after applying capsaicin, as accidental exposure to mucous membranes and the eyes can lead to severe burns.
- **Corn Starch**
  - Over the counter, cornstarch-based powders are recommended instead of the formerly available talc powders, which have been removed from the market.
- **Alcohol Content**
  - Parents should be encouraged to avoid diaper wipes containing fragrance or alcohol to prevent diaper dermatitis recurrence.

High-Yield Core Evidence
- **SPACE**
  - This pragmatic trial randomized patients recruited from Veterans Affairs primary care clinics to compare opioid vs. nonopioid medications (including capsaicin) over 12 months on pain-related function, pain intensity, and adverse effects.
  - Chronic pain diagnoses among eligible patients included moderate to severe chronic back pain or hip or knee osteoarthritis pain despite analgesic use.
  - Whether opioid or nonopioid, analgesic therapy followed a treat-to-target strategy to improve pain and function and included a stepwise process in an escalation of analgesic therapy.
  - According to the BPI severity scale, there was no significant difference in the primary outcome of pain-related function over 12 months and the main secondary outcome of pain intensity.
  - However, the patient reported pain intensity was significantly better in the nonopioid group over 12 months than in the opioid group.
  - Furthermore, there was a higher incidence of adverse medication-related symptoms in the opioid group over 12 months.
  - The authors concluded that treatment with opioids was not superior to treatment with nonopioid medications for improving pain-related function over 12 months. (JAMA. 2018 Mar 6;319(9):872-882.)

High-Yield Fast-Fact
- **Talc Removed**
  - In 2020, Johnson & Johnson voluntarily discontinued talc-based baby powder production due to its classification as carcinogenic to humans.

HIGH-YIELD BOARD EXAM ESSENTIALS
- **CLASSIC AGENTS:** Aluminum acetate (Burow Solution), calamine, capsaicin, coal tar, lanolin, selenium sulfide, silver sulfadiazine, urea, zinc oxide
- **DRUG CLASS:** Miscellaneous Agents
- **INDICATIONS:** Analgesia (capsaicin), dandruff (coal tar, selenium sulfide), seborrhea (coal tar), skin irritation (aluminum acetate, calamine), protective coating for skin irritations (zinc oxide), pruritus (odevixibat), psoriasis (coal tar)
- **MECHANISM:**
  - Aluminum Acetate, Calamine, Lanolin - Topical soothing effect on the skin.
  - Capsaicin - Agonist of the transient receptor potential vanilloid (TRPV1) receptor modulating noxious stimulation and the sensation of heat.
  - Coal Tar - Anti-inflammatory, antimicrobial, and antipruritic activity as a result of suppression of DNA synthesis.
  - Selenium sulfide - Slows the production of corneocytes and skin flaking on the epidermis and epithelium through a cytostatic activity.
  - Silver sulfadiazine - Silver ions complex with chloride in tissues to form silver chloride, causing cellular protein coagulation and an eschar's formation.
  - Zinc oxide - Mild astringent and antiseptic activity.
- **SIDE EFFECTS:** Dry skin, skin discoloration, burning sensation (capsaicin)
- **CLINICAL PEARLS:**
  - Patients must be instructed to wash their hands before and after applying topical skin products to avoid oral ingestion. This is particularly important after applying capsaicin, as accidental exposure to mucous membranes and the eyes can lead to severe burns.

Table: Drug Class Summary

| | Miscellaneous Agents - Drug Class Review
High-Yield Med Reviews |

	**Mechanism of Action:** Aluminum Acetate, Calamine, Lanolin - Topical soothing effect on the skin. Capsaicin - Agonist of the transient receptor potential vanilloid (TRPV1) receptor, modulates noxious stimulation and heat sensation. Coal Tar - Antiinflammatory, antimicrobial, and antipruritic activity due to suppression of DNA synthesis. Selenium sulfide - Slows the production of corneocytes and skin flaking on the epidermis and epithelium through a cytostatic activity. Silver sulfadiazine - Silver ions complex with chloride in tissues to form silver chloride, causing cellular protein coagulation and an eschar's formation. Zinc oxide - Mild astringent and antiseptic activity.
	**Class Effects:** Commonly available over-the-counter topical skin products can be used with or without concomitant topical corticosteroids.

Generic Name	Brand Name	Main Indication(s) or Uses	Notes

Aluminum acetate	Boro-Packs, Pedi-Boro Soak	- Skin irritation	- **Dosing (Adult):**
			  – Soak affected area in solution for 15-30 minutes as needed
			- **Dosing (Peds):**
			  – Soak affected area in solution for 15-30 minutes as needed
			- **CYP450 Interactions:** None
			- **Renal or Hepatic Dose Adjustments:** None
			- **Dosage Forms:** Topical (packet, solution)

Calamine	Caladryl, Calagesic	- Skin irritation	- **Dosing (Adult):**
			  – Topical: application as often as needed
			- **Dosing (Peds):**
			  – Topical: application as often as needed
			- **CYP450 Interactions:** None
			- **Renal or Hepatic Dose Adjustments:** None
			- **Dosage Forms:** Topical (lotion, suspension)

Capsaicin	Numerous brand products, including Capzasin, Flexin, Neuvaxin, Releevia, Salonpas, Trixaicin, Zostrix	- Analgesia	- **Dosing (Adult):**
			  – Topical application: 3 to 4 times daily, as needed
			  – Topical: 1 to 4 patches to affected area for up to 8 hours
			- **Dosing (Peds):**
			  – Topical application: 3 to 4 times daily, as needed
			  – Topical: 1 to 4 patches to affected area for up to 8 hours
			- **CYP450 Interactions:** Substrate CYP2E1
			- **Renal or Hepatic Dose Adjustments:** None
			- **Dosage Forms:** Topical (cream, gel, liquid, lotion, patch)

Miscellaneous Agents - Drug Class Review
High-Yield Med Reviews

Generic Name	Brand Name	Main Indication(s) or Uses	Notes
Coal Tar	Beta Care Betatar, DHS Tar, Ionil-T, PC-Tar, Scytera, TeraGel, Theraplex, X-Seb	<ul><li>Seborrhea</li><li>Dandruff</li><li>Psoriasis</li></ul>	<ul><li>**Dosing (Adult):**<ul><li>Topical application: 1 to 4 times daily</li><li>Bath - add 60 to 90mL to bathwater</li></ul></li><li>**Dosing (Peds):**<ul><li>Topical application: 1 to 4 times daily</li></ul></li><li>**CYP450 Interactions:** None</li><li>**Renal or Hepatic Dose Adjustments:** None</li><li>**Dosage Forms:** Topical (foam, ointment, shampoo, solution)</li></ul>
Lanolin	HPA Lanolin, Lan-O-Soothe	<ul><li>Skin protectant</li></ul>	<ul><li>**Dosing (Adult):**<ul><li>Topical application: as needed several times daily</li></ul></li><li>**Dosing (Peds):**<ul><li>Topical application: as needed several times daily</li></ul></li><li>**CYP450 Interactions:** None</li><li>**Renal or Hepatic Dose Adjustments:** None</li><li>**Dosage Forms:** Topical (cream)</li></ul>
Odevixibat	Bylvay	<ul><li>Pruritus due to progressive familial intrahepatic cholestasis</li></ul>	<ul><li>**Dosing (Adult):**<ul><li>Oral: 40 mcg/kg daily, titrated up to 120 mcg/kg daily.</li><li>Maximum 6 mg/day</li></ul></li><li>**Dosing (Peds):**<ul><li>Oral: 40 mcg/kg daily, titrated up to 120 mcg/kg daily.</li><li>Maximum 6 mg/day</li></ul></li><li>**CYP450 Interactions:** P-gp substrate</li><li>**Renal or Hepatic Dose Adjustments:**<ul><li>Hepatic impairment during therapy, slow titration</li></ul></li><li>**Dosage Forms:** Topical (cream)</li></ul>
Selenium Sulfide	Anti-Dandruff, SelRx, Tersi	<ul><li>Dandruff</li></ul>	<ul><li>**Dosing (Adult):**<ul><li>Topical application: to wet scalp and leave for 2-3 minutes, then rinse scalp thoroughly</li></ul></li><li>**Dosing (Peds):**<ul><li>Topical application: to wet scalp and leave for 2-3 minutes, then rinse scalp thoroughly</li></ul></li><li>**CYP450 Interactions:** None</li><li>**Renal or Hepatic Dose Adjustments:** None</li><li>**Dosage Forms:** Oral (capsule)</li></ul>

| \multicolumn{4}{c}{**Miscellaneous Agents - Drug Class Review**} |
| | | | |

Generic Name	Brand Name	Main Indication(s) or Uses	Notes
Silver sulfadiazine	Silvadene, SSD	• Burn treatment	• **Dosing (Adult):** – Topical: apply to a thickness of 1/16th inch once or twice daily, until healing has occurred • **Dosing (Peds):** – Topical: apply to a thickness of 1/16th inch once or twice daily, until healing has occurred • **CYP450 Interactions:** None • **Renal or Hepatic Dose Adjustments:** None • **Dosage Forms:** Topical (cream))
Urea	Numerous brand products, including Aquaphilic, Beta Care, Carb-O-Lac, Carmol, Gordons Urea, Rea Lo, Rynoderm, Umecta	• Hyperkeratotic conditions	• **Dosing (Adult):** – Topical application: 1-3 times daily • **Dosing (Peds):** – Not routinely used • **CYP450 Interactions:** None • **Renal or Hepatic Dose Adjustments:** None • **Dosage Forms:** Topical (cream, emulsion, foam, gel, kit, lotion, ointment, shampoo, solution, stick, suspension)
Zinc oxide	Numerous brand products, including: AmeriDerm, Ammens, Balmex, Boudreaux's Butt Paste, Desitin, Dr. Smith's Diaper Rash, Triple paste	• Protective coating for skin irritations	• **Dosing (Adult):** – Topical application as needed several times daily • **Dosing (Peds):** – Topical application as needed several times daily • **CYP450 Interactions:** None • **Renal or Hepatic Dose Adjustments:** None • **Dosage Forms:** Topical (cream, paste, stick, powder)

DERMATOLOGY – NON-STEROIDAL ANTIINFLAMMATORY DRUGS (NSAIDS) - TOPICAL

Drug Class
- NSAIDs (Topical)
- Agents:
    - Acute Care
        - Diclofenac

Main Indications or Uses
- Acute Care
    - Analgesia
    - Antipyresis
        - Diclofenac
    - Closure of patent ductus arteriosus (infants only)
        - Indomethacin
    - Dysmenorrhea
    - Ischemic stroke or transient ischemic attack
- Chronic Care
    - Anti-inflammatory
    - Cardiovascular disease primary and secondary prevention

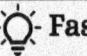

Fast Facts
- ✓ Diclofenac is also available in oral and ophthalmic dosage forms.
- ✓ It is also formulated with misoprostol to help reduce the NSAID gastritis but is associated with more GI side effects.

Mechanism of Action
- Inhibit the conversion of arachidonic acid to prostaglandins by inhibiting COX-1 and/or COX-2 either reversibly (NSAIDs) or irreversibly (aspirin).

Primary Net Benefit
- NSAIDs produce dose-dependent analgesia, anti-inflammatory, and antiplatelet effects, devoid of CNS effects but are associated with GI bleeding, adverse cardiac effects (other than aspirin), and may be nephrotoxic.
- Main Labs to Monitor:
    - No routine lab monitoring

High-Yield Basic Pharmacology
- **Prostaglandin Products**
    - NSAID inhibition of cyclooxygenase decreases the production of prostaglandins, thromboxane, and prostacyclin production.
        - Prostaglandin H2 typically produces prostacyclins, Prostaglandin D, E, and F, and thromboxanes.
    - Thromboxanes stimulate platelet aggregation and decrease renal blood flow.
        - Thus, inhibition of thromboxane (typically TXA2) by NSAIDs decreases platelet aggregation and may augment renal blood flow.
    - Prostaglandin inhibition may also produce vasoconstriction and bronchoconstriction.
- **Central Vs. Peripheral Prostaglandin Inhibition**
    - The anti-inflammatory properties of NSAIDs are attributed to their inhibition of peripherally located prostaglandins.
    - The analgesic properties of NSAIDs result from the inhibition of prostaglandins located in the CNS.
- **Analgesic Properties**
    - Upon tissue injury and the accompanying inflammation contributing pain is caused by the release of prostaglandins by cytokines such as bradykinin.
    - Local or systemic inhibition of COX and prostaglandins by salicylates contribute to analgesia, which may be combined with other pain management strategies.

High-Yield Clinical Knowledge
- **Cardiovascular Risk**
  - Inhibition of COX-2 by NSAIDs inhibits endothelial-derived prostacyclin I2 and lacks a potent TXA2 inhibitory effect on platelets, leading to an increased risk of cardiovascular adverse events.
  - COX-2 selective inhibitors were developed to reduce the risk of GI and cardiac adverse events. Still, rofecoxib and valdecoxib were removed from the market due to their association with increased cardiac events.
    - Celecoxib remains in the market but carries a black boxed warning concerning this cardiovascular risk.
  - Aspirin is the exception to this class effect, as it has a net clinical benefit in reducing cardiovascular morbidity and mortality.
- **GI Bleeds**
  - Inhibition of COX-1 by NSAIDs prevents PGE2 and PGI2, which leads to a decline in the production of the protective mucous lining in the GI mucosal lining, exposing the underlying tissue to gastric acid.
    - Normal coagulation may be impaired due to NSAIDs due to their inhibition of TXA2 and direct cytotoxic and irritating effects.
  - The most common ulcers formed by NSAIDs are located in the duodenum.
- **Kidney Injury**
  - Renal perfusion and glomerular filtration rate are partially regulated by COX-1 and PGI2, PGE2, and PGD2.
  - Inhibition of COX-1 can decrease renal blood flow and counteract renal hemodynamics by causing increased sodium reabsorption and decreased renin synthesis.
- **Closing Patent Ductus Arteriosus**
  - Ibuprofen and indomethacin can be used intravenously in preterm infants for the closure of patent ductus arteriosus.
    - Other parenteral NSAIDs include ketorolac and meloxicam, although these are only used in adult patients.
- **NSAIDs in Pregnancy**
  - NSAIDs during pregnancy are associated with premature closure of the ductus arteriosus, which impairs fetal circulation in utero.
    - This was observed among patients who were given indomethacin to terminate preterm labor.

High-Yield Core Evidence
- **Diclofenac Systematic Review**
  - This was a systematic review of topical diclofenac's efficacy and safety in acute and chronic musculoskeletal pain in adults.
  - From a total of twenty-three studies included, there were 5170 participants in this systematic review.
  - Diclofenac formulations included gel, a solution with or without DMSO, emulsion, and plaster.
  - Compared to placebo, diclofenac significantly improved pain compared to placebo.
  - There was no difference concerning local adverse events between diclofenac and placebo.
  - The authors concluded that topical diclofenac is effective for acute pain, such as sprains, with minimal adverse events. (Curr Med Res Opin. 2020 Apr;36(4):637-650.)

High-Yield Fast-Fact
- **NSAIDs and Methotrexate**
  - Although patients with Rheumatoid Arthritis may take both, NSAIDs may increase the serum levels of methotrexate, potentially leading to toxicity.
  - NSAIDs are believed to decrease the renal excretion of methotrexate by inhibiting its renal transport and a decreased renal perfusion.

> **HIGH-YIELD BOARD EXAM ESSENTIALS**
> - **CLASSIC AGENTS:** Diclofenac
> - **DRUG CLASS:** NSAIDs
> - **INDICATIONS:** Analgesia
> - **MECHANISM:** Inhibit the conversion of arachidonic acid to prostaglandins by inhibition of COX-1 and/or COX-2 either reversibly (NSAIDs) or irreversibly (aspirin).
> - **SIDE EFFECTS:** Dry skin, red skin, scaling or hardening of skin
> - **CLINICAL PEARLS:**
>   - Although patients with Rheumatoid Arthritis may take both, NSAIDs may increase the serum levels of methotrexate, potentially leading to toxicity.
>   - NSAIDs are believed to decrease the renal excretion of methotrexate by inhibiting its renal transport and a decreased renal perfusion.

Table: Drug Class Summary

NSAIDs - Drug Class Review High-Yield Med Reviews			
Mechanism of Action: *Inhibit the conversion of arachidonic acid to prostaglandins by inhibiting COX-1 and/or COX-2 either reversibly (NSAIDs) or irreversibly (aspirin).*			
Class Effects: *NSAIDs produce dose-dependent analgesia, anti-inflammatory, and antiplatelet effects, devoid of CNS effects but are associated with GI bleeding, adverse cardiac effects (other than aspirin), and may be nephrotoxic.*			
Generic Name	**Brand Name**	**Indication(s) or Uses**	**Notes**

Diclofenac	Diclo Gel, Diclozor, EnovaRX, Flector, Klofensaid, Licart, Pennsaid, Rexaphenac, Solaraze, Venn Gel, Voltaren, Xrylix	- Actinic keratosis
		- Analgesia
			- **Dosing (Adult):**
			  - Patch: apply 1 patch twice daily to the painful area
			  - Gel: apply 2 to 4 g to the painful area 3 to 4 times daily for up to 7 days
			- **Dosing (Peds):**
			  - Patch: apply 1 patch twice daily to the painful area
			  - Gel: apply 2 to 4 g to the painful area 3 to 4 times daily for up to 7 days
			- **CYP450 Interactions:** Substrate CYP1A2, 2B6, 2C19, 2C9, 2D6, 3A4; Inhibits UGT 1A6
			- **Renal or Hepatic Dose Adjustments:** None (for topical use)
			- **Dosage Forms:** Topical (cream, gel, kit, patch, solution, therapy pack)

2025

A COMPREHENSIVE *RAPID REVIEW*

NAPLEX

Pharmacology & Drug Classes

Electrolytes

ELECTROLYTES – MAGNESIUM

Drug Class
- Magnesium
- Agents:
    - Acute Care
        - Magnesium sulfate
    - Chronic Care
        - Magnesium carbonate
        - Magnesium chloride
        - Magnesium citrate
        - Magnesium gluconate
        - Magnesium hydroxide
        - Magnesium L-aspartate hydrochloride
        - Magnesium L-lactate
        - Magnesium oxide

> **Accelerate Your Knowledge**
> - Patients with low magnesium (Mg) levels can also experience hypokalemia. In order to allow for proper replacement of K+, you must replace the Mg first.
> - IV magnesium can be used to facilitate bronchodilation by competing with calcium binding with actin and myosin.
> - Patients with low magnesium will commonly exhibit prolongation of the QT interval.

Main Indications or Uses
- Acute Care
    - Magnesium Sulfate (only)
        - Acute severe asthma
        - Cardiac arrest/Ventricular arrhythmias/QT prolongation
        - Eclampsia
- Chronic Care
    - Dietary supplementation
    - Laxative

Mechanism of Action
- Essential element involved in basic cellular functions, protein synthesis, cardiac and skeletal muscle contractility, neurotransmission, and parathyroid secretion.

Primary Net Benefit
- Distributed primarily in bone and muscle tissue, magnesium is the second most abundant intracellular cation supporting a wide range of physiologic functions.
- Main Labs to Monitor:
    - Serum calcium, magnesium

High-Yield Basic Pharmacology
- **Intracellular Cation**
    - Magnesium is primarily located intracellularly.
- **Smooth Muscle Relaxation and Cardiac Contractility**
    - Magnesium produces smooth muscle relaxation by displacing calcium from actin/myosin and also as by blocking calcium entry into synaptic terminals.
- **CNS Effects**
    - Magnesium has also been suggested to act in the CNS to inhibit excitatory NMDA receptors.
    - This mechanism informs the effect of magnesium on seizures in eclampsia.

High-Yield Clinical Knowledge
- **Hypomagnesemia Risk Factors**
    - Patients with a history of GI disease involving small bowel (where magnesium is absorbed) or who have an increased renal elimination of magnesium (due to diuretic therapy) are at risk of hypomagnesemia.

- **Acute Care Uses**
  - Magnesium sulfate is used acutely for acute severe asthma (in combination with bronchodilators and steroids), for the treatment of cardiac arrhythmias (primarily ventricular tachycardia/fibrillation and QT interval prolongation), and in the management of eclampsia and preeclampsia.
- **Hypermagnesemia**
  - Although rare, hypermagnesemia can occur during the use of high-dose magnesium sulfate infusions in pregnant women with eclampsia or preeclampsia.
  - While serum magnesium levels are kept below 4 mEq/L, signs of hypermagnesemia, primarily loss of deep tendon reflexes, may be more rapidly recognized.
  - Without rapid correction (with calcium and decreased magnesium doses), loss of deep tendon reflexes can extend to loss of skeletal and smooth muscle activity.
- **Nutritional Intake**
  - The normal recommended daily intake of magnesium ranges from 310 mg/day for healthy women to 400 mg/day for healthy men.
- **Diarrhea**
  - Excessive magnesium supplementation or doses above 800 mg/dose, are associated with diarrhea.
  - In fact, magnesium citrate is used primarily as a laxative, and these dose ranges should be considered when determining a magnesium supplementation regimen.
- **Administration**
  - For patients receiving magnesium sulfate for an acute care indication, the rate of IV administration is considerably faster than for normal magnesium supplementation.
  - For eclampsia/preeclampsia, initial loading doses of 10 g (5 g IM per buttock) or 1-6 g/hour infusion are standard doses for this indication.
  - For acute severe asthma or cardiac indications, 2 g may be rapidly administered over 10 minutes.
  - In cardiac arrest, 2 g of magnesium sulfate 50% can be administered via IV push.

High-Yield Core Evidence
- **MAGPIE**
  - This was a multi-center, placebo-controlled trial of pregnant women who had not given birth or were less than 24 hours postpartum with hypertension and proteinuria and where clinical uncertainty of the benefit of magnesium sulfate were randomized to receive either magnesium sulfate IV or placebo.
  - Women who were randomized to magnesium sulfate experienced a 58% lower risk of eclampsia, which was statistically significantly better than those receiving placebo.
  - However, in women who were randomized prior to delivery, there was no clear difference in the risk of neonatal death, but there was an observed risk reduction in the risk of placental abruption among patients receiving magnesium sulfate.
  - The authors concluded that magnesium sulfate halves the risk of eclampsia and probably reduces the risk of maternal death. There do not appear to be substantive harmful effects to mother or baby in the short term. (Lancet. 2002 Jun 1;359(9321):1877-90.)
- **Magnesium for Asthma**
  - This was a meta-analysis of randomized clinical trials of adults treated in the emergency department for exacerbations of asthma, comparing intravenous magnesium sulfate with placebo.
  - A total of fourteen studies were included, accounting for 2313 patients and otherwise met the predefined inclusion criteria and were primarily double-blinded trials comparing a single infusion of 1.2 g or 2 g IV magnesium sulfate over 15 to 30 minutes versus matching placebo.
  - Patients receiving IV magnesium sulfate experienced significantly fewer hospital admissions compared with placebo, translating to a reduction of seven hospital admissions for every 100 adults treated with IV magnesium sulfate.
  - The authors noted there was no statistical heterogeneity between the three severity subgroups, or between the four studies that administered nebulized ipratropium bromide as a co-medication and those that did not.
  - Furthermore, a sensitivity analysis in which unpublished data and studies at high risk for blinding were removed from the primary analysis did not change conclusions.

- The authors concluded that a single infusion of 1.2 g or 2 g IV magnesium sulfate over 15 to 30 minutes reduces hospital admissions and improves lung function in adults with acute asthma who have not responded sufficiently to oxygen, nebulized short-acting beta-2-agonists and IV corticosteroids. (Cochrane Database Syst Rev. 2014 May 28;(5):CD010909.)

High-Yield Fast-Fact
- **Nebulized Magnesium**
    - Although magnesium can be nebulized, the ideal route of administration for the treatment of acute severe asthma is intravenous.

HIGH-YIELD BOARD EXAM ESSENTIALS
- **CLASSIC AGENTS:** Magnesium carbonate, magnesium chloride, magnesium citrate, magnesium gluconate, magnesium hydroxide, magnesium l-aspartate hydrochloride, magnesium l-lactate, magnesium sulfate, magnesium oxide
- **DRUG CLASS:** Magnesium salts
- **INDICATIONS:** Acute severe asthma, cardiac arrest/ventricular arrhythmias/QT prolongation, dietary supplement, eclampsia.
- **MECHANISM:** Essential element involved in basic cellular functions, protein synthesis, cardiac and skeletal muscle contractility, neurotransmission, and parathyroid secretion. It is a divalent cation (like calcium) and thus competes with calcium to result in a decreased muscle contraction.
- **SIDE EFFECTS:** Smooth muscle relaxation/paralysis, diarrhea
- **CLINICAL PEARLS:**
    - Patients with a history of GI disease involving small bowel (where magnesium is absorbed) or who have an increased renal elimination of magnesium (due to diuretic therapy) are at risk of hypomagnesemia.
    - Magnesium works like a calcium-antagonist to cause bronchodilation of small airways and reduce neurotransmitter release in pre-eclampsia or eclampsia.

Table: Drug Class Summary

	Magnesium - Drug Class Review High-Yield Med Reviews		
Mechanism of Action: *Essential element involved in basic cellular functions, protein synthesis, cardiac and skeletal muscle contractility, neurotransmission, and parathyroid secretion.*			
Class Effects: *Distributed primarily in bone and muscle tissue, magnesium is the second most abundant intracellular cation supporting a wide range of physiologic functions.*			
Generic Name	**Brand Name**	**Main Indication(s) or Uses**	**Notes**

Magnesium carbonate	Magonate	- Dietary supplementation	- **Dosing (Adult):**
			  – Oral: 5 mL 3 times daily
			- **Dosing (Peds):**
			  – Oral: (elemental magnesium) 10 to 20 mg/kg/dose q6-24h
			- **CYP450 Interactions:** None
			- **Renal or Hepatic Dose Adjustments:**
			  – Should be avoided in PEDIATRICS with renal impairment
			- **Dosage Forms:** Oral (liquid, powder)

Magnesium chloride	Chloromag
	Magdelay
	Nu-Mag
	Slow-Mag
		- Dietary supplementation	- **Dosing (Adult):**
			  – Oral: 2 tablets daily
			  – IV: 8 to 20 mEq/day
			- **Dosing (Peds):**
			  – IV: (elemental magnesium) 2.5 to 5 mg/kg/dose q6h
			  – Oral: (elemental magnesium) 10 to 20 mg/kg/dose q6-24h
			- **CYP450 Interactions:** None
			- **Renal or Hepatic Dose Adjustments:**
			  – Should be avoided in PEDIATRICS with renal impairment
			- **Dosage Forms:** Oral (tablet), IV (solution)

Magnesium citrate	Citroma	- Laxative	- **Dosing (Adult):**
			  – 1 to 1.5 bottles (300 to 450 mL) 8 hours prior to procedure
			- **Dosing (Peds):**
			  – Age 2 to 6 years: 60 to 90 mL once or in divided doses
			  – Age 6 to < 12 years: 100 to 150 mL once or in divided doses
			- **CYP450 Interactions:** None
			- **Renal or Hepatic Dose Adjustments:**
			  – Should be avoided in PEDIATRICS with renal impairment
			- **Dosage Forms:** Oral (solution, tablet)

Magnesium - Drug Class Review
High-Yield Med Reviews

Generic Name	Brand Name	Main Indication(s) or Uses	Notes
Magnesium gluconate	Mag-G Magonate	- Dietary supplement	- **Dosing (Adult):** 　- Oral 550 mg once or twice daily - **Dosing (Peds):** 　- Oral (elemental magnesium) 10 to 20 mg/kg/dose q6-24h - **CYP450 Interactions:** None - **Renal or Hepatic Dose Adjustments:** 　- Should be avoided in PEDIATRICS with renal impairment - **Dosage Forms:** Oral (tablet)
Magnesium hydroxide	Milk of Magnesia Pedia-Lax Phillips Milk of Magnesia	- Antacid - Laxative	- **Dosing (Adult):** 　- Oral: 400 to 1,200 mg as needed up to 4 times daily 　　- Maximum 4,800 mg/day - **Dosing (Peds):** 　- Oral: 400 to 1,200 mg as needed up to 4 times daily 　　- Age 2 to 6 years maximum 1,200 mg/day 　　- Age 6 to < 12 years: maximum 2,400 mg/day - **CYP450 Interactions:** None - **Renal or Hepatic Dose Adjustments:** 　- Should be avoided in PEDIATRICS with renal impairment - **Dosage Forms:** Oral (suspension, tablet)
Magnesium L-aspartate hydrochloride	Maginex	- Dietary supplementation	- **Dosing (Adult):** 　- Oral: 2 tablets daily 　- Oral: 1 packet up to three times daily - **Dosing (Peds):** 　- Oral: (elemental magnesium) 10 to 20 mg/kg/dose q6-24h - **CYP450 Interactions:** None - **Renal or Hepatic Dose Adjustments:** 　- Should be avoided in PEDIATRICS with renal impairment - **Dosage Forms:** Oral (granules, tablet)
Magnesium L-lactate	Mag-Tab SR	- Dietary supplementation	- **Dosing (Adult):** 　- Oral: 1 to 2 caplets q12h - **Dosing (Peds):** 　- Oral: (elemental magnesium) 10 to 20 mg/kg/dose q6-24h - **CYP450 Interactions:** None - **Renal or Hepatic Dose Adjustments:** 　- GFR < 30 mL/minute: use with caution - **Dosage Forms:** Oral (tablet)

Magnesium - Drug Class Review
High-Yield Med Reviews

Generic Name	Brand Name	Main Indication(s) or Uses	Notes

Magnesium oxide	Mag-Oxide
	Magox
	Uro-Mag
		• Antacid
		• Dietary supplementation
			• **Dosing (Adult):**
			  – Oral: 400 mg twice daily
			• **Dosing (Peds):**
			  – Extra info if needed
			    – Extra info if needed
			• **CYP450 Interactions:** None
			• **Renal or Hepatic Dose Adjustments:**
			  – Should be avoided in PEDIATRICS with renal impairment
			• **Dosage Forms:** Oral (capsule, packet, tablet)

Magnesium sulfate	Epsom Salt
	Magnacaps
		• Asthma
		• Constipation
		• Eclampsia/preeclampsia
		• Hypomagnesemia
		• Torsades de pointes
			• **Dosing (Adult):**
			  – Oral: 10 to 20 g dissolved in 240 mL water, maximum 2 doses/day
			  – IV: 1 to 2 g IV push over 1-2 minutes
			  – IV: 1 to 6 g IV over 1-30 minutes, followed by 1 to 4 g/hour infusion (if necessary)
			  – IM: 10 g (2x 5g in each buttock) at onset of labor, followed by 5 g q4h
			• **Dosing (Peds):**
			  – IV: (elemental magnesium) 2.5 to 5 mg/kg/dose q6h
			  – Oral: (elemental magnesium) 10 to 20 mg/kg/dose q6-24h
			• **CYP450 Interactions:** None
			• **Renal or Hepatic Dose Adjustments:**
			  – Severe renal impairment
			    – IV: 4-6 g loading dose over 15-30 min, then 1 g/hour infusion (maximum 10 g/24h)
			• **Dosage Forms:** Oral (capsule, granules), IV (solution)

ELECTROLYTES – POTASSIUM

Drug Class
- Potassium
- Agents:
    - Acute & Chronic Care
        - Potassium acetate
        - Potassium bicarbonate
        - Potassium chloride
        - Potassium citrate
        - Potassium gluconate
        - Potassium iodide
        - Potassium phosphate
        - Potassium P-aminobenzoate

> **Accelerate Your Knowledge**
>
> ✓ In patients found to have hypokalemia, check the magnesium level. If the Mg is low, replace first as it will be necessary to replace the total body potassium since Mg is used as a co-factor my transporters moving K+ back into the cell.
> ✓ Patients with hypokalemia can experience QT prolongation (just like in patients with low Mg and low Ca). They can also demonstrate U-waves.
> ✓ Hypokalemia (even mild cases) has been associated with worse control of hypertension.

Main Indications or Uses
- Acute Care
    - Antidote (potassium iodide)
    - Alkalinization (potassium citrate)
    - Dietary supplement (potassium gluconate)
    - Expectorant (potassium iodide)
    - Hypokalemia (potassium acetate, potassium bicarbonate, potassium chloride)
    - Hypophosphatemia (potassium phosphate)
    - Urine acidification (potassium phosphate)

Mechanism of Action
- **Potassium acetate, potassium bicarbonate, potassium chloride, potassium gluconate**
    - Replaces potassium for necessary physiologic functions.
- **Potassium citrate**
    - Undergoes hepatic metabolism to produce bicarbonate, contributing to establishing alkalemia
- **Potassium iodide**
    - Specific and competitive inhibitor of iodine uptake into the thyroid and inhibit thyroglobulin proteolysis, inhibiting thyroid hormone release.
- **Potassium phosphate**
    - Supplements and replaces phosphate.
- **Potassium P-aminobenzoate**
    - P-aminobenzoate is a B vitamin complex, providing dietary supplementation.

Primary Net Benefit
- Potassium is the principal intracellular cation responsible for numerous physiologic functions. Potassium salts provide supplementation but are limited in dose GI adverse events, tolerability of IV infusion, and cardiac conduction effects.
- Main Labs to Monitor:
    - 12-lead ECG
    - Venous blood gas (if acid – base disturbance is present)
    - Basic or Complete metabolic panel (BMP or CMP)
    - CBC with differential

High-Yield Basic Pharmacology
- **Normal Serum Potassium**
    - Normal serum concentrations of potassium typically range from 3.5 to 5.5 mEq/L.
    - It is the principal intracellular cation with approximately 98% of its total body load existing intracellularly, with 2% in the extracellular space.

- Approximately 75% of intracellular potassium is found in muscle cells.
- **SSKI, Lugol's, or Tablets**
    - Potassium iodide is available as either a supersaturated potassium iodide (SSKI) containing 38 mg iodide/drop, a less concentrated solution (Lugol's) of 6.3 mg/drop of potassium iodide, and tablets which are available as 130 mg.

High-Yield Clinical Knowledge
- **Potassium Replacement**
    - For every 0.3 mEq decrease in serum potassium, there is approximately 100 mEq total body deficit.
    - For each 10 mEq of potassium that is replaced, the serum potassium should increase by 0.1 mEq/L.
    - Before replacing potassium, reversible or modifiable causes should be addressed to avoid continued potassium loss.
        - Magnesium should be considered, as failure to correct hypomagnesemia can fail to restore potassium.
        - This is a result of a failure of the sodium-potassium-ATPase pump function.
- **Potassium Administration**
    - For mild to moderate hypokalemia (2.5 to 3.5 mEq/L), oral potassium replacement should be considered.
    - For most patients, the maximum tolerated oral dose of potassium chloride is 40 mEq every 4 hours.
    - In contrast, the maximum concentration for administering potassium chloride via peripheral IV access is 10 mEq/100 mL per 1 hour.
        - A typical administration cocktail for select patients is administering 40 mEq oral while beginning an infusion of 10 mEq/100 mL per 1 hour for four doses.
- **Regulation**
    - The potassium gradient that exists across cell membranes is maintained by the sodium-potassium-ATPase pump and also regulated by renal handling of potassium.
        - Other systems that contribute to potassium regulation include the renin-angiotensin-aldosterone system, pH, certain medications (ACE inhibitors, diuretics, catecholamines), and the GI tract.
- **Organ Systems**
    - Cardiac tissue is sensitive to potassium concentration changes as conduction abnormalities will occur in hyper or hypokalemia scenarios.
    - Skeletal muscle is also dependent on potassium for normal function and can lead to weakness, paresthesias, paralysis, among other symptoms, if concentrations are above or below normal reference ranges.
- **Hypokalemia**
    - Hypokalemia is very common in clinical practice, existing in approximately 20% of hospitalized patients and patients taking diuretics (thiazide and loop).
    - Other causes of hypokalemia include osmotic diuresis, increased mineralocorticoid activity, kidney injury, GI losses from vomiting or diarrhea, skin loss through perspiration or burns, inadequate dietary intake, transcellular shifts, and certain genetic disorders.

High-Yield Core Evidence
- **Potassium Supplementation Meta-Analysis**
    - This meta-analysis was conducted to assess oral potassium supplementation on blood pressure in patients with primary hypertension.
    - The authors included randomized placebo-controlled clinical trials addressing the effect of potassium supplementation on primary hypertension for a minimum of 4 weeks.
    - When compared to placebo, potassium supplementation resulted in modest but significant reductions in both systolic and diastolic blood pressure.
    - The authors concluded that potassium supplementation is a safe medication with no substantial adverse effects that has a modest but significant impact on blood pressure and may be recommended as an adjuvant antihypertensive agent for patients with essential hypertension. (PLoS One. 2017 Apr 18;12(4):e0174967.)

High-Yield Fast-Fact
- **Sialadenitis**
    - Supplementation with potassium iodide is associated with sialadenitis, otherwise known as iodide mumps.
    - Other common adverse effects include acneiform rash, mucous membrane ulceration, conjunctivitis, and bleeding disorders.

HIGH-YIELD BOARD EXAM ESSENTIALS
- **CLASSIC AGENTS:** Potassium acetate, potassium bicarbonate, potassium chloride, potassium citrate, potassium gluconate, potassium iodide, potassium phosphate, potassium p-aminobenzoate
- **DRUG CLASS:** Potassium
- **INDICATIONS:** Antidote (potassium iodide), Alkalinization (potassium citrate), Dietary supplement (potassium gluconate), Expectorant (potassium iodide), Hypokalemia (potassium acetate, potassium bicarbonate, potassium chloride), Hypophosphatemia (potassium phosphate), Urine acidification (potassium phosphate)
- **MECHANISM:**
    - Potassium acetate, potassium bicarbonate, potassium chloride, potassium gluconate - Replaces potassium for necessary physiologic functions.
    - Potassium citrate - Undergoes hepatic metabolism to produce bicarbonate, contributing to establishing alkalemia.
    - Potassium iodide – Specific and competitive inhibitor of iodine uptake into the thyroid and inhibit thyroglobulin proteolysis, inhibiting thyroid hormone release.
    - Potassium phosphate - Supplements and replaces phosphate.
    - Potassium P-aminobenzoate - P-aminobenzoate is a B vitamin complex, providing dietary supplementation.
- **SIDE EFFECTS:** Infusion reactions, diarrhea, cardiac toxicity (SA node depression)
- **CLINICAL PEARLS:** Potassium is the principal intracellular cation responsible for numerous physiologic functions. Potassium salts provide supplementation but are limited in dose due to GI adverse events, tolerability of IV infusion, and cardiac conduction effects.

Table: Drug Class Summary

Potassium - Drug Class Review High-Yield Med Reviews			
Mechanism of Action: *Potassium acetate, potassium bicarbonate, potassium chloride, potassium gluconate - Replaces potassium for necessary physiologic functions.* *Potassium citrate - Undergoes hepatic metabolism to produce bicarbonate, contributing to establishing alkalemia.* *Potassium iodide - Specific and competitive inhibitor of iodine uptake into the thyroid and inhibit thyroglobulin proteolysis, inhibiting thyroid hormone release.* *Potassium phosphate - Supplements and replaces phosphate.* *Potassium P-aminobenzoate - P-aminobenzoate is a B vitamin complex, providing dietary supplementation.*			
Class Effects: *Potassium is the principal intracellular cation responsible for numerous physiologic functions. Potassium salts provide supplementation but are limited in dose due to GI adverse events, tolerability of IV infusion, and cardiac conduction effects.*			
Generic Name	**Brand Name**	**Main Indication(s) or Uses**	**Notes**
Potassium acetate	Brand Name (if available)	• Hypokalemia	• **Dosing (Adult):** — IV: 10 mEq/hour up to 400 mEq/24 hours • **Dosing (Peds):** — IV: 1 to 4 mEq/kg/day, maximum 40 mEq/dose • **CYP450 Interactions:** None • **Renal or Hepatic Dose Adjustments:** None • **Dosage Forms:** IV (solution)
Potassium bicarbonate	Effer-K, K-Prime, K-Vescent, Klor-Con/EF	• Hypokalemia	• **Dosing (Adult):** — Oral: 20 to 100 mEq/day in 1 to 4 divided doses • **Dosing (Peds):** — Not routinely used • **CYP450 Interactions:** None • **Renal or Hepatic Dose Adjustments:** None • **Dosage Forms:** Oral (tablet)
Potassium chloride	K-tab, Klor-Con, K-Dur	• Hypokalemia	• **Dosing (Adult):** — Oral: 10 to 40 mEq 3-4 times daily — IV: 10 to 20 mEq/hour • **Dosing (Peds):** — Oral: 2 to 5 mEq/kg/day, maximum 2 mEq/kg/dose — IV: 2 to 4 mEq/kg/day, maximum 0.5 mEq/kg/hour • **CYP450 Interactions:** None • **Renal or Hepatic Dose Adjustments:** None • **Dosage Forms:** Oral (capsule, packet, solution, tablet), IV (solution)

Magnesium - Drug Class Review
High-Yield Med Reviews

Generic Name	Brand Name	Main Indication(s) or Uses	Notes
Potassium citrate	Urocit-K	• Alkalinization	• **Dosing (Adult):** – Oral: 10 to 30 mEq 2-3 times daily • **Dosing (Peds):** – Not routinely used • **CYP450 Interactions:** None • **Renal or Hepatic Dose Adjustments:** – GFR < 0.7 mL/kg/minute: Contraindicated • **Dosage Forms:** Oral (tablet)
Potassium gluconate	K-99	• Dietary supplement	• **Dosing (Adult):** – Oral: one capsule daily • **Dosing (Peds):** – Oral: 2 to 5 mEq/kg/day, maximum 2 mEq/kg/dose • **CYP450 Interactions:** None • **Renal or Hepatic Dose Adjustments:** None • **Dosage Forms:** Oral (capsule, tablet)
Potassium iodide	iOSTAT, SSKI, ThyroSafe	• Antidote • Expectorant	• **Dosing (Adult):** – Antidote: Oral: 130 mg daily for 10-14 days – Expectorant: Oral: 300 to 600 mg 3-4 times daily – Thyrotoxicosis (SSKI): 250 mg q6h • **Dosing (Peds):** – Infants and children younger than 3 years, 32.5 mg daily – Age 3 to 12 years, oral 65 mg daily • **CYP450 Interactions:** None • **Renal or Hepatic Dose Adjustments:** None • **Dosage Forms:** Oral (solution, tablet)
Potassium Phosphate	K-Phos	• Hypophosphatemia • Urine acidification	• **Dosing (Adult):** – IV: 0.16 to 1 mmol/kg over 4 to 12 hours – Oral: 1,000 mg q6h • **Dosing (Peds):** – IV: 0.16 to 1 mmol/kg over 4 to 12 hours • **CYP450 Interactions:** None • **Renal or Hepatic Dose Adjustments:** – GFR < 30 mL/minute: ORAL contraindicated • **Dosage Forms:** Oral (tablet), IV (solution)
Potassium P-aminobenzoate	Potaba	• Scleroderma	• **Dosing (Adult):** – Oral: 12 g/day divided 4-6 doses • **Dosing (Peds):** – Oral: 1 g/4.54 kg body weight per day • **CYP450 Interactions:** None • **Renal or Hepatic Dose Adjustments:** None • **Dosage Forms:** Oral (capsule, packet)

ELECTROLYTES – SODIUM

Drug Class
- **Sodium**
- **Agents:**
  - Acute Care
    - Sodium bicarbonate
    - Sodium citrate
    - Sodium chloride
    - Sodium phosphate
    - Sodium nitrite
    - Sodium stibogluconate

Main Indications or Uses
- **Acute Care**
  - Sodium bicarbonate
    - Sodium channel blocker toxicity, salicylate overdose, phenobarbital overdose, methotrexate overdose
  - Sodium citrate
    - Alkalization
  - Sodium chloride
    - Restores sodium and volume
  - Sodium phosphate
    - Hypophosphatemia
    - Parenteral nutrition
    - Laxative
  - Sodium nitrate
    - Cyanide poisoning
  - Sodium stibogluconate
    - Leishmaniasis

Mechanism of Action
- **Sodium bicarbonate**
  - Increases plasma and urine bicarbonate, buffering excess hydrogen ions.
  - Increases sodium and changes the proportion of sodium channel blocking xenobiotic that is ionized, displacing it from binding sites.
- **Sodium citrate**
  - Citrate chelates free ionized calcium, preventing its use in the coagulation cascade, thereby causing an anticoagulation effect.
- **Sodium chloride**
  - Supports numerous physiologic functions, including volume regulation, osmotic pressure control, and electrolyte balance.
- **Sodium phosphate**
  - Produces osmotic effect in the small intestine, stimulating distention and peristalsis.
- **Sodium nitrate**
  - Induces the formation of methemoglobin.
- **Sodium stibogluconate**
  - Converted to trivalent antimony, which affects glucose homeostasis, fatty acid beta-oxidation, and ATP formation.

Primary Net Benefit
- Sodium is an essential element, with numerous salt preparations that possess unique indications and pharmacologic actions.

- Main Labs to Monitor:
  - ECG
  - Venous blood gas
  - Complete metabolic panel
  - CBC with differential

High-Yield Basic Pharmacology
- **Osmolarity**
  - Under most circumstances, the maximum osmolarity of intravenous fluid for peripheral administration is 900 mOsmol.
  - Sodium bicarbonate is commonly available 8.4% solution has an osmolarity of 2,000 mOsmol but is routinely administered via peripheral IV access.
  - "Normal Saline," which is sodium chloride 0.9%, has a serum osmolarity of 308 mOsmol, and sodium chloride 3%'s osmolarity is 1028 mOsmol.
- **Antimony**
  - Sodium stibogluconate is a pentavalent antimony preparation that is used for the treatment of cutaneous or visceral leishmaniasis.
  - Upon absorption, antimony is converted to trivalent antimony, affecting glucose homeostasis, fatty acid beta-oxidation, and ATP formation.

High-Yield Clinical Knowledge
- **Corrected Sodium Formula**
  - Among patients with hyperglycemia, serum sodium concentrations may be falsely low on basic or complete metabolic panels.
  - To correct for hyperglycemia, the observed serum sodium should be increased by 1.6 mEq/L for every 100 mg/dL of glucose over 100 to 400 mg/dL.
    - For glucose above 400 mg/dL, the observed serum sodium should be increased by 4.0 for every 100 mg/dL over 400 mg/dL.
- **Clinical Presentation of Hyponatremia**
  - The clinical manifestations of hyponatremia depend on how rapid the change in serum sodium, not just how low serum sodium levels reach.
  - Nonspecific symptoms of hyponatremia include anorexia, nausea and vomiting, and weakness.
  - Severe acute reductions in serum sodium can cause altered mental status, seizures, coma, cerebral edema, and brainstem herniation.
- **Treatment Strategies of Hyponatremia**
  - The management of hyponatremia depends on the presenting symptoms, the onset of hyponatremia, and the degree of hyponatremia.
  - Euvolemic hyponatremia likely attributed to SIADH, can be managed with free water restriction and treatment of the underlying disease or with "vaptans," otherwise known as vasopressin V2 receptor antagonists (conivaptan, tolvaptan)
  - Hypervolemic hyponatremia is managed with water restriction and treatment of the underlying cause, often excess free water intake.
  - Hypovolemic hyponatremia is treated with sodium replacement, but depending on the clinical sequelae, the concentration and rate of administration of sodium changes.
- **Hyponatremia Types**
  - Hyponatremia can be described as hypovolemic, euvolemic, hypervolemic or pseudohyponatremia.
- **Emergent Sodium Correction**
  - In hyponatremic patients presenting with seizures or severe mental status changes, hypertonic saline (typically NaCl 3%) is rapidly administered to increase serum sodium by 4 to 6 mEq/L within 6 hours until seizures stop.
  - Once symptoms have been controlled, sodium chloride is administered at 1-2 mEq/L/hour with the goal of 10 to 12 mEq/24hour replacement.

- **Rapid Sodium Correction Consequences**
  - Osmotic demyelination results from correcting serum sodium too rapidly, as fluid is pulled from the neurons into extracellular space, causing paralysis and death.
  - Risk factors of osmotic demyelination include overcorrection of sodium (more than 12 mEq/24 hours or 18 mEq/48 hours), patients with a history of alcoholism, malnourishment, and the elderly.
- **Renal Tubular Acidosis**
  - In combination with citric acid and potassium citrate, sodium citrate is used to manage both type 1 and type 2 renal tubular acidosis.
- **Cyanide Antidote Kit**
  - Sodium nitrite is a component of the former cyanide antidote kit and was used in combination with sodium thiosulfate.
  - Sodium nitrite is intended to induce methemoglobin, which has a more favorable oxygen dissociation compared to cyanohemoglobin.
- **Sodium Phosphate**
  - Sodium phosphate has broad therapeutic applications, including acute hypophosphatemia management, as a component of parenteral nutrition and as a laxative.

High-Yield Core Evidence

- **BICAR-ICU**
  - This was a multicenter, open-label, phase 3 trial that randomized patients admitted within 48 hours to an ICU with severe acidemia with a total SOFA score of 4 or more and an arterial lactate of 2 mmol/L or more to receive either no sodium bicarbonate (control group) or 4·2% of intravenous sodium bicarbonate infusion (bicarbonate group) to maintain the arterial pH above 7·30.
  - There was no significant difference between groups in the primary outcome of a composite of death from any cause by day 28 and the presence of at least one organ failure at day 7.
  - However, patients with acute kidney injury receiving sodium bicarbonate had a significantly higher 28-day survival than control.
  - The authors concluded that sodium bicarbonate in patients with severe metabolic acidemia did not affect the primary composite outcome (Lancet. 2018 Jul 7;392(10141):31-40.)
- **SALT-ED**
  - This was a single-center, pragmatic, multiple-crossover trial comparing balanced crystalloids (lactated Ringer's solution or Plasma-Lyte A) with saline among adults treated with intravenous crystalloids in the emergency department and were subsequently hospitalized outside an ICU.
  - There was no difference in the primary outcome of the number of hospital-free days between the balanced-crystalloids and saline groups.
  - However, balanced crystalloids resulted in a lower incidence of major adverse kidney events within 30 days than saline.
  - The authors concluded that there was no difference in hospital-free days between treatment with balanced crystalloids and treatment with saline among noncritically ill adults treated with intravenous fluids in the emergency department. (N Engl J Med. 2018 Mar 1;378(9):819-828.)

High-Yield Fast-Fact

- **ICP Elevation**

As an alternative to hypertonic sodium chloride, sodium bicarbonate 8.4% can be rapidly administered to reduce intracranial pressure and is routinely available in many emergency departments and critical care areas.

HIGH-YIELD BOARD EXAM ESSENTIALS

- **CLASSIC AGENTS:** Sodium (bicarbonate, citrate, chloride, phosphate, nitrite, stibogluconate)
- **DRUG CLASS:** Sodium
- **INDICATIONS:** Sodium replacement, management of metabolic acidosis, sodium channel blocker toxicity, urine alkalinization
- **MECHANISM:**
    - **Sodium bicarbonate** - Sodium channel blocker toxicity, salicylate overdose, phenobarbital overdose, methotrexate overdose.
    - **Sodium citrate** – Alkalization. Sodium chloride – Restores sodium and volume.
    - **Sodium phosphate** - Hypophosphatemia, Parenteral nutrition, Laxative.
    - **Sodium nitrate** - Cyanide poisoning. Sodium stibogluconate - Leishmaniasis
- **SIDE EFFECTS:** Hypernatremia, volume overload, diarrhea
- **CLINICAL PEARLS:** In hyponatremic patients presenting with seizures or severe mental status changes, hypertonic saline (typically NaCl 3%) is rapidly administered to increase serum sodium by 4 to 6 mEq/L within 6 hours until seizures stop.

Table: Drug Class Summary

Sodium - Drug Class Review High-Yield Med Reviews	
Mechanism of Action: Sodium bicarbonate - Sodium channel blocker toxicity, salicylate overdose, phenobarbital overdose, methotrexate overdose Sodium citrate - Alkalization Sodium chloride - Restores sodium and volume. Sodium phosphate - Hypophosphatemia, Parenteral nutrition, Laxative Sodium nitrate - Cyanide poisoning Sodium stibogluconate - Leishmaniasis	
Class Effects: Sodium is an essential element, with numerous salt preparations that possess unique indications and pharmacologic actions.	

Generic Name	Brand Name	Main Indication(s) or Uses	Notes
Sodium Bicarbonate	Neut	- Management of metabolic acidosis - Sodium channel blocker toxicity - Urine alkalinization	- **Dosing (Adult):** – IV/IO: 1 mEq/kg/dose repeated as necessary with or without 0.5 to 1 mEq/kg/hour infusion - **Dosing (Peds):** – IV/IO: 1 mEq/kg/dose repeated as necessary with or without 0.5 to 1 mEq/kg/hour infusion - **CYP450 Interactions:** None - **Renal or Hepatic Dose Adjustments:** None - **Dosage Forms:** IV (solution), Oral (powder, tablet)
Sodium citrate (with citric acid, and/or potassium citrate)	Cytra-2, Oracit, Cytra-3	- Systemic alkalization	- **Dosing (Adult):** – Oral: 10 to 30 mL four times daily - **Dosing (Peds):** – Oral: 2 to 4 mL/kg/day - **CYP450 Interactions:** None - **Renal or Hepatic Dose Adjustments:** None - **Dosage Forms:** Oral (solution)
Sodium chloride	Normal Saline	- Restores sodium and volume	- **Dosing (Adult):** – Inhalation/Nebulized: 1 to 4 mL 2 to 4 times daily – Irrigation: 1 to 3 L/day – IV: 10 to 20 mL/kg bolus (0.9% NaCl) – Ophthalmic 1-2 drops in affected eyes q3-4h - **Dosing (Peds):** – See adult dosing - **CYP450 Interactions:** None - **Renal or Hepatic Dose Adjustments:** None - **Dosage Forms:** Nasal (aerosol, gel), IV (solution), Inhalation (solution), Oral (tablet), Ophthalmic (solution)

| \multicolumn{4}{c}{**Sodium - Drug Class Review**} |
Generic Name	**Brand Name**	**Main Indication(s) or Uses**	**Notes**
Sodium phosphate	Fleet enema, OsmoPrep	<ul><li>Constipation</li><li>Bowel cleansing</li><li>Hypophosphatemia</li></ul>	<ul><li>**Dosing (Adult):**<ul><li>IV: 0.16 to 1 mmol/kg over 4 to 12 hours</li><li>Parenteral Nutrition: 10 to 15 mmol/1,000 kcal</li><li>Rectal: 4.5 ounces once</li><li>Oral: 15 to 45 mL once</li></ul></li><li>**Dosing (Peds):**<ul><li>IV: 0.16 to 1 mmol/kg over 4 to 12 hours</li><li>Parenteral nutrition 0.5 to 2 mmol/kg/day Rectal: 4.5 ounces once</li><li>Oral: 7.5 to 45 mL once</li></ul></li><li>**CYP450 Interactions:** None</li><li>**Renal or Hepatic Dose Adjustments:**<ul><li>GFR < 30 mL/minute: avoid oral solution</li></ul></li><li>**Dosage Forms:** IV (solution), Oral (solution, tablet), Rectal (solution)</li></ul>
Sodium nitrite	Cyanide antidote kit	<ul><li>Cyanide poisoning</li></ul>	<ul><li>**Dosing (Adult):**<ul><li>IV: 300 mg, or 0.19 to 0.39 mL/kg of 3% solution</li></ul></li><li>**Dosing (Peds):**<ul><li>IV: 6 mg/kg, maximum 300 mg</li></ul></li><li>**CYP450 Interactions:** None</li><li>**Renal or Hepatic Dose Adjustments:** None</li><li>**Dosage Forms:** IV (solution)</li></ul>
Sodium stibogluconate	Pentostam	<ul><li>Leishmaniasis</li></ul>	<ul><li>**Dosing (Adult):**<ul><li>IM/IV: 20 mg/kg/day for 28 days</li></ul></li><li>**Dosing (Peds):**<ul><li>IM/IV: 20 mg/kg/day for 28 days</li></ul></li><li>**CYP450 Interactions:** None</li><li>**Renal or Hepatic Dose Adjustments:** None</li><li>**Dosage Forms:** IV (solution)</li></ul>

2025

A COMPREHENSIVE *RAPID REVIEW*

NAPLEX

Pharmacology & Drug Classes

Endocrinology

ENDOCRINE – ANDROGEN REPLACEMENT THERAPY

Drug Class
- Androgen

Main Indications or Uses
- Hypogonadism
- Hormone therapy (female-to-male)

Mechanism of Action
- Androgens are responsible for male sexual organ growth and development.

Primary Overall Net Benefit
- Replaces androgen to achieve an adequate testosterone level.
- Main Labs to Monitor:
  - Testosterone
    - Total: every 3 to 6 months until at goal, then every 6 to 12 months after that.
      - May differ depending on the dosage form selected.
    - Free: consider if total testosterone is in borderline amount.
  - BP, CBC, LFTs, lipid panel, and PSA

High-Yield Basic Pharmacology
- **Therapy Considerations**
  - Oral testosterone has a low bioavailability; non-oral dosage forms are generally preferred.
  - Undergoes hepatic metabolism
  - Highly protein-bound

High-Yield Core Knowledge
- **Hypogonadism**
  - Routine screening of total testosterone for hypogonadism for cisgender males is not recommended.
  - Screening should be completed for men with symptoms of hypogonadism.
  - Total testosterone level must be drawn fasting x 2 separate days due to influencing variables.
- **Dosage Form Selection**
  - Injectable therapies are generally the most cost-effective.
  - Use topical preparations with caution due to potential effects on pets, children, or females.
- **Potential Adverse Reactions**
  - Can have many adverse effects, including sodium retention, polycythemia (hematocrit > 55%), hepatotoxicity, dyslipidemia, VTE, BPH, depression, priapism, gynecomastia
  - Data regarding the increased risk of prostate cancer is controversial.
- **Boxed Warnings**
  - BP increases may occur that can lead to CV events with any agent, but testosterone undecanoate and testosterone enanthate carry greater risk.
  - Secondary exposure can cause virilization in children who are exposed to testosterone products.
  - Pulmonary oil microembolism may occur with IM testosterone undecanoate.

High-Yield Clinical Knowledge
- **Androgen Therapy Initiation**
  - Total testosterone of < 200 – 300 ng/dL is consistently considered androgen deficient.
  - Initiate in patients with symptoms and those with an understanding of the risks and benefits of therapy.
  - Testosterone replacement in the elderly is not generally recommended due to the increased risk of fluid retention, prostatic hyperplasia, LFT elevations, and prostate cancer

- **Androgen Therapy Contraindications**
  - The upcoming desire for fertility
  - Breast or prostate cancer
  - PSA >4 ng/mL (>3 ng/mL with high-risk prostate cancer)
  - Untreated severe obstructive sleep apnea
  - Elevated hematocrit or thrombophilia
  - Uncontrolled HF or stroke or MI within 6 months.
- **Differentiation from Erectile Dysfunction**
  - Androgen deficiency symptoms: fatigue, muscle wasting, low libido.
    - The patient does not have an adequate response to stimulation.
  - Erectile dysfunction symptoms: inadequate erection (quality and quantity).
    - The patient has a response to stimulation but the inability to achieve an adequate erection.

High-Yield Core Evidence
- **Testosterone and Prostate Outcomes**
  - Androgens play a role in prostate cancer, but the evidence is controversial as to whether testosterone replacement therapies increase the risk of prostate cancer in men without a history.
  - J Natl Cancer Inst. 2008;100(3):170–183.; J Clin Oncol. 2000;18(4):847–853.
- **Testosterone and Cardiovascular Outcomes**
  - Low testosterone has consistently been proven to correlate with worsened CV outcomes. However, in recent years, evidence has been controversial regarding testosterone replacement therapy's role in worsening CV outcomes.
  - Expert Opin Drug Saf 2014;13:1327.; N Engl J Med 2010;363:109.; J Clin Endocrinol Metab 2011;96(10):3007-2019.; Am Coll Cardiol 2011;58(16):1674-1681.

High-Yield Fast-Fact
- **Anabolic Steroids**
  - Commonly used for performance enhancement, anabolic steroids can result in secondary hypogonadism due to suppression of the hypothalamic-pituitary-gonadal axis.
  - Potency and inactive ingredients in anabolic steroid preparations are unknown as the substances are not regulated or FDA-approved.
  - Testosterone preparations have a potential for abuse, misuse, or diversion. Consider in patients with CV or psychiatric adverse events.
- **Female-to-Male Androgen Replacement Therapy**
  - Lab values in electronic health records will match the patient's assigned gender. For example, if testosterone labs are drawn for a transgender male with an assigned gender of female in the electronic health record, the normal lab value will be that of a female. Be mindful of actual hormone targets as opposed to the lab's normal/reference range.

HIGH-YIELD BOARD EXAM ESSENTIALS
- **CLASSIC AGENTS:** Testosterone
- **DRUG CLASS:** Androgen replacement therapy
- **INDICATIONS:** Hypogonadism (testosterone deficiency), female-to-male hormone therapy
- **MECHANISM:** Responsible for male sexual organ growth and development.
- **SIDE EFFECTS:** Hepatotoxicity, hypernatremia, polycythemia, potential for prostate cancer, BP increase.
- **CLINICAL PEARLS:** Routine screening of total testosterone for hypogonadism for cisgender males is not recommended. Have potential for abuse or diversion.

Table: Drug Class Summary

| | Androgen Replacement Therapy Drug Class Review
High-Yield Med Reviews |

Mechanism of Action: Androgens are responsible for male sexual organ growth and development.			
Class Effects: *Replacement of androgen to achieve adequate testosterone level.*			
Generic Name	Brand Name	Indication(s) or Uses	Notes
Testosterone Intramuscular Injection	Depo-Testosterone Aveed	▪ Hypogonadism (testosterone deficiency), female-to-male hormone therapy	▪ **Dosing (Adult):** – Testosterone enanthate, cypionate: 75-100mg once weekly or 150-200mg every 2 weeks – Testosterone undecanoate: 750mg every 4 weeks x 2, then 750mg every 10 weeks after that ▪ **Dosing (Peds):** various regimens – Testosterone enanthate, cypionate: approved ≥12 years of age ▪ **CYP450 Interactions:** minor substrate of CYP2B6, CYP2C19, CYP2C9, CYP3A4 ▪ **Renal or Hepatic Dose Adjustments:** Testosterone cypionate contraindicated in hepatic failure ▪ **Dosage forms:** Injection (solution)
Testosterone Subcutaneous Injection	Xyosted	▪ Hypogonadism (testosterone deficiency), female-to-male hormone therapy	▪ **Dosing (Adult):** – 75mg once weekly ▪ **Dosing (Peds):** not approved ▪ **CYP450 Interactions:** minor substrate of CYP2B6, CYP2C19, CYP2C9, CYP3A4 ▪ **Renal or Hepatic Dose Adjustments:** Testosterone cypionate contraindicated in hepatic failure ▪ **Dosage forms:** Injection (subcutaneous solution)
Testosterone Oral	Jatenzo	▪ Hypogonadism (testosterone deficiency), female-to-male hormone therapy	▪ **Dosing (Adult):** – Testosterone enanthate, cypionate: 75-100mg once weekly or 150-200mg every 2 weeks – Testosterone undecanoate: 750mg every 4 weeks x 2, then 750mg every 10 weeks after that ▪ **Dosing (Peds):** various regimens – Testosterone enanthate, cypionate: approved ≥12 years of age ▪ **CYP450 Interactions:** minor substrate of CYP2B6, CYP2C19, CYP2C9, CYP3A4 ▪ **Renal or Hepatic Dose Adjustments:** Testosterone cypionate contraindicated in hepatic failure ▪ **Dosage forms:** Oral (capsule)

| \multicolumn{4}{c}{**Androgen Replacement Therapy Drug Class Review**} |
| \multicolumn{4}{c}{High-Yield Med Reviews} |

Generic Name	Brand Name	Indication(s) or Uses	Notes
Testosterone Nasal	Natesto	▪ Hypogonadism (testosterone deficiency), female-to-male hormone therapy	▪ **Dosing (Adult):** 11mg (2 pumps) three times daily ▪ **Dosing (Peds):** not approved ▪ **CYP450 Interactions:** minor substrate of CYP2B6, CYP2C19, CYP2C9, CYP3A4 ▪ **Renal or Hepatic Dose Adjustments:** Testosterone cypionate contraindicated in hepatic failure ▪ **Dosage forms:** Intranasal (gel)
Testosterone Pellet	Testopel	▪ Hypogonadism (testosterone deficiency), female-to-male hormone therapy	▪ **Dosing (Adult):** 150 to 450 mg implanted every 3 to 6 months ▪ **Dosing (Peds):** approved ≥12 years of age, various regimens, consider weight-based dosing ▪ **CYP450 Interactions:** minor substrate of CYP2B6, CYP2C19, CYP2C9, CYP3A4 ▪ **Renal or Hepatic Dose Adjustments:** Testosterone cypionate contraindicated in hepatic failure ▪ **Dosage forms:** Pellet (non-oral)
Testosterone Transdermal Gel and Solution	AndroGel Fortesta Vogelxo Axiron	▪ Hypogonadism (testosterone deficiency), female-to-male hormone therapy	▪ **Dosing (Adult):** variable doses depending on the product selected, approximately 40mg – 60mg once daily ▪ **Dosing (Peds):** not approved ▪ **CYP450 Interactions:** minor substrate of CYP2B6, CYP2C19, CYP2C9, CYP3A4 ▪ **Renal or Hepatic Dose Adjustments:** Testosterone cypionate contraindicated in hepatic failure ▪ **Dosage forms:** Topical (gel solution)
Testosterone Transdermal Patch	Androderm	▪ Hypogonadism (testosterone deficiency), female-to-male hormone therapy	▪ **Dosing (Adult):** 4mg patch once daily ▪ **Dosing (Peds):** not approved ▪ **CYP450 Interactions:** minor substrate of CYP2B6, CYP2C19, CYP2C9, CYP3A4 ▪ **Renal or Hepatic Dose Adjustments:** Testosterone cypionate contraindicated in hepatic failure ▪ **Dosage forms:** Topical (patch)

ENDOCRINE – ANTIDIABETIC AGENTS - ALPHA-GLUCOSIDASE INHIBITORS

Drug Class

- Alpha-glucosidase inhibitors (AGIs)
- Agents: acarbose, miglitol

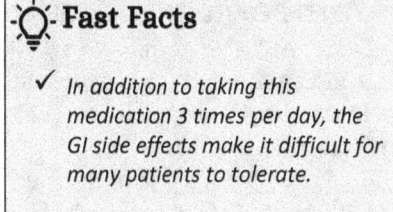

Fast Facts

✓ In addition to taking this medication 3 times per day, the GI side effects make it difficult for many patients to tolerate.

Main Indications or Uses
- Type 2 diabetes (T2DM) management as an adjunct to diet and exercise

Mechanism of Action
- Pancreatic alpha-amylase and intestinal brush border alpha-glucosidase inhibitor, which delays hydrolysis of complex carbohydrates and disaccharides and glucose absorption.

Primary Net Benefit
- Delays absorption of glucose that results in postprandial glucose reductions.
- Main Labs to Monitor:
    - A1c every 3-6 months, depending on whether the patient is at goal.
    - Monitor SCr and LFTs every 3 months for 1 year, then periodically.

High-Yield Basic Pharmacology
- Acts locally in GI tract.
- Peaks in 1 hour with a half-life of 2 hours.

High-Yield Clinical Knowledge
- Doses should be titrated slowly over 4-8 weeks.
    - May start with 1 meal and increase to other meals, then increase the dose, or start with low doses at all 3 meals.
    - Max dose for ≤60 kg = 50 mg TID; >60 kg = 100 mg TID
        - Minimal efficacy gained at 100 mg but increased adverse effects.
    - Dosing is the same for pediatrics (acarbose only), but evidence in this population is largely experiential.
- GI adverse effects, most prominently flatulence, diarrhea, bloating, and/or abdominal pain, occur frequently and limit use. Effects are transient if tolerated.
    - Avoid a diet high in sugar because of the increased risk of significant GI effects.
    - If GI effects occur despite a low carbohydrate diet, reduce the dose and consider whether titration can be retried.
- Administer with the first bite of each meal.
- Has low risk of hypoglycemia.
    - Use dextrose instead of sucrose (cane sugar) to treat hypoglycemia since hydrolysis of sucrose to glucose/fructose is inhibited.
- Any weight loss is not clinically meaningful.
- Contraindicated in cirrhosis, IBD, and other GI diseases.
- Discontinue therapy with LFT elevations.
- Generics are available at low cost, but despite this, the class is rarely utilized in practice due to GI intolerability.

High-Yield Fast-Fact
- Has off-label use for postprandial hyperinsulinemic hypoglycemia post-gastric bypass surgery.
- Patients do not favor this class of medications because of the social implications of the adverse effects.

> **HIGH-YIELD BOARD EXAM ESSENTIALS**
> - **CLASSIC AGENTS:** Acarbose, miglitol
> - **DRUG CLASS:** Alpha-glucosidase inhibitors
> - **INDICATIONS:** Type 2 diabetes (T2DM)
> - **MECHANISM:** Delays absorption of carbohydrates from the small intestine.
> - **SIDE EFFECTS:** High rate of GI adverse effects (flatulence, diarrhea, bloating, and/or abdominal pain)
> - **CLINICAL PEARLS:** Has low risk of hypoglycemia. Use dextrose instead of sucrose (cane sugar) to treat hypoglycemia since hydrolysis of sucrose to glucose/fructose is inhibited.

Table: Drug Class Summary

Alpha-Glucosidase Inhibitors Drug Class Review High-Yield Med Reviews			
Mechanism of Action: *delays absorption of carbohydrates from the small intestine.*			
Class Effects: *Decrease A1c 0.6-0.8%, CV neutral, no beneficial effect on weight, high rate of GI adverse effects.*			
Generic Name	**Brand Name**	**Indication(s) or Uses**	**Notes**
Acarbose	Precose	• Type 2 diabetes as adjunct to diet and exercise	• **Dosing (Adult):** 25 mg TID with first bite of each meal – Increase every 4 weeks to 50-100 mg TID as tolerated. – Max dose ≤60 kg = 50 mg TID; >60 kg = 100 mg TID. • **Dosing (Peds):** ≥10 yo 25 mg TID with first bite of each meal – Increase every 4 weeks to 50-100 mg TID as tolerated. – Max dose ≤60 kg = 50 mg TID; >60 kg = 100 mg TID. • **CYP450 Interactions:** N/A • **Renal Dose Adjustments:** SCr>2 mg/dL or CrCl<25 mL/min not recommended • **Dosage Forms:** 25 mg, 50 mg, 100 mg tablets
Miglitol	Glyset	• Type 2 diabetes as adjunct to diet and exercise	• **Dosing (Adult):** 25 mg TID with first bite of each meal – Increase in 4 weeks to 50 mg TID, then 100 mg TID in 3 months. • **Dosing (Peds):** None • **CYP450 Interactions:** N/A • **Renal or Hepatic Dose Adjustments:** SCr>2 mg/dL or CrCl<25 mL/min not recommended • **Dosage Forms:** 25 mg, 50 mg, 100 mg tablets

Endocrinology

ENDOCRINE – AMYLIN ANALOGS

Drug Class
- **Amylin Mimetic**
  - **Agents:** Pramlintide

Main Indications or Uses
- Type 1 and 2 diabetes adjunct therapy with prandial insulin use

Mechanism of Action
- Amylin analog that is secreted with insulin from pancreatic beta cells
  - Delays gastric emptying, decreases post-prandial glucagon secretion, and reduces appetite through a centrally mediated mechanism.

> **Warnings & Alerts**
> ✓ Since pramlintide will delay glucose absorption, this can result in delaying the rise in serum glucose when insulin is starting to peak. As such, patients need to consider reductions in insulin dose.

Primary Overall Net Benefit
- Decreases post-prandial glucose while promoting weight loss.
- Main Labs to Monitor:
  - A1c every 3-6 months depending on whether the patient is at goal.

High-Yield Basic Pharmacology
- Time to peak: approximately 20 min
- Duration: 3 hours

High-Yield Clinical Knowledge
- Causes nausea (transient), weight loss (1-2 kg), hypoglycemia, and injection site reactions.
  - Hypoglycemia is due to combination with insulin, not pramlintide alone.
  - Severe hypoglycemia may occur within 3 hours when administered with insulin. Consider high-risk activities when severe hypoglycemia may cause serious injury (i.e., driving, operating machinery, etc.).
- Avoid in gastroparesis and hypoglycemia unawareness.
- Room temperature injections may decrease injection site reactions; injections are stable at room temperature or refrigeration for 30 days after initial use.
- **Administration**
  - Must reduce prandial and mixed insulin 50% when initiating pramlintide.
  - Can be administered with basal insulin alone as an alternative to prandial insulin.
    - Consider reducing basal dose if close to goal or high risk for hypoglycemia.
  - Cannot be mixed with insulin; requires additional injections, which is often a barrier to effective use due to noncompliance.
  - Administer SC into abdomen or thigh; do not inject in the arm due to erratic absorption.
  - If rapid absorption of other medications is needed, administer them 1 h before or 2 h after pramlintide.

High-Yield Core Evidence
- **Pramlintide in T1DM Trial**
  - Multicenter, RCT in 651 T1DM patients on insulin given pramlintide or placebo demonstrated pramlintide was safe and effective for glycemic control and beneficial to weight loss after 1 year.
    - A1c reduced approx. 0.4%; weight reduced approx. 1.3 kg; insulin doses reduced approx. 8 units.
    - Severe hypoglycemia approx. increased by 3-7%. Important to reduce prandial insulin 50%.
  - Diabet Med 2004; 21(11):1204-12.
- **Pramlintide in T2DM Trial**
  - Multicenter, RCT in 656 T2DM patients on various insulin +/- oral agent regimens plus pramlintide or placebo demonstrated pramlintide was safe and effective for glycemic control and beneficial to weight loss after 1 year.

- A1c reduced approx. 0.6%, weight reduced 1.4 kg; no significant increase in severe hypoglycemia.
- Diabetes Care 2003; 26(3):784-90.

High-Yield Fast-Fact
- Some providers utilize pramlintide in combination with basal insulin as an alternative to basal plus prandial insulin to promote improved post-prandial glucose control and weight loss.

HIGH-YIELD BOARD EXAM ESSENTIALS
- **CLASSIC AGENTS:** Pramlintide
- **DRUG CLASS:** Amylin mimetic
- **INDICATIONS:** Type 1 and 2 diabetes as adjunct therapy with prandial insulin use
- **MECHANISM:** Decreases post-prandial glucose by delaying gastric emptying, decreasing post-prandial glucagon secretion, and centrally mediated appetite suppression.
- **SIDE EFFECTS:** Causes nausea, weight loss, hypoglycemia, and injection site reactions.
- **CLINICAL PEARLS:** If rapid absorption of other medications is needed, administer them 1 h before or 2 h after pramlintide.

Table: Drug Class Summary

Amylin Mimetic Drug Class Review				
High-Yield Med Reviews				
Mechanism of Action: Decreases post-prandial glucose by delaying gastric emptying, decreasing post-prandial glucagon secretion, and centrally-mediated appetite suppression.			
Class Effects: Decreases A1c 0.2-0.7% by post-prandial glucose control, weight loss, hypoglycemia, nausea, injection site reactions			
Generic Name	**Brand Name**	**Indication(s) or Uses**	**Notes**

Pramlintide	SymlinPen	• Type 1 and 2 diabetes adjunct therapy with prandial insulin use	• **Dosing (Adult):** decrease prandial/mixed insulin 50% when initiating
			  – Type 1 DM
			    – 15 mcg immediately prior to major meals
			    – Titrate by 15 mcg every 3 days to 30-60 mcg
			    – Consider DC if intolerant to $\geq$30 mcg
			  – Type 2 DM
			    – 60 mcg immediately prior to major meals
			    – Titrate to 120 mcg in 3 days if nausea is insignificant
			• **Dosing (Peds):** None
			• **CYP450 Interactions:** None
			• **Renal or Hepatic Dose Adjustments:** None
			• **Dosage Forms:** 60 pen (1500 mcg/1.5 mL), 120 pen (2700 mcg/2.7 mL)

ENDOCRINE – ANTIDIABETIC AGENTS - BIGUANIDES

Drug Class

- Biguanide
- Agent:
  - Metformin

> **Fast Facts**
>
> ✓ Metformin is a cost-effective treatment option that can cause weight loss, sustained reductions in HgbA1C, very low risk for causing hypoglycemia, and no clear beta-cell burn out that worsens type 2 DM.

Main Indications or Uses
- T2DM management as an adjunct to diet and exercise (first-line agent)
- Common off-label uses:
  - Prediabetes
  - GDM
  - PCOS
  - Antipsychotic-induced weight gain

Mechanism of Action
- Decreases insulin resistance, hepatic glucose production, and intestinal absorption of glucose.

Primary Net Benefit
- Lowers A1C up to 2% without causing beta-cell burnout while also offering weight loss and limited risk for drug interactions.
- Labs to Monitor:
  - A1c every 3-6 months depending on whether patient is at goal
  - eGFR every 3-12 months depending on value (3 months eGFR 30-45 mL/min/1.73m^2, 6 months 46-60 mL/min/1.73m^2, 12 months eGFR>60 mL/min/1.73m^2)
  - Vitamin B-12 (with chronic use every 2-3 years)

High-Yield Basic Pharmacology
- Renal dose adjustments are recommended based on eGFR:
  - eGFR 46-60 mL/min/1.73m^2 – none, or may consider max 1500 mg/daily
  - eGFR 30-45 mL/min/1.73m^2 – 500 mg BID if started; if already taking metformin, decrease to 500 mg BID
  - eGFR <30 mL/min/1.73m^2 – contraindicated
- Potential drug interactions include iodinated contrast dye and carbonic anhydrase inhibitors, as well as other drugs that may potentiate lactic acidosis.

High-Yield Clinical Knowledge
- Metformin remains a potential first-line choice for T2DM therapy, but others may be considered for monotherapy or in combination with metformin based on patient-specific factors (i.e., CVD, CKD).
- Side Effects
  - Diarrhea and other GI adverse effects are most common.
    - GI adverse effects may be mitigated by utilizing metformin ER formulations, taking metformin with food, and slowly titrating doses (i.e., increase by 500 mg weekly).
  - Metformin is minimally weight neutral and may promote weight loss.
  - Has no hypoglycemia risk with monotherapy.
  - Peripheral neuropathy and anemia may indicate vitamin B12 deficiency.
- Formulations
  - May see ER tablet shells in stools.
  - Use metformin IR post-bariatric surgery due to reduction in absorption with ER formulations.
- Hypoglycemic Risk
  - This agent has a low risk of hypoglycemia.
- Special Populations or Clinical Situations

- May increase the risk of lactic acidosis in patients with renal or hepatic dysfunction, taking other drugs causing lactic acidosis, $\geq$ 65 years old, undergoing radiologic study with contrast dye, having surgery or other procedures, with excessive alcohol use, and with hypoxic states (acute HF).
- Hold metformin at or before iodinated contrast imaging procedures if patients have eGFR 30-60 mL/min/1.73m^2, history of hepatic disease, alcoholism, HF, or intra-arterial iodinated contrast use; reevaluate eGFR 48 hours post-procedure and restart if renal function is stable.
- Hold metformin on day of surgery and restart when stable post-op due to risk of hypotension or blood loss that may decrease renal perfusion because of the surgery.

High-Yield Core Evidence
- Evidence of metformin's potential CV and mortality benefit: Han et al. Cardiovascular Diabetology 2019;18:96; UKPDS 34 Lancet 1998;352:854-65.

High-Yield Fast-Facts
- **Type 1 Diabetics**
    - Is utilized off-label in T1DM, especially if overweight, obese, or demonstrating insulin resistance.
- **CVD and Events**
    - Metformin may improve CV risk and mortality in T2DM.
- **Dosage Formulations for Special Populations**
    - Metformin is available in liquid form for pediatric patients.

HIGH-YIELD BOARD EXAM ESSENTIALS
- **CLASSIC AGENTS:** Metformin
- **DRUG CLASS:** Biguanides
- **INDICATIONS:** T2DM; Off-Label: Prediabetes, PCOS, Gestational DM
- **MECHANISM:** Decreases insulin resistance, hepatic glucose production, and intestinal absorption of glucose without increasing the workload on the pancreas to cause beta-cell burnout.
- **SIDE EFFECTS:** Weight loss, GI side effects (diarrhea, bloating)
- **CLINICAL PEARLS:**
    - A first-line therapy for T2DM along with lifestyle changes.
    - Low risk of hypoglycemia
    - Unlike sulfonylureas, A1c reductions with metformin are sustained with diet and lifestyle changes.
    - There is a small risk for lactic acidosis that can occur with worsening renal function.

Table: Drug Class Summary

Biguanide Drug Class Review			
High-Yield Med Reviews			
Mechanism of Action: *Decreases insulin resistance, hepatic glucose production, and intestinal absorption of glucose.*			
Class Effects: *Decreases A1c, promotes weight neutrality or loss, causes low hypoglycemic risk, causes GI side effects.*			
Generic Name	**Brand Name**	**Main Indication(s) or Uses**	**Notes**
Metformin	Glucophage	<ul><li>T2DM as an adjunct to diet and exercise</li><li>Off-label: Prediabetes, PCOS, GDM, antipsychotic-induced weight gain</li></ul>	<ul><li>**Note:** A1c reduction: 0.7-1.6%</li><li>**Dosing (Adult):** − 500 mg PO daily with food; increase by 500 mg weekly up to 2000 mg daily</li><li>**Dosing (Peds):** − $\geq$6 years (obesity) and $\geq$10 years (DM) same as adult</li><li>**CYP450 Interactions:** None</li><li>**Renal or Hepatic Dose Adjustments:** − 45-60 mL/min/1.73m^2 increase monitoring − 30-45 mL/min/1.73m^2 500 mg BID with close monitoring; 30 mL/min/1.73m^2 contraindicated</li><li>**Dosage Forms:** 500 mg, 750 mg, 850 mg, 1000 mg tablets (IR and ER, except 850 mg IR only); 500 mg/5mL solution and ER suspension</li></ul>

ENDOCRINE – DPP-4 INHIBITORS

Drug Class
- **Dipeptidyl peptidase-4 inhibitors**
- **Agents:**
    - Sitagliptin, saxagliptin, linagliptin, alogliptin

Main Indications or Uses
- T2DM management as an adjunct to diet and exercise

Mechanism of Action
- Inhibits the dipeptidyl peptidase-4 enzyme that is responsible for the inactivation of incretin hormones, allowing greater availability of native hormones.

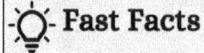

Fast Facts

✓ These agents are weight neutral, overall are well tolerated, do not increase the progression of the disease, and have low risk for hypoglycemia. However, they do have some clinical issues worth considering in some patients, including cost.

Primary Net Benefit
- Increases availability of GLP-1 approximately 2-fold but does not increase the concentration of GLP-1.
- Main effect is on post-prandial glucose in a glucose-dependent manner.
- Main Labs to Monitor:
    - A1c every 3-6 months depending on whether patient is at goal
    - Alogliptin: baseline LFTs and evaluate if signs/symptoms of hepatic injury develop.

High-Yield Basic Pharmacology
- **Drug Interactions with Saxagliptin and Linagliptin**
    - Linagliptin and saxagliptin may have significant drug interactions due to being major substrates of CYP 3A4 and p-glycoprotein/ABCB1; check drug interactions to assess.

High-Yield Clinical Knowledge
- **Weight Gain/Loss**
    - Have weight neutral effects, which is beneficial to overweight or obese patients with T2DM.
- **Adverse Events**
    - Cause low risk of hypoglycemia due to glucose-dependent effects.
    - Class is neutral regarding CV and renal benefits.
    - Generally, are well-tolerated; most common clinical adverse effect may be transient nasopharyngitis.
    - May cause reversible arthralgias at any point in therapy. Discontinue and evaluate pain, then restart to determine if DPP-4s are the etiology.
    - May cause pancreatitis; caution in patients with a history of or risk factors for pancreatitis.
    - May cause bullous pemphigoid; patients should report blisters or erosions, discontinue therapy, and seek referral to dermatologist.
        - Cases normally resolve with discontinuation of DPP-4 inhibitor and topical or systemic immunosuppressive therapy.
- **Hospitalization Risk**
    - Saxagliptin and alogliptin may increase risk of hospitalizations for HF. Others have not been implicated.
- **Hepatotoxicity**
    - Alogliptin may cause hepatotoxicity; monitor LFTs prior to initiation and if signs/symptoms of hepatic injury occur.
        - If LFTs elevated at baseline, consider alternative agent in class.
    - If LFT elevations are clinically significant or worsening, discontinue until alternative etiology is determined.

- **Other**
    - Linagliptin may be clinically preferred due to lack of renal or hepatic adjustments.
    - Consider in patients who need improved post-prandial control, low hypoglycemia risk (elderly), and oral therapy.
    - Alogliptin may decrease A1c up to 1%, but clinical relevance is uncertain based on lack of other benefits and relatively similar A1c lowering with other agents in class.

High-Yield Core Evidence
- **CARMELINA (JAMA 2019;321:69-79), EXAMINE (NEJM 2013;369:1327-35), and TECOS (NEJM 2015;373:232-42)**
    - Large, multicenter, RCT designed to determine CV benefit with linagliptin, alogliptin, and sitagliptin, respectively.
    - Demonstrated noninferiority to placebo for 3-point MACE of either linagliptin, alogliptin, or sitagliptin in patients with established CVD (CARMELINA, EXAMINE, TECOS) or high risk of CVD (CARMELINA).
- **CAROLINA**
    - Large, multicenter, RCT with active-comparator that assessed 3-point MACE in patients with ASCVD or multiple CV risk factors between linagliptin and glimepiride.
    - Demonstrated glimepiride is noninferior to linagliptin.
    - Of note, glimepiride is often considered the preferred SU regarding CV risk.
    - JAMA 2019;322(12):1155-66.
- **SAVOR-TIMI 53**
    - Large, multicenter RCT trial designed to determine the CV benefit with saxagliptin in established CVD or high risk of CVD.
    - Demonstrated noninferiority to placebo for 3-point MACE with saxagliptin.
    - Found 0.7% increased risk for hospitalizations for HF (289 saxagliptin vs 228 placebo).
        - Has not been demonstrated as a class effect; Increased risk for hospitalizations for HF is also unexplained.
    - NEJM 2013; 369(14):1317-26.

High-Yield Fast Facts
- Avoid DPP-4 inhibitors in combination with GLP-1 agonists since there is a lack of additional benefit.

HIGH-YIELD BOARD EXAM ESSENTIALS
- **CLASSIC AGENTS:** Sitagliptin, saxagliptin, linagliptin, alogliptin
- **DRUG CLASS:** Dipeptidyl peptidase-4 inhibitors
- **INDICATIONS:** Type 2 diabetes (T2DM) management as adjunct to diet and exercise
- **MECHANISM:** Inhibits the dipeptidyl peptidase-4 enzyme that is responsible for the inactivation of incretin hormones, allowing greater availability of native hormones.
- **SIDE EFFECTS:** Low hypoglycemia risk, neutral regarding weight and CV/renal benefits
- **CLINICAL PEARLS:**
    - May cause reversible arthralgias at any point in therapy. Discontinue and evaluate pain, then restart.

Table: Drug Class Summary

| | **Dipeptidyl Peptidase-4 Inhibitors Drug Class Review** High-Yield Med Reviews |

Mechanism of Action: *Inhibits the dipeptidyl peptidase-4 enzyme that is responsible for the inactivation of incretin hormones, allowing greater availability of native hormones.*			
Class Effects: *Decrease A1c 0.5-0.9%, low hypoglycemia risk, neutral regarding weight and CV/renal benefits*			
Generic Name	**Brand Name**	**Indication(s) or Uses**	**Notes**
Alogliptin	Nesina	▪ Type 2 diabetes (T2DM) management as adjunct to diet and exercise	▪ **Dosing (Adult):** 25 mg daily ▪ **Dosing (Peds):** None ▪ **CYP450 Interactions:** text ▪ **Renal or Hepatic Dose Adjustments:** CrCl≥30-60 mL/min 12.5 mg daily; CrCl≥15-30 mL/min 6.25 mg daily; CrCl<15 mL/min or HD 6.25 mg daily; if persistent or worsening LFTs without alternative etiology, discontinue. ▪ **Dosage Forms:** 6.25 mg, 12.5 mg, 25 mg
Linagliptin	Tradjenta	▪ Type 2 diabetes (T2DM) management as adjunct to diet and exercise]	▪ **Dosing (Adult):** 5 mg daily − Check drug interactions for required dose reductions to 2.5 mg. ▪ **Dosing (Peds):** None ▪ **CYP450 Interactions:** CYP3A4 inducers, P-glycoprotein/ABCB1 inducers ▪ **Renal or Hepatic Dose Adjustments:** text ▪ **Dosage Forms:** 5 mg
Saxagliptin	Onglyza	▪ Type 2 diabetes (T2DM) management as adjunct to diet and exercise	▪ **Dosing (Adult):** 2.5-5 mg daily − Check drug interactions for required dose reductions to 2.5 mg. ▪ **Dosing (Peds):** None ▪ **CYP450 Interactions:** CYP3A4 inhibitors, P-glycoprotein/ABCB1 inhibitors ▪ **Renal or Hepatic Dose Adjustments:** eGFR<45 mL/min/1.73m^2 2.5 mg daily; HD 2.5 mg daily post-dialysis ▪ **Dosage Forms:** 2.5 mg, 5 mg
Sitagliptin	Januvia	▪ Type 2 diabetes (T2DM) management as adjunct to diet and exercise	▪ **Dosing (Adult):** 100 mg daily ▪ **Dosing (Peds):** None ▪ **CYP450 Interactions:** text ▪ **Renal or Hepatic Dose Adjustments:** eGFR≥30-45 mL/min/1.73m^2 50 mg daily; eGFR<30 mL/min/1.73m^2 or intermittent HD 25 mg daily ▪ **Dosage Forms:** 25 mg, 50 mg, 100 mg

ENDOCRINE – GIP/GLP-1 AGONIST

Drug Class
- **Glucose-Dependent Insulinotropic Polypeptide (GIP) / GLP-1 agonist**
- **Agents**: tirzepatide

Main Indications or Uses
- T2DM management as an adjunct to diet and exercise

Mechanism of Action
- Increases glucose-dependent insulin secretion, decreases glucagon secretion, and delays gastric emptying.
    - GIP is another incretin hormone produced by the K cells of the intestine and is released in response to mainly carbohydrates and lipids to stimulate glucose-dependent insulin secretion.
    - GIP has dual functions related to glucagon; it is glucagonotropic in normo- or hypoglycemia and is glucagonostatic in hyperglycemia.
    - GIP also reduces food intake and increases energy expenditure to add to the effects of GLP-1.

Primary Net Benefit
- Demonstrates high efficacy with glucose control and low risk of hypoglycemia. Promotes clinically meaningful weight loss in patients with T2DM.
- Main Labs to Monitor:
    - A1c every 3-6 months depending on whether the patient is at goal and/or the time since titration.

High-Yield Basic Pharmacology
- Affects the absorption of orally administered drugs due to delayed gastric emptying. Separate from medications that have a narrow therapeutic index.
- Tirzepatide is highly albumin-bound (99%), which results in its longer half-life (5 days) and weekly dosing.
- Consider the half-life and dose titration to determine the appropriate timing for rechecking A1c and follow-up. The 2.5 mg initial dose is not considered therapeutic and should not be factored into the monitoring interval.

High-Yield Clinical Knowledge
- **Secondary Benefit Consideration**
    - GIP/GLP-1 agonists promote weight loss and should be considered in obese patients with T2DM.
- **GI Effects**
    - Nausea, vomiting, diarrhea, decreased appetite, and other GI adverse effects (dyspepsia, constipation, abdominal pain) are the most common adverse effects.
    - Tirzepatide has a titration schedule to manage transient GI adverse effects in which the lowest dose is not therapeutic.
- **Hypoglycemic Risk**
    - Hypoglycemia risk is low due to glucose-dependent insulin secretion, but when added to insulin or sulfonylureas, consider decreasing the doses depending on the patient.
- **Pancreatitis**
    - May increase the risk of pancreatitis. Use caution if the patient has a history of pancreatitis and if other conditions may predispose to pancreatitis (obesity, TG$\geq$500 mg/dL, excessive alcohol consumption).
- **Boxed Warning**
    - Contraindicated in patients with a personal or family history of MTC or in patients with MEN2.

- **Other Warnings**
  - Avoid in patients with gastroparesis or other severe GI diseases, especially those that affect motility, since they have not been studied with GIP/GLP1 agonists.
  - Acute renal failure and chronic renal failure exacerbations may occur; monitor closely for clinical situations affecting hydration, such as nausea, vomiting, or diarrhea that may occur with tirzepatide.
  - May increase the risk for gallbladder and bile duct disease.
  - Advise females to change to a non-oral contraceptive method or add a barrier method 4 weeks after starting or dose escalations due to potential conflict with absorption of oral contraceptives.
- **Bariatric Surgery**
  - GLP-1 agonists may be used post-bariatric surgery if volume status has been restored and maintained to avoid acute renal failure.
  - Monitor for pancreatitis post-gastric bypass or sleeve gastrectomy since these procedures result in increases in endogenous GLP-1, and therapy may be redundant.

High-Yield Core Evidence
- SURPASS 1-5 evaluated tirzepatide as monotherapy and in combination with metformin, sulfonylureas, SGLT2 inhibitors, and/or basal insulin. Tirzepatide was compared to placebo, semaglutide 1 mg, insulin degludec, and/or insulin glargine.
  - A1c reduction as monotherapy was approximately 1.5-2%. A1c reduction as combination therapy reached > 2%.
  - Weight loss as monotherapy was approximately 5-7 kg. Weight loss as combination therapy could be up to 10-11 kg.
  - Compared to semaglutide 1 mg, tirzepatide reduced A1c by 0.5% and weight by 5.5 kg more than semaglutide.
  - Compared to insulin degludec or insulin glargine, tirzepatide reduced A1c by approximately 1% and weight by 12-13 kg more than these basal insulins.
  - Lancet 2021;398:143-155; NEJM 2021;385:503-515; Diabetes 2021;70:78-LB; Lancet 2021;398:1811-1824; JAMA 2022;327:534-545.
- SURPASS-4 demonstrated significant reductions in macroalbuminuria with tirzepatide compared to insulin glargine in a prespecified subanalysis.
  - Lancet 2021;398:1811-1824.

High-Yield Fast-Facts
- Anti-tirzepatide antibodies do not cause clinically meaningful effects.
- Tirzepatide is being studied for obesity (SURMOUNT 1-4) and has demonstrated weight loss up to 24 kg (22.5%) in SURMOUNT-1 and 15.6 kg (15.7%) in SURMOUNT-2.
- GIP/GLP-1 agonists are also called "twincretins."

HIGH-YIELD BOARD EXAM ESSENTIALS
- **CLASSIC AGENTS:** Tirzepatide
- **DRUG CLASS:** GIP / GLP-1 agonist
- **INDICATIONS:** T2DM management as adjunct to diet and exercise
- **MECHANISM:** Increases glucose-dependent insulin secretion, decreases glucagon secretion, increases satiety, and delays gastric emptying
- **SIDE EFFECTS:** Nausea, vomiting, GI intolerance, weight loss, low hypoglycemia risk
- **CLINICAL PEARLS:** Demonstrates high efficacy with A1c and weight reductions. Consider in obese patients with T2DM. Contraindicated with MEN2 or personal or family history of MTC. May increase risk of pancreatitis. Advise patients when to use additional oral contraceptives. Tirzepatide 2.5 mg is for titration and not therapeutic; consider this and the 4-week titration intervals when determining the timing of A1c monitoring.

Table: Drug Class Summary

GIP / GLP-1 Agonist Drug Class Review High-Yield Med Reviews			
Mechanism of Action: *Increases glucose-dependent insulin secretion, decreases glucagon secretion, increases satiety, and delays gastric emptying.*			
Class Effects: *Decreases A1c (approx. 1.5-2%), promotes weight loss (approx. 5-7 kg), low hypoglycemic risk, GI adverse effects*			
Generic Name	**Brand Name**	**Main Indication(s) or Uses**	**Notes**
Tirzepatide	Mounjaro	▪ Type 2 diabetes as adjunct to diet and exercise	▪ **A1c reduction**: 1.7-1.8% (>2% combination) ▪ **Dosing (Adult):** — Initial 2.5 mg SC weekly, then increase to 5 mg weekly. Titrate by 2.5 mg every 4 weeks up to 15 mg if needed. ▪ **Dosing (Peds):** N/A ▪ **CYP450 Interactions**: N/A ▪ **Renal or Hepatic Dose Adjustments**: N/A ▪ **Dosage Forms:** Single-dose pens (2.5, 5, 7.5, 10, 12.5, 15 mg)

ENDOCRINE – GLP-1 AGONISTS

Drug Class
- GLP-1 agonists
- **Agents**: dulaglutide, exenatide, exenatide ER, liraglutide, lixisenatide, semaglutide

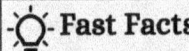

Fast Facts

✓ While GLP-1 agonists are expensive and can cause relevant GI adverse effects, they promote sustained A1C reductions and weight loss, have convenient dosing options, and do not cause T2DM progression.

Main Indications or Uses
- T2DM management as an adjunct to diet and exercise
- Risk reduction of major CV events in T2DM and established CVD (liraglutide, semaglutide SC)
- Risk reduction of major CV events in T2DM and established CVD or multiple CV risk factors (dulaglutide)

Mechanism of Action
- Mimics human GLP-1 hormone to increase glucose-dependent insulin secretion, decrease glucagon secretion, increase satiety, and delay gastric emptying.

Primary Net Benefit
- Increases glucose-dependent insulin secretion to lower glucose with CV and weight-loss benefits.
- Main Labs to Monitor:
  - A1c every 3-6 months depending on whether the patient is at goal and which GLP-1 agonist is utilized (based on half-life AND titration of GLP-1 agonist)

High-Yield Basic Pharmacology
- Consider the half-life and dose titration of once-weekly agents to determine the appropriate timing for rechecking A1c and follow-up.
  - Approximate time to efficacy:
  - Dulaglutide – 2 weeks
  - Exenatide ER – 6-10 weeks
  - Semaglutide SC – 4-5 weeks
- Drug interactions may exist with the slowing of gastric emptying.

High-Yield Clinical Knowledge
- **Secondary Benefit Considerations**
  - Liraglutide, semaglutide SC, or dulaglutide should be considered when a patient has CVD.
  - Dulaglutide can be considered in patients requiring or desiring primary CV prevention.
  - GLP-1 agonists promote weight loss and should be considered in obese patients with T2DM.
- **GI Effects**
  - Nausea, vomiting, and other GI adverse effects (diarrhea, constipation, reflux) are the most common adverse effects. Headaches and injection site reactions may also occur.
  - Liraglutide, lixisenatide, and semaglutide PO/SC have a titration schedule to manage transient GI adverse effects in which the lowest dose is not therapeutic. Exenatide and dulaglutide should also be started with a lower dose and increased to avoid GI adverse effects. Exenatide ER is the only GLP-1 agonist without the potential for dose titration or escalation.
- **Hypoglycemic Risk**
  - Hypoglycemia risk is low due to glucose-dependent insulin secretion.
- **Antibody Development**
  - Antibodies can develop with exenatide (Byetta), liraglutide, and lixisenatide, but ONLY exenatide and lixisenatide antibodies may affect therapeutic efficacy that requires therapy modification.
- **Pancreatitis**
  - May increase the risk of pancreatitis. Use caution if the patient has a history of pancreatitis and if other conditions may predispose to pancreatitis (obesity, TG ≥ 500 mg/dL, excessive alcohol consumption).

- **Pediatric Use**
  - Dulaglutide, exenatide ER, and liraglutide are approved for use in pediatric patients with T2DM. Monitor closely for hypoglycemia and dehydration regardless of concomitant therapies.
- **Combination Products**
  - Two products are combinations of GLP-1 agonists and basal insulins: liraglutide/insulin degludec (Xultophy) and lixisenatide/insulin glargine (Soliqua®).
- **Other Clinical Pearls**
  - Semaglutide PO MUST be taken with ≤4 oz of WATER only and NO other food, drink, or medication for 30-60 minutes to be effective.
  - GLP-1 agonists are contraindicated in patients with a personal or family history of MTC or MEN2, except exenatide (Byetta) and lixisenatide.
  - Acute renal failure and chronic renal failure exacerbations have occurred; monitor closely for scenarios affecting hydration.
  - May increase the risk for gallbladder and bile duct disease.
  - Use caution or avoid it in patients with gastroparesis as this has not been studied, and GLP-1s slow GI motility.
  - GLP-1 agonists may be used in patients who have undergone bariatric surgery. Avoid using if patients are not adequately hydrated. Monitor for pancreatitis due to increased endogenous post-prandial GLP-1 concentrations post-gastric bypass or sleeve gastrectomy.
  - Caution with semaglutide in patients with retinopathy as there may be increased complications.
  - Do not take more than 1 tablet of Rybelsus for dosing (i.e., two 3 mg tablets).
  - Lixisenatide (Adlyxin) is not typically prescribed as monotherapy but may be utilized in lixisenatide/insulin glargine (Soliqua).

High-Yield Core Evidence
- LEADER (NEJM 2016;375(4):311-22), SUSTAIN-6 (NEJM 2016;375(19)1834-44), and REWIND (Lancet 2019;394:121-30) were multi-center, RCTs that resulted in liraglutide, semaglutide SC, and dulaglutide obtaining secondary CV prevention indications.
  - Dulaglutide also is indicated for primary prevention in patients with multiple CV risk factors.

High-Yield Fast-Facts
- Liraglutide (Saxenda dosed up to 3 mg daily) and semaglutide (Wegovy dosed up to 2.4 mg weekly) are also marketed and indicated for obesity in patients ≥ 12 years.
- GLP-1 agonists have evidence for benefit in CKD patients with albuminuria and HF patients to reduce HF hospitalizations, but none have indications.
- Avoid GLP-1 agonists in combination with DPP-4 inhibitors since there is a lack of additional benefits.
- Liraglutide and semaglutide can be dosed by "clicks" to further mitigate GI adverse effects by slowing titration.
- Consider dulaglutide for a patient with visual disabilities due to its ease of dosing and administration with its device.
- Semaglutide (Ozempic) comes with pen needles. No additional prescription for needles is needed.
- Exenatide is a synthetic form of a protein that mimics GLP-1 from a Gila monster.

HIGH-YIELD BOARD EXAM ESSENTIALS
- **CLASSIC AGENTS:** Dulaglutide, exenatide, exenatide ER, liraglutide, lixisenatide, semaglutide
- **DRUG CLASS:** GLP-1 agonists
- **INDICATIONS:** T2DM management as adjunct to diet and exercise; risk reduction of major CV events in T2DM and established CVD (liraglutide, semaglutide SC); risk reduction of major CV events in T2DM and established CVD or multiple CV risk factors (dulaglutide)
- **MECHANISM:** Mimics glucagon-like peptide-1 and increases glucose-dependent insulin secretion, decreases glucagon secretion, increases satiety, and delays gastric emptying
- **SIDE EFFECTS:** Nausea, vomiting, GI intolerance, weight loss, low hypoglycemia risk
- **CLINICAL PEARLS:** Liraglutide, lixisenatide, and semaglutide PO/SC have a titration schedule to manage transient GI adverse effects in which the lowest dose is not therapeutic. Exenatide ER is the only GLP-1 agonist without potential for dose titration or escalation. Semaglutide PO should be taken with a sip of water 30-60 minutes before breakfast.

Table: Drug Class Summary

\<GLP-1 Agonist Drug Class Review\>			
High-Yield Med Reviews			
Mechanism of Action: *Mimics glucagon-like peptide-1 and increases glucose-dependent insulin secretion, decreases glucagon secretion, increases satiety, and delays gastric emptying.*			
Class Effects: *Decreases A1c (approx. 1-2%), promotes weight loss (approx. 2-6 kg), low hypoglycemic risk, GI adverse effects, CV benefit (drug-dependent)*			
Generic Name	**Brand Name**	**Main Indication(s) or Uses**	**Notes**
Dulaglutide	Trulicity	<ul><li>Type 2 diabetes as adjunct to diet and exercise</li><li>Risk reduction of major CV events in type 2 diabetes and established CVD or multiple CVD risk factors</li></ul>	<ul><li>**Note:** A1c reduction: 0.7-1.6%</li><li>**Dosing (Adult):** 0.75 mg SC weekly; may increase every 4 weeks to 1.5 mg, 3 mg, and up to 4 mg weekly if needed</li><li>**Dosing (Peds):** ≥10 years, same as adult</li><li>**CYP450 Interactions:** None</li><li>**Renal or Hepatic Dose Adjustments:** None</li><li>**Dosage Forms:** 0.75 mg pen, 1.5 mg pen, 3 mg pen, 4.5 mg pen</li></ul>
Exenatide	Byetta	<ul><li>Type 2 diabetes as adjunct to diet and exercise</li></ul>	<ul><li>A1c reduction: 0.5-0.9% (>1% with insulin)</li><li>**Dosing (Adult):** 5 mcg SC BID within 60 min before 2 main meals; may increase to 10 mcg if needed after 4 weeks</li><li>**Dosing (Peds):** ER only: ≥10 years, same as adult</li><li>**CYP450 Interactions:** None</li><li>**Renal or Hepatic Dose Adjustments:** Caution when initiating/increasing at CrCl 30-50 mL/min; Not recommended CrCl<30 mL/min</li><li>**Dosage Forms:** 5 mcg pen, 10 mcg pen</li></ul>
Exenatide ER	Bydureon BCise	<ul><li>Type 2 diabetes as adjunct to diet and exercise</li></ul>	<ul><li>A1c reduction: 0.9-1.6%</li><li>**Dosing (Adult):** 2 mg SC weekly</li><li>**Dosing (Peds):** ≥10 years, same as adult</li><li>**CYP450 Interactions:** None</li><li>**Renal or Hepatic Dose Adjustments:** Not recommended eGFR<45 mL/min/1.73m^2</li><li>**Dosage Forms:** 2 mg pen</li></ul>
Liraglutide	Victoza Saxenda (obesity only)	<ul><li>Type 2 diabetes as adjunct to diet and exercise in patients ≥10 years</li><li>Risk reduction of major CV events in type 2 diabetes and established CVD</li><li>Obesity as adjunct to diet and exercise in adults with BMI ≥30 kg/m^2 or ≥27 kg/m^2 with 1 obesity-related comorbidity; pediatric patients >60 kg</li></ul>	<ul><li>A1c reduction: 0.8-1.5%</li><li>Weight reduction (Saxenda only): 9-10%</li><li>**Dosing (Adult):** 0.6 mg SC daily x 7 days, then increase by 0.6 mg x 7 days up to 1.8 mg daily if needed (Saxenda may increase by 0.6 mg up to 3 mg daily)</li><li>**Dosing (Peds):** Victoza: ≥10 years, same as adult; Saxenda: ≥12 years, same as adult</li><li>**CYP450 Interactions:** None</li><li>**Renal or Hepatic Dose Adjustments:** None, but use caution when initiating or titrating</li><li>**Dosage Forms:** 18 mg/3mL pen</li></ul>

Liraglutide/insulin degludec	Xultophy	with BMI corresponding to adult BMI ≥30 kg/m²	- **Dosing (Adult):** Naïve to GLP-1 agonist or basal – 10 units SC daily; Current GLP-1 agonist or basal – 16 units daily; titrate by 2 units q3-4 days with max dose 50 units - **Dosage Forms:** 100 units/3.6 mg/mL
Lixisenatide	Adlyxin (discontinued as monotherapy)	- Type 2 diabetes as adjunct to diet and exercise	- **A1c reduction:** 0.5-0.9% - **CYP450 Interactions:** None - **Renal or Hepatic Dose Adjustments:** No dose adjustment eGFR 15-89 mL/min/1.73m² but monitor for conditions predisposing to dehydration; levels increased from eGFR 15-29 mL/min/1.73m²; not recommended eGFR<15 mL/min/1.73m²
Lixisenatide/insulin glargine	Soliqua		- **Dosing (Adult):** Naïve, current GLP-1, or current insulin users at <30 units - 15 units SC daily; titrate by 2-4 units weekly with max dose 60 units - **Dosage Forms:** 100 units/33 mcg/mL
Semaglutide PO	Rybelsus	- Type 2 diabetes as adjunct to diet and exercise	- **A1c reduction:** 0.9-1.4% - **Dosing (Adult):** 3 mg PO daily x 30 days, then 7 mg daily x 30 days; may increase to 14 mg daily if needed; MUST be taken with ≤4 oz WATER AND 30-60 min BEFORE ANY food, drink, or medication. - **Dosing (Peds):** N/A - **CYP450 Interactions:** None - **Renal or Hepatic Dose Adjustments:** None - **Dosage Forms:** 3 mg, 7 mg, 14 mg
Semaglutide SC	Ozempic Wegovy (obesity only)	- Type 2 diabetes as adjunct to diet and exercise - Risk reduction of major CV events in type 2 diabetes and established CVD - Obesity as adjunct to diet and exercise in adults with BMI ≥30 kg/m² or ≥27 kg/m² with 1 obesity-related comorbidity; pediatric patients with BMI ≥95th percentile	- **A1c reduction:** 1.2-1.7% - **Weight reduction (Wegovy only):** 15% - **Dosing (Adult):** Initial 0.25 mg SC weekly, then increase to 0.5 mg, 1 mg, and up to 2 mg weekly by titrating every 4 weeks (follow same titration schedule for Wegovy with its respective pen strengths up to 2.4 mg weekly) - **Dosing (Peds):** Wegovy only: ≥12 years, same as adult - **CYP450 Interactions:** None - **Renal or Hepatic Dose Adjustments:** None - **Dosage Forms (Ozempic):** 0.25 mg/0.5 mg/DOSE pen, 1 mg/DOSE pen, 2 mg/DOSE pen - **Dosage Forms (Wegovy):** 0.25 mg/DOSE pen, 0.5 mg/DOSE pen, 1 mg/DOSE pen, 1.7 mg/DOSE pen, 2.4 mg/DOSE pen

ENDOCRINE – MEGLITINIDES

Drug Class
- **Meglitinides**
- **Agents:** Nateglinide, repaglinide

Main Indications or Uses
- T2DM management as adjunct to diet and exercise

Mechanism of Action
- Blocks ATP-dependent K^+ channels, which depolarizes the membrane and causes Ca^{2+} influx that stimulates insulin release.

Primary Net Benefit
- Stimulates insulin release in a glucose-dependent manner.
- Main Labs to Monitor:
  - A1c every 3-6 months depending on whether patient is at goal
  - Lipids periodically

High-Yield Basic Pharmacology
- Absorption is decreased when taken with food; take 30 min prior to meals.
- **Nateglinide**
  - Active metabolite can increase risk of hypoglycemia, especially in severe renal impairment.

High-Yield Core Knowledge
- **Class Benefits**
  - Low cost, oral option to target post-prandial glucose.
    - Should only take if eating a meal.
    - May take with each meal, which can vary between patients (typically 2-4 meals daily).
- **Adverse Events**
  - May result in weight gain (1-3 kg) and upper respiratory infections.
  - Has low risk of hypoglycemia due to glucose-dependent effects.

High-Yield Fast-Fact
- This class is rarely utilized because of compliance issues and the development of other drug classes with benefits beyond glycemia for T2DM.

 Fast Facts

✓ These agents function largely like sulfonylureas but have a shorter half-life and thus have to be administered more frequently. Their use in clinical practice is limited.

HIGH-YIELD BOARD EXAM ESSENTIALS
- **CLASSIC AGENTS:** Nateglinide, repaglinide
- **DRUG CLASS:** Meglitinides
- **INDICATIONS:** Type 2 diabetes (T2DM) management as adjunct to diet and exercise
- **MECHANISM:** Stimulates insulin release in a glucose-dependent manner through influx of Ca^{2+}.
- **SIDE EFFECTS:** Weight gain, upper respiratory tract infection, hypoglycemia
- **CLINICAL PEARLS:** Has low risk of hypoglycemia due to glucose-dependent effects when utilized with non-insulin modulating agents.

Table: Drug Class Summary

| \multicolumn{4}{c}{**Meglitinides Drug Class Review**} |
| \multicolumn{4}{c}{High-Yield Med Reviews} |

Mechanism of Action: *Stimulates insulin release in a glucose-dependent manner through influx of Ca^{2+}.*

Class Effects: *Decreases A1c 0.4-0.9%, CV neutral, weigh gain, low risk hypoglycemia.*

Generic Name	Brand Name	Indication(s) or Uses	Notes

Nateglinide	Starlix	- T2DM) management as adjunct to diet and exercise	- **Dosing (Adult):**
			  - 60-120 mg TID 30 min prior to meals
			- **Dosing (Peds):** N/A
			- **CYP450 Interactions:**
			  - CYP3A4 and CYP2C9 substrate
			- **Renal Dose Adjustments:**
			  - eGFR<30 mL/min/1.73m² start at 60 mg TIDAC
			- **Hepatic Dose Adjustments:**
			  - None, but Child Pugh B/C may increase risk of hypoglycemia
			- **Dosage Forms:** 60 mg, 120 mg tablets

Repaglinide	Prandin	- T2DM management as adjunct to diet and exercise	- **Dosing (Adult):** 0.5-2 mg TID 30 min prior to meals
			  - Titrate weekly
			  - Start 0.5 mg if close to goal.
			  - 16 mg/d max
			- **Dosing (Peds):** N/A
			- **CYP450 Interactions:**
			  - CYP3A4 and CYP2C8 inhibitors/inducers
			- **Renal Dose Adjustments:**
			  - CrCl 20-40 mL/min start 0.5 mg and titrate
			  - CrCl<20 mL/min not studied
			- **Dosage Forms:** 0.5 mg, 1 mg, 2 mg tablets

ENDOCRINE – SGLT2 INHIBITORS

Drug Class
- Sodium-Glucose Cotransporter 2 (SGLT2) Inhibitors
- Agents:
  - Canagliflozin, dapagliflozin, empagliflozin, ertugliflozin, sotagliflozin

Main Indications or Uses
- Type 2 DM
  - Adjunct to diet and exercise (except sotagliflozin)
  - Canagliflozin – risk reduction of major CV events in T2DM and established CVD
  - Empagliflozin – risk reduction of CV mortality in T2DM with established CVD
  - Dapagliflozin – risk reduction of heart failure (HF) hospitalization in T2DM and established CVD or multiple risk factors
  - Canagliflozin – risk reduction of end-stage kidney disease, doubling of SCr, CV death, and HF hospitalization in T2DM and DM nephropathy with UAE>300 mg/d
- Chronic Kidney Disease
  - Dapagliflozin – risk reduction of sustained eGFR decline, end-stage kidney disease, CV death, and HF hospitalization in patients at risk of progression
- Heart Failure
  - Dapagliflozin and empagliflozin - risk reduction of CV death and hospitalization for HF (dapagliflozin – reduction in urgent HF visits)
  - Sotagliflozin - risk reduction of CV death, HF hospitalization, and urgent HF visits in patients with HF or T2DM, CKD, and other CV risk factors

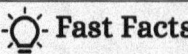

Fast Facts

✓ The "weight loss" and use for heart failure are due to the prevention of glucose reabsorption within the nephron, which results in increased diuresis. This is also why patients are at increased risk of UTIs and mycotic infections.

Mechanism of Action
- Inhibits reabsorption of filtered glucose in the proximal renal tubules by blocking SGLT2 receptors (~90% reabsorption), causing increased urinary glucose elimination and decreasing the renal threshold for glucose.
- Many mechanisms are hypothesized for the SGLT2 benefits in HF, including stimulation of natriuresis and osmotic diuresis, reduction in preload/afterload, and changes in remodeling.
- Sotagliflozin – inhibits SGLT1 and SGLT2; the mechanism of CV benefits is not established, but SGLT2 inhibition decreases renal reabsorption of glucose and sodium that may reduce preload and afterload and downregulate sympathetic activity. SGLT1 inhibition decreases intestinal glucose and sodium absorption.

Primary Net Benefit
- Decreases renal glucose reabsorption in a glucose-dependent manner with benefits for cardiovascular, renal, and/or heart failure outcomes.
- Main Labs to Monitor:
  - A1c every 3-6 months, depending on whether the patient is at goal
  - BP, SCr, eGFR, and K^+ periodically
  - Urinary ketones and bicarbonate if DKA is suspected; consider blood ketones and arterial pH.

High-Yield Basic Pharmacology
- Result in 30-50% less glucose reabsorption
- Lower the renal threshold for glucose reabsorption
- May improve post-prandial glucose when taken before the first meal by delaying intestinal glucose absorption

High-Yield Clinical Knowledge
- **Recommended Populations for Use**
  - Independent of metformin or A1c target, patients with the following comorbidities can be considered candidates for SGLT2 inhibitor therapy

- CKD - dapagliflozin
- CVD - canagliflozin or empagliflozin
- DKD with albuminuria – canagliflozin
- HF – dapagliflozin, empagliflozin, sotagliflozin
- DM2 – empagliflozin is indicated in patients > 10 years and older
- **Genital Mycotic Infections or UTIs**
  - Mainly occurs in patients with a history of GU infections, females, or uncircumcised males.
  - Most clinicians will tolerate 1 infection before considering alternate therapy since the pathophysiology is closely related to initial glucose wasting through the urine.
- **Renal Disease**
  - Initial decreases in eGFR can occur in weeks, but decreasing eGFR over time is slowed.
    - AKI may occur.
  - Contraindicated in patients on dialysis.
    - Canagliflozin can be used except in patients on dialysis.
  - Most can be continued at lower eGFRs, but initiating therapy is not recommended.
  - Glycemic benefit decreases as eGFR decreases.
- **DKA**
  - Can occur in T1DM and T2DM, although more common in T1DM patients, and may be euglycemic.
    - Euglycemic DKA can occur when insulin is decreased or absent, and SGLT2 inhibitor is causing glucose excretion in the urine, which results in lower glucose at presentation of DKA.
    - Do not abruptly discontinue insulin when initiating or while on an SGLT2 inhibitor. Adjust insulin doses slowly to avoid DKA.
  - Caution if patients cannot maintain hydration to avoid DKA.
    - Discontinue 3-5 days before surgery.
    - Discontinue with acute illness or other conditions that may predispose to dehydration (GI illness, influenza).
- **Fracture Risk**
  - Increased fracture risk has been seen with canagliflozin mainly from the CANVAS trial data, but meta-analyses have not extrapolated that risk to others in the class.
- **History of Amputations/PVD**
  - Increased risk of lower limb amputations was observed with canagliflozin (CANVAS, CANVAS-R), but others in the class have not consistently demonstrated the same risk.
  - Consider risk factors of prior amputation, PVD, neuropathy, and DM foot ulcers.
  - Discontinue therapy if signs/symptoms occur.
- **Fournier's Gangrene** (necrotizing fasciitis of the perineum)
  - Consider if the patient presents with fever, erythema, pain, tenderness, and edema in the genital or perianal area, but the occurrence is rare.
- **Elevated LDL**
  - May elevate LDL via reduced clearance but have not demonstrated increased CV risk due to this potential.
- **Adverse Effects**
  - Weight loss of 1-2 kg is a potentially beneficial effect.
  - Consider as low risk for hypoglycemia when given as monotherapy or combination therapy with drugs that do not modulate insulin release.
  - Monitor for signs/symptoms of orthostatic hypotension, especially in those predisposed (i.e., elderly).
  - Sotagliflozin may cause diarrhea as a result of SGLT1 inhibition.
- **Concomitant Medication Considerations**
  - Consider reducing the loop diuretic dose when starting (up to 50%).
  - Caution with loop diuretics, ACEIs, ARBs, NSAIDs, and other drugs that can precipitate AKI.
- Maximum doses typically cause the most weight loss with modest additional glycemic control.
- Since ertugliflozin has not demonstrated superiority in CV outcomes and renal outcomes have only been analyzed from VERTIS-CV, clinicians do not commonly utilize this agent.

High-Yield Core Evidence
- **CVD Evidence**
  - CANVAS/CANVAS-R (NEJM 2017;377:64-57), DECLARE-TIMI 58 (NEJM 2019;380:347-57), EMPA-REG (NEJM 2015;373:2117-28), VERTIS CV (NEJM 2020;383:1425-35.
    - Multicenter, large RCTs between canagliflozin, dapagliflozin, empagliflozin, and ertugliflozin, respectively, were designed to determine the superiority of the SGLT2-inhibitor to placebo in preventing 3-point MACE.
      - Populations included patients with established CVD or multiple risk factors for CVD, except EMPA-REG and VERTIS CV (established CVD only).
    - CANVAS and EMPA-REG
      - Superiority to placebo for 3-point MACE that led to indication for secondary CVD prevention with 14% reduction for both.
        - EMPA-REG was driven by reduced CV death.
      - Demonstrated reduced hospitalization for HF.
    - DECLARE-TIMI 58 population was investigated in primary and secondary prevention.
      - Noninferiority to placebo for 3-point MACE.
      - Decreased CV death or hospitalization for HF.
  - VERTIS-CV
    - Noninferiority to placebo for 3-point MACE and decreased CV death or hospitalization for HF.
    - Results are largely unexplained, except for possibly more aggressive secondary prevention measures in recent years and/or class differences related to SGLT1 or 2 specificity.
  - CANVAS
    - Demonstrated increased risk of amputations (97%) and fractures (26%).
      - Amputations are mostly at the toe/metatarsal, with the highest risk in those with previous amputations or PVD.
  - CVD Real
    - Multicenter, large retrospective analysis reviewing patients on SGLT2 inhibitors or other glucose-lowering drugs
      - Most were on canagliflozin and dapagliflozin.
    - Reduced hospitalizations for HF, all-cause mortality, and hospitalizations for HF and death.
    - Circulation 2017;377:644-57.
- **HF Evidence**
  - DAPA-HF
    - First trial designed with the primary outcome to evaluate worsening HF (unplanned hospitalization or urgent visit for IV therapy for HF) or CV death.
    - 26% reduction in primary outcome with dapagliflozin, which was driven by both worsening HF and CV death endpoints.
    - Effective in T2DM patients and those without T2DM, leading to indication for T2DM and HF without T2DM.
    - NEJM 2019;381:1995-2008.
  - EMPEROR-Reduced
    - Multicenter RCT in 3730 patients with class II-IV heart failure and EF $\leq 40\%$ given empagliflozin 10 mg daily. Patients were enrolled with and without diabetes.
    - 25% reduction in the primary outcome of CV death and hospitalization for worsening HF. Outcome was driven by HF hospitalization.

- NEJM 2020;383:1413-24.
- EMPEROR-Preserved
    - Multicenter RCT in 5988 patients with class II-IV heart failure and EF > 40% given empagliflozin 10 mg daily. Patients were enrolled with and without diabetes.
    - 21% reduction in the primary outcome of CV death and HF hospitalization. Outcome was driven by HF hospitalization.
    - NEJM 2021;385:1451-61.
- SOLOIST-WHF
    - Multicenter RCT in 1222 patients with recent worsening HF (majority EF < 50%) and evidence of T2DM given sotagliflozin 200-400 mg daily, depending on response.
    - 33% reduction in the primary outcome of CV death, HF hospitalizations, and urgent HF visits (NNT = 4). Outcome was mainly driven by HF hospitalization and urgent HF visit reductions.
    - Trial was stopped early due to funding loss, and the primary endpoint was changed to be based on investigator-defined events. Events were not adjudicated as originally planned.
    - NEJM 2021;384:117-28.
- SCORED
    - Multicenter RCT in 10,584 patients with T2DM, CKD, and risk for CVD given sotagliflozin 200-400 mg daily, depending on response.
    - 25% reduction in the primary outcome of CV death, HF hospitalizations, and urgent HF visits.
    - Primary endpoint changed during the trial to the composite of CV death, HF hospitalizations, and urgent HF visits.
    - Trial was stopped early due to funding loss.
    - NEJM 2021;384:129-39.
- **Renal Evidence**
    - CREDENCE
        - Multicenter, large, RCT in patients with T2DM and nephropathy defined by eGFR 30 to <90 mL/min/1.73m^2 and albumin:Cr >300-5000 mg/g.
        - Primary outcome was ESKD, doubling SCr, renal death, or CV death.
            - Reduced 30% with canagliflozin when the trial stopped early due to benefits.
        - All stratified outcomes, at a minimum, trended toward benefit with canagliflozin.
    - CANVAS-R also demonstrated benefits in primary renal outcomes, but these results could not be considered significant due to the prespecified hypothesis testing sequence.
    - DAPA-CKD
        - Multicenter, large, RCT in patients with or without T2DM, eGFR 25-75 mL/min/1.73m^2 and albumin:Cr 200-5000 mg/g, and ACEi/ARB if not contraindicated or not tolerated.
        - Primary outcome was sustained decline in eGFR$\geq$50%, ESKD, renal or CV death and showed a 39% reduction. All subgroup analyses showed significant benefits of dapagliflozin except geographically in Asia, which trended toward benefit in this population.
    - EMPA-REG Empagliflozin and Progression of Kidney Disease in T2DM
        - The prespecified secondary objective of the CV outcomes trial.
        - Primary renal outcome was progression to macroalbuminuria, doubling SCr with eGFR$\leq$45 mL/min/1.73m^2, initiation of renal replacement therapy, or death from renal disease.
            - Significant RRR = 39% with consistent benefits across subgroups.
    - VERTIS CV Data
        - Evaluation of renal data found a significant 34% reduction in sustained eGFR reduction of 40%, dialysis or transplant, or renal death for ertugliflozin.

High-Yield Fast-Facts
- Empagliflozin is indicated for type 2 diabetes in pediatric patients ≥ 10 years.
- Consider a patient's occupation, ability to maintain hydration, and risks related to the occurrence of orthostatic hypotension at work (i.e., a roofer with low-normal BP).
- SGLT2 inhibitors are not indicated for T1DM but are utilized in these patients to potentially reduce insulin doses or promote weight loss.
- Bexagliflozin (Brenzavvy) is also an SGLT2 inhibitor that is FDA-approved as an adjunct to lifestyle changes to improve glycemic control in T2DM.

HIGH-YIELD BOARD EXAM ESSENTIALS
- **CLASSIC AGENTS:** Canagliflozin, dapagliflozin, empagliflozin, ertugliflozin, sotagliflozin
- **DRUG CLASS:** SGLT2 Inhibitors (sotagliflozin also inhibits SGLT1)
- **INDICATIONS:** Type 2 DM, HF patients, CKD, Diabetic kidney disease
- **MECHANISM:** Inhibits reabsorption of filtered glucose in the proximal renal tubules by blocking SGLT2 receptors (~90% reabsorption), causing increased urinary glucose elimination and decreasing the renal threshold for glucose.
- **SIDE EFFECTS:** GU/UTI infections, euglycemic ketoacidosis, increased fracture risk, orthostatic hypotension
- **CLINICAL PEARLS:**
    - The weight loss manifested is a loss in "water weight" due to increased diuresis, not fat. This may be helpful to a patient with HF and evidence of fluid overload.
    - The increase in glucose in the urine can increase the risk of UTIs and yeast infections.
    - May elevate LDL via reduced clearance but have not demonstrated increased CV risk due to this potential.

Table: Drug Class Summary

	SGLT2-Inhibitors Drug Class Review High-Yield Med Reviews		
Mechanism of Action: inhibits glucose reabsorption in the proximal renal tubule by blocking SGLT2 receptors			
Class Effects: Decreases A1c 1% (except sotagliflozin), weight loss 1-2 kg, low hypoglycemia risk, GU infections, CV and renal benefits (drug-dependent), orthostatic hypotension, euglycemic DKA, amputations, fracture risk, Fournier's gangrene, AKI, elevated LDL			
Generic Name	**Brand Name**	**Main Indication(s) or Uses**	**Notes**
Canagliflozin	Invokana	<ul><li>Type 2 diabetes as adjunct to diet and exercise</li><li>Risk reduction of major CV events in T2DM and established CVD</li><li>Risk reduction of ESRD, doubling SCr, CV death, and hospitalization for HF in T2DM and DM nephropathy with UAE>300 mg/d</li></ul>	<ul><li>**Dosing (Adult):** 100 mg daily before first meal<ul><li>Increase to 300 mg daily after 4-12 weeks if needed</li></ul></li><li>**Dosing (Peds):** N/A</li><li>**CYP450 Interactions:** N/A</li><li>**Renal or Hepatic Dose Adjustments:** eGFR 30-60 mL/min/1.73m^2 100 mg daily; eGFR<30 mL/min/1.73m^2 do not initiate, but if established, may continue 100 mg daily</li><li>**Dosage Forms:** 100 mg, 300 mg</li></ul>
Dapagliflozin	Farxiga	<ul><li>Type 2 diabetes as adjunct to diet and exercise</li><li>Risk reduction of HF hospitalization in T2DM and established CVD or multiple CV risk factors</li><li>risk reduction of CV death, HF hospitalization, and urgent HF visits</li><li>Risk reduction of sustained eGFR decline, ESRD, CV death, and HF hospitalization with chronic kidney disease at risk of progression</li></ul>	<ul><li>**Dosing (Adult):** 5 mg daily in AM<ul><li>Increase to 10 mg daily after 4-12 weeks if needed</li><li>HF: 10 mg daily</li></ul></li><li>**Dosing (Peds):** N/A</li><li>**CYP450 Interactions:** N/A</li><li>**Renal or Hepatic Dose Adjustments:**<ul><li>Hyperglycemia: eGFR <45 mL/min/1.73m^2: not recommended</li><li>CKD, HF, diabetic kidney disease: eGFR <25 mL/min/1.73m^2 – if established may continue 10 mg</li></ul></li><li>**Dosage Forms:** 5 mg, 10 mg</li></ul>
Empagliflozin	Jardiance	<ul><li>Type 2 diabetes as adjunct to diet and exercise in patients ≥ 10 years</li><li>Risk reduction of CV mortality in T2DM and established CVD</li><li>Risk reduction of CV mortality and HF hospitalization in HF</li></ul>	<ul><li>**Dosing (Adult):** 10 mg daily in AM<ul><li>Increase to 25 mg daily after 4-12 weeks if needed.</li><li>HF: 10 mg daily</li></ul></li><li>**Dosing (Peds):** ≥ 10 years, same as adult</li><li>**CYP450 Interactions:** N/A</li><li>**Renal or Hepatic Dose Adjustments:** eGFR <30 mL/min/1.73m^2: not recommended for glycemic control<ul><li>Previously on empagliflozin: 10 mg daily for renal disease (off-label)</li><li>eGFR≥20: HF and renal benefits</li></ul></li><li>**Dosage Forms:** 10 mg, 25 mg</li></ul>

SGLT2-Inhibitors Drug Class Review </br> High-Yield Med Reviews			
Generic Name	**Brand Name**	**Main Indication(s) or Uses**	**Notes**
Ertugliflozin	Steglatro	• Type 2 diabetes as adjunct to diet and exercise	• **Dosing (Adult):** 5 mg daily in AM – Increase to 15 mg daily if needed • **Dosing (Peds):** N/A • **CYP450 Interactions:** N/A • **Renal or Hepatic Dose Adjustments:** eGFR<45 mL/min/1.73m^2: not recommended • **Dosage Forms:** 5 mg, 15 mg
Sotagliflozin	Inpefa	• Risk reduction of CV mortality, HF hospitalization, and urgent HF visit in HF • Risk reduction of CV mortality, HF hospitalization, and urgent HF visit in T2DM, CKD, and other CV risk factors	• **Dosing (Adult):** 200-400 mg daily • **Dosing (Peds):** N/A • **CYP450 Interactions:** N/A • **Renal or Hepatic Dose Adjustments:** eGFR<30 mL/min/1.73m^2: not recommended – Moderate-severe hepatic impairment: not recommended • **Dosage Forms:** 200 mg, 400 mg

ENDOCRINE – SULFONYLUREAS

Drug Class
- Sulfonylureas
- Agents:
  - Glimepiride
  - Glipizide
  - Glyburide

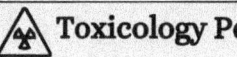
Toxicology Pearl
- ✓ Out of all of the agents in this class, the one most commonly associated with toxicity (symptomatic hypoglycemia) is glyburide.

Main Indications or Uses
- T2DM management as an adjunct to diet and exercise

Mechanism of Action
- Stimulates pancreatic insulin secretion (primary); also reduces hepatic glucose output and improves peripheral insulin sensitivity (to a lesser degree).

Primary Net Benefit
- Increases insulin secretion to lower A1c
- Main Labs to Monitor:
  - A1c every 3-6 months, depending on whether the patient is at goal

High-Yield Basic Pharmacology
- Special Considerations for Glyburide
  - Glyburide has active metabolites that increase the risk of hypoglycemia.
  - Avoid glyburide in CKD.

High-Yield Clinical Knowledge
- Administration Considerations
  - Take with the first meal daily. Morning administration will assist in avoiding nocturnal hypoglycemia.
  - Titrate weekly to the next dose until control is achieved.
  - May split doses BID when at the highest doses for improved control.
  - Glimepiride 8 mg may offer little benefit compared to 4 mg daily. Can divide dose.
- Warnings
  - Secondary failure may occur due to decreased beta-cell function (i.e., beta-cell burnout) with T2DM progression.
  - Avoid glyburide in the elderly due to an active metabolite that may increase the risk of hypoglycemia (Beers List).
  - Consider potential CV risk; glimepiride may be preferred.
    - Evidence on CV safety or risk with SUs is controversial. Some data demonstrate the least risk with glimepiride and the greatest risk with glyburide.
    - ADA recommends alternative agents in patients with CVD or at high risk for CVD.
  - Glyburide may have efficacy in pregnancy but crosses the placenta and increases risk of neonatal hypoglycemia.
  - Caution is advised with sulfonamide allergies, although cross-reactivity is unlikely.
  - Consider alternatives in patients with G6PD deficiency due to increased risk of hemolytic anemia.
- May cause weight gain, hypoglycemia, or rash.
- Micronized glyburide (Glynase) is not bioequivalent to conventional glyburide.

High-Yield Core Evidence
- UKPDS 33
  - Large, prospective trial of 10 years duration that demonstrated SU efficacy at 0.9-1.6% A1c reduction in diabetes patients with a reduction in microvascular complications but neutral effects on macrovascular outcomes.

- Lancet 1998;352:837-53.
- **CAROLINA**
  - Multicenter, RCT with active-comparator in 6042 patients that assessed 3-point MACE in patients with ASCVD or multiple CV risk factors between linagliptin and glimepiride.
    - Demonstrated glimepiride is noninferior to linagliptin in established or high CV risk patients for CVD.
    - Of note, glimepiride is often considered the preferred SU regarding CV risk.
  - JAMA 2019;322(12):1155-66.

High-Yield Fast-Fact
- **Cost-Effectiveness**
  - Cost limitations and fear of injections are the primary reasons to consider using SUs due to lack of secondary benefits.

HIGH-YIELD BOARD EXAM ESSENTIALS
- **CLASSIC AGENTS:** Glimepiride, glipizide, glyburide
- **DRUG CLASS:** Sulfonylureas
- **INDICATIONS:** T2DM management as adjunct to diet and exercise
- **MECHANISM:** Stimulates pancreatic insulin secretion (primary); also reduces hepatic glucose output and improves peripheral insulin sensitivity (to a lesser degree).
- **SIDE EFFECTS:** Weight gain, high hypoglycemic risk
- **CLINICAL PEARLS:**
  - Can lower HgbA1c by up to 2% from baseline but unfortunately is not sustained.
  - This class of drugs is initially cost-effective but also causes beta-cell burnout that results in disease progression.
  - Since SUs increase insulin release, hypoglycemia and weight gain are adverse effects.
  - Avoid glyburide in elderly due to active metabolite that may increase risk of hypoglycemia (Beers List).

Table: Drug Class Summary

	Sulfonylureas Drug Class Review High-Yield Med Reviews

Mechanism of Action: Stimulates pancreatic insulin secretion (primary); also reduces hepatic glucose output and improves peripheral insulin sensitivity.			
Class Effects: Decreases A1c 1-2%, weight gain, high hypoglycemic risk, secondary failure			
Generic Name	**Brand Name**	**Indication(s) or Uses**	**Notes**
Glimepiride	Amaryl	• Type 2 diabetes as adjunct to diet and exercise	• **Dosing (Adult):** 1-2 mg daily – Titrate weekly up to 8 mg daily • **Dosing (Peds):** None • **CYP450 Interactions:** None • **Renal or Hepatic Dose Adjustments:** Start 1 mg daily; consider alternative if eGFR<15 mL/min/1.73m² • **Dosage Forms:** 1 mg, 2 mg, 4 mg
Glipizide	Glucotrol, Glucotrol XL	• Type 2 diabetes as adjunct to diet and exercise	• **Dosing (Adult):** 2.5 mg daily – Titrate weekly by 2.5-5 mg up to 20 mg daily • **Dosing (Peds):** None • **CYP450 Interactions:** None • **Renal or Hepatic Dose Adjustments:** Start 2.5 mg daily • **Dosage Forms:** 5 mg, 10 mg; ER 2.5 mg, 5 mg, 10 mg

Glyburide	Glynase	• Type 2 diabetes as adjunct to diet and exercise	• **Dosing (Adult):**
			  – Micronized: 1.5-3 mg daily
			    – Titrate weekly by 1.5 mg up to 12 mg daily
			• **Dosing (Peds):** None
			• **CYP450 Interactions:** None
			• **Renal or Hepatic Dose Adjustments:** Avoid in CKD
			• **Dosage Forms (micronized):** 1.25 mg, 1.5 mg, 2.5 mg, 3 mg, 5 mg, 6 mg

ENDOCRINE – THIAZOLIDINEDIONES

Drug Class
- Thiazolidinediones (TZDs)
    - **Agents:** pioglitazone, rosiglitazone

Main Indications or Uses
- T2DM management as an adjunct to diet and exercise

Mechanism of Action
- Decreases insulin resistance as a peroxisome proliferator-activated receptor-gamma (PPARgamma) agonist, affecting genetic production in glucose metabolism.

Primary Net Benefit
- Decreases insulin resistance to lower A1c by 1-1.5%
- Main Labs to Monitor:
    - A1c every 3-6 months, depending on whether the patient is at goal
    - LFTs at initiation and periodically

> **Warnings & Alerts**
> ✓ Avoid these agents in patients with known NYHA Class III/IV heart failure as they are known to increase the plasma volume and cause edema.

High-Yield Basic Pharmacology
- **Drug Interactions**
    - Strong CYP2C8 inhibitors (i.e., gemfibrozil)
        - Pioglitazone 15 mg daily maximum dose with these.

High-Yield Clinical Knowledge
- **Warnings**
    - Contraindicated in patients with NYHA Class III/IV HF.
        - Caution with NYHA Class I/II HF, or in patients on insulin due to increase in edema.
        - May cause new HF.
    - May cause hepatic failure; LFT monitoring required.
    - May increase the risk of fractures.
    - Avoid use in patients with bladder cancer, and caution with a history of bladder cancer.
        - Formal dosing limitations have been removed due to controversial evidence.
- **Special Populations**
    - May improve insulin resistance in NAFLD and fibrosis in NASH.
- **Edema and Weight Gain**
    - Edema and weight gain are common because of visceral fat being converted to SC fat.
- **Vision Changes**
    - Monitor any vision changes due to potential macular edema and refer to an ophthalmologist.
- **Lipid Effects**
    - Decrease TG and raise HDL, but data has been inconsistent with the class.
        - Rosiglitazone demonstrated potential CV risk and was under a REMS program, but this barrier has been removed; however, most clinicians now utilize pioglitazone as a result.
    - Pioglitazone may provide CV benefits, although this is not a common reason for utilizing in practice.

High-Yield Core Evidence
- **PROactive**
    - A multicenter RCT in 5238 T2DM patients to determine secondary macrovascular disease prevention potential of pioglitazone.
    - Pioglitazone reduced the risk of all all-cause mortality, nonfatal MI, and nonfatal stroke in patients with DM and high CV risk as a secondary endpoint by a 16% reduction. Lancet 2005;366:1279-89.

Endocrinology

- **RECORD**
    - A multicenter, randomized, open-label trial in 4447 T2DM patients to assess CV hospitalization or CV death with pioglitazone.
        - Rosiglitazone did not increase risk of the primary outcome but did approximately double the risk of HF admission or death.
        - Also, found increased risk of lower limb fractures in women. Lancet 2009;373:2125-35.
    - A meta-analysis by Nissen and Wolski that ultimately included 42 trials found an overall 43% increased risk of MI and 64% increased risk of CV death with rosiglitazone, recognizing the small number of events overall that could have affected these results. NEJM 2007;356:2457-71.
    - Rosiglitazone was deemed not to increase CV risk, as was found in Nissen and Wolski's meta-analysis, which resulted in the REMS program being subsequently ended in 2015.

High-Yield Fast-Fact
- Anecdotally, TZDs have been used short-term (8-12 weeks) to reduce visceral fat and improve insulin resistance in patients on insulin therapy, with the hope of improving the response to insulin even after discontinuation.
- Cost is the main reason for use in clinical practice with the lack of secondary benefits from TZDs.

HIGH-YIELD BOARD EXAM ESSENTIALS
- **CLASSIC AGENTS:** Pioglitazone, rosiglitazone
- **DRUG CLASS:** Thiazolidinediones (TZDs)
- **INDICATIONS:** T2DM management as adjunct to diet and exercise
- **MECHANISM:** Decreases insulin resistance as a PPARgamma agonist
- **SIDE EFFECTS:** Edema, weight gain, low hypoglycemic risk
- **CLINICAL PEARLS:** Contraindicated in patients with NYHA Class III/IV HF. Caution with NYHA Class I/II HF or in patients on insulin due to increase in edema. May cause new HF.

Table: Drug Class Summary

	Thiazolidinediones Drug Class Review High-Yield Med Reviews		
Mechanism of Action: *Decreases insulin resistance as a peroxisome proliferator-activated receptor-gamma (PPARgamma) agonist.*			
Class Effects: *Decreases A1c 1-1.5%, edema, weight gain, low hypoglycemic risk.*			
Generic Name	**Brand Name**	**Indication(s) or Uses**	**Notes**
Pioglitazone	Actos	- T2DM as an adjunct to diet and exercise	- **Dosing (Adult):** 15-45 mg daily – Limit to lower dose if NYHA Class I/II HF - **Dosing (Peds):** None - **CYP450 Interactions:** Strong CYP2C8 inhibitors - **Renal or Hepatic Dose Adjustments:** If LFTs >3xULN after initiating therapy and pioglitazone is suspected, do not restart. - **Dosage Forms:** 15 mg, 30 mg, 45 mg
Rosiglitazone	Avandia	- T2DM as adjunct to diet and exercise	- **Dosing (Adult):** 4-8 mg daily – May divide BID - **Dosing (Peds):** None - **CYP450 Interactions:** Strong CYP2C8 inhibitors - **Renal or Hepatic Dose Adjustments:** DC if ALT consistently >3xULN - **Dosage Forms:** 2 mg, 4 mg, 8 mg

ENDOCRINE – BASAL INSULIN

Drug Class
- Basal Insulin
- Agents:
  - Intermediate-acting – NPH, U-500
  - Long-acting – insulin degludec (U-100, U-200), detemir, glargine (U-100, U-300)

> **Fast Facts**
> ✓ Insulin degludec and glargine are the only basal or long-acting insulins that can be administered once-a-day and provide 24-hour coverage.

Main Indications or Uses
- Treatment of T1DM and T2DM in adult and pediatric patients

Mechanism of Action
- Replaces endogenous insulin due to pancreatic beta-cell deficiency or insufficiency; insulin normally regulates carbohydrate, protein, and fat metabolism, stimulates hepatic glycogen synthesis, decreases lipolysis, and increases uptake of triglycerides.

Primary Net Benefit
- Improves glycemic control by replacing insulin and reducing fasting glucose.
- Main Labs to Monitor:
  - A1c every 3-6 months depending on whether the patient is at goal
  - Urinary ketones and bicarbonate if DKA suspected; consider blood ketones and arterial pH.

High-Yield Basic Pharmacology
- TZDs can increase risk of edema and/or HF when used with insulin.

Intermediate-Acting Insulin*

Insulin Type	Brand Names	Concentrations	Onset	Peak	Duration
NPH	Novolin N, Humulin N	U-100	2-4 hours	4-6 hours	8-12 hours
Insulin regular	Humulin R	U-500	30-60 min	2-3 hours	13-24 hours

*Mixed insulin also available as Humulin 70/30, Novolin 70/30, Humalog 50/50, 75/25, and NovoLog Mix 70/30.

Long-Acting Insulin

Insulin Type	Brand Names	Concentrations	Onset	Peak	Duration
Degludec	Tresiba	U-100, U-200	30-90 min	Relatively peakless action	42 hours
Detemir	Levemir	U-100	2-4 hours	8-12 hours	14-24 hours
Glargine	Basaglar, Lantus, Semglee	U-100	2-4 hours	Relatively peakless action	22-24 hours
Glargine	Toujeo, Toujeo Max	U-300	6 hours	Relatively peakless action	24-30 hours

High-Yield Clinical Knowledge
- Adverse Events
  - Causes hypoglycemia, weight gain and/or edema, and injection-site reactions.
    - Patients with renal or hepatic disease may be more susceptible to hypoglycemia.
    - Beta-blockers can mask hypoglycemic effects.
- Basal Insulin Dosing
  - Insulin pens should be primed with 2-4 units before use.
  - Basal/Bolus is usually divided in approximately a 50/50% ratio.
  - T1DM

- Dosing is initially weight-based, but should be adjusted in a patient-specific manner.
- 0.4-1 units/kg/d total daily insulin dose
- T2DM
  - Dosing should be patient-specific.
  - Start 10 units daily or 0.1-0.2 units/kg/d in insulin-naïve, or 1:1 if converting from another basal insulin for most.
- Adjust basal insulin by 2-4 units every 3-4 days depending on patient goals and response.
- Decrease dose for hypoglycemia by 10-40% depending on severity.
- Doses should be empirically reduced when adding other DM medications and/or those that predispose to hypoglycemia depending on current glycemic control and/or goals.
- Conversions between basal insulins can generally be changed 1:1, but there are exceptions.
  - Insulin Glargine Conversions (1:1 unless otherwise specified below)
    - Use 80% TDD NPH BID dose when converting to glargine.
    - Use 80% TDD detemir BID when converting to Toujeo.
    - Use 80% Toujeo dose when converting to Lantus.
    - Toujeo may require a higher dose than Lantus to maintain control.
- Insulin glargine U-300 (Toujeo Max) and degludec U-200 are able to deliver single doses up to 160 units by 2 unit increments.
- Insulin detemir, glargine, and NPH may be divided into BID dosing.
  - NPH can be divided 50/50, or 2/3 in AM and 1/3 in PM. Some evidence supports NPH divided 3-4 times daily to reduce hypoglycemia risk.
  - Detemir and glargine are typically divided when basal dose is >50 units.
  - Consider administering 80% of the previous basal insulin dose as NPH if changing agents to avoid hypoglycemia.
- Insulin degludec can be administered up to 8 hours before the next scheduled dose if a patient misses a dose without affecting efficacy or safety.
- Insulin detemir is the only insulin that is pregnancy category B.
- May need to discontinue prior to some procedures and surgeries.

- **Administration**
  - May inject SC only into the back of the arm, outer thigh, buttocks, or abdomen.
    - Site rotation should be advised to avoid lipodystrophy.
  - Insulin should be clear, except insulin containing NPH, which is cloudy.
    - Need to invert or roll NPH in hands to resuspend.
  - Do not mix any long-acting insulins.
  - Clean site; do not pinch unless the patient is very thin; inject at a 90° angle; hold needle in skin for a count of 5-10 to ensure insulin does not leak out of injection site.
  - Do not draw insulin out of pen devices, especially with different concentrations.
  - Avoid injecting cold insulin to avoid increased pain.
  - Consider device when choosing insulin for patients who are visually impaired (pen vs. vial) or with dexterity problems (FlexTouch vs. FlexPens or other insulin pens).
  - Do not use basal insulin in insulin pumps, except for U-500.

- **Storage and Expiration**
  - Insulin expires according to the package date if refrigerated.
  - Insulin expires at varying times once at room temperature and/or used for the first time.
    - Typically, expiration is 28 days once used/at room temperature.
      - Insulin detemir expires after 42 days.
      - Insulin degludec and insulin glargine U-300 expire after 56 days.

- **Generic Substitution**
  - Semglee can be substituted for Lantus without a prescription change.

- **U-500**
    - U-500 regular insulin is utilized in patients (mostly T2DM) requiring >200 units daily to improve absorption by decreasing the injected volume.
        - U-500 is the only concentrated insulin that accomplishes this effect.
    - Used off-label in insulin pumps.
    - Causes significant weight gain.
    - Dosing and Administration
        - Discontinue all other insulins.
        - Start 80% of the total daily dose of the previous regimen divided at 60/40% BID or 40/30/30% TID 30 min prior to meals.
        - Use only U-500 syringes or Humalog KwikPen U-500. Dosed in 5-unit increments.

High-Yield Core Evidence

- **DCCT**
    - Multicenter, large, RCT trial of approx. 6.5 years duration in T1DM that demonstrated intensive insulin therapy compared to conventional insulin therapy decreased microvascular outcomes.
        - Severe hypoglycemia was increased with intensive insulin.
    - NEJM 1993;329(14)977-86.
- **DCCT/EDIC**
    - Patients (97%) from DCCT continued or changed to intensive insulin therapy and were followed approx. 17 years
        - Demonstrated 42% CV event reduction in patients initially managed with intensive insulin therapy.
    - NEJM 2005;353(25)2643-53.
- **UKPDS 33**
    - Multicenter, large, prospective trial of 10 years duration that demonstrated intensive insulin therapy in new T2DM resulted in a reduction in microvascular complications but neutral effects on macrovascular outcomes with increased risk of hypoglycemia.
    - Lancet 1998;352:837-53.
- **ORIGIN**
    - Multicenter, large, RCT of approx. 6 years duration that compared insulin glargine to standard care in patients with high CV risk and IFG, IGT, or T2DM for 3-point MACE and 3-point MACE plus revascularization or hospitalization for HF.
        - CV outcomes were neutral but demonstrated greater hypoglycemia and weight gain.
        - No increase in the risk of cancers.
    - NEJM 2012;367:319-328.
- **DEVOTE**
    - Multicenter, large RCT compared insulin degludec to insulin glargine U-100 in patients with T2DM and high risk for CV events (most established CVD).
        - Primary outcome was 3-point MACE (noninferior); prespecified secondary outcome was severe hypoglycemia (superior with absolute 1.7% reduction in degludec).
        - 53% decrease in severe nocturnal hypoglycemia with degludec.
    - NEJM 2017;377:723-32.

High-Yield Fast-Facts

- Do not use basal insulin when treating DKA. Must use rapid or regular insulin.
- Insulin was found to be produced in the pancreas by 2 German researchers in 1889 who observed when dogs' pancreas glands were removed that they developed diabetes. Insulin was first discovered by Frederick Banting, Charles Best, John McLeod, and James Collip in 1921 and successfully utilized in trials in 1922.
- Bovine and porcine insulins are not utilized due to higher potential antibody formation or allergic reactions.

Table: Drug Class Summary

Basal Insulin Drug Class Review			
High-Yield Med Reviews			
Mechanism of Action: Replaces endogenous insulin due to pancreatic beta-cell deficiency or insufficiency.			
Class Effects: Decrease A1c 1.5-2%, hypoglycemia, weight gain/edema, injection site reactions			
Generic Name	**Brand Name**	**Main Indication(s) or Uses**	**Notes**

Insulin Degludec	Tresiba (U-100, U-200)	▪ Treatment of T1DM and T2DM in adult and pediatric patients	▪ **Dosing:** Approx. 1/3-1/2 total daily dose in basal insulin; dosing should be patient-specific.
			   − T1DM: 0.4-1 unit/kg/d total daily insulin dose
			   − T2DM: 0.1-0.2 units/kg/d total daily insulin or 10 units daily
			▪ **Dosing (Peds):** 0.4-1 units/kg/d in insulin-naïve depending on developmental stage and history
			   − Start 80% of current basal dose when converting to degludec
			▪ **CYP450 Interactions:** N/A
			▪ **Renal or Hepatic Dose Adjustments:** N/A
			▪ **Dosage Forms:** U-100 pen, U-200 pen, U-100 vial

Insulin Detemir	Levemir	▪ Treatment of T1DM and T2DM in adult and pediatric patients	▪ **Dosing (Adult):** Approx. 1/3-1/2 total daily dose in basal insulin; dosing should be patient-specific.
			   − T1DM: 0.4-1 unit/kg/d total daily insulin dose
			   − T2DM: 0.1-0.2 units/kg/d total daily insulin or 10 units daily
			▪ **Dosing (Peds):** ≥2 yo – 0.4-1 units/kg/d depending on developmental stage and history
			▪ **CYP450 Interactions:** N/A
			▪ **Renal or Hepatic Dose Adjustments:** N/A
			▪ **Dosage Forms:** U-100 pen, U-100 vial

Insulin Glargine	Basaglar (U-100)
	Lantus (U-100)
	Semglee (U-100)
	Toujeo (U-300)
	Toujeo Max (U-300)
		▪ Treatment of T1DM and T2DM in adult and pediatric patients	▪ **Dosing (Adult):** Approx. 1/3-1/2 total daily dose in basal insulin; dosing should be patient-specific.
			   − T1DM: 0.4-1 unit/kg/d total daily insulin dose
			   − T2DM: 0.1-0.2 units/kg/d total daily insulin or 10 units daily
			▪ **Dosing (Peds):** ≥6 yo – 0.4-1 unit/kg/d total daily dose depending on developmental stage and history
			▪ **CYP450 Interactions:** N/A
			▪ **Renal or Hepatic Dose Adjustments:** N/A
			▪ **Dosage Forms:** U-100 pen (Basaglar, Lantus, Semglee), U-300 pen (Toujeo, Toujeo Max), U-100 vial (Lantus, Semglee)

| GLP-1 Agonist Drug Class Review ||||
| High-Yield Med Reviews ||||
Generic Name	Brand Name	Main Indication(s) or Uses	Notes

Insulin NPH	Humulin N
	Novolin N
		• Treatment of T1DM and T2DM in adult and pediatric patients	• **Dosing (Adult):** Approx. 1/3-1/2 total daily dose in basal insulin; give 2/3 NPH in AM, 1/3 in PM; dosing should be patient-specific.
			   – T1DM: 0.4-1 unit/kg/d total daily insulin dose
			      – May consider lower to avoid hypoglycemia
			   – T2DM: 0.1-0.2 units/kg/d total daily insulin or 10 units daily or divided BID
			• **Dosing (Peds):** 0.4-1 unit/kg/d total daily dose depending on developmental stage and history
			• **CYP450 Interactions:** N/A
			• **Renal or Hepatic Dose Adjustments:** N/A
			• **Dosage Forms:** U-100 pen, U-100 vial

HIGH-YIELD BOARD EXAM ESSENTIALS

- **CLASSIC AGENTS:** NPH, U-500, insulin degludec (U-100, U-200), detemir, glargine (U-100, U-300)
- **DRUG CLASS:** Basal insulin
- **INDICATIONS:** Treatment of T1DM and T2DM in adult and pediatric patients
- **MECHANISM:** Replaces endogenous insulin due to pancreatic beta-cell deficiency or insufficiency
- **SIDE EFFECTS:** Hypoglycemia, weight gain, edema, injection site pain
- **CLINICAL PEARLS:**
    - Insulin degludec and glargine are typically better basal insulins that can be administered once a day whereas detemir typically requires twice a day dosing and can result in dose increases over time.
    - The basal agents should not be mixed with other insulins (e.g., glargine is acidic).
    - U-500 regular insulin is utilized in patients (mostly T2DM) requiring >200 units daily to improve absorption by decreasing the injected volume.

ENDOCRINE – INSULIN – SHORT ACTING

Drug Class
- Prandial Insulin
- Agents:
  - **Short-Acting**
    - Insulin regular
  - **Rapid-Acting**
    - Insulin aspart (Fiasp, Novolog), glulisine, lispro, lispro-aabc

> **Fast Facts**
> ✓ If regular insulin is used, its timing of the dose is more relevant in the context of when the patient plans to eat versus the rapid acting options can be given right before they sit down to eat.

Main Indications or Uses
- Label
  - Treatment of T1DM and T2DM in adult and pediatric patients
- Common Off-Label
  - Gestational DM
  - Diabetic ketoacidosis (DKA) and hyperosmolar hyperglycemic state (HHS)
  - Hyperglycemia in critical illness
  - Hyperkalemia

Mechanism of Action
- Replaces endogenous insulin due to pancreatic beta-cell deficiency or insufficiency; insulin normally regulates carbohydrate, protein, and fat metabolism, stimulates hepatic glycogen synthesis, decreases lipolysis, and increases uptake of triglycerides.

Primary Net Benefit
- Improves glycemic control by replacing insulin and reducing post-prandial glucose.
- Main Labs to Monitor:
  - A1c every 3-6 months depending on whether patient is at goal
  - K^+ with inpatient continuous infusion
  - Urinary ketones and bicarbonate if DKA suspected; consider blood ketones and arterial pH

High-Yield Basic Pharmacology
- TZDs can increase the risk of edema and/or HF when used with insulin.

Short-Acting Insulin

Insulin Type	Brand Names	Onset	Peak	Duration
Regular	Humulin R Novolin R	15-30 min	2-5 hours	SC: 4-12 hours IV: 2-6 hours

Rapid-Acting Insulin

Insulin Type	Brand Names	Onset	Peak	Duration
Aspart	Fiasp (ultra-rapid) Novolog	5-20 min 15-30 min	1-2 hours	3-5 hours
Glulisine	Apidra	15-30 min	1-2 hours	3-5 hours
Inhaled insulin	Afrezza	12-15 min	1-2 hours	2.5-3 hours
Lispro (U-100, U-200)	Humalog Admelog	15-30 min	1-2 hours	3-5 hours
Lispro-aabc	Lyumjev (ultra-rapid)	15-30 min	1 hour	4-7 hours

Endocrinology

High-Yield Clinical Knowledge
- Causes hypoglycemia, weight gain and/or edema, and injection-site reactions.
    - Patients with renal or hepatic disease may be more susceptible to hypoglycemia.
    - Beta-blockers can mask hypoglycemic effects.
- Rapid insulins are considered to cause less risk of hypoglycemia than regular insulin because of their shorter duration of action.
- Ultra-rapid insulins have demonstrated some potential to improve post-prandial excursions, but further investigation is needed to define their use.
- Generics are available for insulin aspart, insulin aspart 70/30, insulin lispro, insulin lispro 75/25, and insulin glargine.
- Insulin approved for pump use includes insulin regular, insulin aspart, insulin lispro, and insulin glulisine.
- Humalog Jr Kwikpen is designed for pediatric patients but can be useful for any patient needing insulin dosing in 0.5 unit increments.
- **Prandial Insulin Dosing**
    - Insulin pens should be primed with 2 units before use.
    - Basal/Bolus is usually divided in approximately a 50/50% ratio.
    - T1DM
        - Dosing is initially weight-based, but should be adjusted in a patient-specific manner.
        - 0.4-1 units/kg/d total daily insulin dose
    - T2DM
        - Dosing should be patient specific.
        - Start 4-5 units or 10% of basal dose daily prior to largest meal. Add to other meals as needed.
    - Adjust prandial insulin by 1-2 units every 3-4 days, depending on patient goals and response.
    - Decrease dose for hypoglycemia by 10-40% depending on severity.
    - Doses should be empirically reduced when adding other DM medications and/or those that predispose to hypoglycemia depending on current glycemic control and/or goals.
    - Do not administer if fasting (i.e., before surgical procedure).
- **DKA Dosing**
    - Insulin regular preferred; insulin glulisine also has off-label use.
    - Bolus: 0.1 units/kg (optional)
    - Infusion:
        - Bolus – 0.1 units/kg/h
        - No Bolus – 0.14 units/kg/h
    - When glucose is <200 mg/dL, decrease infusion to 0.02-0.05 units/kg/h or switch to SC rapid-acting 0.1 units/kg every 2 hours.
    - Administer dextrose-containing fluids with goal glucose 150-200 mg/dL until resolution.
    - Administer K^+ based on K^+ levels and monitor every 2 hours.
    - Resolution considered when glucose <200 mg/dL and 2 of the following: bicarbonate $\geq$15, venous pH >7.3, anion gap $\leq$12.
- **Administration**
    - Dose timing depends on the type of prandial insulin.
        - Rapid
            - Admelog, Humalog, or Novolog – 5-15 min prior to meal start or immediately after meal
            - Apidra – 15 min prior to meal start or within 20 min after starting meal
            - Fiasp, Lyumjev – at start of meal or within 20 min after starting meal
        - Regular
            - Insulin regular – 30 min prior to meals
    - May inject SC only into back of the arm, outer thigh, buttocks, or abdomen.
        - Abdomen results in the most consistent absorption.
        - Site rotation should be advised to avoid lipodystrophy.
    - Clean site; do not pinch unless the patient is very thin; inject at a 90° angle; hold needle in the skin for a count of 5-10 to ensure insulin does not leak out of the injection site.
    - Prandial insulins should be clear.

- Do not draw insulin out of pen devices, especially with higher concentrations.
- Mixing Prandial Insulins
    - Do not mix Admelog, Apidra, Fiasp, Lyumjev, or any concentrated insulins.
    - Novolog and Humalog may be mixed from a vial only. Draw into syringe before NPH to assess clarity.
- Avoid injecting cold insulin, which can be painful.
- **IV Insulin**
    - May cause hypokalemia and should be monitored during therapy as it can cause significant complications.
    - IV insulin infusion is preferred in critically ill patients; basal-bolus therapy is preferred in non-critically ill.
    - Flush IV tubing with a priming solution of 20 mL from the insulin infusion to minimize insulin adsorption to IV tubing whenever a new tubing set is added.
- **Storage and Expiration**
    - Insulin expires according to the package date if refrigerated.
    - Insulin expires at varying times once at room temperature and/or used for the first time.
        - Typically, expiration is 28 days once used/at room temperature.
- **Inhaled Insulin (Afrezza)**
    - Short-acting inhaled dosage form available in 4, 8, or 12 unit cartridges.
    - Contraindicated in chronic lung disease, such as COPD and asthma, as well as patients who smoke or recently quit.
    - Spirometry should be performed prior to and after starting therapy to assess for lung disease.
    - Has not been heavily utilized in clinical practice due to modest benefits, adverse effects (cough, sore throat), and difficulty with compliance, unless in patients with injection fatigue.

High-Yield Core Evidence
- **FullSTEP Study**
    - Multicenter, RCT in 401 T2DM patients to determine noninferiority of stepwise addition of bolus insulin aspart with full basal-bolus regimens.
        - Both groups experienced approx. 1% A1c reductions
        - 42% reduction in hypoglycemic episodes and greater patient satisfaction in the stepwise group, which led to guideline recommendations to consider the stepwise addition of bolus insulin.
    - Lancet Diabetes Endocrinol 2014;2(1):30-7. 96 ref ADA 2021
- **GLP-1 Agonist vs. Bolus in T2DM**
    - Multicenter, RCT in 627 T2DM patients to determine noninferiority of adding exenatide to 3x daily prandial lispro both added to insulin glargine and metformin.
        - Exenatide was noninferior to lispro with beneficial weight loss (-2.5 kg), lower nocturnal hypoglycemic events, and greater satisfaction.
        - GI effects were more common with exenatide.
    - Diabetes Care 2014;37:2763-73.

High-Yield Fast-Facts
- Insulin was found to be produced in the pancreas by 2 German researchers in 1889 who observed when dogs' pancreas glands were removed that they developed diabetes. Insulin was first discovered by Frederick Banting, Charles Best, John McLeod, and James Collip in 1921 and successfully utilized in trials in 1922.
- Bovine and porcine insulins are not utilized due to higher potential antibody formation or allergic reactions.

HIGH-YIELD BOARD EXAM ESSENTIALS
- **CLASSIC AGENTS:** Insulin regular, aspart (Fiasp, Novolog), glulisine, lispro (Humalog, Admelog), lispro-aabc
- **DRUG CLASS:** Prandial insulin
- **INDICATIONS:** Treatment of T1DM and T2DM in adult and pediatric patients
- **MECHANISM:** Replaces endogenous insulin due to pancreatic beta-cell deficiency or insufficiency.
- **SIDE EFFECTS:** Hypoglycemia, weight gain, injection site pain
- **CLINICAL PEARLS:** Rapid insulins are considered to cause less risk of hypoglycemia than regular insulin because of their shorter duration of action.

Table: Drug Class Summary

	Prandial Insulin Drug Class Review High-Yield Med Reviews		
Mechanism of Action: *Replaces endogenous insulin due to pancreatic beta-cell deficiency or insufficiency.*			
Class Effects: *Decrease A1c 0.5-1%, hypoglycemia, weight gain/edema, injection site reactions*			
Generic Name	**Brand Name**	**Main Indication(s) or Uses**	**Notes**
Insulin Aspart	Fiasp Novolog	<ul><li>Treatment of T1DM and T2DM in adult and pediatric patients</li><li>Off-label: Gestational DM, DKA, HHS, hyperglycemia in critical illness, hyperkalemia</li></ul>	<ul><li>**Dosing (Adult):** Approx. 50-60% total daily dose in prandial insulin; dosing should be patient-specific.<ul><li>T1DM: 0.4-1 unit/kg/d total daily insulin dose</li><li>T2DM: 4-5 units or 10% of basal dose daily prior to largest meal; add to other meals as needed</li></ul></li><li>**Dosing (Peds):** Approx. 50-60% total daily dose in prandial insulin; dosing should be patient-specific.<ul><li>T1DM: 0.4-1 unit/kg/d total daily insulin dose</li><li>T2DM: 4-5 units or 10% of basal dose daily prior to largest meal; add to other meals as needed</li></ul></li><li>**CYP450 Interactions:** N/A</li><li>**Renal or Hepatic Dose Adjustments:** N/A</li><li>**Dosage Forms:** U-100 pen, vial</li></ul>
Insulin Glulisine	Apidra	<ul><li>Treatment of T1DM and T2DM in adult and pediatric patients</li><li>Off-label: Gestational DM, DKA, HHS, hyperglycemia in critical illness, hyperkalemia</li></ul>	<ul><li>**Dosing (Adult):** Approx. 50-60% total daily dose in prandial insulin; dosing should be patient-specific.<ul><li>T1DM: 0.4-1 unit/kg/d total daily insulin dose</li><li>T2DM: 4-5 units or 10% of basal dose daily prior to largest meal; add to other meals as needed</li></ul></li><li>**Dosing (Peds):** Approx. 50-60% total daily dose in prandial insulin; dosing should be patient-specific.<ul><li>T1DM: 0.4-1 unit/kg/d total daily insulin dose</li><li>T2DM: 4-5 units or 10% of basal dose daily prior to largest meal; add to other meals as needed</li></ul></li><li>**CYP450 Interactions:** N/A</li><li>**Renal or Hepatic Dose Adjustments:** N/A</li><li>**Dosage Forms:** U-100 pen, vial</li></ul>

| \multicolumn{4}{c}{**Prandial Insulin Drug Class Review**} |
| \multicolumn{4}{c}{High-Yield Med Reviews} |

Generic Name	Brand Name	Main Indication(s) or Uses	Notes
Insulin Lispro	Admelog Humalog	▪ Treatment of T1DM and T2DM in adult and pediatric patients ▪ Off-label: Gestational DM, DKA, HHS, hyperglycemia in critical illness, hyperkalemia	▪ **Dosing (Adult):** Approx. 50-60% total daily dose in prandial insulin; dosing should be patient-specific. – T1DM: 0.4-1 unit/kg/d total daily insulin dose – T2DM: 4-5 units or 10% of basal dose daily prior to largest meal; add to other meals as needed ▪ **Dosing (Peds):** Approx. 50-60% total daily dose in prandial insulin; dosing should be patient-specific. – T1DM: 0.4-1 unit/kg/d total daily insulin dose – T2DM: 4-5 units or 10% of basal dose daily prior to largest meal; add to other meals as needed ▪ **CYP450 Interactions:** N/A ▪ **Renal or Hepatic Dose Adjustments:** N/A ▪ **Dosage Forms:** Admelog (U-100 pen, vial); Humalog (U-100 pen, vial; U-200 pen)
Insulin Lispro-aabc	Lyumjev	▪ Treatment of T1DM and T2DM in adult and pediatric patients ▪ Off-label: Gestational DM, DKA, HHS, hyperglycemia in critical illness, hyperkalemia	▪ **Dosing (Adult):** Approx. 50-60% total daily dose in prandial insulin; dosing should be patient-specific. – T1DM: 0.4-1 unit/kg/d total daily insulin dose – T2DM: 4-5 units or 10% of basal dose daily prior to largest meal; add to other meals as needed ▪ **Dosing (Peds):** Approx. 50-60% total daily dose in prandial insulin; dosing should be patient-specific. – T1DM: 0.4-1 unit/kg/d total daily insulin dose – T2DM: 4-5 units or 10% of basal dose daily prior to largest meal; add to other meals as needed ▪ **CYP450 Interactions:** N/A ▪ **Renal or Hepatic Dose Adjustments:** N/A ▪ **Dosage Forms:** U-100 pen, vial

Prandial Insulin Drug Class Review
High-Yield Med Reviews

Generic Name	Brand Name	Main Indication(s) or Uses	Notes

Insulin Regular	Humulin R
	Novolin R
		▪ Treatment of T1DM and T2DM in adult and pediatric patients
		▪ Off-label: Gestational DM, DKA, HHS, hyperglycemia in critical illness, hyperkalemia
			▪ **Dosing (Adult):** Approx. 50-60% total daily dose in prandial insulin; dosing should be patient-specific.
			  − T1DM: 0.4-1 unit/kg/d total daily insulin dose
			  − T2DM: 4-5 units or 10% of basal dose daily prior to largest meal; add to other meals as needed
			  − DKA: Bolus: 0.1 units/kg (optional)
			    − Infusion:
			      − Bolus − 0.1 units/kg/h
			      − No Bolus − 0.14 units/kg/h
			▪ **Dosing (Peds):** Approx. 50-60% total daily dose in prandial insulin; dosing should be patient-specific.
			  − T1DM: 0.4-1 unit/kg/d total daily insulin dose
			  − T2DM: 4-5 units or 10% of basal dose daily prior to largest meal; add to other meals as needed
			▪ **CYP450 Interactions:** N/A
			▪ **Renal or Hepatic Dose Adjustments:** N/A
			▪ **Dosage Forms:** Humulin R (vial); Novolin R (U-100 pen, vial)

ENDOCRINE – ANTIGOUT AGENTS

Drug Class
- **Antigout Agents**
- **Agents:**
    - **Acute Care**
        - Colchicine
        - Rasburicase
    - **Chronic Care**
        - Colchicine
        - Pegloticase
        - Probenecid

> **Knowledge Integration**
> - Colchicine can be used for acute or recurrent cases of pericarditis, but if used should be given with aspirin or an NSAID. If the later cannot be used, then corticosteroids can be used.
> - Avoid rasburicase and pegloticase in patients with G6PD deficiency due to risk of hemolysis.

Main Indications or Uses
- **Acute Care**
    - Acute gout (colchicine)
    - Hyperuricemia associated with malignancy (rasburicase)
    - Pericarditis (colchicine)
- **Chronic Care**
    - Gout (colchicine, pegloticase, probenecid)
    - Familial Mediterranean fever (colchicine)
    - Stable ischemic Heart Disease, Prevention of ACVD (low-dose colchicine)

Mechanism of Action
- **Colchicine**
    - Inhibits polymerization of intracellular tubulin into microtubules, inhibiting leukocyte migration and phagocytosis.
- **Pegloticase, Rasburicase**
    - A recombinant form of uricase that converts uric acid to the more water-soluble allantoin.
- **Probenecid**
    - Inhibits the reabsorption of uric acid in the proximal convoluted tubule to reduce uric acid levels

Primary Net Benefit
- Colchicine aids in relieving acute gouty attacks and has recently been developed as an adjunct for post-myocardial infarction and chronic CAD.
- Pegloticase is reserved for severe cases where patients can't tolerate alternative agents.
- Main Labs to Monitor:
    - CBC
    - Liver enzymes (AST/ALT, alk phos)
    - Liver function (INR/PT, albumin, protein, bilirubin)
    - Serum creatinine

High-Yield Basic Pharmacology
- **Microtubule Formation**
    - Colchicine's inhibition of microtubule formation affects cells and tissues throughout the body.
    - While its effects on leukocytes benefit gout and other diseases, colchicine also inhibits neutrophil and synovial cell-mediated chemotaxis and phagocytosis.
- **GABA Effects**
    - Colchicine is a competitive GABA-A receptor antagonist which can potentiate seizures.
- **Rasburicase and Plasma Uric Acid**
    - Patients receiving rasburicase must have blood samples of uric acid transported to the lab with special handling to prevent falsely low plasma uric acid levels due to ex-vivo enzymatic degradation of uric acid.
- **Colchicine Drug Interactions**

- Colchicine is a substrate of CYP3A4 and requires dose adjustment for patients taking CYP3A4 inhibitors (amiodarone, clarithromycin, diltiazem, protease inhibitors, statins, verapamil, and others) or P-glycoprotein inhibitors (amiodarone, cyclosporine, tacrolimus, and others).

High-Yield Clinical Knowledge
- **Colchicine Toxicity**
    - Colchicine is a narrow therapeutic agent with the potential for fatal drug overdoses.
    - Toxic and potentially lethal doses are between 0.5 to 0.8 mg/kg, so for small children, a single tablet of 0.6 mg can be fatal.
    - Patients on concomitant potent CYP3A4 inhibitors or P-glycoprotein inhibitors or those with renal dysfunction can experience toxic effects at much lower doses.
    - Colchicine poisoning presents in three phases:
        - Early GI distress and severe volume distribution persisting 12-24 hours after ingestion.
        - Multiorgan dysfunction and failure, including bone marrow suppression, begins 24 hours after ingestion and lasts for several days.
        - Death or recovery occurs within one week of ingestion or exposure.
- **Uricosuric Therapy**
    - Probenecid is indicated in gout patients where allopurinol or febuxostat are contraindicated or if tophaceous gout is present.
    - Alternatively, probenecid can be added to either allopurinol or febuxostat, but patients must be educated to maintain adequate hydration to avoid the development of uric acid renal stones.
        - Urine pH should also be maintained above 6.0 while taking probenecid, which can be achieved by administering agents such as sodium bicarbonate.
- **Colchicine Myopathy, Neuropathy, and Myoneuropathy**
    - Although colchicine can produce myopathy (made worse by concomitant statin therapy) and neuropathies, myoneuropathies are frequent sequelae of chronic colchicine therapy.
- **Pegloticase and Gout Flares**
    - Early in the course of pegloticase treatment and usually within the first six months of therapy, patients may experience more frequent gout flares requiring NSAID or colchicine therapy.
    - Additionally, with long-term pegloticase therapy, anti-pegloticase antibodies form that shorten its half-life and lead to a significantly diminished efficacy.
        - Trending of plasma uric acid levels is a surrogate marker for anti-pegloticase antibody development.
- **Pegloticase Anaphylaxis**
    - An alarmingly high proportion of patients receiving pegloticase develop anaphylaxis (up to 15%).

High-Yield Core Evidence
- **COLCOT**
    - This was a multicenter, double-blind trial of patients who experienced an acute MI within 30 days to be randomized to receive either colchicine 0.5 mg daily or placebo.
    - Patients randomized to receive colchicine experienced a significantly lower rate of death from cardiovascular causes, resuscitated cardiac arrest, MI, stroke, or urgent hospitalization for angina leading to coronary revascularization.
    - This outcome was driven by a reduced risk of stroke and urgent rehospitalization for angina leading to coronary revascularization.
    - Three was no difference in diarrhea, but pneumonia was more frequent with colchicine than placebo.
    - The authors concluded that colchicine 0.5 mg daily significantly reduced the risk of ischemic CV events than placebo among patients with recent MI. (N Engl J Med. 2019 Dec 26;381(26):2497-2505.)
- **LoDoCo2**
    - This was a multicenter, placebo-controlled, double-blind trial that randomized patients with chronic coronary disease to receive either colchicine 0.5 mg daily or placebo.
    - Patients randomized to receive colchicine experienced a significant reduction in the rate of the primary composite outcome of CV death, spontaneous MI, ischemic stroke, or ischemia-driven coronary revascularization.

- Both the secondary composite endpoint and endpoint, ischemia-driven coronary revascularization, and spontaneous MI were also significantly lower with colchicine than with placebo.
- However, colchicine was associated with an increased incidence of death from noncardiovascular causes compared to placebo.
- The authors concluded that in a randomized trial involving patients with chronic coronary disease, the risk of CV events was significantly lower among those who received colchicine 0.5 mg once daily compared to placebo. (N Engl J Med. 2020 Nov 5;383(19):1838-1847.)

High-Yield Fast-Facts
- Probenecid can be used as a pharmacokinetic enhancer to prolong beta-lactam levels, especially in STDs.
- Colchicine is found in numerous plants. The colchicum autumnale (autumn crocus) was used historically as a poison.
- Benjamin Franklin was a reported user of colchicine for gout treatment and was credited with its introduction to the United States.

HIGH-YIELD BOARD EXAM ESSENTIALS
- **CLASSIC AGENTS:** Colchicine, pegloticase, probenecid, rasburicase
- **DRUG CLASS:** Anti-gout agents
- **INDICATIONS:** Gout (colchicine, pegloticase, probenecid), hyperuricemia associated with malignancy (rasburicase)
- **MECHANISM:** Colchicine inhibits microtubules, leukocyte migration and phagocytosis. Pegloticase and rasburicase convert uric acid to the more water-soluble allantoin. Probenecid inhibits the reabsorption of uric acid to reduce uric acid levels.
- **SIDE EFFECTS:** Diarrhea, myopathy, neuropathy, and myoneuropathy (colchicine), anaphylaxis (pegloticase)
- **CLINICAL PEARLS:**
    - Colchicine is most commonly used for acute gout flares. On rare occasions, colchicine can be used for chronic gout but carries a small risk of bone marrow suppression.
    - Colchicine has been developed as an adjunct post-MI and in chronic CAD.
    - Pegloticase is reserved for severe cases of gout when patients cannot tolerate alternative agents but should be avoided in patients with G6PD deficiency.
    - Rasburicase is indicated for hyperuricemia of malignancy, not gout.

Table: Drug Class Summary

Antigout Agents - Drug Class Review High-Yield Med Reviews			
Mechanism of Action: Colchicine - Inhibits microtubules, leukocyte migration, and phagocytosis. Pegloticase, Rasburicase - Converts uric acid to the more water-soluble allantoin. Probenecid – inhibits reabsorption of uric acid in the proximal convoluted tubule.			
Class Effects: Acute gout treatment, chronic gout treatment limited by adverse effects, potential for toxicity with drug interactions and renal or hepatic impairment, adjunct post-MI			
Generic Name	Brand Name	Main Indication(s) or Uses	Notes
Colchicine	Colcrys, Gloperba, Lodoco, Mitigare	<ul><li>Gout</li><li>Familial Mediterranean fever</li><li>Stable ischemic Heart Disease, Prevention of ACVD</li></ul>	<ul><li>**Dosing (Adult):**<ul><li>Oral: 0.5 - 0.6 mg once or twice daily<ul><li>Maximum 1.2 mg/day</li></ul></li><li>Oral: 1.2 mg at first sign of flare, then 0.6 mg in 1 hour x 1 with 3 dose max for 1 day OR 0.6 mg TID on first day of flare; then 0.6 mg BID until flare resolves<ul><li>Maximum 1.8 mg/day</li></ul></li></ul></li><li>**Dosing (Peds):**<ul><li>Not routinely used</li></ul></li><li>**CYP450 Interactions:** Substrate CYP3A4, P-gp</li><li>**Renal or Hepatic Dose Adjustments:**<ul><li>GFR < 30 mL/minute: consider alternate therapy or 0.3 mg/day</li><li>Hepatic impairment: use with caution</li></ul></li><li>**Dosage Forms:** Oral (capsule, solution, tablet)</li></ul>
Pegloticase	Krystexxa	<ul><li>Gout</li></ul>	<ul><li>**Dosing (Adult):**<ul><li>IV: 8 mg q2weeks</li></ul></li><li>**Dosing (Peds):**<ul><li>Not routinely used</li></ul></li><li>**CYP450 Interactions:** None</li><li>**Renal or Hepatic Dose Adjustments:** None</li><li>**Dosage Forms:** IV (solution)</li></ul>
Probenecid	Benemid, Probalan	<ul><li>Gout</li></ul>	<ul><li>**Dosing (Adult):**<ul><li>Oral: 250 to 500 mg q6-12h<ul><li>Maximum 2,000 mg/day</li></ul></li></ul></li><li>**Dosing (Peds):**<ul><li>Oral: 25 to 40 mg/kg/day divided q6-12h<ul><li>Maximum 500 mg/dose</li></ul></li></ul></li><li>**CYP450 Interactions:** None</li><li>**Renal or Hepatic Dose Adjustments:**<ul><li>GFR < 30 mL/minute: avoid use</li></ul></li><li>**Dosage Forms:** Oral (tablet)</li></ul>

| Antigout Agents - Drug Class Review ||||
High-Yield Med Reviews			
Generic Name	**Brand Name**	**Main Indication(s) or Uses**	**Notes**

Rasburicase	Elitek	- Hyperuricemia associated with malignancy	- **Dosing (Adult):**
			  - IV 0.05 mg to 0.2 mg/kg once daily for up to 7 days
			- **Dosing (Peds):**
			  - IV 0.2 mg/kg/dose once daily for up to 5 days
			- **CYP450 Interactions:** None
			- **Renal or Hepatic Dose Adjustments:** None
			- **Dosage Forms:** IV (solution)

ENDOCRINE – XANTHINE OXIDASE INHIBITORS

Drug Class
- Xanthine Oxidase Inhibitors
- Agents:
    - **Acute Care**
        - Allopurinol
    - **Chronic Care**
        - Allopurinol
        - Febuxostat

Main Indications or Uses
- Acute Care
    - Tumor Lysis Syndrome
- Chronic Care
    - Gout
    - Nephrolithiasis prophylaxis

> **Drug Interaction Pearl**
> ✓ Use extreme caution with the coadministration of allopurinol in a patient already taking azathioprine (mercaptopurine or Imuran) due to the risk of life-threatening bone marrow suppression. In most cases this is contraindicated.

Mechanism of Action
- Inhibit xanthine oxidase to prevent the conversion of hypoxanthine to uric acid.

Primary Net Benefit
- Allopurinol is a first-line treatment for chronic gout but can precipitate gout during the initiation of therapy. Febuxostat also inhibits xanthine oxidase but carries an increased risk of cardiovascular death in some patients.
- Main Labs to Monitor:
    - CBC
    - Liver enzymes (AST/ALT, alk phos)
    - Liver function (INR/PT, albumin, protein, bilirubin)
    - Serum creatinine, BUN
    - Serum urate

> **Pharmacogenetics Tip**
> ✓ In patients with the genetic polymorphism, HLA-B*5801 due to the risk of allopurinol hypersensitivity syndrome.

High-Yield Basic Pharmacology
- Alloxanthine
    - Allopurinol is metabolized to oxypurinol (alloxanthine), which is also active and inhibits xanthine oxidase.
- Purine Analog
    - Allopurinol is a purine analog, whereas febuxostat is a non-purine agent.
- Renal Adjustment
    - Allopurinol dose must be reduced in patients with GFR < 60 mL/minute, which may significantly limit effectiveness.
    - Febuxostat does not typically require renal dose adjustment.

High-Yield Clinical Knowledge
- Allopurinol Vs. Febuxostat
    - Allopurinol inhibits xanthine oxidase and may also inhibit purine nucleoside phosphorylase (PNP) and orotidine-5'-monophosphate decarboxylase (OMPDC).
        - PNP and OMPDC are necessary for the synthesis of pyrimidines required for RNA and DNA synthesis.
    - Febuxostat only inhibits xanthine oxidase.
- Allopurinol Hypersensitivity Syndrome (AHS)
    - AHS is a potentially fatal reaction to allopurinol characterized by reactions ranging from Stevens-Johnson syndrome to toxic epidermal necrolysis, as well as multiorgan injury (liver, renal, bone marrow).
    - The highest risk of AHS occurs within 2 to 4 weeks of starting allopurinol.

- Other risk factors include HLA-B*5801 genotype (prevalent among Han Chinese, Korean, or Thai patients), concomitant diuretic, amoxicillin, or ampicillin use.
    - Allopurinol should immediately be discontinued if a rash occurs during this timeframe.
- **Tumor Lysis Syndrome**
    - Allopurinol is a therapy component for tumor lysis syndrome as its xanthine oxidase inhibition reduces purine conversion to uric acid.
    - As tumors rapidly lyse, large quantities of purines are released, which can precipitate urate nephropathy or calcium-phosphate nephropathy.
    - Alternatively, rasburicase can be used to promote uric acid metabolism to allantoin.
- **Allopurinol Toxicity**
    - Aside from a risk of precipitating gout early in treatment, allopurinol is associated with peripheral neuritis, necrotizing vasculitis, hematologic toxicities (bone marrow suppression, aplastic anemia), hepatotoxicity, renal injury, and skin reactions.
- **Drug Interactions**
    - Allopurinol inhibition of xanthine oxidase can lead to increased azathioprine exposure due to reduced xanthine oxidase activity, which is partially responsible for inactivating 6-mercaptopurine.
        - Allopurinol may also inhibit a secondary metabolic pathway of 6-MP, thiopurine methyltransferase.
    - Without appropriate dose reduction of allopurinol (reduce by 75%), life-threatening bone marrow suppression may occur.
- **Initiating Allopurinol**
    - Allopurinol may precipitate gout flares early in therapy, so prophylaxis may be needed.
    - If initiating allopurinol therapy close to an acute gout flare, either colchicine, NSAIDs, or corticosteroids must be given with allopurinol to avoid acutely worsening gout flare or initiating a new flare.
    - NSAIDs or colchicine should also be started with febuxostat to reduce the risk of gout flares.
- **Cardiovascular Death Risk Boxed Warning**
    - Febuxostat has been associated with an increased risk of CV death among patients with preexisting CVD.
    - Allopurinol does not impact CV death risk.

High-Yield Core Evidence
- **Allopurinol Vs. Febuxostat**
    - This was a multicenter, prospective, randomized trial among patients with gout and serum urate concentrations of at least 8.0 mg/dL.
    - Patients were randomized to either febuxostat 80 mg or 120 mg or allopurinol 300 mg daily for 52 weeks.
    - A significantly higher proportion of subjects randomized to either dose of febuxostat achieved a serum urate concentration of less than 6.0 mg/dL compared to allopurinol.
    - However, there was no difference between groups concerning the overall incidence of acute gout flares or median reduction in tophus area.
    - The authors concluded that febuxostat led to lower serum urate levels than allopurinol but was not different when considering reductions in gout flares and tophus area. (N Engl J Med. 2005;353:2450–2461.)
- **CARES**
    - This was a multicenter, double-blind, noninferiority trial of patients with gout and CVD who were randomized to receive either allopurinol or febuxostat, stratified according to baseline renal function.
    - Both study drugs were discontinued in more than half of the study population, and approximately 45% were lost to follow-up.
    - Allopurinol was non-inferior to febuxostat in the modified ITT analysis with the primary endpoint of a composite of CV death, nonfatal MI, nonfatal stroke, or unstable angina with urgent revascularization.
    - However, all-cause and CV mortality were higher in the febuxostat group than in the allopurinol group.
    - The authors concluded that for patients with gout and major CV coexisting conditions, febuxostat was non-inferior to allopurinol concerning rates of adverse CV events. All-cause mortality and CV mortality were higher with febuxostat than with allopurinol. (N Engl J Med. 2018;310:1200–1210.)

High-Yield Fast-Facts
- **Diet Considerations**
  - A low purine diet may assist in preventing gout flares. Foods high in purine include beer and other alcoholic beverages, red meat or other fatty meats, shellfish and other seafood, organ meats, and foods with high fructose corn syrup.
- **IBS and Crohn's**
  - Allopurinol may be used in patients with IBS or Crohn's disease who do not respond to conventional thiopurine therapy.
- **Hydrochlorothiazide Induced Gout**
  - Patients who develop acute gout flares after starting hydrochlorothiazide should discontinue hydrochlorothiazide rather than allopurinol.

HIGH-YIELD BOARD EXAM ESSENTIALS
- **CLASSIC AGENTS:** Allopurinol, febuxostat
- **DRUG CLASS:** Xanthine oxidase inhibitors
- **INDICATIONS:** Tumor lysis syndrome, gout, nephrolithiasis prophylaxis
- **MECHANISM:** Prevent the conversion of hypoxanthine to uric acid by inhibiting xanthine oxidase.
- **SIDE EFFECTS:** CV death risk (febuxostat), AHS, precipitating gout (allopurinol)
- **CLINICAL PEARLS:**
  - Febuxostat is a "cleaner" xanthine oxidase inhibitor compared to allopurinol thereby causing less side effects.
  - Aside from a risk of precipitating gout early in acute treatment, allopurinol is associated with peripheral neuritis, necrotizing vasculitis, hematologic toxicities (bone marrow suppression, aplastic anemia), hepatotoxicity, renal injury, and skin reactions.
  - Avoid allopurinol in patients with HLA-B*5801 genotype due to risk of hypersensitivity reaction.
  - Both agents should be avoided in almost every scenario with the co-administration of azathioprine or 6-mercaptopurine due to risk of BMS.

Table: Drug Class Summary

Xanthine Oxidase Inhibitors - Drug Class Review High-Yield Med Reviews			
Mechanism of Action: Prevent the conversion of hypoxanthine to uric acid by inhibiting xanthine oxidase.			
Class Effects: First-line treatment for chronic gout, may precipitate gout when initiated, febuxostat may cause fewer adverse effects but increases the risk of CV death, rash should prompt discontinuation			
Generic Name	**Brand Name**	**Indication(s) or Uses**	**Notes**
Allopurinol	Aloprim, Zyloprim	<ul><li>Gout</li><li>Nephrolithiasis prophylaxis</li><li>Tumor Lysis Syndrome</li></ul>	<ul><li>**Dosing (Adult):**<ul><li>Oral: 100-800 mg daily</li><li>Oral (for TLS): 10 mg/kg/day or 300 mg/m2/day divided q8h (max 800 mg/day)</li><li>IV: 200 to 400 mg/m2/day (max 600 mg/day)</li></ul></li><li>**Dosing (Peds):**<ul><li>Oral (for TLS): 10 mg/kg/day or 300 mg/m2/day divided q8h (max 800 mg/day)</li><li>IV: 200-400 mg/m2/day (max 600 mg/day)</li></ul></li><li>**CYP450 Interactions:** None</li><li>**Renal or Hepatic Dose Adjustments:**<ul><li>GFR 30-60 mL/minute: 50 mg daily</li><li>GFR 15-30 ml/minute: 50 mg q48h</li><li>GFR 5-15 mL/minute: 50 mg twice weekly</li><li>GFR < 5 mL/minute: 50 mg weekly</li></ul></li><li>**Dosage Forms:** IV (solution), Oral (tablet)</li></ul>
Febuxostat	Uloric	<ul><li>Gout</li></ul>	<ul><li>**Dosing (Adult):**<ul><li>Oral: 40-120 mg daily</li></ul></li><li>**Dosing (Peds):**<ul><li>Not routinely used</li></ul></li><li>**CYP450 Interactions:** Substrate CYP1A2, 2C8, 2C9</li><li>**Renal or Hepatic Dose Adjustments:**<ul><li>GFR < 30 mL/minute: 40 mg/day</li></ul></li><li>**Dosage Forms:** Oral (tablet)</li></ul>

ENDOCRINE – LONG-ACTING CORTICOSTEROIDS

Drug Class
- Long-Acting Corticosteroids (Glucocorticoids)
- Agents:
    - Acute & Chronic Care
        - Betamethasone
        - Deflazacort
        - Dexamethasone
        - Fludrocortisone

Main Indications or Uses
- Acute & Chronic Care
    - Antenatal fetal maturation
    - Acne vulgaris
    - Acute hypersensitivity/allergy
    - Asthma
    - Atopic dermatitis
    - Bronchiolitis
    - Cancer (hematologic malignancies, prostate cancer)
    - Cluster headache
    - COPD
    - Croup (dexamethasone)
    - Gout and hyperuricemia
    - Immunosuppression after solid organ transplant
    - Meningitis
    - Nausea and vomiting
    - Osteoarthritis
    - Systemic lupus erythematosus
    - Tuberculosis

> **Fast Facts**
> - Of the long-acting corticosteroids, betamethasone and dexamethasone have the least amount of mineralocorticoid activity whereas fludrocortisone has the most.
> - Dexamethasone is the preferred steroid from this group listed for bacterial meningitis and croup.
> - Approximately 0.75 mg of dexamethasone is equivalent to 5 mg of prednisone.

Mechanism of Action
- Corticosteroids possess numerous mechanisms of action, including regulation of gene expression, modulation of carbohydrate, fat, and protein metabolism, and fluid and electrolyte homeostasis.

Primary Net Benefit
- Glucocorticoids have a wide range of therapeutic uses that require specific dosing targeting the desired physiological effects these agents can wield, including regulation of intermediary metabolism, cardiovascular function, growth, and Immunity.
- Main Labs to Monitor:
    - Complete metabolic panel
    - Blood pressure
    - Weight
    - Growth (in pediatrics)
    - Bone mineral density
    - ACTH stimulation test

High-Yield Basic Pharmacology
- Mineralocorticoid Vs Glucocorticoid
    - Corticosteroids are mineralocorticoids or glucocorticoids, depending on their relative potency, sodium and water retention, and carbohydrate metabolism.
    - The anti-inflammatory of a given steroid mirrors its impact on glucose metabolism.

High-Yield Clinical Knowledge
- **Withdrawal**
  - Abrupt discontinuation of corticosteroid therapy can cause acute withdrawal syndrome and an acute worsening of the underlying disease for which corticosteroids were indicated.
  - Acute adrenal insufficiency is a complication of acute corticosteroid withdrawal due to the suppression of the hypothalamic-pituitary-adrenal (HPA) axis suppression.
  - A gradual decrease in dose over days to weeks reduces the risk of withdrawal syndromes for discontinuation of corticosteroids.
- **Taper**
  - Typically, courses of 5-7 days or less do not require tapering.
  - Individualized patient evaluation of the exact dose reduction and schedule depends mainly on the duration of steroid therapy and the steroid dose.
  - However, despite tapering, the recovery of the HPA axis may require several months, and underlying minor but potentially clinically relevant HPA axis suppression may be present for as long as several months after a course of as few as 10-14 days.
- **Equivalent**
  - Dosing of glucocorticoids is often expressed in prednisone dosing, where clinical guidance can select an alternative agent, using a dose conversion to deliver the same glucocorticoid effect.
  - Prednisone 5 mg is equivalent to:
    - Betamethasone 0.6 mg
    - Cortisone 25 mg
    - Dexamethasone 0.75 mg
    - Fludrocortisone 2 mg
    - Hydrocortisone 20 mg
    - Methylprednisolone 4 mg
    - Prednisolone 5mg
    - Triamcinolone 4 mg
- **Lung Maturation**
  - Betamethasone is administered to mothers where delivery is anticipated before 34 weeks gestation and is used to promote lung maturation by stimulating the fetal cortisol secretion.
  - As a result of lower proportional maternal protein binding and decreased placental metabolism compared to other steroids, betamethasone is the preferred agent.
- **Croup**
  - Dexamethasone is administered as a single dose therapy for croup treatment, an acute upper airway infection causing inflammation and characteristic barking cough.
  - A single dose of 0.15 to 0.6 mg/kg of dexamethasone is appropriate. The parenteral dosage form is often administered orally as tablets are difficult to swallow due to the characteristic upper airway swelling croup.
- **Mineralocorticoid**
  - Although it possesses glucocorticoid properties, fludrocortisone is used primarily for its mineralocorticoid effects.
  - Fludrocortisone is primarily used to manage primary adrenal insufficiency and congenital adrenal hyperplasia.

High-Yield Core Evidence
- **Antenatal Glucocorticoids**
  - This was a systematic review of randomized trials to assess the effectiveness and safety of one or more repeat doses of antenatal glucocorticoids for women at risk of preterm birth seven or more days after an initial course.
  - Patients receiving treatment with repeat doses compared with no-repeat treatment reduced the risk of respiratory distress syndrome and serious neonatal morbidity.
  - There was no evidence of significant benefit or harm after at least two and three-year follow-ups.

- The authors concluded that repeat doses of glucocorticoids should be considered in women at risk of preterm birth seven or more days after an initial course because of the neonatal benefits. (Am J Obstet Gynecol, 2012, 206:187–194.)
- **Dexamethasone in Hospitalized COVID**
    - This was a multicenter, open-label trial comparing a range of possible treatments in hospitalized patients with Covid-19.
    - Patients were randomized to receive oral or dexamethasone 6 mg IV daily for up to 10 days or receive usual care alone.
    - Dexamethasone was associated with a significantly lower 28-day mortality rate compared to placebo.
    - The benefit of dexamethasone on mortality was observed among patients receiving oxygen without invasive mechanical ventilation but not among those receiving no respiratory support at randomization.
    - The authors concluded that dexamethasone's use for patients hospitalized with COVID-19 resulted in lower 28-day mortality among those receiving invasive mechanical ventilation or oxygen alone at randomization but not among those receiving no respiratory support. (N Engl J Med. 2021 Feb 25;384(8):693-704.)

High-Yield Fast-Fact
- **Deflazacort Cost**
    - Deflazacort is a recently approved steroid for use in treating Duchenne muscular dystrophy that may cost up to $90,000 per year. Still, it is available from other countries (including Canada) for roughly $1 per day.

HIGH-YIELD BOARD EXAM ESSENTIALS
- **CLASSIC AGENTS:** Betamethasone, deflazacort, dexamethasone, fludrocortisone
- **DRUG CLASS:** Long-acting corticosteroids (glucocorticoids)
- **INDICATIONS:** Antenatal fetal maturation, acne vulgaris, acute hypersensitivity/allergy, asthma, atopic dermatitis. bronchiolitis, cancer (hematologic malignancies, prostate cancer), cluster headache, COPD, gout and hyperuricemia, immunosuppression after solid organ transplant, meningitis, nausea and vomiting, osteoarthritis, systemic lupus erythematosus, tuberculosis
- **MECHANISM:** Corticosteroids possess numerous mechanisms of action, including regulation of gene expression, modulation of carbohydrate, fat, and protein metabolism, fluid and electrolyte homeostasis.
- **SIDE EFFECTS:** Electrolyte abnormalities, volume overload, hyperglycemia
- **CLINICAL PEARLS:** Although it possesses glucocorticoid properties, fludrocortisone is used primarily for its mineralocorticoid effects. Fludrocortisone is primarily used in the management of primary adrenal insufficiency and congenital adrenal hyperplasia.

Table: Drug Class Summary

\multicolumn{4}{c}{**Long-Acting Corticosteroids - Drug Class Review**}
\multicolumn{4}{c}{High-Yield Med Reviews}

\multicolumn{4}{l}{**Mechanism of Action:** *Corticosteroids possess numerous mechanisms of action, including regulation of gene expression, modulation of carbohydrate, fat, and protein metabolism, and fluid and electrolyte homeostasis.*}
\multicolumn{4}{l}{**Class Effects:** *Reductions in inflammation, accumulation of fluid/edema, elevated glucose, CNS stimulation, decreased bone mineral density with chronic use, and increases in gastric acid production.*}

Generic Name	Brand Name	Main Indication(s) or Uses	Notes
Betamethasone	BSP 0820, Celestone Soluspan, Pod-Care, ReadySharp	<ul><li>Antenatal fetal maturation</li><li>Bursitis</li><li>Dermatologic conditions</li><li>Foot disorders</li><li>Multiple sclerosis</li><li>Rheumatoid and osteoarthritis</li><li>Tenosynovitis</li></ul>	<ul><li>**Dosing (Adult):** — IM: 0.25 to 12 mg/day — Intra-articular: 3 to 12 mg once</li><li>**Dosing (Peds):** — IM: 0.02 to 0.3 mg/kg/day</li><li>**CYP450 Interactions:** Substrate of CYP3A4</li><li>**Renal or Hepatic Dose Adjustments:** None</li><li>**Dosage Forms:** Injection suspension</li></ul>
Deflazacort	Emflaza	<ul><li>Duchenne muscular dystrophy</li></ul>	<ul><li>**Dosing (Adult):** — Oral: 0.9 mg/kg once daily</li><li>**Dosing (Peds):** — Oral: 0.9 mg/kg once daily</li><li>**CYP450 Interactions:** Substrate of CYP3A4</li><li>**Renal or Hepatic Dose Adjustments:** None</li><li>**Dosage Forms:** Oral (suspension, tablet)</li></ul>
Dexamethasone	Decadron	<ul><li>Allergic states</li><li>Dermatologic diseases</li><li>Endocrine disorders</li><li>GI diseases</li><li>Hematologic disorders</li><li>Neoplastic diseases</li><li>Ophthalmic diseases</li><li>Renal diseases</li><li>Respiratory diseases</li><li>Rheumatic disorders</li></ul>	<ul><li>**Dosing (Adult):** — Oral/IV/IM: 4 to 20 mg/day divided q6-24h</li><li>**Dosing (Peds):** — Oral/IV/IM: 0.02 to 0.3 mg/kg/day divided q6-24h</li><li>**CYP450 Interactions:** Substrate of CYP3A4</li><li>**Renal or Hepatic Dose Adjustments:** None</li><li>**Dosage Forms:** Oral (concentrate, elixir, solution, tablet), IV (solution)</li></ul>
Fludrocortisone	Florinef	<ul><li>Addison disease (primary adrenal insufficiency)</li><li>Congenital adrenal hyperplasia</li></ul>	**Dosing (Adult):** — Oral: 0.05 to 0.1 mg daily **Dosing (Peds):** — Oral: 0.05 to 0.2 mg daily — Maximum 0.3 mg/day **CYP450 Interactions:** Substrate of CYP3A4 **Renal or Hepatic Dose Adjustments:** None **Dosage Forms:** Oral (tablet)

ENDOCRINE – SHORT TO MEDIUM ACTING CORTICOSTEROIDS

Drug Class
- Short To Medium Acting Glucocorticoids
- Agents:
    - Acute & Chronic Care
        - Cortisone
        - Hydrocortisone
        - Methylprednisolone
        - Prednisone
        - Prednisolone

> **Fast Facts**
> - Of the shorter acting corticosteroids listed, methylprednisolone has less mineralocorticoid effect compared to the other agents.
> - Most adults produce the equivalent of 5-7.5 mg of prednisone per day. Therefore, when the daily dose exceeds this the risk for HPA suppression can occur.

Main Indications or Uses
- Acute & Chronic Care
    - Acne vulgaris
    - Acute hypersensitivity/allergy
    - Asthma
    - Atopic dermatitis
    - Bronchiolitis
    - Cancer (hematologic malignancies, prostate cancer)
    - Cluster headache
    - COPD
    - Gout and hyperuricemia
    - Immunosuppression after solid organ transplant
    - Meningitis
    - Nausea and vomiting
    - Osteoarthritis
    - Systemic lupus erythematosus
    - Tuberculosis

Mechanism of Action
- Corticosteroids possess numerous mechanisms of action, including regulation of gene expression, modulation of carbohydrate, fat, and protein metabolism, and fluid and electrolyte homeostasis.

Primary Net Benefit
- Glucocorticoids have a wide range of therapeutic uses that require specific dosing targeting the desired physiological effects these agents can wield, including regulation of intermediary metabolism, cardiovascular function, growth, and immunity.
- Main Labs to Monitor:
    - Complete metabolic panel
    - Blood pressure
    - Weight
    - Growth (in pediatrics)
    - Bone mineral density
    - ACTH stimulation test

High-Yield Basic Pharmacology
- **Mineralocorticoid Vs Glucocorticoid**
    - Corticosteroids are mineralocorticoids or glucocorticoids, depending on their relative potencies at sodium and water retention and carbohydrate metabolism.
    - The anti-inflammatory of a given steroid mirrors its impact on glucose metabolism.

High-Yield Core Knowledge

- **Withdrawal**
    - Abrupt discontinuation of corticosteroid therapy can cause acute withdrawal syndrome and an acute worsening of the underlying disease for which corticosteroids were indicated.
    - Acute adrenal insufficiency is a complication of acute corticosteroid withdrawal due to the suppression of the hypothalamic-pituitary-adrenal (HPA) axis suppression.
    - For discontinuation of corticosteroids, a gradual decrease in dose over days to weeks reduces the risk of withdrawal syndromes.
- **Taper**
    - Typically, courses of 5-7 days or less do not require tapering.
    - Individualized patient evaluation of the exact dose reduction and schedule depends mainly on the duration of steroid therapy and the steroid dose.
    - However, despite tapering, the recovery of the HPA axis may require several months, and underlying minor but potentially clinically relevant HPA axis suppression may be present for as long as several months after a course of as few as 10-14 days.
- **Equivalent**
    - Dosing of glucocorticoids is often expressed in prednisone dosing, where clinical guidance can select an alternative agent, using a dose conversion to deliver the same glucocorticoid effect.
    - Prednisone 5 mg is equivalent to:
        - Betamethasone 0.6 mg
        - Cortisone 25 mg
        - Dexamethasone 0.75 mg
        - Fludrocortisone 2 mg
        - Hydrocortisone 20 mg
        - Methylprednisolone 4 mg
        - Prednisolone 5mg
        - Triamcinolone 4 mg
- **Inflammation**
    - Glucocorticoids effectively counteract inflammation caused by a wide range of clinical scenarios by preventing extravasation and infiltration of leukocytes into the affected tissue.
    - Suppress polymorphonuclear leukocyte migration, and decrease capillary permeability, thereby reducing inflammation.
    - Inflammation is also inhibited through phospholipase A2 inhibition, reducing the synthesis of arachidonic acid and reducing the release of cyclooxygenase 2 and inducible nitric oxide synthase.
    - The long-term suppression of prostaglandin synthesis may also impact GI epithelial function, leading to peptic ulcers.
- **Immunosuppression**
    - The immunosuppressive effects of glucocorticoids are similar in mechanism to the anti-inflammatory effects.
    - Although there may be increases in the circulating number of neutrophils due to increased influx from the bone and decreased migration from blood vessels, there is ultimately a reduced number at the active sites.
        - Increases in white blood cell counts are approximately 4,000/mm3 and can exceed levels of 20,000/mm3 in some patients.
        - The demargination of neutrophils from the endovascular lining has primarily attributed to this increase and delayed migration of polymorphonuclear leukocytes.
    - Other antigen-presenting cells are also inhibited, including dendritic cells and macrophages, which cannot kill microorganisms and produce TNF-alfa, IL-1, IL-12, interferon-gamma, T-helper cells metalloproteinases, and plasminogen activator.

- **Glucose**
  - The effect of glucocorticoids on glucose homeostasis is clinically significant and varied.
  - Glucocorticoids increase glucose levels by stimulating hepatic gluconeogenesis and glycogen synthesis and storage and inhibit the uptake of glucose by muscle cells despite insulin release and increase the synthesis of glutamine and increase lipolysis.
    - This insulin release also stimulates lipogenesis, inhibits lipolysis, increases fat deposition, and releases fatty acids and glycerol.
- **Lipid Metabolism**
  - Chronic glucocorticoids may cause a redistribution of adipose tissue manifesting as decreased fat in the extremities but increased fat deposition on the back of the neck and around the face, causing the characteristic buffalo hump, or moon face, respectively.
- **Renal**
  - Sodium and water retention are characteristic effects of mineralocorticoids due to their actions on the renal distal tubules and collecting ducts.
  - Mineralocorticoids also increase the urinary excretion of both hydrogen and potassium.
  - Glucocorticoids cause excess free water retention due to increased secretion of arginine vasopressin (antidiuretic hormone), causing the kidney to reabsorb water.
- **Cardiovascular**
  - Mineralocorticoid-induced primary aldosteronism causing decreased sodium elimination may cause hypertension, but other mineralocorticoid effects include interstitial cardiac fibrosis and enhanced vascular response to vasoactive substances.
- **Anabolic and Catabolic Effects**
  - Glucocorticoids cause an anabolic and catabolic effect in connective tissue, skin, fat, and muscle.
  - As a result, clinical sequelae associated with high-dose glucocorticoids include decreased muscle mass, weakness, thinning of the skin, osteoporosis, and reduced growth in children.
- **CNS/Psychiatric**
  - Glucocorticoids may impair sleep quality, causing insomnia and other behavioral disturbances or psychosis.
  - These agents also produce Cushing's syndrome, dose-dependent suppression of ACTH, growth hormone, thyroid-stimulating hormone, and luteinizing hormone.
- **Bone and Skeletal Muscle**
  - Hypokalemia due to mineralocorticoids may cause a depressive effect on skeletal muscle function.
  - Steroid myopathy is an effect of chronic glucocorticoid excess leading to muscle weakness and muscle wasting.
  - Acute vascular necrosis is associated with high-dose glucocorticoid therapy, generally with therapies exceeding prednisone 20 mg per day for extended periods.
    - Risk factors for acute vascular necrosis include patients with underlying systemic lupus erythematosus, renal transplant, and disproportionately occurring post total hip arthroplasties.

High-Yield Core Evidence
- **Steroids Adjunct and CAP**
  - This was a double-blind, multicentre, placebo-controlled trial that randomized adult patients with community-acquired pneumonia within 24 hours of presentation to receive prednisone 50 mg daily for seven days or a placebo.
  - Patients randomized to receive placebo were significantly more likely to achieve the primary outcome of the time to clinical stability, defined as the time (days) until stable vital signs for at least 24 hours and analyzed by intention to treat.
  - Although there was no difference in pneumonia-associated complications until day 30, prednisone was associated with a higher incidence of in-hospital hyperglycemia needing insulin treatment.
  - The authors concluded that prednisone treatment for seven days in patients with community-acquired pneumonia admitted to the hospital shortens the time to clinical stability without increasing complications. This finding is relevant from a patient perspective and an important determinant of hospital costs and efficiency. (Lancet. 2015. 385(9977):1511-1518.)

- **CORTICUS**
  - This landmark multicenter, double-blind, placebo-controlled trial randomized patients with septic shock who remained hypotensive after fluid and vasopressor resuscitation to receive either hydrocortisone 50 mg IV q6h for five days or placebo.
  - There was no significant difference concerning the primary outcome of 28-day mortality among patients who did not have a response to a corticotropin test.
  - However, in patients receiving hydrocortisone, the shock was reversed more quickly than in the placebo group, but this was offset by more episodes of superinfection, including new sepsis and septic shock because of hydrocortisone.
  - The authors concluded that hydrocortisone did not improve survival or reversal of shock in patients with septic shock, either overall or in patients who did not respond to corticotropin. However, hydrocortisone hastened the reversal of shock in patients in whom shock was reversed. (N Engl J Med. 2008 Jan 10;358(2):111-24.)

High-Yield Fast-Fact
- **Glycyrrhizic Acid**
  - The inhibition of 11-beta-hydroxylase may be caused by glycyrrhizic acid, a component of licorice.

HIGH-YIELD BOARD EXAM ESSENTIALS
- **CLASSIC AGENTS:** Cortisone, hydrocortisone, methylprednisolone, prednisone, prednisolone
- **DRUG CLASS:** Short to medium acting glucocorticoids
- **INDICATIONS:** Acne vulgaris, acute hypersensitivity/allergy, asthma, atopic dermatitis. bronchiolitis, cancer (hematologic malignancies, prostate cancer), cluster headache, COPD, gout and hyperuricemia, immunosuppression after solid organ transplant, meningitis, nausea and vomiting, osteoarthritis, systemic lupus erythematosus, tuberculosis
- **MECHANISM:** Corticosteroids possess numerous mechanisms of action, including regulation of gene expression, modulation of carbohydrate, fat, and protein metabolism, fluid and electrolyte homeostasis.
- **SIDE EFFECTS:** Electrolyte abnormalities, volume overload, hyperglycemia, avascular necrosis of hip (rare, more common with high doses)
- **CLINICAL PEARLS:** The effect of glucocorticoids on glucose homeostasis is clinically significant and varied. Glucocorticoids are known to increase glucose levels by stimulating hepatic gluconeogenesis and glycogen synthesis and storage and inhibit the uptake of glucose by muscle cells despite insulin release and increase the synthesis of glutamine and increase lipolysis.

Table: Drug Class Summary

	Short To Medium Acting Glucocorticoids - Drug Class Review High-Yield Med Reviews		
Mechanism of Action: *Corticosteroids possess numerous mechanisms of action, including regulation of gene expression, modulation of carbohydrate, fat, and protein metabolism, and fluid and electrolyte homeostasis.*			
Class Effects: *Glucocorticoids have a wide range of therapeutic uses that require specific dosing targeting the desired physiological effects these agents can wield, including regulation of intermediary metabolism, cardiovascular function, growth, and immunity.*			
Generic Name	**Brand Name**	**Main Indication(s) or Uses**	**Notes**
Cortisone	Brand Name (if available)	<ul><li>Allergic states</li><li>Dermatologic diseases</li><li>Endocrine disorders</li><li>GI diseases</li><li>Hematologic disorders</li><li>Neoplastic diseases</li><li>Ophthalmic diseases</li><li>Renal diseases</li><li>Respiratory diseases</li><li>Rheumatic disorders</li></ul>	<ul><li>**Dosing (Adult):**<ul><li>Oral: 25 to 300 mg/day</li></ul></li><li>**Dosing (Peds):**<ul><li>Oral: 0.7 to 10 mg/kg/day<ul><li>Usual range 25 to 300 mg/day</li></ul></li></ul></li><li>**CYP450 Interactions:** Substrate CYP3A4</li><li>**Renal or Hepatic Dose Adjustments:** None</li><li>**Dosage Forms:** Oral (tablet)</li></ul>
Hydrocortisone	Solu-Cortef	<ul><li>Allergic states</li><li>Dermatologic diseases</li><li>Endocrine disorders</li><li>GI diseases</li><li>Hematologic disorders</li><li>Neoplastic diseases</li><li>Ophthalmic diseases</li><li>Renal diseases</li><li>Respiratory diseases</li><li>Rheumatic disorders</li></ul>	<ul><li>**Dosing (Adult):**<ul><li>IV: 50 to 100 mg q6-8h</li><li>Oral: 10 to 240 mg/day divided q8-12h</li><li>IM/SQ: 100 to 500 mg q6-12h</li></ul></li><li>**Dosing (Peds):**<ul><li>IV: 50 to 100 mg/m2/day q6-8h</li><li>Oral: 2.5 to 10 mg/kg/day divided q6-8h</li><li>IM/SQ: 20 to 240 mg/m2/day q6-8h</li></ul></li><li>**CYP450 Interactions:** Substrate CYP3A4, P-gp</li><li>**Renal or Hepatic Dose Adjustments:** None</li><li>**Dosage Forms:** Oral (capsule, tablet), IV solution</li></ul>
Methylprednisolone	Solu-Medrol	<ul><li>Allergic states</li><li>Dermatologic diseases</li><li>Endocrine disorders</li><li>GI diseases</li><li>Hematologic disorders</li><li>Neoplastic diseases</li><li>Ophthalmic diseases</li><li>Renal diseases</li><li>Respiratory diseases</li><li>Rheumatic disorders</li></ul>	<ul><li>**Dosing (Adult):**<ul><li>IV: 1 to 2 mg/kg/day</li><li>Oral: 16 to 64 mg/day</li><li>IM: 40 to 60 mg/dose</li><li>Intra-articular 10 to 80 mg</li></ul></li><li>**Dosing (Peds):**<ul><li>IV/Oral: 1 to 2 mg/kg/day<ul><li>Maximum 60 mg/day</li></ul></li><li>IM: 7.5 mg/kg/day<ul><li>Maximum 240 mg/day</li></ul></li></ul></li><li>**CYP450 Interactions:** Substrate CYP3A4</li><li>**Renal or Hepatic Dose Adjustments:** None</li><li>**Dosage Forms:** Oral (tablet), Injection (solution, suspension)</li></ul>

Short To Medium Acting Glucocorticoids - Drug Class Review High-Yield Med Reviews				
Generic Name	**Brand Name**	**Main Indication(s) or Uses**	**Notes**
Prednisone	Brand Name (if available)	<ul><li>Allergic states</li><li>Dermatologic diseases</li><li>Endocrine disorders</li><li>GI diseases</li><li>Hematologic disorders</li><li>Neoplastic diseases</li><li>Ophthalmic diseases</li><li>Renal diseases</li><li>Respiratory diseases</li><li>Rheumatic disorders</li></ul>	<ul><li>**Dosing (Adult):**<ul><li>Oral: 2.5 to 80 mg/day once or divided q6-12h</li></ul></li><li>**Dosing (Peds):**<ul><li>Oral: 0.25 to 2 mg/kg/day divided 1 to 2 times daily<ul><li>Maximum 60 mg/day</li></ul></li></ul></li><li>**CYP450 Interactions:** Substrate CYP3A4</li><li>**Renal or Hepatic Dose Adjustments:** None</li><li>**Dosage Forms:** Oral (concentrate, solution, tablet)</li></ul>
Prednisolone	Omnipred, Pred Forte, Pred Mild	<ul><li>Allergic states</li><li>Dermatologic diseases</li><li>Endocrine disorders</li><li>GI diseases</li><li>Hematologic disorders</li><li>Neoplastic diseases</li><li>Ophthalmic diseases</li><li>Renal diseases</li><li>Respiratory diseases</li><li>Rheumatic disorders</li></ul>	<ul><li>**Dosing (Adult):**<ul><li>Oral: 5 to 60 mg/day</li><li>Ophthalmic: Instill 1 to 2 drops to affected eye(s) 2 to 4 times daily</li></ul></li><li>**Dosing (Peds):**<ul><li>Oral: 0.25 to 2 mg/kg/day divided 1 to 2 times daily<ul><li>Maximum 60 mg/day</li></ul></li><li>Ophthalmic: Instill 1 to 2 drops to affected eye(s) 2 to 4 times daily</li></ul></li><li>**CYP450 Interactions:** Substrate CYP3A4</li><li>**Renal or Hepatic Dose Adjustments:** None</li><li>**Dosage Forms:** Oral (solution, syrup, tablet), Ophthalmic ointment</li></ul>
Triamcinolone	Kenalog	<ul><li>Allergic states</li><li>Dermatologic diseases</li><li>Endocrine disorders</li><li>GI diseases</li><li>Hematologic disorders</li><li>Neoplastic diseases</li><li>Ophthalmic diseases</li><li>Renal diseases</li><li>Respiratory diseases</li><li>Rheumatic disorders</li></ul>	<ul><li>**Dosing (Adult):**<ul><li>IM: 40 to 160 mg once</li><li>Intra-articular: 2.5 to 80 mg once</li><li>Intravitreal: 1 to 4 mg once</li></ul></li><li>**Dosing (Peds):**<ul><li>Intra-articular: 0.5 to 2 mg/kg/dose</li></ul></li><li>**CYP450 Interactions:** Substrate CYP3A4</li><li>**Renal or Hepatic Dose Adjustments:** None</li><li>**Dosage Forms:** Injection suspension</li></ul>

ENDOCRINE – CORTICOSTEROID CHART

Drug	Equivalent Potency (mg)	Na+/Water Retaining Potency	Plasma Half-life (min)	Biological Half-life (hr); effect of drug
Long Acting				
Dexamethasone	0.75	0	110-210	≥ 36
Budesonide	0.6	0	200+	≥ 20-35
Betamethasone	0.6	0	300+	≥ 35
Short Acting				
Cortisone	25	2+	30	≥ 8
Hydrocortisone	20	2+	80-118	≥ 8
Prednisone	5	1+	60	≥ 18
Prednisolone	5	1+	115-212	≥ 18
Methylprednisolone	4	0.5+	78-188	≥ 18
Triamcinolone	4	0	200	≥ 12

ENDOCRINE – GLUCAGON

Drug Class
- Glucagon
- Agents: glucagon

Main Indications or Uses
- Acute
  - Acute beta-blocker or calcium channel blocker toxicity
  - Hypoglycemia

Mechanism of Action
- Increases hepatic glycogenolysis and gluconeogenesis, causing an increase in blood glucose.

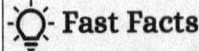

Fast Facts
✓ Glucagon is preferred in the treatment of symptomatic hypoglycemia when patients cannot take anything by mouth due to altered mental status and when IV administration of dextrose is not feasible because it can be given IM or intranasally.

Primary Net Benefit
- Glucagon may rapidly increase blood glucose in patients who cannot take oral glucose or in patients whose IV access has not been established.
- Main Labs to Monitor:
  - Blood glucose

High-Yield Basic Pharmacology
- **Recombinant Glucagon**
  - The pharmacologic glucagon product is a recombinant form of the single-chain 29 amino acid polypeptide.
- **Hepatic Glycogen**
  - The effect of glucagon on increasing blood glucose requires sufficient existing hepatic glycogen stores.
- **Hepatocyte Action**
  - Glucagon increases intracellular cAMP via the Gs-cAMP-PKA pathway and binds to a specific glucagon binding site (GTP-Gs).

High-Yield Clinical Knowledge
- **Glucagon Rescue**
  - Glucagon should be prescribed to all patients who take insulin, have a history of severe hypoglycemia, or are at a high risk of hypoglycemia.
  - Additionally, the family members or caretakers should be educated on the preparation and administration of glucagon since the patient will unlikely be able to self-administer the dose.
- **Onset**
  - The increasing glucose effect of glucagon is delayed and may take up to 15 minutes.
  - This is a result of the action of glucagon in mobilizing hepatic glucose stores.
- **Nausea and Vomiting**
  - Glucagon is associated with a dose-dependent effect of nausea and vomiting due to reduced GI motility.
  - Patients, caretakers, and family members should be educated to position the patient on their side with the head tilted downwards to avoid aspiration should vomiting occur.
- **Glucagon Uses**
  - Glucagon has a wide range of acute uses, including hypoglycemia, anaphylaxis refractory to epinephrine, TCA overdose refractory to sodium bicarbonate, and BB overdose.
  - In BB toxicity, glucagon can improve both chronotropy, inotropy, and coronary blood flow.
  - The initial dose of 50 mcg/kg (3-5 mg) is recommended via slow IV push over 10 minutes.
    - Lower doses can paradoxically worsen bradycardia and hypotension.
    - The slow administration is essential to avoid dose and rate-dependent nausea and vomiting, which may compromise the patient's airway leading to aspiration and requiring advanced airway support.
  - Continuous infusion of 2-5 mg/hr is used if a positive clinical response is observed.

- Tachyphylaxis can occur; increasing the infusion rate may be necessary.
- Administration: Slow IV administration over 10 minutes
- **Preferred Route**
    - Although glucagon may be administered via IV, SQ, or IM injection, the IM route is preferred for hypoglycemic patients as the onset of effect is similar but associated with a lower risk of nausea and vomiting.

High-Yield Core Evidence
- **Nasal Glucagon**
    - This was a multicenter, open-label, prospective, phase III study that randomized adults with type 1 diabetes to receive nasal glucagon to treat moderate/severe hypoglycemic events.
    - Both patients and caregivers were educated on the administration technique for nasal glucagon and instructed to record the time taken to awaken or return to normal status and measure blood glucose levels over time.
    - Among patients who experienced a hypoglycemic event, hypoglycemia resolved within 30 minutes of nasal glucagon administration.
    - Concerning the 12 severe hypoglycemic events, patients awakened or returned to normal status within 15 minutes of nasal glucagon administration without additional external medical help.
    - Most caregivers reported that nasal glucagon was easy to use.
    - The authors concluded that a single 3 mg dose of nasal glucagon demonstrated real-life effectiveness in treating moderate and severe hypoglycemic events in adults with type 1 diabetes. (Diabetes Obes Metab. 2018 May;20(5):1316-1320.)

High-Yield Fast-Fact
- Patients with inadequate glycogen stores may include those experiencing starvation, adrenal insufficiency, or chronic hypoglycemia. Give these patients glucose.
- **Hypoglycemia Classification**
    - Hypoglycemia is classified into levels:
        - Level 1: glucose 54-70 mg/dL
        - Level 2: glucose < 54 mg/dL
        - Level 3: severe event causing altered mental and/or physical status that requires assistance

HIGH-YIELD BOARD EXAM ESSENTIALS
- **CLASSIC AGENTS:** Glucagon
- **DRUG CLASS:** Glucagon
- **INDICATIONS:** Hypoglycemia, acute beta-blocker or calcium channel blocker toxicity, anaphylaxis
- **MECHANISM:** Increases hepatic glycogenolysis and gluconeogenesis causing an increase in blood glucose.
- **SIDE EFFECTS:** Nausea and vomiting (dose-dependent)
- **CLINICAL PEARLS:** Although glucagon may be administered via IV, SQ, or IM injection, the IM route is preferred for hypoglycemic patients as the onset of effect is similar but associated with a lower risk of nausea and vomiting.

Table: Drug Class Summary

Glucagon - Drug Class Review			
High-Yield Med Reviews			
Mechanism of Action: *Increases hepatic glycogenolysis and gluconeogenesis causing an increase in blood glucose.*			
Class Effects: *Increase glucose, dose-dependent nausea/vomiting*			
Generic Name	**Brand Name**	**Indication(s) or Uses**	**Notes**
Glucagon	Baqsimi, GlucaGen, Gvoke	<ul><li>Anaphylaxis</li><li>BB or CCB overdose</li><li>Hypoglycemia</li></ul>	<ul><li>Dosing (Adult):<ul><li>IV: Initial dose of 50 mcg/kg (3-10 mg)<ul><li>Continuous infusion of 3-5 mg/hr if positive clinical response.</li></ul></li><li>IM/SQ: 1 mg once, may repeat in 15 minutes.</li><li>Intranasal: 3 mg once, may repeat in 15 minutes.</li></ul></li><li>Dosing (Peds):<ul><li>IV: Initial dose of 50 mcg/kg (3-5 mg)<ul><li>Continuous infusion of 0.05 to 0.1 mg/kg/hr if positive clinical response.</li></ul></li><li>IM/SQ: 0.5 mg once, may repeat in 15 minutes.</li><li>Intranasal (≥ 4 years): 3 mg in single nostril once, then repeat in 15 min if no response</li></ul></li><li>CYP450 Interactions: None</li><li>Renal or Hepatic Dose Adjustments: None</li><li>Dosage Forms: IV (solution), Nasal powder</li></ul>

ENDOCRINE – GLUCAGON RECEPTOR AGONIST

Drug Class
- **Glucagon Receptor Agonist**
- **Agents:** dasiglucagon

Main Indications or Uses
- **Acute and Chronic**
    - Hypoglycemia

Mechanism of Action
- Dasiglucagon is a glucagon receptor agonist that causes glycogenolysis and hepatic gluconeogenesis to increase glucose levels. Action requires hepatic glycogen stores.

Primary Net Benefit
- Treats hypoglycemia in a ready-to-use device with slightly faster action.
- Main Labs to Monitor:
    - Blood glucose

High-Yield Basic Pharmacology
- **Pharmacokinetics**
    - Onset of action is approximately 10 minutes, which is overall similar to glucagon IM and SC.
    - Half-life and peak effect are approximately 30 minutes (20 min peak in peds).

High-Yield Clinical Knowledge
- **Adverse Effects**
    - Nausea and vomiting are the most common adverse effects resulting from decreased GI motility from glucagon.
- **Administration**
    - Does not require reconstitution and is ready-to-use.
    - May inject SC into upper arm, lower abdomen, thighs, or buttocks.
    - Lay the patient in the lateral recumbent position to prevent choking with vomiting.
    - Give fast- and long-acting carbohydrates post-treatment.
    - Prefilled syringe: pinch skin and inject at 45-degree angle.
    - Auto-injector: push the device straight down until the needle guard is fully depressed, then hold for a 10-count or until the device window is red.
- **Hypoglycemia Rescue**
    - Patients who take insulin, have a history of severe hypoglycemia, or are at high risk of hypoglycemia should be prescribed a method of glucagon rescue.
    - Additionally, the family members or caretakers should be educated on the preparation and administration since the patient will unlikely be able to self-administer the dose.

High-Yield Core Evidence
- A randomized, double-blind trial in 170 adults with type 1 DM compared dasiglucagon, reconstituted glucagon, or placebo during controlled, insulin-induced hypoglycemia.
- The primary endpoint was time to glucose recovery, which was defined as a $\geq$ 20 mg/dL increase in glucose from baseline without glucose rescue.
    - A significant difference was found in recovery time with dasiglucagon compared to placebo (10 min vs. 40 min, respectively), but there was a similar recovery time with glucagon (12 min).
- Nausea and vomiting were similar between dasiglucagon and glucagon.
- Dasiglucagon provided safe and effective hypoglycemia recovery compared to placebo and was similar to reconstituted glucagon injection.
- Diabetes Care 2021; 44(6):1361-1367.

High-Yield Fast Facts
- Patients with inadequate glycogen stores may include those experiencing starvation, adrenal insufficiency, or chronic hypoglycemia. Give these patients glucose.

HIGH-YIELD BOARD EXAM ESSENTIALS
- **CLASSIC AGENTS:** Dasiglucagon
- **DRUG CLASS:** Glucagon Receptor Agonist
- **INDICATIONS:** Hypoglycemia
- **MECHANISM:** Glucagon receptor agonist that promotes glycogenolysis and hepatic gluconeogenesis to increase glucose
- **SIDE EFFECTS:** Nausea, vomiting
- **CLINICAL PEARLS:** Has similar efficacy and safety to IM and SC glucagon with some possible benefits. Does not require reconstitution.

Table: Drug Class Summary

Glucagon Receptor Agonist - Drug Class Review			
High-Yield Med Reviews			
Mechanism of Action: *Glucagon receptor agonist that promotes glycogenolysis and hepatic gluconeogenesis to increase glucose*			
Class Effects: *Increase glucose; Risk of nausea/vomiting, ready-to-use injection*			
Generic Name	**Brand Name**	**Indication(s) or Uses**	**Notes**

Dasiglucagon	Zegalogue	- Hypoglycemia (Severe)	- **Dosing (Adult):**
			  - 0.6 mg SC, then may repeat in 15 min
			- **Dosing (Peds):**
			  - ≥6 years: same as adults
			- **CYP450 Interactions:** None
			- **Renal or Hepatic Dose Adjustments:** None
			- **Dosage Forms:** Auto-injector, prefilled syringe

ENDOCRINE – INSULIN-LIKE GROWTH FACTOR

Drug Class
- Insulin-Like Growth Factor
- Agents:
  - Chronic Care
    - Mecasermin

Main Indications or Uses
- Chronic Care
  - Primary insulin-like growth factor 1 (IGF-1) deficiency

Mechanism of Action
- A recombinant form of IGF-1, circumventing a lack of growth hormone (GH), stimulated hepatic IGF-1 secretion.

Primary Net Benefit
- Increases growth velocity in children with short stature due to severe primary IGF-1 deficiency.
- Main Labs to Monitor:
  - Pre-prandial glucose
  - IGF-1 level

High-Yield Basic Pharmacology
- Glucose Effects.
  - IGF-1 suppresses hepatic glucose production, promotes peripheral glucose utilization, and inhibits pancreatic insulin secretion.

High-Yield Clinical Knowledge
- Growth Effects
  - Congenital or acquired IGF-1 deficiency causes defects in growth hormone function, causing short stature.
    - Treatment alone with GH may not improve growth.
  - Mecasermin is a recombinant IGF-1, bypassing the role of GH in stimulating IGF-1 release.
    - In addition to improving growth, mecasermin is also associated with adenoidal hypertrophy, lymphoid hypertrophy, and coarsening facial features.
- With Meals
  - Mecasermin must be administered within 20 minutes of a meal or snack.
  - If the patient cannot eat, the dose should be skipped.
  - The next dose should be reduced if hypoglycemia occurs despite adequate food intake.
- Open Epiphyses
  - Mecasermin is contraindicated in patients with close epiphyses.
  - It is also contraindicated in patients with suspected or active cancer and should be stopped if cancer is found.
- Adverse Events
  - Severe adverse reactions associated with mecasermin include intracranial hypertension and anaphylaxis.
- Alternative Indications
  - Mecasermin can also be used in some patients with severe insulin resistance, including muscular dystrophy and HIV-related fat redistribution syndrome.

High-Yield Core Evidence
- Long Term Mecasermin Use
  - This was a long-term open-label, observational trial to examine the safety and efficacy of recombinant IGF-1 (rhIGF-1, mecasermin) 60 and 120 mcg/kg twice daily in children with severe IGF-1 deficiency due to GH insensitivity and were followed from the age of two to up to twelve years.

- rhIGF-1 significantly increased the height velocity, skeletal maturation, and adverse events were measured.
- Height velocities were highest during the first year of treatment and lowered in subsequent years but were maintained above baseline for up to eight years.
- Hypoglycemia was reported in approximately half of the study subjects and observed before and during therapy.
- The authors concluded that treatment with rhIGF-I stimulates linear growth in children with severe IGF-I deficiency due to GH insensitivity. (J Clin Endocrinol Metab. 2007 Mar;92(3):902-10.)

High-Yield Fast-Fact
- Bodybuilding
  - Mecasermin has been used for bodybuilding as a growth agent but is generally avoided due to its hypoglycemic effects.

HIGH-YIELD BOARD EXAM ESSENTIALS
- **CLASSIC AGENTS:** Mecasermin
- **DRUG CLASS:** Insulin-Like Growth Factor
- **INDICATIONS:** Primary insulin-like growth factor 1 (IGF-1) deficiency
- **MECHANISM:** A recombinant form of IGF-1, circumventing a lack of growth hormone (GH), stimulated hepatic IGF-1 secretion.
- **SIDE EFFECTS:** Intracranial hypertension and anaphylaxis.
- **CLINICAL PEARLS:** Mecasermin has been used for bodybuilding as a growth agent but is generally avoided due to its hypoglycemic effects.

Table: Drug Class Summary

Insulin-Like Growth Factor - Drug Class Review				
High-Yield Med Reviews				
Mechanism of Action: *A recombinant form of IGF-1, circumventing a lack of growth hormone (GH), stimulated hepatic IGF-1 secretion.*				
Class Effects: *Increases growth velocity in children with short stature due to severe primary IGF-1 deficiency.*				
Generic Name	**Brand Name**	**Indication(s) or Uses**	**Notes**	

Mecasermin	Increlex	• Primary insulin-like growth factor 1 deficiency	• **Dosing (Adult):**
			  – Not routinely used
			• **Dosing (Peds):**
			  – SQ: 0.04 to 0.08 mg/kg/dose BID, increasing by 0.04 mg/kg/dose q7days to maximum 0.12 mg/kg/dose
			• **CYP450 Interactions:** None
			• **Renal or Hepatic Dose Adjustments:** None
			• **Dosage Forms:** Subcutaneous solution	

ENDOCRINE – NONSTEROIDAL MINERALOCORTICOID RECEPTOR ANTAGONIST

Drug Class
- **Nonsteroidal Mineralocorticoid Receptor Antagonist (NMRA)**
- **Agents:** finerenone

Main Indications or Uses
- **Chronic**
    - CKD in patients with T2DM

Mechanism of Action
- Decreases fibrosis and inflammation by selectively blocking mineralocorticoid receptors in the epithelial (kidney) and nonepithelial (blood vessels, heart) tissues

Primary Net Benefit
- Reduces the progression of CKD and CV events in patients with T2DM
- Main Labs to Monitor:
    - K^+ (baseline, 4 weeks after initiation or dose adjustments, then periodically)
    - eGFR (baseline, periodically)

High-Yield Basic Pharmacology
- **Drug Interactions**
    - Avoid strong CYP3A4 inducers and inhibitors since finerenone is a major CYP3A4 substrate.
    - Use caution with other drugs that increase potassium, including ACE inhibitors, ARBs, potassium-sparing diuretics, and potassium salts.

High-Yield Clinical Knowledge
- **Initiation and Dosing**
    - Do not start if potassium > 5 mEq/L.
    - May start with potassium 4.8 – 5 mEq/L and increased monitoring for 4 weeks.
    - Starting dose based on eGFR:
        - ≥ 60 mL/min/1.73m^2: 20 mg daily
        - ≥ 25 to < 60 mL/min/1.73m^2: 10 mg daily
        - < 25 mL/min/1.73m^2: not recommended
- **Maintenance Dose**
    - Determined by potassium measured 4 weeks after initiation
    - If eGFR decreases by > 30%, maintain 10 mg dose

Current K$^+$ (mEq/L)	Current Dose 10 mg	Current Dose 20 mg
≤ 4.8	Increase to 20 mg	Continue 20 mg
> 4.8 – 5.5	Continue 10 mg	Continue 20 mg
≥ 5.5	Hold, consider restarting 10 mg when K$^+ \leq 5$	Hold, consider restarting 10 mg when K$^+ \leq 5$

- **Adverse Effects**
    - Hyperkalemia is the most common adverse effect.
    - May also cause hypotension.

High-Yield Core Evidence
- **FIDELIO-DKD Trial**
    - This was a double-blind, placebo-controlled, multicenter trial that randomized 5734 patients with T2DM and CKD (UACR 30 to < 300 or UACR ≥ 300 – 5000, all eGFR between 25 to 75 mL/min/1.73m^2) to finerenone or placebo while on concomitant RAS therapy.
    - Primary outcome was kidney failure, a sustained decrease of at least 40% eGFR from baseline, or death from renal causes, and was significantly reduced with finerenone.
    - Secondary outcome was death from CV causes, nonfatal MI, nonfatal stroke, or HF hospitalization, and was significantly reduced with finerenone.
    - Safety was similar, but finerenone was discontinued more due to hyperkalemia.
    - Concluded that finerenone reduced the risk of CKD progression and CV events compared to placebo. (NEJM 2020;383:2219-2229.)
- **FIGARO-DKD Trial**
    - This was a double-blind, placebo-controlled, multicenter, event-driven trial that randomized patients with T2DM and CKD (UACR 30 to < 300 or UACR ≥ 300 – 5000, all eGFR between 25 to 90 mL/min/1.73m^2) to finerenone or placebo while on RAS therapy. Patients with UACR ≥ 300 had eGFR ≥ 60.
    - Primary outcome was death from CV causes, nonfatal MI, nonfatal stroke, or HF hospitalizations, which was significant and mainly driven by a reduction in HF hospitalizations.
    - Secondary outcome was kidney failure, 40% sustained decrease in eGFR from baseline, or death from renal causes, which was not significant.
    - Safety was similar, but finerenone was discontinued more due to hyperkalemia.
    - Concluded that finerenone improved CV outcomes compared to placebo in T2DM patients with CKD Stage 2-4 and moderate albuminuria or CKD Stage 1-2 and severe albuminuria. (NEJM 2021;385:2252-2263.)

High-Yield Fast Facts
- Advise patients to avoid salt substitutes to avoid potential hyperkalemia from potassium replacing sodium in these products.

HIGH-YIELD BOARD EXAM ESSENTIALS
- **CLASSIC AGENTS:** Finerenone
- **DRUG CLASS:** NMRA
- **INDICATIONS:** Reduce risk of CKD progression and CV events in T2DM
- **MECHANISM:** Decreases fibrosis and inflammation by selectively blocking mineralocorticoid receptors in the epithelial (kidney) and nonepithelial (blood vessels, heart) tissues
- **SIDE EFFECTS:** Hyperkalemia
- **CLINICAL PEARLS:** Initial dose is based on potassium and eGFR, then subsequent dosing and maintenance dose is determined by potassium, eGFR, and starting dose.

Table: Drug Class Summary

	**Nonsteroidal Mineralocorticoid Receptor Antagonist - Drug Class Review** High-Yield Med Reviews
	**Mechanism of Action:** *Decreases fibrosis and inflammation by selectively blocking mineralocorticoid receptors in the epithelial (kidney) and nonepithelial (blood vessels, heart) tissues*
	**Class Effects:** Reduce the risk of CKD progression and CV events in T2DM, hyperkalemia, dosing based on initial dose, eGFR, and potassium.
Generic Name	Brand Name	Indication(s) or Uses	Notes
Finerenone	Kerendia	• Reduce the risk of CKD progression and CV events in T2DM	• **Dosing (Adult):** 　– 10-20 mg daily. Do not start with K^+ > 5 mEq/L. 　– Starting dose based eGFR and K^+ 　– Subsequent and maintenance dose based on starting dose, K^+ at 4 weeks, and eGFR • **Dosing (Peds):** N/A • **CYP450 Interactions:** CYP3A4, CYP2C8 substrate • **Renal or Hepatic Dose Adjustments (Initial):** 　– eGFR ≥ 60 mL/min/1.73m^2: 20 mg 　– eGFR ≥ 25 – 60 mL/min/1.73m^2: 10 mg 　– eGFR < 25 mL/min/1.73m^2: Not recommended 　– If eGFR decreases > 30%, maintain 10 mg dose • **Dosage Forms:** Oral (tablet)

ENDOCRINE – PANCREATIC ENZYMES

Drug Class
- Pancreatic Enzymes
- Agents:
  - Chronic Care
    - Pancrelipase

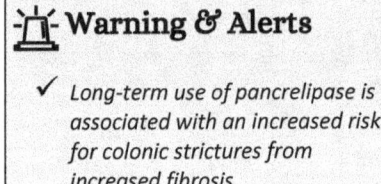

Warning & Alerts
- ✓ Long-term use of pancrelipase is associated with an increased risk for colonic strictures from increased fibrosis.

Main Indications or Uses
- Chronic Care
  - Exocrine pancreatic insufficiency

Mechanism of Action
- Supplements pancreatic activity through supplementation of pancreatic enzymes amylase, lipase, and protease.

Primary Net Benefit
- Pancrelipase prompts weight maintenance or weight gain by aiding the absorption of fat, protein, and fat-soluble vitamin absorption and reduces the incidence of steatorrhea, azotorrhea, and weight loss.
- Main Labs to Monitor:
  - No routine laboratory monitoring, however, monitor weight and stools

High-Yield Basic Pharmacology
- Pancreatic Enzyme Supplement
  - Pancreatin is an over-the-counter pancreatic enzyme supplement derived from the porcine pancreas and has relatively low concentrations of lipase and proteolytic enzymes.
  - Pancrelipase is an enriched preparation of pancreatic enzymes and is the pharmacologically relevant pancreatic enzyme supplement.
- Enteric Coating
  - As gastric acids rapidly inactivate pancrelipase enzymes, most dosage forms are prepared in an enteric coating, or concomitant acid suppression therapy is necessary for adequate absorption.

High-Yield Clinical Knowledge
- Brand Names
  - Pancrelipase is available in numerous dosage forms under a wide range of brand names.
  - Depending on the formulation, different amylase, lipase, and protease concentrations are present but are not always reflected by the clinical enzymatic activity of a given product.
  - Products are not equivalent, and one product's substitution for another should prompt close monitoring, including for patients admitted where formularies may not contain their particular dosage form.
- Dosage Forms
  - Available oral dosage forms include conventional tablets, bicarbonate-buffered enteric-coated tablets, enteric-coated tablets, beads, minitablets, or microtablets.
- Administration Schedule
  - Pancrelipase must be administered with each meal or snack, but dosing is individualized to patient-specific factors, including age, weight, pancreatic insufficiency, and dietary fat intake.
- Do Not Chew
  - Decreased clinical responses to enteric-coated agents may result from inadequate mixing of the granules with food.
  - Patients must be instructed that capsules must be swallowed, not chewed, which increases the risk of mucositis.

- **NPO Administration**
  - For patients who cannot swallow or have feeding tubes, pancrelipase microspheres can be mixed with enteral feeding formula products for administration.
    - However, these microspheres must be administered with food or solutions with a pH of 4.5 or less.
- **Long Term Use**
  - Patients with cystic fibrosis who require long-term pancrelipase therapy are at risk of fibrosing colonopathy leading to colon strictures.

High-Yield Core Evidence
- **Creon For Chronic Pancreatitis or Pancreatic Surgery**
  - This was a multicenter, double-blind, parallel-group, placebo-controlled trial that randomized adult patients with exocrine pancreatic insufficiency due to chronic pancreatitis or pancreatic surgery to receive either pancrelipase delayed-release capsules (Creon) 72,000 units/meal or 36,000 units/snack or placebo for seven days.
  - Pancrelipase-treated patients experience a significantly more change in baseline fat absorption from baseline to the end of the double-blind period than placebo.
  - Active treatment with pancrelipase was also associated with more significant improvements from baseline in stool frequency, stool consistency, abdominal pain, and flatulence observed with pancrelipase vs. placebo.
  - There was no difference between groups in treatment-emergent adverse events, and no treatment discontinuations occurred due to adverse events.
  - The authors concluded that pancrelipase delayed-release 12,000-lipase unit capsules effectively treated fat and nitrogen maldigestion with a treatment-emergent adverse events rate similar to placebo in patients with exocrine pancreatic insufficiency due to chronic pancreatitis or pancreatic surgery. (Am J Gastroenterol. 2010 Oct;105(10):2276-86.)

High-Yield Fast-Fact
- **FDA Mandate**
  - In 2004, the FDA mandated that any pancrelipase product undergo approval, as numerous unapproved products existed.

HIGH-YIELD BOARD EXAM ESSENTIALS
- **CLASSIC AGENTS:** Pancrelipase
- **DRUG CLASS:** Pancreatic Enzymes
- **INDICATIONS:** Exocrine pancreatic insufficiency
- **MECHANISM:** Supplements pancreatic activity through supplementation of pancreatic enzymes amylase, lipase, and protease.
- **SIDE EFFECTS:** Abdominal pain, diarrhea, itching, headache
- **CLINICAL PEARLS:** Decreased clinical responses to enteric-coated agents may be a result of inadequate mixing of the granules with food. Patients must be instructed that capsules must be swallowed, not chewed, which increases the risk of mucositis.

Table: Drug Class Summary

Pancreatic Enzymes - Drug Class Review High-Yield Med Reviews			
Mechanism of Action: *Supplements pancreatic activity through supplementation of pancreatic enzymes amylase, lipase, and protease.*			
Class Effects: *Pancrelipase prompts weight maintenance or weight gain by aiding the absorption of fat, protein, and fat-soluble vitamin absorption and reduces the incidence of steatorrhea, azotorrhea, and weight loss.*			
Generic Name	**Brand Name**	**Indication(s) or Uses**	**Notes**
Pancrelipase	Creon, Pancreaze, Pancrelipase, Pertzye, Viokace, Zenpep	• Pancreatic insufficiency	• **Dosing (Adult):** – Oral: 500 to 2,500 units/kg/meal • **Dosing (Peds):** – Infants: Oral 2,000 to 5,000 units per feeding – Maximum 10,000 units/kg/day – Ages 1 to 4 year: Oral 1,000 to 2,5000 units/kg/meal – Maximum 10,000 units/kg/day – Ages 4 and older: Oral 500 to 2,500 units/kg/meal • **CYP450 Interactions:** None • **Renal or Hepatic Dose Adjustments:** None • **Dosage Forms:** Oral (capsule, tablet)

ENDOCRINE – PHOSPHATE BINDING AGENTS

Drug Class
- Phosphate Binding Agents
- Agents:
    - Chronic Care
        - Aluminum hydroxide
        - Calcium acetate
        - Calcium carbonate
        - Ferric citrate
        - Magnesium carbonate
        - Lanthanum
        - Sevelamer
        - Sucroferric oxyhydroxide

> **Knowledge Integration**
> ✓ Non-calcium containing phosphate binders are less likely to deposit in the endovascular lining causing vascular calcifications with long-term use in patients with CKD but are more expensive.
> ✓ While aluminum hydroxide is an effective phosphate binder for patients with CKD, the Al can accumulate over time and cause renal bone disease.

Main Indications or Uses
- Chronic Care
    - Antacid (calcium acetate)
    - Calcium supplementation (calcium acetate, calcium carbonate)
    - Hyperphosphatemia (calcium acetate, calcium carbonate, ferric citrate, lanthanum, sevelamer, sucroferric oxyhydroxide)
    - Hypoparathyroidism (calcium carbonate)
    - Iron deficiency anemia (ferric citrate)

Mechanism of Action
- Form insoluble compounds with phosphate in the GI by binding to dietary phosphorus.

Primary Net Benefit
- Oral calcium phosphate binders are first-line agents, followed by sevelamer, which may reduce the risk of coronary artery calcification associated with long-term calcium use. Lanthanum is an alternative with a lower hypercalcemia risk, and more recent iron-based binders lower phosphorus with a lower pill burden.
- Main Labs to Monitor:
    - Serum calcium, phosphorus
    - Parathyroid hormone
    - Liver function (INR/PT, albumin, protein, bilirubin)

High-Yield Basic Pharmacology
- Calcium Carbonate or Acetate
    - Although calcium carbonate contains more elemental calcium, calcium acetate is preferred in patients with CKD due to the lower elemental calcium content.
    - For every 1 g of calcium acetate, 45 mg of phosphorus is bound.
    - Calcium carbonate 1 g binds approximately 39 mg of phosphorus.
- Relevant Interactions
    - Numerous interactions exist with oral phosphate binders, and patients must be counseled to separate other medications by at least 1-2 hours before or 3 hours after phosphate binder administration.
    - Sevelamer may reduce the absorption of fluoroquinolones and mycophenolate resulting in the risk of clinical failure.
    - Lanthanum may reduce the absorption of fluoroquinolones, tetracyclines, and levothyroxine.
    - Iron-based binding agents may result in the chelation of numerous medications due to their iron content.

- **Phosphate Binding Equivalence**
  - Dosing equivalents are compared to the phosphate binding capacity of calcium carbonate 1g:
    - Aluminum hydroxide 500 mg = 0.75
    - Calcium carbonate 1,000 mg = 1
    - Calcium acetate 667 mg = 0.67
    - Ferric citrate 210 mg = 0.64
    - Lanthanum 500 mg = 1.0
    - Sevelamer carbonate 800 mg = 0.6
    - Sucroferric oxyhydroxide 500 mg = 1.6

High-Yield Clinical Knowledge
- **Hyperphosphatemia**
  - Hyperphosphatemia occurs in patients with chronic kidney disease due to decreased phosphorus elimination and may cause secondary hyperparathyroidism and increased osteoclast activity.
- **Serum Iron**
  - Iron-based phosphate binders may increase serum iron, ferritin, and iron saturation, thus increasing iron overload risk.
  - Patients should be educated that dark color stools are expected, but if there is a concern for GI bleeding, seek healthcare provider advice.
- **Aluminum and HD**
  - Aluminum hydroxide used as a phosphate binder has diminished due to the availability of suitable alternatives and aluminum toxicity risk, to include negative impact on the bone.
    - Aluminum may inhibit delta-aminolaevulinic acid dehydrogenase leading to the accumulation of erythrocyte protoporphyrin, which manifests as microcytic hypochromic anemia resistant to iron.
      - This anemia precedes more serious toxic manifestations of aluminum of encephalopathy, myoclonus, and seizures.
- **Vascular Calcifications**
  - Chronic use of calcium-based phosphate binders contributes to increased vascular calcification in patients with chronic kidney disease.
- **Cholesterol-Lowering Effect**
  - Sevelamer reduces LDL cholesterol, providing an added benefit in patients with underlying cardiovascular disease.
- **Chewable Dosage Forms**
  - Patients must be instructed to chew lanthanum and sucroferric oxyhydroxide tablets to reduce the risk of the tablets themselves accumulating in the gut, leading to severe constipation or GI obstruction and perforation.

High-Yield Core Evidence
- **COSMOS**
  - This was a 3-year, multicenter, open-cohort, prospective study in adult chronic hemodialysis patients who were followed to assess the association of serum phosphorus, calcium, and PTH with relative mortality risk.
  - The study investigators observed that high and low serum phosphorus, calcium, and PTH were associated with higher mortality risk.
  - The most significant benefit was observed among patients with baseline phosphorus levels between 3.6 and 5.2 mg/dL, calcium between 7.9 and 9.5 mg/dL, and PTH between 168 to 674 pg/mL.
  - Decreases in serum phosphorus and calcium with baseline elevated levels, and increases in serum PTH below baseline levels, respectively, were associated with improved survival.
  - The authors concluded that there is an association between serum phosphorus, calcium, and PTH and mortality and suggest survival benefits of controlling chronic kidney disease-mineral and bone disorder biochemical parameters in CKD5D patients. (Nephrol Dial Transplant. 2015 Sep;30(9):1542-51.)

- **Phos, PTH, and Calcium Meta-Analysis**
  - This was a systematic review and meta-analysis to assess the association between serum phosphorus levels, parathyroid hormone, calcium, and risks of death, cardiovascular mortality, and nonfatal cardiovascular events in individuals with chronic kidney disease.
  - A total of forty-seven cohort studies were included in the final meta-analysis.
  - The study authors observed a statistically significant 18% increased risk of death for every 1 mg/dL increase in serum phosphorus.
  - However, there was no significant association between all-cause mortality and serum PTH or serum calcium levels. Still, data for the association between serum levels of phosphorus, parathyroid hormone, and calcium and cardiovascular death were available in only one adequately adjusted cohort study.
  - The study authors concluded that there appears to be an association between higher serum levels of phosphorus and this population's mortality. (JAMA. 2011 Mar 16;305(11):1119-27.)

High-Yield Fast-Fact
- **Bicarbonate Vs. Hydrochloride**
  - Sevelamer carbonate and sevelamer hydrochloride are considered interchangeable therapeutically, but the hydrochloride may be absorbed and poses a risk of metabolic acidosis.

HIGH-YIELD BOARD EXAM ESSENTIALS
- **CLASSIC AGENTS:** Aluminum hydroxide, calcium acetate, calcium carbonate, ferric citrate, magnesium carbonate, lanthanum, sevelamer, sucroferric oxyhydroxide
- **DRUG CLASS:** Phosphate Binding Agents
- **INDICATIONS:** Antacid (calcium acetate), calcium supplementation (calcium acetate, calcium carbonate), hyperphosphatemia (calcium acetate, calcium carbonate, ferric citrate, lanthanum, sevelamer, sucroferric oxyhydroxide), hypoparathyroidism (calcium carbonate), iron deficiency anemia (ferric citrate)
- **MECHANISM:** Form insoluble compounds with phosphate in the GI by binding to dietary phosphorus
- **SIDE EFFECTS:** Metallic taste, constipation, diarrhea
- **CLINICAL PEARLS:**
  - Chronic use of calcium-based phosphate binders contributes to increased vascular calcification in patients with chronic kidney disease.
  - Aluminum-based phosphate binders are very effective at binding phosphate, but aluminum can accumulate with chronic use and lead to bone disease.

Table: Drug Class Summary

	Phosphate Binding Agents - Drug Class Review High-Yield Med Reviews		
Mechanism of Action: *Form insoluble compounds with phosphate in the GI by binding to dietary phosphorus*			
Class Effects: *Oral calcium phosphate binders are first-line agents, followed by sevelamer, which may reduce the risk of coronary artery calcification associated with long-term calcium use. Lanthanum is an alternative with a lower hypercalcemia risk, and more recent iron-based binders lower phosphorus with a lower pill burden.*			
Generic Name	**Brand Name**	**Main Indication(s) or Uses**	**Notes**
Aluminum hydroxide	AlternaGel	• Hyperphosphatemia	• **Dosing (Adult):** — Oral: 300 to 600 mg qmeal • **Dosing (Peds):** — Oral: 150 to 300 mg qmeal • **CYP450 Interactions:** None • **Renal or Hepatic Dose Adjustments:** None • **Dosage Forms:** Oral (capsule, solution, tablet)
Calcium acetate	Calphron Eliphos PhosLo Phoslyra	• Hyperphosphatemia	• **Dosing (Adult):** — Oral: 1,334 to 2,668 mg qmeal • **Dosing (Peds):** — Oral: 667 to 1,000 mg qmeal • **CYP450 Interactions:** None • **Renal or Hepatic Dose Adjustments:** None • **Dosage Forms:** Oral (capsule, solution, tablet)
Calcium carbonate	Antacid Cal-Carb Caltrate Florical Maalox Oysco Tums	• Antacid • Calcium supplementation • Hyperphosphatemia • Hypoparathyroidism	• **Dosing (Adult):** — Oral: 500 to 8,000 mg per day — Maximum for CKD 2,000 mg/day • **Dosing (Peds):** — Oral: 375 to 7,500 mg/day — Maximum for CKD 2,000 mg/day • **CYP450 Interactions:** None • **Renal or Hepatic Dose Adjustments:** None • **Dosage Forms:** Oral (capsule, powder, suspension, tablet)
Ferric citrate	Auryxia	• Hyperphosphatemia • Iron deficiency anemia	• **Dosing (Adult):** — Oral: 210 to 420 mg TID — Maximum 2,520 mg/day • **Dosing (Peds):** — Not routinely used • **CYP450 Interactions:** None • **Renal or Hepatic Dose Adjustments:** None • **Dosage Forms:** Oral (tablet)
Lanthanum	Fosrenol	• Hyperphosphatemia	• **Dosing (Adult):** — Oral: 1,500 to 4,500 mg daily • **Dosing (Peds):** — Not routinely used • **CYP450 Interactions:** None • **Renal or Hepatic Dose Adjustments:** None • **Dosage Forms:** Oral (packet, tablet)

Endocrinology

Phosphate Binding Agents - Drug Class Review
High-Yield Med Reviews

Generic Name	Brand Name	Main Indication(s) or Uses	Notes

Magnesium carbonate	Magonate	• Dietary supplementation	• **Dosing (Adult):**
			  − Oral: 5 mL 3 times daily
			• **Dosing (Peds):**
			  − Oral (elemental magnesium): 10 to 20 mg/kg/dose q6-24h
			• **CYP450 Interactions:** None
			• **Renal or Hepatic Dose Adjustments:**
			  − Should be avoided in PEDIATRICS with renal impairment
			• **Dosage Forms:** Oral (liquid, powder)

Sevelamer	Renagel, Renvela	• Hyperphosphatemia	• **Dosing (Adult):**
			  − Oral: 600 to 1,600 mg TID with meals
			• **Dosing (Peds):**
			  − Oral: 400 to 800 mg TID with meals
			• **CYP450 Interactions:** None
			• **Renal or Hepatic Dose Adjustments:** None
			• **Dosage Forms:** Oral (packet, tablet)

Sucroferric oxyhydroxide	Velphoro	• Hyperphosphatemia	• **Dosing (Adult):**
			  − Oral: 500 to 2,000 mg TID with meals
			• **Dosing (Peds):**
			  − Not routinely used
			• **CYP450 Interactions:** None
			• **Renal or Hepatic Dose Adjustments:** None
			• **Dosage Forms:** Oral (tablet)

ENDOCRINE – POTASSIUM BINDING AGENTS

Drug Class
- Potassium Binding Agents
- Agents:
  - Acute Care
    - Patiromer
    - Sodium Polystyrene Sulfonate
    - Sodium Zirconium Cyclosilicate

> **Warning & Facts**
> ✓ Sodium polystyrene sulfonate is associated with colonic necrosis which has contributed to its decline in clinical practice and replacement with other options.

Main Indications or Uses
- Acute Care
  - Hyperkalemia

Mechanism of Action
- Cation exchange resins reduce potassium absorption from the gut.

Primary Net Benefit
- Potassium lowering agents are used for chronic management of hyperkalemia in patients with chronic kidney disease.
- Main Labs to Monitor:
  - Serum potassium, sodium

High-Yield Basic Pharmacology
- **Sorbitol Suspension**
  - SPS is a suspension in sorbitol to promote excretion of the bound potassium but frequently is associated with diarrhea.
  - Patiromer also contains sorbitol but in a significantly lower quantity than in SPS.
- **Sodium Content**
  - SPS also contains a considerable amount of sodium, 100 mg per 1 g of SPS.
    - For a given dose of 15 to 60 g, patients may be exposed to 1,500 to 6,000 mg of sodium, and when administered q4h, this can significantly exceed the recommended daily intake of sodium.
  - Each 10 g dose of sodium zirconium cyclosilicate contains 800 mg of sodium, for a total daily intake of 2,400 mg of sodium from this drug alone.

High-Yield Clinical Knowledge
- **Colonic Necrosis**
  - Sorbitol has also been associated with colonic necrosis, particularly in preparations with 70% sorbitol.
  - There is a lower risk of colonic necrosis with the 33% sorbitol SPS formulation.
- **SPS Potassium Lowering**
  - Although 1 mEq of SPS will exchange 1 mEq of potassium, this exchange occurs in the intestines and does not equate to SPS's plasma potassium lowering effect.
  - SPS may lower plasma potassium by approximately 0.5 mEq/L and may do so within 3 to 4 hours of an oral or rectal dose.
    - Therefore, SPS should not be used to rapidly lower potassium in patients with severe or symptomatic hyperkalemia.
  - Patiromer is not appropriate for the rapid potassium lowering effect.
  - Sodium zirconium cyclosilicate has a much more rapid onset within 1 hour after administration; however, clinical experience is lacking, and more clinically essential interventions in hyperkalemia should be prioritized (calcium, insulin, diuresis/dialysis, beta-agonists).

- **Chronic SPS Vs. Alternatives**
  - Patients with chronic kidney disease receiving RAAS inhibitor therapy can receive SPS to maintain normal serum potassium.
  - However, due to the significant sodium content, associated diarrhea, and risk of colonic necrosis, alternative cation exchange resins (patiromer, sodium zirconium cyclosilicate) can be used.
- **Drug Interactions**
  - Any of these cation exchange agents will bind numerous oral medications and must be administered at least 3 hours before or after any other medication.
- **Potassium Exchange Location**
  - SPS and sodium zirconium cyclosilicate exchange sodium for potassium across the length of the intestinal tract.
  - Conversely, patiromer only exchanges calcium for potassium in the distal colon.

High-Yield Core Evidence
- **HARMONIZE**
  - This was a multicenter, double-blind, placebo-controlled, phase 3 clinical trial.
  - Study subjects were outpatients with hyperkalemia and randomized to receive sodium zirconium cyclosilicate 10 g three times daily in a 48-hour open-label phase to achieve normokalemia, followed by either sodium zirconium cyclosilicate 5 g, 10 g, 15 g, or placebo daily for 28 days.
  - Each group randomized to receive sodium zirconium cyclosilicate experienced a significantly lower mean serum potassium level on days 8 through 29.
  - Similarly, the proportion of patients with mean potassium less than 5.1 mEq/L during days 8 through 29 was significantly higher among patients receiving sodium zirconium cyclosilicate dose.
  - More edema was observed in the sodium zirconium cyclosilicate 15 g group than placebo, and more hypokalemia developed in the 10 g and 15 g sodium zirconium cyclosilicate to none in the 5 g or placebo groups.
  - The authors concluded that open label followed by sodium zirconium cyclosilicate daily among outpatients with hyperkalemia resulted in lower potassium levels and a higher proportion of patients with normal potassium levels for up to 28 days. (JAMA. 2014 Dec 3;312(21):2223-33.)
- **OPAL-HK**
  - This prospective multicenter trial was in patients with chronic kidney disease receiving a RAAS inhibitor with 5.1 to 6.5 mmol/L potassium levels.
  - In the first phase of the study, patients received patiromer 4.2 to 8.4 g twice daily for four weeks, followed by randomization to either continue patiromer or switch to placebo among patients who responded clinically for another eight weeks.
  - Of the 237 patients who received the initial four-week run-in phase patiromer, 107 subjects were randomized to either patiromer or placebo.
  - Patients randomized to placebo experienced a significant increase in potassium level from baseline, and recurrent hypokalemia occurred in 60% of subjects receiving placebo and 15% receiving patiromer.
  - The authors concluded that in patients with chronic kidney disease who were receiving RAAS inhibitors and who had hyperkalemia, patiromer treatment was associated with a decrease in serum potassium levels and a reduction in the recurrence of hyperkalemia compared with placebo. (N Engl J Med. 2015 Jan 15;372(3):211-21.)

High-Yield Fast-Fact
- **Foul Taste**
  - Oral SPS has a foul taste which negatively impacts compliance.

Table: Drug Class Summary

Potassium Binding Agents - Drug Class Review High-Yield Med Reviews			
Mechanism of Action: *Cation exchange resins reduce potassium absorption from the gut.*			
Class Effects: *Potassium lowering agents used for chronic management of hyperkalemia in patients with chronic kidney disease.*			
Generic Name	**Brand Name**	**Indication(s) or Uses**	**Notes**
Patiromer	Veltassa	• Hyperkalemia	• **Dosing (Adult):** — Oral: 8.4 to 25.2 g once daily • **Dosing (Peds):** — Not routinely used • **CYP450 Interactions:** None • **Renal or Hepatic Dose Adjustments:** None • **Dosage Forms:** Oral (packet)
Sodium Polystyrene Sulfonate	Kayexalate, Kionex	• Hyperkalemia	• **Dosing (Adult):** — Oral: 15 to 60 g 1 to 4 times daily — Rectal: 30 to 50 g q6h • **Dosing (Peds):** — Oral: 1g/kg/dose q6h — Maximum 15 g/dose — Rectal: 1 g/kg/dose retained for 15-60 minutes q2-6h — Maximum 50 g/dose • **CYP450 Interactions:** None • **Renal or Hepatic Dose Adjustments:** None • **Dosage Forms:** Oral (powder, suspension), Rectal (suspension)
Sodium Zirconium Cyclosilicate	Lokelma	• Hyperkalemia	• **Dosing (Adult):** — Oral: 5 to 15 g TID for up to 48 hours • **Dosing (Peds):** — Not routinely used • **CYP450 Interactions:** None • **Renal or Hepatic Dose Adjustments:** None • **Dosage Forms:** Oral (packet)

HIGH-YIELD BOARD EXAM ESSENTIALS
- **CLASSIC AGENTS:** Patiromer, sodium polystyrene sulfonate, sodium zirconium cyclosilicate
- **DRUG CLASS:** Potassium binding agents
- **INDICATIONS:** Hyperkalemia
- **MECHANISM:** Cation exchange resins that reduce potassium absorption from the gut.
- **SIDE EFFECTS:** Hypernatremia, edema, diarrhea
- **CLINICAL PEARLS:** Patients with chronic kidney disease receiving RAAS inhibitor therapy can receive SPS to maintain normal serum potassium. However, due to the significant sodium content, associated diarrhea, and risk of colonic necrosis, alternative cation exchange resins (patiromer, sodium zirconium cyclosilicate) can be used.

ENDOCRINE – IODIDES

Drug Class
- Iodides
- Agents:
  - **Acute Care**
    - Potassium iodide
  - **Chronic Care**
    - Sodium iodide

Main Indications or Uses
- **Acute Care**
  - Potassium iodide
    - Antidote (radioactive iodine)
    - Expectorant
- **Chronic Care**
  - Sodium iodide
    - Iodine supplement

Mechanism of Action
- Specific and competitive inhibitor of iodine uptake into the thyroid.
- Inhibit thyroglobulin proteolysis, which inhibits thyroid hormone release.

Primary Net Benefit
- Iodides are dietary supplements. Most importantly, they are used for thyroid protection after radiologic exposure, rapid establishment of the euthyroid state in thyrotoxicosis, or before thyroid surgery.
- Main Labs to Monitor:
  - TSH, T4

High-Yield Basic Pharmacology
- **Iodine Vs. Iodide**
  - Iodine is the chemical element and is caustic.
  - Iodide refers to the negatively charged state, forming inorganic compounds like sodium and potassium iodide.
- **Thyroid Effects**
  - Iodides inhibit organification and hormone release from thyroid tissue and can also decrease the gland's size and vascularity.
  - Iodides can precipitate either hyperthyroidism or hypothyroidism.
- **SSKI, Lugol's, or Tablets**
  - Potassium iodide is available as either a supersaturated potassium iodide (SSKI) containing 38 mg iodide/drop, a less concentrated solution (Lugol's) of 6.3 mg/drop of potassium iodide, and tablets which are available as 130 mg.

High-Yield Clinical Knowledge
- **Radiologic Exposure**
  - Potassium iodide is used for post-exposure prophylaxis after radiation exposure to competitively inhibit radioactive iodine uptake into the thyroid.
    - Exposure usually occurs from inhalation of radioactive iodine or ingestion of contaminated food.
  - It has been used in Pacific Islanders exposed to nuclear weapon testing in the 1950s to reduce thyroid exposure to radioactive iodine.
  - More recently, nuclear incidents in Ukraine (Chernobyl) and Japan (Fukushima) have prompted the public at risk of exposure to take potassium iodide.

- Among children with radiologic exposure from Chernobyl, children in Poland who had access to potassium iodide have a significantly lower risk of thyroid cancer than Ukrainian children who were largely not given potassium iodide.
- **Iodine Allergy**
    - A true iodine allergy is incompatible with life.
    - There has been no evidence to suggest IgE antibody development to small molecules, including either iodine or iodide.
        - Radiocontrast media, which often contains iodine, is associated with anaphylactoid reactions due to osmolarity or other high molecular weight components but is not a result of its iodine content.
    - Patients who experience allergic responses to povidone-iodine do not exhibit adverse reactions to potassium iodide.
- **Pregnant Women and Children**
    - Children and pregnant women are at high risk of radioactive iodine's toxic effects compared to men and adult women.
    - However, pregnant women must only receive a single dose as the risk of the Wolff-Chaikoff effect (where iodine inhibits the synthesis of thyroid hormones) may be catastrophic in fetal neurologic development.
- **Physiologic Function**
    - Iodine is an essential element required to synthesize thyroid hormones triiodothyronine (T3) and thyroxine (T4).
        - If the synthesis of T3 or T4 is absent, supplementation is necessary for life.
- **Sialadenitis**
    - Supplementation with potassium iodide is associated with sialadenitis, otherwise known as iodide mumps.
    - Other common adverse effects include acneiform rash, mucous membrane ulceration, conjunctivitis, and bleeding disorders.

High-Yield Core Evidence
- **Iodide Prophylaxis in Poland After Chernobyl**
    - This was an observational pilot and field study of over 34,000 subjects with known or suspected exposure to radiologic iodine following the Chernobyl radiologic incident. They were also enrolled in a long-term follow-up research study.
    - Of the 34,000 questionnaire respondents, approximately 12,000 children received iodide, and over 5,000 adults received iodide.
    - There were no acute intrathyroidal adverse effects in study subjects, except for transient thyroid blockade observed in newborn infants to mothers who had taken potassium iodide.
    - This study supported the efficacy of delayed administration of potassium iodide to individuals exposed to radioactive iodine beyond 36 hours after exposure.
    - Additionally, this study supported prolonging the shelf-life of potassium iodide products, which can significantly expand the available doses for radiologic disaster victims. (Am J Med 1993 May;94(5):524-532.)

High-Yield Fast-Fact
- **Iodine Radiation**
    - Radioactive iodine emits beta-radiation and gamma-radiation.

Endocrinology

> ## HIGH-YIELD BOARD EXAM ESSENTIALS
> - **CLASSIC AGENTS:** Sodium iodide, potassium iodide
> - **DRUG CLASS:** Iodides
> - **INDICATIONS:** Antidote (radioactive iodine), expectorant, iodine supplement
> - **MECHANISM:** Specific and competitive inhibitor of iodine uptake into the thyroid. Inhibit thyroglobulin proteolysis, which inhibits thyroid hormone release.
> - **SIDE EFFECTS:** Sialadenitis, acneiform rash, mucous membrane ulceration, conjunctivitis, and bleeding disorders.
> - **CLINICAL PEARLS:**
>   - Can precipitate hyperthyroidism or hypothyroidism
>   - Since these agents in higher doses can not only suppress thyroid hormone release but can also reduce blood flow to the thyroid gland and inhibit the delivery of other drugs to the thyroid gland, the order of drug administration in certain conditions can be relevant.
>   - Children and pregnant women are at high risk of radioactive iodine's toxic effects compared to men and adult women. However, pregnant women must only receive a single dose as the risk of the Wolff-Chaikoff effect may be catastrophic in fetal neurologic development.

Table: Drug Class Summary

Iodides - Drug Class Review High-Yield Med Reviews			
Mechanism of Action: Specific and competitive inhibitor of iodine uptake into the thyroid.			
Class Effects: *Iodide dietary supplements, thyroid protection after radiologic exposure, rapid establishment of a euthyroid state in thyrotoxicosis or before thyroid surgery.*			
Generic Name	**Brand Name**	**Indication(s) or Uses**	**Notes**
Potassium iodide	iOSTAT, SSKI, Thyrosafe	- Antidote - Expectorant	- **Dosing (Adult):** – Antidote: 130 mg daily for 10-14 days – Expectorant: 300-600 mg 3-4 times daily – Thyrotoxicosis (SSKI): 250 mg q6h - **Dosing (Peds):** – Infants and children < 3 years: 32.5 mg daily – Age 3-12 years: 65 mg daily - **CYP450 Interactions:** None - **Renal or Hepatic Dose Adjustments:** None - **Dosage Forms:** Oral (solution, tablet)
Sodium iodide	Iodopen	- Iodine supplement	- **Dosing (Adult):** – IV: 1-3 mcg/kg/day administered in parenteral nutrition - **Dosing (Peds):** – IV: 1-3 mcg/kg/day administered in parenteral nutrition - **CYP450 Interactions:** None - **Renal or Hepatic Dose Adjustments:** None - **Dosage Forms:** IV (solution)

ENDOCRINE – THIOAMIDES

Drug Class
- Thioamide
- **Agents:** methimazole, propylthiouracil

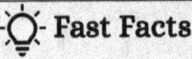
Fast Facts
- ✓ Propylthiouracil is more commonly used in acute thyrotoxicosis or thyroid storm due to its ability to inhibit the peripheral conversion of T4 to the more biological active form, T3.

Main Indications or Uses
- **Acute Care**
  - Management of thyroid storm
    - Methimazole, propylthiouracil
- **Chronic Care**
  - Treatment of hyperthyroidism in patients with Graves disease or toxic multinodular goiter when surgery or radioactive iodine is not recommended
    - Methimazole is preferred.
  - Management of hyperthyroidism as preparation for thyroidectomy or radioactive iodine
    - Methimazole is preferred.
  - Iodine-induced and type I amiodarone-induced thyrotoxicosis
    - Off-label: methimazole

Mechanism of Action
- Block thyroid hormone synthesis by inhibiting thyroid peroxidase; does not inactivate existing T3 or T4.
  - Propylthiouracil: also, inhibits peripheral conversion of T4 to T3.
- Do not interfere with orally or parenterally administered thyroid hormones.

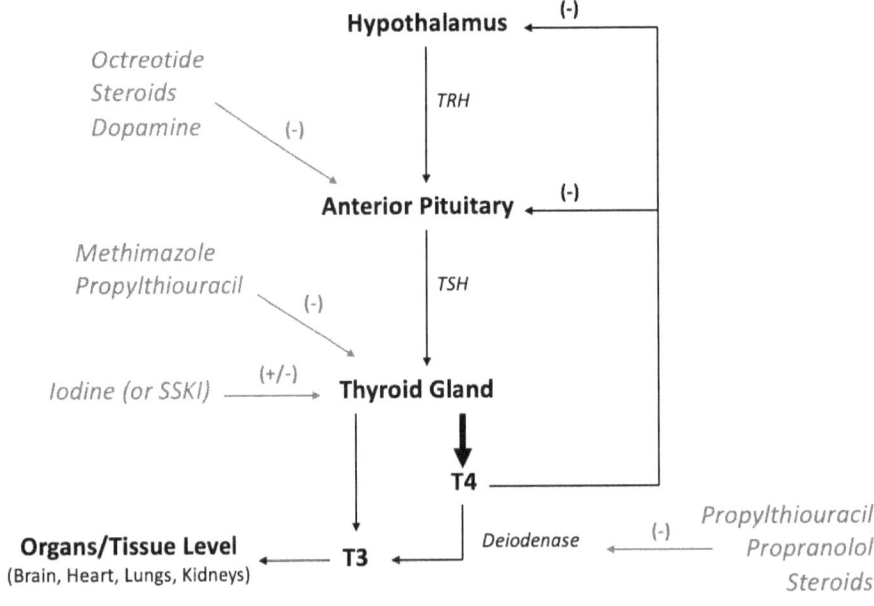

Primary Net Benefit
- Main Labs to Monitor:
  - Free T4 and total T3 every 4-6 weeks when titrating, then every 2-3 months when euthyroid.
    - Needed to determine initial response.
    - Graves' disease: if thyrotropin receptor antibodies are negative, monitor thyroid function tests every 2-3 months for 6 months, 4-6 months for 6 months, then every 6-12 months.
  - TSH 6-8 weeks after initiation or dose changes.
  - CBC w/differential and LFTs at baseline, then if symptoms if adverse effects occur.
  - PT before surgical procedures.

High-Yield Basic Pharmacology
- **Onset**
  - Propylthiouracil provides significant therapeutic effects in 24-36 hours.
- **Distribution**
  - Concentrated in thyroid gland.
- **Drug Interactions**
  - Monitor INR with concomitant warfarin use, especially with starting (INR may decrease) or stopping (INR may increase) antithyroid medications.
  - Monitor with myelosuppressive agents.

High-Yield Clinical Knowledge
- **General Clinical Pearls**
  - Hypothyroid symptoms may occur with over treatment.
  - May be used in combination with beta-blockers for symptom management.
  - Propylthiouracil may be preferred in thyroid storm because it inhibits peripheral conversion of T4 to T3, unless the patient has liver disease or is in the 2nd/3rd trimester of pregnancy.
  - May divide methimazole doses to mitigate GI effects.
  - Can be administered rectally if needed.
- **Radioactive Iodide Treatments**
  - Discontinue antithyroid agents 3 days before sodium iodide, I-131 administration.
  - May resume 2-3 days after treatment.
- **Bone Marrow Suppression**
  - May cause bone marrow suppression, including agranulocytosis, thrombocytopenia, and aplastic anemia.
  - Usually occurs within first 3 months.
  - With methimazole, risk increases with doses $\geq$40 mg daily.
- **Hepatic Toxicity**
  - May cause acute and/or fatal liver failure.
  - Propylthiouracil demonstrates greater risk than methimazole. Recommended only in patients intolerant to methimazole or who are not candidates for surgery and radioactive iodine.
  - Discontinue therapy if signs/symptoms of liver failure occur, or LFTs $\geq$2-3 times ULN.
- **Other Warnings**
  - Bleeding, fever, dermatologic toxicities, pneumonitis, nephritis, lupus-like syndrome, and vasculitis (risk increases with duration) may occur.
- **Pediatric Patients**
  - Methimazole is preferred; propylthiouracil should be used only in patients who have experienced adverse effects with methimazole or are not candidates for surgery or radioactive iodine treatment due to hematologic and hepatic toxicities.
- **Pregnancy**
  - 1st Trimester
    - Avoid methimazole in 1st trimester due to teratogenesis.
    - Use propylthiouracil.
  - 2nd/3rd Trimester
    - Methimazole is preferred due to increased risk of adverse effects with propylthiouracil to the mother.
  - Monitor and adjust doses as pregnancy progresses to maintain response.
    - Thyroid function can improve with pregnancy progression, leading to potential discontinuation 2-3 months prior to birth with careful monitoring.

- **Lactation**

- Thioamides are compatible with breastfeeding.
    - Methimazole recommended at 20-30 mg daily in divided doses taken after breastfeeding sessions.
    - Propylthiouracil is acceptable at ≤450 mg daily.
    - Monitor infant's thyroid function, growth, and development.

High-Yield Core Evidence
- **Comparison of Acute Changes with Antithyroid Agents**
    - Demonstrated that propylthiouracil inhibited peripheral conversion of T4 to T3 based on acute decreases in T3 with propylthiouracil compared to methimazole within the first 5 days of therapy.
    - J Clin Invest 1974;54:201-208.

- **Comparison of Therapies for Graves' Hyperthyroidism Systematic Review**
    - Demonstrated increased hepatotoxicity with propylthiouracil compared to methimazole (2.7% vs 0.4%, respectively), in addition to dermatologic toxicities (6% vs 3%).
    - J Clin Endocrinol Metab 2013;98:3671-77.

High-Yield Fast-Fact
- Common abbreviations for thioamides are MMI (methimazole) and PTU (propylthiouracil).

HIGH-YIELD BOARD EXAM ESSENTIALS
- **CLASSIC AGENTS:** Methimazole, propylthiouracil
- **DRUG CLASS:** Thioamide
- **INDICATIONS:** Hyperthyroidism/thyrotoxicosis
- **MECHANISM:** Blocks thyroid hormone synthesis. Propylthiouracil inhibits conversion of peripheral T4 to T3.
- **SIDE EFFECTS:** Hepatotoxicity (propylthiouracil>methimazole), bone marrow suppression, hypothyroid symptoms.
- **CLINICAL PEARLS:**
    - PTU is utilized in the 1st trimester of pregnancy, then methimazole is utilized for 2nd and 3rd trimesters.
    - Propylthiouracil may be preferred in thyroid storm because it inhibits peripheral conversion of T4 to T3, unless the patient has liver disease or is in the 2nd/3rd trimester of pregnancy.

Table: Drug Class Summary

Thyroid Replacements Drug Class Review High-Yield Med Reviews			
Mechanism of Action: Blocks thyroid hormone synthesis. Propylthiouracil also inhibits conversion of peripheral T4 to T3.			
Class Effects: Hepatotoxicity (propylthiouracil>methimazole), bone marrow suppression, hypothyroid symptoms			
Generic Name	**Brand Name**	**Indication(s) or Uses**	**Notes**
Methimazole	Tapazole	<ul><li>Hyperthyroidism</li><li>Thyroid storm</li><li>Iodine and amiodarone-induced thyrotoxicosis</li></ul>	<ul><li>**Dosing (Adult):** 5-40 mg daily<ul><li>Free T4 1-1.5x ULN: 5-10 mg; 1.5-2x ULN: 10-20 mg; 2-3x ULN: 30-40 mg</li><li>May divide in 2-3 doses >30 mg daily; may mitigate GI effects.</li><li>Adjust dose and duration based on definitive therapy and thyroid function tests.</li></ul></li><li>**Dosing (Peds):** 0.4 mg/kg/d divided Q8h, then 0.2 mg/kg/d divided Q8h<ul><li>Can also follow fixed dosing by age</li></ul></li><li>**CYP450 Interactions:** N/A</li><li>**Renal or Hepatic Dose Adjustments:** None</li><li>**Dosage Forms:** 5 mg, 10 mg</li></ul>
Propylthiouracil		<ul><li>Hyperthyroidism</li><li>Thyroid storm (preferred)</li></ul>	<ul><li>**Dosing (Adult):** 300 mg daily divided Q8h<ul><li>Doses up to 900 mg daily may be given.</li><li>Thyroid storm: 500-1000 mg, then 250 mg Q4h, then reduce to maintenance dosage</li></ul></li><li>**Dosing (Peds):** Initial 6-10 yrs: 50-150 mg/d divided Q8h; >10 yrs: 150-300 mg/d divided Q8h<ul><li>Maintenance 50 mg BID</li></ul></li><li>**CYP450 Interactions:** N/A</li><li>**Renal or Hepatic Dose Adjustments:** None</li><li>**Dosage Forms:** 50 mg</li></ul>

ENDOCRINE – THYROID HORMONE REPLACEMENTS

Drug Class
- Thyroid Replacements
- Agents: desiccated thyroid, levothyroxine, liothyronine
    - Acute Care
        - Levothyroxine, liothyronine
    - Chronic Care
        - Desiccated thyroid, levothyroxine, liothyronine

Main Indications or Uses
- Acute Care
    - Myxedema coma
        - Levothyroxine +/- liothyronine
- Chronic Care
    - Hypothyroidism
        - Desiccated thyroid, levothyroxine, liothyronine
    - Pituitary thyrotropin-stimulating hormone suppression
        - Levothyroxine

> **Fast Facts**
> - Synthetic T4 (or levothyroxine) is the drug of choice in the management of hypothyroidism. Dose adjustments should occur every 6-7 weeks when the TSH is at steady state for that dose.
> - The dose of levothyroxine should be increased by 20% to 30% on the same day the patient with hypothyroidism is found to be pregnant to prevent the risk of miscarriage or poor neurologic outcomes.

Mechanism of Action
- Ultimately, agents result in thyroid replacement.
- Desiccated thyroid: primarily T3, but also contains T4 and iodine.
- Levothyroxine: synthetic T4 (thyroxine) that is converted to its active metabolite T3 (triiodothyronine).
- Liothyronine: T3 hormone as replacement.

Primary Net Benefit
- Utilized to replace thyroid hormone in a hypothyroid state.
- Main Labs to Monitor:
    - Signs and symptoms of under or overtreatment.
    - TSH 6-8 weeks after initiation or dose changes, BMD periodically, and vital signs and cardiac symptoms at each visit.
    - Myxedema coma: TFTs every 1-2 days along with clinical response.
    - Pediatrics: TSH and free or total T4 at 2 and 4 weeks after initiation, every 1-2 months until 12 months, every 2-3 months from 1-3 years, then every 3-12 months; every 2 weeks after dose changes; monitor brain and growth development.
    - Pregnancy: TSH every 4 weeks until midgestation and once near 30 weeks, TSH every 2-4 weeks after initiation or dose changes

High-Yield Basic Pharmacology
- Liothyronine Only
    - Well-absorbed with a half-life of 0.75 days, which results in a faster steady state.
- Absorption
    - Erratic unless in a fasting state, which allows up to 80% oral absorption.
- Half-life Elimination
    - 6-10 days depending on thyroid state
    - Steady state achieved approximately 6 weeks after initiation or dose changes.
- Protein Binding
    - >99% protein bound to plasma proteins
- Metabolism
    - Hepatically metabolized to T3
- Drug Interactions

- Sucralfate, bile acid sequestrants, raloxifene, and calcium- or iron-containing products may reduce thyroid absorption and decrease the effect of replacement. Consider separating by 4 hours.
- Amiodarone, iodine-containing medications, estrogen derivatives, and lithium may decrease the effect of thyroid hormone replacement.
- Rifampin, phenobarbital, phenytoin, and carbamazepine can increase the metabolism of thyroxine.
- Furosemide, mefenamic acid, and salicylates can displace thyroid hormone from protein binding.
- Warfarin effects may be increased (elevated INR).
- Cardiac glycoside and theophylline concentrations may be reduced.
- Sodium iodide I131 effects may be decreased by thyroid replacement; discontinue T3 2 weeks before and T4 4 weeks before administration.

High-Yield Clinical Knowledge
- **General Clinical Pearls**
    - Levothyroxine is recommended as first-line therapy for hypothyroidism and in other hypothyroid states.
    - Current practice does not recommend combinations of levothyroxine/T3 over levothyroxine monotherapy for managing hypothyroidism.
    - Liothyronine is utilized off-label for improving mood in treatment-resistant depression.
- **Desiccated Thyroid**
    - Contains variable amounts of T4, T3, and other compounds more likely to cause cardiac toxicities.
    - It is porcine-derived, so there is a low potential risk for contamination with viruses.
- **Cardiovascular Disease**
    - Dosage forms containing active T3 increase potential for cardiac toxicities.
    - Initiate reduced doses and increase doses cautiously. Overtreatment can increase risk of adverse cardiac events in all patient populations.
    - Reduce dose or hold for 7 days if signs or symptoms occur.
- **Diabetes**
    - May worsen glycemic control with treatment due to increased elimination of insulin.
- **Osteoporosis**
    - Long-term treatment may reduce BMD and is likely dose-related. Use caution especially in postmenopausal women.
- **Benign Thyroid Nodules**
    - T4 use for suppression of TSH is not recommended.
    - Treatment should never be fully suppressive.
    - Avoid in postmenopausal women, elderly, CVD patients, osteoporosis patients, large thyroid nodules or long-standing goiters, or with low-normal TSH levels.
- **Adrenal Insufficiency**
    - Contraindicated in uncorrected adrenal insufficiency.
    - In adrenal insufficiency, glucocorticoid treatment should precede levothyroxine.
- **Obesity**
    - Should not be utilized for weight reduction due to potential toxicities, especially with larger doses
    - Normal daily dosing will not result in effective weight loss in euthyroid patients.
- **Geriatric Considerations**
    - Use lower doses in elderly because of increased risk of atrial fibrillation, other cardiac toxicities, and CV mortality.
    - T3 concentrations decrease in elderly, but it is not treated as a deficiency, which requires a lower starting dose.
- **Pregnancy**
    - Levothyroxine is preferred and recommended in pregnancy to avoid adverse outcomes.
    - If hypothyroid prior to pregnancy, increase dose 20-30% immediately and adjust dose every 4 weeks with close monitoring.
- **Lactation**
    - Levothyroxine is first-line, compatible with breastfeeding, and allows maintenance of supply.
- **Dosing**
    - Dosing should be patient-specific and based on clinical response in combination with TSH and/or T4 levels.

- Caution when interpreting orders to avoid 1000-fold overdose due to potential errors with mcg and mg units.
- T4 requirements correlate with lean body mass more so than total body weight.
- IV doses should be 70-80% of the oral dose (ATA recommends 75%).
- When converting to liothyronine from desiccated thyroid or levothyroxine, start a low dose and increase slowly, as other thyroid preparations will be present for several weeks.
  - **Administration**
    - PO should be administered in the morning 30-60 min before meals or at night 3-4 hours after the last meal.
    - IV can be administered at a maximum rate of 100 mcg/min.
  - **Bioequivalence**
    - Thyroid replacements are narrow therapeutic index drugs; any change in manufacturer or from brand to generic or vice versa should be followed up with monitoring.

High-Yield Core Evidence
- **Dosing Recommendations**
  - Demonstrated 25 mcg daily dose adjustments are often too much or too little; dosage forms were created in between to manage.
  - Clin Endocrinol 1988;28:325.
- **Pregnancy Recommendations**
  - Thyroid replacement in pregnant patients requires dose adjustments.
  - NEJM 1990;323:91.
- **T4/T3 Combination**
  - T4/T3 combination has mainly demonstrated more adverse effects compared to T4 monotherapy, but clinically, some patients benefit.
  - Major associations have recommended additional trials and outlined appropriate methods.
  - Thyroid Res 2018;11:1-11.
  - Thyroid 2021;31:156-182.

High-Yield Fast-Facts
- Levothyroxine can really be taken with or without food as long as the patient takes the dose consistently in the same way to avoid fluctuations.
- Levothyroxine can be administered IM as an off-label route.
- Levothyroxine can be given off-label for deceased organ donor management for hormonal resuscitation.
- Desiccated thyroid can be measured in grains (1 grain=65 mg).

HIGH-YIELD BOARD EXAM ESSENTIALS
- **CLASSIC AGENTS:** Desiccated thyroid, levothyroxine, liothyronine
- **DRUG CLASS:** Thyroid Replacements
- **INDICATIONS:** Hypothyroidism, myxedema coma, pituitary thyrotropin-stimulating hormone suppression
- **MECHANISM:** Replaces thyroid hormone in hypothyroid state.
- **SIDE EFFECTS:** Cardiac toxicity, glucose intolerance, BMD changes, hyperthyroid symptoms
- **CLINICAL PEARLS:**
  - Synthetic T4 hormone replacement is the drug of choice in hypothyroidism. Upon starting, change in dosage, or change in manufacturer, a TSH lab check will be needed in 6-7 weeks to determine control.
  - Dosage forms containing active T3 increase potential for cardiac toxicities. Initiate reduced doses and increase doses cautiously. Overtreatment can increase risk of adverse cardiac events (i.e., AF or high output HF) in some patient populations.
  - Pregnant patients will need much higher doses of levothyroxine immediately to avoid risk of miscarriage, pre-term delivery, or poor CNS development of the baby.

Table: Drug Class Summary

Thyroid Replacements Drug Class Review			
High-Yield Med Reviews			
Mechanism of Action: replaces thyroid hormone in hypothyroid state.			
Class Effects: cardiac toxicities, BMD changes, monitor dosage forms for bioequivalence, T4 preferred			
Generic Name	**Brand Name**	**Main Indication(s) or Uses**	**Notes**

Desiccated thyroid	Armour Thyroid	• Hypothyroidism	• **Dosing (Adult):** 30-32.5 mg/d
			  – Increase 15-16.25 mg/d every 2-3 weeks
			  – With CVD: 15-16.25 mg/d
			• **Dosing (Peds):** 1.2-6 mg/kg/dose based on age from 1 month-17 years
			• **CYP450 Interactions:** None
			• **Renal or Hepatic Dose Adjustments:** None
			• **Dosage Forms:** 15, 30, 60, 90, 120, 180, 240, 300 mg

Levothyroxine	Euthyrox
	Levoxyl
	Synthroid
	Tirosint
	Tirosint-SOL
	Unithroid
		• Hypothyroidism
		• Pituitary TSH suppression
		• Myxedema coma (IV)
			• **Dosing (Adult):** 1.6 mcg/kg/d, including new diagnosis in pregnancy
			  – >60 yrs or with CVD: 12.5-50 mcg/d
			  – Increase by 12.5 mcg-25 mcg every 4-6 weeks
			  – Myxedema coma (concomitant glucocorticoid +/-liothyronine): 200-400 mcg IV slow bolus, then 50-100 mcg daily
			• **Dosing (Peds):** 4-15 mcg/kg/dose based on age from 1 month-12 years; higher doses at younger ages; >12 years: use adult dosing
			• **CYP450 Interactions:** None
			• **Renal or Hepatic Dose Adjustments:** None
			• **Dosage Forms:** Capsules & PO solution (13, 25, 50, 75, 88, 100, 112, 125, 137, 150, 175, 200 mcg); IV (100 mcg/5mL, 200 mcg/5mL, 500 mcg/5mL); Tablets (25, 50, 75, 88, 100, 112, 125, 137 150, 175, 200, 300 mcg)

Liothyronine	Cytomel
	Triostat
		• Hypothyroidism	• **Dosing (Adult):** 25 mcg daily; increase by 25 mcg every 1-2 weeks
			  – CVD: 5 mcg daily, then increase by 5 mcg every 2 weeks
			  – Myxedema coma in combination with levothyroxine: 5-20 mcg LD, then 2.5-10 mcg Q8H
			  – Changing from desiccated thyroid or levothyroxine: stop other agent; start low dose liothyronine and increase slowly.
			• **Dosing (Peds):** 20-75 mcg daily based on age from infant-17 years; doses increase with age.
			• **CYP450 Interactions:** None
			• **Renal or Hepatic Dose Adjustments:** None
			• **Dosage Forms:** IV (10 mcg/mL); Tablet (5, 25, 50 mcg)

ENDOCRINE – VASOPRESSIN RECEPTOR ANTAGONISTS AND DEMECLOCYCLINE

Drug Class
- Demeclocycline and Vasopressin Receptor Antagonists
- Agents:
  - Acute & Care
    - Demeclocycline
    - Conivaptan
    - Tolvaptan

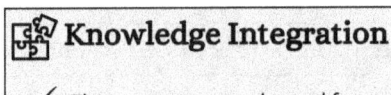

Knowledge Integration
- ✓ These agents are only used for SIADH when other treatments (e.g., free water restriction) fail to correct the problem.

Main Indications or Uses
- Acute & Chronic Care
  - Autosomal dominant polycystic kidney disease
  - Euvolemic or hypervolemic hyponatremia
  - SIADH

Mechanism of Action
- Demeclocycline
  - Tetracycline antibiotic but inhibits renal tubular arginine vasopressin activity, increasing free water excretion.
- Conivaptan and Tolvaptan
  - Vasopressin 2 (aquaporin 2) receptor antagonists.

Primary Net Benefit
- AVP receptor antagonists effectively correct hyponatremia, but their effects are short-lived and present safety concerns related to rapid sodium correction, hepatic injury, and drug interactions.
- Main Labs to Monitor:
  - Serum sodium (baseline, q1-4hours during the acute phase, then daily, weekly)
  - Liver enzymes (AST/ALT, alkaline phosphatase) (baseline then at 2 and 4 weeks)
  - Liver function (INR/PT, albumin, protein, bilirubin) (baseline then at 2 and 4 weeks)

High-Yield Basic Pharmacology
- Vasopressin Receptor Selectivity
  - Vasopressin receptor antagonism produces free-water loss (aquaresis) and increases serum sodium concentrations.
  - Conivaptan is a nonselective V1a and V2 receptor antagonist.
  - Tolvaptan is a selective V2 receptor antagonist.
- Hepatic Oxidation
  - Tolvaptan is extensively metabolized by CYP3A4 and is a substrate of and inhibits P-glycoprotein.
  - Conivaptan is a substrate and inhibitor of CYP3A4.
  - Numerous medications may lead to drug-drug interactions, including potent CYP3A4 inhibitors (clarithromycin, protease inhibitors, and ketoconazole), CYP3A4 inducers (phenytoin, phenobarbital, St. John's Wort), and P-glycoprotein substrates (cyclosporine, digoxin, diltiazem, tacrolimus).

High-Yield Clinical Knowledge
- Chronic Management
  - Demeclocycline, conivaptan, and tolvaptan should not be used to immediately manage acute hyponatremia.
  - Tolvaptan's onset of action is up to 4 hours and has not been evaluated thoroughly in serum sodium concentrations below 120 mEq/L.
- Limited Duration and Effects
  - Tolvaptan and conivaptan are effective interventions to correct hyponatremia in euvolemic or hypovolemic scenarios.

- Furthermore, their effects are short-lived as tolvaptan is limited to 30 days of therapy, and hyponatremia returns with drug discontinuation.
- Conivaptan is only available as an IV dosage form and should not be used for more than four days.
- Vaptan therapy is limited due to the increased risk of liver injury with continued therapy beyond the recommended time.
- **Gradual Sodium Replacement**
    - Correction of sodium levels in patients with hyponatremia should not exceed 10 to 12 mEq/L in a 24-hour period.
        - In patients with symptomatic hyponatremia (altered mental status, seizures, or neurological deficits), rapid correction of sodium at a rate of 2 mEq/L/hour of the sodium deficit can be replaced until control of seizures, resolution of neurological deficit or more than 12 to 15 mEq/L replaced per 24-hour period.
    - A black boxed warning exists with tolvaptan, as there is a risk of rapid sodium correction.
    - The clinical sequelae of rapid sodium correction are central pontine demyelination.
    - Tolvaptan must only be started or resumed in an acute care setting where serum sodium can be readily monitored.
- **Demeclocycline Induced DI**
    - The action of demeclocycline on the inhibition of renal tubular vasopressin activity is essentially a drug-induced nephrogenic diabetes insipidus used to treat SIADH.
    - Other causes of drug-induced nephrogenic diabetes insipidus include cisplatin, clozapine, colchicine, foscarnet, and lithium.
- **Anuric Patients**
    - Conivaptan and tolvaptan are contraindicated in stage 4 or 5 chronic kidney disease patients.
- **Adverse Events**
    - As a result of the potent free-water losses, patients on conivaptan or tolvaptan therapy are at risk of dehydration, volume depletion, hypotension, pyrexia, and xerostomia.
    - Conivaptan and tolvaptan have also been associated with hyperkalemia and hyperglycemia due to free-water losses.

High-Yield Core Evidence
- **SALT 1 & SALT 2**
    - This was a single publication of two multicenter, double-blind, placebo-controlled trials that randomized patients with euvolemic or hypovolemic hyponatremia to receive either oral tolvaptan 15 mg daily (and increased to 30 mg then 60 mg daily, if necessary) or placebo.
    - Tolvaptan led to a significant improvement in the primary outcome of the change in the average daily area under the curve for the serum sodium concentration from baseline to day four and the change from baseline to day 30.
    - This correlated clinically with the improvement of patients with mild or marked hyponatremia who received tolvaptan therapy.
    - However, within one week of tolvaptan discontinuation, hyponatremia recurred.
    - Tolvaptan was associated with an increased incidence of adverse effects, including thirst, dry mouth, and increased urination.
    - The authors concluded that among patients with euvolemic or hypervolemic hyponatremia, tolvaptan, an oral vasopressin V2-receptor antagonist, effectively increased serum sodium concentrations at day four and day thirty. (N Engl J Med. 2006;355:2099–2112.)
- **EVEREST**
    - This was a single publication of two multicenter, double-blind, event-driven, placebo-controlled trials of hospitalized patients with heart failure who were randomized to receive either tolvaptan 30 mg daily or placebo in addition to standard therapy.
    - There was no difference between groups concerning all-cause mortality and cardiovascular death or hospitalization for heart failure.
    - Tolvaptan was non-inferior to placebo concerning all-cause mortality.
    - There was no difference in any secondary outcome, including cardiovascular mortality, cardiovascular death or hospitalization, and worsening heart failure.

- However, tolvaptan significantly improved day one patient-assessed dyspnea, day one bodyweight, and day seven edema.
- The authors concluded that tolvaptan initiated for acute treatment of patients hospitalized with heart failure did not affect long-term mortality or heart failure-related morbidity. (JAMA. 2007 Mar 28;297(12):1319-31.)

High-Yield Fast-Fact
- **Lithium**
    - Lithium affects sodium, similar to demeclocycline, by increasing free water excretion.
    - However, it should not be used to treat hyponatremia due to its narrow therapeutic index, safety, and availability of suitable alternatives.

HIGH-YIELD BOARD EXAM ESSENTIALS
- **CLASSIC AGENTS:** Demeclocycline, conivaptan, tolvaptan
- **DRUG CLASS:** Demeclocycline and Vasopressin Receptor Antagonists
- **INDICATIONS:** Autosomal dominant polycystic kidney disease, euvolemic or hypervolemic hyponatremia, SIADH
- **MECHANISM:** Demeclocycline - inhibits renal tubular arginine vasopressin activity, increasing free water excretion. Conivaptan and Tolvaptan - Vasopressin 2 (aquaporin-2) receptor antagonists.
- **SIDE EFFECTS:** Hyperkalemia, hyperglycemia, dehydration, volume depletion, hypotension, pyrexia, xerostomia
- **CLINICAL PEARLS:**
    - These agents should only be considered in patients who have failed free water restriction when managing SIADH.
    - The action of demeclocycline (an old tetracycline antibiotic) on the inhibition of renal tubular vasopressin activity is essentially a drug-induced nephrogenic diabetes insipidus used to treat SIADH.

Table: Drug Class Summary

| | Demeclocycline and Vasopressin Receptor Antagonists - Drug Class Review
High-Yield Med Reviews |

Mechanism of Action:
Demeclocycline - inhibits renal tubular arginine vasopressin activity, increasing free water excretion.
Conivaptan and Tolvaptan - Vasopressin 2 (aquaporin-2) receptor antagonists.

Class Effects: *AVP receptor antagonists are effective means of correcting hyponatremia, but their effects are short-lived and present safety concerns related to rapid sodium correction, hepatic injury, and drug interactions.*

Generic Name	Brand Name	Main Indication(s) or Uses	Notes
Demeclocycline	Detravis, Meciclin, Mexocine, Clortetrin	• SIADH	• **Dosing (Adult):** – Oral: 600 to 1,200 mg/day divided q6h • **Dosing (Peds):** – Oral: 7 to 13 mg/kg/day divided q6-12h • **CYP450 Interactions:** None • **Renal or Hepatic Dose Adjustments:** None • **Dosage Forms:** Oral (tablet)
Conivaptan	Vaprisol	• Euvolemic or hypervolemic hyponatremia	• **Dosing (Adult):** – IV: 20 mg over 30 minutes, then 0.83 to 1.7 mg/hour for 2-4 days – Maximum 40 mg/24hours • **Dosing (Peds):** – Not routinely used • **CYP450 Interactions:** Substrate CYP3A4; Inhibits CYP3A4 • **Renal or Hepatic Dose Adjustments:** – GFR < 30 mL/minute: not recommended – Anuria: Contraindicated – Child-Pugh class C: Use with caution • **Dosage Forms:** IV (solution)
Tolvaptan	Jynarque Samsca	• Autosomal dominant polycystic kidney disease • Euvolemic or hypervolemic hyponatremia	• **Dosing (Adult):** – Oral: 60 mg/day in divided doses, titrated to 120 mg/day in divided doses to urine osmolality less than 300 mOsm/kg – Oral: 15 to 60 mg daily for maximum 30 days • **Dosing (Peds):** – Not routinely used • **CYP450 Interactions:** Substrate CYP3A4, P-gp • **Renal or Hepatic Dose Adjustments:** – GFR < 10 mL/minute: not recommended – AST/ALT > 3x upper limit of normal, or underlying liver disease: not recommended • **Dosage Forms:** Oral (tablet)

2025

A COMPREHENSIVE *RAPID REVIEW*

NAPLEX

Pharmacology & Drug Classes

Gastroenterology

GASTROENTEROLOGY – 5-ASA DERIVATIVES

Drug Class
- 5-Aminosalicylic Acid (5-ASA) Derivatives
- Agents
  - Active Form of 5-ASA
    - Mesalamine
  - Prodrugs Converted to 5-ASA
    - Azo-Bonded = Balsalazide, olsalazine
    - Non-Azo-Bonded = Sulfasalazine

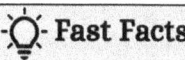 **Fast Facts**

✓ The most common 5-ASA used in clinical practice is mesalamine. This is due, in part, to the availability of a wide variety of dosage forms to provide the patient with treatment options specific to their symptoms and degree of disease.

Main Indications or Uses
- Inflammatory Bowel Diseases:
  - Crohn's Disease
  - Ulcerative Colitis
- Rheumatoid Arthritis (only sulfasalazine)

Mechanism of Action
- 5-ASA has localized or targeted anti-inflammatory effects within the colonic mucosa within the lumen of the GI tract by modulating the formation of pro-inflammatory mediators derived from arachidonic acid.
  - The release of 5-ASA or topical application of the 5-ASA is highly influenced by the dosage formulation being used.
    - For example, mesalamine has different types of coating to facilitate the release of the medication in specific locations within the large intestine, where patients are known to have areas of inflammation. In addition, the release of 5-ASA from the dosage formulation can, in part, be influenced by the changes in pH of the intestinal lumen.

Primary Net Benefit
- Reduce the symptoms of inflammatory bowel disorder with significant systemic effects by providing localized, topical effects within the GI tract.

High-Yield Basic Pharmacology
- The location and severity of intestinal inflammation may influence which dosage forms a patient can take. The location of lesions is typically determined by EGD, pill endoscopy, and/or colonoscopy.
  - Oral dosage forms:
    - Administered by mouth but are formulated with coatings to affect the release of 5-ASA to a specific target or location within the intestine.
  - Enema dosage formulations:
    - Administered rectally (lying in lateral position), which can provide treatment up to the splenic flexure.
  - Suppositories:
    - Administered rectally and can provide topical treatment to the rectum only.
- The azo-bonded prodrugs must have the azo bond cleaved so that the 5-ASA (active product) can provide an anti-inflammatory effect. The breaking or cleavage of this bond can occur by bacteria specifically located in the colon.
  - Olsalazine consists of two 5-ASA moieties linked by an azo bond, whereas balsalazide has an inert carrier molecule linked to 5-ASA.
  - Sulfasalazine is 5-ASA linked to sulfapyridine but not by an azo-bond.

High-Yield Clinical Knowledge
- **Which IBD Benefits More?**
  - 5-ASA derivatives are considered first-line therapy for mild Crohn's disease or mild to moderate UC, traditionally defined as fewer than 4-6 bowel movements per day, mild-moderate rectal bleeding, absence of systemic symptoms, and low overall inflammatory burden.

- They can help with active flares as well as inducing remission for UC. Compliance with 5-ASA products during remission is essential for preventing flares (i.e., this is a chronic treatment, not intermittent use).
- Most patients with mild to moderate UC respond to 5-ASA products and gain clinical remission with their use. However, the remaining are more complicated cases warranting other immunomodulating treatments.
- 5-ASA derivatives that have azo-bonds (i.e., balsalazide and olsalazine) work primarily in the colon or large intestine, which is why they are more effective and approved for UC treatment and not Crohn's disease.
- **Side Effects of 5-ASA Products**
    - The sulfapyridine carrier molecule of sulfasalazine has no therapeutic benefit in IBD and instead contributes to most of the side effects experienced by patients. Common side effects include GI intolerance, male infertility due to a reversible decrease in sperm production, and interference of folate absorption. Furthermore, patients with "sulfa" allergies should avoid this drug.
        - For this reason, mesalamine does not contain a sulfa group and is the active drug only (i.e., 5-ASA) and is more commonly used.
        - Women of child-bearing age who want to get pregnant and take sulfasalazine should take 2 mg of folate per day.
        - If GI side effects result in intolerance, consider reducing the dose of sulfasalazine by 50%.
- **Dosage Formulations and UC**
    - Enemas and suppository dosage formulations are primarily helpful for UC, given the dosage forms' ability to get to the site of inflammation. In addition, since the inflammation in UC starts at the rectum and moves proximally in the large intestine, they can be helpful. In contrast, Crohn's disease occurs as skip lesions anywhere from the oropharynx to the rectum.
        - Formulations of mesalamine include Canasa (rectal suppositories) and Rowasa (rectal suspension).
- **Rheumatoid Arthritis**
    - Only sulfasalazine is used in the treatment of Rheumatoid arthritis. Ironically, the sulfapyridine component exerts the therapeutic effect, which may be why the other 5-ASA products are not used.

High-Yield Core Evidence
- One of the original articles aiding in the severity definition of UC was the Truelove and Witt's criteria.
    - Br Med J 1955;2:1041-8.

High-Yield Fast-Facts
- The underlying cause of IBD is not fully known. What is known is that immunomodulating drugs help control the disease. However, what is causing the immune system to be overly aggravated in the colonic mucosa is unknown.
- Patients with UC are at risk of toxic megacolon, whereas Crohn's disease is only associated with the formation of fistulas.
- Patients with UC are at increased risk of colon cancer and need colonoscopies sooner than patients without UC.

HIGH-YIELD BOARD EXAM ESSENTIALS
- **CLASSIC AGENTS:** Balsalazide, mesalamine, olsalazine
- **DRUG CLASS:** 5-ASA Derivatives
- **INDICATIONS:** Crohn's Disease, Ulcerative Colitis
- **MECHANISM:** Intestinal mucosal inflammation by reducing the release of pro-inflammatory mediators.
- **SIDE EFFECTS:** GI side effects, infertility due to reversible reduced sperm production (sulfasalazine only)
- **CLINICAL PEARLS:** These agents have greater efficacy at lower doses in ulcerative colitis because of how these drugs work to provide targeted topical therapy. With Crohn's disease having skip lesions and involvement outside of the large intestine where these agents work, the overall efficacy is less. Several agents come in multiple dosage formulations that allow for patient specific use based on the extent of disease, especially in patients with ulcerative colitis.

Table: Drug Class Summary

5-Aminosalicylic Acid (5-ASA) Drug Class Review High-Yield Med Reviews			
Mechanism of Action: *Intestinal mucosal inflammation by reducing the release of pro-inflammatory mediators.*			
Class Effects: *The dosage formulation used in part is influenced by intestinal inflammation location.*			
Active Drugs of 5-ASA			
Generic Name	**Brand Name**	**Main Indication(s) or Uses**	**Notes**
Mesalamine	Apriso Asacol HD Canasa Delzicol Lialda Pentasa Rowasa	▪ Crohn's Disease ▪ Ulcerative Colitis	▪ No carrier or linked molecule. Active form only. ▪ **Dosing (Adult):** Dose depends on dosage formulation used, but doses up to 4.8 g/day ▪ **Dosing (Peds):** Dose depends on dosage formulation. ▪ **CYP450 Interactions:** None ▪ **Renal or Hepatic Dose Adjustments:** None ▪ **Dosage Forms:** Capsule (Delayed & Extended Release), Enema, Rectal Kit, Suppository, Tablets
Prodrugs Converted to 5-ASA			
Azo Bonded *(also called "diazo-bonded" to allow for release in the colon)*			
Balsalazide	Colazal	▪ Ulcerative Colitis	▪ Inert carrier molecule azo-bound to 5-ASA ▪ **Dosing (Adult):** 1.5 to 3.3 g twice a day ▪ **Dosing (Peds):** 2.25 g three times per day or 750 mg three times per day. ▪ **CYP450 Interactions:** None ▪ **Renal or Hepatic Dose Adjustments:** None ▪ **Dosage Forms:** Capsule, Tablets
Olsalazine	Dipentum	▪ Ulcerative Colitis	▪ Two 5-ASA moieties linked by an azo bond ▪ **Dosing (Adult):** 1 to 3 g per day in 2-4 divided doses ▪ **Dosing (Peds):** None ▪ **CYP450 Interactions:** None ▪ **Renal or Hepatic Dose Adjustments:** None ▪ **Dosage Forms:** Capsule
Non-Azo Bonded			
Sulfasalazine	Azulfidine	▪ Crohn's Disease ▪ Ulcerative Colitis ▪ Rheumatoid Arthritis ▪ Psoriasis / Psoriatic Arthritis	▪ Sulfapyridine linked to 5-ASA without an azo-bond. ▪ Avoid in patients allergic to sulfa ▪ **Classic Side Effects:** Infertility in men, reduction in folate absorption, and GI intolerance. ▪ **Dosing (Adult):** 2-4 g/d in 3-4 divided doses. If GI intolerance, decrease dose by 50%. ▪ **Dosing (Peds):** 30-70 mg/kg/day in 3-6 divided doses ▪ **CYP450 Interactions:** None ▪ **Renal or Hepatic Dose Adjustments:** None ▪ **Dosage Forms:** Tablet (Regular & Delayed Release)

GI – ADSORBENTS AND ANTISECRETORY AGENTS

Drug Class
- **Adsorbents and Antisecretory Agents**
- **Agents:**
  - **Acute Care**
    - Bismuth subsalicylate
    - Bismuth subcitrate
  - **Chronic Care**
    - Crofelemer
    - Methylcellulose
    - Polycarbophil
    - Psyllium

> **Fast Facts**
> ✓ Bismuth subsalicylate can turn the surface of the tongue and stool black in color. Both are reversible upon discontinuation.

Main Indications or Uses
- **Acute Care**
  - Constipation
    - Bismuth subsalicylate
    - Bismuth subcitrate
    - Polycarbophil
    - Psyllium
  - Diarrhea
    - Bismuth subsalicylate
    - Bismuth subcitrate
    - Polycarbophil
    - Psyllium
  - Dyspepsia
    - Bismuth subsalicylate
    - Bismuth subcitrate
  - Helicobacter pylori eradication
    - Bismuth subsalicylate
    - Bismuth subcitrate
- **Chronic Care**
  - HIV related diarrhea
    - Crofelemer
  - Soluble fiber supplementation
    - Methylcellulose
    - Polycarbophil
    - Psyllium

Mechanism of Action
- **Bismuth Compounds**
  - Bismuth counteracts pepsin and gastric acid's effects on ulcers and erosions by increasing bicarbonate (increasing pH) and stimulating prostaglandin and mucus production.
  - Although it inhibits intestinal and gastric prostaglandin secretion, salicylates also increase chloride secretion.
- **Crofelemer**
  - Inhibitor of cystic fibrosis transmembrane conductance regulator (CFTR) causing inhibition of chloride-rich secretion into the GI tract and a slowing of intestinal transit.
- **Methylcellulose, Polycarbophil, Psyllium**
  - Forms of soluble fiber that absorb water into the intestine, promoting peristalsis.

Primary Net Benefit
- Over-the-counter products are used for GI disorders, including constipation and diarrhea.
- Main Labs to Monitor:
    - No routine monitoring

High-Yield Basic Pharmacology
- **Formulation**
    - Bismuth subsalicylate is a suspension of trivalent bismuth and salicylate in a mixture of aluminum silicate clay.
    - An alternative, bismuth subcitrate potassium, is also available but is a prescription-only product.
- **Bulk Forming Agents**
    - Methylcellulose, polycarbophil, and psyllium are natural or synthetic agents that increase stool water content, increasing fecal bulk.

High-Yield Clinical Knowledge
- **Stool Discoloration**
    - Bismuth compounds cause a darkening of stools, including blackening of the stool.
    - This discoloration may be confused with GI (melena), but patients on anticoagulants should be educated on other signs and symptoms of GI bleeding.
    - A similar discoloration of the tongue can also occur.
- **Cardiovascular Risk Reduction**
    - Psyllium dietary supplementation may reduce cardiovascular disease risk and can be added to most patients with primary or secondary cardiac disease.
    - The daily target dose is 30 g of soluble fiber, challenging to ingest and tolerate if initial slow titration is not followed.
    - Dietary supplementation of psyllium fiber products does not affect the absorption of most medications.
- **Antimicrobial Action**
    - Bismuth possesses direct antimicrobial activity, particularly against Helicobacter pylori, and binding effectively to enterotoxins associated with traveler's diarrhea pathogens.
- **Helicobacter pylori Treatment**
    - Bismuth-containing compounds are a component of triple or quadruple therapy for H. pylori infection.
        - Prolonged therapy with excessive doses may result in salicylate toxicity and rarely in encephalopathy.

High-Yield Core Evidence
- **Psyllium on LDL**
    - This was a meta-analysis of the effect of psyllium on LDL cholesterol, non-HDL cholesterol, and apolipoprotein B (apo B).
    - The analysis included 28 trials with 1924 study subjects.
    - Psyllium supplementation of 10.2 g (median dose) significantly reduced LDL cholesterol, non-HDL cholesterol, and apoB.
    - The authors concluded that psyllium fiber effectively improves conventional and alternative lipids markers, potentially delaying the process of atherosclerosis-associated CVD risk in those with or without hypercholesterolemia. (Am J Clin Nutr. 2018 Nov 1;108(5):922-932.)

High-Yield Fast-Facts
- **Psyllium Origin**
    - Psyllium was once derived from the Plantago herb's seed, whereas most modern products contain a component of the Plantago herb.
- **Erythema of the 9th Day**
    - Bismuth has been associated with the so-called "Erythema of the 9th day," a self-resolving rash first attributed to arsphenamine used to treat syphilis in the early 1910s.

Table: Drug Class Summary

Adsorbents and Antisecretory Agents - Drug Class Review
High-Yield Med Reviews

Mechanism of Action:
Bismuth increases bicarbonate (thus increasing pH) and stimulates prostaglandin and mucus production.
Crofelemer - Inhibitor of CFTR and a slowing of intestinal transit.
Methylcellulose, Polycarbophil, Psyllium - Absorbs water into the intestine, promoting peristalsis.

Class Effects: Over-the-counter products are used for GI disorders, including constipation and diarrhea.

Generic Name	Brand Name	Main Indication(s) or Uses	Notes

Bismuth subsalicylate	Bismatrol
	Diotame
	Pepto-Bismol
		- Diarrhea
		- Dyspepsia
		- Helicobacter pylori eradication
			- **Dosing (Adult):**
			  – Oral: 300 to 1,050 mg q30-60 minutes
			  – Maximum 4,200 mg/day
			- **Dosing (Peds):**
			  – Oral: 87 to 262 mg q30-60 minutes up to 1,050 mg/dose (age and weight dependant)
			  – Maximum 8 doses/day
			- **CYP450 Interactions:** None
			- **Renal or Hepatic Dose Adjustments:** None
			- **Dosage Forms:** Oral (suspension, tablet)

Bismuth subcitrate	Pylera (bismuth subcitrate, metronidazole, tetracycline)	- H. pylori-associated duodenal ulcer	- **Dosing (Adult):**
			  – Oral: 3 capsules 4 times daily after meals and at bedtime x 10 days
			- **Dosing (Peds):**
			  – Not routinely used
			- **CYP450 Interactions:** None
			- **Renal or Hepatic Dose Adjustments:**
			  – Child-Pugh class C – Not recommended
			- **Dosage Forms:** Oral (suspension, tablet)

Crofelemer	Mytesi	- HIV related diarrhea	- **Dosing (Adult):**
			  – Oral: 125 mg BID
			- **Dosing (Peds):**
			  – Not routinely used
			- **CYP450 Interactions:** None
			- **Renal or Hepatic Dose Adjustments:** None
			- **Dosage Forms:** Oral (tablet)

Methylcellulose	Citrucel	- Constipation	- **Dosing (Adult):**
			  – Oral: 2 g in 240 mL water as needed up to 3 times daily
			- **Dosing (Peds):**
			  – Oral: 1 g in 240 mL water as needed up to 3 times daily
			- **CYP450 Interactions:** None
			- **Renal or Hepatic Dose Adjustments:** None
			- **Dosage Forms:** Oral (powder, tablet)

| \multicolumn{4}{c}{**Adsorbents and Antisecretory Agents - Drug Class Review**} |
| \multicolumn{4}{c}{High-Yield Med Reviews} |
Generic Name	Brand Name	Main Indication(s) or Uses	Notes

Polycarbophil	Fiber Laxative, FiberCon	- Constipation or Diarrhea	- **Dosing (Adult):**
			  - Oral: 1,250 mg q6-24h
			- **Dosing (Peds):**
			  - Oral: 625 mg q6-24h
			- **CYP450 Interactions:** None
			- **Renal or Hepatic Dose Adjustments:** None
			- **Dosage Forms:** Oral (tablet)

Psyllium	Konsyl, Metamucil, Mucilin, Natural Fiber	- Constipation or Diarrhea	- **Dosing (Adult):**
			  - Oral: 2.5 to 30 g per day in divided doses
			- **Dosing (Peds):**
			  - Oral: 1.25 to 30 g per day in divided doses
			- **CYP450 Interactions:** None
			- **Renal or Hepatic Dose Adjustments:** None
			- **Dosage Forms:** Oral (capsule, packet, powder, wafer)

HIGH-YIELD BOARD EXAM ESSENTIALS

- **CLASSIC AGENTS:** Bismuth subsalicylate, bismuth subcitrate, crofelemer, methylcellulose, polycarbophil, psyllium
- **DRUG CLASS:** Adsorbents and antisecretory agents
- **INDICATIONS:** Constipation, diarrhea, dyspepsia, Helicobacter pylori eradication, HIV related diarrhea, soluble fiber supplementation
- **MECHANISM:** Bismuth increases bicarbonate (thus increasing pH) and stimulating prostaglandin and mucus production. Crofelemer - Inhibitor of CFTR and a slowing of intestinal transit. Methylcellulose, Polycarbophil, Psyllium - Absorbs water into the intestine, promoting peristalsis.
- **SIDE EFFECTS:** Stool discoloration, constipation, flatulence
- **CLINICAL PEARLS:**
  - Bismuth compounds cause a darkening of stools, including blackening of the stool. This discoloration may be confused with GI (melena), but patients on anticoagulants should be educated or other signs and symptoms of GI bleeding.
  - A similar, reversible, discoloration of the tongue can also occur.

GI – HISTAMINE H2 RECEPTOR ANTAGONISTS

Drug Class
- Histamine H2 Receptor Antagonists
- Agents:
    - **Acute & Chronic Care**
        - Cimetidine
        - Famotidine
        - Nizatidine

Main Indications or Uses
- **Acute & Chronic**
    - Dyspepsia
    - Gastroesophageal reflux disease
    - Helicobacter pylori
    - Peptic ulcer disease

 Fast Facts
- Unlike PPIs, tolerance, resulting in breakthrough of acid secretion, can develop with the use of H2 receptor antagonists.
- In general, these drugs are dosed twice a day, require renal dosing, and are less effective compared to PPI at raising the pH > 4 where gastric healing occurs most.
- Ranitidine (Zantac) is no longer on the market due to risk of possible carcinogen exposure.

Mechanism of Action
- Competitive inhibition of the parietal cell histamine-2 receptor, preventing gastric acid secretion.

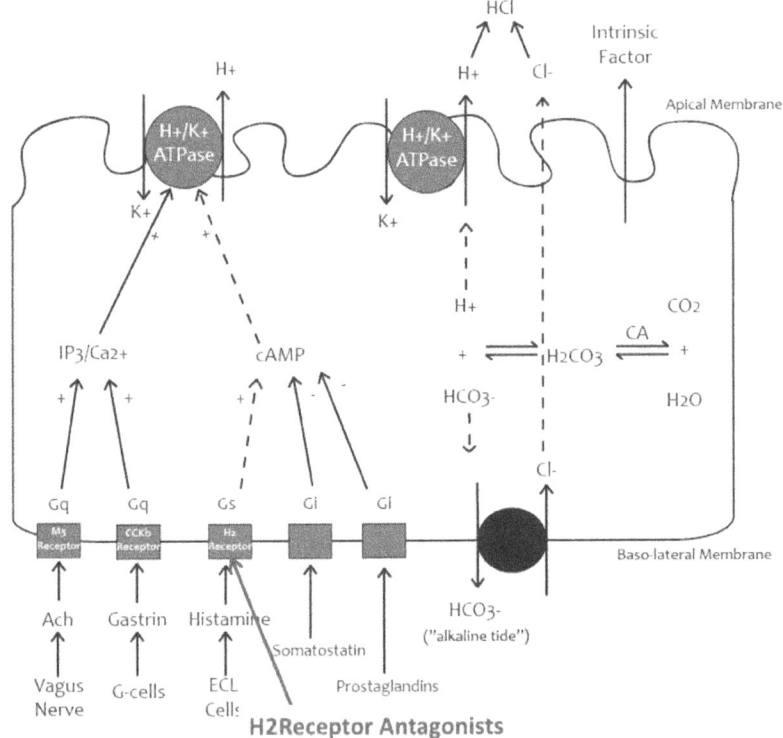

Primary Net Benefit
- Cornerstone therapy for gastroesophageal reflux disease and available as over-the-counter agents for dyspepsia.
- Main Labs to Monitor:
    - CBC (if signs or symptoms of thrombocytopenia, anemia, neutropenia)
    - SCr
    - Vitamin B12 (with long-term use ≥ 2 years.

Gastroenterology

High-Yield Basic Pharmacology
- **H2 Blockade**
  - H2RAs are highly selective and competitive inhibitors of parietal cell histamine-2 receptors responsible for both basal and meal-stimulated acid secretion.
- **Gastric Acid Suppression**
  - All H2RAs reduce gastric acid secretion by between 60 – 70% in a given 24-hour period.
    - However, nocturnal gastric acid secretion is inhibited to a more considerable degree since this gastric acid secretion is dependent on histamine.
  - Requires separation of doses for drugs requiring an acidic pH for efficacy.
- **Renal Clearance in Elderly**
  - Elderly patients have up to 50% reduced clearance of H2RAs independent of renal clearance.

High-Yield Clinical Knowledge
- **Renal Dose Adjustment**
  - All available H2RAs require dose adjustments in the setting of renal impairment.
    - Independent of renal function, elderly patients (over the age of 65 years) also have a decrease in H2RA drug clearance by as much as 50%.
  - These patients may be at increased risk of Clostridoides difficile infection and CNS effects (confusion).
  - Patients are also at risk of QT prolongation.
- **Cimetidine Drug Interactions**
  - Cimetidine is a potent inhibitor of P-glycoprotein and an inhibitor of CYP 1A2, 2C19, 2D6, and 3A4.
  - Numerous clinically relevant interactions exist, including narrow therapeutic agents such as theophylline, phenytoin, warfarin, phenytoin, calcium channel blockers, and beta-blockers.
  - Furthermore, cimetidine, as with all H2RAs, can decrease the absorption of protease inhibitors, requiring separation of drug administration to facilitate adequate absorption.
- **Common Indications**
  - H2RAs are used for a wide range of indications that span both prescription use and OTC use.
    - OTC indications - Dyspepsia
    - Rx indications - H. pylori infection/Peptic ulcer disease, GERD, stress ulcer prophylaxis.
- **Alcohol Dehydrogenase Inhibition**
  - Cimetidine inhibits alcohol dehydrogenase and can significantly decrease the rate of elimination of alcohol.
  - In the case of ethanol, alternative metabolic pathways via CYP2E1 are limited in capacity, and patients can quickly experience the toxic and inebriating effects of ethanol at much lower doses/volumes than their average perceived tolerance level.
- **Duration of Therapy**
  - For GERD treatment, H2RAs may be continued for a prolonged duration of therapy, whereas for duodenal ulcer treatment, treatment is limited to 6 weeks.
  - Patients taking OTC products for extended periods or at excessive doses should be referred to primary care for re-evaluation of their dyspepsia.
- **Serum Creatinine Changes with Cimetidine**
  - Cimetidine is associated with an increase in SCr and, therefore, CrCl due to the competitive inhibition of cimetidine with creatinine for active tubular secretion.
  - The actual underlying renal function is not changed, and serum creatinine elevations return to baseline after cimetidine discontinuation.
- **Gastritis and Tolerance**
  - Other pathways of acid secretion can lead to escape acid production leading to gastritis and tolerance with H2RAs; these do not occur with PPIs.

High-Yield Core Evidence
- **FAMOUS Trial**

- This was a multicenter, double-blind, placebo-controlled phase III trial that randomized adult patients taking aspirin 75–325 mg/day with or without other cardioprotective drugs and without ulcers or erosive esophagitis on endoscopy at baseline to either famotidine 20 mg twice daily or placebo.
- Patients randomized to famotidine experienced significantly fewer new ulcers in the stomach or duodenum or erosive esophagitis at 12 weeks after randomization than patients randomized to placebo.
- There were fewer adverse events in the famotidine group than in the placebo group.
- The authors concluded that famotidine is useful in preventing gastric and duodenal ulcers and erosive esophagitis in patients taking low-dose aspirin. (Lancet. 2009;374(9684):119–125.)

- **PEPTIC**
  - This was a multicenter, open-label, cluster cross-over, institution-level intervention, registry trial that randomized patients requiring invasive mechanical ventilation within 24 hours of ICU admission to receive either PPI or H2RA prophylaxis strategies.
  - There was no difference between groups concerning the primary outcome of all-cause mortality within 90 days during the index hospitalization.
  - However, the 95% confidence interval included 1.0, and the p-value of this difference was 0.054, favoring PPI use.
  - Furthermore, there was a significantly lower incidence of clinically meaningful upper gastrointestinal bleeding among patients receiving a PPI than an H2RA.
  - There was no difference in the rates of Clostridioides difficile infection and ICU and hospital lengths of stay.
  - The authors concluded that among ICU patients requiring mechanical ventilation, a strategy of stress ulcer prophylaxis with PPI vs. H2RA resulted in in-hospital mortality rates of 18.3% vs. 17.5%, respectively. The difference did not reach statistical significance. (JAMA. 2020 Feb 18;323(7):616-626.)

High-Yield Fast-Fact
- **Ranitidine Removal**
  - In 2020, the FDA removed ranitidine products from the market after determining the risk of exposure to N-Nitrosodimethylamine in ranitidine, a possible carcinogen.
  - The degree of exposure to N-Nitrosodimethylamine may increase when the product is stored at higher than room temperatures.

HIGH-YIELD BOARD EXAM ESSENTIALS
- **CLASSIC AGENTS:** Cimetidine, famotidine, nizatidine
- **DRUG CLASS:** Histamine H_2 receptor antagonists
- **INDICATIONS:** Dyspepsia, gastroesophageal reflux disease, Helicobacter pylori, peptic ulcer disease
- **MECHANISM:** Competitive inhibition of the parietal cell histamine-2 receptor, preventing gastric acid secretion
- **SIDE EFFECTS:** Confusion, C. difficile infection
- **CLINICAL PEARLS:**
  - Available OTC. This could be a problem if patients are taking medications that require an acidic environment for absorption and do not consult with you or their prescribing provider.
  - Due to other pathways of acid production, many patients will experience escape acid production (gastritis) and tolerance over time, which do not occur with PPIs.
  - All available H2RAs require dose adjustments in the setting of renal impairment. Independent of renal function, elderly patients (over the age of 65 years) also have a decrease in H2RA drug clearance by as much as 50%.
  - Cimetidine has significant drug interactions.

Table: Drug Class Summary

Histamine H2 Receptor Antagonists - Drug Class Review High-Yield Med Reviews			
Mechanism of Action: *Competitive inhibition of the parietal cell histamine-2 receptor, preventing gastric acid secretion.*			
Class Effects: Cornerstone therapy for GERD, available OTC, drug administration interactions, renal dose adjustments, C. diff infections			
Generic Name	**Brand Name**	**Main Indication(s) or Uses**	**Notes**
Cimetidine	Tagamet	<ul><li>Dyspepsia</li><li>Gastroesophageal reflux disease</li></ul>	<ul><li>**Dosing (Adult):**<ul><li>Oral: 200 to 400 mg q6h or 800 mg q12h</li></ul></li><li>**Dosing (Peds):**<ul><li>Oral: 20 to 40 mg/kg/day in 3-4 divided doses<ul><li>Maximum 2,400 mg/day</li></ul></li></ul></li><li>**CYP450 Interactions:** Substrate P-gp; Inhibits CYP 1A2, 2C19, 2D6, 3A4</li><li>**Renal or Hepatic Dose Adjustments:**<ul><li>GFR 10 to 50 mL/minute: Administer 50% of normal dose</li><li>GFR < 10 mL/minute: 300 mg q12h</li></ul></li><li>**Dosage Forms:** Oral (solution, tablet)</li></ul>
Famotidine	Pepcid	<ul><li>Dyspepsia</li><li>Gastroesophageal reflux disease</li><li>Helicobacter pylori</li><li>Peptic ulcer disease</li></ul>	<ul><li>**Dosing (Adult):**<ul><li>IV: 20 to 40 mg q12h</li><li>Oral: 10 to 20 mg q12h</li></ul></li><li>**Dosing (Peds):**<ul><li>Oral: 0.5 to 1 mg/kg/dose<ul><li>Maximum 40 mg/dose</li></ul></li><li>IV: 0.25 mg/kg/dose q12-24h<ul><li>Maximum 40 mg/day</li></ul></li></ul></li><li>**CYP450 Interactions:** None</li><li>**Renal or Hepatic Dose Adjustments:**<ul><li>CrCl 30 to 60 mL/minute: Administer q24h</li><li>CrCl < 30 mg: 10 mg q24-48h</li></ul></li><li>**Dosage Forms:** Oral (suspension, tablet), IV (solution)</li></ul>
Nizatidine	Axid	<ul><li>Dyspepsia</li><li>Gastroesophageal reflux disease</li><li>Peptic ulcer disease</li></ul>	<ul><li>**Dosing (Adult):**<ul><li>Oral: 150 to 300 mg q12-24h, maximum 8 weeks</li></ul></li><li>**Dosing (Peds):**<ul><li>Oral: 5 mg/kg/dose q12h<ul><li>Maximum 300 mg/day</li></ul></li></ul></li><li>**CYP450 Interactions:** text</li><li>**Renal or Hepatic Dose Adjustments:**<ul><li>CrCl 20 to 50 mL/minute: 150 mg q24h</li><li>CrCl < 20 mL/minute: 150 mg q48h</li></ul></li><li>**Dosage Forms:** Oral (capsule, solution)</li></ul>

GI – PROTON PUMP INHIBITORS

Drug Class
- **Proton Pump Inhibitors (PPI)**
- **Agents:**
    - Dexlansoprazole
    - Esomeprazole
    - Lansoprazole
    - Omeprazole
    - Pantoprazole
    - Rabeprazole

> **Fast Facts**
> - Unlike with H2 receptor antagonists, tolerance does not develop with PPIs.
> - PPIs are able to maintain the gastric pH > 4 longer than H2 receptor antagonists to facilitate healing of ulcers.
> - Their irreversible inhibition of the H/K ATPase pump allows for once-a-day dosing.
> - There are many drug-drug interactions with PPIs that can be clinically relevant. See text.

Main Indications or Uses
- **Acute Care**
    - Acute gastrointestinal bleeding: (esomeprazole & pantoprazole)
- **Chronic Care**
    - Duodenal ulcer
    - Erosive esophagitis
    - Gastroesophageal reflux disease
    - Helicobacter pylori eradication
    - Peptic ulcer disease
    - Zollinger-Ellison Syndrome

Mechanism of Action
- Inhibit acid secretion by binding covalently to sulfhydryl groups of the H/K-ATPase (aka proton pump), causing irreversible inhibition.

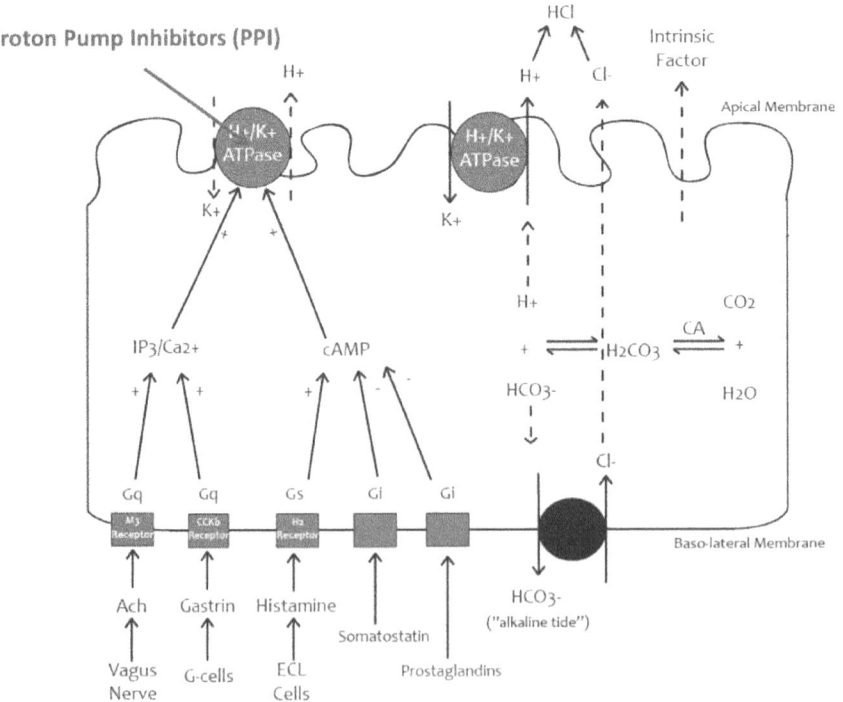

Primary Net Benefit
- PPIs are associated with the most meaningful GI symptom improvement, improved gastric ulcer healing rates, and low risk of clinically relevant adverse events.
- Main Labs to Monitor:

Gastroenterology

- Mg^{2+} (especially with digoxin, diuretics, or others causing hypomagnesemia)
- Ca^{2+} (especially with patients at risk)

High-Yield Basic Pharmacology
- **Prodrugs**
  - All PPIs are prodrugs that are converted to their active form in the acidic secretory canaliculi of the parietal cell.
- **Irreversible Inhibition**
  - As a result of their covalent binding to sulfhydryl groups of the proton pump, PPIs irreversibly inhibit its activity.
  - New proton pumps are formed in the interstitial gastric membrane, then moved to the luminal membrane after 24-48 hours.
- **Gastric pH Target**
  - PPIs are an effective means of achieving sustained gastric pH above 4 in patients on oral therapy and gastric pH above 6 (facilitating platelet aggregation) in patients with gastric bleeding.

High-Yield Clinical Knowledge
- **Drug Interactions**
  - PPIs have numerous clinically relevant pharmacokinetic and pharmacodynamic interactions.
  - Omeprazole and esomeprazole inhibit CYP2C19 and can induce CYP1A2.
    - Inhibition of CYP2C19 can prevent the activation of clopidogrel from its prodrug to the active compound.
      - Pantoprazole is the least likely to cause changes in clopidogrel activation.
    - Induction of CYP1A2 can increase the clearance of numerous antipsychotic agents, imipramine and theophylline.
  - PPIs compete for elimination with methotrexate, and therefore, increase the risk of methotrexate toxicity.
  - Medications such as atazanavir, itraconazole capsules, and erlotinib require an acidic environment for adequate absorption.
  - Avoid concomitant use of PPIs and H2RAs, prostaglandin analogues, or somatostatin analogues due to decreased acid inhibition effects.
    - Separate administration of these agents, i.e., one agent in the morning and one in the evening.
- **Chronic Use Adverse Events**
  - PPIs are associated with an increased risk of pneumonia, including hospital-acquired pneumonia and Clostridoides difficile infection.
  - In patients with underlying hepatic disease and ascites, PPIs increase the risk for spontaneous bacterial peritonitis.
  - Bone fractures have also been associated with long-term use of PPIs, attributed to decreased absorption of calcium and magnesium.
- **Enteric Coatings**
  - All PPIs are susceptible to degradation in acidic environments like the stomach, necessitating formulation in delayed-release capsules or tablets.
  - Patients must be instructed not to split, crush or chew tablets and not to open capsules.
  - In patients unable to swallow oral dosage forms whole, capsules may be opened and taken with sodium bicarbonate (omeprazole), water (esomeprazole), or applesauce (rabeprazole).
    - Dexlansoprazole and lansoprazole are available as an orally disintegrating tablet.

- **Time to Maximum Onset**
  - PPIs will only inhibit the active proton pumps' activity, requiring repetitive dosing (given once per day) over approximately 2 to 5 days.
  - More frequent dosing intervals, including every 12-hours, or give as an IV infusion, can reduce this time to maximum onset.
- **Vitamin B12 Deficiency**
  - May occur with chronic use of PPIs and is associated with decreased absorption of vitamin B12. May have greater risk in elderly or malnourished patients.

- **Acute GI Bleeding**
  - In patients with acute gastric bleeding or undifferentiated upper gastrointestinal bleeding, an IV bolus of esomeprazole or pantoprazole 80 mg is followed by an infusion of 8 mg/hour to target a gastric pH of 6-7 and continued for 72 hours.
  - Alternative dosing of 80 mg IV q12h achieves similar gastric pH and may be a reasonable alternative to continuous infusions.

High-Yield Core Evidence

- **Omeprazole in Peptic Ulcer Bleeding**
  - This was a single-center, double-blinded, parallel-group, placebo-controlled trial that randomized patients with actively bleeding ulcers or ulcers with nonbleeding visible vessels that underwent thermocoagulation to either omeprazole 80 mg bolus followed by an 8 mg/hour infusion for 72 hours or placebo, followed by omeprazole 20 mg orally daily for eight weeks in all patients.
  - Omeprazole infusion significantly reduced the risk of recurrent bleeding within 30 days after endoscopy.
  - Most episodes of recurrent bleeding occurred during the first three days.
  - The authors concluded that after endoscopic treatment of bleeding peptic ulcers, a high-dose infusion of omeprazole substantially reduces the risk of recurrent bleeding. (N Engl J Med. 2000 Aug 3;343(5):310-6.)
- **PPI Prophylaxis in ICU**
  - This was a multicenter, parallel-group, blinded trial, that randomized critical care patients at risk for gastrointestinal bleeding to either pantoprazole 40 mg IV daily or placebo.
  - There was no difference between groups regarding the primary outcome of death by 90 days after randomization.
  - There was also no significant difference between groups regarding the occurrence of clinically important events, including gastrointestinal bleeding, pneumonia, Clostridoides difficile infection, or myocardial ischemia.
  - However, numerically fewer patients in the pantoprazole group experienced clinically significant gastrointestinal bleeding than the placebo group.
  - The authors concluded that among adult patients in the ICU who were at risk for gastrointestinal bleeding, mortality at 90 days and the number of clinically significant events were similar in those assigned to pantoprazole and those assigned to placebo. (N Engl J Med. 2018 Dec 6;379(23):2199-2208.)

High-Yield Fast-Facts

- **Iron Absorption**
  - PPIs will decrease the absorption of oral iron products by allowing higher gastric pH to oxidize ferrous iron to the poorly absorbed ferric iron.

HIGH-YIELD BOARD EXAM ESSENTIALS
- **CLASSIC AGENTS:** Dexlansoprazole, esomeprazole, lansoprazole, omeprazole, pantoprazole, rabeprazole
- **DRUG CLASS:** Proton pump inhibitors
- **INDICATIONS:** Acute gastrointestinal bleeding, duodenal ulcer, erosive esophagitis, GERD, Helicobacter pylori eradication, peptic ulcer disease, Zollinger-Ellison syndrome
- **MECHANISM:** Inhibit acid secretion by binding covalently to sulfhydryl groups of the H/K-ATPase (aka proton pump), causing an irreversible inhibition
- **SIDE EFFECTS:** Infections (pneumonia, spontaneous bacterial peritonitis, C. difficile),
- **CLINICAL PEARLS:**
  - Unlike H2RAs, there is no development of tolerance to gastric acid suppression. PPIs can maintain the gastric pH > 4 for a longer duration thereby conferring a greater ability of gastric ulcers to heal.
  - All PPIs are susceptible to degradation in acidic environments, such as the stomach, necessitating formulation in delayed-release capsules or tablets. Patients must be instructed not to split, crush or chew tablets and not open capsules.
  - Pantoprazole may be less likely to interfere with clopidogrel activation and overall activity, whereas lansoprazole and omeprazole are more likely to inhibit the functional activation of clopidogrel.

Table: Drug Class Summary

Proton Pump Inhibitors Drug Class Review High-Yield Med Reviews			
Mechanism of Action: *Inhibit acid secretion by binding covalently to sulfhydryl groups of the / K-ATPase (aka proton pump), causing an irreversible inhibition.*			
Class Effects: *Largest improvement in GI symptoms, improved gastric ulcer healing rates, and low risk of clinically relevant adverse events, possible infections include pneumonia and C. diff., possible risk of fracture*			
Generic Name	**Brand Name**	**Main Indication(s) or Uses**	**Notes**
Dexlansoprazole	Dexilant	<ul><li>Erosive esophagitis</li><li>Gastroesophageal reflux disease</li></ul>	<ul><li>**Dosing (Adult):**<ul><li>Oral: 60 mg daily for up to 8 weeks</li><li>Oral: 30 mg daily<ul><li>Max 4 weeks for GERD</li></ul></li></ul></li><li>**Dosing (Peds):**<ul><li>Oral: 30-60 mg daily for 8 weeks</li><li>Max 4 weeks for GERD</li></ul></li><li>**CYP450 Interactions:** Substrate CYP2C19</li><li>**Renal or Hepatic Dose Adjustments:**<ul><li>Child-Pugh class C: not recommended</li></ul></li><li>**Dosage Forms:** Oral (capsule)</li></ul>
Esomeprazole	Nexium	<ul><li>Gastroesophageal reflux disease</li><li>Helicobacter pylori eradication</li><li>Peptic ulcer disease</li></ul>	<ul><li>**Dosing (Adult):**<ul><li>Oral/IV: 20-40 mg q12-24h</li><li>IV: 80 mg bolus followed by 8 mg/hour infusion</li></ul></li><li>**Dosing (Peds):**<ul><li>Oral: 2.5-10 mg daily for up to 6 weeks</li><li>IV: 0.5-3.3 mg/kg/dose daily, max 40 mg/dose</li></ul></li><li>**CYP450 Interactions:** CYP2C19, 3A4 substrate; CYP2C19 inhibitor</li><li>**Renal or Hepatic Dose Adjustments:**<ul><li>Child-Pugh class B: Lower infusion rate to 6 mg/hour</li><li>Child-Pugh class C: Max 20 mg/day; Lower infusion rate to 4 mg/hour</li></ul></li><li>**Dosage Forms:** Oral (capsule, kit, packet, tablet), IV (solution)</li></ul>
Lansoprazole	Prevacid	<ul><li>Gastroesophageal reflux disease</li><li>Hypersecretory conditions</li><li>Peptic ulcer disease</li></ul>	<ul><li>**Dosing (Adult):**<ul><li>Oral: 15-60 mg daily</li><li>Oral: 30 mg up to TID (H. pylori)</li></ul></li><li>**Dosing (Peds):**<ul><li>Oral: 0.7-3 mg/kg/day</li><li>Max 30 mg/day</li></ul></li><li>**CYP450 Interactions:** CYP2C19, 2C9, 3A4 substrate</li><li>**Renal or Hepatic Dose Adjustments:**<ul><li>Child-Pugh class C - Max 30 mg/day</li></ul></li><li>**Dosage Forms:** Oral (capsule, tablet)</li></ul>

Proton Pump Inhibitors Drug Class Review High-Yield Med Reviews			
Generic Name	**Brand Name**	**Main Indication(s) or Uses**	**Notes**

Omeprazole	Prilosec	- Gastroesophageal reflux disease
		- Helicobacter pylori eradication
		- Peptic ulcer disease
		- Zollinger-Ellison Syndrome
			- **Dosing (Adult):**
			   - Oral: 10-40 mg q12-24h
			- **Dosing (Peds):**
			   - Oral: 2.5-10 mg daily for up to 6 weeks
			      - Maximum 20 mg/day
			- **CYP450 Interactions:** CYP2A6, 2C19, 2D6, 3A4 substrate; CYP2C19 inhibitor
			- **Renal or Hepatic Dose Adjustments:**
			   - Child-Pugh class A-C: Max 20 mg/day
			- **Dosage Forms:** Oral (capsule, packet, tablet)

Pantoprazole	Protonix	- Gastroesophageal reflux disease
		- Helicobacter pylori eradication
		- Peptic ulcer disease
		- Zollinger-Ellison Syndrome
			- **Dosing (Adult):**
			   - Oral/IV: 20 to 40 mg q12-24h
			   - IV: 80 mg bolus followed by 8 mg/hour infusion
			- **Dosing (Peds):**
			   - Oral: 2.5-10 mg daily for up to 6 weeks
			   - IV: 0.5-3.3 mg/kg/dose daily, max 40 mg/dose
			- **CYP450 Interactions:** CYP2C19, 2D6, 3A4 substrate
			- **Renal or Hepatic Dose Adjustments:** None
			- **Dosage Forms:** Oral (packet, tablet), IV (solution)

Rabeprazole	Aciphex	- Duodenal ulcers
		- Gastroesophageal reflux disease
		- Helicobacter pylori eradication
			- **Dosing (Adult):**
			   - Oral: 20-40 mg q12-24h
			- **Dosing (Peds):**
			   - Oral: 2.5-10 mg daily for up to 6 weeks
			      - Max 20 mg/day
			- **CYP450 Interactions:** CYP 2C19, 3A4 substrate
			- **Renal or Hepatic Dose Adjustments:**
			   - Child-Pugh class C: Avoid use
			- **Dosage Forms:** Oral (capsule, packet, tablet)

ANTIEMETICS – DOPAMINE ANTAGONIST ANTIEMETICS

Drug Class
- Dopamine antagonist antiemetics
- Agents:
  - Acute & Chronic Care
    - Droperidol
    - Haloperidol
    - Metoclopramide
    - Trimethobenzamide
    - Chlorpromazine
    - Perphenazine
    - Prochlorperazine
    - Promethazine

Fast Facts

✓ Metoclopramide is unique within this drug class because it can also be used as a promotility agent with gastroparesis or to tighten the lower esophageal sphincter to aid in the treatment of GERD.

Main Indications or Uses
- Acute & Chronic Care
  - Nausea and/or vomiting

Mechanism of Action
- Block dopamine receptors in the chemoreceptor trigger zone (CTZ).

Primary Net Benefit
- Provide relief for nausea and/or vomiting
- Main Labs to Monitor:
  - SCr, EKG (for small risk of QT prolongation)

High-Yield Basic Pharmacology
- Grouped by Chemical Structure
  - Butyrophenone Antipsychotics
    - Includes droperidol and haloperidol. In addition to dopaminergic blockade in the CTZ, they also blocker alpha-adrenergic receptors and can cause peripheral vascular dilation and reduce the pressor effect of epinephrine, resulting in hypotension and decreased peripheral vascular resistance.
  - Phenothiazine Antipsychotics
    - Includes chlorpromazine, perphenazine, prochlorperazine, and promethazine. In addition to dopaminergic blockade in the CTZ, they also possess alpha-adrenergic blocking and anticholinergic effects.
  - Substituted Benzamides
    - Includes metoclopramide and trimethobenzamide. At higher doses, metoclopramide also blocks serotonin receptors in the CTZ. Trimethobenzamide possesses weak antihistaminic activity.

High-Yield Clinical Knowledge
- Antipsychotic Agents as Antiemetics
  - Chlorpromazine, droperidol, haloperidol, and prochlorperazine are all considered first-generation antipsychotic agents and can be utilized for other indications. Antiemetic effects of these agents are attributed to the blockade of dopamine subtype 2 receptors in the CTZ.
    - In 2005, the FDA informed healthcare professionals and the public about the increased risk of mortality in elderly patients receiving atypical antipsychotic drugs to treat dementia-related psychosis. This statement was based on a meta-analysis of 17 placebo-controlled trials that enrolled 5377 elderly patients with dementia-related behavioral disorders. The meta-analysis result revealed an increased risk of death in the drug-treated patients between 1.6 to 1.7 times

seen in placebo-treated patients. Many agents in this category have a black box warning for this reason. The agents in meta-analyses were primary utilized for behavioral-related indications. When used infrequently as antiemetics, this warning may carry less clinical relevance.

- **Extrapyramidal Side Effects**
  - Extrapyramidal symptoms (EPS) is an umbrella term used to describe antipsychotic-induced movement side effects due to excess dopamine blockade in the nigrostriatal pathway. Symptoms include dystonia, akathisia, pseudoparkinsonism, and tardive dyskinesia.
    - Extrapyramidal effects appear to occur more commonly in children and young adults and at higher doses.
    - Prochlorperazine can cause EPS after a one-time dose. Metoclopramide has a lower risk of EPS compared to prochlorperazine.
- **Unique Administration Considerations**
  - Chlorpromazine: Intravenous administration associated with a high rate of hypotension. If given intravenously, the solution should be diluted and administered no faster than 1 mg/minute.
  - Haloperidol: Injectable solution available in two salt forms: lactate and decanoate. The decanoate formulation is intended for intramuscular injection only.
  - Metoclopramide: Rapid IV administration has been associated with a transient but intense feeling of anxiety and restlessness, often followed by drowsiness. Doses less than 10 mg can be given undiluted over 1 to 2 minutes; doses greater than 10 mg should be diluted into 50 mL of a compatible solution and administered over 15 minutes.
  - Prochlorperazine: Lower risk of EPS when administered as a 15-minute infusion versus rapid IV bolus. Intravenous administration has been associated with a high rate of hypotension.
  - Promethazine: Injectable promethazine is a vesicant and has been associated with severe cases of tissue necrosis. The Institute for Safe Medical Practices (ISMP) discourages using any form of injectable promethazine due to the risk of severe tissue damage.
  - Trimethobenzamide: Injectable solution is intended for intramuscular injection only. It should be injected into the upper outer quadrant of the gluteal muscle.
- **QT Interval Prolongation**
  - Many antipsychotic agents can also block potassium currents in the myocardium, leading to a prolonged QT interval. The smaller doses of antipsychotic agents utilized for their antiemetic effects decrease the clinical risk of QT prolongation.
  - In 2001, the FDA issued a black box warning for QT prolongation effects caused by droperidol based on 274 cases of adverse effects reported to MedWatch. There is a lack of robust data supporting this claim. The manufacturing labeling still recommends EKG monitoring before droperidol initiation and 2 to 3 hours after therapy to monitor for arrhythmias.
- **Patient Population Considerations**
  - **Avoid in Patients with Parkinson Disease**
    - Dopamine antagonism can reduce levodopa's efficacy due to direct dopamine antagonism and exacerbate symptoms of Parkinson's disease. These agents should be avoided in this patient population. Parkinson's disease is a contraindication to haloperidol therapy.
  - **Pediatric Considerations**
    - Dopamine receptor antagonists are not considered the preferred agents for treating nausea and/or vomiting in pediatric patients due to the side effect profile and risk of EPS. Use has generally been replaced by agents that are more effective with fewer adverse events. If used, employ extreme caution and utilize the lowest effective dose.
    - Promethazine should not be used in pediatric patients younger than two years because of the potential for fatal respiratory depression. It carries a black box warning for this reason.
    - Droperidol and prochlorperazine lack black box warnings for use in pediatric populations but should not be utilized for patients younger than two years of age.

High-Yield Core Evidence
- **Prophylactic Anticholinergics to Decrease EPS**
    - A meta-analysis of four randomized control trials of patients receiving dopamine-receptor antagonists
    - Results: Prophylactic diphenhydramine reduced EPS in patients who received a D2 antagonist as a rapid bolus (2 minutes) but not when administered slowly (15-minute infusion).
    - Conclusion: Because of significantly greater sedation with diphenhydramine, the most effective strategy is to administer the D2 antagonist antiemetic as a 15-minute infusion without prophylaxis.
    - (Emerg Med J. 2018 May;35(5):325-331.)
- **Droperidol verses ondansetron**
    - A multi-center, randomized, placebo-controlled trial compared ondansetron 4 mg IV, droperidol 0.625 mg IV, and droperidol 1.25 mg IV in adult surgical outpatients at high risk for PONV. Study drugs were administered before anesthesia induction in combination with a barbiturate.
    - Results: In the 0 to 2-hour postoperative period, complete response (no emesis or rescue antiemetic) was seen in 46% of the placebo group, 62% of the ondansetron group, 63% of the droperidol 0.625 mg group, and 69% of the droperidol 1.25 mg group. No significant differences in complete response were found in the 0 to 24-hour post-operative period between ondansetron and either droperidol group. The proportion of patients without nausea in the 0 to 24-hour period was more significant in the droperidol 1.25 mg group when compared with ondansetron and droperidol 0.625 mg (43% vs. 29% vs. 29%, respectively).
    - (Anesth Analg. 1998 Apr;86(4):731-8.)

High-Yield Fast-Facts
- The substituted benzamides are derivatives of para-aminobenzoic acid and are structurally related to the antiarrhythmic procainamide.
- Dopaminergic stimulation of the glottis is postulated as one of the potential pathophysiological mechanisms of hiccups. Many dopamine receptor antagonists have been utilized to treat intractable hiccups. Chlorpromazine is even FDA-approved for this indication. The longest recorded case of intractable hiccups in medical history can be credited to Charles Osborne, a farmer who continuously hiccupped for 68 years!

HIGH-YIELD BOARD EXAM ESSENTIALS
- **CLASSIC AGENTS:** Droperidol, haloperidol, metoclopramide, trimethobenzamide, chlorpromazine, perphenazine, prochlorperazine, promethazine
- **DRUG CLASS:** Dopamine antagonist antiemetics
- **INDICATIONS:** Nausea and/or vomiting
- **MECHANISM:** Block dopamine receptors in the chemoreceptor trigger zone (CTZ)
- **SIDE EFFECTS:** QT prolongation, dystonia, akathisia, pseudoparkinsonism, and tardive dyskinesia.
- **CLINICAL PEARLS:** Chlorpromazine, droperidol, haloperidol, and prochlorperazine are all considered first-generation antipsychotic agents and can be utilized for other indications. Antiemetic effects of these agents are attributed to the blockade of dopamine subtype 2 receptors in the CTZ.

Table: Drug Class Summary

\multicolumn{4}{c}{**Dopamine Antagonist Antiemetics - Drug Class Review**}
\multicolumn{4}{c}{High-Yield Med Reviews}
Mechanism of Action: Block dopamine receptors in the chemoreceptor trigger zone (CTZ)			
Class Effects: Provide relief for nausea and/or vomiting			
Generic Name	**Brand Name**	**Main Indication(s) or Uses**	**Notes**
Chlorpromazine	Compazine (DSC)	• Nausea and/or vomiting	• **Dosing (Adult):** — PO: 10 to 25 mg Q4-8H PRN — IM, IV: 25 to 50 mg once PRN • **Dosing (Peds), >2 years:** — IM, IV: 0.01 to 0.015 mg/kg/dose (Max dose = 1.25 mg/dose) • **CYP450 Interactions:** Substrate of CYP1A2, CYP2D6, CYP3A4 • **Renal or Hepatic Dose Adjustments:** None • **Dosage Forms:** PO (tablet), Injectable
Droperidol	Brand Name (if available)	• Nausea and/or vomiting	• **Dosing (Adult):** — IM, IV: 0.625 to 2.5 mg • **Dosing (Peds), >2 years:** — IM, IV: 0.01 to 0.015 mg/kg/dose (Max dose = 1.25 mg/dose) • **CYP450 Interactions:** None • **Renal or Hepatic Dose Adjustments:** None • **Dosage Forms:** Injectable
Haloperidol	Haldol	• Nausea and/or vomiting	• **Dosing (Adult):** — PO, IV: 0.5 to 2 mg q6hr — Cont SubQ: 1 to 5 mg per 24 hours • **Dosing (Peds):** Not routinely used for this indication • **CYP450 Interactions:** Substrate of CYP1A2, CYP2D6, CYP3A4 • **Renal or Hepatic Dose Adjustments:** None • **Dosage Forms:** PO (tablet, solution), Injectable
Metoclopramide	Reglan Gimoti (nasal)	• Nausea and/or vomiting	• **Dosing (Adult):** — PO: 10 mg Q4-6H PRN — IV: 10 to 20 mg PRN • **Dosing (Peds):** — IV: 0.1 to 0.25 mg/kg/dose q6-8hr (Max dose= 10 mg) • **CYP450 Interactions:** Substrate of CYP1A2, CYP2D6 • **Renal or Hepatic Dose Adjustments:** — CrCl 10-60 mL/min: Reduce dose by 50% — Child-Pugh Class C or D: Use not recommended • **Dosage Forms:** PO (tablet, ODT, solution), Nasal, Injectable

\multicolumn{4}{c}{**Dopamine Antagonist Antiemetics - Drug Class Review**}
\multicolumn{4}{c}{High-Yield Med Reviews}
Generic Name	**Brand Name**	**Main Indication(s) or Uses**	**Notes**
Perphenazine	N/A	• Nausea and/or vomiting	• **Dosing (Adult):** – PO: 8-24 mg/day • **Dosing (Peds):** Not used • **CYP450 Interactions:** Substrate of CYP2D6 • **Renal or Hepatic Dose Adjustments:** None • **Dosage Forms:** Oral (tablet, concentrate)
Prochlorperazine	Compazine, Compro (rectal)	• Nausea and/or vomiting	• **Dosing (Adult):** – PO/IM/IV: 2.5-10 mg Q6H PRN – Max daily dose: 40 mg – PR: 25 mg BID • **Dosing (Peds), >2 yrs and >9 kg:** – PO: 2.5 mg Q6-24H PRN – Frequency and maximum daily doses vary by weight – IM/IV: 0.1-0.15 mg/kg/dose – Maximum single dose: 10 mg/dose • **CYP450 Interactions:** None • **Renal or Hepatic Dose Adjustments:** None • **Dosage Forms:** Oral (tablet), Injectable, Rectal
Promethazine	Phenergan	• Nausea and/or vomiting	• **Dosing (Adult):** – PO/IM/IV/PR: 12.5-25 mg Q4-6H PRN **Dosing (Peds), >2 yrs:** – PO/IM/IV/PR: 0.25-1 mg/kg/dose Q4-6H PRN – Maximum dose: 25 mg/dose • **CYP450 Interactions:** None • **Renal or Hepatic Dose Adjustments:** text • **Dosage Forms:** Oral (tablet, solution, syrup), Injectable, Rectal
Trimethobenzamide	Tigan	• Nausea and/or vomiting	• **Dosing (Adult):** – PO: 300 mg TID-QID – IM: 300 mg TID-QID – Extra info if needed • **Dosing (Peds):** – PO: 100-200 mg Q6H PRN – Use is strongly discouraged due to risk of EPS • **CYP450 Interactions:** None • **Renal or Hepatic Dose Adjustments:** CrCl < 70 mL/min: reduce dose or increase interval • **Dosage Forms:** Oral (capsule), Injection

ANTIEMETICS – MISCELLANEOUS ANTIEMETICS

Drug Class
- **Miscellaneous Antiemetics**
- **Agents**:
  - Acute & Chronic
    - Anticholinergics
      - Hyoscyamine
      - Scopolamine
    - Antihistamines
      - Dimenhydrinate
      - Diphenhydramine
      - Meclizine
    - Cannabinoids
      - Dronabinol
      - Nabilone

> **Fast Facts**
> - Use caution in elderly patients where the risk of side effects can be worse.
> - Diphenhydramine at high doses can inhibit sodium channels in the heart and cause QRS widening.
> - Dimenhydrinate, meclizine is commonly used for peripheral vertigo like symptoms.

Main Indications or Uses
- Nausea and/or vomiting
- Vertigo

Mechanism of Action
- **Antihistamines** (Dimenhydrinate, diphenhydramine, hydroxyzine, meclizine)
  - Reversibly compete with histamine binding at H_1 receptors to reduce histaminergic stimulation of the vestibular apparatus.
- **Anticholinergics** (Hyoscyamine, scopolamine)
  - Block effects of acetylcholine at muscarinic receptors in the chemoreceptor trigger zone (CTZ).
- **Cannabinoid receptor agonists** (Dronabinol, nabilone)
  - Stimulate CB-1 subtype of cannabinoid receptors on neurons in and around the CTZ and emetic center.

Primary Net Benefi
- Provide relief for nausea and/or vomiting
- Main Labs to Monitor:
  - N/A

High-Yield Basic Pharmacology
- **Anticholinergics**
  - The anticholinergics included in this class act as antagonists at muscarinic subtype-1 (M_1) receptors.
  - These receptors are found on the central nervous system (CNS) neurons, many presynaptic sites, and gastric and salivary glands.
- **H_1-antihistamines**
  - Inverse agonists
    - Although antihistamines are commonly called histamine antagonists, they act as inverse agonists. Inverse agonists preferentially bind to and stabilize the inactivated conformation of receptors and produce the opposite pharmacological effect of an activating ligand.
  - First-generation versus second-generation agents
    - H_1-antihistamines can be divided into first-generation and second-generation agents.
    - The second-generation agents do not cross the blood-brain-barrier and are considered to be nonsedating.
      - Utilized for allergic conditions, not nausea/vomiting.
      - Examples: cetirizine (Zyrtec), loratadine (Claritin), and fexofenadine (Allegra)

- **Cannabinoids**
    - The term cannabinoids encompass a wide variety of compounds. They can be endogenous, derived from plants, or synthetically produced. Dronabinol and nabilone are FDA-approved, synthetically produced analogs of delta-9-tetrahydrocannabinol (THC), a naturally occurring component of *Cannabis sativa* (marijuana).
    - To date, two endogenous cannabinoid receptors have been identified, CB-1 and CB-2. The pharmacological effects of cannabinoids have been attributed to the activation of the CB-1 receptor.

High-Yield Clinical Knowledge
- **Adverse Effects**
    - Anticholinergic Toxidrome:
        - The classic anticholinergic toxidrome can be remembered with the phrase "mad as a hatter" (altered mental status), "blind as a bat" (mydriasis), "red as a beet" (flushed skin), "hot as a hare" (dry skin), "dry as a bone" (dry mucous membranes), and "full as a flask" (urinary retention).
    - CNS effects
        - Euphoria: Cannabinoids
        - Sedation: Anticholinergics, first-generation H_1-antihistamines, and cannabinoids

- **Cannabinoids Are Controlled Substances**
    - Dronabinol is commercially available as two oral formulations, capsules and solution. Both formulations have poor bioavailability (~10%) due to extensive first-pass metabolism.
        - The capsules, marketed under the brand name, Marinol®, are formulated with sesame oil and encapsulated in a gel capsule. It was initially classified as a Schedule II controlled substance but was later rescheduled to Schedule III after the Drug Enforcement Agency (DEA) determined the separation of dronabinol from sesame oil was difficult giving it a lower abuse potential.
        - In 2016, an oral dronabinol solution under the brand name, Syndros® gained FDA approval. Even though this formulation contains the same active pharmaceutical ingredient, Syndros® was classified as a Schedule II controlled substance. The DEA and the Department of Health and Human Services (HHS) stated the solution was more amenable to manipulation. They stated this led to higher abuse potential which necessitated a Schedule II designation.
    - Nabilone is only available as oral capsules and is classified as a Schedule II controlled substance. It has a higher oral bioavailability (~90%) and a longer duration of action than dronabinol due to conversion to active metabolites.
- **Antiemetic Selection and Patient Considerations**
    - Avoid anticholinergics and antihistamines in elderly patients, and those with benign prostatic hypertrophy (BPH), gastrointestinal motility disorders, and narrow or closed-angle glaucoma as these comorbidities can be exacerbated by the side effect profile of anticholinergics.
    - Antihistamines may be beneficial as antiemetics in patients with Parkinson's Disease who are at an increased risk of extrapyramidal symptoms associated with dopaminergic antiemetics.
    - Cannabinoids may be useful in patients with chemotherapy-induced nausea/vomiting or other indications which cause appetite suppression due to their stimulating effect.
- **Antiemetic Selection and Situational Emesis**
    - Postoperative: Scopolamine
    - Motion sickness: Antihistamines, scopolamine
    - Pregnancy: Antihistamines
    - Chemotherapy-induced: Cannabinoids
- **Nonpharmacological Antiemetic Options**
    - <u>Ginger</u>: Studies have shown that constituents of ginger have inhibitory effects at neurokinin-1 (NK-1), serotonin (5-HT_3), and muscarinic receptors. The predominant effect of ginger is located in the gastrointestinal tract, but some evidence has shown that some constituents may have CNS effects.
    - <u>Acupressure wristbands</u>: These wristbands are sold as an over-the-counter product under various brand names. The antiemetic effect is attributed to stimulation of the pericardium 6 (P6) meridian point.

High-Yield Core Evidence
- **Scopolamine Plus Ondansetron Reduced Post-Operative Nausea/Vomiting**
  - The combination of transdermal scopolamine plus intravenous ondansetron resulted in a statistically significant reduction in postoperative nausea/vomiting (PONV) when compared to ondansetron monotherapy in female patients undergoing laparoscopic breast augmentation.
  - Anesthesia & Analgesia 2009; 108(5):1498-1504.

High-Yield Fast-Facts
- **Benzodiazepines as Miscellaneous Antiemetics**
  - While not directly effective as an antiemetic, benzodiazepines are often utilized to reduce anticipatory chemotherapy-induced nausea and/or vomiting.
- **Urine Drug Screening**
  - Dronabinol will produce positive results for THC on a urine drug screen, whereas nabilone will not. This is due to the difference in metabolic byproduct production.
  - Several medications have been reported to produce false-positive results for THC on urine drug screens due to cross-reactivity to immunoassays. Some of these medication classes include proton pump inhibitors (PPIs), nonsteroidal anti-inflammatory drugs (NSAIDs), and efavirenz.

HIGH-YIELD BOARD EXAM ESSENTIALS
- **CLASSIC AGENTS:** Hyoscyamine, scopolamine, dimenhydrinate, diphenhydramine, meclizine, dronabinol, nabilone
- **DRUG CLASS:** Miscellaneous antiemetics
- **INDICATIONS:** Nausea and/or vomiting
- **MECHANISM:** Inverse agonist at H1-receptors (antihistamines), M1-antagonists (anticholinergics), CB-1 agonists (cannabinoids)
- **SIDE EFFECTS:** Anticholinergic effects, euphoria, sedation
- **CLINICAL PEARLS:** Avoid anticholinergics and antihistamines in elderly patients, and those with benign prostatic hypertrophy (BPH), gastrointestinal motility disorders, and narrow or closed-angle glaucoma as these comorbidities can be exacerbated by the side effect profile of anticholinergics.

Table: Drug Class Summary

\multicolumn{4}{c}{**Miscellaneous Antiemetics - Drug Class Review**}

| | **Miscellaneous Antiemetics - Drug Class Review**
 High-Yield Med Reviews |

Mechanism of Action: <u>Antihistamines</u>: Inverse agonist at H_1-receptors; <u>Anticholinergics</u>: M_1-antagonists; <u>Cannabinoids</u>: CB-1 agonists

Class Effects: Provide relief for nausea and/or vomiting

Generic Name	Brand Name	Main Indication(s) or Uses	Notes

Dronabinol	Marinol (capsules)
	
	 Syndros (solution)
		- Nausea and/or vomiting
		 - Anorexia in patients with AIDS
			- **Dosing (Adult):**
			   – PO, capsules: 2.5 to 10 mg TID-QID *or* 5 to 15 mg/m² up to 6 doses/day
			   – PO, solution: 4.2 to 12.6 mg/m² up to 6 doses/day
			 - **Dosing (Peds):** Same as adults
			 - **CYP450 Interactions:** Substrate of CYP2C9, CYP3A4
			 - **Renal or Hepatic Dose Adjustments:** None
			 - **Dosage Forms:** PO (capsules, solution)

Nabilone	N/A	- Nausea and/or vomiting	- **Dosing (Adult):**
			   – PO: 1 to 2 mg BID-TID
			     – Max daily dose=6 mg/day
			 - **Dosing (Peds, ≥ 3 yrs):**
			   – PO: 0.5 to 1 mg BID
			     – Weight-based adjustments
			 - **CYP450 Interactions:** None
			 - **Renal or Hepatic Dose Adjustments:** None
			 - **Dosage Forms:** PO (capsules)

Dimenhydrinate	Driminate (OTC), GoodSense Motion SIckness (OTC)	- Nausea and/or vomiting associated with motion sickness	- **Dosing (Adult):**
			   – PO: 50 to 100 mg Q4-6H PRN
			     – Max daily dose= 400 mg/day
			   – IM/IV: 50 to 100 mg Q4H PRN
			 - **Dosing (Peds, ≥ 2 yrs):**
			   – PO: 12.5 to 25 mg Q6-8H *or* 1 to 1.5 mg/kg/dose Q6H
			     – Max daily dose varies by age group
			   – IM: 1.25 mg/kg/dose QID
			     – Max daily dose=300 mg/day
			 - **CYP450 Interactions:** None
			 - **Renal or Hepatic Dose Adjustments:** text
			 - **Dosage Forms:** PO (tablets, chewable), Injectable

| \multicolumn{4}{c}{**Miscellaneous Antiemetics - Drug Class Review**} |

Generic Name	Brand Name	Main Indication(s) or Uses	Notes

Diphenhydramine	Benadryl
	
	*Multiple OTC brand names
		▪ Nausea and/or vomiting
		▪ Nausea and/or vomiting associated with motion sickness
			▪ **Dosing (Adult):**
			   – PO: 25 to 50 mg Q4-8H PRN
			   – IM/IV: 10 to 50 mg Q6H PRN
			▪ **Dosing (Peds):**
			   – PO: 5 mg/kg/day divided into 3 or 4 doses
			   – IM/IV: 1.25 mg/kg/dose Q6H
			▪ **CYP450 Interactions:** Substrate of CYP1A2, CYP2C9, CYP2D6; Inhibits CYP2D6
			▪ **Renal or Hepatic Dose Adjustments:** None
			▪ **Dosage Forms:** PO (capsules, tablets, chewable, elixir, solution, syrup), Injectable

Meclizine	Bonine (OTC), Dramamine Less Drowsy (OTC), Motion-Time (OTC), Travel-Ease (OTC)	▪ Nausea and/or vomiting associated with motion sickness ▪ Vertigo	▪ **Dosing (Adult):** – PO, PR: 25 mg prn ▪ **Dosing (Peds, ≥ 12 yrs):** Same as adults ▪ **CYP450 Interactions:** Substrate of CYP2D6 ▪ **Renal or Hepatic Dose Adjustments:** text ▪ **Dosage Forms:** PO (tablets, chewable)

Scopolamine	Transderm-Scop	▪ Nausea and/or vomiting associated with motion sickness
		▪ Nausea and/or vomiting associated with preoperative anesthesia
			▪ **Dosing (Adult):**
			   – Topical: 1 patch every 3 days PRN
			▪ **Dosing (Peds):**
			   – Topical: ¼ to 1 patch PRN (varies by age)
			▪ **CYP450 Interactions:** None
			▪ **Renal or Hepatic Dose Adjustments:** None
			▪ **Dosage Forms:** Topical (72 hr-patch) [Injectable formulation available in Canada]

ANTIEMETICS – SELECTIVE SEROTONIN ANTAGONISTS (5-HT$_3$-RA)

Drug Class
- Agents:
  - **Acute & Chronic Care**
    - Alosetron
    - Dolasetron
    - Granisetron
    - Ondansetron
    - Palonosetron

 Fast Facts
- ✓ The 5-HT$_3$-RA can be identified by their shared suffix, -setron and work in both the GI tract and CNS.
- ✓ Alosetron is uniquely indicated for IBS with predominant symptom being diarrhea.

Main Indications or Uses
- **Acute & Chronic Care**
  - Nausea/vomiting
  - Chemotherapy-Induced Nausea and Vomiting Prophylaxis
  - Postoperative Nausea and Vomiting
- **Alosetron only**
  - Women with diarrhea-predominant - irritable bowel syndrome

Mechanism of Action
- Selective serotonin antagonists (5-HT$_3$-RA) selectively block serotonin subtype 3 receptors (5-HT$_3$) both centrally in the chemotherapy trigger and peripherally in the gastrointestinal tract resulting in antiemetic effects.

Primary Net Benefit
- Provide supportive care for nausea and emesis
- Main Labs to Monitor:
  - EKG for high-risk patients (elderly patients or those on concomitant medications that prolong the QTc)

High-Yield Basic Pharmacology
- **Serotonin receptor subtypes**
  - Several serotoninergic receptor subtypes have been identified (5-HT1 (5-HT1A, 5-HT1B, 5-HTID, 5-HTIE, and 5-HT1F), 5-HT2 (5-HT2A, 5-HT2B and 5-HT2C), 5-HT3, 5-HT4, 5-HT5 (5-HT5A, 5-HT5B), 5-HT6/7.
    - 5-HT3 receptors are located in the vomiting center of the brain and the gastrointestinal system
      - Peripheral 5-HT3 receptor antagonism in the gut prevents ACh release, decreasing gut motility and vagal nerve excitation.
      - Central 5-HT3 receptor antagonism reduced chemotherapy trigger zone stimulation.
- **Palonosetron**
  - Palonosetron is unique among the 5-HT$_3$-RA due to its longer half-life of ~40 hours (compared to <10 hours for the other agents in this class), making it useful for preventing delayed CINV.

High-Yield Clinical Knowledge
- **Class Naming Convention**
  - The 5-HT$_3$-RA can be identified by their shared suffix, -setron
- **Use and efficacy**
  - Useful as a single-agent or combination therapy for prophylaxis of chemotherapy-induced nausea/vomiting (CINV) or postoperative nausea/vomiting (PONV)
  - These agents (except for alosetron) are equally efficacious at equivalent doses; thus, agent selection is usually dictated by cost and availability
  - Alosetron (Lotronex) is only indicated for use in women with irritable bowel syndrome; it should not be utilized as an antiemetic agent
- **Contraindications**
  - 5-HT$_3$-RAs are contraindicated with concurrent apomorphine administration due to their ability to cause profound hypotension

- **Alosetron**
  - Alosetron is only approved for women with severe diarrhea-predominant irritable bowel syndrome (IBS)
  - It was briefly withdrawn from the US market due to the high incidence of ischemic colitis, leading to surgery and even death. However, it was reapproved for diarrhea-predominant IBS under a limited distribution system.
  - It may only be dispensed upon presenting a prescription for Alosetron with a sticker for the Prescribing Program for Alosetron attached. No telephone, facsimile, or computerized prescriptions are permitted with this program. Refills are allowed to be written on prescriptions.
- **Serotonin syndrome**
  - Characterized by alterations in mentation and cognition, autonomic nervous system dysfunction, and neuromuscular abnormalities
    - Symptoms include agitation, convulsions, coma, tachycardia, diaphoresis, hyperthermia, hypertension, shivering, myoclonus, tremor, hyperreflexia, and muscle rigidity (esp., of legs).
  - Can presumably result when 5-HT3 receptor antagonists are used with other serotonergic medications.
- **Chemotherapy-induced nausea/vomiting (CINV)**
  - While useful for preventing acute CINV, when 5-HT$_3$-RA are used as monotherapy they have little efficacy for preventing delayed CINV.
  - 5-HT$_3$-RA may be used in combination with other antiemetic classes to prevent CINV depending on the emetogenic potential of the chemotherapeutic regimen being utilized.
- **QT Interval Prolongation**
  - Dolasetron, granisetron, and ondansetron cause a dose-dependent prolongation of the QT interval and are associated with a risk of ventricular arrhythmias.
  - Palonosetron has not been observed to prolong the QT interval, whereas dolasetron carries the highest QT interval prolongation risk.
  - The dose associated with clinically relevant QT interval prolongation is single doses above 16 mg.
  - Since the typical acute care dose of ondansetron is 4 to 8 mg, this is below the threshold where additional ECG monitoring is not always necessary.
    - Historical use of ondansetron for chemotherapy-induced nausea prophylaxis used single doses of 16 and 32 mg and is the setting in which most QT interval prolongation has been observed.

High-Yield Core Evidence
- **Comparative Efficacy**
  - A meta-analysis of 85 studies (15,269 patients) demonstrated that granisetron was significantly better at preventing post-operative nausea/vomiting (PONV, defined as patients experiencing nausea, vomiting, retching, or any combination of these symptoms less than 24 hours after surgery) than ondansetron and dolasetron. However, these agents demonstrated similar efficacy for the prevention of postoperative vomiting itself (defined as patients experiencing vomited, retched, or both less than 24 hours after surgery). Clin Ther 2012;34(2):282-94.

High-Yield Fast-Fact
- **"Zorphine"**
  - Injectable morphine sulfate and ondansetron are syringe compatible. They can be drawn up into the same

HIGH-YIELD BOARD EXAM ESSENTIALS
- **CLASSIC AGENTS:** Alosetron, dolasetron, granisetron, ondansetron, palonosetron
- **DRUG CLASS:** Serotonin Antagonists
- **INDICATIONS:** Nausea/vomiting, chemotherapy-induced nausea and vomiting prophylaxis, postoperative nausea and vomiting, women with diarrhea-predominant - irritable bowel syndrome
- **MECHANISM:** Selective inhibition of 5-HT3 both centrally in the chemotherapy trigger and peripherally in the gastrointestinal tract resulting in antiemetic effects.
- **SIDE EFFECTS:** QT prolongation, serotonin syndrome
- **CLINICAL PEARLS:** Alosetron is only approved for women with severe diarrhea-predominant IBS. It was briefly withdrawn from the US market due to the high incidence of ischemic colitis, leading to surgery and even death. However, it was reapproved for diarrhea-predominant IBS under a limited distribution system.

Table: Drug Class Summary

\multicolumn{4}{c}{**Serotonin Antagonists - Drug Class Review**}
\multicolumn{4}{c}{High-Yield Med Reviews}
Mechanism of Action: Selectively block 5-HT$_3$ serotonin receptors, both peripherally and centrally, resulting in antiemetic effects			
Class Effects: Provide supportive care for nausea and emesis			
Generic Name	**Brand Name**	**Maines**	**Notes**

Alosetron	Lotronex	• Women with diarrhea-predominant irritable bowel syndrome (IBS)	• **Dosing (Women):**
			  – PO: 0.5 to 1 mg BID
			• **Dosing (Peds):** Not used
			• **CYP450 Interactions:** Substrate of CYP1A2, CYP2C9, CYP3A4
			• **Renal or Hepatic Dose Adjustments:**
			  – Child-Pugh C: Contraindicated
			• **Dosage Forms:** Oral (tablets)

Dolasetron	Anzemet	• Nausea and/or vomiting	• **Dosing (Adult):**
			  – PO: 100 mg
			• **Dosing (Peds):**
			  – PO: 1.8 mg/kg
			• **CYP450 Interactions:** Substrate of CYP2C9, CYP3A4
			• **Renal or Hepatic Dose Adjustments:** None
			• **Dosage Forms:** Oral (tablets)

Granisetron	Sancuso (transdermal patch)
	
	Sustol (SubQ)
		• Nausea and/or vomiting	• **Dosing (Adult):**
			  – PO: 1-2 mg daily
			  – IV: 10 **mcg**/kg or 1 mg
			  – SC: 10 mg
			  – Transdermal: 3.1 mg/24hr patch, may be worn for up to 7 days
			• **Dosing (Peds):**
			  – PO: 40 mcg/kg/dose every 12 hours on chemotherapy days
			  – IV: 40 mcg/kg as a single dose prior to chemotherapy
			• **CYP450 Interactions:** Substrate of CYP3A4
			• **Renal or Hepatic Dose Adjustments:**
			  – IV, Oral, Transdermal: No dosage adjustment necessary
			  – SC:
			    – CrCl 30-59 mL/min: 10 mg NMT once every 14 days
			    – CrCl <30: Avoid use
			• **Dosage Forms:** Oral (tablets), subcutaneous, injectable, transdermal

Serotonin Antagonists - Drug Class Review
High-Yield Med Reviews

Generic Name	Brand Name	Maines	Notes

Ondansetron	Zofran
	
	Zuplenz (oral film)
		- Nausea and/or vomiting	- **Dosing (Adult):**
			  - Oral: 4 to 16 mg/day, divided doses
			  - IV, IM: 4 to 8 mg as a single dose
			- **Dosing (Peds):**
			  - Oral: 2 to 8 mg
			  - IV: 0.15 to 0.4 mg/kg/dose (maximum dose: 16 mg/dose)
			- **CYP450 Interactions:** Substrate of CYP1A2, CYP2C9, CYP2D6, CYP2E1, CYP3A4
			- **Renal or Hepatic Dose Adjustments:**
			  - Child-Pugh C: Maximum daily dose 8 mg
			- **Dosage Forms:** Oral (tablet, disintegrating tablet, film, solution), Injectable

Palonosetron	Aloxi (IV)	- Nausea and/or vomiting	- **Dosing (Adult):**
			  - IV: 0.25 mg
			- **Dosing (Peds):**
			  - IV: 20 **mcg**/kg (maximum dose: 1500 **mcg**/dose)
			- **CYP450 Interactions:** Substrate of CYP1A2, CYP2D6, CYP3A4
			- **Renal or Hepatic Dose Adjustments:** None
			- **Dosage Forms:** Injectable (also available as a combo product)

Fosnetupitant/**palonosetron**	Akynzeo (IV)	- Nausea/vomiting	- **Dosing (Adult):**
			  - IV: 235/0.25 mg on day 1 of chemo only
			- **Dosing (Peds):** Not used
			- **CYP450 Interactions:** None
			- **Renal or Hepatic Dose Adjustments:**
			  - CrCl < 30: Avoid
			  - Child-Pugh C: Avoid
			- **Dosage Forms:** Injectable

Netupitant/**palonsetron**	Akynzeo (PO)	- Nausea/vomiting	- **Dosing (Adult):**
			  - PO: 300/0.5 mg on day 1 of chemo
			- **Dosing (Peds):** Not used
			- **CYP450 Interactions:** Substrate of CYP3A4; Inhibits CYP3A4
			- **Renal or Hepatic Dose Adjustments:**
			  - CrCl < 30: Avoid
			  - Child-Pugh C: Avoid
			- **Dosage Forms:** Oral (capsule)

ANTIEMETICS – SUBSTANCE P/ NEUROKININ 1 (NK-1) RECEPTOR ANTAGONISTS

Drug Class
- Substance P/Neurokinin 1 Receptor Antagonist
- Agents:
  - Acute & Chronic Care
    - Aprepitant
    - Fosaprepitant (± palonosetron)
    - Netupitant (± palonosetron)
    - Rolapitant

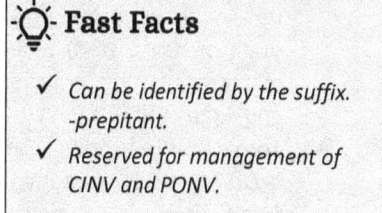

Fast Facts
- ✓ Can be identified by the suffix. -prepitant.
- ✓ Reserved for management of CINV and PONV.

Main Indications or Uses
- Acute & Chronic
  - Prevention of chemotherapy-induced nausea and vomiting (CINV)
  - Prevention of postoperative nausea and vomiting (PONV)

Mechanism of Action
- Selectively inhibit substance P/neurokinin-1 (NK-1) receptors distributed peripherally and centrally to inhibit substance P-mediated responses.

Primary Net Benefit
- Prevents acute and delayed phase CINV
- Main Labs to Monitor:
  - INR (if on concomitant warfarin)

High-Yield Basic Pharmacology
- Prodrugs
  - Fosaprepitant is rapidly (within 30 minutes of the end of the infusion) converted into aprepitant.
  - Fosnetupitant is rapidly converted into netupitant via hydrolysis.
- Hepatic Metabolism
  - All agents are extensively metabolized via the CYP3A4 pathway and are therefore subject to many drug-drug interactions. Aprepitant and fosaprepitant undergo minor metabolism via CYP1A2 and CYP2C19.

High-Yield Clinical Knowledge
- Naming convention
  - Can be identified by the suffix -prepitant
- Chemotherapy-induced nausea/vomiting (CINV)
  - Substance P/NK-1 receptor antagonists are considered to be effective in the prevention of acute and delayed phase CINV.
  - They are used as part of a three- or four-drug combination to prevent CINV, depending on the emetogenic potential of the chemotherapeutic regimen being utilized.
- Dosing schedule
  - All substance P/NK-1 antagonists are single-dose regimens administered on day 1 of chemotherapy only, except for aprepitant, which can be utilized as a three-day regimen.
- Oral contraceptives
  - The efficacy of hormonal contraceptives may be reduced during and for 28 days following the last dose of aprepitant or fosaprepitant. Clinicians should recommend alternative or additional contraceptive methods during treatment and at least one month following treatment.

High-Yield Core Evidence
- **Aprepitant Reduced CINV When Added to a Standard Antiemetic Regimen**
    - Randomized, placebo-controlled phase III trial
    - Patients with multiple myeloma receiving melphalan were randomly assigned at a one-to-one ratio to receive either aprepitant (125 mg orally on day 1 and 80 mg orally on days 2 to 4), granisetron (2 mg orally on days 1 to 4), and dexamethasone (4 mg orally on day 1 and 2 mg orally on days 2 to 3) or matching placebo, granisetron (2 mg orally on days 1 to 4), and dexamethasone (8 mg orally on day 1 and 4 mg orally on days 2 to 3)
    - The primary endpoint (complete response) was defined as no emesis and no rescue therapy within 120 hours of melphalan administration.
    - Significantly more patients receiving aprepitant reached the primary end point (58% v 41%; odds ratio [OR], 1.92; 95% CI, 1.23 to 3.00; P .0042). Absence of major nausea (94% v 88%; OR, 2.37; 95% CI, 1.09 to 5.15; P .026) and emesis (78% v 65%; OR, 1.99; 95% CI, 1.25 to 3.18; P .0036) within 120 hours was increased by aprepitant
    - (J Clin Oncol. 2014 Oct 20;32(30):3413-20.)

High-Yield Fast Facts
- Useful for the prevention, not the treatment, of acute and delayed CINV
- **Fos**aprepitant and **fos**netupitant are the **phos**phoral prodrugs of their parent compounds.
- Rolapitant injectable emulsion (Varubi®) was discontinued in the U.S. after the FDA released postmarketing reports linking administration to severe anaphylactoid reactions and anaphylactoid shock.

HIGH-YIELD BOARD EXAM ESSENTIALS
- **CLASSIC AGENTS:** Aprepitant, fosaprepitant (± palonosetron), netupitant (± palonosetron), rolapitant
- **DRUG CLASS:** Substance P/neurokinin 1 receptor antagonist
- **INDICATIONS:** CNIV, PONV
- **MECHANISM:** Selectively inhibit substance P/neurokinin-1 (NK-1) receptors distributed peripherally and centrally to inhibit substance P-mediated responses.
- **SIDE EFFECTS:** Fatigue, neutropenia, hypotension, bradycardia, headache, constipation
- **CLINICAL PEARLS:** All substance P/NK-1 antagonists are single-dose regimens administered on day 1 of chemotherapy only, except for aprepitant, which can be utilized as a three-day regimen.

Table: Drug Class Summary

Substance P/Neurokinin 1 Receptor Antagonist - Drug Class Review High-Yield Med Reviews			
Mechanism of Action: *Selectively inhibit substance P/neurokinin-1 (NK-1) receptors distributed peripherally and centrally to inhibit substance P-mediated responses*			
Class Effects: *Prevents acute and delayed phase CINV*			
Generic Name	**Brand Name**	**Main Indication(s) or Uses**	**Notes**

Aprepitant	Cinvanti	• Nausea/vomiting	• **Dosing (Adult):**
			  – PO: 40-125 mg or 3 mg/kg
			  – IV: 100-300 mg
			• **Dosing (Peds):**
			  – PO: 2-3 mg/kg/dose
			• **CYP450 Interactions:** Substrate of CYP1A2, CYP2C19, CYP3A4; Inhibits CYP3A4; Induces CYP2c9
			• **Renal or Hepatic Dose Adjustments:** None
			• **Dosage Forms:** Oral (capsule, suspension), injectable

Fosaprepitant	Emend	• Nausea/vomiting	• **Dosing (Adult):**
			  – IV: 150 mg on day 1 of chemo only
			    – Infused over 20-30 min
			• **Dosing (Peds):**
			  – IV: 3-5 mg/kg on day 1 of chemo only
			• **CYP450 Interactions:** Substrate of CYP1A2, CYP2C19, CYP3A4; Inhibits CYP3A4; Induces CYP2C9
			• **Renal or Hepatic Dose Adjustments:** None
			• **Dosage Forms:** Injectable

Rolapitant	Varubi	• Nausea/vomiting	• **Dosing (Adult):**
			  – PO: 180 mg on day 1 of chemo only
			  – IV: 166.5 mg on day 1 of chemo only
			• **Dosing (Peds):** Not used
			• **CYP450 Interactions:** Substrate of CYP1A2, CYP2C19, CYP3A4; Inhibits CYP2B6, CYP2D6, PGP
			• **Renal or Hepatic Dose Adjustments:** None
			• **Dosage Forms:** Oral (tablet), injectable (discontinued in the US)

Fosnetupitant/ palonosetron	Akynzeo (IV)	• Nausea/vomiting	• **Dosing (Adult):**
			  – IV: 235/0.25 mg on day 1 of chemo only
			• **Dosing (Peds):** Not used
			• **CYP450 Interactions:** None
			• **Renal or Hepatic Dose Adjustments:**
			  – CrCl < 30: Avoid
			  – Child-Pugh C: Avoid
			• **Dosage Forms:** Injectable

Substance P/Neurokinin 1 Receptor Antagonist - Drug Class Review High-Yield Med Reviews			
Generic Name	**Brand Name**	**Main Indication(s) or Uses**	**Notes**

Netupitant/
palonosetron
	Akynzeo (PO)	- Nausea/vomiting	- **Dosing (Adult):**
			   – PO: 300/0.5 mg on day 1 of chemo
			- **Dosing (Peds):** Not used
			- **CYP450 Interactions:** Substrate of CYP3A4; Inhibits CYP3A4
			- **Renal or Hepatic Dose Adjustments:**
			   – CrCl < 30: Avoid
			   – Child-Pugh C: Avoid
			- **Dosage Forms:** Oral (capsule)

Gastroenterology

GI – ANTIMOTILITY AGENTS

Drug Class
- Antimotility Agents
- Agents:
    - Acute or Chronic Care
        - Diphenoxylate-Atropine
        - Difenoxin-Atropine
        - Eluxadoline
        - Loperamide
        - Opium tincture
        - Paregoric

> **Fast Facts**
> ✓ Loperamide is available over-the-counter and is relatively easy to use.
> ✓ Loperamide is also the first-line therapy for irinotecan induced diarrhea. Sometimes the doses needed are higher than other situations.

Main Indications or Uses
- Acute or Chronic
    - Diarrhea
    - Eluxadoline – IBS with diarrhea

Mechanism of Action
- Mu and delta-opioid receptor agonists decrease gastrointestinal motility and secretion.
- Eluxadoline
    - Mu-opioid receptor agonist, delta-opioid receptor antagonist, and kappa-opioid receptor agonist acting locally on GI epithelium.

Primary Net Benefit
- OTC and prescription relief for non-infectious diarrhea formulated in abuse-deterrent combinations or limited sale
- Main Labs to Monitor:
    - No routine lab monitoring

High-Yield Basic Pharmacology
- Opioid Receptors
    - The three primary opioid receptors relevant to pharmacotherapy are the delta, kappa, and mu-opioid receptors.
    - Although eluxadoline possesses opioid agonist effects, it is not systemically absorbed, allowing a local opioid action on the GI epithelium.
- Mu Receptor Subtype
    - Mu-2 opioid receptors, although responsible for the diminished ventilatory response to hypoxia, are also located in the GI wall.
    - Agonist activity on GI mu-2 receptors is responsible for constipation from chronic systemic opioid use and the target for opioid-antidiarrheal agents.
    - Eluxadoline is a mixed opioid receptor agonist/antagonist that limits constipating adverse effects.
- Active Metabolite
    - Difenoxin is the active metabolite of diphenoxylate.
    - These agents are structurally related to meperidine.

High-Yield Clinical Knowledge
- Atropine
    - Although diphenoxylate and difenoxin are co-formulated with atropine, the role of atropine is primarily abuse-deterrent rather than therapeutic.
    - If patients surreptitiously administer diphenoxylate or difenoxin in massive quantities orally or parenterally, atropine creates an unpleasant anticholinergic response to offset any opioid-related euphoria.

- Anticholinergic antidiarrheal effects are minimal and not likely contributory to the action of these agents.
- **Inflammatory Bowel Disease**
  - Loperamide should be avoided in patients with IBD that involves the colon due to the high risk of developing toxic megacolon.
- **Opioid Tinctures**
  - Opium tincture contains significantly more morphine than paregoric, leading to significant dosing errors if dosing in drops is miscalculated.
    - Opium tincture contains morphine 10 mg/mL, whereas paregoric contains 0.4 mg/mL of morphine.
  - Both preparations pose a high risk of abuse, diversion, or misuse and have fallen out of favor.
  - Although largely abandoned in clinical practice, updates regarding opium tincture dosing expression have included representing it in morphine dosing units.
  - The concentration of morphine in opium tincture is 10 mg/mL.
  - When converting between doses expressed as drops, milligrams, or units, significant dosing errors are possible.
- **Opioid Antagonists**
  - Conversely, the opioid antagonist methylnaltrexone or naloxone can be used to treat opioid-induced constipation.
    - Oral naloxone doses between 2-6 mg are often ideal for this indication, and doses greater than 6 mg should be avoided due to systemic absorption and potential precipitation of acute systemic opioid withdrawal.
- **Infectious Diarrhea**
  - Infectious causes of diarrhea, particularly diarrhea caused by Clostridoides difficile, should be ruled out before initiating one of these agents.
    - Some infectious diarrhea may be treated using antimotility agents but should be done under an appropriate provider's observation.
- **Pancreatitis with Eluxadoline**
  - The use of eluxadoline is associated with a dose-dependent increased risk of pancreatitis.
  - The risk of pancreatitis is significantly higher in patients who have had their gallbladder removed, sphincter of Oddi disease, or dysfunction.
    - Other independent risk factors that increase pancreatitis risk include pancreatic duct obstruction, alcohol abuse, severe hepatic impairment.

High-Yield Core Evidence
- **OTC Loperamide Safety**
  - This is a case report of two fatalities associated with abuse of OTC loperamide.
  - The first case was a 24-year-old male brought to the ED by EMS after benign found pulseless and apneic following ingestion of approximately 6 boxes of loperamide.
  - This patient attempted to self-treat opioid withdrawal with loperamide as an opioid substitute.
  - Resuscitation and naloxone were ineffective, and the patient was pronounced dead.
  - The second patient was a 39-year-old female presenting to the ED in asystole with EMS-provided CPR en route.
  - Similar to the first patient, this patient was also attempting to self-treat opioid withdrawal with loperamide as an opioid substitute, but resuscitation and naloxone were ineffective, and the patient was pronounced dead
  - The authors urged clinicians to report all loperamide toxicity cases to the Food and Drug Administration's MedWatch. (Ann Emerg Med. 2017 Jan;69(1):83-86.)

High-Yield Fast-Fact
- **Paregoric**
  - Paregoric may also be referred to as camphorated opium tincture.

Table: Drug Class Summary

Antimotility Agents - Drug Class Review High-Yield Med Reviews			
Mechanism of Action: *Mu and delta-opioid receptor agonists decrease gastrointestinal motility and secretion.* *Eluxadoline: Mu-opioid receptor agonist, delta-opioid receptor antagonist, and kappa-opioid receptor agonist acting locally on GI epithelium.*			
Class Effects: *Over-the-counter and prescription relief for non-infectious diarrhea formulated in abuse-deterrent combinations or limited sale to prevent acute toxicity.*			
Generic Name	**Brand Name**	**Main Indication(s) or Uses**	**Notes**

Diphenoxylate-Atropine	Lomotil (C-V)	• Diarrhea	• **Dosing (Adult):**
			  – Oral: 5 mg q6h until control achieved
			    – Maximum 20 mg/day
			• **Dosing (Peds):**
			  – Oral: 0.3 to 0.4 mg/kg/day divided q6h
			    – Maximum 10 mg/day
			• **CYP450 Interactions:** None
			• **Renal or Hepatic Dose Adjustments:** None
			• **Dosage Forms:** Oral (liquid, tablet)

Difenoxin-Atropine	Motofen (C-IV)	• Diarrhea	• **Dosing (Adult):**
			  – Oral: 2 tablets x 1, then 1 tablet after each loose stool or q3-4h
			    – Maximum 8 tablets/day
			• **Dosing (Peds):**
			  – For children 12 years and older only
			    – Use adult dosing
			• **CYP450 Interactions:** None
			• **Renal or Hepatic Dose Adjustments:**
			  – No specific adjustments
			  – Use with caution in patients with renal or hepatic dysfunction
			• **Dosage Forms:** Oral (tablet)

Eluxadoline	Viberzi	• Irritable bowel syndrome	• **Dosing (Adult):**
			  – Oral: 75 to 100 mg BID
			• **Dosing (Peds):**
			  – Not routinely used
			• **CYP450 Interactions:** None
			• **Renal or Hepatic Dose Adjustments:**
			  – GFR < 60 mL/minute: 75 mg BID
			  – Child-Pugh class A or B: 75 mg BID
			  – Child-Pugh class C: Contraindicated
			• **Dosage Forms:** Oral (Tablet)

Antimotility Agents - Drug Class Review
High-Yield Med Reviews

Generic Name	Brand Name	Main Indication(s) or Uses	Notes

Loperamide	Imodium A-D (OTC)	• Diarrhea	• **Dosing (Adult):**
			  − Oral: 4 mg followed by 2 mg after each loose stool
			    − Maximum 16 mg/day
			• **Dosing (Peds):**
			  − Oral: 0.08 to 0.25 mg/kg/day q6-12h as needed after each loose stool
			    − Maximum: age-dependent 3 to 8 mg/day
			• **CYP450 Interactions:** Substrate of CYP2B6, 2C8, 2D6, 3A4, P-gp
			• **Renal or Hepatic Dose Adjustments:** None
			• **Dosage Forms:** Oral (capsule, liquid, solution, suspension, tablet)

Opium tincture	N/A (C-II)	• Diarrhea	• **Dosing (Adult):**
			  − Oral: 6 mg q6h
			• **Dosing (Peds):**
			  − Not routinely used
			• **CYP450 Interactions:** None
			• **Renal or Hepatic Dose Adjustments:** None
			• **Dosage Forms:** Oral tincture

Paregoric	N/A (C-III)	• Diarrhea	• **Dosing (Adult):**
			  − Oral: 5 to 10 mL q6-24h
			    − 1 mL = 0.4 mg morphine
			• **Dosing (Peds):**
			  − Oral: 0.25 to 0.5 mL/kg/dose q6-24h
			    − Maximum 10 mL/dose
			• **CYP450 Interactions:** None
			• **Renal or Hepatic Dose Adjustments:** None
			• **Dosage Forms:** Oral tincture

HIGH-YIELD BOARD EXAM ESSENTIALS
- **CLASSIC AGENTS:** Diphenoxylate-atropine, difenoxin-atropine, loperamide, opium tincture, paregoric
- **DRUG CLASS:** Antimotility agents
- **INDICATIONS:** Diarrhea
- **MECHANISM:** Mu and delta-opioid receptor agonists decreasing gastrointestinal motility and secretion. Eluxadoline: Mu-opioid receptor agonist, delta-opioid receptor antagonist, and kappa-opioid receptor agonist acting locally on GI epithelium.
- **SIDE EFFECTS:** Constipation, GI obstruction
- **CLINICAL PEARLS:**
  - Although diphenoxylate and difenoxin are co-formulated with atropine, its role is primarily abuse-deterrence rather than therapeutic since these agents can stimulate the mu opioid receptors and increase risk of possible abuse.
  - Avoid their use in patients with ulcerative colitis and evidence or risk for toxic megacolon because this could result in bowel perforation.
  - Eluxadoline is associated with a dose-dependent risk of pancreatitis.

Gastroenterology

GI - LAXATIVES (BULK-FORMING, EMOLLIENT, LUBRICANT, OSMOTIC, SALINE, STIMULANT)

Drug Class
- Laxatives (Emollient, Osmotic, Saline, Stimulant)
- Agents:
    - Acute Care
        - Bisacodyl
        - Castor oil
        - Docusate
        - Glycerin
        - Lactulose
        - Magnesium citrate
        - Magnesium hydroxide
        - Magnesium sulfate
        - Methylcellulose
        - Mineral oil
        - Polycarbophil
        - Polyethylene glycol
        - Psyllium
        - Senna
        - Sodium Picosulfate, Magnesium Oxide, and Citric Acid
        - Sodium Sulfate, Magnesium Sulfate, and Potassium Chloride
        - Sodium Sulfate, Potassium Sulfate, and Magnesium Sulfate
        - Sorbito

Main Indications or Uses
- Acute & Chronic Care
    - Bowel preparation
        - Magnesium Citrate
        - Polyethylene glycol
        - Sodium Picosulfate, Magnesium Oxide, and Citric Acid
        - Sodium Sulfate, Magnesium Sulfate, and Potassium Chloride
        - Sodium Sulfate, Potassium Sulfate, and Magnesium Sulfate
    - Constipation
        - Bisacodyl
        - Castor oil
        - Docusate
        - Glycerin
        - Lactulose
        - Magnesium Citrate
        - Magnesium hydroxide
        - Magnesium sulfate
        - Methylcellulose
        - Mineral oil
        - Polycarbophil
        - Polyethylene glycol
        - Psyllium
        - Senna
        - Sorbitol
    - Hepatic encephalopathy
        - Lactulose

Mechanism of Action
- **Bulk-forming agents (methylcellulose, polycarbophil, psyllium)**
    - Increase the water content of the stool, thereby increasing the bulk and weight of the stool.
- **Emollient laxatives (docusate)**
    - Facilitates mixing of aqueous and fatty materials in the GI tract.
- **Lubricant laxative (castor oil, mineral oil)**
    - Improves water content in stool and lubricates the intestine.
- **Osmolar laxatives**
    - Lactulose, sorbitol
        - Colonic bacteria metabolize these agents to low-molecular-weight acids that increase fluid retention in the colon.
    - Glycerin, Polyethylene glycol
        - Creates a hyperosmotic environment without metabolism, different from lactulose or sorbitol.

- **Saline cathartics (Sodium Picosulfate, Sodium Sulfate, Magnesium Hydroxide, Magnesium Oxide, Magnesium Sulfate, Potassium Chloride, Potassium Sulfate)**
  - Promotes osmotic retention of fluid, distending the colon and stimulating peristaltic activity.
- **Stimulant Laxative (bisacodyl, senna)**
  - Stimulates the nerve plexus of the colon to stimulate peristalsis and increases interstitial fluid secretion.

Primary Net Benefit
- Over-the-counter agents for self-care of constipation, as well as bowel preparatory agents, to facilitate endoscopy.
- Main Labs to Monitor:
  - No routine monitoring

High-Yield Basic Pharmacology
- **Castor oil**
  - The castor bean, from which castor oil is derived, also contains ricin.
- **Fiber Supplementation**
  - Dietary or supplemental fiber is fermented in the GI, producing increased intestinal bacterial mass and increased short-chain fatty acids.

High-Yield Clinical Knowledge
- **Cardiovascular Benefits**
  - Fiber supplementation has been associated with improved cardiovascular outcomes, and it is recommended to consume approximately 30 g of fiber daily for most adults.
  - The typical American diet does not contain sufficient fiber, and supplementation using bulk-forming laxatives can consume the target fiber intake.
- **Prevention of Opioid Associated Constipation**
  - Patients receiving acute or chronic opioids should maintain bowel health to avoid intestinal obstructions, which increase the risk of perforation.
  - Combining docusate plus senna is a commonly recommended bowel regimen for patients in acute care facilities receiving opioids.
  - GI obstruction must be ruled out in patients presenting with constipation related to opioid use before using stimulant laxatives, as they are associated with an increased risk of perforation.
- **Stimulant Laxative Duration**
  - Stimulant laxatives, namely bisacodyl, should not be used for more than ten consecutive days.
  - If relief has not been achieved, referral to primary care or GI specialists is required.
- **Dietary Supplement Product**
  - Senna leaf extract syrup is considered a dietary supplement and is not interchangeable with other sennoside-containing products.
- **Docusate Ear Wax Removal**
  - Docusate has been used in some cases to aid in the disimpaction of cerumen in the outer ear.
  - The gel capsules can be opened, with the contents administered in the outer ear.
- **Mineral Oil Ingestion**
  - Mineral oil, taken by mouth to relieve constipation, must be used with caution in patients with difficulty swallowing or altered mental status as the risk of aspiration is very high.
  - If inhaled, lipoid pneumonia can result, leading to unnecessary increased morbidity and mortality.

High-Yield Core Evidence
- **Dietary Fiber and Cardiovascular Disease**
    - This was a systematic review and meta-analysis of prospective studies reporting associations between fiber intake and coronary heart disease or cardiovascular disease, with a minimum follow-up of three years, including searches of the Cochrane Library, Medline, Medline in-process, Embase, CAB Abstracts, ISI Web of Science, BIOSIS, and hand searching.
    - A total of 22 cohort study publications met inclusion criteria which demonstrated that total dietary fiber intake was inversely associated with the risk of cardiovascular disease and coronary heart disease.
    - Fiber sources, including cereal, vegetable, and fruit sources, were inversely associated with cardiovascular disease risk.
    - The authors concluded that greater dietary fiber intake is associated with a lower risk of cardiovascular disease and coronary heart disease. (BMJ. 2013 Dec 19;347:f6879.)

High-Yield Fast-Fact
- **Anthracenes**
    - Sennosides contain a tricyclic anthracene nucleus that is similar to other similar compounds in aloe and cascara.

HIGH-YIELD BOARD EXAM ESSENTIALS
- **CLASSIC AGENTS:** Bisacodyl, castor oil, docusate, glycerin, lactulose, magnesium salts, methylcellulose, mineral oil, polyethylene glycol, senna, sorbitol
- **DRUG CLASS:** Laxatives
- **INDICATIONS:** Constipation
- **MECHANISM:** Bulk-forming agents (methylcellulose, polycarbophil, psyllium), emollient laxatives (docusate), lubricant laxative (castor oil, mineral oil), osmolar laxatives (glycerin, lactulose, polyethylene glycol, sorbitol), saline cathartics (sodium picosulfate, sodium sulfate, magnesium hydroxide, magnesium oxide, magnesium sulfate, potassium chloride, potassium sulfate), stimulant laxative (bisacodyl, senna)
- **SIDE EFFECTS:** Flatulence, diarrhea
- **CLINICAL PEARLS:**
    - Fiber supplementation has been associated with improved cardiovascular outcomes and is recommended to consume approximately 30 g of fiber daily for most adults.
    - The typical American diet does not contain sufficient fiber, and supplementation using bulk-forming laxatives can consume the target fiber intake.
    - Stool softeners (e.g., docusate) alone are not sufficient for preventing opioid induced constipation.

Table: Drug Class Summary

Laxatives (Emollient, Lubricant, Osmotic, Saline, Stimulant) - Drug Class Review High-Yield Med Reviews			
Mechanism of Action: *Bulk-forming agents (methylcellulose, polycarbophil, psyllium)* *Emollient laxatives (docusate)* *Lubricant laxative (castor oil, mineral oil)* *Osmolar laxatives (Glycerin, lactulose, polyethylene glycol, sorbitol)* *Saline cathartics (Sodium Picosulfate, Sodium Sulfate, Magnesium Hydroxide, Magnesium Oxide, Magnesium Sulfate, Potassium Chloride, Potassium Sulfate)* *Stimulant Laxative (bisacodyl, senna)*			
Class Effects: *Over-the-counter agents for self-care of constipation and bowel preparatory agents to facilitate endoscopy.*			
Generic Name	**Brand Name**	**Main Indication(s) or Uses**	**Notes**

Bisacodyl	Biscolax
	Ducodyl
	Ducolax
	Fleet
	Bisacodyl
		- Constipation
		- Ear wax removal (off-label; OTC as a Ceruminolytic)
			- **Dosing (Adult):**
			  – Rectal: 10 mg once
			  – Oral: 5 to 15 mg once daily
			- **Dosing (Peds):**
			  – Rectal: 10 mg once
			  – Oral: 5 to 15 mg once daily
			- **CYP450 Interactions:** None
			- **Renal or Hepatic Dose Adjustments:** None
			- **Dosage Forms:** Oral (tablet), Rectal (enema, suppository)

Castor oil	GoodSense Castor Oil	- Constipation	- **Dosing (Adult):**
			  – Oral: 15 to 60 mL as a single dose
			- **Dosing (Peds):**
			  – Oral: 5 to 60 mL as a single dose
			- **CYP450 Interactions:** None
			- **Renal or Hepatic Dose Adjustments:** None
			- **Dosage Forms:** Oral (oil)

Docusate	Colace
	Stool softener
		- Constipation	- **Dosing (Adult):**
			  – Oral: (sodium salt) 50 to 360 mg daily
			  – Oral: (calcium salt) 240 mg daily
			  – Rectal: 283 mg 1 to 3 times daily
			- **Dosing (Peds):**
			  – Oral: (sodium salt) 5 mg/kg/day in 1-4 divided doses
			  – Rectal: 100 to 283 mg daily
			- **CYP450 Interactions:** None
			- **Renal or Hepatic Dose Adjustments:** None
			- **Dosage Forms:** Oral (capsule, liquid, syrup, tablet), Rectal (enema)

\multicolumn{4}{c}{**Laxatives (Emollient, Lubricant, Osmotic, Saline, Stimulant) - Drug Class Review**}
\multicolumn{4}{c}{High-Yield Med Reviews}
Generic Name	**Brand Name**	**Main Indication(s) or Uses**	**Notes**

Glycerin	Fleet Liquid Glycerin	- Constipation	- **Dosing (Adult):**
			  – Rectal enema or suppository daily as needed
			- **Dosing (Peds):**
			  – Rectal enema or suppository daily as needed
			- **CYP450 Interactions:** None
			- **Renal or Hepatic Dose Adjustments:** None
			- **Dosage Forms:** Rectal (enema, suppository)

Lactulose	Constulose
	Enulose
	Generlac
	Kristalose
		- Constipation
		- Hepatic encephalopathy
			- **Dosing (Adult):**
			  – Oral: 10 to 30 g q1-8h as needed
			  – Rectal: 200 g
			- **Dosing (Peds):**
			  – Extra info if needed
			    – Extra info if needed
			- **CYP450 Interactions:** text
			- **Renal or Hepatic Dose Adjustments:** text
			- **Dosage Forms:** [e.g., basic info]

Magnesium citrate	Citroma	- Bowel preparation prior to colonoscopy	- **Dosing (Adult):**
			  – 1 to 1.5 bottles (300 to 450 mL) 8 hours prior to procedure
			- **Dosing (Peds):**
			  – Age 2 to 6 years : 60 to 90 mL once or in divided doses
			  – Age 6 to < 12 years : 100 to 150 mL once or in divided doses
			- **CYP450 Interactions:** None
			- **Renal or Hepatic Dose Adjustments:**
			  – Should be avoided in PEDIATRICS with renal impairment
			- **Dosage Forms:** Oral (solution, tablet)

Magnesium hydroxide	Milk of Magnesia
	Pedia-Lax
	Phillips Milk of Magnesia
		- Antacid
		- Laxative
			- **Dosing (Adult):**
			  – Oral: 400 to 1,200 mg as needed up to 4 times daily
			    – Maximum 4,800 mg/day
			- **Dosing (Peds):**
			  – Oral: 400 to 1,200 mg as needed up to 4 times daily
			    – Age 2 to 6 years maximum 1,200 mg/day
			    – Age 6 to < 12 years: maximum 2,400 mg/day
			- **CYP450 Interactions:** None
			- **Renal or Hepatic Dose Adjustments:**
			  – Should be avoided in PEDIATRICS with renal impairment
			- **Dosage Forms:** Oral (suspension, tablet)

| Laxatives (Emollient, Lubricant, Osmotic, Saline, Stimulant) - Drug Class Review ||||
High-Yield Med Reviews			
Generic Name	**Brand Name**	**Main Indication(s) or Uses**	**Notes**
Magnesium sulfate	Epsom Salt Magnacaps	<ul><li>Asthma</li><li>Constipation</li><li>Eclampsia/preeclampsia</li><li>Hypomagnesemia</li><li>Torsades de pointes</li></ul>	<ul><li>**Dosing (Adult):**<ul><li>Oral: 10 to 20 g dissolved in 240 mL water, maximum 2 doses/day</li><li>IV: 1 to 2 g IV push over 1-2 minutes</li><li>IV: 1 to 6 g IV over 1-30 minutes, followed by 1 to 4 g/hour infusion (if necessary)</li><li>IM: 10 g (2x 5g in each buttock) at onset of labor, followed by 5 g q4h</li></ul></li><li>**Dosing (Peds):**<ul><li>IV: (elemental magnesium) 2.5 to 5 mg/kg/dose q6h</li><li>Oral: (elemental magnesium) 10 to 20 mg/kg/dose q6-24h</li></ul></li><li>**CYP450 Interactions:** None</li><li>**Renal or Hepatic Dose Adjustments:**<ul><li>Severe renal impairment<ul><li>IV: 4-6 g loading dose over 15-30 min, then 1 g/hour infusion (maximum 10 g/24h)</li></ul></li></ul></li><li>**Dosage Forms:** Oral (capsule, granules), IV (solution)</li></ul>
Methylcellulose	Citrucel	<ul><li>Constipation</li></ul>	<ul><li>**Dosing (Adult):**<ul><li>Oral: 2 caplets 6 times per day, up to 12 caplets/day</li></ul></li><li>**Dosing (Peds):**<ul><li>Oral: 1 caplets 6 times per day, up to 6 caplets/day</li></ul></li><li>**CYP450 Interactions:** None</li><li>**Renal or Hepatic Dose Adjustments:** None</li><li>**Dosage Forms:** Oral (powder, tablet)</li></ul>
Mineral oil	Fleet oil	<ul><li>Constipation</li></ul>	<ul><li>**Dosing (Adult):**<ul><li>Oral: 15 to 45 mL/day (plain) or 30 to 90 mL/day (suspension)</li><li>Rectal: 118 mL once</li></ul></li><li>**Dosing (Peds):**<ul><li>Oral: 5 to 15 mL/day (plain) or 10 to 30 mL/day (suspension)</li><li>Rectal: 59 to 118 mL once</li></ul></li><li>**CYP450 Interactions:** None</li><li>**Renal or Hepatic Dose Adjustments:** None</li><li>**Dosage Forms:** Oral (oil), Rectal (enema)</li></ul>

Laxatives (Emollient, Lubricant, Osmotic, Saline, Stimulant) - Drug Class Review			
High-Yield Med Reviews			
Generic Name	**Brand Name**	**Main Indication(s) or Uses**	**Notes**

Polycarbophil	Fiber Laxative, Fiber-Caps, Fiber-Lax, FiberCon	- Constipation	- **Dosing (Adult):**
			   - Oral: 1250 mg q6-24h
			- **Dosing (Peds):**
			   - Oral: 625 mg q6-24h
			- **CYP450 Interactions:** None
			- **Renal or Hepatic Dose Adjustments:** None
			- **Dosage Forms:** Oral (tablet)

Polyethylene glycol 3350	Gavilax, Gialax, Glycolax, Healthylax, Miralax, PEGylax	- Bowel preparation prior to colonoscopy	- **Dosing (Adult):**
			   - Oral: 17 g in 240 mL q10minutes until 2,000 mL consumed.
			   - Oral: 17g in 240 mL once daily, as needed
			- **Dosing (Peds):**
			   - Oral: 1.5 g/kg/day for 4 days
			      - Maximum 100 g/day
			   - Oral: 0.2 to 1 g/kg once daily
			      - Maximum 17 g/day
			- **CYP450 Interactions:** None
			- **Renal or Hepatic Dose Adjustments:** None
			- **Dosage Forms:** Oral (kit, packet, powder)

Psyllium	Evac, Knsyl, Metamucil, Mucilin, Natural Fiber Therapy, Sorbulax	- Constipation
		- CHD risk reduction
			- **Dosing (Adult):**
			   - Oral: 2.5 to 30 g per day in divided doses
			- **Dosing (Peds):**
			   - Oral: 2.5 to 30 g per day in divided doses
			- **CYP450 Interactions:** None
			- **Renal or Hepatic Dose Adjustments:** None
			- **Dosage Forms:** Oral (capsule, packet, powder)

Senna	Ex-Lax, Geri-kot, Senexon, Senna Lax, Senna-tabs, Senokot	- Constipation	- **Dosing (Adult):**
			   - Oral: 8.6 to 50 mg (of sennosides) 1-2 times/day
			- **Dosing (Peds):**
			   - Oral: 4.4 to 50 mg (of sennosides) 1-2 times/day
			- **CYP450 Interactions:** None
			- **Renal or Hepatic Dose Adjustments:** None
			- **Dosage Forms:** Oral (leaves, liquid, syrup, tablet)

Sodium Picosulfate, Magnesium Oxide, and Citric Acid	Clenpiq Prepopik	- Bowel preparation prior to colonoscopy	- **Dosing (Adult):**
			   - Oral: 150 to 160 mL 12 hours prior to colonoscopy.
			- **Dosing (Peds):**
			   - Extra info if needed
			      - Extra info if needed
			- **CYP450 Interactions:** None
			- **Renal or Hepatic Dose Adjustments:**
			   - GFR < 30 mL/minute - Contraindicated
			- **Dosage Forms:** Oral (powder, solution)

\multicolumn{4}{c}{**Laxatives (Emollient, Lubricant, Osmotic, Saline, Stimulant) - Drug Class Review**}
\multicolumn{4}{c}{High-Yield Med Reviews}
Generic Name	**Brand Name**	**Main Indication(s) or Uses**	**Notes**
Sodium Sulfate, Magnesium Sulfate, and Potassium Chloride	Sutab	• Bowel preparation prior to colonoscopy	• **Dosing (Adult):** – Night before procedure: Take 12 tablets with 16 ounces of water over a 15–20 minute period, followed in 1 hour by an additional 16 oz of water every 30 minutes, twice. – Morning of procedure: repeat the above process, starting 8 hours before the procedure. • **Dosing (Peds):** – Not routinely used • **CYP450 Interactions:** None • **Renal or Hepatic Dose Adjustments:** None • **Dosage Forms:** Oral (tablet)
Sodium Sulfate, Potassium Sulfate, and Magnesium Sulfate	Suprep Bowel Prep Kit	• Bowel preparation prior to colonoscopy	• **Dosing (Adult):** – Oral: 2,888 mL in divided doses prior to the procedure. • **Dosing (Peds):** – Oral: 2,128 mL in divided doses prior to the procedure. • **CYP450 Interactions:** None • **Renal or Hepatic Dose Adjustments:** None • **Dosage Forms:** Oral (solution)
Sorbitol	N/A	• Laxative	• **Dosing (Adult):** – Oral: 30 to 45 mL as 70% solution – Rectal: 120 mL as 25 to 35% solution • **Dosing (Peds):** – Oral: 1 to 3 mL/kg/day in divided doses – Rectal: 30 to 120 mL as needed • **CYP450 Interactions:** None • **Renal or Hepatic Dose Adjustments:** None • **Dosage Forms:** Oral (solution), Rectal (solution)

GI - PROKINETIC AGENTS

Drug Class
- Prokinetic Agents
- Agents:
    - Acute Care
        - Erythromycin
        - Metoclopramide
    - Chronic Care
        - Linaclotide
        - Lubiprostone
        - Plecanatide
        - Prucalopride

Main Indications or Uses
- Acute Care
    - Pre-endoscopy prokinetic adjunct
        - Erythromycin
    - Gastroparesis
        - Metoclopramide
    - Nausea and Vomiting
        - Metoclopramide
- Chronic Care
    - Chronic Idiopathic Constipation
        - Linaclotide
        - Lubiprostone
        - Plecanatide
        - Prucalopride
    - Irritable bowel syndrome
        - Eluxadoline (diarrhea)
        - Linaclotide (constipation)
        - Lubiprostone (constipation)
        - Plecanatide (constipation)
    - Opioid-induced constipation
        - Lubiprostone

Mechanism of Action
- Erythromycin
    - Direct agonist effect on motilin receptors in GI smooth muscle.
- Metoclopramide
    - Dopamine (D-2) receptor antagonists in the GI and chemoreceptor trigger zone, aiding cholinergic smooth muscle stimulation.
- Lubiprostone
    - Activates chloride channels on GI luminal epithelium by binding to the prostanoid receptor (EP4) for prostaglandin E2, stimulating chloride-rich fluid secretion in the intestinal lumen, increasing intraluminal fluid secretion softening the stool, and accelerating GI transit.
- Linaclotide, Plecanatide
    - Activates the intestinal epithelial guanylate cyclase C receptor, increasing intestinal fluid secretion.
- Prucalopride
    - Selective serotonin (5-HT4) receptor agonist that stimulates acetylcholine release and increases GI motility.

Primary Net Benefit
- Management of GI distress (nausea, constipation), largely by increasing motility according to the disease.
- Main Labs to Monitor: No routine labs

High-Yield Basic Pharmacology
- **GI Serotonin Receptors**
  - Serotonin 5HT4 receptors are located throughout the GI tract and enhance acetylcholine release, stimulating motility across the GI tract, including the stomach, small intestine, and colon.
- **Tolerance Effect**
  - Although erythromycin is an effective prokinetic agent, tolerance to motilin's stimulation rapidly develops, diminishing its use.

High-Yield Clinical Knowledge
- **Nausea**
  - Lubiprostone, linaclotide, and plecanatide are associated with a high incidence (up to 30%) of drug-induced nausea.
- **QT Prolongation**
  - This group of medications, except for prucalopride, is associated with QT prolongation.
    - Inhibition of Human Ether-a-go-go-related Gene (hERG) potassium channels is a known cause of QT interval prolongation.
  - Cisapride and tegaserod were GI prokinetic agents used commonly but have been removed from the US market due to the risk of QT prolongation and adverse cardiovascular events.
- **Endoscopy Adjunct Therapy**
  - In patients with acute GI bleeding who require emergent endoscopy, the presence of clots in the stomach makes effective visualization on emergency endoscopy difficult.
  - Erythromycin and metoclopramide have been used for their prokinetic effects to stimulate GI motility, aiding in the clearance of obstructions from the GI tract and improving visualization on an endoscopic exam.
    - As the dose of erythromycin used for this indication is lower than an otherwise therapeutic dose, the safety (QT prolongation, nausea/vomiting) is likely better than metoclopramide, which is dosed at normal therapeutic doses, increasing the risk of extrapyramidal symptoms.
- **Metoclopramide EPS**
  - As a result of its dopamine antagonist properties, metoclopramide is associated with extrapyramidal effects, including akathisia, dystonias, and parkinsonism.
    - With chronic use, metoclopramide is also associated with galactorrhea, gynecomastia, impotence, and menstrual disorders.

High-Yield Core Evidence
- **Lubiprostone Meta-Analysis**
  - This was a systematic review and meta-analysis that examined the efficacy and safety of lubiprostone in treating chronic idiopathic constipation (CIC) and irritable bowel syndrome with constipation (IBS-C).
  - The literature search conducted by these authors included MEDLINE, Cochrane, Google Scholar, and ClinicalTrials.gov databases.
  - The final analysis included nine trials consisting of 1468 patients in the lubiprostone group and 841 in the placebo group.
  - Lubiprostone was associated with a significant improvement in constipation severity, stool consistency, abdominal pain, degree of straining, and abdominal bloating at both one week and one month.
  - There was no difference observed regarding the incidence of abdominal pain at one month vs. placebo.
  - Lubiprostone was associated with only a significant improvement in abdominal bloating at three months.
  - The most commonly observed adverse effects included nausea, vomiting, and diarrhea.
  - The authors concluded that lubiprostone is a safe and efficacious drug for treating chronic idiopathic constipation and irritable bowel syndrome with constipation, with limited adverse effects in 3 months of follow-up. (Mayo Clin Proc. 2016 Apr;91(4):456-68.)

- **Erythromycin Before Endoscopy**
    - This was a single-center, double-blind study of patients with acute upper GI bleeding who were randomized to receive gastric lavage plus either erythromycin 250 mg IVPB or placebo.
    - Patients randomized to erythromycin experienced a significantly improved primary endpoint of stomach cleansing before endoscopy, assessed by both subjective and objective criteria.
    - Erythromycin improved gastric mucosa visualization, the quality of examination of the upper gastrointestinal tract, and identification of clots in the GI.
    - There was no difference observed regarding identifying the source of the bleeding, mean duration of endoscopy, and need for a second-look endoscopy.
    - There was no significant difference in the incidence of adverse events between groups.
    - The authors concluded that intravenous erythromycin before endoscopy improves stomach cleansing and quality of endoscopic examination in patients with upper gastrointestinal bleeding, but the clinical benefit is limited. (Am J Gastroenterol. 2006 Jun;101(6):1211-5.)

High-Yield Fast-Fact
- **Cisapride and Tegaserod**
    - Cisapride and tegaserod were removed from the market because of increased risk of CV adverse events.

HIGH-YIELD BOARD EXAM ESSENTIALS
- **CLASSIC AGENTS:** Erythromycin, metoclopramide, linaclotide, lubiprostone, plecanatide, prucalopride
- **DRUG CLASS:** Prokinetic agents
- **INDICATIONS:** Pre-endoscopy prokinetic adjunct (erythromycin), gastroparesis (metoclopramide), nausea and vomiting (metoclopramide), chronic idiopathic constipation (linaclotide, lubiprostone, plecanatide, prucalopride), irritable bowel syndrome (linaclotide, lubiprostone, plecanatide), opioid-induced constipation (lubiprostone)
- **MECHANISM:**
    - Erythromycin: Direct agonist effect on motilin receptors in GI smooth muscle
    - Metoclopramide: D-2 receptor antagonists in the GI and chemoreceptor trigger zone
    - Lubiprostone: Activates GI chloride channels increasing intraluminal fluid secretion
    - Linaclotide, plecanatide: Intestinal epithelial guanylate cyclase c receptor agonists, increasing intestinal fluid secretion
    - Prucalopride: Selective 5-ht4 receptor agonist
- **SIDE EFFECTS:** Nausea, QT prolongation
- **CLINICAL PEARLS:** Lubiprostone, linaclotide, and plecanatide are associated with a high incidence of drug-induced nausea in up to 30% of patients.

Table: Drug Class Summary

	**Prokinetic Agents - Drug Class Review** High-Yield Med Reviews
	**Mechanism of Action:** *Erythromycin - Direct agonist effect on motilin receptors in GI smooth muscle.* *Metoclopramide - D-2 receptor antagonists in the GI and chemoreceptor trigger zone* *Lubiprostone - Activates GI chloride channels increasing intraluminal fluid secretion.* *Linaclotide, Plecanatide - Intestinal epithelial guanylate cyclase C receptor agonists, increasing intestinal fluid secretion.* *Prucalopride - Selective 5-HT4 receptor agonist*
	**Class Effects:** *Stimulate GI motility, aiding in resolving constipation from various underlying causes.*

Generic Name	Brand Name	Main Indication(s) or Uses	Notes

Erythromycin	Erythrocin	- Bacterial infections
		- Pre-endoscopy prokinetic adjunct
			- **Dosing (Adult):**
			  – IV: 3 mg/kg or 250 mg as a single dose over 30 minutes, 1 hour prior to endoscopy
			- **Dosing (Peds):**
			  – Not used for GI indication
			- **CYP450 Interactions:** Substrate CYP2B6, 3A4, P-gp; Inhibits CYP3A4, P-gp
			- **Renal or Hepatic Dose Adjustments:** None
			- **Dosage Forms:** Oral (capsule, tablet, solution), IV (solution)

Metoclopramide	Reglan	- Chemotherapy-induced nausea and vomiting prophylaxis
		- Gastroparesis
		- Nausea and Vomiting
			- **Dosing (Adult):**
			  – Oral/IV/SQ: 10 mg q4-6h
			- **Dosing (Peds):**
			  – IV: 0.5-2 mg/kg/dose q6-8h
			  – Oral: 0.1-0.2 mg/kg/dose q6-8h
			  – Max 10 mg/dose
			- **CYP450 Interactions:** Substrate CYP1A2
			- **Renal or Hepatic Dose Adjustments:**
			  – CrCl 10-60 mL/minute: Administer 50% of total daily dose
			  – CrCl < 10 mL/minute: Administer 33% of total daily dose
			  – Child-Pugh class B or C: Use not recommended
			- **Dosage Forms:** Oral (solution, tablet), IV (solution), Nasal solution

Linaclotide	Linzess	- Chronic idiopathic constipation
		- Irritable bowel syndrome
			- **Dosing (Adult):**
			  – Oral: 72-290 mcg daily
			- **Dosing (Peds):**
			  – Not routinely used
			- **CYP450 Interactions:** None
			- **Renal or Hepatic Dose Adjustments:** None
			- **Dosage Forms:** Oral (capsules)

\multicolumn{4}{c}{**Prokinetic Agents - Drug Class Review**}
\multicolumn{4}{c}{High-Yield Med Reviews}
Generic Name	**Brand Name**	**Main Indication(s) or Uses**	**Notes**

Lubiprostone	Amitiza	• Chronic idiopathic constipation
		• Irritable bowel syndrome
		• Opioid-induced constipation
			• **Dosing (Adult):**
			  — Oral: 8-24 mcg BID
			• **Dosing (Peds):**
			  — Not routinely used
			• **CYP450 Interactions:** None
			• **Renal or Hepatic Dose Adjustments:**
			  — Child-Pugh class B: 16 mcg BID
			  — Child-Pugh class C: 8 mcg BID
			• **Dosage Forms:** Oral (capsule)

Plecanatide	Trulance	• Chronic idiopathic constipation
		• Irritable bowel syndrome
			• **Dosing (Adult):**
			  — Oral: 3 mg daily
			• **Dosing (Peds):**
			  — Not routinely used
			• **CYP450 Interactions:** None
			• **Renal or Hepatic Dose Adjustments:** None
			• **Dosage Forms:** Oral (tablet)

Prucalopride	Motegrity	• Chronic idiopathic constipation	• **Dosing (Adult):**
			  — Oral: 2 mg daily
			• **Dosing (Peds):**
			  — Not routinely used
			• **CYP450 Interactions:** Substrate of P-gp
			• **Renal or Hepatic Dose Adjustments:**
			  — CrCl < 30 mL/minute: 1 mg daily
			• **Dosage Forms:** Oral (tablet)

2025

A COMPREHENSIVE *RAPID REVIEW*

NAPLEX

Pharmacology & Drug Classes

Genitourinary

GENITOURINARY – 5-ALPHA REDUCTASE INHIBITORS

Drug Class
- 5-Alpha Reductase Inhibitors
- Agents:
  - Acute Care
    - Dutasteride
    - Finasteride

Main Indications or Uses
- Chronic Care
  - Androgenetic alopecia (finasteride)
  - Benign prostatic hyperplasia (dutasteride, finasteride)

Mechanism of Action
- Inhibit 5-alpha-reductase mediated conversion of testosterone to dihydrotestosterone.

> **Counseling Points**
> ✓ Since these agents are contraindicated in pregnancy and the theoretical risk of systemic absorption, those who are pregnant or of child-bearing age should not physically handle the medication and use protective equipment.
> ✓ These agents take several months to exert their clinical effects. As such, patients should not expect acute effects.

Primary Net Benefit
- 5-alpha-reductase inhibitor therapy decreases prostate size and prostate-specific antigen (PSA), but combination therapy with tamsulosin, mirabegron, or a PDE5 inhibitor may be added to improve time to relieve BPH symptoms but does not impact disease progression.
- Main Labs to Monitor:
  - PSA at baseline and after three months of therapy

High-Yield Basic Pharmacology
- Type 1 and 2 5-Alpha-Reductase
  - Dutasteride and finasteride differ slightly in their mechanism as dutasteride inhibits type 1 and 2 5-alpha-reductase, whereas finasteride inhibits type 2 only.

High-Yield Clinical Knowledge
- Pre-Treatment PSA
  - As a result of decreased prostate-specific antigen (PSA) levels from dutasteride or finasteride treatment, a baseline level must be drawn for prostate cancer screening.
  - While taking dutasteride and finasteride, measured PSA levels should be doubled for prostate cancer screening.
- Category X
  - Both dutasteride and finasteride are contraindicated in pregnancy or women of child-bearing age.
  - Furthermore, pregnant women or women of child-bearing age should not handle either medication without appropriate personal protective equipment.
- Combination Treatment
  - Patients with moderate to severe BPH with enlarged prostates greater than 40 g may benefit from dutasteride and tamsulosin combination therapy to improve urinary flow rate and BPH progression.
- Onset of Benefit
  - Dutasteride and finasteride may take days to achieve clinical benefit and provide relief to patients.
  - 5-alpha-reductase inhibitor therapy should continue for 6 to 12 months before determining clinical response.
  - Combination therapy with tamsulosin, mirabegron, or a PDE5 inhibitor may be added to improve time to relieve BPH symptoms but does not impact disease progression.
- Sexual Dysfunction
  - 5-alpha-reductase inhibitor therapy is associated with sexual dysfunction, including decreased libido, impotence, and gynecomastia.

- **Baldness**
  - Finasteride is also commonly used to treat androgenetic alopecia or male pattern baldness but may also treat hirsutism.

High-Yield Core Evidence
- **MTOPS**
  - This was a multicenter, long-term, double-blind trial that randomized male patients to either placebo, doxazosin, finasteride, and combination therapy on measures of the clinical progression of benign prostatic hyperplasia.
  - Dutasteride or finasteride significantly decreased the risk of overall clinical progression, defined as an increase above the baseline of at least 4 points in the American Urological Association symptom score, acute urinary retention, urinary incontinence, renal insufficiency, or recurrent urinary tract infection.
  - Combination therapy significantly reduced the primary outcome's risk (above) compared to doxazosin or finasteride alone.
  - The need for invasive treatment was significantly reduced by combination therapy and finasteride but not by doxazosin.
  - The authors concluded that long-term combination therapy with doxazosin and finasteride was safe and reduced the risk of overall clinical progression of benign prostatic hyperplasia significantly more than treatment with either drug alone. (N Engl J Med. 2003;349(25):2387–2398.)
- **COMBAT**
  - This was a multicenter, double-blind, parallel-group study that included men over the age of 50 years with a clinical diagnosis of BPH, international Prostate Symptom Score of 12 or greater, a prostate volume of 30 cm3 or greater, PSA 1.5-10 ng/mL and a maximum urinary flow rate between 5 and 15 mL/minute with the minimum voided volume of at least 125 mL.
  - Eligible men were randomized to receive either combination therapy (dutasteride plus tamsulosin) or either treatment alone.
  - Combination therapy was significantly superior to tamsulosin but not dutasteride concerning the primary outcome of the relative risk for acute urinary retention, BPH-related surgery, and BPH clinical progression over 4 yr in men at increased risk of progression.
  - Combination therapy provided significantly greater symptom benefit than either monotherapy at 4 yr.
  - The authors concluded that these results support the long-term use of dutasteride and tamsulosin combination therapy in men with moderate-to-severe LUTS due to BPH and prostatic enlargement. (Eur Urol. 2010;57(1):123–131.)

High-Yield Fast-Fact
- **Saw Palmetto**
  - The herbal agent saw palmetto has a mild to moderate effect on reducing BPH symptoms but has failed to show benefit compared to placebo in clinical trials.

HIGH-YIELD BOARD EXAM ESSENTIALS
- **CLASSIC AGENTS:** Dutasteride, finasteride
- **DRUG CLASS:** 5-alpha reductase inhibitors
- **INDICATIONS:** Androgenetic alopecia (finasteride), benign prostatic hyperplasia (dutasteride, finasteride)
- **MECHANISM:** Inhibit 5-alpha-reductase mediated conversion of testosterone to dihydrotestosterone.
- **SIDE EFFECTS:** Teratogenic effects, sexual dysfunction
- **CLINICAL PEARLS:**
  - Finasteride is also commonly used to treat androgenetic alopecia or male pattern baldness but may also be used to treat hirsutism.
  - Pregnant patients should avoid physical contact with these agents to include handling the dosage forms or coming in contact with fluids containing these agents due to the very rare risk of absorbing the drugs that could impact the developing baby.

Table: Drug Class Summary

5-Alpha Reductase Inhibitors - Drug Class Review			
High-Yield Med Reviews			
Mechanism of Action: *Inhibit 5-alpha-reductase mediated conversion of testosterone to dihydrotestosterone.*			
Class Effects: *5-alpha-reductase inhibitor therapy decreases prostate size and prostate-specific antigen (PSA), but combination therapy with tamsulosin, mirabegron, or a PDE5 inhibitor may be added to improve time to relieve BPH symptoms but do not impact disease progression.*			
Generic Name	**Brand Name**	**Indication(s) or Uses**	**Notes**

Dutasteride	Avodart	- Benign prostatic hyperplasia	- **Dosing (Adult):**
			  - Oral: 0.5 mg daily
			- **Dosing (Peds):**
			  - Not routinely used
			- **CYP450 Interactions:** Substrate CYP3A4
			- **Renal or Hepatic Dose Adjustments:** None
			- **Dosage Forms:** Oral (capsule)

Dutasteride and tamsulosin	Jalyn	- Benign prostatic hyperplasia	- **Dosing (Adult):**
			  - Oral: one capsule (0.5 mg / 0.4 mg) daily
			- **Dosing (Peds):**
			  - Not routinely used
			- **CYP450 Interactions:** Substrate CYP2D6, 3A4
			- **Renal or Hepatic Dose Adjustments:** None
			- **Dosage Forms:** Oral (capsule)

Finasteride	Propecia, Proscar	- Androgenetic alopecia
		- Benign prostatic hyperplasia
			- **Dosing (Adult):**
			  - Oral: 1 to 5 mg daily
			- **Dosing (Peds):**
			  - Not routinely used
			- **CYP450 Interactions:** Substrate CYP3A4
			- **Renal or Hepatic Dose Adjustments:** None
			- **Dosage Forms:** Oral (tablet)

GENITOURINARY – ALPHA-1A SELECTIVE BLOCKERS

Drug Class
- Alpha 1a Blockers (Selective)
  - For nonselective alpha 1 blockers, see the Cardiovascular section
- Agents
  - Alfuzosin
  - Silodosin
  - Tamsulosin

Main Indications or Uses
- Acute Care:
  - Ureteral calculi expulsion (off-label use)
- Chronic Care:
  - Benign prostatic hyperplasia (BPH)

> **Fast Facts**
> ✓ The focused concentration of alpha 1a receptors in the bladder helps to reduce the systemic effect where patients might otherwise experience orthostasis. This is especially relevant in older patients where we do not want them to experience orthostasis and potentially fall.

Mechanism of Action
- Alpha-1a receptors are primarily located in the prostate and bladder. When blocked causes a relaxation of the smooth muscle of the bladder neck, and prostate that facilitates the better flow of urine and reduces BPH symptoms.
- Additional Details:
  - The relaxation of this smooth muscle occurs from an inhibition of Gq-protein coupled receptors, which then inhibits the IP3 pathway and ultimately inhibits the release of calcium from the sarcoplasmic reticulum that allows actin and myosin to interact during muscle contraction.

High-Yield Basic Pharmacology
- Knowing that about 75% of the alpha receptors in the bladder are alpha 1a subtype receptors allows for a better-localized effect specific to the bladder and prostate.
  - This means fewer alpha 1 receptors in the systemic vasculature will likely be antagonized, leading to less vasodilation (or changes in blood pressure when it is not desired).

Primary Net Benefit
- In the context of BPH, they improve urinary flow rates, greater emptying of the bladder, and overall symptoms of BPH without causing as much orthosis stasis in older patients. In addition, these agents "may" help relax the ureters to facilitate the expulsion or elimination of a renal stone in kidney stone expulsion.

High-Yield Clinical Knowledge
- Acute Care
  - The smooth relaxation may facilitate ureteral calculi (renal stones located in the ureter) expulsion in the bladder, specifically in the area where the ureter empties into the bladder (e.g., at the ureterovesical junction (UVJ))
- Chronic Care
  - Selective alpha 1a blockers are not indicated for the management of hypertension like the nonselective alpha 1 blockers (e.g., doxazosin, prazosin) due to their focused mechanisms for alpha 1a receptors that reside mainly in the prostate and bladder.
  - Tamsulosin is associated with floppy iris syndrome. Although it has been reported with doxazosin and silodosin, it is more prevalent with tamsulosin.
    - This adverse effect occurs due to the alpha-1a antagonist effects in iris dilator muscles, increasing the likelihood of post-ophthalmologic operative complications, including posterior capsular rupture, retinal detachment, residual retained lens material, or endophthalmitis. In addition, permanent loss of vision can result.

High-Yield Core Evidence
- **Acute Care**
  - To assess the role of tamsulosin in the passage of symptomatic ureteral stones, adult patients presenting to one of 6 emergency departments (ED) in the United States with a symptomatic urinary stone determined by computed tomography (CT) to be < 9 m in diameter and located in the ureter were randomized to tamsulosin 0.4 mg or matching placebo daily for 28 days.
  - There was no statistically significant difference between groups regarding the primary outcome of stone passage based on visualization or capture by the study participant by day 28.
  - This study contrasts with existing urology guidelines that continue to recommend tamsulosin for ureteral colic based on lesser quality data.
  - JAMA Intern Med. 2018 Aug 1;178(8):1051-1057.
- **Chronic Care**
  - The role of tamsulosin in BPH has been extensively assessed throughout the literature. One of the landmark studies (COMBAT Study) examined tamsulosin in combination with dutasteride, a 5-alpha reductase inhibitor, or either agent alone in patients with enlarged prostate glands or elevated PSA levels.
  - This study demonstrated that the combination of the two agents was more effective in reducing symptoms at the study endpoint of 9 months after the start of treatment than either agent alone.
  - Eur Urol. 2010;57(1):123–131.

High-Yield Fast-Facts
- **Alfuzosin and QT prolongation:** Uniquely among alpha-1 antagonists, alfuzosin is associated with QT prolongation, thus caution in patients at risk of Torsades de Pointe and/or other QT prolongation.

HIGH-YIELD BOARD EXAM ESSENTIALS
- **CLASSIC AGENTS:** Alfuzosin, silodosin, tamsulosin
- **DRUG CLASS:** Alpha-1A Selective Blockers
- **INDICATIONS:** Benign Prostatic Hyperplasia, Ureteral Calculi Expulsion)
- **MECHANISM:** Selectively inhibit alpha-1a receptors located in the prostate and bladder thereby causing a relaxation of the smooth muscle of the bladder neck and prostate to improve the flow of urine and a reduction in the symptoms.
- **SIDE EFFECTS:** Minimal, fairly well tolerated
- **CLINICAL PEARLS:**
  - The primary value of these agents in older patients with BPH is in causing less side effects (mainly less orthostasis). However, they cost more than non-selective alpha-1 blockers.
  - While tamsulosin may be helpful to some patients trying to pass a kidney stone, the evidence supporting this indication is not significant.

Table: Drug Class Summary

Selective Alpha-1a Blockers - Drug Class Review		
High-Yield Med Reviews		
Mechanism of Action: *Selectively inhibit alpha-1a receptors primarily located in the prostate and bladder, thereby causing a relaxation of the smooth muscle of the bladder neck, and prostate to improve the flow of urine and a reduction in the symptoms of BPH.*		
Class Effects: *Improved urine flow, lower residuals in the bladder; less orthostasis compared to nonselective agents*		

Generic Name	Brand Name	Main Indication(s) or Uses	Notes
Alfuzosin	Uroxatral	- Benign prostatic hyperplasia - Ureteral calculi expulsion	- **Dosing (Adult):** PO: 10 mg once daily - **Dosing (Peds):** Not used in pediatrics - **CYP450 Interactions:** Substrate of CYP3A4 - **Renal or Hepatic Dose Adjustments:** – Contraindicated for patients with moderate or severe hepatic impairment (Child-Pugh class B or C) - **Dosage Forms:** Extended-release tablet

Silodosin	Rapaflo	- Benign prostatic hyperplasia
		- Ureteral calculi expulsion
			- **Dosing (Adult):** 8 mg once daily
			- **Dosing (Peds):** Not recommended
			- **CYP450 Interactions:** Substrate of CYP3A4, P-gp
			- **Renal or Hepatic Dose Adjustments:**
			   – CrCl 30-50 mL/minute: 4 mg once daily;
			   – CrCl <30 mL/minute: Contraindicated.
			   – Contraindicated for patients with moderate or severe hepatic impairment (Child-Pugh class B or C)
			- **Dosage Forms:** Oral (capsule)

Tamsulosin	Flomax	- Benign prostatic hyperplasia - Ureteral calculi expulsion	- **Dosing (Adult):** 0.4 to 0.8 mg once daily - **Dosing (Peds):** 0.2 or 0.4 mg once daily at bedtime - **CYP450 Interactions:** Substrate of CYP3A4, 2D6 - **Renal or Hepatic Dose Adjustments:** None - **Dosage Forms:** Oral (capsule)

GENITOURINARY – ANTIMUSCARINICS & BETA-3 RECEPTOR ACTIVATOR

Drug Class
- Antimuscarinics
- Agents:
    - Acute & Chronic Care
        - Darifenacin
        - Fesoterodine
        - Methscopolamine
        - Mirabegron
        - Oxybutynin
        - Scopolamine
        - Solifenacin
        - Tolterodine
        - Trospium

Main Indications or Uses
- Acute & Chronic Care
    - Overactive bladder
        - Darifenacin
        - Fesoterodine
        - Oxybutynin
        - Solifenacin
        - Tolterodine
        - Trospium
    - Peptic ulcer
        - Methscopolamine
    - Postoperative and motion sickness induced nausea and vomiting
        - Scopolamine

Mechanism of Action
- Overactive Bladder
    - Darifenacin, fesoterodine, oxybutynin, solifenacin, tolterodine, trospium: Competitive antagonists of acetylcholine on muscarinic receptors to decrease bladder contraction, increase residual urine volume, and decrease detrusor muscle pressure
    - Mirabegron: Beta-3 adrenergic receptor activator, relaxing detrusor muscle during the urinary bladder-fill-void cycle and increasing bladder capacity.
- Peptic Ulcer Disease
    - Methscopolamine is an anticholinergic that reduces the volume and acid content of gastric secretions and inhibits GI motility and salivary secretion.
- Nausea/Vomiting (Motion Sickness and Postoperative)
    - Scopolamine inhibits acetylcholine at parasympathetic sites in smooth muscle, secretory glands, and the CNS.

Primary Net Benefit
- Overactive Bladder
    - Second-line treatment for overactive bladder that provide symptomatic relief of urinary urgency, but older agents' nonspecific antimuscarinic properties may lead to concerning adverse events, particularly in the elderly.
- GI Effects
    - Anticholinergic activity improves secretions and nausea/vomiting.
- Main Labs to Monitor:
    - Postvoid residual volume

High-Yield Basic Pharmacology
- **Muscarinic Specificity**
  - M2 and M3 receptors are primarily expressed in the bladder, but the M3 is responsible for direct activation and contraction.
  - Selective M3 antagonists include oxybutynin and the newer agents trospium, darifenacin, and solifenacin.
  - Tolterodine is selective for M2 and M3.
- **Active Metabolites**
  - The extended-release formulation of oxybutynin is associated with lower concentrations of its active metabolite, thought to be responsible for a lower dry mouth incidence than the immediate-release formulation.
- **Beta-3 Effects**
  - Although mirabegron is beta-3 specific, there are concerns about blood pressure and heart rate changes in patients with CVD or those on beta-blockers and calcium channel blockers.
  - The BP change is less than 1-2 mmHg, and the HR change is less than 2 beats per min.

High-Yield Clinical Knowledge
- **Antimuscarinic (Anticholinergic) Adverse Effects**
  - Antimuscarinic adverse events associated with this class include dry mouth/eyes, constipation, dizziness, drowsiness, altered mental status, hyperpyrexia, vision disturbances, and flushing.
  - These adverse events are particularly concerning in elderly patients because of the increased risk of falls.
  - Newer generation antimuscarinics more specific for M2 and M3 receptors decrease these adverse events.
- **Contraindications**
  - Antimuscarinic agents are contraindicated in patients with a history of narrow-angle glaucoma, urinary or gastric retention, or ileus.
- **Drug Interactions**
  - Antimuscarinic agents have CYP 450 interactions and other pharmacodynamic interactions.
    - Tolterodine combined with CYP3A4 inhibitors may significantly increase tolterodine exposure.
  - Additive antimuscarinic effects can be observed when these agents are combined with antipsychotics, antidepressants, antiparkinsonian agents, or OTC antihistamines.
- **BPH**
  - Although not contraindicated, these agents should be used with caution in patients with BPH due to the risk of acute urinary retention, particularly in patients with poor detrusor contractility.
- **Maximum Benefit**
  - The highest tolerable dose should be targeted for patients to receive maximal benefit from these agents.
  - The maximal benefit's onset may be up to 8 weeks after initiation or dose titration.
- **Quaternary Ammonium**
  - Quaternary ammonium antimuscarinics (trospium and methscopolamine) do not readily cross the blood-brain barrier and carry a lower risk of CNS-related anticholinergic adverse events (confusion, altered mental status.
- **Pediatric Administration**
  - Administer with food in pediatric patients.
  - Shake granules for 1 minute and wait until foam decreases 1-2 min before dosing.
  - If unused for 2 or more days, shake 1 minute for each day missed.

High-Yield Core Evidence
- **Solifenacin Vs OnabotulinumtoxinA**
  - This was a double-blind, double-placebo-controlled trial that randomized women with idiopathic urgency urinary incontinence who had five or more episodes of urgency urinary incontinence per three-day period to daily solifenacin plus one intradetrusor injection of saline (placebo) or one intradetrusor injection of 100 units of onabotulinumtoxinA plus oral placebo.
  - There was no difference between groups concerning the primary outcome of the reduction from baseline in mean episodes of urgency urinary incontinence per day over six months.

- However, within each group, patients experienced complete resolution of urgency urinary incontinence, which improved the quality of life in both groups.
- More patients in the solifenacin group had a higher dry mouth rate but lower catheter use rates at two months and UTIs.
- The authors concluded that oral anticholinergic therapy and onabotulinumtoxinA by injection were associated with similar reductions in the frequency of daily episodes of urgency urinary incontinence. (N Engl J Med. 2012 Nov 8;367(19):1803-13.)
- **Risk Vs. Benefit Systematic Review**
    - This systematic literature review of drugs for urgency urinary incontinence in women searched MEDLINE, the Cochrane Central Register of Controlled Trials, SCIRUS, and Google Scholar for randomized, controlled trials reported in English dating back to 1966.
    - A pooled analysis of the 94 eligible trials revealed that among drugs for urgency urinary incontinence, per 1000 treated women, continence was restored in 130 with fesoterodine, 85 with tolterodine, 114 with oxybutynin, 107 with solifenacin, and 114 with trospium.
    - Corresponding treatment discontinuation rates due to adverse effects were 31 per 1000 treated with fesoterodine, 63 with oxybutynin, 18 with trospium, and 13 with solifenacin.
    - The authors concluded that medications for urgency urinary incontinence showed similar benefits, but individualized treatment could reduce adverse events. (Ann Intern Med. 2012 Jun 19;156(12):861-74, W301-10.)

High-Yield Fast-Fact
- **Botulinum Toxin**
    - OnabotulinumtoxinA has been reported to reduce urinary incontinence and may be an option for patients failing or not tolerating antimuscarinic agents.
- **QT prolongation**
    - Solifenacin, oxybutynin, tolterodine, and fesoterodine can cause associated with QT prolongation.

HIGH-YIELD BOARD EXAM ESSENTIALS
- **CLASSIC AGENTS:** Darifenacin, fesoterodine, methscopolamine, mirabegron, oxybutynin, scopolamine, solifenacin, tolterodine, trospium
- **DRUG CLASS:** Antimuscarinics
- **INDICATIONS:** Overactive bladder (darifenacin, fesoterodine, oxybutynin, solifenacin, tolterodine, trospium), peptic ulcer (methscopolamine), motion sickness and postoperative nausea/vomiting from (scopolamine)
- **MECHANISM:** Antagonists of acetylcholine on muscarinic receptors.
    - Mirabegron: beta-3 agonist, relaxing detrusor muscle during the urinary bladder-fill-void cycle.
- **SIDE EFFECTS:** Dry mouth/eye, constipation, dizziness, drowsiness, altered mental status, hyperpyrexia, vision disturbances, and flushing.
- **CLINICAL PEARLS:** Antimuscarinic agents are contraindicated in patients with a history of narrow-angle glaucoma, urinary or gastric retention, or ileus. Adverse effects are improved with newer agents for overactive bladder.

Table: Drug Class Summary

Antimuscarinics - Drug Class Review High-Yield Med Reviews			
Mechanism of Action: Antagonists of acetylcholine on muscarinic receptors. Mirabegron - Beta-3 adrenergic receptor agonist that relaxes detrusor muscle during the urinary bladder-fill-void cycle.			
Class Effects: Second-line treatment for overactive bladder, treatment of peptic ulcer disease and nausea/vomiting, provides symptomatic relief, anticholinergic adverse effects, caution in elderly			
Generic Name	**Brand Name**	**Main Indication(s) or Uses**	**Notes**
Darifenacin	Enablex	• Overactive bladder	• **Dosing (Adult):** — Oral: 7.5-15 mg daily • **Dosing (Peds):** — Not routinely used • **CYP450 Interactions:** CYP2D6, 3A4 substrate; CYP2D6 inhibitor • **Renal or Hepatic Dose Adjustments:** — Child-Pugh class B: Max 7.5 mg/day — Child-Pugh class C: Not recommended • **Dosage Forms:** Oral (tablet)
Fesoterodine	Toviaz	• Overactive bladder	• **Dosing (Adult):** — Oral: 4-8 mg daily • **Dosing (Peds):** — Not routinely used • **CYP450 Interactions:** Substrate 2D6, 3A4 • **Renal or Hepatic Dose Adjustments:** — CrCl < 30 mL/minute: 4 mg/day — Child-Pugh class C: Not recommended • **Dosage Forms:** Oral (tablet)
Methscopolamine	Pamine	• Peptic ulcer	• **Dosing (Adult):** — Oral: 2.5 mg 30 min before meals and 2.5 to 5 mg at bedtime — Max 30 mg/day • **Dosing (Peds):** — Not routinely used • **CYP450 Interactions:** None • **Renal or Hepatic Dose Adjustments:** None • **Dosage Forms:** Oral (tablet)

Genitourinary

Antimuscarinics - Drug Class Review
High-Yield Med Reviews

Generic Name	Brand Name	Main Indication(s) or Uses	Notes

Mirabegron	Myrbetriq	- Overactive bladder
		- Neurogenic detrusor overactivity
			- **Dosing (Adult):**
			   - Oral: 25-50 mg daily
			- **Dosing (Peds):** use granules for all, tablets once ≥ 35 kg
			   - 11 to <22 kg: Initial 24 mg daily; max 48 mg
			   - 22 to <35 kg: Initial 32 mg daily; max 64 mg
			   - ≥ 35 kg: Granules - Initial 48 mg daily w/ max 80 mg; tablets – 25 mg daily; max 50 mg
			   - Titrate every 4-8 weeks
			- **CYP450 Interactions:** CYP2D6, 3A4, P-gp substrate
			- **Renal or Hepatic Dose Adjustments:**
			   - GFR 15-29 mL/minute/1.73m^2: Max 25 mg/day
			   - GFR < 15 mL/minute/1.73m^2: not recommended
			   - Child-Pugh class B: Max 25 mg/day
			   - Child-Pugh class C: Not recommended
			- **Dosage Forms:** Oral (tablet)

Oxybutynin	Ditropan
	Gelnique
	Oxytrol
		- Overactive bladder	- **Dosing (Adult):**
			   - Oral: ER 5-30 mg daily
			   - Oral: IR 2.5-5 mg q8-12h, maximum 5 mg 4 times daily
			   - Topical gel: apply 1 sachet or 1 actuation of pump once daily
			   - Transdermal patch: 3.9 mg/day q3-4days
			- **Dosing (Peds):**
			   - Oral: 0.1 to 0.2 mg/kg/dose q8-12h
			      - Max 5 mg/dose
			   - Oral: ER 5 mg daily
			- **CYP450 Interactions:** CYP3A4 substrate
			- **Renal or Hepatic Dose Adjustments:** None
			- **Dosage Forms:** Oral (syrup, tablet), Transdermal (gel, patch)

Scopolamine	Transderm Scop	- Nausea and vomiting from motion sickness	- **Dosing (Adult):**
			   - Topical: Apply 1 patch behind ear at least 4 hours prior to exposure q3days as needed
			- **Dosing (Peds):**
			   - Topical: Apply 0.25 to 1 patch q3 days as needed
			- **CYP450 Interactions:** None
			- **Renal or Hepatic Dose Adjustments:** None
			- **Dosage Forms:** Topical (patch)

| Antimuscarinics - Drug Class Review |||||
| High-Yield Med Reviews |||||
Generic Name	Brand Name	Main Indication(s) or Uses	Notes

Solifenacin	Vesicare	- Overactive bladder	- **Dosing (Adult):**
			  - Oral: 5-10 mg daily
			- **Dosing (Peds):**
			  - Not routinely used
			- **CYP450 Interactions:** Substrate CYP2A4
			- **Renal or Hepatic Dose Adjustments:**
			  - CrCl 30 mL/minute: 5 mg/day
			  - Child-Pugh class B: Max 5 mg/day
			  - Child-Pugh class C: Not recommended
			- **Dosage Forms:** Oral (suspension, tablet)

Tolterodine	Detrol, Detrol LA	- Overactive bladder	- **Dosing (Adult):**
			  - Oral: IR 1-2 mg BID
			  - Oral: ER 2-4 mg daily
			- **Dosing (Peds):**
			  - Not routinely used
			- **CYP450 Interactions:** CYP2C9, 2C19, 2D6, 3A4 substrate
			- **Renal or Hepatic Dose Adjustments:**
			  - CrCl 10-30 mL/min: 2 mg/day
			  - CrCl < 10 mL/min: Not recommended
			  - Child-Pugh class B: Maximum 2 mg/day
			  - Child-Pugh class C: Not recommended
			- **Dosage Forms:** Oral (capsule, tablet)

Trospium	Trosec	- Overactive bladder	- **Dosing (Adult):**
			  - Oral: IR 20 mg BID
			  - Oral: ER 60 mg daily
			- **Dosing (Peds):**
			  - Not routinely used
			- **CYP450 Interactions:** None
			- **Renal or Hepatic Dose Adjustments:**
			  - CrCl < 30 mL/min: IR 20 mg daily; ER not recommended
			  - Child-Pugh class B or C: not recommended
			- **Dosage Forms:** Oral (capsule, tablet)

GENITOURINARY – PHOSPHODIESTERASE-5 INHIBITORS

Drug Class
- **Phosphodiesterase-5 Inhibitors**
- **Agents:** Avanafil, sildenafil, tadalafil, vardenafil

Main Indications or Uses
- **Chronic Care**
    - Erectile dysfunction
        - Avanafil, sildenafil, tadalafil, vardenafil
    - Pulmonary arterial hypertension
        - Sildenafil, tadalafil
    - Benign prostatic hyperplasia
        - Tadalafil

> **Drug Interaction Pearl**
> ✓ Avoid the use of these agents within 24 hrs of also using a nitrate (and up to 48 hrs with tadalafil) due to the risk of hypotension.
> ✓ Caution with coadministration of alpha blockers that can also cause orthostasis or hypotension.

Mechanism of Action
- Inhibit the phosphodiesterase-5 inhibitor, which is responsible for degrading cGMP
    - cGMP allows for smooth muscle relaxation and penile blood-filling

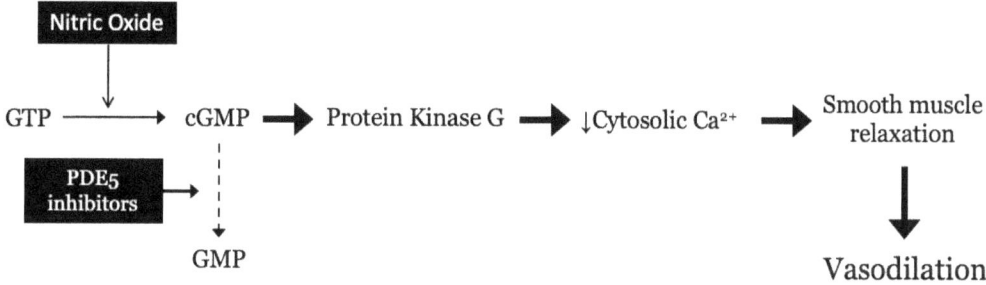

Primary Net Benefit
- Achievement and maintenance of an erection
    - Note: does not affect libido; a male must have adequate libido/sexual desire
- Monitoring Considerations:
    - Erectile Function Questionnaire such as the International Index of Erectile Function (IIEF)
    - Blood pressure

High-Yield Basic Pharmacology
- Onset and duration vary by agent
    - Avanafil, sildenafil, vardenafil
        - Onset within 1 hour (50% achieve erection within 30 minutes)
            - Delayed by high-fat food consumption
        - t ½ = 5 hours
    - Tadalafil
        - Longer onset of 2 hours
        - t ½ = 16 hours
- Hepatic metabolism via CYP3A4
- There are at least 11 phosphodiesterase isoenzymes; inhibition explains therapeutic and adverse effects
    - Phosphodiesterase-1 is found in the peripheral vasculature
        - Therapeutic effect: blood pressure lowering
        - Adverse effects: flushing, tachycardia
    - Phosphodiesterase-6 is found in retinal rods and cones
        - Adverse effects: blurred vision, blue vision

- Phosphodiesterase-11 is found in striated muscle
    - Adverse effect: myalgias

High-Yield Clinical Knowledge
- Up to 40% of patients prescribed a PDE5-i report it to be ineffective
    - Strategies to mitigate perceived and real ineffectiveness of PDE5-i
        - Counsel on timing and interactions that may delay the onset
        - Educate on the need for sexual stimulation
        - Use at least five times before deemed failed intervention
        - Increase dosage
        - Trial another medication in the same class
- Caution against alcohol use
    - Efficacy: contributes to erectile dysfunction
    - Safety: increases risk of orthostasis
- Strong caution/contraindication in combination with other vasodilators
    - Increased risk of orthostasis

High-Yield Core Evidence
- **ICSM 2015: Pharmacotherapy for Erectile Dysfunction**
    - PDE5-inhibitors are recognized as first-line therapy for erectile dysfunction
        - PDE5-i are regarded to be effective, safe, and well-tolerated
        - PDE5-i dose titration is recommended to improve efficacy and patient satisfaction
    - Psychosocial factors should be evaluated in the work-up for erectile dysfunction and taken into consideration regarding interventions
    - *J Sex Med 2016 Apr;13(4):465-88*
- **Undertreatment of Erectile Dysfunction**
    - Despite a high prevalence of diagnosed erectile dysfunction, claims data from this study revealed only 25% of patients received medical treatment
    - The authors cited both patient and provider knowledge as a reason for low medical intervention
    - *J Sex Med 2014 Oct;11(10):2546-53*

High-Yield Fast-Fact
- Before the 1980s, erectile dysfunction was considered by most clinicians to be of mental etiology. However, Dr. Giles Brindley, a British physiologist, shocked the audience at the 1983 American Urological Association Meeting when he revealed his full erection while speaking. Dr. Brindley had injected a vasodilator into his penis before taking the stage as a showcase that erectile dysfunction was not solely a psychiatric diagnosis.
- PDE5-i were discovered accidentally. In a clinical trial investigating sildenafil for angina and hypertension, the adverse effect of erections was identified. Subsequently, Pfizer decided to study the medication for erectile dysfunction. Sildenafil gained FDA approval as the first oral therapy to treat the disease in 1998.

HIGH-YIELD BOARD EXAM ESSENTIALS
- **CLASSIC AGENTS:** Avanafil, sildenafil, tadalafil, vardenafil
- **DRUG CLASS:** Phosphodiesterase-5 inhibitors
- **INDICATIONS:** Erectile dysfunction (avanafil, sildenafil, tadalafil, vardenafil), pulmonary arterial hypertension (sildenafil, tadalafil), benign prostatic hyperplasia (tadalafil)
- **MECHANISM:** Inhibit the phosphodiesterase-5 inhibitor which is responsible for degrading cGMP
- **SIDE EFFECTS:** Hypotension (in combination with nitrates/vasodilators)
- **CLINICAL PEARLS:** The agents in this class are subject to drug interactions when used with other medications that inhibit CYP3A4. Avoid co-administration with nitrates within 24 hrs of each other due to risk of hypotension. High fat meals delay onset of sildenafil and vardenafil, alcohol increases risk of orthostasis and can contribute to erectile dysfunction.

Table: Drug Class Summary

	PDE5 - Inhibitors Drug Class Review High-Yield Med Reviews		
Mechanism of Action: *inhibition of the PDE5 enzyme results in smooth muscle relaxation and subsequently increased blood flow into the penis*			
Class effects: *alpha-blockers should be used cautiously; nitrates are contraindicated within 24 hours of taking avanafil, sildenafil, and vardenafil and within 48 hours of taking tadalafil*			
Generic Name	**Brand Name**	**Indication(s) or Uses**	**Notes**
Avanafil	Stendra	- Erectile dysfunction	- **Dosing (Adult):** 50 to 200 mg - **CYP450 Interactions:** CYP3A4 substrate - **Renal or Hepatic Dose Adjustments:** – Severe hepatic impairment: avoid use - **Dosage Forms:** Oral (tablet)
Sildenafil	Viagra	- Erectile dysfunction - Pulmonary arterial hypertension	- **Dosing (Adult):** 50 to 100 mg - **CYP450 Interactions:** CYP3A4 substrate - **Renal or Hepatic Dose Adjustments:** – Severe hepatic impairment: starting dose 25 mg - **Dosage Forms:** Oral (tablet); Solution for IV

Tadalafil	Cialis	- Erectile dysfunction
		- Pulmonary arterial hypertension
		- Benign prostatic hyperplasia
			- **Dosing:**
			   – As needed: 5 to 20 mg; Daily: 2.5mg
			- **CYP450 Interactions:** CYP3A4 substrate
			- **Renal or Hepatic Dose Adjustments:**
			   – Severe hepatic impairment: avoid use
			   – CrCl 30-50 mL/min: max dose 5mg
			   – CrCl <30 mL/min: avoid use
			- **Dosage Forms:** Oral (tablet)

Vardenafil	Levitra
	Staxyn
		- Erectile dysfunction	- **Dosing:**
			   – Oral tablet (Levitra): 5 to 20 mg
			   – Oral disintegrating tablet (Staxyn): 10mg
			- **CYP450 Interactions:** CYP3A4 substrate
			- **Renal or Hepatic Dose Adjustments:**
			   – Severe hepatic impairment: avoid use
			- **Dosage Forms:** Oral (tablet)

2025

A COMPREHENSIVE *RAPID REVIEW*

NAPLEX
Pharmacology & Drug Classes

Hematology

HEMATOLOGY – ERYTHROPOIESIS STIMULATING AGENTS

Drug Class
- Erythropoiesis Stimulating Agents (ESAs)
- Agents:
  - Chronic Care
    - Darbepoetin alfa
    - Epoetin alfa
    - Methoxy polyethylene glycol-epoetin beta

> **Warnings & Alerts**
> ✓ The risk of cardiovascular, stroke, thromboembolic events, and mortality increases with the use of ESAs when hemoglobin levels are above 11 g/dL.
> ✓ Iron stores in the body must also be adequate for these agents to work.

Main Indications or Uses
- Chronic Care
  - Anemia
    - Darbepoetin alfa, epoetin alfa, methoxy polyethylene glycol-epoetin beta)
  - Reduction of allogeneic RBC transfusion
    - Epoetin alfa

Mechanism of Action
- Synthetic erythropoietin interacts with red cell progenitor erythropoietin receptors to stimulate erythroid proliferation and differentiation.

Primary Net Benefit
- ESAs stimulate red blood cell production and, in combination with appropriate iron intake, are effective for a wide range of anemias but must be balanced with the risk of thromboembolic events and hypertension.
- Main Labs to Monitor:
  - CBC
  - Transferrin saturation
  - Serum ferritin

High-Yield Basic Pharmacology
- **Endogenous Erythropoietin**
  - Most of the body's erythropoietin is usually produced in the kidney and is stimulated in response to tissue hypoxia through an increased rate of erythropoietin gene transcription.
  - In chronic kidney disease, endogenous erythropoietin levels are suppressed as the erythropoietin growth factor production is limited.
    - Conversely, in many other causes of anemia, including bone marrow disorders, secondary anemias, and nutritional deficiencies, endogenous erythropoietin levels are high and do not respond to additional exogenous erythropoietin.
- **ESA Formulations**
  - **Epoetin alfa**
    - Is a recombinant human erythropoietin, whereas darbepoetin alpha and methoxy polyethylene glycol epoetin beta are modified forms.
  - **Darbepoetin alpha**
    - Is a glycosylated from a modified amino acid structure, resulting in a longer duration of action.
  - **Methoxy Polyethylene glycol epoetin beta**
    - Is erythropoietin covalently bound to a polyethylene glycol polymer to prolong its half-life significantly.

High-Yield Clinical Knowledge
- **Thrombosis Risk**
  - The risk of cardiovascular, stroke, thromboembolic events, and mortality increases with the use of ESAs when hemoglobin levels are above 11 g/dL.
  - Rapid increases in hemoglobin, faster than 0.5 g/dL per week, may also contribute to this risk.
    - Hemoglobin levels among patients with chronic kidney disease receiving ESAs should not increase above 11 g/dL.
  - However, in cancer patients, ESAs are associated with increased all-cause mortality and venous thromboembolism.
    - ESAs should be used in cancer patients to avoid transfusion when hemoglobin levels are below 10 g/dL.
    - In cancers where therapeutic interventions are considered to be curative, ESAs are not recommended.
- **Hypertension**
  - Increased blood pressure among patients receiving ESAs is expected and correlates with rapid increases in hematocrit.
  - ESAs should be avoided in patients with uncontrolled hypertension but can be used in patients receiving antihypertensive drug therapy.
- **Iron Intake**
  - Iron is a crucial component of heme and essential during erythropoietin therapy among patients with serum ferritin levels below 100 mcg/L, or transferrin saturation is below 20%.
  - Iron supplementation can be accomplished using oral iron dosage forms targeting 200 mg elemental iron per day or parenteral iron supplementation.
- **ESA in Oncology**
  - ESAs are less commonly used in oncologic applications and reserved for select patients where conservation of blood transfusions is desired.
  - However, methoxy polyethylene glycol-epoetin beta must be avoided in this patient population due to an association with increased mortality in cancer patients.
- **Hypoxia-Inducible Factor (HIF)**
  - HIF is a DNA-regulating factor that becomes activated in hypoxic conditions, resulting in erythropoiesis.
  - HIF is regulated and inactivated by prolyl hydroxylases (PHD) at normal oxygen levels, which has become a new drug therapy target and the action of the oral agent roxadustat.
- **ESAs Vs. Roxadustat**
  - In phase 3 studies (below), roxadustat achieved similar increases in hemoglobin than epoetin alfa in CKD patients on dialysis but is associated with a roughly 30% lower risk of major adverse cardiac events.

High-Yield Core Evidence
- **Roxadustat Vs Epoetin Alfa**
  - This prospective, open-label, placebo-controlled, phase III trial randomized patients undergoing dialysis and receiving ESA therapy with epoetin alfa for at least six weeks were randomized to receive either roxadustat or continue epoetin alfa three times per week for 26 weeks.
  - Roxadustat, compared to epoetin alfa, was non-inferior concerning the primary endpoint of the mean change in hemoglobin level from baseline to the average level during weeks 23 through 27.
  - However, roxadustat was associated with a significant increase in transferrin level, maintained the serum iron level, attenuated decreases in the transferrin saturation, lower total cholesterol, and lower LDL cholesterol than epoetin alfa.
  - Furthermore, roxadustat was associated with a significantly larger mean reduction in hepcidin than epoetin alfa.
  - Roxadustat was associated with more hyperkalemia and upper respiratory infections, but there was a higher incidence of hypertension in the epoetin alfa group.
  - The authors concluded that oral roxadustat was non-inferior to parenteral epoetin alfa as therapy for anemia in Chinese patients undergoing dialysis. (N Engl J Med. 2019 Sep 12;381(11):1011-1022.)

- **Erythropoiesis-stimulating agents - Meta-Analysis**
  - This was a systematic review and meta-analysis to compare the efficacy and safety of ESAs (epoetin alfa, epoetin beta, darbepoetin alfa, or methoxy polyethylene glycol-epoetin beta, and biosimilar ESAs, against each other, placebo, or no treatment) to treat anemia in adults with CKD.
  - All randomized controlled trials (RCTs) that included a comparison of an ESA (epoetin alfa, epoetin beta, darbepoetin alfa, methoxy polyethylene glycol-epoetin beta, or biosimilar ESA) with another ESA, placebo or no treatment in adults with CKD and that reported prespecified patient-relevant outcomes were considered for inclusion.
  - A total of fifty-six studies were identified and included in this analysis.
  - There was no difference between agents concerning preventing blood transfusions compared to placebo.
  - Biosimilar ESA therapy was also no better than a placebo for preventing blood transfusions.
  - All ESAs were associated with hypertension compared to placebo.
  - The authors concluded that there is currently insufficient evidence to suggest the superiority of any ESA formulation based on available safety and efficacy data in the CKD setting. (Cochrane Database Syst Rev. 2014 Dec 8;2014(12):CD010590.)

High-Yield Fast-Fact
- **Blood Doping**
  - ESAs have been used surreptitiously by endurance athletes to enhance performance and are universally banned and routinely tested for in athletic events.

HIGH-YIELD BOARD EXAM ESSENTIALS
- **CLASSIC AGENTS:** Darbepoetin alfa, epoetin alfa, methoxy polyethylene glycol-epoetin beta
- **DRUG CLASS:** Erythropoiesis stimulating agents
- **INDICATIONS:** Anemia, reduction of allogeneic RBC transfusion
- **MECHANISM:** Synthetic erythropoietin interacts with red cell progenitor erythropoietin receptors to stimulate erythroid proliferation and differentiation.
- **SIDE EFFECTS:** Thrombosis, hypertension
- **CLINICAL PEARLS:**
  - Increases in the hemoglobin will also cause an increase in plasma volume which can increase the blood pressure and the viscosity of the vascular space.
  - The risk of cardiovascular, stroke, thromboembolic events, and mortality are all increased with the use of ESAs when hemoglobin levels are above 11 g/dL. Rapid increases in hemoglobin, faster than 0.5 g/dL per week, may also contribute to this risk.

Table: Drug Class Summary

Erythropoiesis Stimulating Agents - Drug Class Review High-Yield Med Reviews			
Mechanism of Action: *Synthetic erythropoietin interacts with red cell progenitor erythropoietin receptors to stimulate erythroid proliferation and differentiation.*			
Class Effects: *ESAs stimulate red blood cell production and, in combination with appropriate iron intake, are effective for a wide range of anemias but must be balanced with the risk of thromboembolic events and hypertension.*			
Generic Name	**Brand Name**	**Indication(s) or Uses**	**Notes**
Darbepoetin alfa	Aranesp	• Anemia (chemotherapy, chronic kidney disease, zidovudine)	• **Dosing (Adult):** – IV/SQ: 0.45 to 0.75 mcg/kg q1-4weeks, adjusted to hemoglobin • **Dosing (Peds):** – IV/SQ: 0.45 to 0.75 mcg/kg q1-4weeks, adjusted to hemoglobin • **CYP450 Interactions:** None • **Renal or Hepatic Dose Adjustments:** None • **Dosage Forms:** Injection solution
Epoetin alfa	Epogen, Procrit, Retacrit	• Anemia (chemotherapy, chronic kidney disease, zidovudine) • Reduction of allogeneic RBC transfusion	• **Dosing (Adult):** – IV/SQ: 50 to 100 mcg/kg three times weekly or q1-2weeks adjusted to hemoglobin • **Dosing (Peds):** – IV/SQ: 50 to 100 mcg/kg three times weekly or q1-2weeks adjusted to hemoglobin • **CYP450 Interactions:** None • **Renal or Hepatic Dose Adjustments:** None • **Dosage Forms:** Injection solution
Methoxy polyethylene glycol-epoetin beta	Mircera	• Anemia	• **Dosing (Adult):** – IV: 0.6 mcg/kg q2weeks, adjusted to hemoglobin • **Dosing (Peds):** – IV: 0.6 mcg/kg q2weeks, adjusted to hemoglobin • **CYP450 Interactions:** None • **Renal or Hepatic Dose Adjustments:** None • **Dosage Forms:** Injection solution

HEMATOLOGY – GRANULOCYTE COLONY STIMULATING FACTOR

Drug Class
- Granulocyte Colony Stimulating Factor
- Agents:
  - Acute Care
    - Filgrastim and Tbo-Filgrastim
    - Sargramostim
    - Pegfilgrastim

Main Indications or Uses
- Acute Care
  - Acute myeloid leukemia
  - Chemotherapy-induced myelosuppression
  - Bone marrow transplant
  - Hematopoietic radiation injury syndrome
  - Peripheral blood progenitor cell collection and therapy
  - Severe chronic neutropenia

Mechanism of Action
- G-CSF (Filgrastim/tbo-filgrastim, pegfilgrastim)
  - Stimulates the proliferation, differentiation, and function of neutrophils.
- GM-CSF (sargramostim)
  - Stimulates the proliferation, differentiation, and function of numerous myeloid cells, including basophils, eosinophils, granulocytes, and monocytes.

Primary Net Benefit
- Reduces neutropenic nadirs and shortens the duration of neutropenia caused by myelosuppressive chemotherapy.
- Main Labs to Monitor:
  - CBC with differential

High-Yield Basic Pharmacology
- G-CSF/GM-CSF Function
  - In addition to stimulating myeloid cell lineages, GM-CSFs may also enhance the antibody-dependent cell-mediated toxicity of neutrophils, eosinophils, and monocytes.
  - G-CSF agents may also interact with IL-3, promoting other cell line production, or reducing inflammation by inhibiting inflammatory cytokines (IL-1, TNF-alfa, interferon-gamma).

High-Yield Clinical Knowledge
- Adverse Events
  - G-CSF/GM-CSF agents are commonly associated with bone pain, flu-like symptoms, rash, diarrhea, dyspnea, supraventricular arrhythmias, elevated serum creatinine, bilirubin, and hepatic enzymes.
- Sargramostim Fever
  - GM-CSF (sargramostim) is more often associated with acute fever, limiting its use in preventing febrile neutropenia.
  - Acute first dose reactions to sargramostim may also occur, including flushing, hypotension, dyspnea, nausea, and vomiting.
    - Oxygen saturation may also decrease acutely due to pulmonary sequestration of granulocytes.
- Acute Myeloid Leukemia
  - G-CSF agents were historically avoided in acute myeloid leukemia (AML), as leukemic cells arose from progenitors that were regulated, in part, by G-CSF and GM-CSF.
  - New evidence suggests these agents are safe following induction and consolidation treatment of AML and acute lymphoblastic leukemia, leading to FDA approvals for these indications.

- **Neutropenia**
  - Absolute neutrophil counts (ANC) of less than 500 cells/mL is associated with significant morbidity and mortality among patients receiving myelosuppressive chemotherapy.
  - The ANC is calculated using the formula = (segmented neutrophils + banded neutrophils)/WBC.
  - G-CSF/GM-CSF agents reduce the incidence, magnitude, and duration of neutropenia and are recommended if the risk of febrile neutropenia of a given chemotherapy regimen is at least 20%.
  - However, these interventions do not impact mortality among cancer patients.
- **Stem Cell Transplant Adjunct**
  - Due to the benefit of G-CSF or GM-CSF-induced mobilization of peripheral hematopoietic stem cells from the marrow to the peripheral blood, these agents have become a common method to enhance donor stem cell products.
- **Alternative Indications**
  - G-CSF/GM-CSF agents may also play a role in neutropenia in patients with congenital neutropenia, cyclic neutropenia, myelodysplasia, and aplastic anemia.

High-Yield Core Evidence
- **Pegfilgrastim Versus Daily Filgrastim**
  - This was a prospective trial of patients receiving myelosuppressive chemotherapy who were randomized to either a single dose of pegfilgrastim 6 mg SQ per cycle of chemotherapy compared with daily filgrastim 5 mg/kg SQ in the provision of neutrophil support after doxorubicin and docetaxel chemotherapy.
  - There was no significant difference between groups concerning the duration of grade 4 neutropenia, depth of neutrophil nadir, the incidence of febrile neutropenia, and time to neutrophil recovery.
  - There was a non-significant trend toward a lower incidence of febrile neutropenia was noted across all cycles with pegfilgrastim compared with filgrastim (13% versus 20%, respectively).
  - The authors concluded that a single fixed dose of pegfilgrastim was as safe and well-tolerated as standard daily filgrastim. (Ann Oncol. 2003 Jan;14(1):29-35.)
- **Primary G-CSF Prophylaxis Meta-Analysis**
  - This was a systematic review and meta-analysis of all reported randomized controlled trials (RCTs) of prophylactic G-CSF compared to placebo or untreated controls in adult solid tumor and malignant lymphoma patients.
  - A total of seventeen RCTs were identified, including 3,493 patients.
  - G-CSF was associated with a significant risk reduction of infection-related mortality, early mortality, and febrile neutropenia.
  - The reactive dose intensity (RDI) was significantly higher in patients who received G-CSF than in control patients.
  - Significantly more patients receiving G-CSF agents complained of bone or musculoskeletal pain.
  - The authors concluded that prophylactic G-CSF reduces the risk of febrile neutropenia and early deaths, including infection-related mortality, while increasing RDI and musculoskeletal pain. (J Clin Oncol. 2007 Jul 20;25(21):3158-67.)

High-Yield Fast-Fact
- **Radiologic Attack**
  - G-CSF and GM-CSF have been identified as agents that can reduce neutropenia's likelihood following radiologic disasters or nuclear explosions.

HIGH-YIELD BOARD EXAM ESSENTIALS

- **CLASSIC AGENTS:** Filgrastim and Tbo-filgrastim, sargramostim, pegfilgrastim
- **DRUG CLASS:** Granulocyte colony stimulating factor
- **INDICATIONS:** AML, chemotherapy-induced myelosuppression, bone marrow transplant, hematopoietic radiation injury syndrome, peripheral blood progenitor cell collection and therapy, severe chronic neutropenia
- **MECHANISM:** G-CSF (Filgrastim/tbo-filgrastim, pegfilgrastim) stimulates the proliferation, differentiation, and function of neutrophils. GM-CSF (sargramostim) stimulates the proliferation, differentiation, and function of numerous myeloid cells, including basophils, eosinophils, granulocytes, and monocytes.
- **SIDE EFFECTS:** Bone pain, flu-like symptoms, rash, diarrhea, dyspnea, supraventricular arrhythmias, and elevations in serum creatinine, bilirubin, and hepatic enzymes.
- **CLINICAL PEARLS:** ANC of less than 500 cells/mL is associated with significant morbidity and mortality among patients receiving myelosuppressive chemotherapy. G-CSF/GM-CSF agents reduce the incidence, magnitude, and duration of neutropenia and are recommended if the risk of febrile neutropenia of a given chemotherapy regimen is at least 20%.

Table: Drug Class Summary

Granulocyte Colony Stimulating Factor - Drug Class Review High-Yield Med Reviews			
Mechanism of Action: *G-CSF - Stimulates the proliferation, differentiation, and function of neutrophils.* *GM-CSF - Stimulates the proliferation, differentiation, and function of numerous myeloid cells, including basophils, eosinophils, granulocytes, and monocytes.* **Class Effects:** *Reduces neutropenic nadirs and shortens the duration of neutropenia caused by myelosuppressive chemotherapy.*			
Generic Name	**Brand Name**	**Main Indication(s) or Uses**	**Notes**
Filgrastim; TBO-filgrastim	Granix, Neupogen, Nivestym, Zarxio	<ul><li>Acute myeloid leukemia</li><li>Chemotherapy-induced myelosuppression</li><li>Bone marrow transplant</li><li>Hematopoietic radiation injury syndrome</li><li>Peripheral blood progenitor cell collection and therapy</li><li>Severe chronic neutropenia</li></ul>	<ul><li>**Dosing (Adult):** − IV/SQ: 5 to 10 mcg/kg/day − SQ: 75 to 300 mcg three times weekly</li><li>**Dosing (Peds):** − IV/SQ: 5 to 10 mcg/kg/day − SQ: 1 to 20 mcg/kg/day mcg three times weekly</li><li>**CYP450 Interactions:** None</li><li>**Renal or Hepatic Dose Adjustments:** None</li><li>**Dosage Forms:** Injection solution, Subcutaneous solution</li></ul>

Sargramostim	Leukine	<ul><li>Acute myeloid leukemia</li><li>Chemotherapy-induced myelosuppression</li><li>Bone marrow transplant</li><li>Hematopoietic radiation injury syndrome</li><li>Peripheral blood progenitor cell collection, therapy, and transplantation</li></ul>	<ul><li>**Dosing (Adult):**
			− IV/SQ: 250 mcg/m2/day
			  − IV: over 2 hours
			  − SQ: immediately following infusion of progenitor cells</li><li>**Dosing (Peds):**
			− IV/SQ: 250 mcg/m2/day
			  − IV: over 2 hours
			  − SQ: immediately following infusion of progenitor cells</li><li>**CYP450 Interactions:** None</li><li>**Renal or Hepatic Dose Adjustments:** None</li><li>**Dosage Forms:** Injection solution</li></ul>

Pegfilgrastim	Fulphila, Neulasta, Udenyca, Ziextenzo	<ul><li>Acute myeloid leukemia</li><li>Chemotherapy-induced myelosuppression</li><li>Bone marrow transplant</li><li>Hematopoietic radiation injury syndrome</li><li>Peripheral blood progenitor cell collection and therapy</li><li>Severe chronic neutropenia</li></ul>	<ul><li>**Dosing (Adult):** − SQ: 6 mg once per chemotherapy cycle</li><li>**Dosing (Peds):** − SQ: 0.1 mg/kg or 1.5 to 6 mg once per chemotherapy cycle</li><li>**CYP450 Interactions:** None</li><li>**Renal or Hepatic Dose Adjustments:** None</li><li>**Dosage Forms:** Injection solution, Subcutaneous solution</li></ul>

HEMATOLOGY – MEGAKARYOCYTE GROWTH FACTOR

Drug Class
- Megakaryocyte Growth Factor
- Agents:
    - Acute & Chronic Care
        - Avatrombopag
        - Eltrombopag
        - Lusutrombopag
        - Romiplostim

Main Indications or Uses
- Acute & Chronic Care
    - Aplastic anemia (eltrombopag)
    - Chronic hepatitis C infection-associated thrombocytopenia (eltrombopag)
    - Chronic liver disease-associated thrombocytopenia (avatrombopag, lusutrombopag)
    - Hematopoietic syndrome of acute radiation syndrome (romiplostim)
    - Immune thrombocytopenia (eltrombopag, romiplostim)

Mechanism of Action
- Thrombopoietin Receptor Agonists (avatrombopag, eltrombopag, lusutrombopag)
    - Thrombopoietin receptor agonists increased platelet production by stimulating the proliferation and differentiation of megakaryocytes from bone marrow progenitor cells.
- Thrombopoietin (TPO) Mimic (romiplostim)
    - Binds with high affinity to the thrombopoietin receptor and mimics the thrombopoietic effect of TPO.

Primary Net Benefit
- Novel agents for managing thrombocytopenia may reduce the need for platelet transfusions.
- Main Labs to Monitor:
    - CBC with differential

High-Yield Basic Pharmacology
- Romiplostim Administration
    - Romiplostim is administered via subcutaneous injection and is a very small volume for the typical dose.
    - The administration must be accomplished using a syringe with 0.01 mL graduations.
- Oral Absorption
    - The thrombopoietin receptor agonists are orally administered agents.

High-Yield Clinical Knowledge
- Thromboembolic Complications
    - Avatrombopag, eltrombopag, lusutrombopag, and romiplostim have been associated with thromboembolic complications.
    - Among patients receiving these agents with concomitant chronic liver disease, portal vein thrombosis may be prevalent.

- Myelodysplastic Syndromes
    - There is a risk of progression from an existing myelodysplastic syndrome to acute myeloid leukemia with romiplostim.
- Hepatic Decompensation
    - Eltrombopag is associated with an increased risk of severe, life-threatening hepatotoxicity.
    - There is an increased risk of hepatic decompensation in patients with chronic hepatitis C receiving eltrombopag with concomitant interferon and ribavirin.
        - The current recommendations are to stop eltrombopag should hepatic decompensation occur.

High-Yield Core Evidence
- **Romiplostim RCT**
  - This was a single publication of two parallel trials that were prospective, blinded, and randomized splenectomized and non-splenectomized patients with ITP to receive either long-term administration of romiplostim or placebo.
  - Among both splenectomized and non-splenectomized patients, romiplostim was associated with a significant improvement in the primary outcome of the durable platelet response.
  - However, 87% of patients given romiplostim reduced or discontinued concurrent therapy compared with only 38% of those given placebo, although adverse events were similar between groups.
  - The authors concluded that romiplostim was well tolerated and increased and maintained platelet counts in splenectomized and non-splenectomized patients with ITP. (Lancet. 2008 Feb 2;371(9610):395-403.)
- **Eltrombopag RCT**
  - This was a multicenter, prospective, blinded, placebo-controlled trial that randomized patients with chronic ITP and platelet count less than 30,000/mL who had relapsed or whose platelet count was refractory to at least one standard treatment for ITP to receive the eltrombopag at a dose of 30, 50, or 75 mg daily or placebo.
  - Significantly more patients randomized to any eltrombopag dose met the primary outcome of a platelet count of 50,000/mL or more on day 43.
  - However, the median platelet counts on day 43 for the groups receiving 30, 50, and 75 mg of eltrombopag were 26,000, 128,000, and 183,000/mL, respectively.
  - Bleeding also decreased during treatment in these two groups, and the incidence and severity of adverse events were similar in the placebo and eltrombopag groups.
  - The authors concluded that eltrombopag increased platelet counts in a dose-dependent manner in patients with relapsed or refractory ITP. (N Engl J Med. 2007 Nov 29;357(22):2237-47.)

High-Yield Fast-Fact
- **Prior Agents**
  - Although no longer available, predecessors to these agents included oprelvekin, a recombinant IL-11, and thrombopoietin were investigated for these indications.

HIGH-YIELD BOARD EXAM ESSENTIALS
- **CLASSIC AGENTS:** Avatrombopag, eltrombopag, lusutrombopag, romiplostim
- **DRUG CLASS:** Megakaryocyte growth factor
- **INDICATIONS:** Aplastic anemia (eltrombopag), chronic hepatitis C infection-associated thrombocytopenia (eltrombopag), chronic liver disease-associated thrombocytopenia (avatrombopag, lusutrombopag), hematopoietic syndrome of acute radiation syndrome (romiplostim), immune thrombocytopenia (eltrombopag, romiplostim)
- **MECHANISM:** Thrombopoietin receptor agonists increased platelet production through the stimulation of proliferation and differentiation of megakaryocytes from bone marrow progenitor cells (avatrombopag, eltrombopag, lusutrombopag). Binds with high affinity to the thrombopoietin receptor and mimicking the thrombopoietic effect of TPO (romiplostim)
- **SIDE EFFECTS:** Thrombosis, progression of myelodysplastic syndrome
- **CLINICAL PEARLS:** Among patients receiving these agents with concomitant chronic liver disease, portal vein thrombosis may be prevalent.

Table: Drug Class Summary

Megakaryocyte Growth Factor - Drug Class Review High-Yield Med Reviews			
Mechanism of Action: *Avatrombopag, eltrombopag, lusutrombopag - Thrombopoietin receptor agonists increased platelet production by stimulating proliferation and differentiation of megakaryocytes bone marrow progenitor cells.* *Romiplostim - Binds with high affinity to the thrombopoietin receptor and mimicking the thrombopoietic effect of TPO.*			
Class Effects: *Novel agents for managing thrombocytopenia that may reduce the need for platelet transfusions.*			
Generic Name	**Brand Name**	**Main Indication(s) or Uses**	**Notes**
Avatrombopag	Doptelet	<ul><li>Chronic immune thrombocytopenia</li><li>Chronic liver disease-associated thrombocytopenia</li></ul>	<ul><li>**Dosing (Adult):** − Oral: 20 mg daily adjusted to "dose-level 1 to 6"</li><li>**Dosing (Peds):** − Not routinely used</li><li>**CYP450 Interactions:** Substrate CYP2C9, 3A4, P-gp</li><li>**Renal or Hepatic Dose Adjustments:** None</li><li>**Dosage Forms:** Oral (tablet)</li></ul>
Eltrombopag	Promacta	<ul><li>Aplastic anemia</li><li>Chronic hepatitis C infection-associated thrombocytopenia</li><li>Immune thrombocytopenia</li></ul>	<ul><li>**Dosing (Adult):** − Oral: 25 to 100 mg daily</li><li>**Dosing (Peds):** − Oral: 2.5 mg/kg/dose − Maximum 37.5 mg/dose</li><li>**CYP450 Interactions:** Substrate CYP1A2, 2C8</li><li>**Renal or Hepatic Dose Adjustments:** − Child-Pugh class A, B, or C: 12.5 mg daily</li><li>**Dosage Forms:** Oral (packet, tablet)</li></ul>
Lusutrombopag	Mulpleta	<ul><li>Chronic liver disease-associated thrombocytopenia</li></ul>	<ul><li>**Dosing (Adult):** − Oral: 3 mg daily for 7 days</li><li>**Dosing (Peds):** − Not routinely used</li><li>**CYP450 Interactions:** None</li><li>**Renal or Hepatic Dose Adjustments:** None</li><li>**Dosage Forms:** Oral (tablet)</li></ul>
Romiplostim	Nplate	<ul><li>Hematopoietic syndrome of acute radiation syndrome</li><li>Immune thrombocytopenia</li></ul>	<ul><li>**Dosing (Adult):** − SQ: 10 mcg/kg once − SQ: 1 to 10 mcg/kg q1week</li><li>**Dosing (Peds):** − SQ: 10 mcg/kg once − SQ: 1 to 10 mcg/kg q1week</li><li>**CYP450 Interactions:** None</li><li>**Renal or Hepatic Dose Adjustments:** None</li><li>**Dosage Forms:** Injection solution</li></ul>

HEMATOLOGY – IRON

Drug Class
- Iron
- Agents:
    - **Chronic Care**
        - Ferric carboxymaltose
        - Ferric citrate
        - Ferric derisomaltose
        - Ferric gluconate
        - Ferric maltol
        - Ferric pyrophosphate citrate
        - Ferrous fumarate
        - Ferrous gluconate
        - Ferrous sulfate
        - Ferumoxytol
        - Iron dextran
        - Iron sucrose
        - Polysaccharide-Iron Complex

Main Indications or Uses
- **Chronic Care**
    - Iron-deficiency anemia

> **Fast Facts**
> - If oral iron replacement is utilized, then the target dose each day should be 200 mg of elemental. Form of oral iron replacement used will influence the amount given to achieve this.
> - It is best to take oral iron on an empty stomach to maximize absorption, however most patients experience nausea doing this.
> - Avoid oral iron with the coadministration of di- or tri-valent cations due to reduction in their absorption.
> - Iron dextran has been associated with allergic reactions with IV administration. This is less with other newer forms of iron.

Mechanism of Action
- Replace physiologic iron stores, which promote appropriate erythropoiesis and erythrocyte maturation.

Primary Net Benefit
- Iron deficiency anemia is the most common cause of chronic anemia but can be treated with available oral or parenteral iron products.
- Main Labs to Monitor:
    - CBC
    - Transferrin saturation
    - Serum ferritin

High-Yield Basic Pharmacology
- **Iron Content**
    - Elemental iron content varies between the different iron salts.
    - Among the available oral iron preparations, the polysaccharide-iron complex contains 46% elemental iron, the highest elemental iron content, and ferrous gluconate contains the least at 12%.
    - Parenteral iron salts contain considerably lower elemental iron, with iron dextran and iron sucrose containing 5%, and 2%, respectively.
- **Absorption**
    - GI absorption of oral iron preparations is generally limited in normal therapeutic dosing but can range between 10-90% bioavailability.
    - After absorption, iron is actively transported into the blood, where transferrin moves iron to active sites where hemoglobin is synthesized or stored as ferritin.
    - If excessive iron is ingested, such as in an overdose, iron-induced oxidative stress results in significantly increased bioavailability, further worsening the disruption of oxidative phosphorylation.
- **Iron Storage and Transfer**
    - Most physiologic iron is stored in hemoglobin or myoglobin but can also be stored in hepatocytes.
    - Transferrin is a plasma protein responsible for iron-transferrin complex receptors' internal exchange of iron and delivered to intracellular sites.

- After dissociation, transferrin is recycled out of the cell, leaving iron to participate in its numerous physiologic functions.

High-Yield Clinical Knowledge
- **Iron Deficiency Anemia**
  - Severe iron deficiency anemia manifests as microcytic, hypochromic anemia, affecting the oxygen-carrying capacity of hemoglobin, myoglobin synthesis, heme enzyme synthesis, function, and other enzymatic processes, including xanthine oxidase.
- **Oral Vs. Parenteral Iron**
  - Oral iron supplementation is preferred, with a target dose of 200 mg of elemental iron daily, which should be taken on an empty stomach (if tolerated).
  - For patients who cannot tolerate oral iron, are non-compliant, or have identified oral iron malabsorption, parenteral iron therapy should be used.
- **Test Doses**
  - A test dose is required before administering the first dose of iron dextran as the risk of hypersensitivity and anaphylaxis is high, specifically with this dosage form.
  - While other iron products suggest test doses, they are not required before administration.
- **IV Complications**
  - Common adverse events associated with parenteral iron products include arthralgias, hypotension, flushing, pruritus, and arrhythmias.
- **Iron Chelation**
  - If serum iron concentrations are above 500 mcg/dL, patients are at high risk of hemodynamic collapse and shock.
  - This toxic iron level is an indication for iron chelation therapy with deferoxamine.
    - Other indications for deferoxamine in iron toxicity include:
      - Repetitive vomiting, toxic appearance, lethargy, hypotension with metabolic acidosis, shock.
  - For each 100 mg of deferoxamine will bind 8.5 mg of ferric ion.
- **Chelation of Other Medications**
  - Oral iron therapy will bind to numerous medications, including fluoroquinolones, tetracyclines, and phenytoin.
  - Proton pump inhibitors cause a decreased absorption of oral iron products by increasing the duodenum's pH, causing oxidation of ferrous iron to ferric iron, which is not readily absorbed.

High-Yield Core Evidence
- **FIND-CKD**
  - This was a 56-week, open-label, multicenter, prospective study that randomized patients with non-dialysis-dependent CKD, anemia, and iron deficiency not receiving ESAs to receive either ferric carboxymaltose (FCM) IV, targeting a higher (400-600 mcg/L) or lower (100-200 mcg/L) ferritin or oral iron therapy.
  - Patients randomized to high- or low-ferritin groups experienced a significantly lower incidence of the primary outcome of time to initiate other anemia management triggers of two consecutive values of hemoglobin levels less than 10 g/dL during weeks 8-52.
  - Consistent with the primary outcome findings, the increase in hemoglobin was more significant with the high-ferritin versus oral iron group, and a greater proportion of patients achieved a hemoglobin increase at least 1 g/dL with high-ferritin.
  - Rates of adverse events and serious adverse events were similar in all groups.
  - The authors concluded that compared with oral iron, IV FCM targeting ferritin of 400-600 mcg/L quickly reached and maintained hemoglobin levels and delayed and/or reduced the need for other anemia management, including ESAs. (Nephrol Dial Transplant. 2014 Nov;29(11):2075-84.)
- **REVOKE**
  - This was an open-label, multicenter, prospective study that randomized patients with stage 3 and 4 CKD and iron-deficiency anemia to either open-label oral ferrous sulfate or intravenous iron sucrose.

- This study was prematurely halted after an interim analysis revealed a higher risk of serious adverse events associated with iron sucrose and no difference in the primary outcome of the between-group difference in slope of measured glomerular filtration rate change over two years.
- The authors concluded that among non-dialyzed patients with CKD, intravenous iron therapy is associated with an increased risk of serious adverse events, including those from cardiovascular causes and infectious diseases. (Kidney Int. 2015 Oct;88(4):905-14.)

High-Yield Fast-Fact
- **Deferoxamine in Aluminum Toxicity**
    - CKD patients receiving dialysis may be at risk of aluminum toxicity from bladder irrigations.
    - Deferoxamine can be used to manage aluminum toxicity as it will bind it in a 1-to-1 ratio.

HIGH-YIELD BOARD EXAM ESSENTIALS
- **CLASSIC AGENTS:** Ferric carboxymaltose, ferric citrate, ferric derisomaltose, ferric gluconate, ferric maltol, ferric pyrophosphate citrate, ferrous fumarate, ferrous gluconate, ferrous sulfate, ferumoxytol, iron dextran, iron sucrose, polysaccharide-iron complex
- **DRUG CLASS:** Iron
- **INDICATIONS:** Iron-deficiency anemia
- **MECHANISM:** Replace physiologic iron stores which promote appropriate erythropoiesis and erythrocyte maturation.
- **SIDE EFFECTS:** Constipation, infusion reactions (IV only), chelation
- **CLINICAL PEARLS:** Severe iron deficiency anemia manifests as microcytic, hypochromic anemia, affecting the oxygen-carrying capacity of hemoglobin, myoglobin synthesis, heme enzyme synthesis, and function, as well as other enzymatic processes, including xanthine oxidase.

Table: Drug Class Summary

\multicolumn{4}{c}{**Iron - Drug Class Review**}
\multicolumn{4}{c}{High-Yield Med Reviews}
Mechanism of Action: *Replace physiologic iron stores which promote appropriate erythropoiesis and erythrocyte maturation.*			
Class Effects: *Iron deficiency anemia is the most common cause of chronic anemia but can be treated with available oral or parenteral iron products.*			
Generic Name	**Brand Name**	**Main Indication(s) or Uses**	**Notes**

Ferric carboxymaltose	Injectafer	- Iron-deficiency anemia	- Dosing (Adult):
			  – IV: 15 mg/kg for two doses separated by 7 days
			    – Maximum 750 mg/dose
			  – IV: 1,000 mg, followed by 500 mg 7 days later
			- Dosing (Peds):
			  – Not routinely used
			- CYP450 Interactions: None
			- Renal or Hepatic Dose Adjustments: None
			- Dosage Forms: Intravenous (solution)

Ferric citrate	Auryxia	- Hyperphosphatemia
		- Iron-deficiency anemia
			- Dosing (Adult):
			  – Oral: 1 to 12 tablets TID
			- Dosing (Peds):
			  – Not routinely used
			- CYP450 Interactions: None
			- Renal or Hepatic Dose Adjustments: None
			- Dosage Forms: Oral tablet

Ferric derisomaltose	Monoferric	- Iron-deficiency anemia	- Dosing (Adult):
			  – IV: 20 mg/kg once
			  – IV: 1,000 mg
			- Dosing (Peds):
			  – Not routinely used
			- CYP450 Interactions: None
			- Renal or Hepatic Dose Adjustments: None
			- Dosage Forms: Intravenous (solution)

Ferric gluconate	Ferrlecit	- Iron-deficiency anemia	- Dosing (Adult):
			  – IV: 125 to 250 mg per dialysis session
			- Dosing (Peds):
			  – IV: 1.5 mg/kg/dose per dialysis sessions for 8 sequential sessions
			    – Maximum 125 mg/dose
			- CYP450 Interactions: None
			- Renal or Hepatic Dose Adjustments: None
			- Dosage Forms: Intravenous (solution)

Iron - Drug Class Review
High-Yield Med Reviews

Generic Name	Brand Name	Main Indication(s) or Uses	Notes
Ferric maltol	Accrufer	- Iron-deficiency anemia	- **Dosing (Adult):** — Oral: 30 mg BID - **Dosing (Peds):** — Not routinely used - **CYP450 Interactions:** None - **Renal or Hepatic Dose Adjustments:** None - **Dosage Forms:** Oral
Ferric pyrophosphate citrate	Triferic	- Iron-deficiency anemia	- **Dosing (Adult):** — Intradialytic admixture into bicarbonate concentrate dialysate for use at each dialysis session - **Dosing (Peds):** — Not routinely used - **CYP450 Interactions:** None - **Renal or Hepatic Dose Adjustments:** None - **Dosage Forms:** Solution for dialysate
Ferrous fumarate	Ferretts, Ferrimin, Hemocyte	- Iron-deficiency anemia	- **Dosing (Adult):** — Oral: 30 to 200 mg elemental iron/day in three divided doses - **Dosing (Peds):** — Oral: 3 to 6 mg/kg/day in 3 divided doses — Maximum 200 mg/day - **CYP450 Interactions:** None - **Renal or Hepatic Dose Adjustments:** None - **Dosage Forms:** Oral (tablet)
Ferrous gluconate	Ferate	- Iron-deficiency anemia	- **Dosing (Adult):** — Oral: 65 to 200 mg elemental iron/day in three divided doses - **Dosing (Peds):** — Oral: 3 to 6 mg/kg/day in 3 divided doses — Maximum 200 mg/day - **CYP450 Interactions:** None - **Renal or Hepatic Dose Adjustments:** None - **Dosage Forms:** Oral (tablet)
Ferrous sulfate	Fe-Vite, Fer-In-Sol, Fer-Iron, FeroSul, Slow Fe, Slow Iron	- Iron-deficiency anemia	- **Dosing (Adult):** — Oral: 65 to 200 mg elemental iron/day in three divided doses - **Dosing (Peds):** — Oral: 3 to 6 mg/kg/day in 3 divided doses — Maximum 200 mg/day - **CYP450 Interactions:** None - **Renal or Hepatic Dose Adjustments:** None - **Dosage Forms:** Oral (elixir, liquid, solution, syrup, tablet)

\multicolumn{4}{c}{**Iron - Drug Class Review**}

Generic Name	Brand Name	Main Indication(s) or Uses	Notes

Ferumoxytol	Feraheme	• Iron-deficiency anemia	• **Dosing (Adult):**
			  − IV: 510 mg over 15 minutes, repeated after 3-8 days later
			  − IV: 1,020 mg over 30 minutes once
			• **Dosing (Peds):**
			  − Not routinely used
			• **CYP450 Interactions:** None
			• **Renal or Hepatic Dose Adjustments:** None
			• **Dosage Forms:** Intravenous (solution)

Iron dextran	Infed	• Iron-deficiency anemia	• **Dosing (Adult):**
			  − IV: 25 mg test dose followed by 75 mg q1week for 2 weeks, then 100 mg per week
			  − IM/IV: Dose (in mL) = 0.0442 (desired hemoglobin - observed hemoglobin) x Lean body weight in kg + (0.26 x LBW)
			• **Dosing (Peds):**
			  − IM/IV: Dose (in mL) = 0.0442 (desired hemoglobin - observed hemoglobin) x Lean body weight in kg + (0.26 x LBW)
			• **CYP450 Interactions:** None
			• **Renal or Hepatic Dose Adjustments:** None
			• **Dosage Forms:** Intravenous (solution)

Iron sucrose	Venofer	• Iron-deficiency anemia	• **Dosing (Adult):**
			  − IV: 100 to 300 mg/dose during dialysis to a total cumulative dose of 1,000 mg
			  − IV: 200 mg once every 3 weeks for 5 doses
			• **Dosing (Peds):**
			  − IV: 0.5 mg/kg/dose every 2-4 weeks for 12 weeks
			    − Maximum 100 mg/dose
			  − IV: 5 to 7 mg/kg/dose q1-7days
			    − Maximum 300 mg/dose
			• **CYP450 Interactions:** None
			• **Renal or Hepatic Dose Adjustments:** None
			• **Dosage Forms:** Intravenous (solution)

Polysaccharide iron complex	EZFE, Ferrex, IFerex, Myferon, NovaFerrum, Nu-Iron, Poly-Iron	• Iron-deficiency anemia	• **Dosing (Adult):**
			  − Oral: 65 to 200 mg elemental iron/day in three divided doses
			• **Dosing (Peds):**
			  − Oral: 3 to 6 mg/kg/day in 3 divided doses
			    − Maximum 200 mg/day
			• **CYP450 Interactions:** None
			• **Renal or Hepatic Dose Adjustments:** None
			• **Dosage Forms:** Oral (capsule, liquid)

2025

A COMPREHENSIVE *RAPID REVIEW*

NAPLEX

Pharmacology & Drug Classes

Immunology

IMMUNOLOGY – ANTIHISTAMINES

Drug Class
- Antihistamines (Oral and Parenteral)
- Agents:
    - Acute & Chronic Care
        - Brompheniramine
        - Carbinoxamine
        - Cetirizine
        - Chlorpheniramine
        - Clemastine
        - Cyproheptadine
        - Desloratadine
        - Dexchlorpheniramine
        - Dexbrompheniramine
        - Dimenhydrinate
        - Diphenhydramine
        - Doxylamine
        - Fexofenadine
        - Hydroxyzine
        - Levocetirizine
        - Loratadine
        - Meclizine
        - Promethazine
        - Triprolidine

> **Fast Facts**
> ✓ First-generation antihistamines cause more sedation than second generation because they can pass through the blood brain barrier more efficiently and have antihistaminic effects that lead to sedation.
> ✓ Cyproheptadine is most commonly used for weight gain due to its appetite stimulant effects. It is also commonly cited as a treatment for serotonin syndrome although not very effective.

> 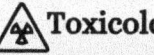 **Toxicology Pearls**
> ✓ Overdoses with diphenhydramine can cause QRS widening due to its Na+ blocking effects at high doses. This is similar to TCA's effect on the heart.

Main Indications or Uses
- **Acute & Chronic Care**
    - Allergies (Brompheniramine, carbinoxamine, cetirizine, chlorpheniramine, clemastine, desloratadine, dexchlorpheniramine, dexbrompheniramine, dimenhydrinate, diphenhydramine, doxylamine, fexofenadine, levocetirizine, loratadine, triprolidine)
    - Anaphylaxis (Diphenhydramine, cetirizine)
    - Angioedema (Cetirizine, clemastine, diphenhydramine)
    - Anxiety (Hydroxyzine)
    - Appetite (Cyproheptadine)
    - Urticaria (Cetirizine, clemastine, desloratadine, diphenhydramine, fexofenadine, hydroxyzine, levocetirizine, loratadine)
    - Extrapyramidal symptoms (Diphenhydramine)
    - Motion sickness (Dimenhydrinate, meclizine, promethazine)
    - Nausea and vomiting (Dimenhydrinate, diphenhydramine, doxylamine, promethazine)
    - Serotonin syndrome (Cyproheptadine)
    - Vertigo (Dimenhydrinate, diphenhydramine, meclizine)
    - Insomnia (Diphenhydramine, doxylamine)
    - Pruritus (Diphenhydramine, hydroxyzine)

Mechanism of Action
- **Histamine-1 Receptor Inverse Agonists**
    - Competes with histamine binding at histamine-1 receptors (H_1) on effector cells in the GI tract, respiratory tract, and blood vessels.
        - This is a distinction from H1 antagonists, which are competitive antagonists of histamine at the H_1 receptor.

Primary Net Benefit

- OTC agents for the management of common allergy-related complaints and acute care use of specific agents for numerous indications that are extensions of their central and peripheral antihistamine effect.
- Main Labs to Monitor:
  - No routine monitoring

High-Yield Basic Pharmacology
- **Generational Antihistamines**
  - First-generation antihistamines are nonselective and are associated with sedation and other anticholinergic effects.
    - First-generation antihistamines include brompheniramine, carbinoxamine, chlorpheniramine, clemastine, dexchlorpheniramine, dexbrompheniramine, dimenhydrinate, diphenhydramine, doxylamine, hydroxyzine, meclizine, and promethazine.
  - Second-generation antihistamines are more H_1 selective and preferred as first-line agents for most indications.
    - Second-generation antihistamines include cetirizine, desloratadine, fexofenadine, levocetirizine, loratadine, and triprolidine.
- **Cyproheptadine**
  - Cyproheptadine is a nonselective antihistamine and possesses 5-HT2A receptor blocking properties, improving autonomic instability observed in serotonin syndrome.
  - For serotonin syndrome, cyproheptadine must be used in combination with benzodiazepines, removal of serotonergic agents, and extravascular/intravascular cooling.
- **Fexofenadine and Terfenadine**
  - Fexofenadine is the active metabolite of the first-generation antihistamine, terfenadine.

High-Yield Clinical Knowledge
- **Angioedema**
  - Parenteral diphenhydramine can be used as a component of the management of angioedema. Cetirizine and clemastine could also be used.
  - However, diphenhydramine alone is unlikely to be beneficial, as angioedema must be aggressively managed with epinephrine, corticosteroids, and airway support, including endotracheal intubation.
- **Anticholinergic Toxicity**
  - First-generation antihistamines may cause excessive sedation in supratherapeutic doses or when combined with other sedative agents.
  - There is also a risk of potentially fatal anticholinergic toxicity in an overdose of first-generation antihistamines with characteristic anticholinergic toxidrome.
  - Classic antimuscarinic toxidrome: "Blind as a bat, Dry as a bone, Hot as a hare, Mad as a hatter, Red as a beet."
  - The anticholinergic toxidrome presents in three phases:
    - Induction phase: peripheral anticholinergic effects
    - Stupor phase: somnolence, restlessness, ataxia, hyperthermia, hypertension.
    - Delirium phase: amnesia, confusion, hallucinations, incoherent speech.
- **Second-Generation Sedation**
  - Although the likelihood of sedative effects due to second-generation antihistamines may be lower than from first-generation agents, there is wide interpatient variability.
  - As the first-generation agents are similarly effective to second-generation agents for the treatment of allergies as OTC agents, patient-specific response and cost play into selecting the appropriate agent.

- **Sleep Aids**
  - As a result of their sedative properties, some first-generation antihistamines are used as over-the-counter night-time sleep aids.
  - Diphenhydramine and doxylamine are commonly used for their sedative properties.
  - Some children, particularly those younger than 2, may experience a paradoxical stimulant response to first-generation antihistamines.

- **Urticaria**
  - The underlying pathophysiologic mechanism of urticaria is histamine, specifically, H_1 receptor-mediated.
  - First-generation antihistamines are preferred for acute management, and second-generation agents can be used for pre-exposure prevention.
- **Nausea and Vomiting in Pregnancy**
  - Doxylamine is commonly used for the treatment of nausea and vomiting in pregnancy.
  - It is formulated with pyridoxine (brand name Bonjesta or Diclegis), which also may have antiemetic properties, but is only available as a prescription agent.
    - Compared to 5-HT3 antagonists (ondansetron), doxylamine plus pyridoxine is similarly effective and does not carry the small (and questionable) risk of birth defects.
  - Dimenhydrinate, diphenhydramine, and promethazine can also be used.
- **Drug Interactions**
  - Cetirizine, chlorpheniramine, fexofenadine, and loratadine are CYP3A4 substrates and should be avoided with potent CYP3A4 inhibitors, including macrolide antibiotics, ketoconazole, and itraconazole.
  - Diphenhydramine is a substrate of CYP1A2, 2C19, 2C9, and 2D6 and inhibits CYP2D6, leading to potentially numerous pharmacokinetic interactions, and in the case of antidepressants (fluoxetine, sertraline, TCAs), it can also have additive anticholinergic effects.
- **Pregnancy Risks**
  - Hydroxyzine and fexofenadine have been associated with teratogenic effects in animal models.
  - The antihistamines chlorpheniramine, cetirizine, diphenhydramine, and loratadine have not been associated with this risk.
- **Geriatric Use**
  - First-generation antihistamines are on the Beers Criteria due to their anticholinergic effects, sedation, urinary retention, and confusion.
  - Second-generation antihistamines are recommended, but caution is advised because of interpatient variability and potential for adverse effects to still occur.

High-Yield Core Evidence
- **Antihistamines and Birth Defects**
  - This is a systematic review of the peer-reviewed epidemiologic literature on the association between prenatal exposure to antihistamines and congenital disabilities.
  - Research including H_1 or H_2-receptor antagonists was included, but studies of doxylamine plus pyridoxine were excluded.
  - The authors did not find an association with the use of antihistamines during pregnancy regarding congenital disabilities.
  - The authors concluded that selected antihistamines had been very well studied, but H2-receptor antagonists require additional study before assessing safety concerning congenital disability risk. (Expert Opin Drug Saf. 2014 Dec;13(12):1667-98.)

High-Yield Fast-Facts
- **Dye Allergies**
  - Patients can have hypersensitivity to the pink dye in many dosage forms of diphenhydramine.
  - Dye-free dosage forms are available.

- **Fexofenadine and Juice**
  - Apple, grapefruit, and orange juice can reduce fexofenadine's efficacy and should be spaced by at least 4 hours.

Table: Drug Class Summary

Antihistamines (Oral and Parenteral) - Drug Class Review High-Yield Med Reviews			
Mechanism of Action: *Competes with histamine binding at histamine-1 receptors (H_1) on effector cells in the GI tract, respiratory tract, and blood vessels.*			
Class Effects: *OTC agents for managing common allergy-related complaints, acute care use for anaphylaxis/angioedema, and nausea/vomiting, may cause drowsiness (especially 1st generation) or anticholinergic effects, indications that are extensions of their central and peripheral antihistamine effect.*			
Generic Name	**Brand Name**	**Main Indication(s) or Uses**	**Notes**

Brompheniramine	Formulated in combinations
	
	 W/phenylephrine: Dimetapp, Glenmax PEB, Rynex PE, Brohist, Ru-Hist D
	
	 W/pseudoephedrine: Lodrane, Rynex PSE
	
	 W/Dextromethorphan and phenylephrine; Dimaphen DM, Enda-Cof DM, Glenmax PEB DM, Rynex DM, LoHist-DM
	
	 W/pseudoephedrine and dextromethorphan: Brotapp-DM, Bromfed DM
		• Cough and upper respiratory symptoms	• **Dosing (Adult):**
			   – Oral: 1-4 mg q4h as needed
			 • **Dosing (Peds):**
			   – Oral: 1-4 mg q4h as needed
			 • **CYP450 Interactions:** None
			 • **Renal or Hepatic Dose Adjustments:** None
			 • **Dosage Forms:** Oral (capsule, liquid, syrup)

Carbinoxamine	Karbinal ER, Ryvent	• Allergic rhinitis	• **Dosing (Adult):**
			   – Oral: IR 4-8 mg q6-8h
			   – Oral: ER 6-16 mg q12h
			 • **Dosing (Peds):**
			   – Oral: 0.2-0.4 mg/kg/day divided q6-8h
			     – Maximum 16 mg/dose
			 • **CYP450 Interactions:** None
			 • **Renal or Hepatic Dose Adjustments:** None
			 • **Dosage Forms:** Oral (ER suspension, tablet)

Antihistamines (Oral and Parenteral) - Drug Class Review High-Yield Med Reviews			
Generic Name	**Brand Name**	**Main Indication(s) or Uses**	**Notes**

Cetirizine	Zyrtec, Zyrtec-D (with pseudoephedrine), Zerviate (ophthalmic), Quzyttir (IV)	- Allergic rhinitis	- **Dosing (Adult):**
			  - Oral: 5-10 mg daily
			  - Ophthalmic 1 drop in affected eye(s) BID
			  - IV: 10 mg q12-24h
			- **Dosing (Peds):**
			  - Oral: 2.5-10 mg daily
			  - Ophthalmic 1 drop in affected eye(s) BID
			- **CYP450 Interactions:** CYP3A4, P-gp substrate
			- **Renal or Hepatic Dose Adjustments:**
			  - CrCl 11 to 30 mL/minute - 5 mg daily
			  - CrCl < 10 mL/minute - not recommended
			  - Child-Pugh class A, B or C - 5 mg daily
			- **Dosage Forms:** Oral (liquid, tablet), ophthalmic solution, IV (solution)

Chlorpheniramine	Chlor-Trimeton (available in numerous combinations under various brand names)	- Allergic pruritus, rhinitis, urticaria	- **Dosing (Adult):**
			  - Oral: IR 4 mg q4-6h
			  - Oral: ER 12 mg q12h
			  - Max 24 mg/day
			- **Dosing (Peds):**
			  - Oral: IR 1-4 mg q4-6h
			  - Maximum 6 to 24 mg/day
			  - Oral: ER: Children older than 12: use adult dosing
			- **CYP450 Interactions:** CYP2D6, 3A4 substrate
			- **Renal or Hepatic Dose Adjustments:** None
			- **Dosage Forms:** Oral (syrup, tablet)

Clemastine	Dayhist, Tavist	- Allergic rhinitis	- **Dosing (Adult):**
			  - Oral: 1.34 mg BID to 2.68 mg TID
			  - Max 8.04 mg/day
			- **Dosing (Peds):**
			  - Children younger than 12 years
			    Oral: 0.67 mg BID
			  - Max 4.02 mg/day
			- **CYP450 Interactions:** None
			- **Renal or Hepatic Dose Adjustments:** None
			- **Dosage Forms:** Oral (tablet)

Cyproheptadine	Periactin	- Decreased appetite from chronic disease
		- Serotonin syndrome
		- Spasticity due to spinal cord damage
			- **Dosing (Adult):**
			  - Oral: 4-20 mg divided q8h
			  - Max 32 mg/day
			  - Oral: 12 mg followed by 2 mg q2h or 4-8 mg q6h
			- **Dosing (Peds):**
			  - Oral: 2-4 mg q8-12h
			  - Max 12-16 mg/day
			- **CYP450 Interactions:** None
			- **Renal or Hepatic Dose Adjustments:** None
			- **Dosage Forms:** Oral (syrup, tablet)

Antihistamines (Oral and Parenteral) - Drug Class Review High-Yield Med Reviews				
Generic Name	**Brand Name**	**Main Indication(s) or Uses**	**Notes**

Desloratadine	Clarinex, Clarinex-D	<ul><li>Allergic rhinitis</li><li>Chronic idiopathic urticaria</li></ul>	<ul><li>**Dosing (Adult):**
			  – Oral: 5 mg daily, up to 10 mg BID</li><li>**Dosing (Peds):**
			  – Oral: 1 to 5 mg daily</li><li>**CYP450 Interactions:** CYP2C8, P-gp substrate</li><li>**Renal or Hepatic Dose Adjustments:** None</li><li>**Dosage Forms:** Oral (syrup, tablet)</li></ul>

Dexchlorpheniramine	RyClora	<ul><li>Hypersensitivity reactions</li><li>Allergic rhinitis (Peds)</li></ul>	<ul><li>**Dosing (Adult):**
			  – Oral: 2 mg q4-6h</li><li>**Dosing (Peds):**
			  – 2-5 years: 0.5 mg q4-6h</li><li>**CYP450 Interactions:** None</li><li>**Renal or Hepatic Dose Adjustments:** None</li><li>**Dosage Forms:** Oral solution</li></ul>

Dexbrompheniramine	W/phenylephrine: Alahist PE, G-Hist PE
	
	W/chlophedianol: Chlo Hist
	
	W/chlophedianol and pseudoephedrine: Chlo Tuss
		<ul><li>Allergic rhinitis</li></ul>	<ul><li>**Dosing (Adult):**
			  – Oral: 2 mg q4-6h</li><li>**Dosing (Peds):**
			  – Oral: 0.5 to 2 mg q4-6h</li><li>**CYP450 Interactions:** None</li><li>**Renal or Hepatic Dose Adjustments:** None</li><li>**Dosage Forms:** Oral (solution)</li></ul>

Dimenhydrinate	Driminate	<ul><li>Motion sickness</li><li>Vertigo</li><li>Postoperative nausea/vomiting</li><li>Radiation sickness</li><li>Pregnancy-related nausea/vomiting</li></ul>	<ul><li>**Dosing (Adult):**
			  – Motion sickness, nausea/vomiting: 50 to 100 mg q4-6h
			    – Max 400 mg/day
			  – IM/IV: 50-100 mg q4h</li><li>**Dosing (Peds):**
			  – Oral: 12.5-100 mg q4-8h
			  – IM: 1.25 mg/kg/dose q6h
			  – Max doses dependent on route and age.</li><li>**CYP450 Interactions:** None</li><li>**Renal or Hepatic Dose Adjustments:** None</li><li>**Dosage Forms:** Oral (tablet), IV (solution)</li></ul>

Antihistamines (Oral and Parenteral) - Drug Class Review
High-Yield Med Reviews

Generic Name	Brand Name	Main Indication(s) or Uses	Notes
Diphenhydramine	Benadryl (numerous other brand names)	<ul><li>Allergies</li><li>Anaphylaxis</li><li>Angioedema</li><li>Extrapyramidal symptoms</li><li>Insomnia</li><li>Motion sickness</li><li>Nausea and vomiting</li><li>Pruritus</li><li>Vertigo</li></ul>	<ul><li>**Dosing (Adult):**<ul><li>Oral: 12.5-50 mg q4-6h as needed</li><li>IV/IM: 10-50 mg q6h as needed</li><li>Topical apply 1% to 2% to affected area up to 3-4 times daily</li></ul></li><li>**Dosing (Peds):**<ul><li>IV/IM/Oral: 0.5-2 mg/kg/dose q6h</li><li>Topical: Apply 1% to 2% to affected area up to 3-4 times daily</li></ul></li><li>**CYP450 Interactions:** CYP1A2, 2C19, 2C9, 2D6 substrate; CYP2D6 inhibitor</li><li>**Renal or Hepatic Dose Adjustments:** None</li><li>**Dosage Forms:** Oral (capsule, elixir, liquid, syrup, tablet), IV (solution), Topical cream</li></ul>
Doxylamine	Sleep Aid W/ pyridoxine: Bonjesta, Diclegis	<ul><li>Insomnia</li><li>Nausea and vomiting associated with pregnancy (w/ pyridoxine)</li></ul>	<ul><li>**Dosing (Adult):**<ul><li>Oral: 10-25 daily</li></ul></li><li>**Dosing (Peds):**<ul><li>Oral: 25 mg at bedtime</li></ul></li><li>**CYP450 Interactions:** None</li><li>**Renal or Hepatic Dose Adjustments:** None</li><li>**Dosage Forms:** Oral (tablet)</li></ul>
Fexofenadine	Allegra	<ul><li>Allergies</li><li>Chronic idiopathic urticaria</li></ul>	<ul><li>**Dosing (Adult):**<ul><li>Once daily formulations<ul><li>Oral: 60 mg q12h</li></ul></li><li>Twice daily formulations<ul><li>Oral: 180 mg daily</li></ul></li></ul></li><li>**Dosing (Peds):**<ul><li>Oral: 15-30 mg q12h</li><li>Max 60 mg/day</li></ul></li><li>**CYP450 Interactions:** Substrate CYP3A4, P-gp</li><li>**Renal or Hepatic Dose Adjustments:**<ul><li>GFR < 10 mL/minute – dose q24h</li></ul></li><li>**Dosage Forms:** Oral (suspension, tablet)</li></ul>
Hydroxyzine	Vistaril	<ul><li>Anxiety</li><li>Pruritus/Urticaria</li></ul>	<ul><li>**Dosing (Adult):**<ul><li>Oral: 10-50 mg up to 4 times daily<ul><li>Max 400 mg/day</li></ul></li><li>IM: 25-50 mg q4-6h as needed</li></ul></li><li>**Dosing (Peds):**<ul><li>Oral: 0.5-2 mg/kg/day q6-8h</li><li>Max 25 mg/dose</li></ul></li><li>**CYP450 Interactions:** None</li><li>**Renal or Hepatic Dose Adjustments:**<ul><li>CrCl < 50 mL/minute: Reduce dose by 50%</li></ul></li><li>**Dosage Forms:** Oral (capsule, syrup, tablet), IM solution</li></ul>

\multicolumn{4}{c}{**Antihistamines (Oral and Parenteral) - Drug Class Review**}
\multicolumn{4}{c}{High-Yield Med Reviews}
Generic Name	**Brand Name**	**Main Indication(s) or Uses**	**Notes**

Levocetirizine	Xyzal	• Allergic rhinitis
		• Chronic idiopathic urticaria
			• **Dosing (Adult):**
			   – Oral: 2.5-5 mg daily
			• **Dosing (Peds):**
			   – Oral: 1.25-5 mg daily
			• **CYP450 Interactions:** None
			• **Renal or Hepatic Dose Adjustments:**
			   – CrCl 50 to 80 mL/minute: 2.5 mg daily
			   – CrCl 30 to 50 mL/minute: 2.5 mg q48h
			   – CrCl 10 to 30 mL/minute: 2.5 mg twice weekly
			   – CrCl < 10 mL/minute: contraindicated
			• **Dosage Forms:** Oral (solution, tablet)

Loratadine	Alavert, Alavert-D Claritin, Claritin-D, Claritin Reditabs	• Allergic rhinitis
		• Urticaria
			• **Dosing (Adult):**
			   – Oral: 10 mg daily or 5 mg BID
			• **Dosing (Peds):**
			   – Children younger than 6 years
			      – Oral: 5 mg daily
			• **CYP450 Interactions:** CYP2D6, 3A4, P-gp substrate
			• **Renal or Hepatic Dose Adjustments:**
			   – CrCl < 30 mL/minute: q48h
			• **Dosage Forms:** Oral (capsule, solution, syrup, tablet, ODT)

Meclizine	Antivert, Bonine, Travel-Ease	• Motion sickness
		• Vertigo
			• **Dosing (Adult):**
			   – Oral: 12.5-50 mg 1 hour before travel
			   – Oral: 12.5-100 mg daily in divided doses
			   – Max 100 mg daily
			• **Dosing (Peds):**
			   – Oral: 25-50 mg 1 hour before travel
			   – Oral: 25-100 mg daily in 3-4 divided doses
			• **CYP450 Interactions:** CYP2D6 substrate
			• **Renal or Hepatic Dose Adjustments:** None
			• **Dosage Forms:** Oral (tablet)

Promethazine	Phenadoz, Phenergan, Promethegan	• Nausea/vomiting (including w/ pregnancy)	• **Dosing (Adult):**
			   – IM/IV/Rectal/Oral: 6.25-25 mg q4-8h as needed
			• **Dosing (Peds):**
			   – IM/IV/Rectal/Oral: 0.25-1.1 mg/kg q4-6h as needed
			      – Max 25 mg/dose
			• **CYP450 Interactions:** CYP2B6, 2D6 substrate
			• **Renal or Hepatic Dose Adjustments:** None
			• **Dosage Forms:** IV solution, Oral (solution, syrup, tablet), Rectal suppository

Antihistamines (Oral and Parenteral) - Drug Class Review High-Yield Med Reviews			
Generic Name	**Brand Name**	**Main Indication(s) or Uses**	**Notes**

Triprolidine	Histex, Histex PD, PediaClear PD	- Allergies	- **Dosing (Adult):**
			  - Oral: 2.5 mg q4-6h
			    - Max 10 mg/day
			- **Dosing (Peds):**
			  - Oral: 0.313-1.25 mg q4-6h as needed
			    - Max 4 doses/24 hours
			- **CYP450 Interactions:** text
			- **Renal or Hepatic Dose Adjustments:** text
			- **Dosage Forms:** Oral (liquid, syrup)

HIGH-YIELD BOARD EXAM ESSENTIALS
- **CLASSIC AGENTS:** Brompheniramine, carbinoxamine, cetirizine, chlorpheniramine, clemastine, cyproheptadine, desloratadine, dexchlorpheniramine, dexbrompheniramine, dimenhydrinate, diphenhydramine, doxylamine, fexofenadine, hydroxyzine, levocetirizine, loratadine, meclizine, promethazine, triprolidine
- **DRUG CLASS:** Antihistamines
- **INDICATIONS:** Allergies, anaphylaxis, angioedema, extrapyramidal symptoms, insomnia, motion sickness, nausea and vomiting (including pregnancy), pruritus, vertigo
- **MECHANISM:** Competes with histamine binding at histamine-1 receptors (H_1) on effector cells in the GI tract, respiratory tract, and blood vessels.
- **SIDE EFFECTS:** Dry mucous membranes, restlessness, ataxia, hyperthermia, hypertension
  - Some have anticholinergic and sedative effects as well.
- **CLINICAL PEARLS:**
  - Although the likelihood of sedative effects due to second-generation antihistamines may be lower than from first-generation agents, there is wide interpatient variability.
  - Cyproheptadine is more commonly used for appetite stimulant for weight gain and is one of the historical "antidotes" for the treatment of serotonin syndrome.
  - At high doses or in toxicology cases, diphenhydramine can inhibit Na+ channels in the heart and cause QRS widening.

IMMUNOSUPPRESSANTS – ANTI-CD52 MONOCLONAL ANTIBODY

Drug Class
- Anti-CD52 Monoclonal Antibody
- Agents:
    - Acute Care
        - Alemtuzumab

Main Indications or Uses
- Acute & Chronic Care
    - Acute graft-versus-host disease
    - B-cell chronic lymphocytic leukemia
    - Relapsing Multiple sclerosis

> **Fast Facts**
> ✓ PJP prophylaxis is recommended for at least two months after the last dose of alemtuzumab or until the patient's CD4+ count is 200 cells/microL or higher.

Mechanism of Action
- Removes both B and T lymphocytes from the blood, bone marrow, and organs by binding to the CD52 surface antigen and inducing antibody-dependent cell lysis.

Primary Net Benefit
- Used for induction of immunosuppression for an organ transplant as an alternative to antithymocyte globulins.
- Main Labs to Monitor:
    - CBC with differential (baseline, weekly)
    - Serum creatinine (baseline, monthly until 48 months after the last dose)
    - Liver function (bilirubin), liver enzyme (ALT/AST) (baseline, monthly until 48 months after the last dose)
    - TSH (baseline, every three months until 48 months after the last dose)
    - CD4+ lymphocyte counts (until recovery)
    - CMV antigen

High-Yield Basic Pharmacology
- **Deceiving Half-life**
    - Despite a half-life of 11 hours to 6 days after 12 weeks of therapy, the duration of effect of alemtuzumab is profound.
    - After one to two doses, alemtuzumab causes complete lymphocyte depletion, which persists for more than one year.
        - The extent of alemtuzumab's effect is due to the presence of CD52 surface antigen found on eosinophils, macrophages, and monocytes.
- **B/T-Cell Action**
    - The precise mechanism of alemtuzumab is unknown, but leading hypotheses point towards induction of complement and antibody-dependent cytotoxicity.

High-Yield Clinical Knowledge
- **Infusion Reactions**
    - Alemtuzumab must be administered as an IV infusion over 2 hours, not via IV push.
    - Rare infusion-related reactions include rigors, hypotension, fever, shortness of breath, bronchospasms, and chills.
        - The risk of these adverse events can be minimized by using premedications such as acetaminophen, corticosteroids, and diphenhydramine.
- **Pneumocystis Jiroveci Prophylaxis**
    - PJP prophylaxis is recommended for at least two months after the last dose of alemtuzumab or until the patient's CD4+ count is 200 cells/microL or higher.
    - Prophylaxis for herpes is recommended for as long as PJP prophylaxis is administered.

- **Alemtuzumab or Anithymocyte Globulins**
  - Alemtuzumab has been compared with antithymocyte globulins for induction of immunosuppression therapy.
  - The long-term immunosuppression observed with alemtuzumab is weighed against the safety and tolerability of antithymocyte globulins in the acute phase of transplant care (see INTAC study below).
- **Subcutaneous Administration**
  - Although administered via IV infusion in most cases, some indications allow for subcutaneous administration of alemtuzumab.
  - With subQ administration, the risk of infusion reactions is minimal, if not absent altogether.

High-Yield Core Evidence
- **INTAC Study**
  - This prospective study compared alemtuzumab or conventional induction therapy (basiliximab or rabbit antithymocyte globulin) for induction regimens in patients with high or low immunologic risk after renal transplant.
  - All patients received tacrolimus and mycophenolate mofetil and underwent a 5-day glucocorticoid taper in a regimen of early steroid withdrawal.
  - Patients randomized to alemtuzumab saw a significantly lower risk of the primary endpoint of biopsy-confirmed acute rejection at 6 months and 12 months compared to placebo.
  - This risk reduction was maintained at 3 years in the biopsy-confirmed acute rejection in low-risk patients, but no significant difference was observed among high-risk patients.
  - Adverse-event rates were similar among all four treatment groups.
  - The authors concluded that alemtuzumab's apparent superiority concerning early biopsy-confirmed acute rejection was restricted to patients at low risk for transplant rejection; among high-risk patients, alemtuzumab and rabbit antithymocyte globulin had similar efficacy. N Engl J Med. 2011 May 19;364(20):1909-19.

High-Yield Fast-Fact
- **Free Drug**
  - The manufacturer provided alemtuzumab at a very small or no cost through its US Campath Distribution program for a short period.

HIGH-YIELD BOARD EXAM ESSENTIALS
- **CLASSIC AGENTS:** Alemtuzumab
- **DRUG CLASS:** Anti-CD52 monoclonal antibody
- **INDICATIONS:** Acute graft-versus-host disease, B-cell chronic lymphocytic leukemia, relapsing Multiple sclerosis
- **MECHANISM:** Removes both B and T lymphocytes from the blood, bone marrow, and organs by binding to the CD52 surface antigen and inducing antibody-dependent cell lysis.
- **SIDE EFFECTS:** Infusion-related reactions (rigors, hypotension, fever, shortness of breath, bronchospasms, and chills)
- **CLINICAL PEARLS:** PJP prophylaxis is recommended for at least two months after the last dose of alemtuzumab or until the patient's CD4+ count is 200 cells/microL or higher.

Table: Drug Class Summary

Anti-CD52 Monoclonal Antibody - Drug Class Review			
High-Yield Med Reviews			
Mechanism of Action: *Removes B and T lymphocytes from the blood, bone marrow, and organs by binding to the CD52 surface antigen and inducing antibody-dependent cell lysis.*			
Class Effects: *Used for induction of immunosuppression for an organ transplant as an alternative to antithymocyte globulins.*			
Generic Name	**Brand Name**	**Indication(s) or Uses**	**Notes**
Alemtuzumab	Campath Lemtrada	<ul><li>Acute graft-versus-host disease</li><li>B-cell chronic lymphocytic leukemia</li><li>Relapsing Multiple sclerosis</li></ul>	<ul><li>**Dosing (Adult):**<ul><li>B-CLL:<ul><li>Initial IV: 3 mg q24h, increasing to 30 mg IV/SQ three times weekly</li></ul></li><li>Transplant:<ul><li>IV: 10 mg daily x 5 days, then 10 mg weekly until symptom resolution</li><li>IV/SQ: 30 mg immediately before transplant, then repeated for 1-2 doses q24h</li></ul></li><li>MS:<ul><li>IV: 12 mg daily x 5 days, then 12 months later 12 mg daily for 3 days</li></ul></li></ul></li><li>**Dosing (Peds):**<ul><li>IV: 0.2 mg/kg/dose x 10 days<ul><li>Maximum 10 mg/dose</li></ul></li></ul></li><li>**CYP450 Interactions:** None</li><li>**Renal or Hepatic Dose Adjustments:** None</li><li>**Dosage Forms:** IV (solution)</li></ul>

IMMUNOSUPPRESSANTS – ANTITHYMOCYTE GLOBULIN

Drug Class
- **Antithymocyte Globulin**
- **Agents:**
    - Acute Care
        - Antithymocyte Globulin (Equine)
        - Antithymocyte Globulin (Rabbit)

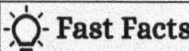

Fast Facts

✓ *Since these agents are not from human sources patients can develop antibodies against them and also cause infusion-related reactions known as cytokine release syndrome.*

Main Indications or Uses
- **Acute Care**
    - Acute/Chronic graft-versus-host disease
    - Aplastic anemia
    - Transplant induction therapy
    - Transplant rejection

Mechanism of Action
- Antithymocyte globulins bind to CD2, CD3, CD4, CD8, CD 11a, CD18, CD25, CD 44, CD45 receptors, and HLA class I and II molecules on the surface of lymphocytes, causing complement-mediated lymphocyte lysis leading to lymphocyte depletion (including B-cells, T-cells, and leukocytes) and blocking lymphocyte function.

Primary Net Benefit
- Induction of immunosuppression agents for transplant recipients with significant toxicities related to immunosuppression/myelosuppression and infusion reactions.
- Main Labs to Monitor:
    - CBC with differential
    - Absolute DC3 count

High-Yield Basic Pharmacology
- **Onset and Duration**
    - The onset of immunosuppression and T-cell depletion for either agent is approximately 24 hours.
    - However, the duration of effect is prolonged, where lymphopenia may persist for up to 2 years.
- **Antiequine Antibodies**
    - Antibody development to anti-thymocyte globulin frequently occurs in 78% of patients receiving equine and up to 68% receiving rabbit formulations.
        - The clinical impact is not fully understood; however, many patients who begin therapy with equine formulations are ultimately converted to the rabbit formulation due to intolerances or adverse events.

High-Yield Clinical Knowledge
- **Administration & Pre-Medication**
    - Infusion-related febrile events frequently occur with the administration of either antithymocyte globulin preparation.
        - This is otherwise known as the "cytokine release syndrome," causing a range of events, including fever, headache, chills, rigors, dyspnea, hyper OR hypotension, rash, and nausea/vomiting/diarrhea.
    - All patients should receive acetaminophen, diphenhydramine, and corticosteroids before administering either antithymocyte product.
    - Administration via central IV catheters and/or slowing the infusion over 4-6 hours can also reduce these reactions.
- **Delayed Calcineurin Inhibitor**
    - In renal transplant recipients, antithymocyte globulins are administered to recover from ischemic reperfusion injuries and avoid early therapy with the nephrotoxic calcineurin inhibitors (cyclosporin and tacrolimus).

- **Atgam Test Dose**
  - Before administering antithymocyte globulin (equine), a test dose is recommended to screen for anaphylaxis reactions.
    - Testing may be accomplished using an escalating exposure technique from epicutaneous prick to an intradermal injection of the dilute drug with saline control.
    - Although they predict an increased risk of anaphylaxis, positive tests are not a contraindication; but additional precautions should be taken (crash cart, airway support, epinephrine, close by).
- **CMV Screening**
  - Screening for CMV before transplant and for patients in whom CMV screening is seropositive at the time of transplant should receive antiviral prophylaxis.
    - CMV-seronegative, but receiving organ tissue from a CMV-seropositive donor should also receive antiviral prophylaxis.

High-Yield Core Evidence

- **Thymoglobulin Induction Study**
  - This was a multicenter, prospective study that randomized patients at high risk for acute rejection or delayed graft function who received a renal transplant from a deceased donor to either antithymocyte globulin (rabbit) or basiliximab-based therapy.
  - There was no difference in the primary outcome of the composite of acute rejection, delayed graft function, graft loss, and death between study groups.
  - In examining the composite independently, antithymocyte globulin was associated with a lower incidence of acute rejection and acute rejection requiring antibody treatment.
  - Patients receiving antithymocyte globulin had a greater incidence of infection but a lower incidence of cytomegalovirus disease.
  - The authors concluded that among patients at high risk for acute rejection or delayed graft function who received a renal transplant from a deceased donor, induction therapy consisting of a 5-day course of antithymocyte globulin, as compared with basiliximab, reduced the incidence and severity of acute rejection but not the incidence of delayed graft function. (N Engl J Med. 2006 Nov 9;355(19):1967-77.)
- **STAT Trial**
  - This was a multicenter, double-blind/double-dummy study comparing single-dose vs. traditional antithymocyte globulin (rabbit) induction-based therapy among renal transplant recipients.
  - There was no difference between groups regarding the primary outcome of the composite of fever, hypoxia, hypotension, cardiac complications, and delayed graft function.
  - The authors concluded that single-dose induction therapy is non-inferior to double-dose induction in terms of early tolerability and equivalent in 12-month safety in adult renal transplantation (Am J Transplant. 2016 Jun;16(6):1858-67.)

High-Yield Fast-Fact

- **Malignancy Risk**
  - Both antithymocyte globulins are associated with an increased risk of malignancies.

HIGH-YIELD BOARD EXAM ESSENTIALS
- **CLASSIC AGENTS:** Antithymocyte globulin (equine), antithymocyte globulin (rabbit)
- **DRUG CLASS:** Antithymocyte globulin
- **INDICATIONS:** Acute/chronic graft-versus-host disease, aplastic anemia, transplant induction therapy, transplant rejection
- **MECHANISM:** Bind to numerous CD* receptors and HLA class I and II molecules on lymphocytes, causing complement-mediated lymphocyte lysis leading to lymphocyte depletion and blocking lymphocyte function.
- **SIDE EFFECTS:** Infusion-related fever, cytokine release syndrome, anaphylaxis
- **CLINICAL PEARLS:** In renal transplant recipients, antithymocyte globulins are administered to recover from ischemic reperfusion injuries and avoid early therapy with the nephrotoxic calcineurin inhibitors (cyclosporin and tacrolimus).

Table: Drug Class Summary

\multicolumn{4}{c}{**Antithymocyte Globulin – Drug Class Review**}
\multicolumn{4}{c}{High-Yield Med Reviews}
\multicolumn{4}{l}{**Mechanism of Action:** *Bind to numerous CD* receptors and HLA class I and II molecules on lymphocytes, causing complement-mediated lymphocyte lysis leading to lymphocyte depletion and blocking lymphocyte function.*}
\multicolumn{4}{l}{**Class Effects:** *Induction of immunosuppression agents for transplant recipients with significant toxicities related to immunosuppression/myelosuppression and infusion reactions.*}
Generic Name	**Brand Name**	**Indication(s) or Uses**	**Notes**
Antithymocyte Globulin (Equine)	Atgam	<ul><li>Aplastic anemia</li><li>Transplant induction therapy</li><li>Transplant rejection</li></ul>	<ul><li>**Dosing (Adult):** − IV: 5 to 40 mg/kg q24h x 3 to 14 days</li><li>**Dosing (Peds):** − IV: 5 to 40 mg/kg q24h x 3 to 14 days</li><li>**CYP450 Interactions:** None</li><li>**Renal or Hepatic Dose Adjustments:** None</li><li>**Dosage Forms:** IV (solution)</li></ul>
Antithymocyte Globulin (Rabbit)	Thymoglobulin	<ul><li>Renal transplant rejection</li><li>Transplant induction therapy</li></ul>	<ul><li>**Dosing (Adult):** − IV: 0.5 to 2.5 mg/kg q24h for 5 to 7 days</li><li>**Dosing (Peds):** − IV: 0.5 to 3.5 mg/kg q24h for 5 to 7 days</li><li>**CYP450 Interactions:** None</li><li>**Renal or Hepatic Dose Adjustments:** None</li><li>**Dosage Forms:** IV (solution)</li></ul>

IMMUNOSUPPRESSANTS – CALCINEURIN INHIBITORS

Drug Class
- **Calcineurin Inhibitors**
- **Agents:**
  - **Acute & Chronic Care**
    - Cyclosporine
    - Tacrolimus

> 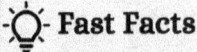 **Fast Facts**
> ✓ Not only do these drugs require drug level monitoring, but other labs have to be monitored due to the risk of nephrotoxicity, metabolic disturbances (elevated glucose), and hyperlipidemia.

Main Indications or Uses
- **Acute & Chronic Care**
  - Psoriasis
    - Cyclosporine
  - Rheumatoid arthritis
    - Cyclosporine
  - Transplant rejection prophylaxis
    - Cyclosporine, tacrolimus

Mechanism of Action
- Bind to cyclophilin (cyclosporine) or FKBP12 (tacrolimus), which inhibits calcineurin, halting the transcription of numerous key cytokines (specifically IL-2) necessary for T-cell activation.

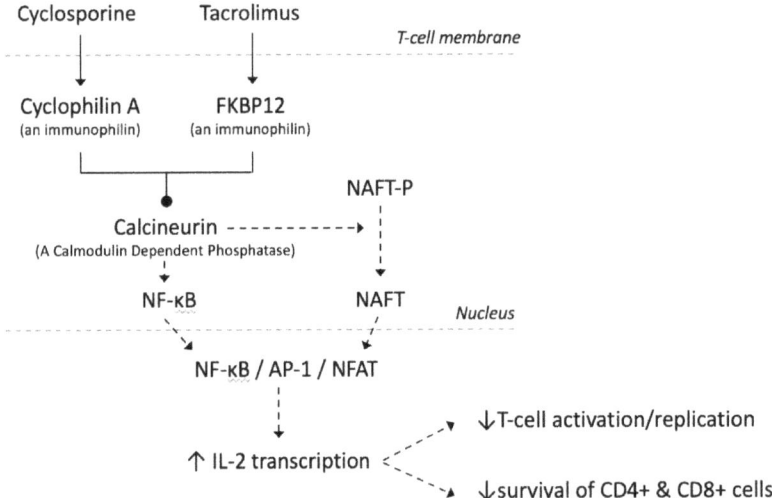

Primary Net Benefit
- A core component of immunosuppression post-transplant with clinically relevant drug interactions, therapeutic drug level monitoring, and nephrotoxicity.
- Main Labs to Monitor:
  - CBC with differential
  - Complete metabolic
    - Electrolytes, renal function
    - Liver function (albumin, bilirubin, PT/INR), liver enzyme (ALT/AST)
  - Therapeutic drug monitoring (whole blood)
  - Serum cholesterol and triglycerides

High-Yield Basic Pharmacology
- **Cyclosporine Modified Vs. Non-Modified**
  - Oral dosage forms of cyclosporine exist in either a "modified" or "non-modified" format, which are not bioequivalent.
    - To convert between dosage forms that are not bioequivalent, patients should have a trough concentration drawn 7 days before conversion, then every 5-7 days afterward, with appropriate adjustments made.
  - The FDA has deemed the generic formulations of both Neoral and Sandimmune bioequivalent.
- **Calcineurin Inhibition**
  - Calcineurin is normally responsible for the dephosphorylation and then the movement of a component of the nuclear factor of activated T lymphocytes, which induces cytokine genes for IL-2.
    - Thus, blocking calcineurin activity (calcineurin inhibitor) or its secondary downstream effects (everolimus, sirolimus) prevents the activation of IL-2.
- **Castor Oil**
  - Cyclosporine is not water-soluble, so to permit absorption, the oral and IV formulations contain castor oil, alcohol (ethanol), or cremophor to ensure solubilization.
    - The IV must be diluted before administration since it contains an ethanol and castor oil vehicle.

High-Yield Clinical Knowledge
- **Glucose Intolerance**
  - New-onset diabetes after transplantation is observed frequently with tacrolimus as it impairs pancreatic beta-cell response to glucose.
  - However, the combination of cyclosporine plus corticosteroids may cause diabetes more frequently.
- **Nephrotoxicity**
  - Dose-dependent nephrotoxicity complicates the use of calcineurin inhibitors, particularly after renal transplants.
    - This effect is dose/concentration-dependent; therefore, close therapeutic drug monitoring may limit the degree of nephrotoxicity.
    - Also, reducing exposure to other nephrotoxins (aminoglycosides, loop diuretics, NSAIDs, etc.) can control the risk of nephrotoxicity.
- **Cardiovascular Adverse Events**
  - Cyclosporine is associated with a high incidence of hyperlipidemia, and hypertension, which could increase cardiovascular events.
    - Furthermore, therapy with statins to counterbalance the risk of CYP3A4 interaction requires careful selection of the appropriate agent and dose (rosuvastatin dose limited to 5 mg, atorvastatin use contraindicated).
    - Other common adverse events include tremor, hirsutism, gum hyperplasia, and hyperuricemia.
  - Tacrolimus is not associated with hyperlipidemia and may be more ideal in patients where cardiovascular disease risk is high and/or continuing high-intensity statin therapy.
- **Tacrolimus Dosing**
  - Tacrolimus therapeutic drug monitoring should use trough concentrations to guide acute and post-transplant therapy.
  - Target tacrolimus trough concentrations in the acute post-transplant phase range from 10 to 15 ng/mL and increase to 100 to 200 ng/mL 3 months post-transplant.
- **Oral Tacrolimus Formulations**
  - Like cyclosporine, the modified release preparations of tacrolimus are not interchangeable with any other immediate or modified release dosage form.
  - If conversions are clinically necessary, increased drug level monitoring should occur until troughs are maintained in the therapeutic range.
- **Cyclosporine Absorption and Monitoring**
  - The gold standard cyclosporine drug level is drawn two hours after dose administration, known as C2 levels.

- Although absorption is limited (approximately 20-25%), further absorption limits occur when cyclosporine is administered with food.
- Individualized dosing regimens are key, and patients should be encouraged to maintain consistent medication administration/eating patterns.

High-Yield Core Evidence
- **ELITE-Symphony Study**
  - This was a landmark multicenter, open-label, parallel-group, controlled trial comparing the four groups of standard-dose cyclosporine, daclizumab induction with either low dose cyclosporine, low dose sirolimus, or low dose tacrolimus (all with mycophenolate mofetil, and corticosteroids) to assess the efficacy and relative toxic effects of these regimens.
  - Patients receiving low-dose tacrolimus-based therapy saw a significantly improved primary endpoint (eGFR, Cockcroft-Gault formula, 12 months after transplantation) compared to any other regimen.
  - The low-dose tacrolimus group also saw improved secondary endpoints, including higher graft survival rates and lower rejection rates at 12 months.
  - Serious adverse events were more common in the low-dose sirolimus group than in the other groups.
  - However, a similar proportion of patients in each group had at least one adverse event during treatment.
  - The authors concluded that a regimen of daclizumab, mycophenolate mofetil, and corticosteroids combined with low-dose tacrolimus might be advantageous for renal function, allograft survival, and acute rejection rates, as compared with regimens containing daclizumab induction plus either low-dose cyclosporine or low-dose sirolimus or with standard-dose cyclosporine without induction. (N Engl J Med. 2007 Dec 20;357(25):2562-75.)
- **Three-Year Symphony Follow Up**
  - This was an observational follow-up study of patients in the ELITE-Symphony Study, followed for an additional two years.
  - Low-dose tacrolimus-based therapy continued to see significantly higher eGFRs than cyclosporine regimens and higher graft survival rates, reducing differences between groups over time.
  - The authors concluded that over 3 years, daclizumab induction, mycophenolate, corticosteroids, and low-dose tacrolimus proved highly efficacious, without the negative effects on renal function commonly reported for standard cyclosporine regimens. (Am J Transplant. 2009 Aug;9(8):1876-85.)

High-Yield Fast-Facts
- **Castor Oil**
  - Aside from castor oil, the castor bean also produces the toxin ricin.
  - Rosary peas contain a similar toxin to ricin, known as abrin.
- **Cyclosporine and Eye Color**
  - Ophthalmic cyclosporine administration has been associated with both eyelash growth and iris color change.
  - This adverse event has been used for cosmetic purposes.

HIGH-YIELD BOARD EXAM ESSENTIALS
- **CLASSIC AGENTS:** Cyclosporine, tacrolimus
- **DRUG CLASS:** Calcineurin inhibitors
- **INDICATIONS:** Psoriasis, rheumatoid arthritis, transplant rejection prophylaxis
- **MECHANISM:** Bind to cyclophilin (cyclosporine) or FKBP12 (tacrolimus), which inhibits calcineurin, halting the transcription of numerous key cytokines (specifically IL-2) necessary for T-cell activity.
- **SIDE EFFECTS:** Nephrotoxicity, hyperlipidemia, hypertension, glucose intolerance
- **CLINICAL PEARLS:** New-onset diabetes after transplantation is observed frequently with tacrolimus as it impairs pancreatic beta-cell response to glucose. However, the combination of cyclosporine plus corticosteroids may cause diabetes more frequently.

Table: Drug Class Summary

	Calcineurin Inhibitors – Drug Class Review High-Yield Med Reviews		
Mechanism of Action: *Bind to cyclophilin (cyclosporine) or FKBP12 (tacrolimus), which inhibits calcineurin, halting the transcription of numerous key cytokines (specifically IL-2) necessary for T-cell activation.*			
Class Effects: *A core component of immunosuppression post-transplant with clinically relevant drug interactions, therapeutic drug level monitoring, and nephrotoxicity.*			
Generic Name	**Brand Name**	**Main Indication(s) or Uses**	**Notes**
Cyclosporine	Gengraf Neoral Sandimmune	<ul><li>Psoriasis</li><li>Rheumatoid arthritis</li><li>Transplant rejection prophylaxis</li></ul>	<ul><li>**Dosing (Adult):**<ul><li>Modified: Oral: 4 to 12 mg/kg/day in two divided doses</li><li>Non-modified: IV: 3 to 7.5 mg/kg/day continuous or intermittent infusion</li></ul></li><li>**Dosing (Peds):**<ul><li>Modified: Oral: 4 to 12 mg/kg/day in two divided doses</li><li>Non-modified: IV: 3 to 7.5 mg/kg/day continuous or intermittent infusion</li></ul></li><li>**CYP450 Interactions:** Substrate of CYP3A4, P-gp; Inhibits CYP2C9, CYP3A4, P-gp</li><li>**Renal or Hepatic Dose Adjustments:**<ul><li>Dose adjustments for non-transplant indications (psoriasis, rheumatoid arthritis, and nephritic syndrome)<ul><li>Reduce dose by 25 to 50% for serum creatinine levels more than 25-30% above baseline</li></ul></li></ul></li><li>**Dosage Forms:**<ul><li>Modified (capsule, oral solution)</li><li>Non-modified (capsule, oral solution)</li><li>IV (solution)</li></ul></li></ul>
Tacrolimus	Astagraf XL, Envarsus, Prograf	<ul><li>Transplant rejection prophylaxis</li></ul>	<ul><li>**Dosing (Adult):**<ul><li>Oral: 0.1 to 0.2 mg/kg/day in 2 divided doses</li><li>IV: 0.03 to 0.05 mg/kg/day continuous infusion</li></ul></li><li>**Dosing (Peds):**<ul><li>Extra info if needed<ul><li>Extra info if needed</li></ul></li></ul></li><li>**CYP450 Interactions:** Substrate of CYP3A4, P-gp</li><li>**Renal or Hepatic Dose Adjustments:** No empiric adjustments</li><li>**Dosage Forms:** Oral (capsule, packet, tablet), IV (solution)</li></ul>

IMMUNOSUPPRESSION – INTERFERON

Drug Class
- Interferon
- Agents:
  - **Acute & Chronic Care**
    - Interferon-Alfa-2b
    - Interferon-Gamma-1b
    - Peginterferon-Alfa-2a
    - Peginterferon-Alfa-2b
    - Interferon-Alfa-n3
    - Interferon-Beta-1a
    - Interferon-Beta-1b
    - Peginterferon-Beta-1a

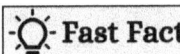

Fast Facts
- ✓ These agents can activate various aspects of the immune response thereby leading to a wide variety of side effects that mimic the flu or other viral infections.

Main Indications or Uses
- **Acute & Chronic Care**
  - AIDS-related Kaposi sarcoma
    - Interferon-Alfa-2b
  - Chronic granulomatous disease
    - Interferon-Gamma-1b
  - Chronic hepatitis B
    - Interferon-Alfa-2b
    - Peginterferon-Alfa-2a
  - Chronic hepatitis C
    - Interferon-Alfa-2b
    - Peginterferon-Alfa-2a
    - Peginterferon-Alfa-2b
  - Condylomata acuminata
    - Interferon-Alfa-2b
    - Interferon-Alfa-n3
  - Follicular lymphoma
    - Interferon-Alfa-2b
  - Hairy cell leukemia
    - Interferon-Alfa-2b
  - Malignant melanoma
    - Interferon-Alfa-2b
    - Peginterferon-Alfa-2b
  - Malignant osteopetrosis
    - Interferon-Gamma-1b
  - Relapsing multiple sclerosis
    - Interferon-Beta-1a
    - Interferon-Beta-1b
    - Peginterferon-Beta-1a

Mechanism of Action
- **Tyle 1 Interferons**
  - Interferon-Alfa and interferon-Beta
    - Produce intracellular antimicrobial effects by producing interferon-stimulated genes in hepatitis B or C infected cells and neighboring cells.
    - Enhance adaptive immune responses by amplifying antigen presentation, macrophage, NK cell, and cytotoxic T-lymphocyte activation by innate immune cells.
- **Type 2 Interferons**

- Interferon-gamma
  - Exerts an immune-enhancing effect by augmenting antigen presentation and macrophage, NK cell, and cytotoxic T-lymphocyte activation.
  - Enhances increased expression of class II MHC molecules on cell surfaces.

Primary Net Benefit
- Conveys antiviral, antiproliferative, and immunomodulatory functions onto target cells yet comes with significant toxicities and intolerances that preclude completion of the full course of treatment.
- Main Labs to Monitor:
  - Baseline chest x-ray, serum creatinine, albumin, prothrombin time, triglycerides
  - Ongoing through therapy:
    - CBC with differential, complete metabolic panel, liver function tests, TSH, ophthalmic exam, ECG, LDH, bodyweight, and neuropsychiatric changes during and 6 months after therapy.

High-Yield Basic Pharmacology
- Pegylation
  - Several interferon products exist as conventional or pegylated products.
  - The addition of a PEG (polyethylene glycol) polymer chain to the interferon drug molecule enhances pharmacokinetic half-life, permitting less frequent dosing.
  - However, toxicities are not necessarily improved with the PEG modification of the interferon product.
- Interferon-Beta
  - Interferon-beta may decrease blood-brain barrier permeability and T-cell proliferation from its actions on decreasing matrix metalloproteinases.
- Endogenous Interferon-Gamma
  - Interferon-gamma, produced by activated T helper cells and natural killer cells, augments macrophage-induced nitric oxide synthase's antimicrobial activity and increases nitric oxide production and its intracellular antimicrobial capacity.

High-Yield Clinical Knowledge
- Toxicities and Adverse Events
  - Therapy with interferon products is complicated by common injection site reactions, flu-like syndrome (lasting up to 24 hours after injection), thrombocytopenia, neutropenia (in up to 90% of patients) hepatic injury/failure.
    - There are numerous other serious and therapy complicating adverse reactions ranging from fatigue, chills, and depression to alopecia, myalgias, and insomnia.
  - Many patients cannot tolerate the adverse events therapy the duration, prompting discontinuation and selection of alternative regimens.
    - There are numerous antiviral therapeutics for hepatitis B and C that have now largely replaced Interferons for this indication.
- Pregnancy Safety
  - Interferons have been associated with spontaneous abortion in pregnant patients and are not recommended for this population.
  - Sexually active pregnant patients should be counseled to use appropriate contraception while taking interferon products.
- Relapsing-Remitting Multiple Sclerosis
  - Interferon-beta 1-a, interferon-beta-1b, and peginterferon-beta-1a are vital medications for managing relapsing-remitting multiple sclerosis.
    - Head-to-head data is lacking, but these agents can be selected based on patient-specific criteria.
- Avonex Titration
  - While initiating interferon-beta-1a therapy, although the initial IM dosing is 30 mcg once weekly, most patients cannot tolerate this starting dose due to flu-like symptoms.
  - An initial lower starting dose of 7.5 mcg administered IM every week with 7.5 mcg incremental dose increases every 2-4 weeks is recommended to mitigate this adverse reaction.
- Adaptive Immune Augmentation

- Interferon-gamma enhances the adaptive immune system's activity through Ig-isotype switching in B cells and T helper cell 1 differentiation.
- **Evolution in Safety and Efficacy**
  - With the development of alternative agents to treat hepatitis infections and multiple sclerosis, interferon therapy has been relegated as a non-preferred therapy, finding clinical use among patients who fail or otherwise are not candidates for these newer interventions.
  - As a result, rarer adverse events are becoming more prevalent, specifically pulmonary arterial hypertension.
  - PAH secondary to interferon therapy appears to be irreversible, and its risk increases with prolonged therapy.

High-Yield Core Evidence
- **PRISMS**
  - This was a multicenter, double-blind, placebo-controlled study in relapsing/remitting multiple sclerosis comparing subcutaneous interferon beta-1a (22 mcg or 44 mcg) placebo.
  - After a follow-up period of 2 years, patients randomized to interferon beta-1a saw a significantly lower relapse rate than patients receiving placebo.
  - Within the interferon groups, patients receiving the 44 mcg dose had a longer time to first relapse of 5 months than patients receiving 22 mcg (3 months), which was statistically significantly different.
  - Interferon therapy also delayed progression in disability and decreased accumulated disability during the study.
  - The authors concluded that interferon beta-1a is an effective treatment for relapsing/remitting multiple sclerosis in terms of relapse rate, defined disability, and all MRI outcome measures in a dose-related manner, and it is well tolerated. (Lancet 1999 Feb 20;353(9153):678.)
- **ADVANCE**
  - This was a multicenter, double-blind, parallel-group, phase 3 study that randomized patients with relapsing-remitting multiple sclerosis to receive peginterferon beta-1a or placebo.
  - Patients randomized to receive peginterferon beta-1a experienced a significant improvement in the primary endpoint of the annualized relapse rate at 48 weeks.
  - Significantly more patients receiving peginterferon beta-1a reported adverse events, including injection site reactions, influenza-like symptoms, pyrexia, headache, multiple sclerosis relapse, pneumonia, and urinary tract infections.
  - The authors concluded that peginterferon beta-1a significantly reduced relapse rate compared with placebo. (Lancet Neurol. 2014;13:657–665.)

High-Yield Fast-Facts
- **HCV Antivirals**
  - HCV treatment with newer antiviral regimens such as ledipasvir-sofosbuvir and sofosbuvir-velpatasvir have largely replaced interferon-based therapy.
- **Cytokine Family**
  - Interferons belong to the larger group known as cytokines, including TNF-alpha, Interleukin 2, and GCSF.
- **Interferon Delta, Epsilon, And Omega**
  - Other interferons exist, including interferons delta, epsilon, and omega.
  - Interferon epsilon and omega belong to the Type 1 interferon family, whereas interferon delta is a type three interferon.

Table: Drug Class Summary

colspan Interferon - Drug Class Review
Interferon - Drug Class Review High-Yield Med Reviews
Mechanism of Action: *Type 1 Interferons - Produce interferon-stimulated genes in hepatitis B or C infected cells and neighboring cells and enhances adaptive immune responses.* *Type 2 Interferons - Immune-enhancement by augmenting antigen presentation and macrophage, NK cell, and cytotoxic T-lymphocyte activation.*
Class Effects: *Conveys antiviral, antiproliferative, and immunomodulatory functions onto target cells yet comes with significant toxicities and intolerances that preclude completion of the full course of treatment.*

Generic Name	Brand Name	Main Indication(s) or Uses	Notes

Interferon-Alfa-2b	Intron A	- AIDS-related Kaposi sarcoma
		- Chronic hepatitis B
		- Chronic hepatitis C infection
		- Condylomata acuminata
		- Follicular lymphoma
		- Hairy cell leukemia
		- Malignant melanoma
			- **Dosing (Adult):**
			  – IM/SQ: 5 million units daily
			  – IM/SQ: 2 to 30 million units/m² three times weekly
			  – IV: 20 million units/m² daily x 5 days for 4 weeks, then SQ 10 million units/m² three times weekly x 48 weeks
			- **Dosing (Peds):**
			  – IM/SQ: 3 million units/m² three times weekly for 1 week, then 6 million units/m² three times weekly
			    – Maximum 10 million units/dose
			- **CYP450 Interactions:** Inhibits CYP1A2
			- **Renal or Hepatic Dose Adjustments:**
			  – ASL/ALT: 5 to 10x ULN: temporarily hold, then resume at 50% previous dose
			  – ASL/ALT: > 10x ULN: discontinue
			- **Dosage Forms:** Injection (solution, powder for solution)

Peginterferon-Alfa-2a	Pegasys	- Chronic hepatitis B
		- Chronic hepatitis C
			- **Dosing (Adult):**
			  – SQ: 180 mcg qweek x48 weeks
			    – Extra info if needed
			- **Dosing (Peds):**
			  – SQ: 65 to 180 mcg/dose (based on BSA)
			  – SQ: 104 mcg/m² qweek
			    – Maximum 180 mcg/dose
			- **CYP450 Interactions:** Inhibits CYP1A2
			- **Renal or Hepatic Dose Adjustments:**
			  – GFR: < 30 mL/minute: 135 mcg qweek
			  – ALT 5x ULN: temporarily hold, then resume at 135 mcg dose
			  – ALT > 10x ULN: discontinue
			- **Dosage Forms:** Injection (solution)

Interferon - Drug Class Review
High-Yield Med Reviews

Generic Name	Brand Name	Main Indication(s) or Uses	Notes

Peginterferon-Alfa-2b	PegIntron, Sylatron	- Chronic hepatitis C
		- Melanoma adjuvant treatment
			- **Dosing (Adult):**
			  - SQ: 6 mcg/kg/week x8 doses, then 3 mcg/kg/week for up to 5 years
			- **Dosing (Peds):**
			  - SQ: 60 mcg/m2 qweek
			- **CYP450 Interactions:** Inhibits CYP1A2
			- **Renal or Hepatic Dose Adjustments:**
			  - GFR: 30 to 50 mL/min/1.73 m²: 4.5 mcg/kg/week, then 2.25 mcg/kg/week
			  - GFR: < 30 mL/min/1.73 m²: 3 mcg/kg/week, then 1.5 mcg/kg/week
			- **Dosage Forms:** IV (powder for solution)

Interferon-Alfa-n3	Alferon N	- Condylomata acuminata	- **Dosing (Adult):**
			  - Intralesional 250,000 units per wart twice weekly
			    - Maximum dose per session of 2.5 million units, maximum duration 8 weeks
			- **Dosing (Peds):** Not routinely used
			- **CYP450 Interactions:** None
			- **Renal or Hepatic Dose Adjustments:** None
			- **Dosage Forms:** Injection (solution)

Interferon-Gamma-1b	Actimmune	- Chronic granulomatous disease
		- Malignant osteopetrosis
			- **Dosing (Adult):**
			  - SQ: 50 mcg/m² three times weekly
			- **Dosing (Peds):**
			  - BSA: 0.5 m² or less: 1.5 mcg/kg/dose three times weekly
			    - Maximum 50 mcg/m²
			- **CYP450 Interactions:** None
			- **Renal or Hepatic Dose Adjustments:** None
			- **Dosage Forms:** Injection (solution)

Interferon-Beta-1a	Avonex, Rebif	- Relapsing multiple sclerosis	- **Dosing (Adult):**
			  - IM: 30 mcg qweek
			  - SQ: 8.8 mcg three times weekly x2 weeks, then 22 mcg three times weekly x2 weeks, then 44 mcg three times weekly
			- **Dosing (Peds):** Not routinely used
			- **CYP450 Interactions:** None
			- **Renal or Hepatic Dose Adjustments:**
			  - ALT 5x ULN: temporarily hold, then resume at 50% previous dose
			- **Dosage Forms:** Injection (solution)

Interferon - Drug Class Review
High-Yield Med Reviews

Generic Name	Brand Name	Main Indication(s) or Uses	Notes

Interferon-Beta-1b	Betaseron, Extavia	• Relapsing multiple sclerosis	• **Dosing (Adult):**
			  – SQ: 2 million units every other day, titrated up q2weeks
			    – Target dose 8 million units every other day
			• **Dosing (Peds):** Not routinely used
			• **CYP450 Interactions:** None
			• **Renal or Hepatic Dose Adjustments:** None
			• **Dosage Forms:** Injection (solution)

Peginterferon-Beta-1a	Plegridy	Relapsing multiple sclerosis	• **Dosing (Adult):** – SQ: 63 mcg on day 1, 94 mcg on day 15, then 125 mcg q2weeks on day 29 • **Dosing (Peds):** Not routinely used • **CYP450 Interactions:** None • **Renal or Hepatic Dose Adjustments:** None • **Dosage Forms:** Injection (solution)

HIGH-YIELD BOARD EXAM ESSENTIALS
- **CLASSIC AGENTS:** Interferon-alfa-2b, interferon-gamma-1b, peginterferon-alfa-2a, peginterferon-alfa-2b, interferon-alfa-n3, interferon-beta-1a, interferon-beta-1b, peginterferon-beta-1a
- **DRUG CLASS:** Interferon
- **INDICATIONS:** AIDS-related Kaposi sarcoma, chronic hepatitis B, chronic hepatitis C infection, condylomata acuminata, follicular lymphoma, hairy cell leukemia, malignant melanoma, relapsing multiple sclerosis
- **MECHANISM:** Produce interferon-stimulated genes in hepatitis B or C infected cells and neighboring cells and enhances adaptive immune responses (Type 1 Interferons); Immune-enhancement by augmenting antigen presentation and macrophage, NK cell, and cytotoxic T-lymphocyte activation (Type 2 Interferons)
- **SIDE EFFECTS:** Injection site reactions, flu-like syndrome, thrombocytopenia, neutropenia, hepatic injury/failure.
- **CLINICAL PEARLS:** With the development of alternative agents to treat hepatitis infections and multiple sclerosis, interferon therapy has been relegated as a non-preferred therapy, finding clinical use among patients who fail or otherwise are not candidates for these newer interventions. As a result, rarer adverse events are becoming more prevalent, specifically pulmonary arterial hypertension.

IMMUNOSUPPRESSANTS – ANTIMETABOLITES

Drug Class
- Antimetabolites
- Agents:
  - Acute & Chronic Care
    - Azathioprine
    - Mycophenolate mofetil
    - Mycophenolate sodium

> **Fast Facts**
> ✓ The different MPA formulations, mycophenolate mofetil and mycophenolate sodium, are not dose equivalent.
>
> ✓ Use caution with the coadministration of a xanthine oxidase inhibitor along with azathioprine due to the risk of severe bone marrow suppression.

Main Indications or Uses
- Acute & Chronic Care
  - Prophylaxis of organ rejection
  - Rheumatoid arthritis
  - Lupus nephritis

Mechanism of Action
- **Azathioprine**
  - A prodrug metabolized to 6-mercaptopurine (6-MP), then to 6-thioguanine nucleotides, ultimately disrupting de novo and salvaging the synthesis of DNA and RNA proteins, preventing cellular proliferation.
- **Mycophenolic acid (MPA) derivatives (mycophenolate mofetil and mycophenolate sodium)**
  - Non-competitive inhibitor of inosine monophosphate dehydrogenase (IMPDH) I and II prevents de novo guanosine nucleotide synthesis, diminishes DNA polymerase activity, and reduces lymphocyte proliferation.

Primary Net Benefit
- Azathioprine is used in combination with corticosteroids for immunosuppression after organ transplant, but due to dose-limiting toxicities, it has been reserved for patients intolerant to alternative medications.
- MPA derivatives combined with calcineurin inhibitors produce targeted immunosuppression and improved tolerability and safety post-transplant with expanding roles in other diseases.
- Main Labs to Monitor:
  - CBC with differential
  - Serum creatinine
  - Liver function (albumin, bilirubin, PT/INR), liver enzyme (ALT/AST)
  - Opportunistic infections

High-Yield Basic Pharmacology
- **Prodrug**
  - Mycophenolate mofetil is a prodrug form that MPA produced after hepatic-first pass metabolism.
  - Mycophenolate sodium uses an enteric coating to preserve MPA from gastric pH but allows for direct absorption of MPA from the small intestine.
    - Both are metabolized hepatically to the inactive metabolite MPAG, which is excreted in the bile and urine.
- **MPAG Deconjugation**
  - MPAG can undergo deconjugation after enterohepatic recirculation, contributing to the total therapeutic effect of MPA and potentially a second peak 6 to 12 hours after administration.
- **Azathioprine Activation**
  - Azathioprine is better thought of as a prodrug to 6-MP, which has numerous metabolic fates:
    - Xanthine oxidase metabolism of 6-MP to 6-thiouric acid (inactive).
    - Thiopurine S-methyltransferase (TPMT) methylates 6-MP to 6-methylmercaptophurine (inactive).
    - Hypoxanthine-guanine phosphoribosyltransferase converts 6-MP to several different 6-thioguanine nucleotides (6-TGNs).

- 6-TGNs are then metabolized by xanthine oxidase and TPMT to their inactive products.

High-Yield Clinical Knowledge
- **Azathioprine Dose Limiting Toxicity**
    - The use of azathioprine is limited by hematologic toxicities, including anemia, leukopenia, and thrombocytopenia.
    - Other common adverse events include alopecia, hepatotoxicity, and pancreatitis.
- **Xanthine-Oxidase and Its Inhibitors**
    - Coadministration of azathioprine (or 6-MP) increases 6-TGN production, resulting in an increased risk of bone marrow toxicity and pancytopenia.
        - Empiric dose reductions by 5- to 75 % are recommended when allopurinol is added to azathioprine.
- **MPA Oral Forms Not Equivalent**
    - The different MPA formulations, mycophenolate mofetil and mycophenolate sodium, are not equivalent concerning the dose.
        - The approximate equivalence is mycophenolate mofetil 250 mg is equivalent to mycophenolate sodium 180 mg.
- **IMPDH I and II**
    - MPA derivatives non competitively inhibit both IMPDH I and II.
    - These agents are more specific to IMPDH II, expressed only in B and T lymphocytes, whereas IMPDH I is expressed in cells throughout the body.
        - Additionally, B/T lymphocytes are dependent upon the de novo nucleotide synthesis pathway, where IMPDH expressing cells are capable of alternative synthesis pathways for nucleotides.
- **MPA Drug Interactions**
    - Acyclovir competes with MPAG for renal tubular secretion, resulting in increased AUC of both, accompanying increased risk of adverse events, particularly bone marrow suppression.
    - Cyclosporine can decrease MPA trough concentrations by 40-50% compared to therapy with tacrolimus due to cyclosporine's inhibition of MPAG enterohepatic recycling.
        - Cyclosporine specifically inhibits multidrug-resistance-associated protein 2 (MRP-2), responsible for inhibition of enterohepatic cycling of MPAG.
        - Antibiotics have also affected MPAG recycling and should be used with caution in combination with MPA agents.
- **Pharmacogenomics**
    - Azathioprine dosing based on specific genotypes of TPMT activity has been suggested to reduce the risk of severe pancytopenia.
        - In patients with at least two nonfunctional alleles of TPMT, representing low or absent activity should be considered at higher risk of hematologic toxicity and may benefit from alternative therapy.

High-Yield Core Evidence
- **MYSS**
    - The MYSS trial was a multicenter, prospective, randomized, parallel-group trial that compared acute rejections and adverse events in recipients of cadaver-kidney transplants over 6-month treatment with mycophenolate mofetil or azathioprine along with cyclosporine microemulsion and steroids (phase A), and over 15 more months without steroids (phase B).
    - There was no difference between treatment arms for the primary endpoint of acute rejection episodes in both treatment phases (A and B).
    - The authors concluded that in recipients of cadaver kidney transplants, mycophenolate mofetil offers no advantages over azathioprine in preventing acute rejections and is about 15 times more expensive. (Lancet. 2004 Aug 7-13;364(9433):503-12.)

- **MAINTAIN**
  - This was an investigator-initiated randomized trial comparing mycophenolate mofetil to azathioprine as maintenance treatment in patients with proliferative lupus nephritis with a primary endpoint of time to renal flare.
  - There was no difference in the primary outcome of time to renal flares between treatment groups, including no difference in time to renal flare, severe systemic flare, benign flare, and renal remission.
  - Significantly more patients receiving azathioprine experienced hematological cytopenias but led only one patient dropped out.
  - The authors concluded fewer renal flares were observed in patients receiving MMF, but the difference did not reach statistical significance. (Ann Rheum Dis. 2010 Dec;69(12):2083-9.)

High-Yield Fast-Facts
- **Pregnancy**
  - MPA derivatives should be avoided in pregnant patients due to the risk of pregnancy loss and congenital malformations.
  - Patients of childbearing potential should follow appropriate contraception during MPA treatment and 6 weeks after.
- **Cell Phase**
  - The specific cell cycle azathioprine disrupts the G2-M phase.
- **MPA Oral dosage form**
  - In pediatric patients, mycophenolate mofetil may be preferred because of an oral suspension, where mycophenolate sodium is only available as a tablet.

HIGH-YIELD BOARD EXAM ESSENTIALS
- **CLASSIC AGENTS:** Azathioprine, mycophenolate mofetil, mycophenolate sodium
- **DRUG CLASS:** Antimetabolites
- **INDICATIONS:** Prophylaxis of organ rejection, rheumatoid arthritis, Lupus nephritis
- **MECHANISM:** Azathioprine - Metabolized to 6-MP, then to 6-thioguanine nucleotides, disrupting DNA and RNA synthesis, preventing cellular proliferation. MPA derivatives prevent de novo guanosine nucleotide synthesis, diminished DNA polymerase activity, and reduced lymphocyte proliferation.
- **SIDE EFFECTS:** Anemia, leukopenia, thrombocytopenia, alopecia, hepatotoxicity, and pancreatitis.
- **CLINICAL PEARLS:** Coadministration of azathioprine (or 6-MP for that matter) increases 6-TGN production, resulting in an increased risk of bone marrow toxicity and pancytopenia. Empiric dose reductions by 5- to 75 % are recommended when allopurinol is added to azathioprine.

Table: Drug Class Summary

Antimetabolites - Drug Class Review High-Yield Med Reviews			
Mechanism of Action: Azathioprine - Metabolized to 6-MP, then to 6-thioguanine nucleotides, disrupting DNA and RNA synthesis and preventing cellular proliferation. MPA derivatives prevent de novo guanosine nucleotide synthesis, diminish DNA polymerase activity, and reduce lymphocyte proliferation.			
Class Effects: After an organ transplant, azathioprine is used in combination with corticosteroids but has been reserved for patients intolerant to alternative medications. MPA derivatives combined with calcineurin inhibitors produce targeted immunosuppression and improved tolerability and safety post-transplant with expanding roles in other diseases.			
Generic Name	**Brand Name**	**Main Indication(s) or Uses**	**Notes**

Azathioprine	Azasan, Imuran	▪ Kidney transplantation
		▪ Rheumatoid arthritis
			▪ **Dosing (Adult):**
			  – IV/Oral: 2 to 5 mg/kg once followed by 1 to 3 mg/kg by mouth daily
			    – Normal dose range 50 to 150mg/day
			▪ **Dosing (Peds):**
			  – IV/Oral: 2 to 5 mg/kg once followed by 1 to 3 mg/kg by mouth daily
			▪ **CYP450 Interactions:** None
			▪ **Renal or Hepatic Dose Adjustments:**
			  – GFR: 10 to 50 mL/minute: Reduce dose by 25%
			  – GFR: < 10 mL/minute: Reduce dose by 50%
			▪ **Dosage Forms:** IV (solution), Oral (tablet)

Mycophenolate mofetil	CellCept	▪ Organ transplantation	▪ **Dosing (Adult):**
			  – IV/Oral: 1 to 1.5 g q12h
			▪ **Dosing (Peds):**
			  – Oral: 600 mg/m^2/dose divided q12h
			    – Maximum 2,000 mg/day
			▪ **CYP450 Interactions:** None
			▪ **Renal or Hepatic Dose Adjustments:** None
			▪ **Dosage Forms:** IV (solution), Oral (capsule, tablet, suspension)

Mycophenolate sodium	Myfortic	Organ transplantation	▪ **Dosing (Adult):**
			  – Oral: 360 to 1080 mg BID
			    – Extra info if needed
			▪ **Dosing (Peds):**
			  – Oral: 400 mg/mg/m^2/dose divided q12h
			    – Maximum 1,440 mg/day
			▪ **CYP450 Interactions:** None
			▪ **Renal or Hepatic Dose Adjustments:** None
			▪ **Dosage Forms:** Oral (tablet)

IMMUNOSUPPRESSANTS – ANTIPROLIFERATIVE AGENTS (mTOR INHIBITORS)

Drug Class
- Antiproliferative Agents (mTOR Inhibitors)
- Agents:
  - Acute & Chronic Care
    - Everolimus
    - Sirolimus

Main Indications or Uses
- Acute & Chronic Care
  - Everolimus
    - Breast cancer
    - Neuroendocrine tumors
    - Liver, renal transplant
    - Renal cell carcinoma
  - Sirolimus
    - Renal transplant
    - Lymphangioleiomyomatosis

> **Fast Facts**
> ✓ Similar to other medications used for organ transplantation, drug levels need to be monitored. They are also associated with lipid abnormalities and renal toxicity where additional labs are warranted.
>
> ✓ These agents are also associated with drug-interactions due to being substrates of CYP3A4.

Mechanism of Action
- Complex with FKBP12 to form a complex that binds to and inhibits the protein kinase mTOR and thus prevents cell cycle progression at the G1 to S phase transition.

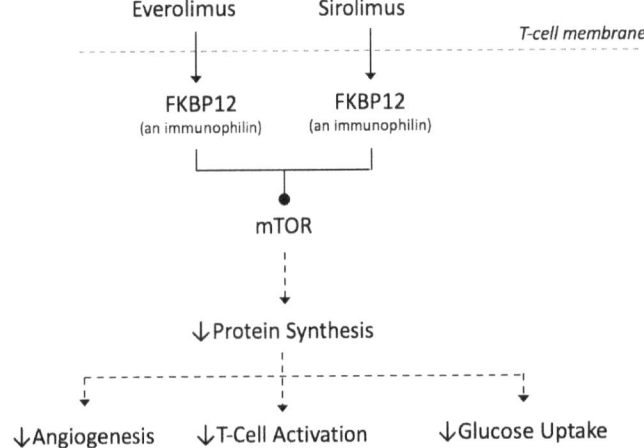

Primary Net Benefit
- Similar efficacy but improved safety compared to calcineurin-inhibitor-based therapy post-transplant.
- Main Labs to Monitor:
  - CBC with differential
  - Serum creatinine
  - Liver function (albumin, bilirubin, PT/INR), liver enzyme (ALT/AST)
  - Therapeutic drug monitoring (trough)
  - Serum cholesterol and triglycerides

High-Yield Basic Pharmacology
- **Everolimus Origin**
  - Everolimus is a synthetic derivative of sirolimus but carries a much shorter half-life than sirolimus (30 hours vs. 62 hours).

- **Oral Absorption**
  - A high-fat meal decreases exposure of both everolimus and sirolimus by 23-35%.
  - Patients should be instructed to keep a consistent diet, which will allow appropriate titration to therapeutic targets.

High-Yield Clinical Knowledge
- **Delayed Wound Healing**
  - The initiation of sirolimus is delayed 3 months after transplant (or once surgical wounds are healed) due to sirolimus delayed wound healing.
  - Everolimus has a lower risk of delayed wound healing, with some providers beginning therapy before the 3-month time frame associated with sirolimus.
- **Cholesterol and Triglycerides**
  - The mTOR inhibitors are associated with hypercholesterolemia and hypertriglyceridemia due to the overproduction of lipoproteins and lipoprotein lipase inhibition.
  - These effects are managed via dose reduction or the initiation of a statin or fibrate.
- **Mouth Ulcers**
  - Mouth ulcers are a dose-dependent adverse event associated with sirolimus and can occur in 60% of patients.
- **Drug Interactions**
  - Sirolimus and cyclosporine are CYP3A4 substrates and inhibitors; thus, when combined, they cause increased AUC and trough concentrations of each.
    - The risk of neurotoxicity and nephrotoxicity is significant without appropriate dose adjustments.
  - The combination of sirolimus tacrolimus is associated with an increased risk of nephrotoxicity.
    - Everolimus has not demonstrated this increased risk when combined with cyclosporine or tacrolimus.
  - Grapefruit and grapefruit juice may affect the absorption of sirolimus and everolimus, and its consumption should be discouraged.
- **Dose-Dependent Myelosuppression**
  - Both everolimus and sirolimus are associated with dose-dependent myelosuppression that is often transient.
  - Thrombocytopenia typically occurs within 2 weeks of sirolimus initiation and is associated with higher trough concentrations (above 15 ng/mL).
- **Combination Therapy**
  - The role of sirolimus is limited to preventing rejection in kidney transplant patients in combination with cyclosporine, tacrolimus, or mycophenolate.
  - Compared with cyclosporine or tacrolimus, the combination of sirolimus and mycophenolate can be similarly effective but reduce the risk of nephrotoxicity.

High-Yield Core Evidence
- **Everolimus With High or Low Dose Tacrolimus**
  - This prospective, multicenter, open-label, exploratory study was conducted in de novo renal transplant patients who received everolimus (plus steroids and basiliximab) with high or low dose tacrolimus.
  - There was no difference in the primary objective of renal function at 6 months after transplant measured by mean serum creatinine.
  - Biopsy-proven acute rejection occurred similarly between groups and was no statistically different.
  - The authors concluded that tacrolimus exposure reduction in the presence of everolimus, steroids, and basiliximab induction results in good efficacy in de novo renal transplant recipients with very well-preserved renal function. (Transplantation. 2008 Mar 27;85(6):821-6.)

- **Heart Transplant Everolimus Therapy**
  - This was an open-labeled, multicenter study of maintenance thoracic transplant patients who were at least 1-year post-transplant.
  - Patients were randomized to continue their current calcineurin inhibitor (CNI)-based immunosuppression or start everolimus with predefined CNI exposure reduction.
  - Everolimus-based therapy was associated with a significant improvement in the primary endpoint, mean change in measured glomerular filtration rate from baseline to month 12.
  - There was no difference in biopsy-proven treated acute rejection between treatment arms.
  - However, more patients receiving everolimus experienced a severe adverse event than controls.
  - The authors concluded that everolimus with CNI reduction offers a significant renal function improvement in maintenance heart and lung transplant recipients. (Transplantation. 2010 Apr 15;89(7):864-72.)

High-Yield Fast-Facts
- **IL-2 Antagonism**
  - The mTOR inhibitors do not directly inhibit IL-2; they diminish the cellular response to IL-2 stimulation.
  - Thus, we can link the understanding of mTOR inhibition to understanding the therapeutic role of IL-2 antagonists such as basiliximab or daclizumab.
- **Aka Rapamycin**
  - Sirolimus may be referred to as rapamycin in some literature.

HIGH-YIELD BOARD EXAM ESSENTIALS
- **CLASSIC AGENTS:** Everolimus, sirolimus
- **DRUG CLASS:** Antiproliferative agents (mTOR inhibitors)
- **INDICATIONS:** Breast cancer, neuroendocrine tumors, liver, renal transplant, renal cell carcinoma, renal transplant
- **MECHANISM:** Complex with FKBP12 to form a complex that binds to and inhibits the protein kinase mTOR and prevents cell cycle progression at the G1 to S phase transition.
- **SIDE EFFECTS:** Delayed wound healing, mouth ulcers, hypercholesterolemia and hypertriglyceridemia
- **CLINICAL PEARLS:**
  - Impaired renal function, glucose regulation, and lipid metabolism are common with this drug class and requiring lab monitoring.
  - Sirolimus and cyclosporine are both CYP3A4 substrates and inhibitors and are associated with drug interactions.
  - Both everolimus and sirolimus are associated with dose-dependent myelosuppression that is often transient. Thrombocytopenia typically occurs within 2 weeks of sirolimus initiation and is associated with higher trough concentrations (above 15 ng/mL).

Table: Drug Class Summary

Antiproliferative Agents (mTOR Inhibitors) - Drug Class Review High-Yield Med Reviews			
Mechanism of Action: *Complex with FKBP12 to form a complex that binds to and inhibits the protein kinase mTOR and prevents cell cycle progression at the G1 to S phase transition.*			
Class Effects: *Similar efficacy but improved safety compared to calcineurin-inhibitor-based therapy post-transplant.*			
Generic Name	**Brand Name**	**Main Indication(s) or Uses**	**Notes**
Everolimus	Afinitor, Zortress	<ul><li>Breast cancer</li><li>Neuroendocrine tumors</li><li>Liver, renal transplant</li><li>Renal cell carcinoma</li></ul>	<ul><li>**Dosing (Adult):**<ul><li>Oral: 5 to 10 mg daily</li><li>Oral: 1 mg BID with tacrolimus</li></ul></li><li>**Dosing (Peds):**<ul><li>Oral: 0.8 to 4.5 mg/m2/dose once to twice daily. Max dose 1.5 mg/dose (transplant indication)</li></ul></li><li>**CYP450 Interactions:** Substrate & inhibits CYP3A4</li><li>**Renal or Hepatic Dose Adjustments:**<ul><li>Child-Pugh Class A: Reduce dose by ⅓</li><li>Child-Pugh Class B: Reduce dose by ½</li><li>Child-Pugh Class C: Reduce dose by ½ to ¾</li></ul></li><li>**Dosage Forms:** Oral (tablet, soluble tablet)</li></ul>
Sirolimus	Rapamune	<ul><li>Renal transplant</li></ul>	<ul><li>**Dosing (Adult):**<ul><li>< 40kg: 3 mg/m^2 x1 followed by 1 mg/m^2 daily</li><li>40 kg or over: 6 to 15 mg x 1 followed by 2 to 5 mg daily. Max loading dose of 40 mg</li></ul></li><li>**Dosing (Peds):**<ul><li>3 mg/m^2 x1 followed by 1 mg/m^2 daily<ul><li>Maximum daily dose of 40 mg</li></ul></li></ul></li><li>**CYP450 Interactions:** Substrate of CYP3A4</li><li>**Renal or Hepatic Dose Adjustments:**<ul><li>Child-Pugh Class A: Reduce dose by ⅓</li><li>Child-Pugh Class B/C: Reduce dose by ½</li></ul></li><li>**Dosage Forms:** Oral (solution, tablet)</li></ul>

IMMUNOSUPPRESSANTS – DISEASE-MODIFYING ANTIRHEUMATIC DRUGS

Drug Class
- Disease-Modifying Antirheumatic Drugs
- Agents:
    - Chronic Care
        - Hydroxychloroquine
        - Leflunomide
        - Methotrexate
        - Sulfasalazine
        - Tofacitinib

Main Indications or Uses
- Chronic Care
    - Polyarticular course juvenile idiopathic arthritis
        - Tofacitinib
    - Psoriatic arthritis
        - Methotrexate
        - Tofacitinib
    - Lupus erythematosus
        - Methotrexate
        - Hydroxychloroquine
    - Rheumatoid arthritis
        - Methotrexate
        - Leflunomide
        - Sulfasalazine
        - Tofacitinib
    - Ulcerative colitis
        - Methotrexate
        - Sulfasalazine
        - Tofacitinib

> **Fast Facts**
>
> ✓ DMARDs can take 2-3 months for the full clinical benefit to be known.
>
> ✓ The most common DMARD used for RA is methotrexate. While methotrexate is a chemotherapeutic agent, the dose used in RA is significantly lower than in treating cancer.
>
> ✓ Hydroxychloroquine has limited utility in clinical practice but if it is to be used, there is a small risk of retinopathy (especially at higher doses) and thus periodical eye exams are recommended.
>
> ✓ Leflunomide undergoes extensive enterohepatic recirculation and stay in the body for months after discontinuation.

Mechanism of Action
- Hydroxychloroquine
    - Poorly understood mechanisms may include interference with antigen processing in macrophages and other antigen-presenting cells.
- Leflunomide
    - A prodrug converted in the GI and blood to an active metabolite (A77 1726) stops cellular growth by inhibiting dihydroorotate dehydrogenase and decreasing ribonuclease synthesis.
- Methotrexate (low-dose)
    - Inhibits inflammation via different pathways:
        - Inhibits lymphocyte, macrophage, neutrophil, and dendritic cell function via amino-imidazole-carboxamide-ribonucleotide (AICAR) transformylase and thymidylate synthetase inhibition and extracellular AMP accumulation.
        - Impairs polymorphonuclear chemotaxis and function.
- Sulfasalazine
    - Converted to 5-aminosalicylic (5-ASA) acid and sulfapyridine, impair B-cell and T-cell response and proliferation and inhibit the production of inflammatory cytokines including IL-1, IL-6, IL-12, and TNF-alpha.
- Tofacitinib
    - Selectively inhibits Janus Kinase 3 (JAK3) and JAK1, which then prevents the JAK3/JAK1 complex from activating the signal transduction and activators of transcription (STATs), impairing cytokine and growth

factor-mediated gene expression and intracellular activity of B and T lymphocytes, CD- natural killer cells, and immune globulins.

Primary Overall Benefit
- Recently designated conventional synthetic DMARDs (csDMARDs) impact disease severity and quality of life in autoimmune diseases but carry significant toxicities and intolerances.
- Main Labs to Monitor:
    - CBC with differential
    - Complete metabolic
        - Electrolytes, renal function
        - Liver function (albumin, bilirubin, PT/INR), liver enzyme (ALT/AST)
    - Serum cholesterol and triglyceride

High-Yield Basic Pharmacology
- **Leflunomide Broad Effect**
    - The mechanism of leflunomide's active metabolite leads to broad inhibition of numerous mediators of inflammation, including inhibiting B-cell antibody production, inhibiting T-cell proliferation, increasing IL-10 receptor mRNA, decreasing IL-8 receptor mRNA, and decreasing TNF-alpha–dependent NFK-beta activation.
- **But Folic Acid?**
    - Although methotrexate is widely known as a structural analog of folic acid that inhibits dihydrofolate reductase at doses used for autoimmune and rheumatic disease, this effect is relatively minor and of limited clinical relevance.
        - Of course, through its dihydrofolate reductase inhibition, methotrexate inhibits dihydrofolic acid reduction to folinic acid, thus inhibiting DNA synthesis and repair.
- **Sulfasalazine Absorption**
    - Sulfasalazine undergoes enterohepatic recirculation, which can be an advantage for inflammatory GI disorders (Crohn's disease and ulcerative colitis) as this increases the GI concentration of 5-ASA, which is not absorbed.
        - So with each recirculation, more 5-ASA is produced in the GI, where it can continue its GI effect.

High-Yield Clinical Knowledge
- **Hepatotoxicity**
    - Leflunomide has been associated with mitochondrial toxicity, directly related to its mechanism inhibiting dihydroorotate dehydrogenase, which is also essential for Coenzyme Q's oxidation complex III of the electron transport chain.
        - The electron transport chain's inhibition may cause a shutdown of glycolysis, ATP production, and a shift to lipolysis, proteolysis, oxidative stress, and necrosis.
    - Liver tissue, particularly zone three hepatocytes, are at high risk of this oxidative damage, and their damage or loss can lead to hepatic injury and failure.
- **Methotrexate Dosing**
    - For rheumatoid arthritis and other autoimmune disorders, methotrexate is typically dosed on a weekly schedule.
        - Typical starting doses of methotrexate are 7.5 mg weekly.
    - Severe toxicity can occur through prescribing, dispensing, or administration errors in the daily delivery of the required weekly dose.
- **Tofacitinib Cancer Risk**
    - JAK inhibitors have been associated with increased lymphomas and other malignancies, including breast cancer.
        - This risk is the subject of one of the Black Box Warnings for tofacitinib.

- **Methotrexate Adverse Events**
  - Nausea and stomatitis are common adverse events with methotrexate.
  - More severe events such as anemia, leukopenia, alopecia, and GI ulceration are rarely observed with typical dosing for autoimmune or rheumatic diseases.
    - Should these occur, drug interactions or dosing errors should be sought as possible contributing factors.
- **Sulfasalazine Intolerance**
  - Many patients, up to 30% started on sulfasalazine, cannot continue due to intolerances, and alternative agents must be selected.
    - Most common events leading to discontinuation include nausea, vomiting, headache, and rash, but rare serious adverse events can occur, including hemolytic anemia or methemoglobinemia.
    - Patients with HLA-B*08-01 and HLA-A*31-01 are at high risk of neutropenia from sulfasalazine.
- **Tofacitinib With or Without Methotrexate**
  - In patients who have failed or are intolerant to methotrexate, tofacitinib is indicated as monotherapy or other conventional DMARD agents.
    - Still, it should not be combined with bDMARDs due to the increased risk of immunosuppression.
  - Tofacitinib can be used in combination with methotrexate in select patients.
  - Tofacitinib has also been associated with dose-dependent increases in cholesterol (LDL, HDL, and TC) and has been associated with a dose-dependent risk of pulmonary embolism.

High-Yield Core Evidence
- **ORAL Solo**
  - This was a phase 3, double-blind, placebo-controlled, parallel-group, 6-month study that randomized patients with rheumatoid arthritis to tofacitinib 5 mg BID, 10 mg BID, placebo for three months, then tofacitinib 5 mg BID, or placebo for three months, then tofacitinib 10 mg BID.
  - Tofacitinib was more effective than placebo groups in the primary outcome of the percentage of patients with at least a 20% improvement in the American College of Rheumatology scale (ACR 20), the change from baseline in Health Assessment Questionnaire-Disability Index (HAQ-DI) scores (which range from 0 to 3, with higher scores indicating significant disability), and the percentage of patients with a Disease Activity Score for 28-joint counts based on the erythrocyte sedimentation rate (DAS28-4[ESR]) of less than 2.6 (with scores ranging from 0 to 9.4 and higher scores indicating more disease activity).
  - More patients receiving tofacitinib experienced severe infections, and tofacitinib treatment was associated with elevated LDL cholesterol levels and reductions in neutrophil counts.
  - The authors concluded that in patients with active rheumatoid arthritis, tofacitinib monotherapy was associated with reductions in signs and symptoms of rheumatoid arthritis and improvement in physical function. (N Engl J Med. 2012 Aug 9;367(6):495-507.)
- **OPAL Broaden**
  - This was a double-blind, active-controlled, and placebo-controlled phase 3 trial that randomized patients to tofacitinib 5 mg BID, 10 mg BID, adalimumab 40 mg SQ every two weeks, placebo for three months, then tofacitinib 5 mg BID, or placebo for three months then tofacitinib 10 mg BID.
  - Significantly more patients receiving tofacitinib saw an improvement in the primary outcome of the proportion of patients who had an American College of Rheumatology 20 (ACR20) response (≥20% improvement from baseline in the number of tender and swollen joints and at least three of five other important domains) at month 3 and the change from baseline in the Health Assessment Questionnaire–Disability Index (HAQ-DI) score (scores range from 0 to 3, with higher scores indicating greater disability) at month 3.
  - More patients receiving tofacitinib experience adverse events, including four cases of cancer, three serious infections, and four cases of herpes zoster.
  - The authors concluded that tofacitinib was superior to that of placebo at month 3 in patients with psoriatic arthritis who had previously had an inadequate response to conventional synthetic DMARDs. In addition, adverse events were more frequent with tofacitinib than with placebo. (N Engl J Med 2017; 377:1537-1550).

High-Yield Fast-Facts
- **Gold**
  - Gold salts were used to treat RA but have fallen out of favor due to significant toxicity and unproven benefits.
- **Biologic DMARDs (bDMARDs)**
  - bDMARDs are large-molecule medications and can be further divided into the biological original (boDMARD) and biosimilar DMARDs (bsDMARDs).
- **Genomic Prediction**
  - Patients with CYP450 mutations, specific solute carrier genes, or mitochondrial aldehyde dehydrogenase genes are at higher risk of methotrexate toxicity.
- **Hydroxychloroquine and COVID**
  - The use of hydroxychloroquine for COVID-19 was the subject of much controversy, but available evidence suggested no significant improvement on the pandemic-causing virus.

HIGH-YIELD BOARD EXAM ESSENTIALS
- **CLASSIC AGENTS:** Hydroxychloroquine, Leflunomide, Methotrexate, Sulfasalazine, Tofacitinib
- **DRUG CLASS:** DMARD
- **INDICATIONS:** Lupus erythematosus, polyarticular course juvenile idiopathic arthritis, psoriatic arthritis, rheumatoid arthritis, ulcerative colitis
- **MECHANISM:**
  - Interferences with antigen processing in macrophages and other antigen-presenting cells (hydroxychloroquine)
  - Its active metabolite (A77 1726) stops cellular growth by inhibiting dihydroorotate dehydrogenase and decreased ribonuclease synthesis (leflunomide)
  - Inhibits lymphocyte, macrophage, neutrophil, and dendritic cell function via AICAR transformylase and thymidylate synthetase inhibition and extracellular AMP accumulation (methotrexate)
  - Impairs B-cell and T-cell response and proliferation and inhibits inflammatory cytokines production, including IL-1, IL-6, IL-12, and TNF-alfa (sulfasalazine)
  - Selectively JAK inhibitor, impairing cytokine and growth factor-mediated gene expression and intracellular activity of B and T lymphocytes, CD- natural killer cells, and immune globulins (tofacitinib)
- **SIDE EFFECTS:** Nausea, stomatitis, anemia, leukopenia, alopecia, rash
- **CLINICAL PEARLS:** Patients with HLA-B*08-01 and HLA-A*31-01 are at high risk of neutropenia from sulfasalazine.

Table: Drug Class Summary

DMARDs – Drug Class Review High-Yield Med Reviews			
Mechanism of Action: *Hydroxychloroquine* - Interferences with antigen processing in macrophages and other antigen-presenting cells. *Leflunomide* - Its active metabolite (A77 1726) stops cellular growth by inhibiting dihydroorotate dehydrogenase and decreased ribonuclease synthesis. *Methotrexate (low-dose)* - Inhibits lymphocyte, macrophage, neutrophil, and dendritic cell function via AICAR transformylase and thymidylate synthetase inhibition and extracellular AMP accumulation. *Sulfasalazine* - Impairs B-cell and T-cell response and proliferation and inhibits inflammatory cytokines production, including IL-1, IL-6, IL-12, and TNF-alfa. *Tofacitinib* - Selectively JAK inhibitor, impairing cytokine and growth factor-mediated gene expression and intracellular activity of B and T lymphocytes, CD- natural killer cells, and immune globulins.			
Class Effects: Recently designated conventional synthetic DMARDs (csDMARDs) impact disease severity and quality of life in autoimmune disease but carry significant toxicities and intolerances.			
Generic Name	**Brand Name**	**Main Indication(s) or Uses**	**Notes**

Hydroxy-chloroquine	Plaquenil	• Lupus erythematosus	• **Dosing (Adult):**
			  – Oral: 200 to 400 mg daily
			• **Dosing (Peds):**
			  – Oral: 5 mg/kg/day in 1-2 divided doses
			    – Maximum 400 mg/day
			• **CYP450 Interactions:** Substrate CYP2D6
			• **Renal or Hepatic Dose Adjustments:** None
			• **Dosage Forms:** Oral (tablet)

Leflunomide	Arava	• Rheumatoid arthritis	• **Dosing (Adult):**
			  – Oral: 100 mg daily x 3 days, then 20 mg daily
			• **Dosing (Peds):**
			  – < 20 kg - 100 mg x 1 then 10 mg every other day
			  – 20 to 40 kg - 100 mg daily x 2, then 10 mg daily
			• **CYP450 Interactions:** Inhibits CYP2C8, Induces CYP1A2
			• **Renal or Hepatic Dose Adjustments:**
			  – Discontinue if ALT elevations more than 3 times ULN
			• **Dosage Forms:** Oral (tablet)

Methotrexate	Otrexup
	Rasuvo
	Trexall
	Xatmep
		• Polyarticular course juvenile idiopathic arthritis
		• Psoriatic arthritis
		• Rheumatoid arthritis
		• Ulcerative colitis
			• **Dosing (Adult):** Rheumatic/DMARD Dosing only
			  – IM/SQ/Oral: 7.5 to 25 mg weekly
			• **Dosing (Peds):**
			  – Oral/SQ: 10 to 30 mg/m^2
			    – Maximum 25 mg/week
			• **CYP450 Interactions:** P-gp substrate
			• **Renal or Hepatic Dose Adjustments:**
			  – GFR: 10 to 50 mL/minute - Reduce dose by 50%
			  – GFR: < 10 mL/minute - avoid use
			• **Dosage Forms:** Oral (tablet, solution), Injection (solution)

DMARDs – Drug Class Review High-Yield Med Reviews			
Generic Name	**Brand Name**	**Main Indication(s) or Uses**	**Notes**
Sulfasalazine	Azulfidine	<ul><li>Rheumatoid arthritis</li><li>Ulcerative colitis</li></ul>	<ul><li>**Dosing (Adult):**<ul><li>Oral: 500 to 2000 mg/day in 1-2 divided doses<ul><li>Maximum 3 g/day</li></ul></li></ul></li><li>**Dosing (Peds):**<ul><li>Oral: 40 to 70 mg/kg/day in 3 to 6 divided doses<ul><li>Maximum 4 g/day</li></ul></li></ul></li><li>**CYP450 Interactions:** None</li><li>**Renal or Hepatic Dose Adjustments:** None</li><li>**Dosage Forms:** Oral (tablet)</li></ul>
Tofacitinib	Xeljanz	<ul><li>Polyarticular course juvenile idiopathic arthritis</li><li>Psoriatic arthritis</li><li>Rheumatoid arthritis</li><li>Ulcerative colitis</li></ul>	<ul><li>**Dosing (Adult):**<ul><li>Oral: IR tablet 5 to 10 mg BID</li><li>Oral: ER tablet 11 to 22 mg daily</li></ul></li><li>**Dosing (Peds):** IR only<ul><li>10 to < 20 kg: Oral 3.2 mg BID</li><li>20 to < 40 kg: Oral 4 mg BID</li></ul></li><li>**CYP450 Interactions:** Substrate CYP2C19, CYP3A4</li><li>**Renal or Hepatic Dose Adjustments:**<ul><li>Moderate to severe impairment - reduce dose by half</li></ul></li><li>**Dosage Forms:** Oral (tablet)</li></ul>

IMMUNOSUPPRESSANTS – IL-1 ANTAGONISTS

Drug Class
- IL-1 Antagonists
- Agents:
    - **Chronic Care**
        - Anakinra
        - Canakinumab
        - Rilonacept

> **Fast Facts**
> ✓ Anakinra has been around the longest as an adjunct to DMARD therapy for RA.

Main Indications or Uses
- **Chronic Care**
    - Adult-onset Still's disease
        - Canakinumab
    - Cryopyrin-associated periodic syndromes
        - Rilonacept
    - Deficiency of IL-1 receptor antagonist
        - Anakinra
        - Rilonacept
    - Neonatal-onset multisystem inflammatory disease
        - Anakinra
    - Periodic fever syndromes
        - Canakinumab
    - Rheumatoid arthritis
        - Anakinra
    - Systemic juvenile idiopathic arthritis
        - Canakinumab

Mechanism of Action
- IL-1 receptor antagonists competitively inhibit the proinflammatory IL-1-alpha and IL-1-beta
    - Anakinra decreases immune-inflammatory response by its actions as a recombinant version of IL-1 receptor agonists and blocks the effects of IL-1-alpha and IL-1-beta on this receptor.
    - Canakinumab and rilonacept complex with IL-1-beta, preventing its binding to IL-1 receptors.
        - The follow-up CIRT Trial, with low dose methotrexate, failed to improve secondary cardiac events after MI.

Primary Net Benefit
- High IL-1 levels are correlated with active inflammatory processes, sparking IL-1 receptor antagonists' development, but their use has been limited due to costs and efficacy compared to conventional DMARDs.
- Main Labs to Monitor:
    - CBC with differential
    - Complete metabolic
        - Electrolytes, renal function
        - Liver function (albumin, bilirubin, PT/INR), liver enzyme (ALT/AST)
    - Tuberculosis screening at baseline

High-Yield Basic Pharmacology
- **Bone and Joint Effects**
    - IL-1 receptor antagonism can decrease or stop cartilage degradation from loss of proteoglycans and halts bone resorption.
- **Antibody Vs. Recombinant Receptor**
    - Anakinra and rilonacept are recombinant forms of the IL-1 receptor and the IL-1 receptor ligand-binding domain, respectively.

- Canakinumab is a human monoclonal antibody against IL-1-beta specifically.

High-Yield Clinical Knowledge
- **Injection Reactions**
    - These agents are all administered via subcutaneous injection, associated with a high prevalence of injection site reactions.
    - Injection site reactions are self-limiting and do not frequently require intervention.
- **Infection Risk**
    - Upper respiratory tract infections are a frequent adverse event following IL-1 antagonist therapy, affecting 55% of patients.
    - Mycoplasma tuberculosis infection is also possible and requires TB screening before initiation of these agents.
- **Cryopyrin**
    - Cryopyrin is a protein regulated by a collection of specific genes (NLR, NLRP-3, and CIAS1), but importantly, it regulates IL-1-beta activation.
    - In patients with cryopyrin-associated periodic syndromes (CAPS) where cryopyrin deficiencies result in excessive inflammation, IL-1-beta antagonism can reduce the accompanying inflammatory response.
- **Cardiovascular Effect**
    - IL-1-beta inhibition has been proposed to improve the inflammatory pathway after acute myocardial infarctions, particularly C-reactive protein and IL-6.
        - This effect has been supported with canakinumab in the CANTOS trial, further described below.

High-Yield Core Evidence
- **CANTOS Trial**
    - This was a double-blind trial that randomized patients with previous myocardial infarction and elevated high-sensitivity C-reactive protein placebo or canakinumab (doses of 50 mg, 150 mg, or 300 mg) to assess their impact on the incidence of nonfatal myocardial infarction, nonfatal stroke, or cardiovascular death.
    - Canakinumab doses at 150 mg and 300 mg (but not 50 mg) significantly improved the composite endpoint of the incidence of nonfatal myocardial infarction, nonfatal stroke, or cardiovascular death.
    - Interestingly, canakinumab, at any dose, did not reduce lipid levels from baseline.
    - The 150-mg dose, but not the other doses, met the prespecified multiplicity-adjusted threshold for statistical significance for the primary endpoint, and the secondary endpoint additionally included hospitalization for unstable angina that led to urgent revascularization.
    - However, canakinumab was associated with a higher incidence of fatal infection than was placebo, and there was no significant difference in all-cause mortality.
    - The authors concluded that canakinumab at a dose of 150 mg every 3 months led to a significantly lower rate of recurrent cardiovascular events than placebo, independent of lipid-level lowering. (N Engl J Med. 2017 Sep 21;377(12):1119-1131.)
- **Anakinra for RA**
    - This was a multicenter, double-blind trial in patients with active RA despite methotrexate therapy who were randomized to etanercept alone, etanercept full dose plus anakinra, or half-dose etanercept plus anakinra.
    - There was no difference among treatment groups in patient response as measured by the American College of Rheumatology core set criteria and the Disease Activity Score.
    - More patients were experiencing serious infections in the combination therapy groups, compared to single-drug therapy.
    - The authors concluded that combination therapy with etanercept and anakinra provides no added benefit and an increased risk than etanercept alone and is not recommended to treat patients with RA. (Arthritis Rheum. 2004 May;50(5):1412-9.)

High-Yield Fast-Facts
- **Off-Label Uses**
  - Anakinra, canakinumab, and rilonacept have been used for various off-label indications, including gout, and familial Mediterranean fever.
- **HIT and Recurrent Stroke**
  - Anakinra has been suggested as an alternative agent for treating heparin-induced thrombocytopenia or preventing recurrent stroke or TIA.

HIGH-YIELD BOARD EXAM ESSENTIALS
- **CLASSIC AGENTS:** Anakinra, canakinumab, rilonacept
- **DRUG CLASS:** IL-1 Antagonists
- **INDICATIONS:** Deficiency of IL-1 receptor antagonist (anakinra, rilonacept), neonatal-onset multisystem inflammatory disease, rheumatoid arthritis (anakinra), adult-onset still's disease, periodic fever syndromes, systemic juvenile idiopathic arthritis (canakinumab), cryopyrin-associated periodic syndromes (rilonacept)
- **MECHANISM:** Competitively inhibit proinflammatory interleukins IL-1-alpha and IL-1-beta.
- **SIDE EFFECTS:** Injection site reactions, upper respiratory tract infections
- **CLINICAL PEARLS:** IL-1-beta inhibition has been proposed to improve the inflammatory pathway after acute myocardial infarctions, particularly C-reactive protein and IL-6. This effect has been supported with the use of canakinumab in the CANTOS trial, further described below.

Table: Drug Class Summary

IL-1 Antagonists - Drug Class Review High-Yield Med Reviews			
Mechanism of Action: *Competitively inhibit proinflammatory interleukins IL-1-alpha and IL-1-beta.*			
Class Effects: *High IL-1 levels are correlated with active inflammatory processes, sparking IL-1 receptor antagonists' development, but their use has been limited due to costs and efficacy compared to conventional DMARDs.*			
Generic Name	**Brand Name**	**Main Indication(s) or Uses**	**Notes**
Anakinra	Kineret	<ul><li>Deficiency of IL-1 receptor antagonist</li><li>Neonatal-onset multisystem inflammatory disease</li><li>Rheumatoid arthritis</li></ul>	<ul><li>**Dosing (Adult):**<ul><li>SQ: 1 to 4 mg/kg q24h or 100 mg q24h</li><li>Maximum 200 mg/day</li></ul></li><li>**Dosing (Peds):**<ul><li>SQ: 1 to 4 mg/kg q24h</li><li>Maximum: 200 mg/day</li></ul></li><li>**CYP450 Interactions:** None</li><li>**Renal or Hepatic Dose Adjustments:**<ul><li>GFR: < 30 mL/minute - Administer every other day</li></ul></li><li>**Dosage Forms:** Prefilled syringe</li></ul>
Canakinumab	Ilaris	<ul><li>Adult-onset Still's disease</li><li>Periodic fever syndromes</li><li>Systemic juvenile idiopathic arthritis</li></ul>	<ul><li>**Dosing (Adult):**<ul><li>SQ: 2 to 8 mg/kg every 4 weeks</li><li>Maximum 8 mg/kg/day</li></ul></li><li>**Dosing (Peds):**<ul><li>SQ: 2 to 4 mg/kg q24h</li><li>Maximum: 8 mg/kg/day</li></ul></li><li>**CYP450 Interactions:** None</li><li>**Renal or Hepatic Dose Adjustments:** None</li><li>**Dosage Forms:** Solution for subcutaneous injection</li></ul>
Rilonacept	Arcalyst	<ul><li>Cryopyrin-associated periodic syndromes</li><li>Deficiency of IL-1 receptor antagonist</li></ul>	<ul><li>**Dosing (Adult):**<ul><li>Initial: SQ 320 mg as two injections at two different sites on the same day</li><li>Maintenance: SQ 160 mg a week</li></ul></li><li>**Dosing (Peds):**<ul><li>Initial: SQ 4.4 mg/kg (maximum 320 mg) as two injections at two different sites on the same day</li><li>Maintenance: SQ 2.2 mg/kg (maximum 160 mg) a week</li></ul></li><li>**CYP450 Interactions:** None</li><li>**Renal or Hepatic Dose Adjustments:** None</li><li>**Dosage Forms:** Solution for subcutaneous injection</li></ul>

IMMUNOSUPPRESSION – IL-2 RECEPTOR ANTAGONIST

Drug Class
- IL-2 Antagonists
- Agents:
  - Acute Care
    - Basiliximab
    - Daclizumab (removed from the market on 3/2/18)

Main Indications or Uses
- Acute Care
  - Acute rejection prophylaxis
  - Acute graft-versus-host disease

Mechanism of Action
- Binds to the alpha chain of IL-2 - CD25 receptor complex on the surface of activated T-cells, preventing IL-2 activation and proliferation of T-cells.

Primary Net Benefit
- Compared with other immunosuppressant induction agents, antithymocyte globulins, and alemtuzumab, basiliximab has a safer adverse event profile and similar efficacy but lacks robust data to support widespread use.
- Main Labs to Monitor:
  - Signs of infection or acute transplant rejection

High-Yield Basic Pharmacology
- IL-2 Receptor Binding
  - The degree of IL-2 receptor binding accomplished by basiliximab is extensive, occurs rapidly, and persists for an extended time, typically 4 to 6 weeks after administration.

High-Yield Clinical Knowledge
- Improved Safety
  - Compared with other immunosuppression induction agents, basiliximab is not associated with infusion reactions.
    - Of course, immunosuppression is a class effect and the desired clinical outcome.
- Antimurine Antibodies
  - Basiliximab is not a fully human monoclonal antibody but contains approximately 20% murine monoclonal antibodies.
  - As a result, there is a risk of developing human anti murine antibodies.
- Renal And Liver Transplant
  - Although approved for renal transplants, basiliximab has been used in other organ transplants, including liver, lung, and heart.
  - The use of basiliximab can delay the initiation of calcineurin inhibitor therapy and delay their associated toxicities.

High-Yield Core Evidence
- The 3C Study
  - This was a multicenter, randomized trial comparing alemtuzumab-based induction treatment compared with basiliximab-based induction treatment in patients receiving kidney transplants.
  - Significantly fewer patients treated with alemtuzumab-based regimens experienced the primary outcome of biopsy-proven acute rejection at 6 months, analyzed by intention to treat.
  - There was no between-group difference in treatment effect on transplant failure during the first 6 months or serious infection.

- The authors concluded that alemtuzumab-based induction therapy reduced the risk of biopsy-proven acute rejection in a broad range of patients receiving a kidney transplant. (Lancet. 2014 Nov 8;384(9955):1684-90.)
- **Basiliximab Vs. Daclizumab**
    - This prospective, open-label, single-center study randomized patients receiving kidney transplants that randomized patients to basiliximab (plus triple immunosuppression) or daclizumab (plus triple immunosuppression).
    - There was no difference between treatment arms concerning the intent-to-treat analysis of the incidence of acute rejections, graft function, patient and graft survival, and safety.
    - Similarly, no secondary endpoints were significantly different between either treatment group, including biopsy-confirmed first acute rejection, estimated glomerular filtration rate, survival, and graft survival.
    - The authors concluded that either basiliximab or daclizumab combined with triple therapy was an efficient and safe immunosuppression strategy, demonstrated by a low incidence of acute rejections, excellent graft function, and high survival rates, and acceptable adverse event profile in adult recipients within the 1st year after deceased donor renal transplantation. (Transplantation. 2010 Apr 27;89(8):1022-7.)

High-Yield Fast-Fact
- **Tacrolimus Interaction**
    - According to drug-interaction software programs, the concomitant use of basiliximab and tacrolimus is contraindicated.
    - Since basiliximab is used immediately around transplant and calcineurin inhibitors are typically started 1-3 months after the transplant, this interaction's clinical significance is questionable.

HIGH-YIELD BOARD EXAM ESSENTIALS
- **CLASSIC AGENTS:** Basiliximab
- **DRUG CLASS:** IL-2 Antagonists
- **INDICATIONS:** Acute rejection prophylaxis, acute graft-versus-host disease
- **MECHANISM:** Binds to the alpha chain of IL-2 - CD25 receptor complex on the surface of activated T-cells, preventing IL-2 activation and proliferation of T-cells.
- **SIDE EFFECTS:** Immunosuppression, anti-murine antibody development
- **CLINICAL PEARLS:** The use of basiliximab can delay the initiation of calcineurin inhibitor therapy and delaying their associated toxicities.

Table: Drug Class Summary

IL-2 Antagonist - Drug Class Review High-Yield Med Reviews			
Mechanism of Action: *Binds to the alpha chain of IL-2 - CD25 receptor complex on the surface of activated T-cells, preventing IL-2 activation and proliferation of T-cells.*			
Class Effects: *Compared with other immunosuppressant induction agents, antithymocyte globulins, and alemtuzumab, basiliximab has a safer adverse event profile, and similar efficacy but lacks robust data to support widespread use.*			
Generic Name	**Brand Name**	**Main Indication(s) or Uses**	**Notes**

Basiliximab	Simulect	• Acute rejection prophylaxis	• **Dosing (Adult):**
			  – IV: 20 mg within 2 hours before transplant surgery, then 20 mg 4 days after transplant
			  – IV: 20 mg on days 1 and 4
			• **Dosing (Peds):**
			  – < 35 kg: IV: 10 mg within 6 hours before surgery, then 10 mg 4 days after surgery
			• **CYP450 Interactions:** None
			• **Renal or Hepatic Dose Adjustments:** None
			• **Dosage Forms:** IV (solution)

IMMUNOSUPPRESSION – IL-6 RECEPTOR ANTAGONIST

Drug Class
- IL-6 Receptor Antagonist
- Agents:
    - Chronic Care
        - Sarilumab
        - Tocilizumab

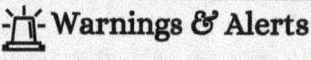

> **Warnings & Alerts**
> ✓ IL-6 antagonists should not be initiated before drawing absolute neutrophil counts (ANC), platelets, and hepatic enzyme levels.

Main Indications or Uses
- Chronic Care
    - Sarilumab
        - Rheumatoid arthritis
    - Tocilizumab
        - Cytokine release syndrome, severe or life-threatening
        - Giant cell arteritis
        - Polyarticular juvenile idiopathic arthritis
        - Rheumatoid arthritis
        - Systemic juvenile idiopathic arthritis

Mechanism of Action
- Inhibits IL-6 mediated inflammation by binding to both soluble and membrane-bound IL-6 receptors.

Primary Net Benefit
- Considered non-TNF biologic DMARD (bDMARD) and counteracts proinflammatory cytokines active in the pathogenesis of rheumatoid arthritis.
- Main Labs to Monitor:
    - CBC with differential
    - Complete metabolic
        - Electrolytes, renal function
        - Liver function (albumin, bilirubin, PT/INR), liver enzyme (ALT/AST)
    - Serum cholesterol and triglyceride
    - Mycoplasma tuberculosis screening

High-Yield Basic Pharmacology
- **Alternative CYP Induction**
    - IL-6 inhibition can cause an increase in the activity of cytochrome P450, leading to numerous interactions.
    - Current evidence suggests IL-6 inhibitors inhibit CYP3A4, but there may also be an induction of other isoenzymes, including CYP2C9, CYP2C19, and CYP2D6.
- **Antibody Development**
    - Approximately 2% of patients receiving tocilizumab and up to 9% of patients taking sarilumab develop antibodies to the drug, causing hypersensitivity reactions and prompting drug discontinuation.
        - This observation may be counterintuitive fully human MABs are considered to have a lower risk of neutralizing antibodies and allergic reactions. Still, tocilizumab is a humanized anti-IL-6 receptor antibody, whereas sarilumab is a fully human monoclonal antibody.

High-Yield Clinical Knowledge
- **Infection Risk**
    - Boxed warnings for infections exist for IL-6 antagonists, specifically tuberculosis (pulmonary or extrapulmonary) or other infections, including invasive fungal, bacterial, viral, protozoal, and other opportunistic infections.
    - Patients should have tuberculosis screening completed before initiation of IL-6 antagonist therapy and to monitor for the development of other infections continually.

- **ANC and ALT Screening**
  - IL-6 antagonists should not be initiated before drawing absolute neutrophil counts (ANC), platelets, and hepatic enzyme levels
  - IL-6 antagonists should not be initiated if ANC is less than 2,000/mm^3, platelets are less than 100,000/mm^3, or if ALT is greater than 1.5 times ULN.
- **Guideline Recommendation**
  - In patients with rheumatoid arthritis and experiencing disease progression despite therapy with a conventional DMARD, bDMARDs, including IL-6 antagonists, are recommended.
    - If subsequent treatment failures occur, alternative bDMARDs can be substituted.

High-Yield Core Evidence
- **MOBILITY**
  - This was a multicenter, prospective, blinded study comparing the efficacy and safety of sarilumab combined with methotrexate to treat rheumatoid arthritis.
  - Co-primary endpoints were the proportion of patients achieving American College of Rheumatology 20% improvement responses at week 24, change from baseline in the Health Assessment Questionnaire Disability Index at week 16, and change from baseline in the modified Sharp/van der Heijde score of radiographic damage at week 52.
  - Sarilumab significantly improved each of the three co-primary endpoints compared to placebo at week 24.
  - Serious infections, neutropenia, elevations in cholesterol, and ALT elevations occurred more frequently in the sarilumab group and did so more frequently with increasing doses.
  - The authors concluded that rheumatoid arthritis patients treated with sarilumab combined with methotrexate provided sustained clinical efficacy, as shown by significant improvements in symptomatic, functional, and radiographic outcomes. (Arthritis Rheumatol. 2015;67(6):1424–1437.)
- **ADACTA**
  - This was a multicenter, double-blind, parallel-group, phase 4 superiority study that randomized patients with rheumatoid arthritis to tocilizumab monotherapy or adalimumab monotherapy to assess the efficacy and safety of these treatments.
  - Patients randomized to tocilizumab therapy had a significantly improved primary endpoint of the change in disease activity score using 28 joints (DAS28) from baseline to week 24 compared to adalimumab.
  - Serious adverse events occurred with similar frequency between either treatment group to reduce signs and symptoms of rheumatoid arthritis in patients for whom methotrexate was deemed inappropriate. (Lancet. 2013;381(9877):1541–1550.)

High-Yield Fast-Fact
- **COVID-19**
  - Sarilumab and tocilizumab were investigated early on as a possible therapeutic intervention for COVID-19 infection; however, they were found not to have a significantly positive effect, but further research in the REMAP-CAP trial suggested a benefit and an NNT of 12.

HIGH-YIELD BOARD EXAM ESSENTIALS
- **CLASSIC AGENTS:** Sarilumab, tocilizumab
- **DRUG CLASS:** IL-6 receptor antagonist
- **INDICATIONS:** Cytokine release syndrome, giant cell arteritis, polyarticular juvenile idiopathic arthritis, rheumatoid arthritis, systemic juvenile idiopathic arthritis
- **MECHANISM:** Inhibits IL-6 mediated inflammation by binding to both soluble and membrane-bound IL-6 receptors.
- **SIDE EFFECTS:** Antibody development/hypersensitivity reaction, infections
- **CLINICAL PEARLS:** IL-6 antagonists should not be initiated before drawing absolute neutrophil counts (ANC), platelets, and hepatic enzyme levels.

Table: Drug Class Summary

| | IL-6 Receptor Antagonist - Drug Class Review
High-Yield Med Reviews |

	**Mechanism of Action:** *Inhibits IL-6 mediated inflammation by binding to both soluble and membrane-bound IL-6 receptors.*
	**Class Effects:** *Considered non-TNF biologic DMARD (bDMARD) and counteracts proinflammatory cytokines active in the pathogenesis of rheumatoid arthritis.*
Generic Name	**Brand Name**	**Indication(s) or Uses**	**Notes**

Sarilumab	Kevzara	• Rheumatoid arthritis	• **Dosing (Adult):**
			  – SQ: 200 mg q2weeks
			• **Dosing (Peds):** Not routinely used
			• **CYP450 Interactions:** None
			• **Renal or Hepatic Dose Adjustments:**
			  – ALT elevation 3x to < 5x ULN: interrupt therapy until ALT < 3x ULN, then 150 mg q2weeks
			  – ALT more than 5x ULN: discontinue
			• **Dosage Forms:** Solution for subcutaneous injection, prefilled syringe

Tocilizumab	Actemra	• Cytokine release syndrome, severe or life-threatening
		• Giant cell arteritis
		• Polyarticular juvenile idiopathic arthritis
		• Rheumatoid arthritis
		• Systemic juvenile idiopathic arthritis
			• **Dosing (Adult):**
			  – IV: 4 mg/kg once, maximum 800 mg/dose
			  – SQ: 162 mg q1week
			• **Dosing (Peds):**
			  – IV: 8 to 12 mg/kg/dose q1-4weeks
			  – SQ: 162 mg q2-3weeks
			    – Extra info if needed
			• **CYP450 Interactions:** Induces CYP3A4, possibly CYP2C9, CYP2C19, and CYP2D6
			• **Renal or Hepatic Dose Adjustments:**
			  – ALT elevation 3x to less than 5x ULN: interrupt therapy until ALT less than 3x ULN, then resume at 150 mg q2weeks
			  – ALT more than 5x ULN: discontinue
			• **Dosage Forms:** Solution for IV and subcutaneous injection, prefilled syringe

IMMUNOSUPPRESSION – IL-17 RECEPTOR ANTAGONISTS

Drug Class
- IL-17 Receptor Antagonists
- Agents:
  - Chronic Care
    - Brodalumab
    - Ixekizumab
    - Secukinumab

Main Indications or Uses
- Chronic Care
  - Brodalumab
    - Plaque psoriasis
  - Ixekizumab and Secukinumab
    - Ankylosing spondylitis
    - Plaque psoriasis
    - Psoriatic arthritis
  - Ixekizumab
    - Nonradiographic axial spondyloarthritis

Mechanism of Action
- Selectively binds to IL-17A and blocks its action on IL-17 receptors, thus inhibiting its release of pro-inflammatory cytokines and chemokines.

Primary Net Benefit
- IL-17 antagonists prevent the inflammatory process associated with plaque psoriasis and psoriatic arthritis and appear to be superior to other bDMARDs for this indication.
- Main Labs to Monitor:
  - Mycoplasma tuberculosis and inflammatory bowel disease screening

High-Yield Basic Pharmacology
- Plaque Psoriasis
  - The action of IL-17 antagonists can specifically bind to keratinocytes, halting their pro-inflammatory response and preventing characteristic psoriatic plaques.
- Neutralizing Antibodies
  - Like other IL antagonists (such as the IL-6 antagonists), there is evidence of the development of neutralizing antibodies that can cause reduced serum concentrations of the biologic and reduced efficacy.

High-Yield Clinical Knowledge
- Infection Risk
  - Patients taking IL-17 antagonists are at increased risk of infection, similar to other IL antagonists.
  - The most commonly observed infection with IL-17 antagonists is mucocutaneous Candida infections.
- Inflammatory Bowel Disease
  - Patients starting IL-17 antagonists who have a history of IBD may worsen their IBD or develop Crohn's disease and ulcerative colitis.
  - The use of these drugs in the context of IBD is discouraged.
- Brodalumab Psychiatric Risk
  - Suicidal ideation or behavior was observed in clinical trials, prompting a black boxed warning of this effect.
  - Furthermore, brodalumab is contraindicated in patients with suicidal ideation, recent suicidal behavior, or a history of suicidal ideation.
  - Brodalumab is also exclusively available through a risk evaluation and mitigation strategy program.

- **Adverse Events**
    - Other common adverse events associated with IL-17 antagonists include injection site reactions, nasopharyngitis, cellulitis, and major cardiac adverse events.

High-Yield Core Evidence
- **ERASURE and FIXTURE**
    - This was a single publication of two phase 3, double-blind trials that randomized patients with moderate-to-severe plaque psoriasis to either secukinumab, etanercept, or placebo.
    - Patients randomized to either secukinumab dose in both studies showed a significant reduction of 75% or more from baseline in the psoriasis area-and-severity index score and a score of 0 or 1 on a 5-point modified investigator's global assessment, compared to either etanercept or placebo.
    - However, the infection rates were higher with secukinumab than with placebo in both studies and were similar to those with etanercept.
    - The authors concluded that secukinumab was effective for psoriasis in two randomized trials, validating IL-17A as a therapeutic target. (New Engl J Med. 2014;371(4):326–338.)
- **UNCOVER-2 and UNCOVER-3**
    - This was a single publication of two prospective, double-blind, multicentre, phase 3 studies that randomized patients with widespread moderate-to-severe psoriasis to either ixekizumab, etanercept, or placebo to assess the safety and efficacy of specifically targeting IL-17A.
    - Ixekizumab significantly improved the co-primary efficacy endpoints in each study of proportions of patients achieving sPGA score 0 or 1 and 75% or greater improvement in PASI at week 12, compared to either etanercept or placebo.
    - Serious adverse events were reported similarly between treatment groups.
    - In two independent studies, the authors concluded that either ixekizumab dose regimens had greater efficacy than placebo and etanercept over 12 weeks. (Lancet. 2015;386(9993):541–551.)

High-Yield Fast-Fact
- **Humanized MAB**
    - All three IL-17 antagonists, brodalumab, ixekizumab, and secukinumab, are fully humanized IgG monoclonal antibodies.

HIGH-YIELD BOARD EXAM ESSENTIALS
- **CLASSIC AGENTS:** Brodalumab, ixekizumab, secukinumab
- **DRUG CLASS:** IL-17 receptor antagonists
- **INDICATIONS:** Ankylosing spondylitis, nonradiographic axial spondyloarthritis, plaque psoriasis, psoriatic arthritis
- **MECHANISM:** Selectively binds to IL-17A and blocks its action on IL-17 receptors, thus inhibiting its release of pro-inflammatory cytokines and chemokines.
- **SIDE EFFECTS:** Increased risk of infection, suicide (brodalumab), injection site reactions, nasopharyngitis, cellulitis, MACE
- **CLINICAL PEARLS:** Patients taking IL-17 antagonists are at increased risk of infection, similar to other IL antagonists. The most commonly observed infection with IL-17 antagonists is mucocutaneous Candida infections.

Table: Drug Class Summary

IL-17 Antagonists - Drug Class Review High-Yield Med Reviews			
Mechanism of Action: *Selectively binds to IL-17A and blocks its action on IL-17 receptors, thus inhibiting its release of pro-inflammatory cytokines and chemokines.*			
Class Effects: *IL-17 antagonists prevent the inflammatory process associated with plaque psoriasis, and psoriatic arthritis and appear to be superior to other bDMARDs for this indication.*			
Generic Name	**Brand Name**	**Indication(s) or Uses**	**Notes**
Brodalumab	Siliq	• Plaque psoriasis	• **Dosing (Adult):** — SQ: 210 mg qweek for 3 weeks, then 210 mg q2weeks • **Dosing (Peds):** Not routinely used • **CYP450 Interactions:** None • **Renal or Hepatic Dose Adjustments:** None • **Dosage Forms:** Solution prefilled syringe
Ixekizumab	Taltz	• Ankylosing spondylitis • Nonradiographic axial spondyloarthritis • Plaque psoriasis • Psoriatic arthritis	• **Dosing (Adult):** — SQ: 160 mg once, then 80 mg q2-4weeks • **Dosing (Peds):** — < 25 kg: SQ 40 mg once, then 20 mg q4weeks — 25 to 50 kg: SQ 80 mg once, then 40 mg q4weeks • **CYP450 Interactions:** None • **Renal or Hepatic Dose Adjustments:** None • **Dosage Forms:** Solution prefilled syringe
Secukinumab	Cosentyx	• Ankylosing spondylitis • Plaque psoriasis • Psoriatic arthritis	• **Dosing (Adult):** — SQ: 150 mg a week for 4 weeks then 150 to 300 mg q4weeks • **Dosing (Peds):** Not routinely used • **CYP450 Interactions:** None • **Renal or Hepatic Dose Adjustments:** None • **Dosage Forms:** Solution prefilled syringe

IMMUNOSUPPRESSION – IL-23 RECEPTOR ANTAGONISTS

Drug Class
- IL-23 Receptor Antagonists
- Agents:
    - Chronic Care
        - Guselkumab
        - Risankizumab
        - Tildrakizumab
        - Ustekinumab (also IL-12 antagonist)

Main Indications or Uses
- Chronic Care
    - Crohn's disease
        - Ustekinumab
        - Risankizumab
    - Plaque psoriasis
        - Guselkumab
        - Risankizumab
        - Tildrakizumab
        - Ustekinumab
    - Psoriatic arthritis
        - Guselkumab
        - Ustekinumab
    - Ulcerative colitis
        - Ustekinumab

Mechanism of Action
- Guselkumab, Risankizumab, Tildrakizumab
    - Bind to the p19 subunit of IL-23 on CD4 cells and NK cells, inhibiting proinflammatory cytokines and chemokine release.
- Ustekinumab
    - Inhibits IL-12 and IL-23 by preventing the binding of the p40 subunit, suppressing the formation of inflammatory T helper cells.

Primary Net Benefit
- IL-12/IL-23 inhibitors are safe and effective options for treating plaque psoriasis that require less frequent dosing than alternative classes and carry a lower risk of candidiasis or inflammatory bowel disease.
- Main Labs to Monitor:
    - Mycoplasma tuberculosis screening
    - Screening for inflammatory bowel disease

High-Yield Basic Pharmacology
- IL-12 and IL-23 Blockade
    - The inhibition of cellular signaling produced by IL-12 and IL-23 receptor antagonists block cytokine production and gene activation and inhibits T helper cell 1 and T helper cell 17 mediated responses.
    - Ustekinumab, an IL-12 and IL-23 inhibitor, was initially developed based on the hypothesis of IL-12 activating T helper 1 cells, which are then linked to the production of TNF-alpha interferon-gamma.
    - However, further research questioned this model and found a T helper cell subtype, T helper 1 and 17, and its production of IL-17 and IL-22 as central components to psoriasis pathophysiology.
    - IL-23 promoted differentiation and proliferation of T helper 17 cells and was identified as a therapeutic target, leading to the IL-23 specific agents, guselkumab, risankizumab, and tildrakizumab.

High-Yield Clinical Knowledge

- **Tildrakizumab Administration**
  - Although tildrakizumab has a similar administration and dosing schedule to the other IL-23 antagonists, it may only be administered by a healthcare provider.
- **bDMARD Conversion**
  - Switching between bDMARDs is possible and likely necessary with long-term treatment as neutralizing antibodies develop after 3 years of treatment.
  - Conversion between agents in the same class is acceptable.
    - Some experts suggest using a four-to-twelve-week washout period (or the dosing interval) before and the planned date of a new biologic initiation.
  - Alternatively, using concomitant methotrexate may increase the bDMARD life-span.
- **Difference Between IL Antagonists**
  - The class of IL-23 antagonists may possess specific long-term advantages compared with IL-17 inhibitors, specifically with long-term efficacy.
  - Combination with other IL antagonists does not offer specific therapeutic advantages, as demonstrated in the UltiMMa studies described below.
- **Lower Infection Risk**
  - The proposed mechanism by which IL-23 antagonists lead to a lower incidence of infections involves the conservation of T helper 1 response activation by IL-12, which preserves interferon-gamma protection against intracellular pathogens Mycobacterium species, Salmonella, Pneumocystis jirovecii, and Toxoplasmosis gondii.

High-Yield Core Evidence

- **reSURFACE 1 and reSURFACE 2**
  - This was a single publication of two three-part phase 3, parallel-group, double-blind, randomized controlled studies comparing tildrakizumab to placebo and etanercept in treating chronic plaque psoriasis.
  - Tildrakizumab treatment groups had a significantly higher proportion of patients achieving the co-primary endpoints of Psoriasis Area and Severity Index and Physician's Global Assessment response at week 12, compared to placebo plus etanercept.
  - Serious adverse events were similar and low in all groups in both trials.
  - The authors concluded that tildrakizumab at 200 mg and 100 mg doses were efficacious compared with placebo and etanercept and were well tolerated in treating patients with moderate-to-severe chronic plaque psoriasis. (Lancet. 2017;390(100091):276–288.)
- **UltiMMa-1 and UltiMMa-2**
  - This was a single publication of two phases 3, randomized, double-blind, placebo-controlled, and active comparator-controlled trials that assessed the efficacy and safety of risankizumab compared with placebo plus ustekinumab in patients with moderate-to-severe chronic plaque psoriasis.
  - In each trial, risankizumab significantly improved the co-primary endpoints of proportions of patients achieving a 90% improvement in the Psoriasis Area Severity Index and a static Physician's Global Assessment at week 16, compared to treatment with placebo plus ustekinumab.
  - There was no difference in safety endpoints between treatment arms in either study.
  - The authors concluded that risankizumab is superior to placebo plus ustekinumab in treating moderate-to-severe plaque psoriasis. (Lancet. 2018 Aug 25;392(10148):650–661.)

High-Yield Fast-Facts

- **IL-23 Antagonist Comparison**
  - Although the data are emerging, guselkumab and risankizumab appear to be associated with better Psoriasis Area Severity Index and a static Physician's Global Assessment scores compared to tildrakizumab and ustekinumab.

- **Major Adverse Cardiac Events**
  - MACE has been a subject of debate surrounding IL-12/23 antagonists; some developmental agents have failed to come to market due to excessive risk in this category, namely briakinumab.
- **Pregnancy**
  - Ustekinumab has the most data in pregnant patients and carries a pregnancy category B.

HIGH-YIELD BOARD EXAM ESSENTIALS
- **CLASSIC AGENTS:** Guselkumab, risankizumab, tildrakizumab, ustekinumab (also IL-12 antagonist)
- **DRUG CLASS:** IL-23 receptor antagonists
- **INDICATIONS:** Crohn's disease, plaque psoriasis, psoriatic arthritis, ulcerative colitis
- **MECHANISM:** Bind to the p19 subunit of IL-23 on CD4 cells and NK cells, resulting in inhibiting the release of proinflammatory cytokines and chemokine
- **SIDE EFFECTS:** Infections, injection site reactions, MACE
- **CLINICAL PEARLS:** The proposed mechanism by which IL-23 antagonists lead to a lower incidence of infections involves the conservation of T helper 1 response activation by IL-12, which preserves interferon-gamma protection against intracellular pathogens Mycobacterium species, Salmonella, Pneumocystis jirovecii, and Toxoplasmosis gondii.

Table: Drug Class Summary

IL-23 Receptor Antagonists Drug Class Review High-Yield Med Reviews			
Mechanism of Action: *Guselkumab, Risankizumab, Tildrakizumab* - Bind to the p19 subunit of IL-23 on CD4 cells and NK cells, resulting in inhibiting the release of proinflammatory cytokines and chemokine. *Ustekinumab* - Inhibits IL-12 and IL-23 by preventing the binding of the p40 subunit, suppressing the formation of inflammatory T helper cells.			
Class Effects: *IL-12/IL-23 inhibitors are safe and effective options for treating plaque psoriasis that require less frequent dosing than alternative classes and carry a lower risk of candidiasis or inflammatory bowel disease.*			
Generic Name	**Brand Name**	**Main Indication(s) or Uses**	**Notes**
Guselkumab	Tremfya	• Plaque psoriasis • Psoriatic arthritis	• **Dosing (Adult):** – SQ: 100 mg at weeks 0, 4, then q8weeks • **Dosing (Peds):** N/A • **CYP450 Interactions:** None • **Renal or Hepatic Dose Adjustments:** None • **Dosage Forms:** Subcutaneous prefilled syringe
Risankizumab	Skyrizi	• Crohn's disease • Plaque psoriasis	• **Dosing (Adult):** – SQ: 150 mg (as 2 separate injections) at weeks 0, 4, then q12weeks – Crohn's: 600 mg IV week 0, 4, 8, then 360 mg SC week 12 then q8weeks • **Dosing (Peds):** N/A • **CYP450 Interactions:** None • **Renal or Hepatic Dose Adjustments:** None • **Dosage Forms:** Subcutaneous prefilled syringe
Tildrakizumab	Ilumya	• Plaque psoriasis	• **Dosing (Adult):** – SQ: 100 mg at weeks 0, 4, then q12weeks • **Dosing (Peds):** N/A • **CYP450 Interactions:** None • **Renal or Hepatic Dose Adjustments:** None • **Dosage Forms:** Subcutaneous prefilled syringe
Ustekinumab	Stelara	• Crohn's disease • Plaque psoriasis • Psoriatic arthritis • Ulcerative colitis	• **Dosing (Adult):** – Induction: IV: 260 to 520 mg x 1 – Maintenance: SQ: 80 mg q8weeks – SQ: 45 to 90 mg at weeks 0, 4, then q12weeks • **Dosing (Peds):** – SQ: 0.75 mg/kg at 0 and 4 weeks, then q12weeks – Max 90 mg/dose • **CYP450 Interactions:** None • **Renal or Hepatic Dose Adjustments:** None • **Dosage Forms:** IV (solution), Subcutaneous prefilled syringe

IMMUNOSUPPRESSION – JANUS KINASE INHIBITOR

Drug Class
- Janus Kinase Inhibitor
- Agents:
    - Chronic Care
        - Baricitinib
        - Tofacitinib
        - Upadacitinib

Fast Facts

✓ Despite having multiple uses, tofacitinib is associated with increases in LDL, HDL, and total cholesterol, worsened cardiovascular mortality, and risk of both arterial and venous thrombosis.

Main Indications or Uses
- Chronic Care
    - Polyarticular course juvenile idiopathic arthritis
        - Tofacitinib
    - Psoriatic arthritis
        - Tofacitinib
    - Rheumatoid arthritis
        - Baricitinib
        - Tofacitinib
        - Upadacitinib
    - Ulcerative colitis
        - Tofacitinib

Mechanism of Action
- Inactivation of Janus kinase (JAK), JAK inhibitors prevent the recruitment, phosphorylation, and activation of STATs, halting the pro-inflammatory cytokine signaling from reaching the cell nucleus, thus stopping the pro-inflammatory process.

Primary Net Benefit
- Targeted synthetic small molecule disease-modifying antirheumatic drugs (tsDMARDs) produce targeted anti-inflammatory effects and can be combined with other DMARDs or monotherapy.
- Main Labs to Monitor:
    - CBC with differential
    - Complete metabolic panel
        - Liver function tests
        - Electrolytes
    - Lipid panel

High-Yield Basic Pharmacology
- **Baricitinib JAK Selectivity**
    - Baricitinib has demonstrated JAK selectivity by reversibly inhibiting JAK1 and JAK3 greater than JAK2.
- **Tofacitinib JAK Selectivity**
    - Tofacitinib has a higher specificity of JAK3 than JAK1, possibly providing enhanced interruption of the JAK-STAT signaling pathway.
- **Upadacitinib JAK Selectivity**
    - Upadacitinib has a greater inhibitory potency for JAK1 compared to JAK2 or JAK3.

High-Yield Clinical Knowledge
- **Viral and Mycobacterial infections**
    - The combination of baricitinib, tofacitinib, or upadacitinib plus prednisone increases the risk of herpes zoster infection, reactivation of herpes virus infections, and invasive fungal or bacterial infections.
    - Similarly, these agents' use is associated with mycobacteria tuberculosis infectious; thus, screening for active or latent tuberculosis is necessary before treatment.

- **Cardiovascular Mortality**
  - Patients receiving tofacitinib for rheumatoid arthritis 50 years of age or older with at least 1 cardiovascular risk factor have a dose-dependent risk of all-cause mortality, including sudden cardiovascular death.
- **Gastrointestinal Perforations**
  - The use of baricitinib has been associated with GI perforations in patients with a history of diverticulitis, prompting caution regarding its use in this population or selecting an alternative agent.
- **Thrombosis Risk**
  - Venous and arterial thrombosis have been observed in patients treated with JAK inhibitors, but the strongest evidence lies with tofacitinib.
  - Like the cardiovascular mortality risk, patients 50 years of age or older with at least 1 cardiovascular risk factor have a higher risk of thrombotic events.
- **Rheumatoid Arthritis**
  - tsDMARDs can be used alone or combined with methotrexate (or other csDMARDs) to manage rheumatoid arthritis.
  - As a result of the increased risk of infection with tsDMARDs, including JAK inhibitors, they should not be used with potent immunosuppressants such as azathioprine, cyclosporine, or biologic DMARDs.
- **Cholesterol**
  - Tofacitinib is associated with increases in LDL, HDL, and total cholesterol.
    - This may be used to partially explain the dose-dependent increase in cardiovascular death risk associated with this agent.

High-Yield Core Evidence
- **SELECT-NEXT**
  - This was a double-blind, placebo-controlled trial comparing two doses of upadacitinib to placebo in patients with inadequate response to conventional synthetic disease-modifying antirheumatic drugs (csDMARDs).
  - Upadacitinib, at either dose studied, significantly improved American College of Rheumatology criteria (ACR20) and a 28-joint disease activity score using C-reactive protein after 12 weeks of therapy.
  - More patients randomized to upadacitinib experienced adverse events than placebo, including serious adverse events such as infection, herpes zoster infections, malignancies, and cardiovascular events.
  - The authors concluded that patients with moderately to severely active rheumatoid arthritis who received upadacitinib (15 mg or 30 mg) combined with csDMARDs showed significant improvements in clinical signs and symptoms compared to placebo. (Lancet 2018;391(10139):2503–2512.)
- **SELECT-CHOICE**
  - This phase 3, double-blind, controlled trial randomized patients with rheumatoid arthritis refractory to biologic disease-modifying antirheumatic drugs (DMARDs) to either oral upadacitinib or intravenous abatacept, each in combination with stable synthetic DMARDs.
  - Patients randomized to upadacitinib experienced a significant improvement in the primary outcome of the change from baseline in the composite Disease Activity Score for 28 joints based on the C-reactive protein level at week 12 compared to abatacept.
  - Furthermore, more patients receiving upadacitinib achieved remission than patients randomized to abatacept.
  - The authors concluded that upadacitinib was superior to abatacept in the change from baseline in the DAS28-CRP and remission achievement at week 12 but was associated with more serious adverse events. (N Engl J Med 2020; 383:1511-1521.)

High-Yield Fast-Fact
- **COVID**
  - The JAK inhibitors were investigated as a potential intervention for COVID-19 but did not significantly improve patient-oriented outcomes.

HIGH-YIELD BOARD EXAM ESSENTIALS
- **CLASSIC AGENTS:** Baricitinib, Tofacitinib, Upadacitinib
- **DRUG CLASS:** Janus Kinase Inhibitor
- **INDICATIONS:** Polyarticular course juvenile idiopathic arthritis, psoriatic arthritis, rheumatoid arthritis, ulcerative colitis
- **MECHANISM:** Prevent the recruitment, phosphorylation, and activation of STATs, halting the pro-inflammatory cytokine signaling form reaching the cell nucleus, thus stopping the pro-inflammatory process.
- **SIDE EFFECTS:** Increased CV death risk, infection risk, increased risk of VTE and arterial thrombosis, increases in LDL, HDL, and total cholesterol
- **CLINICAL PEARLS:** As a result of the increased risk of infection with tsDMARDs, including JAK inhibitors, they should not be used with potent immunosuppressants such as azathioprine, cyclosporine, or biologic DMARDs.

Table: Drug Class Summary

Janus Kinase Inhibitor - Drug Class Review High-Yield Med Reviews			
Mechanism of Action: *Inactivation of Janus kinase (JAK), JAK inhibitors prevent the recruitment, phosphorylation, and activation of STATs, halting the pro-inflammatory cytokine signaling from reaching the cell nucleus, thus stopping the pro-inflammatory process.*			
Class Effects: *Targeted synthetic small molecule disease-modifying antirheumatic drugs (tsDMARDs) produce targeted anti-inflammatory effects and can be combined with other DMARDs or monotherapy.*			
Generic Name	**Brand Name**	**Main Indication(s) or Uses**	**Notes**
Baricitinib	Olumiant	• Rheumatoid arthritis	• **Dosing (Adult):** – Oral: 2 to 4 mg daily • **Dosing (Peds):** – Oral: 2 to 4 mg daily • **CYP450 Interactions:** Substrate of CYP3A4, P-gp • **Renal or Hepatic Dose Adjustments:** – GFR: 30 to 60 mL/min/1.73 m2: 1 mg daily – GFR: < 30 mL/min/1.73 m^2: not recommended • **Dosage Forms:** Oral (tablet)
Tofacitinib	Xeljanz	• Polyarticular course juvenile idiopathic arthritis • Psoriatic arthritis • Rheumatoid arthritis • Ulcerative colitis	• **Dosing (Adult):** – Oral: IR tablet 5 to 10 mg BID – Oral: ER tablet 11 to 22mg daily • **Dosing (Peds):** – Oral: solution 3.2 to 5 mg BID – Extra info if needed • **CYP450 Interactions:** text • **Renal or Hepatic Dose Adjustments:** – Moderate to severe renal impairment: reduce starting dose by 50% – Child-Pugh class C hepatic impairment: use not recommended • **Dosage Forms:** Oral (IR and ER tablet)
Upadacitinib	Rinvoq	• Rheumatoid arthritis	• **Dosing (Adult):** – Oral: 15 mg daily • **Dosing (Peds):** – Not routinely used • **CYP450 Interactions:** text • **Renal or Hepatic Dose Adjustments:** – Child-Pugh class C hepatic impairment - use not recommended • **Dosage Forms:** Oral (tablet)

IMMUNOSUPPRESSION – SELECTIVE T-CELL COSTIMULATION BLOCKER

Drug Class
- Selective T-Cell Costimulation Blocker
- Agents:
    - Acute Care
        - Belatacept
    - Chronic Care
        - Abatacept

Main Indications or Uses
- Acute Care
    - Belatacept
        - Prophylaxis of organ rejection
- Chronic Care
    - Abatacept
        - Psoriatic arthritis
        - Rheumatoid arthritis

Mechanism of Action
- Prevents activation of T-cells by binding to CD80 and CD86 on antigen-presenting cells (APC), blocking the T cell interaction with CD28 and the APCs.

Primary Net Benefit
- Unique therapeutic targets of abatacept and belatacept offer advantages over conventional DMARDs and prevent organ rejection, respectively.
- Main Labs to Monitor:
    - EBV screening (Belatacept)
    - Hepatitis screening
    - Tuberculosis screening

High-Yield Basic Pharmacology
- T-Cell-CD28-APC Interaction
    - Blocking the T-Cell-CD28-APC Interaction, abatacept and belatacept prevent activation of T-cells in synovial fluid (in the case of abatacept and rheumatoid arthritis), preventing T-cell activation post-kidney transplantation from mediators of acute immunologic organ rejection.
- CD28 Signaling
    - The interaction of CD80 and CD86 with CD28 initiates the so-called "signal 2" that produces calcineurin, protein kinases, and NFkB, thus producing activation of T-cells.

High-Yield Clinical Knowledge
- Epstein Barr Virus Screening
    - Patients who may be candidates for belatacept must undergo EBV screening and test negative to be eligible for the drug.
        - Patients with EBV had a higher incidence of posttransplant lymphoproliferative disease (PTLD) than no such cases in EBV-negative patients.
- Progressive multifocal leukoencephalopathy (PML)
    - PML has been reported using belatacept and is a black box warning.
    - A REMS program has been developed, ensuring screening and education for PTLD and PML.
- COPD Risk
    - Abatacept has been associated with increased COPD exacerbations and should be used with caution in this population.

- **Calcineurin Sparing**
  - Belatacept has been proposed as a calcineurin-sparing regimen following renal and liver transplants.
- **Rheumatoid Arthritis (RA)**
  - Abatacept is used to manage RA after conventional DMARDs are not tolerated or fail or can be used in combination with methotrexate.
- **Infection Risk**
  - Patients receiving abatacept are at higher risk of infections, with more than 50% of patients developing an infection in some clinical trials.
    - However, serious infections are rare but may include viral (EBV, HSV), mycobacterial, or fungal.

High-Yield Core Evidence
- **Abatacept Vs. Adalimumab**
  - This was a multicenter, prospective, blinded trial that randomized patients with rheumatoid arthritis to either abatacept or adalimumab, both administered with background methotrexate (MTX).
  - Abatacept demonstrated noninferiority to adalimumab concerning the primary endpoint of the proportion of patients achieving a 20% American College of Rheumatology improvement response (ACR20) at 1 year.
  - Significantly more patients receiving adalimumab experienced injection site reactions than patients receiving abatacept.
  - The authors concluded that abatacept and adalimumab have comparable efficacy in patients with RA, as shown by similar kinetics of response and comparable inhibition of radiographic progression over 1 year of treatment. (Arthritis Rheum. 2013;65(1):28–38.)
- **BENEFIT**
  - This phase III trial compared a more intensive (MI) or less intensive (LI) regimen of belatacept versus cyclosporine in adults receiving a kidney transplant from living or standard criteria deceased donors.
  - There was no difference in patient/graft survival at 12 months.
  - However, belatacept was associated with superior renal function as measured by the composite renal impairment endpoint.
  - However, more patients receiving belatacept patients experienced acute rejection episodes and a higher incidence of a posttransplant lymphoproliferative disorder.
  - The authors concluded that belatacept was associated with superior renal function and similar patient/graft survival versus cyclosporine at 1-year post-transplant, despite a higher rate of early acute rejection. (Am J Transplant. 2010 Mar;10(3):535-46.)

High-Yield Fast-Fact
- **Abatacept/Belatacept Formation**
  - These drugs are products of recombinant fusion proteins composed of the extracellular domain of cytotoxic T-lymphocyte-associated antigen 4, then fused to the Fc domain of human IgG1.

HIGH-YIELD BOARD EXAM ESSENTIALS
- **CLASSIC AGENTS:** Abatacept, belatacept
- **DRUG CLASS:** Selective T-cell costimulation blocker
- **INDICATIONS:** Psoriatic arthritis, rheumatoid arthritis (abatacept), prophylaxis of organ rejection (belatacept)
- **MECHANISM:** Prevents activation of T-cells by binding to CD80 and CD86 on antigen-presenting cells (APC), blocking the T cell interaction with CD28 and the APCs.
- **SIDE EFFECTS:** Increased risk of infections, PML, COPD
- **CLINICAL PEARLS:** Patients receiving abatacept are at higher risk of infections, with more than 50% of patients developing an infection in some clinical trials. However, serious infections are rare but may include viral (EBV, HSV), mycobacterial, or fungal.

Table: Drug Class Summary

\multicolumn{4}{c}{**Selective T-Cell Costimulation Blocker - Drug Class Review**}
\multicolumn{4}{c}{High-Yield Med Reviews}

Mechanism of Action: *Prevents activation of T-cells by binding to CD80 and CD86 on antigen-presenting cells (APC), blocking the T cell interaction with CD28 and the APCs.*

Class Effects: *Unique therapeutic targets of abatacept and belatacept offer advantages over conventional DMARDs and prevent organ rejection, respectively.*

Generic Name	Brand Name	Indication(s) or Uses	Notes

Abatacept	Orencia	• Psoriatic arthritis
		• Rheumatoid arthritis
			• **Dosing (Adult):**
			  – IV: 500 to 1000 mg at 0, 2, 4 weeks, then q4weeks
			  – SQ: 125 mg once weekly
			• **Dosing (Peds):**
			  – IV: 10 mg/kg at 0, 2, 4 weeks, then q4weeks
			    – Maximum 1000 mg/dose
			  – SQ: 50 to 125 mg weekly
			• **CYP450 Interactions:** None
			• **Renal or Hepatic Dose Adjustments:** None
			• **Dosage Forms:** IV (solution), prefilled syringes

Belatacept	Nulojix	• Prophylaxis of organ rejection	• **Dosing (Adult):**
			  – Induction: IV: 10 mg/kg on day 1, 15, 29, 43, and 57 following transplant
			  – Maintenance: IV: 5 mg/kg q4weeks on day 1, 15, 29, 43, and 57 following transplant
			• **Dosing (Peds):** Not routinely used
			• **CYP450 Interactions:** None
			• **Renal or Hepatic Dose Adjustments:** None
			• **Dosage Forms:** IV (solution)

IMMUNOSUPPRESSION – SPHINGOSINE 1-PHOSPHATE (S1P) RECEPTOR MODULATOR

Drug Class
- **Sphingosine 1-Phosphate (S1P) Receptor Modulator**
- **Agents:**
  - Chronic Care
    - Fingolimod
    - Ozanimod
    - Ponesimod
    - Siponimod

Main Indications or Uses
- **Chronic Care**
  - Multiple Sclerosis
    - Ponesimod
    - Siponimod
  - Relapsing multiple sclerosis
    - Fingolimod
    - Ozanimod

Mechanism of Action
- Specifically isolates lymphocytes into the lymph nodes and Peyer patches, away from the circulation, preventing lesions and grafts from T-cell-mediated attacks.

Primary Net Benefit
- Oral medications for relapsing multiple sclerosis management, with significantly improved safety profiles with newer agents in this class.
- Main Labs to Monitor:
  - CBC
  - Liver enzyme and liver function tests
  - Ophthalmologic examination
  - ECG (to evaluate for QT prolongation)

High-Yield Basic Pharmacology
- **T-Cell Sequestration**
  - In addition to its effect on T-cells in the peripheral circulation, fingolimod may also provide a neuroprotective effect by reducing T-lymphocytes' infiltration and macrophages into the CNS.
- **B and T Cell Function**
  - Although these agents sequester t cells, there is no B cell or T cell function impairment.
- **S1P Function**
  - The S1P receptor is normally responsible for controlling lymphocyte release from lymph nodes and the thymus.
  - S1P receptors are also expressed on neurons, particularly in neurodegeneration and repair mechanisms, identified as the S1P receptor modulators' therapeutic target for multiple sclerosis.

High-Yield Clinical Knowledge
- **First Dose Bradycardia**
  - Fingolimod is associated with first dose bradycardia, including bradyarrhythmias such as AV block.
  - Patients must be observed for at least 6 hours after the first dose and longer periods in patients at high risk (pre-existing cardiac disease).
    - Ozanimod does not appear to cause bradycardia or heart block in patients receiving this drug in clinical studies.

- **QT Prolongation**
  - Fingolimod has been associated with QT interval prolongation and risk of torsades de pointes.
  - Concomitant QT-prolonging drugs should be avoided, including amiodarone, dronedarone, dofetilide, ibutilide, sotalol, procainamide, quinidine, and disopyramide.
- **Pre-existing Cardiac Disease**
  - Patients with type II or III heart block, recent myocardial infarction, or heart failure should also not receive fingolimod due to excessive risk of cardiac toxicity.
    - The bradycardia associated with fingolimod further increases the risk of arrhythmias due to QT interval prolongation.
- **Adverse Events**
  - Other common adverse events include infections, macular edema, decreased FEV1 in patients with respiratory disease, liver enzyme elevations, increases in blood pressure, and lymphoma.
- **Ulcerative Colitis**
  - Ozanimod may also play a role in the disease management of Ulcerative Colitis, with evidence front the TOUCHSTONE trial supporting its increased remission incidence compared to placebo.
- **Ozanimod Selectivity**
  - Ozanimod is also an S1P receptor modulator but specifically binds to the subtypes 1 and 5, whereas fingolimod and siponimod appear less selective.
  - The clinical relevance of S1P subtype selectivity has yet to be fully elucidated.

High-Yield Core Evidence
- **TRANSFORMS Study**
  - This prospective, double-blind, double-dummy, phase 3 study of patients with relapsing-remitting multiple sclerosis who had a recent history of at least one relapse was randomized to receive either oral fingolimod (studied at two different doses) or intramuscular interferon beta-1.
  - Patients receiving either dose of fingolimod experienced significant improvements in the primary outcome of the annualized relapse rate and fewer or enlarged lesions on T(2)-weighted magnetic resonance imaging scans at 12 months and progression of disability sustained for at least 3 months.
  - However, two fatal infections occurred in the group that received the 1.25-mg dose of fingolimod and nonfatal herpesvirus infections, bradycardia, atrioventricular block, hypertension, macular edema, skin cancer, and elevated liver enzyme levels.
  - The authors concluded that oral fingolimod was superior to interferon therapy concerning relapse rates and MRI outcomes in patients with multiple sclerosis. (N Engl J Med. 2010 Feb 4;362(5):402-15.)
- **RADIANCE**
  - This was a multicenter, double-blind, double-dummy, phase 3 trial that randomized patients with relapsing multiple sclerosis to either ozanimod (studied at two different doses) or interferon beta-1a.
  - Patients receiving either ozanimod dose experienced significant improvements in the primary outcome of the annualized relapse rate compared to patients receiving interferon beta-1a.
  - More patients randomized to interferon experienced treatment-emergent adverse events, including serious adverse events, than in the ozanimod at either dose studied.
  - There were no cases of ozanimod-related symptomatic reduction in heart rate, and no second-degree or third-degree cases of the atrioventricular block were reported.
  - The authors concluded that in patients with relapsing multiple sclerosis, ozanimod was well tolerated and associated with a significantly lower clinical relapses rate than intramuscular interferon beta-1a. (Lancet Neurol. 2019 Nov;18(11):1021-1033.)

High-Yield Fast-Fact
- **Comparison Data**
  - While ozanimod's potential benefits may improve safety with S1P receptor modulator therapy of MS, there is a lack of robust head-to-head data comparing other agents in this class, such as fingolimod and siponimod.

HIGH-YIELD BOARD EXAM ESSENTIALS
- **CLASSIC AGENTS:** Fingolimod, ozanimod, siponimod
- **DRUG CLASS:** Sphingosine 1-phosphate receptor modulator
- **INDICATIONS:** Relapsing multiple sclerosis
- **MECHANISM:** Specifically isolates lymphocytes into the lymph nodes and Peyer patches, away from the circulation, preventing lesions and grafts from T-cell-mediated attacks.
- **SIDE EFFECTS:** Bradycardia (first dose), QT prolongation, infections, macular edema, decreased FEV1 in patients with respiratory disease, liver enzyme elevations, increases in blood pressure, and lymphoma
- **CLINICAL PEARLS:** Fingolimod is associated with first dose bradycardia, which may include bradyarrhythmias such as AV block. Patients must be observed for at least 6 hours after the first dose and longer periods of time in patients at high risk (pre-existing cardiac disease).

Table: Drug Class Summary

Sphingosine 1-Phosphate (S1P) Receptor Modulator - Drug Class Review				
High-Yield Med Reviews				
Mechanism of Action: *Specifically isolates lymphocytes into the lymph nodes and Peyer patches away from the circulation, preventing lesions and grafts from T-cell-mediated attacks.*				
Class Effects: *Oral medications for relapsing multiple sclerosis management, with significantly improved safety profiles with newer agents in this class.*				
Generic Name	**Brand Name**	**Indication(s) or Uses**	**Notes**	

Fingolimod	Gilenya	• Relapsing multiple sclerosis	• **Dosing (Adult):**
			   – Oral: 0.5 mg daily
			• **Dosing (Peds):**
			   – 40 kg or less: 0.25 mg daily
			• **CYP450 Interactions:** Substrate of CYP3A4, CYP4F2
			• **Renal or Hepatic Dose Adjustments:** None
			• **Dosage Forms:** Oral (capsule)	

Ozanimod	Zeposia	• Relapsing multiple sclerosis	• **Dosing (Adult):**
			   – Oral: 0.23 mg daily on days 1-4, then 0.46 mg daily on days 5-7, then 0.92 mg starting day 8
			• **Dosing (Peds):**
			   – Not routinely used
			• **CYP450 Interactions:** Substrate of CYP2C8, CYP3A4
			• **Renal or Hepatic Dose Adjustments:** None
			• **Dosage Forms:** Oral (capsule)	

Ponesimod	Ponvory	• Multiple sclerosis	• **Dosing (Adult):**
			   – Oral: initial titration day 1 – 20, start at 2 mg increasing to target 20 mg/day
			• **Dosing (Peds):**
			   – Not routinely used
			• **CYP450 Interactions:** Substrate CYP2C9
			• **Renal or Hepatic Dose Adjustments:** Child-Pugh class B or C, avoid use
			• **Dosage Forms:** Oral (tablet)	

Siponimod	Mayzent	• Multiple sclerosis	• **Dosing (Adult):**
			   – Oral: 0.25 mg daily x2, then 0.5 mg x1, 0.75 mg x1, then 1.25 mg daily
			      – Dosing adjusted based on CYP2C9 genotype
			• **Dosing (Peds):**
			   – Not routinely used
			• **CYP450 Interactions:** Substrate CYP2C9
			• **Renal or Hepatic Dose Adjustments:** None
			• **Dosage Forms:** Oral (tablet)	

IMMUNOSUPPRESSANTS – TNF-ALPHA INHIBITORS

Drug Class
- TNF-Alpha Inhibitors
- Agents:
    - Chronic Care
        - Adalimumab
        - Certolizumab
        - Etanercept
        - Golimumab
        - Infliximab

Main Indications or Uses
- Chronic Care
    - Ankylosing spondylitis
        - Adalimumab
        - Certolizumab
        - Etanercept
        - Golimumab
        - Infliximab
    - Axial spondyloarthritis
        - Certolizumab
    - Crohn's disease
        - Adalimumab
        - Certolizumab
        - Etanercept
        - Infliximab
    - Hidradenitis suppurativa
        - Adalimumab
    - Juvenile idiopathic arthritis
        - Adalimumab
        - Etanercept
        - Golimumab
    - Plaque psoriasis
        - Adalimumab
        - Certolizumab
        - Etanercept
        - Infliximab
    - Psoriatic arthritis
        - Adalimumab
        - Certolizumab
        - Etanercept
        - Golimumab
        - Infliximab
    - Rheumatoid arthritis
        - Adalimumab
        - Certolizumab
        - Etanercept
        - Golimumab
        - Infliximab
    - Ulcerative colitis
        - Adalimumab
        - Golimumab

Warnings & Alerts

✓ It is important to test for the presence of latent TB because failure to do prior to initiation of any TNF-alpha antagonist as it could result in the activation of TB. There are cases of disseminated TB that can lead to death.

✓ Avoid the use of TNF-alpha antagonists in patients with class III or IV heart failure.

Dosing Pearls

✓ Golimumab and infliximab can be given by IV infusion whereas as most TNF-alpha antagonists are given by SQ injection.

- Infliximab
- Uveitis
  - Adalimumab

Mechanism of Action
- Anti-TNF-alpha drugs complex with TNF-alpha prevent interaction with the cell surface receptors p55 and/or p75 that ultimately down-regulate macrophage and T-cell function.

Primary Net Benefit
- TNF-alpha inhibitors are primarily used for rheumatoid arthritis generally after disease activity remains moderate or high despite conventional DMARD therapy, and cost and safety may limit its use.
- Main Labs to Monitor:
  - CBC with differential
  - Screening for tuberculosis
  - Hepatitis B screening
  - Signs/symptoms of malignancy and serious infections

High-Yield Basic Pharmacology
- **MAB Source**
  - Adalimumab, certolizumab, and golimumab are fully-humanized monoclonal antibodies, but subtle differences may confer different pharmacologic or pharmacokinetic actions.
    - Certolizumab is a humanized antibody Fab fragment that lacks the Fc region, potentially leading to decreased antibody-dependent cell-mediated cytotoxicity and reduced complement response.
- **Chimeric Antibody**
  - Infliximab is a chimeric monoclonal antibody of mouse and human origin.
    - This chimeric nature increases the risk and incidence of adverse immunologic reactions, potentially limiting therapy.
- **Fusion Protein**
  - Etanercept is not a monoclonal antibody like the other agents in this class.
  - Instead, it is a recombinant fusion protein of two TNF p75 receptor site moieties joined to the Fc portion of human IgG1.
    - Etanercept is capable of binding to both TNF-alpha and lymphotoxin-alpha.

High-Yield Clinical Knowledge
- **Heart Failure Warning**
  - TNF-alpha inhibitor initiation has been associated with new-onset or acute worsening of existing heart failure.
    - As a result, these agents should be avoided in patients with a New York Heart Association class III/IV heart failure history.
- **Infliximab Infusion Reaction and Antibodies**
  - A high proportion of patients (up to 15%) receiving infliximab develop antibodies to infliximab.
  - Antibody development is associated with a higher risk of infusion reactions, more rapid infliximab clearance, and decreased efficacy.
  - The risk of antibody development can be reduced with the concomitant use of methotrexate.
  - Infusion reactions can be mitigated using pre-infusion antihistamines, acetaminophen, and corticosteroids.
- **Skin Cancer Risk**
  - The TNF-alpha inhibitor agents' increased risk of skin cancer and melanoma is a class effect.
    - Patients should undergo routine skin examinations to closely monitor these cancer types in patients at high risk.
- **Infection Risk**
  - All TNF-alpha inhibitors are associated with an increased risk of infections in patients prescribed these agents.

- Infections of concern related to TNF-alpha agents include opportunistic bacterial infections, tuberculosis, viral (hepatitis), or fungal infections.
- **TNF-Alpha Inhibitor in Pregnancy**
  - Careful selection of TNF-alpha agents for pregnant patients is necessary, but certolizumab demonstrated a safer experience in pregnancy patients.
  - Certolizumab is associated with minimal to no placental transfer to the fetus.
  - Similarly, there is no too small transfer from plasma to breast milk.
- **Neutropenias and Demyelinating Disorders**
  - The TNF-alpha inhibitors are associated with an increased risk of neutropenias, leukopenia, thrombocytopenia, or pancytopenia.
  - These agents have been rarely associated with new-onset or acute worsening of demyelinating disorders (multiple sclerosis).

High-Yield Core Evidence
- **Certolizumab Plus Methotrexate**
  - This phase III, multicenter, double-blind, placebo-controlled, parallel-group trial randomized patients with rheumatoid arthritis with an inadequate response to MTX therapy alone to either certolizumab plus methotrexate or placebo plus methotrexate.
  - Certolizumab plus methotrexate led to a significantly improved co-primary endpoint of the response rate at week 24 using the American College of Rheumatology 20% criteria for improvement and the mean change from baseline in the modified total Sharp score at week 52.
  - These observed differences were significant as fast as one week after therapy initiation and were sustained through the study period.
  - Certolizumab also led to a reduction in mean radiographic progression from baseline compared with that in placebo-treated patients.
  - The authors concluded that certolizumab plus methotrexate resulted in a rapid and sustained reduction in rheumatoid arthritis signs and symptoms, inhibited the progression of structural joint damage, and improved physical function compared with placebo plus methotrexate treatment. (Arthritis Rheum. 2008 Nov;58(11):3319-29.)
- **NORD-STAR**
  - This investigator-initiated, open-label, blinded assessor, multiarm, phase IV study randomized patients with early treatment-naive rheumatoid arthritis to either active conventional treatment (with either prednisolone or sulfasalazine plus hydroxychloroquine and intra-articular corticosteroids), certolizumab pegol, abatacept, or tocilizumab.
  - At 24 weeks, abatacept was the only therapy associated with a significant improvement in the primary outcome of adjusted clinical disease activity index remission (CDAI) at 24 weeks with active conventional treatment as the reference.
  - The observed differences in CDAI remission rates for active conventional treatment versus certolizumab and tocilizumab, but not abatacept, remained within the prespecified non-inferiority margin of 15%.
  - Numerically fewer patients receiving abatacept or tocilizumab experienced severe adverse events and/or stopped treatment early due to adverse events.
  - The authors concluded that each of the four treatments achieved high remission rates. Still, a higher CDAI remission rate was observed for abatacept versus active conventional treatment, but not for certolizumab pegol or tocilizumab versus active traditional treatment. In addition, the non-inferiority analysis indicated that active conventional treatment was non-inferior to certolizumab pegol and tocilizumab but not to abatacept. (BMJ. 2020 Dec 2;371:m4328.)

High-Yield Fast-Fact
- **Dubious Natural TNF Inhibition**
  - Some natural compounds have been suggested to have TNF-alpha inhibitor effects, including curcumin, catechins, and cannabinoids.
  - The clinical relevance of this effect in commonly available products is not currently known.

HIGH-YIELD BOARD EXAM ESSENTIALS
- **CLASSIC AGENTS:** Adalimumab, certolizumab, etanercept, golimumab, infliximab
- **DRUG CLASS:** TNF-alpha inhibitors
- **INDICATIONS:** Ankylosing spondylitis, axial spondyloarthritis, Crohn's disease, hidradenitis suppurativa, juvenile idiopathic arthritis, plaque psoriasis, psoriatic arthritis, rheumatoid arthritis, ulcerative colitis, uveitis
- **MECHANISM:** Complex with TNF-alpha, preventing its interaction with the cell surface receptors p55 and/or p75 that ultimately down-regulate macrophage and T-cell function.
- **SIDE EFFECTS:** Increased risk of infection, neutropenia, leukopenia, thrombocytopenia, pancytopenia, demyelinating disorders
- **CLINICAL PEARLS:**
  - TNF-alpha inhibitor initiation has been associated with new-onset or acute worsening of existing heart failure. As a result, these agents should be avoided in patients with a history of New York Heart Association class III/IV heart failure.
  - In addition, patients should be screened for the presence of latent TB and started on TB therapy prior to initiating these agents due to conversion to an active infection.

Table: Drug Class Summary

TNF-Alpha Inhibitors - Drug Class Review			
High-Yield Med Reviews			
Mechanism of Action: *Anti-TNF-alpha drugs complex with TNF-alpha prevent interaction with the cell surface receptors p55 and/or p75 that ultimately down-regulate macrophage and T-cell function.*			
Class Effects: *TNF-alpha inhibitors are used mainly for rheumatoid arthritis generally after disease activity remains moderate or high despite conventional DMARD therapy but may be limited by cost and safety.*			
Generic Name	**Brand Name**	**Main Indication(s) or Uses**	**Notes**
Adalimumab	Humira	<ul><li>Ankylosing spondylitis</li><li>Crohn's disease</li><li>Hidradenitis suppurativa</li><li>Juvenile idiopathic arthritis</li><li>Plaque psoriasis</li><li>Psoriatic arthritis</li><li>Rheumatoid arthritis</li><li>Ulcerative colitis</li><li>Uveitis</li></ul>	<ul><li>**Dosing (Adult):** − SQ: 80 to 160 mg once, then 40 mg q1-2weeks</li><li>**Dosing (Peds):** − 17 to < 40 kg: SQ 80 mg once, then 20 to 40 mg q1-2weeks</li><li>**CYP450 Interactions:** None</li><li>**Renal or Hepatic Dose Adjustments:** None</li><li>**Dosage Forms:** Prefilled syringe kit</li></ul>
Certolizumab	Cimzia	<ul><li>Ankylosing spondylitis</li><li>Axial spondyloarthritis</li><li>Crohn's disease</li><li>Plaque psoriasis</li><li>Psoriatic arthritis</li><li>Rheumatoid arthritis</li></ul>	<ul><li>**Dosing (Adult):** − SQ: 400 mg repeat dose 2 and 4 weeks after initial dose, followed by 200 mg q2weeks or 400 mg q4weeks</li><li>**Dosing (Peds):** Not routinely used</li><li>**CYP450 Interactions:** None</li><li>**Renal or Hepatic Dose Adjustments:** None</li><li>**Dosage Forms:** Prefilled syringe kit</li></ul>
Etanercept	Enbrel	<ul><li>Ankylosing spondylitis</li><li>Juvenile idiopathic arthritis</li><li>Plaque psoriasis</li><li>Psoriatic arthritis</li><li>Rheumatoid arthritis</li></ul>	<ul><li>**Dosing (Adult):** − SQ: 25-50 mg twice weekly or 50 mg weekly</li><li>**Dosing (Peds):** − < 63 kg: 0.8 mg/kg/dose weekly; Max: 50 mg/dose</li><li>**CYP450 Interactions:** None</li><li>**Renal or Hepatic Dose Adjustments:** None</li><li>**Dosage Forms:** Prefilled syringe kit, solution for subcutaneous injection</li></ul>
Golimumab	Simponi	<ul><li>Ankylosing spondylitis</li><li>Juvenile idiopathic arthritis</li><li>Psoriatic arthritis</li><li>Rheumatoid arthritis</li><li>Ulcerative colitis</li></ul>	<ul><li>**Dosing (Adult):** − IV: 2 mg/kg at weeks 0, 4, then q8weeks − SQ: 50 mg q1month</li><li>**Dosing (Peds):** − IV: 80 mg/m^2/dose at week 0, 4, then q8weeks − SQ: 90-200 mg/m2 at week 0 then 45 mg/m2 at week 2 and 1 month thereafter</li><li>**CYP450 Interactions:** None</li><li>**Renal or Hepatic Dose Adjustments:** None</li><li>**Dosage Forms:** IV (solution), Prefilled syringe kit</li></ul>
Infliximab	Avsola Inflectra Remicade Renflexis	<ul><li>Ankylosing spondylitis</li><li>Crohn's disease</li><li>Plaque psoriasis</li><li>Psoriatic arthritis</li><li>Rheumatoid arthritis</li><li>Ulcerative colitis</li></ul>	<ul><li>**Dosing (Adult):** − IV: 5 mg/kg at 0, 2 and 6 weeks, then 5 mg/kg q6weeks</li><li>**Dosing (Peds):** − IV: 5 mg/kg at 0, 2, & 6 weeks; 5 mg/kg q6weeks</li><li>**CYP450 Interactions:** None</li><li>**Renal or Hepatic Dose Adjustments:** None</li><li>**Dosage Forms:** IV (solution)</li></ul>

PULMONOLOGY – LEUKOTRIENE MODIFIERS

Drug Class
- Leukotriene Modifiers
- Agents:
  - Chronic Care
    - Montelukast
    - Zafirlukast
    - Zileuton

> 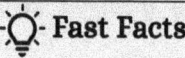 **Fast Facts**
> - ✓ Montelukast is the most common agent in this class used in clinical practice due to easy dosing, once-a-day administration, and least amount of drug interactions.
> - ✓ These agents are for maintenance or prevention of asthma, not acute treatment.

Main Indications or Uses
- Chronic Care
  - Allergic rhinitis (montelukast)
  - Asthma (montelukast, zafirlukast, zileuton)
  - Exercise-induced bronchoconstriction (montelukast, zafirlukast, zileuton)

Mechanism of Action
- Montelukast, Zafirlukast
  - Inhibit the binding of leukotriene D4 to its receptor on target tissues.
- Zileuton
  - Inhibit 5-Lipoxygenase, reducing arachidonic acid synthesis.

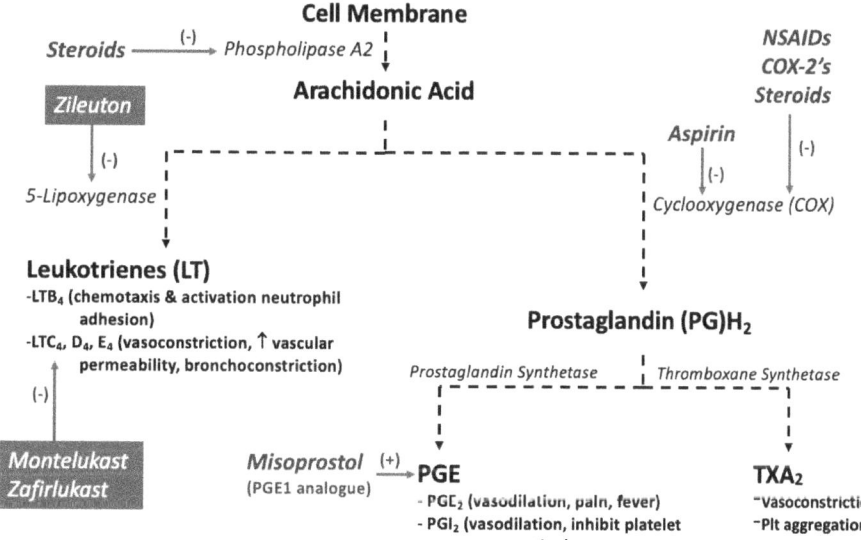

Primary Net Benefit
- Improve asthma control in poorly controlled asthma and reduce the frequency of asthma exacerbations but are less effective than inhaled corticosteroids in mild asthma.
- Main Labs to Monitor:
  - Liver enzymes (AST/ALT)
  - Liver function (INR/PT, albumin, protein, bilirubin)
  - FEV1, FVC (if using as part of the management of asthma)

High-Yield Basic Pharmacology

- **Leukotriene Effects**
  - Leukotriene modifiers reduce the impact of leukotrienes on the respiratory tract by limiting bronchospasm and airway hyperresponsiveness.
  - As airway leukotrienes are also responsible for plasma exudation, mucus secretion, and eosinophilic inflammation, inhibitors of leukotrienes improve airway function by limiting their production.
- **Drug Interactions**
  - Zafirlukast is an inhibitor of CYP2C9 and, as a result, can decrease the elimination of narrow therapeutic index drugs, including warfarin or theophylline.
    - Increased INR monitoring should occur when starting or titrating zafirlukast in the presence of a CYP2C9 substrate.

High-Yield Clinical Knowledge

- **Cardiac and Hepatic Injury**
  - Hepatic injury is a rare effect secondary to leukotriene modifiers and necessitates routine liver-enzyme monitoring.
    - Zileuton carries the highest risk of hepatic injury, occurring within three months after starting therapy.
  - Leukotriene modifiers have been associated with new-onset eosinophilic vasculitis targeting cardiac, peripheral nerves, and renal tissue, known as Churg-Strauss syndrome.
- **Taken with Food**
  - In some children with poor compliance with inhaled LABA or ICS therapy, oral leukotriene modifiers can improve asthma control.
  - Montelukast is available as a once-daily oral preparation that can be taken without regard to food but has only a modest effect on pulmonary function improvements.
  - Zafirlukast must be taken on an empty stomach, as food significantly decreases absorption.
- **Add-On Therapy**
  - Leukotriene modifiers are unsuitable for monotherapy and should not replace LABA or ICS therapy in asthma.
  - Asthma control must be achieved in severe asthma patients before adding leukotriene modifiers.
- **Aspirin-Exacerbated Respiratory Disease (AERD)**
  - As a result of the shifting arachidonic acid metabolism in AERD to the leukotriene pathway, montelukast, zafirlukast, and zileuton have been shown to reduce this response to aspirin and improve asthma control.
    - AERD does not involve immune sensitization to aspirin, as it is not a true allergy, but it can produce severe bronchospasm due to arachidonic acid activation.
- **COPD**
  - Leukotriene modifiers should not be used in patients with COPD.
- **Neuropsychiatric Effects**
  - Children receiving montelukast are 12 times more likely to experience adverse neuropsychiatric effects than children receiving ICS.
    - Neuropsychiatric symptoms associated with montelukast include irritability, aggressiveness, and sleep disturbances.

High-Yield Core Evidence

- **Leukotriene Modifier Cochrane Review**
  - This was a systematic review and meta-analysis to determine if adding a leukotriene receptor antagonist (LTRA) produces a beneficial effect in children and adults with acute asthma who are currently receiving inhaled bronchodilators and systemic corticosteroids.
  - Studies were included if they were randomized trials comparing antileukotrienes and standard acute asthma care versus placebo and standard care in people with acute asthma of any age.
  - The authors observed no significant difference in hospital admission between LTRAs and control.
  - Adult study subjects receiving LTRAs showed improvement in forced expiratory volume in one second (FEV1), but not in children.

- The authors concluded that the available evidence does not support the routine use of oral LTRAs in acute asthma. (Cochrane Database Syst Rev. 2012 May 16;2012(5): CD006100.)

High-Yield Fast-Fact
- **Exercise-Induced Bronchospasm**
  - Montelukast can be used to prevent exercise-induced bronchospasm and, for this indication, should be taken at least 2 hours before physical exertion.

HIGH-YIELD BOARD EXAM ESSENTIALS
- **CLASSIC AGENTS:** Montelukast, zafirlukast, zileuton
- **DRUG CLASS:** Leukotriene modifiers
- **INDICATIONS:** Asthma, COPD
- **MECHANISM:** Montelukast, Zafirlukast - Inhibit the binding of leukotriene D4 to its receptor on target tissues. Zileuton - Inhibit 5-Lipoxygenase, reducing arachidonic acid synthesis.
- **SIDE EFFECTS:** Irritability, aggressiveness, and sleep disturbances
- **CLINICAL PEARLS:**
  - Hepatic injury is a rare effect secondary to leukotriene modifiers and necessitates routine liver-enzyme monitoring.
  - Leukotriene modifiers have been associated with new-onset eosinophilic vasculitis targeting cardiac, peripheral nerves, and renal tissue known as Churg-Strauss syndrome.

Table: Drug Class Summary

Leukotriene Modifiers - Drug Class Review High-Yield Med Reviews			
Mechanism of Action: *Montelukast, Zafirlukast - Inhibit the binding of leukotriene D4 to its receptor on target tissues.* *Zileuton - Inhibit 5-Lipoxygenase, reducing arachidonic acid synthesis.*			
Class Effects: *Improve asthma control in poorly controlled asthma and reduce the frequency of asthma exacerbations but are less effective than inhaled corticosteroids in mild asthma.*			
Generic Name	**Brand Name**	**Main Indication(s) or Uses**	**Notes**

Zileuton	Zyflo	• Asthma	• **Dosing (Adult):**
			   – Oral: IR 600 mg q6h
			   – Oral: ER 1,200 mg q12h
			 • **Dosing (Peds):**
			   – Oral: IR 600 mg q6h
			   – Oral: ER 1,200 mg q12h
			     – Maximum 2,400 mg/day
			 • **CYP450 Interactions:** Substrate CYP1A2, 2C9, 3A4; Inhibits CYP1A2
			 • **Renal or Hepatic Dose Adjustments:**
			   – Active liver disease or AST/ALT greater than 3x upper limit of normal - Contraindicated
			 • **Dosage Forms:** Oral (Tablet)

Montelukast	Singulair	• Allergic rhinitis
		 • Asthma
		 • Exercise-induced bronchoconstriction
			• **Dosing (Adult):**
			   – Oral: 10 mg daily
			 • **Dosing (Peds):**
			   – Oral: 4 to 10 mg daily
			 • **CYP450 Interactions:** Substrate CYP2C8, 2C9, 3A4
			 • **Renal or Hepatic Dose Adjustments:** None
			 • **Dosage Forms:** Oral (packet, tablet)

Zafirlukast	Accolate	• Asthma	• **Dosing (Adult):**
			   – Oral: 20 mg BID
			 • **Dosing (Peds):**
			   – Oral: 10 to 20 mg BID
			 • **CYP450 Interactions:** Substrate CYP2C9; Inhibits CYP2C9
			 • **Renal or Hepatic Dose Adjustments:**
			   – Hepatic impairment - Contraindicated
			 • **Dosage Forms:** Oral (tablet)

VACCINES – GENERAL CONCEPTS

Drug Class
- Agents:
  - **Diphtheria**
    - Diphtheria and tetanus toxoids adsorbed, DT (TDVax)
    - Diphtheria and tetanus toxoids and acellular pertussis vaccine adsorbed, DTaP (Daptacel, Infanrix)
    - Diphtheria and tetanus toxoids and acellular pertussis adsorbed, hepatitis B and inactivated poliovirus vaccine, DTaP-HepB-IPV (Pediarix)
    - Diphtheria and tetanus toxoids and acellular pertussis adsorbed and inactivated poliovirus vaccine, DTaP-IPV (Kinrix, Quadracel)
    - Diphtheria and tetanus toxoids and acellular pertussis adsorbed, inactivated poliovirus and Haemophilus influenzae type b conjugate vaccine, DTaP-IPV/Hib (Pentacel)
  - **Haemophilus b**
    - Haemophilus b conjugate vaccine, Hib (PedvaxHIB, Hiberix, ActHIB)
    - Haemophilus influenzae type b conjugate and hepatitis B vaccine, Hib-HepB (Comvax)
  - **Hepatitis**
    - Hepatitis A vaccine, HepA (Havrix, Vaqta)
    - Hepatitis B vaccine, HepB (Engerix-B, Recombivax HB)
    - Hepatitis B vaccine, HepB-CpG (HEPLISAV-B)
    - Hepatitis A inactivated and hepatitis B vaccine, HepA-HepB (Twinrix)
  - **Herpes zoster**
    - Zoster vaccine live, ZVL (Zostavax)
    - Zoster vaccine recombinant, RZV (Shingrix)
  - **Human papillomavirus**
    - Human papillomavirus 9-valent, 9vHPV (Gardasil 9)
    - Human papillomavirus quadrivalent, 4vHPV (Gardasil)
    - Human papillomavirus bivalent, 2vHPV (Cervarix)
  - **Influenza**
    - Trivalent inactivated influenza vaccine, IIV3 (Afluria, Fluad, Fluarix, Flucelvax, FluLaval, Fluzone)
    - Quadrivalent inactivated influenza vaccine, IIV4 (Fluarix)
    - Live attenuated influenza vaccine, LAIV (FluMist)
  - **Measles, mumps, and rubella vaccine**
    - Measles, mumps, and rubella vaccine, MMR (MMR II)
    - Measles, mumps, rubella, and varicella vaccine, MMRV (ProQuad)
  - **Meningococcal**
    - Quadrivalent meningococcal conjugate vaccine, MenACWY, MenACWY-D, MenACWY CRM (Menactra, Menveo)
    - Serogroup B meningococcal vaccines, MenB, MenB-4c, MenB-FHbp (Bexsero, Trumenba)
    - Bivalent meningococcal conjugate vaccine and Haemophilus influenza type b conjugate vaccine, Hib-MenCY (MenHibrix)
    - Meningococcal polysaccharide vaccine, MPSV4 (Menomune)
  - **Pneumococcal**
    - Pneumococcal conjugate vaccine 13 valent, PCV13 (Prevnar 13)
    - Pneumococcal polysaccharide vaccine 23 valent, PPSV23 (Pneumovax 23)
  - **Poliovirus**
    - Inactivated poliovirus vaccine, IPV (Ipol)
  - **Rotavirus**
    - Rotavirus vaccine monovalent, RV1 (Rotarix)
    - Rotavirus vaccine pentavalent, RV5 (RotaTeq)
  - **SARS-CoV-2**
    - AstraZeneca Oxford

- Johnson & Johnson's Janssen
- Moderna
- Pfizer-BioNTech
- **Tetanus**
    - Tetanus and diphtheria toxoids adsorbed, Td (Decavac, Tenivac)
    - Tetanus toxoid adsorbed, TT
    - Tetanus toxoid, reduced diphtheria toxoid, and acellular pertussis vaccine, adsorbed, Tdap (Adacel, Boostrix)
- **Varicella**
    - Varicella vaccine, VAR (Varivax)
- **Immunoglobulins**
    - Hepatitis B immune globulin
    - Rho(D) immune globulin
    - Tetanus immune globulin
    - Varicella-zoster immune globulin

Primary Net Benefit
- Induce an active immune response to numerous diseases that improve morbidity, mortality, and public health.
- Main Labs to Monitor:
    - No routine monitoring

High-Yield Basic Pharmacology
- **Live Attenuated Vaccines**
    - Intranasal influenza, MMR, rotavirus, varicella vaccine (Varivax), and zoster vaccine (ZVL, Zostavax) are live attenuated vaccines.
    - Certain vaccines use a weakened form of a virus that contains antigens directed to stimulate an immune response.
    - Viruses used in such vaccines have been manipulated to reduce virulence but maintain immunogenic antigens capable of eliciting humoral and cellular responses sufficient for memory cell development.
    - Viruses of live attenuated vaccines can mutate in vivo and possibly become virulent, leading to disease.
    - Live attenuated viruses cannot be used in pregnant patients, immunocompromised patients, such as those with active cancer or HIV
- **Inactivated Vaccines**
    - Influenza, polio, and rabies are examples of inactivated vaccines.
    - Inactivated vaccines are developed using chemicals, heat, or radiation to inactivate pathogens that produce antigenic responses.
    - These vaccine types induce an immune response similar, although much weaker than the natural infection, and require multiple doses to sustain immunity to the pathogen.
- **Subunit Vaccines**
    - Vaccines contain components of the microorganism to elicit an antigenic response that mimics the organism's response.
    - These vaccines contain surface proteins or toxins but elicit a less-robust immune response than live attenuated viruses.
    - Subunit vaccines can be polysaccharide subunits, surface protein subunits, or toxoids.
        - Polysaccharide vaccines (Hib, PCV13) are often bound to carrier proteins (diphtheria) to elicit sustained disease protection.
        - Surface protein subunits such as acellular pertussis (DTaP, Tdap) and hepatitis B vaccines utilize purified proteins from the pathogen to induce an immune response.
        - Toxoids elicit an immune response to the toxin produced by Clostridium tetani (tetanus) or Corynebacterium diphtheria (diphtheria).
            - Toxoids are often formulated with aluminum salts that induce an inflammatory response and enhance their antigenicity.

- **DNA Vaccines**
  - DNA vaccines such as the SARS-CoV-2 vaccines (AstraZeneca Oxford or Johnson & Johnson's Janssen), Zika virus vaccine, or CMV vaccines use encapsulated viral DNA expressing a target protein and introducing it to the host cell cytoplasm. The host nucleus then utilizes host enzymes to convert the delivered viral DNA component into RNA to produce ribosomes to develop proteins (translation) to express either MHC-1 or 2 proteins.
- **Immunoglobulins**
  - Vaccinations confer B-cell expansion and differentiation to memory cells that maintain long-term protection.
  - Immunoglobulins provide passive immunity by providing human-derived Ig antibodies that the host does not produce.

Table: Drug Class Summary

\multicolumn{4}{c}{**Vaccines - Drug Class Review**}

Generic Name	**Brand Name**	**Vaccine Format**	**Notes**
\multicolumn{4}{c}{Diphtheria}
Diphtheria and tetanus toxoids adsorbed, DT	TDVax	• Toxoid	• **Dosing (Adult):** – IM: 0.5 mL every 10 years if pertussis vaccine contraindicated • **Dosing (Peds):** – For children at least 6 weeks old to 7 years old, or if pertussis vaccine contraindicated – IM: 0.5 mL for 5 doses • **Contraindications & Allergies:** – Anaphylaxis to previous DT or any other vaccine containing any similar component • **Dosage Forms:** Intramuscular suspension
Diphtheria and tetanus toxoids and acellular pertussis vaccine adsorbed, DTaP	Daptacel, Infanrix	• Toxoid • Inactivated (bacterial)	• **Dosing (Adult):** – Not routinely used • **Dosing (Peds):** – For children at least 6 weeks old to 7 years old – IM: 0.5 mL for 5 doses • **Contraindications & Allergies:** – Anaphylaxis to previous DTaP or any other vaccine containing any similar component – Encephalopathy within 7 days of pertussis vaccine • **Dosage Forms:** Intramuscular suspension
Diphtheria and tetanus toxoids and acellular pertussis adsorbed, hepatitis B and inactivated poliovirus vaccine, DTaP-HepB-IPV	Pediarix	• Toxoid • Inactivated (bacterial) • Inactivated (viral)	• **Dosing (Adult):** – Not routinely used • **Dosing (Peds):** – For children at least 6 weeks old to 7 years old – IM: 0.5 mL for 3 doses • **Contraindications & Allergies:** – Anaphylaxis to any other vaccine containing any similar component – Encephalopathy within 7 days of pertussis vaccine – Progressive neurologic disorders • **Dosage Forms:** Intramuscular suspension

Vaccines - Drug Class Review
High-Yield Med Reviews

Generic Name	Brand Name	Vaccine Format	Notes
Diphtheria and tetanus toxoids and acellular pertussis adsorbed and inactivated poliovirus vaccine, DTaP-IPV	Kinrix, Quadracel	<ul><li>Toxoid</li><li>Inactivated (bacterial)</li><li>Inactivated (viral)</li></ul>	<ul><li>**Dosing (Adult):**<ul><li>Not routinely used</li></ul></li><li>**Dosing (Peds):**<ul><li>For children at least 6 weeks old to 7 years old</li><li>IM: 0.5 mL once</li></ul></li><li>**Contraindications & Allergies:**<ul><li>Anaphylaxis to any other vaccine containing any similar component</li><li>Encephalopathy within 7 days of pertussis vaccine</li><li>Progressive neurologic disorders</li></ul></li><li>**Dosage Forms:** Intramuscular suspension</li></ul>
Diphtheria and tetanus toxoids and acellular pertussis adsorbed, inactivated poliovirus and Haemophilus influenzae type b conjugate vaccine, DTaP-IPV/Hib	Pentacel	<ul><li>Toxoid</li><li>Inactivated (bacterial)</li><li>Inactivated (viral)</li></ul>	<ul><li>**Dosing (Adult):**<ul><li>Not routinely used</li></ul></li><li>**Dosing (Peds):**<ul><li>For children at least 6 weeks old to 7 years old</li><li>IM: 0.5 mL for 4 doses</li></ul></li><li>**Contraindications & Allergies:**<ul><li>Anaphylaxis to any other vaccine containing any similar component</li><li>Encephalopathy within 7 days of pertussis vaccine</li><li>Progressive neurologic disorders</li></ul></li><li>**Dosage Forms:** Intramuscular suspension</li></ul>

| Vaccines - Drug Class Review ||||
| High-Yield Med Reviews ||||
Generic Name	Brand Name	Vaccine Format	Notes
Haemophilus b			

Haemophilus b conjugate vaccine, Hib	PedvaxHIB, Hiberix, ActHIB	• Inactivated (bacterial)	• **Dosing (Adult):**
			  − IM: 0.5 mL once
			• **Dosing (Peds):**
			  − For children at least 6 weeks old
			  − IM: 0.5 mL for 3 doses (ActHIB, Hiberix); or 2 doses (PedvaxHIB)
			• **Contraindications & Allergies:**
			  − Anaphylaxis to any other vaccine containing any similar component
			• **Dosage Forms:** Injection powder for reconstitution, Injection suspension

Haemophilus influenzae type b conjugate and hepatitis B vaccine, Hib-HepB	Comvax	• Inactivated (bacterial)
		• Inactivated (viral)
			• **Dosing (Adult):**
			  − Not routinely used
			• **Dosing (Peds):**
			  − For children at least 6 weeks old to 7 years old
			  − IM: 0.5 mL for 3 doses
			• **Contraindications & Allergies:**
			  − Anaphylaxis to any other vaccine containing any similar component
			  − Not intended for initial (birth) dose of HepB vaccine
			• **Dosage Forms:** Injection suspension

Vaccines - Drug Class Review High-Yield Med Reviews			
Generic Name	**Brand Name**	**Vaccine Format**	**Notes**
Hepatitis			
Hepatitis A vaccine, HepA	Havrix, Vaqta	• Inactivated (viral)	• **Dosing (Adult):** — IM: 1 mL for two doses • **Dosing (Peds):** — For children 12 to 23 months — IM: 0.5 mL for two doses • **Contraindications & Allergies:** — Anaphylaxis to previous HepA or any other vaccine containing any similar component including neomycin • **Dosage Forms:** Injection suspension
Hepatitis B vaccine, HepB	Engerix-B, Recombivax HB	• Inactivated (viral)	• **Dosing (Adult):** — IM: 1 mL for 3 doses • **Dosing (Peds):** — IM: 0.5 mL for 3 doses • **Contraindications & Allergies:** — Anaphylaxis to previous HepB or any other vaccine containing any similar component • **Dosage Forms:** Injection suspension
Hepatitis B vaccine, HepB-CpG	HEPLISAV-B	• Inactivated (viral)	• **Dosing (Adult):** — IM: 0.5 mL for two doses • **Dosing (Peds):** — Not routinely used • **Contraindications & Allergies:** — Anaphylaxis to previous HepB-CpG or any other vaccine containing any similar component • **Dosage Forms:** Injection suspension, prefilled syringe
Hepatitis A inactivated and hepatitis B vaccine, HepA-HepB	Twinrix	• Inactivated (viral)	• **Dosing (Adult):** — IM: 1 mL for 3 doses • **Dosing (Peds):** — Indicated for 18 years and older • **Contraindications & Allergies:** — Anaphylaxis to previous HepA or HepB or any other vaccine containing any similar component • **Dosage Forms:** Injection suspension

Vaccines - Drug Class Review
High-Yield Med Reviews

Generic Name	Brand Name	Vaccine Format	Notes
Hepatitis B immune globulin	HepaGam B, HyperHEP B S/D, Nabi-HB	• Immune Globulin	• **Dosing (Adult):** 　— IM: 0.06 mL/kg as soon as possible after exposure, may repeat dose 28-30 days later • **Dosing (Peds):** 　— Infants - IM 0.5 mL as soon as possible after exposure 　— Children 12 months and older - IM 0.06 mL/kg as soon as possible after exposure, may repeat dose 28-30 days later • **Contraindications & Allergies:** 　— Anaphylaxis to previous human globulin preparations. 　— IgA deficiency • **Dosage Forms:** Injection solution

Vaccines - Drug Class Review High-Yield Med Reviews				
Generic Name	Brand Name	Vaccine Format	Notes
Herpes zoster			

Zoster vaccine live, ZVL	Zostavax	- Live (viral)	- **Dosing (Adult):**
			  - SQ: 0.65 mL once
			- **Dosing (Peds):**
			  - Not routinely used
			- **Contraindications & Allergies:**
			  - Anaphylaxis to gelatin, neomycin, or any other vaccine component
			  - Immunosuppressed or immunodeficiency patients
			  - Pregnancy
			- **Dosage Forms:** Injection suspension

Zoster vaccine recombinant, RZV	Shingrix	- Inactivated (viral)	- **Dosing (Adult):**
			  - IM: 0.5 mL for two doses
			- **Dosing (Peds):**
			  - Not routinely used
			- **Contraindications & Allergies:**
			  - Anaphylaxis to any vaccine component
			- **Dosage Forms:** Injection suspension

| Vaccines - Drug Class Review || ||
| High-Yield Med Reviews || ||
Generic Name	Brand Name	Vaccine Format	Notes
Human papillomavirus			

Human papillomavirus 9-valent, 9vHPV	Gardasil 9	• Inactivated (viral)	• **Dosing (Adult):**
			   – IM: 0.5 mL for 3 doses
			• **Dosing (Peds):**
			   – For children at least 9 years old
			   – IM: 0.5 mL for 2 or 3 doses
			• **Contraindications & Allergies:**
			   – Anaphylaxis to previous HPV vaccine or any vaccine component
			• **Dosage Forms:** Injection suspension

Human papillomavirus quadrivalent, 4vHPV	Gardasil	• Inactivated (viral)	• **Dosing (Adult):**
			   – IM: 0.5 mL for 3 doses
			• **Dosing (Peds):**
			   – For children at least 9 years old
			   – IM: 0.5 mL for 2 or 3 doses
			• **Contraindications & Allergies:**
			   – Anaphylaxis to previous HPV vaccine or any vaccine component
			• **Dosage Forms:** Injection suspension

Human papillomavirus bivalent, 2vHPV	Cervarix	• Inactivated (viral)	• **Dosing (Adult):**
			   – IM: 0.5 mL for 3 doses
			• **Dosing (Peds):**
			   – For children at least 9 years old
			   – IM: 0.5 mL for 2 or 3 doses
			• **Contraindications & Allergies:**
			   – Anaphylaxis to previous HPV vaccine or any vaccine component
			• **Dosage Forms:** Injection suspension

Vaccines - Drug Class Review High-Yield Med Reviews			
Generic Name	**Brand Name**	**Vaccine Format**	**Notes**
Influenza			
Trivalent inactivated influenza vaccine, IIV3	Afluria, Fluad, Flucelvax, FluLaval, Fluzone	• Inactivated (viral)	• **Dosing (Adult):** – IM: 0.5 to 0.7 mL once per flu season • **Dosing (Peds):** – For children 6 months and older – IM: 0.25 to 0.5 mL once per flu season • **Contraindications & Allergies:** – Anaphylaxis to previous influenza or any other vaccine containing any similar component including egg protein • **Dosage Forms:** Injection suspension
Quadrivalent inactivated influenza vaccine, IIV4	Fluarix	• Inactivated (viral)	• **Dosing (Adult):** – IM: 0.5 to 0.7 mL once per flu season • **Dosing (Peds):** – For children 6 months and older – IM: 0.25 to 0.5 mL once per flu season • **Contraindications & Allergies:** – Anaphylaxis to previous influenza or any other vaccine containing any similar component including egg protein • **Dosage Forms:** Injection suspension
Live attenuated influenza vaccine, LAIV	FluMist	• Live, attenuated (viral)	• **Dosing (Adult):** – Intranasal 0.2 mL per flu season • **Dosing (Peds):** – Children at least 2 years old – Intranasal 0.2 mL per flu season • **Contraindications & Allergies:** – Anaphylaxis to previous flu vaccine or any other vaccine containing any similar component – 50 years of age or older • **Dosage Forms:** Nasal suspension

Vaccines - Drug Class Review
High-Yield Med Reviews

Generic Name	Brand Name	Vaccine Format	Notes
Measles, mumps, and rubella vaccine			
Measles, mumps, and rubella vaccine, MMR	MMR II	• Live (viral)	• **Dosing (Adult):** – SQ: 0.5 mL for 2 doses • **Dosing (Peds):** – For children at least 12 months old – SQ: 0.5 mL for two doses • **Contraindications & Allergies:** – Anaphylaxis to previous MMR or any other vaccine containing any similar component – Active febrile illness – Active untreated tuberculosis – Immunosuppressed or immunodeficiency patients – Pregnancy • **Dosage Forms:** Injection reconstituted
Measles, mumps, rubella, and varicella vaccine, MMRV	ProQuad	• Live (viral)	• **Dosing (Adult):** – SQ: 0.5 mL for 2 doses • **Dosing (Peds):** – For children at least 12 months old – SQ: 0.5 mL for two doses • **Contraindications & Allergies:** – Anaphylaxis to previous MMR or any other vaccine containing any similar component – Active febrile illness – Active untreated tuberculosis – Immunosuppressed or immunodeficiency patients – Pregnancy • **Dosage Forms:** Injection reconstituted

Vaccines - Drug Class Review High-Yield Med Reviews				
Generic Name	**Brand Name**	**Vaccine Format**	**Notes**
Meningococcal				

Quadrivalent meningococcal conjugate vaccine, MenACWY, MenACWY-D, MenACWY-CRM	Menactra, MenQuadfi Menveo	- Inactivated (bacterial)	- **Dosing (Adult):**
			  - IM: 0.5 mL for one to two doses
			- **Dosing (Peds):**
			  - Children 11 to 12 years
			    - IM: 0.5 mL for one to two doses
			  - Infants at least 2 months to 2 years
			    - IM: 0.5 mL for 2 to 4 doses
			- **Contraindications & Allergies:**
			  - Anaphylaxis to previous vaccine or any vaccine containing any similar component (diphtheria)
			- **Dosage Forms:** Injection solution

Serogroup B meningococcal vaccines, MenB, MenB-4c, MenB-FHbp	Bexsero, Trumenba	- Inactivated (bacterial)	- **Dosing (Adult):**
			  - IM: 0.5 mL for 2 to 3 doses
			- **Dosing (Peds):**
			  - For children at least 10 years old
			  - IM: 0.5 mL for 2 to 3 doses
			- **Contraindications & Allergies:**
			  - Anaphylaxis to previous vaccine or any vaccine containing any similar component
			- **Dosage Forms:** Injection suspension

Bivalent meningococcal conjugate vaccine and Haemophilus influenza type b conjugate vaccine, Hib-MenCY	MenHibrix	- Inactivated (bacterial)	- **Dosing (Adult):**
			  - Not routinely used
			- **Dosing (Peds):**
			  - For children at least 6 weeks old to 18 months old
			  - IM: 0.5 mL for 4 doses
			- **Contraindications & Allergies:**
			  - Anaphylaxis to previous vaccine or any vaccine containing any similar component
			- **Dosage Forms:** Injection solution

Meningococcal polysaccharide vaccine, MPSV4	Menomune	- Inactivated (bacterial)	- **Dosing (Adult):**
			  - IM: 0.5 mL once
			- **Dosing (Peds):**
			  - Not routinely used
			- **Contraindications & Allergies:**
			  - Anaphylaxis to previous vaccine or any vaccine containing any similar component
			- **Dosage Forms:** Injection solution

		Pneumococcal	
Pneumococcal conjugate vaccine 13 valent, PCV13	Prenvar 13	• Inactivated (bacterial)	• **Dosing (Adult):** 　− IM: 0.5 mL once • **Dosing (Peds):** 　− For children at least 6 weeks old to 15 months old 　− IM: 0.5 mL for 4 doses • **Contraindications & Allergies:** 　− Anaphylaxis to previous pneumococcal vaccine or any other vaccine containing any similar component (diphtheria toxoid) • **Dosage Forms:** Injection suspension
Pneumococcal polysaccharide vaccine 23 valent, PPSV23	Pneumovax 23	• Inactivated (bacterial)	• **Dosing (Adult):** 　− IM/SQ: 0.5 mL once • **Dosing (Peds):** 　− For children at least 2 years old 　− IM/SQ: 0.5 mL once • **Contraindications & Allergies:** 　− Anaphylaxis to previous pneumococcal vaccine or any other vaccine containing any similar component (diphtheria toxoid) • **Dosage Forms:** Injection suspension

\multicolumn{4}{c	}{**Vaccines - Drug Class Review**}
\multicolumn{4}{c	}{High-Yield Med Reviews}
Generic Name	**Brand Name**	**Vaccine Format**	**Notes**
\multicolumn{4}{c	}{Poliovirus}
Inactivated poliovirus vaccine, IPV	Ipol	• Inactivated (virus)	• **Dosing (Adult):** 　– IM/SQ: 0.5 mL for 3 doses • **Dosing (Peds):** 　– For children at least 6 weeks old 　– IM: 0.5 mL for 3 doses • **Contraindications & Allergies:** 　– Anaphylaxis to previous IPV or any other vaccine containing any similar component (neomycin, formaldehyde, 2-phenoxyethanol, streptomycin, polymyxin B) 　– Acute, febrile illness • **Dosage Forms:** Injection suspension)

Vaccines - Drug Class Review
High-Yield Med Reviews

Generic Name	Brand Name	Vaccine Format	Notes
Rabies			

Rabies Vaccine	Imovax Rabies, RabAvert	• Inactivated (virus)	• **Dosing (Adult):**
			  − IM: 1 mL for 4 doses
			• **Dosing (Peds):**
			  − IM: 1 mL for 4 doses
			• **Contraindications & Allergies:**
			  − Anaphylaxis to previous human globulin preparations.
			• **Dosage Forms:** Injection suspension

Rabies immunoglobulin	HyperRAB, HyperRAB S/D, Imogam Rabies-HT, Kedrab	• Immune Globulin	• **Dosing (Adult):**
			  − Local infiltration or IM 20 units/kg once
			• **Dosing (Peds):**
			  − Local infiltration or IM 20 units/kg once
			• **Contraindications & Allergies:**
			  − Anaphylaxis to previous human globulin preparations (risks vs. benefits)
			• **Dosage Forms:** Injection solution

Vaccines - Drug Class Review			
High-Yield Med Reviews			
Generic Name	Brand Name	Vaccine Format	Notes
RhO(D)			

RhO(D)	HyperRHO S/D, MICRhoGam, Rhophylac, WinRho	- Immune Globulin	- **Dosing (Adult):**
			    − IV: 25 to 60 mcg/kg once
			    − IM: 300 mcg once at week 26-28 gestation, or within 72 hours of delivery
			- **Dosing (Peds):**
			    − Infants: IV: 50 to 75 mcg/kg once
			- **Contraindications & Allergies:**
			    − Anaphylaxis to previous human globulin preparations.
			    − IgA deficiency
			- **Dosage Forms:** Injection solution

Vaccines - Drug Class Review			
High-Yield Med Reviews			
Generic Name	Brand Name	Vaccine Format	Notes
Rotavirus			

Rotavirus vaccine monovalent, RV1	Rotarix	• Live (virus)	• **Dosing (Adult):**
			   – Not routinely used
			• **Dosing (Peds):**
			   – For children at least 6 to 24 weeks old
			   – Oral: 1 mL/dose for 2 doses
			• **Contraindications & Allergies:**
			   – Anaphylaxis to previous Rotavirus or any other vaccine containing any similar component
			   – History of uncorrected congenital malformation of the GI
			   – History of intussusception
			   – Severe combined immunodeficiency disease
			• **Dosage Forms:** Oral powder for suspension

Rotavirus vaccine pentavalent, RV5	RotaTeq	• Live (virus)	• **Dosing (Adult):**
			   – Not routinely used
			• **Dosing (Peds):**
			   – For children at least 6 to 32 weeks old
			   – Oral: 2 mL/dose for 3 doses
			• **Contraindications & Allergies:**
			   – Anaphylaxis to previous Rotavirus or any other vaccine containing any similar component
			   – History of uncorrected congenital malformation of the GI
			   – History of intussusception
			   – Severe combined immunodeficiency disease
			• **Dosage Forms:** Oral solution

| Vaccines - Drug Class Review ||||
| High-Yield Med Reviews ||||
Generic Name	Brand Name	Vaccine Format	Notes
SARS-CoV-2			

AstraZeneca Oxford	N/A	- SARS-CoV-2 infection	- **Dosing (Adult):**
			  - IM: 0.5 mL with the first and second doses separated by 28 to 84 days.
			- **Dosing (Peds):**
			  - Extra info if needed
			    - Extra info if needed
			- **Contraindications:**
			  - Anaphylaxis to first dose
			  - Allergy to polyethylene glycol
			- **Allergies:** No relevant concerns
			- **Dosage Forms:** Intramuscular suspension

Johnson & Jonson's Janssen	N/A	- SARS-CoV-2 infection	- **Dosing (Adult):**
			  - IM: 0.5 mL once
			- **Dosing (Peds):**
			  - IM: 0.5 mL once
			- **Contraindications:**
			  - Anaphylaxis to first dose
			  - Allergy to polyethylene glycol
			- **Allergies:** No relevant concerns
			- **Dosage Forms:** Intramuscular suspension

Moderna	N/A	- SARS-CoV-2 infection	- **Dosing (Adult):**
			  - IM: 0.5 mL once, followed by a second 0.5 mL dose separated by 28 days.
			- **Dosing (Peds):**
			  - IM: 0.5 mL once, followed by a second 0.5 mL dose separated by 28 days.
			- **Contraindications:**
			  - Anaphylaxis to first dose
			  - Allergy to polyethylene glycol
			- **Allergies:** No relevant concerns
			- **Dosage Forms:** Intramuscular suspension

Pfizer-BioNTech	N/A	- SARS-CoV-2 infection	- **Dosing (Adult):**
			  - IM: 0.3 mL once, followed by a second 0.3 mL dose separated by 21 days.
			- **Dosing (Peds):**
			  - IM: 0.3 mL once, followed by a second 0.3 mL dose separated by 21 days.
			- **Contraindications:**
			  - Anaphylaxis to first dose
			  - Allergy to polyethylene glycol
			- **Allergies:** No relevant concerns
			- **Dosage Forms:** Intramuscular suspension

Vaccines - Drug Class Review
High-Yield Med Reviews

Generic Name	Brand Name	Vaccine Format	Notes
Tetanus			

Tetanus and diphtheria toxoids adsorbed, Td	Decavac, Tenivac	• Toxoid	• **Dosing (Adult):**
			  – IM: 0.5 mL every 10 years if pertussis vaccine contraindicated
			• **Dosing (Peds):**
			  – IM: 0.5 mL once (booster) for children at least 7 years old
			• **Contraindications & Allergies:** Anaphylaxis to previous Td or any other vaccine containing any similar component
			• **Dosage Forms:** Injection suspension

Tetanus toxoid adsorbed, TT		• Toxoid	• **Dosing (Adult):**
			  – IM: 0.5 mL every 10 years if pertussis vaccine contraindicated
			• **Dosing (Peds):**
			  – IM: 0.5 mL once (booster) for children at least 7 years old
			• **Contraindications & Allergies:** Anaphylaxis to previous TT or any other vaccine containing any similar component
			• **Dosage Forms:** Injection suspension

Tetanus toxoid, reduced diphtheria toxoid, and acellular pertussis vaccine, adsorbed, Tdap	Adacel, Boostrix	• Toxoid
		• Inactivated (bacterial)
			• **Dosing (Adult):**
			  – IM: 0.5 mL every 10 years
			• **Dosing (Peds):**
			  – IM: 0.5 mL once (booster) for children at least 7 years old
			• **Contraindications & Allergies:** Anaphylaxis to previous Tdap or any other vaccine containing any similar component
			• **Dosage Forms:** Injection suspension

Tetanus immune globulin	HyperTET	• Immune Globulin	• **Dosing (Adult):**
			  – IM: 250 units administered with tetanus toxoid containing vaccine
			• **Dosing (Peds):**
			  – IM: 250 units, or 4 units/kg, administered with tetanus toxoid containing vaccine
			• **Contraindications & Allergies:**
			  – None
			• **Dosage Forms:** Injection solution

Vaccines - Drug Class Review High-Yield Med Reviews			
Generic Name	**Brand Name**	**Vaccine Format**	**Notes**
Varicella			
Varicella vaccine, VAR	Varivax	• Live	• **Dosing (Adult):** — SQ: 0.5 mL for two doses • **Dosing (Peds):** — For children at least 12 months old — SQ: 0.5 mL for two doses • **Contraindications & Allergies:** — Anaphylaxis to previous varicella or any other vaccine containing any similar component — Active untreated tuberculosis — Active febrile illness — Pregnancy or planning pregnancy within the next 3 months — Immunosuppressed or immunodeficient patients • **Dosage Forms:** Injection suspension
Varicella-zoster immune globulin	Varizig	• Immune Globulin	• **Dosing (Adult):** — IM: 625 units once • **Dosing (Peds):** — IM: 62.5 to 625 units once • **Contraindications & Allergies:** — Anaphylaxis to previous human globulin preparations. — IgA deficiency • **Dosage Forms:** Injection solution

VACCINES – ADULT SCHEDULE

Drug Class
- **Adult Schedule**
- **Agents:**
    - Hepatitis
        - Hepatitis A vaccine, HepA (Havrix, Vaqta)
        - Hepatitis B vaccine, HepB (Engerix-B, Recombivax HB)
        - Hepatitis B vaccine, HepB-CpG (HEPLISAV-B)
        - Hepatitis A inactivated and hepatitis B vaccine, HepA-HepB (Twinrix)
    - Herpes zoster
        - Zoster vaccine live, ZVL (Zostavax)
        - Zoster vaccine recombinant, RZV (Shingrix)
    - Human papillomavirus
        - Human papillomavirus 9-valent, 9vHPV (Gardasil 9)
        - Human papillomavirus quadrivalent, 4vHPV (Gardasil)
        - Human papillomavirus bivalent, 2vHPV (Cervarix)
    - Influenza
        - Trivalent inactivated influenza vaccine, IIV3 (Afluria, Fluad, Fluarix, Flucelvax, FluLaval, Fluzone)
        - Quadrivalent inactivated influenza vaccine, IIV4 (Fluarix)
        - Live attenuated influenza vaccine, LAIV (FluMist)
    - Measles, mumps, and rubella vaccine
        - Measles, mumps, and rubella vaccine, MMR (MMR II)
        - Measles, mumps, rubella, and varicella vaccine, MMRV (ProQuad)
    - Meningococcal
        - Quadrivalent meningococcal conjugate vaccine, MenACWY, MenACWY-D, MenACWY-CRM (Menactra, Menveo)
        - Serogroup B meningococcal vaccines, MenB, MenB-4c, MenB-FHbp (Bexsero, Trumenba)
        - Bivalent meningococcal conjugate vaccine and Haemophilus influenza type b conjugate vaccine, Hib-MenCY (MenHibrix)
        - Meningococcal polysaccharide vaccine, MPSV4 (Menomune)
    - Pneumococcal
        - Pneumococcal conjugate vaccine 13 valent, PCV13 (Prevnar 13)
        - Pneumococcal polysaccharide vaccine 23 valent, PPSV23 (Pneumovax 23)
    - SARS-CoV-2
        - AstraZeneca Oxford
        - Johnson & Johnson's Janssen
        - Moderna
        - Pfizer-BioNTech
    - Tetanus
        - Tetanus and diphtheria toxoids adsorbed, Td (Decavac, Tenivac)
        - Tetanus toxoid adsorbed, TT
        - Tetanus toxoid, reduced diphtheria toxoid, and acellular pertussis vaccine, adsorbed, Tdap (Adacel, Boostrix)
    - Immunoglobulins
        - Hepatitis B immune globulin
        - Rho(D) immune globulin
        - Tetanus immune globulin
        - Varicella-zoster immune globulin

Primary Net Benefit
- Induce an active immune response to numerous diseases that improve morbidity, mortality, and public health.
- Main Labs to Monitor:

- No routine monitoring

High-Yield Basic Pharmacology
- **Live Attenuated Vaccines**
  - Intranasal influenza, MMR, rotavirus, varicella vaccine (Varivax), and zoster vaccine (ZVL, Zostavax) are live attenuated vaccines.
  - Certain vaccines use a weakened form of a virus that contains antigens directed to stimulate an immune response.
  - Viruses used in such vaccines have been manipulated to reduce virulence but maintain immunogenic antigens capable of eliciting humoral and cellular responses sufficient for memory cell development.
  - Viruses of live attenuated vaccines can mutate in vivo and possibly become virulent, leading to disease.
  - Live attenuated viruses cannot be used in pregnant patients, immunocompromised patients, such as those with active cancer or HIV
- **Inactivated Vaccines**
  - Influenza, polio, and rabies are examples of inactivated vaccines.
  - Inactivated vaccines are developed using chemicals, heat, or radiation to inactivate pathogens that produce antigenic responses.
  - These vaccine types induce an immune response similar, although much weaker than the natural infection, and require multiple doses to sustain immunity to the pathogen.
- **Subunit Vaccines**
  - Vaccines contain components of the microorganism to elicit an antigenic response that mimics the organism's response.
  - These vaccines contain surface proteins or toxins but elicit a less-robust immune response than live attenuated viruses.
  - Subunit vaccines can be polysaccharide subunits, surface protein subunits, or toxoids.
    - Polysaccharide vaccines (Hib, PCV13) are often bound to carrier proteins (diphtheria) to elicit sustained disease protection.
    - Surface protein subunits such as acellular pertussis (DTaP, Tdap) and hepatitis B vaccines utilize purified proteins from the pathogen to induce an immune response.
    - Toxoids elicit an immune response to the toxin produced by Clostridium tetani (tetanus) or Corynebacterium diphtheria (diphtheria).
      - Toxoids are often formulated with aluminum salts that induce an inflammatory response and enhance their antigenicity.
- **DNA Vaccines**
  - DNA vaccines such as the SARS-CoV-2 vaccines (AstraZeneca Oxford or Johnson & Johnson's Janssen), Zika virus vaccine, or CMV vaccines use encapsulated viral DNA expressing a target protein and introducing it to the host cell cytoplasm. The host nucleus then utilizes host enzymes to convert the delivered viral DNA component into RNA to produce ribosomes to develop proteins (translation) to express either MHC-1 or 2 proteins.
- **Immunoglobulins**
  - Vaccinations confer B-cell expansion and differentiation to memory cells that maintain long-term protection.
  - Immunoglobulins provide passive immunity by providing human-derived Ig antibodies that the host does not produce.

High-Yield Clinical Knowledge
- **Administration of multiple vaccines or simultaneous administration of vaccines**
  - Live vaccines that are not administered during the same visit must be delayed for at least 30 days following the measles or MMR vaccine.
  - Inactivated and live attenuated vaccines can be administered at the same visit but must be given at separate sites.
    - If not given at the same visit, inactivated vaccines must be separated from live vaccines by at least three weeks.

- If other live vaccines are not given together at the same visit, their administration must be separated by at least four weeks.
- **Routes of Administration**
  - Vaccines can be administered via intramuscular (IM), nasal (IN), subcutaneous (SQ), or oral routes (PO).
  - IM administration should be delivered at a 90-degree angle to the deltoid for most adult patients.
    - For pediatrics, IM administration in the anterolateral thigh should be considered.
  - SQ administration of vaccines should utilize a ⅝ inch needle with the needle inserted at a 45-degree angle in the outer aspect of the triceps.
  - FluMist, a nasal vaccine, should be administered as 0.1 mL administrations to each nostril.
  - Oral vaccines such as rotavirus are administered to infants using an oral dropper/syringe.
- **Vaccines in Special Populations**
  - Immunocompromised patients
    - Live vaccines should be avoided in patients with severe immunocompromised states who may receive killed vaccines or toxoids.
    - Live vaccines should be given at least three months before chemotherapy for patients with cancer and planned chemotherapy.
    - In patients with HIV and CD4 counts below 200 c/mL, MMR, varicella, and zoster vaccines should be avoided until CD4 counts recover to above 200 c/mL.
    - Influenza vaccines should be administered two weeks before chemotherapy or in between cycles.
    - Chronic glucocorticoid administration of prednisone 20 mg/day or equivalent for at least two weeks is considered an immunosuppressive dose.
  - Stem Cell Transplant
    - Patients who have undergone a hematopoietic stem cell transplant require reimmunization with inactivated vaccines beginning six months after transplantation.
    - MMR should be delayed 24 months after the transplant and varicella if indicated.
  - Pregnant patients
    - Live vaccines are not recommended in pregnant women due to the risk of transmitting the given organism to the fetus.
      - Should a pregnant patient receive Rh(D) immune globulin, there is a risk that live vaccines may not produce a sufficient immune response.
      - However, the CDC recommends that post-partum doses of Rh(D) immune globulins do not appear to interact with rubella or MMR vaccines.
- **Vaccine Adverse Event Reporting System (VAERS)**
  - All vaccines' adverse events requiring medical attention must be reported to VAERS within 30 days.
  - VAERS is a public health tool to survey changes in the frequency of adverse events and establish the risk for adverse events, including rarely reported events.
- **Hepatitis B Immune Globulin**
  - Post-exposure prophylaxis to hepatitis b can be accomplished by administering hepatitis B immune globulin.
  - Common sources of exposure include perinatal exposure of infants born to mothers who are hepatitis B surface antigen-positive, sexual exposure to hepatitis B surface antigen-positive individuals, or household exposure to individuals with active acute hepatitis B infection.
- **Rabies Immunoglobulins**
  - Rabies is a potentially fatal infection with close to a 99% mortality rate.
  - Pre-exposure prophylaxis with annual rabies vaccination occurs in individuals who work with animals (veterinarians, laboratory workers, wildlife officers, etc.).
  - Post-exposure prophylaxis requires first administering rabies immune globulin around the site of exposure (bite, scratch, wound, etc.), followed by a four-dose series of rabies vaccines for most individuals.
    - Special consideration for the site of administration should occur as the gluteal tissue cannot be used as a site of administration for rabies vaccine, as this has been associated with failures of the immune response.

- **Tetanus Immunoglobulins**
  - Tetanus immunoglobulin should be given to patients with wounds who have not received tetanus immunization or have not completed tetanus toxoid immunizations.
  - The immunoglobulin must be administered in a separate site from tetanus vaccines.
- **Varicella-Zoster Immunoglobulin**
  - Post-exposure prophylaxis of varicella-zoster infection provided passive immunizations in patients who were not adequately immunized, immunocompromised, or otherwise at high risk of complications.
  - Indications for post-exposure varicella-zoster immunoglobulin include:
    - Severe immunocompromised patients
    - Neonates are born to mothers with varicella diagnosed within five days of delivery or two days after delivery.
    - Hospitalized premature infants born to mothers with no evidence of immunity or who weigh less than 1 kg.
- **RhO(D) Immunoglobulin**
  - Mothers who are RhO(D) negative but exposed to fetal erythrocytes expressing RhO(D) are at risk of Rh antibody development.
  - Without intervention, the maternal antibodies cause erythroblastosis fetalis and hemolytic anemia in the fetus, leading to fetal demise.

High-Yield Fast-Fact
- **Cold Chain**
  - Vaccine cold chain describes documenting the maintenance of appropriate vaccination storage at refrigerated or frozen temperatures.
  - This is most relevant when vaccines are transported to resource-poor areas.

HIGH-YIELD BOARD EXAM ESSENTIALS
- **CLASSIC AGENTS:** Quadrivalent inactivated influenza vaccine, IIV4 (Fluarix), Pneumococcal polysaccharide vaccine 23 valent, PPSV23 (Pneumovax 23)
- **DRUG CLASS:** Adult vaccination schedule
- **INDICATIONS:** Various indications based on CDC vaccination guidelines
- **MECHANISM:** Induce an active immune response to numerous diseases that improve morbidity, mortality, and public health.
- **SIDE EFFECTS:** Injection site reaction
- **CLINICAL PEARLS:** In patients with severe immunocompromised states, live vaccines should be avoided but may receive killed vaccines or toxoids. Among patients with cancer and planned chemotherapy, live vaccines should be given at least three months before chemotherapy if possible.

VACCINES – INFANT AND CHILDREN SCHEDULE

Drug Class
- **Infant and Child Vaccine Schedule**
- **Agents:**
  - Diphtheria
    - Diphtheria and tetanus toxoids adsorbed, DT (TDVax)
    - Diphtheria and tetanus toxoids and acellular pertussis vaccine adsorbed, DTaP (Daptacel, Infanrix)
    - Diphtheria and tetanus toxoids and acellular pertussis adsorbed, hepatitis B and inactivated poliovirus vaccine, DTaP-HepB-IPV (Pediarix)
    - Diphtheria and tetanus toxoids and acellular pertussis adsorbed and inactivated poliovirus vaccine, DTaP-IPV (Kinrix, Quadracel)
    - Diphtheria and tetanus toxoids and acellular pertussis adsorbed, inactivated poliovirus and Haemophilus influenzae type b conjugate vaccine, DTaP-IPV/Hib (Pentacel)
  - Haemophilus b
    - Haemophilus b conjugate vaccine, Hib (PedvaxHIB, Hiberix, ActHIB)
    - Haemophilus influenzae type b conjugate and hepatitis B vaccine, Hib-HepB (Comvax)
  - Hepatitis
    - Hepatitis A vaccine, HepA (Havrix, Vaqta)
    - Hepatitis B vaccine, HepB (Engerix-B, Recombivax HB)
    - Hepatitis B vaccine, HepB-CpG (HEPLISAV-B)
    - Hepatitis A inactivated and hepatitis B vaccine, HepA-HepB (Twinrix)
  - Influenza
    - Trivalent inactivated influenza vaccine, IIV3 (Afluria, Fluad, Fluarix, Flucelvax, FluLaval, Fluzone)
    - Quadrivalent inactivated influenza vaccine, IIV4 (Fluarix)
    - Live attenuated influenza vaccine, LAIV (FluMist)
  - Measles, mumps, and rubella vaccine
    - Measles, mumps, and rubella vaccine, MMR (MMR II)
    - Measles, mumps, rubella, and varicella vaccine, MMRV (ProQuad)
  - Pneumococcal
    - Pneumococcal conjugate vaccine 13 valent, PCV13 (Prevnar 13)
  - Poliovirus
    - Inactivated poliovirus vaccine, IPV (Ipol)
  - Rotavirus
    - Rotavirus vaccine monovalent, RV1 (Rotarix)
    - Rotavirus vaccine pentavalent, RV5 (RotaTeq)
  - Varicella
    - Varicella vaccine, VAR (Varivax)
  - Immunoglobulins
    - Hepatitis B immune globulin
    - Tetanus immune globulin
    - Varicella-zoster immune globulin

Primary Net Benefit
- Induce an active immune response to numerous diseases that improve morbidity, mortality, and public health.
- Main Labs to Monitor:
  - No routine monitoring

High-Yield Basic Pharmacology
- **Diphtheria Toxoid Big D and Little d**
  - Vaccines containing diphtheria toxoid are codified using either a "D," denoting pediatric strength, or a "d" for adult strength with less antigen.

High-Yield Clinical Knowledge
- **Hepatitis Vaccines**
  - Hepatitis A vaccine series begins at the age 12 months with a minimum of 6 months between doses.
  - All newborn infants should receive the monovalent HepB vaccine within 24 hours of birth.
  - Hepatitis B immune globulin should be administered to infants within 12 hours of birth who were born to hepatitis B surface antigen-positive mothers.
    - Follow-up hepatitis B surface antigen screening should occur at 9 to 12 months of age.
- **Rotavirus Vaccines**
  - RV1 (Rotarix) is a two-dose series starting at age 2 months, with a second dose at 4 months.
  - RV5 (RotaTeq) is a three-dose series at 2, 4, and 6 months.
    - If there is a loss of information or unknown which product was used for the first dose, infants should receive three doses of RotaTeq.
- **Diphtheria And Tetanus Toxoids And Acellular Pertussis (DTaP)**
  - DTaP is a five-dose series beginning at age 2 months through 18 months.
  - Additional booster doses should be administered at age 4 through 6 years.
  - Numerous products exist, including DTaP combined with inactivated polio (IPV), Haemophilus influenzae type B (HiB), Pentacel, and DTaP-HepB-IPV, known as Pediarix.
  - Tdap vaccination begins at the age of 11 years but can be administered to children as young as 7 years old.
- **Pneumococcal Vaccines**
  - PCV13 vaccinations should occur as a four-dose series from the ages of 2 months through 15 months.
  - PPSV23 may be administered to children who've previously received PCV13, are aged 2 through 5 years with chronic heart, lung, or renal disease, diabetes mellitus, cerebrospinal fluid leak, cochlear implant, sickle cell disease, anatomic or functional asplenia, HIV, or receiving immunosuppression.
    - Children with anatomic or functional asplenia, sickle cell disease, HIV, or persistent complement deficiency should also receive meningococcal conjugate ACWY vaccination (with either Menveo, MenHibrix, Menactra) and meningococcal B vaccination with Bexsero or Trumenba.
- **MMR and MMRV**
  - The MMR and varicella vaccines are not recommended until 12 months of age or older due to circulating maternal antibodies that inhibit the immune response to live vaccines.
    - MMR and varicella vaccination typically begin after 12 months, but the MMR vaccine can start as early as 6 months of age in infants who travel outside the US.
- **Administration of multiple vaccines or simultaneous administration of vaccines**
  - Live vaccines that are not administered during the same visit must be delayed for at least 30 days following the measles or MMR vaccine.
  - Inactivated and live attenuated vaccines can be administered at the same visit but must be given at separate sites.
    - If not given at the same visit, inactivated vaccines must be separated from live vaccines by at least three weeks.
    - If other live vaccines are not given together at the same visit, their administration must be separated by at least 4 weeks.

High-Yield Fast-Fact
- **Autism and SIDS**
  - There has been no definitive association between vaccinations and the development of autism or SIDS.
  - Furthermore, the risks of preventable diseases, both to the patient or public health, are outweighed mainly by the threats of routine vaccination complications.

HIGH-YIELD BOARD EXAM ESSENTIALS

- **CLASSIC AGENTS:** Diphtheria and tetanus toxoids and acellular pertussis adsorbed, hepatitis B and inactivated poliovirus vaccine, DTaP-HepB-IPV (Pediarix), Measles, mumps, rubella, and varicella vaccine, MMRV (ProQuad), Varicella vaccine, VAR (Varivax)
- **DRUG CLASS:** Infant and Child Vaccine Schedule
- **INDICATIONS:** Immunizations based on the CDC vaccination schedule
- **MECHANISM:** Induce an active immune response to numerous diseases that improve morbidity, mortality, and public health.
- **SIDE EFFECTS:** There has been no definitive association between vaccinations and the development of autism or SIDS.
- **CLINICAL PEARLS:** Live vaccines that are not administered during the same visit must be delayed for at least 30 days following the measles or MMR vaccine. Inactivated and live attenuated vaccines can be administered at the same visit but must be given at separate sites.

VACCINES – PRETEEN & TEEN SCHEDULE

Drug Class
- Preteen and Teen Schedule
- Agents:
    - Human papillomavirus
        - Human papillomavirus 9-valent, 9vHPV (Gardasil 9)
        - Human papillomavirus quadrivalent, 4vHPV (Gardasil)
        - Human papillomavirus bivalent, 2vHPV (Cervarix)
    - Influenza
        - Trivalent inactivated influenza vaccine, IIV3 (Afluria, Fluad, Fluarix, Flucelvax, FluLaval, Fluzone)
        - Quadrivalent inactivated influenza vaccine, IIV4 (Fluarix)
        - Live attenuated influenza vaccine, LAIV (FluMist)
    - Meningococcal
        - Quadrivalent meningococcal conjugate vaccine, MenACWY, MenACWY-D, MenACWY-CRM (Menactra, Menveo)
        - Serogroup B meningococcal vaccines, MenB, MenB-4c, MenB-FHbp (Bexsero, Trumenba)
        - Bivalent meningococcal conjugate vaccine and Haemophilus influenza type b conjugate vaccine, Hib-MenCY (MenHibrix)
        - Meningococcal polysaccharide vaccine, MPSV4 (Menomune)
    - Pneumococcal
        - Pneumococcal conjugate vaccine 13 valent, PCV13 (Prevnar 13)
    - SARS-CoV-2
        - AstraZeneca Oxford
        - Johnson & Johnson's Janssen
        - Moderna
        - Pfizer-BioNTech
    - Tetanus
        - Tetanus and diphtheria toxoids adsorbed, Td (Decavac, Tenivac)
        - Tetanus toxoid adsorbed, TT
        - Tetanus toxoid, reduced diphtheria toxoid, and acellular pertussis vaccine, adsorbed, Tdap (Adacel, Boostrix)

Primary Net Benefit
- Induce an active immune response to numerous diseases that improve morbidity, mortality, and public health.
- Main Labs to Monitor:
    - No routine monitoring

High-Yield Clinical Knowledge
- **Human Papillomavirus (HPV)**
    - HPV is the most common sexually transmitted disease, potentially leading to genital warts or cervical, vaginal, and vulvar cancers.
    - However, many individuals infected with HPV are asymptomatic.
    - HPV vaccination is recommended for individuals aged 9 to 26 years.
        - Routine vaccination for HPV occurs at age 11 to 12 years, with numerous catch-up regimens for individuals aged 13 to 26.
        - For adolescents starting HPV vaccination series between 9 and 14 years old, a two-dose series can be administered.
        - A three-dose series is recommended for vaccination series beginning at age 15 or older.
- **Meningococcal Vaccines**
    - Meningitis caused by Neisseria meningitidis may be more prevalent in children, adolescents, and young adults, who are also more likely to be in group settings where transmission is expected.
    - Group settings where N. meningitidis transmission is likely to include classrooms, dormitories, or prisons.

- All first-year college (freshman) students living in residence halls should receive MenACWY vaccination, even if they'd received a meningitis immunization before their 16th birthday, and continued every five years for individuals with continued high risk.
  - Serogroup B meningococcal vaccines are also recommended for college students.
- **Influenza Vaccine**
  - Two seasonal influenza vaccine categories exist, the inactivated influenza vaccine (IIV) and the live-attenuated influenza vaccine (LAIV).
  - IIV are either trivalent or quadrivalent formulations, whereas the LAIV is a quadrivalent product and produced in embryonated hen eggs.
    - Flublok and Flucelvax are the currently available influenza vaccine products considered to be egg-free.
  - These vaccines contain influenza A subtypes H3N2, H1N1, and influenza B virus.
    - Specific strains in the annual vaccine are based on antigenic drift data.
- **Thimerosal**
  - Multidose vials containing vaccines, including IIV products, include the mercury-containing preservative thimerosal.
  - The risk of adverse events from thimerosal exposure from vaccines, including Guillen-Barre syndrome, autism, or any other complication, appears markedly low, and no high-quality evidence exists to suggest harm.
  - However, a growing supply of thimerosal-free vaccines is becoming available.
- **Administration of multiple vaccines or simultaneous administration of vaccines**
  - Live vaccines that are not administered during the same visit must be delayed for at least 30 days following the measles or MMR vaccine.
  - Inactivated and live attenuated vaccines can be administered at the same visit but must be given at separate sites.
    - If not given at the same visit, inactivated vaccines must be separated from live vaccines by at least three weeks.
    - If other live vaccines are not given together at the same visit, their administration must be separated by at least four weeks.

High-Yield Fast-Fact
- **Smallpox**
  - The smallpox vaccine is unique in many ways from other vaccines, as it contains live vaccinia virus, not a killed or weakened virus like many other vaccines, and it is administered after dipping the bifurcated needle into the vaccine vial then prick the skin rapidly with the needle 15 times with the pricks within an area approximately 5 mm in diameter.

HIGH-YIELD BOARD EXAM ESSENTIALS
- **CLASSIC AGENTS:** Human papillomavirus quadrivalent, 4vHPV (Gardasil), Quadrivalent meningococcal conjugate vaccine, MenACWY, MenACWY-D, MenACWY-CRM (Menactra, Menveo), Tetanus toxoid, reduced diphtheria toxoid, and acellular pertussis vaccine, adsorbed, Tdap (Adacel, Boostrix)
- **DRUG CLASS:** Preteen and teen vaccine schedule
- **INDICATIONS:** Population vaccination based on CDC guidelines
- **MECHANISM:** Induce an active immune response to numerous diseases that improve morbidity, mortality, and public health.
- **SIDE EFFECTS:** Injection site reactions,
- **CLINICAL PEARLS:** Meningitis caused by Neisseria meningitidis may be more prevalent in children, adolescents, and young adults, who are also more likely to be in group settings where transmission is expected.

VACCINES – SARS COV-2 VACCINES

Drug Class
- SARS-CoV-2 Vaccines
- Agents:
    - AstraZeneca Oxford
    - Johnson & Johnson's Janssen
    - Moderna
    - Pfizer-BioNTech

Main Indications or Uses
- Acute Care
    - SARS-CoV-2

Mechanism of Action
- Moderna and Pfizer-BioNTech
    - Consists of an mRNA fragment of the SARS-CoV-2 S-protein encapsulated in a carrier molecule to direct the host to mount an adaptive immune response based on the protein created from the RNA.
- AstraZeneca - Oxford and Johnson and Johnson's Janssen
    - Recombinant adenovirus vector expressing SARS-CoV-2 S-protein incapable of viral propagation but induces a host adaptive immune response.

Primary Overall Net Benefit
- Novel vaccine technology provides genetic information to mount an adaptive immune response to several genetic targets beyond infectious diseases and holds the potential for other genetic targets, including certain cancers.

High-Yield Basic Pharmacology
- Moderna and Pfizer-BioNTech
    - Contains an mRNA component of the S-protein "aka spike protein" of the SARS-CoV-2 virus contained in a lipid nanoparticle that functions as a carrier molecule.
    - The lipid nanoparticle fuses with the host cell allowing the mRNA to induce host cell ribosomes to begin translation proteins and express on the cell membrane as MHC-1 or MHC-2 proteins.
        - MHC-2 cells induce cytokine-mediated T-helper cell immune response, including T-cell receptor development, T-helper cell development, and CD4+ cell recruitment.
        - This causes the activation of T-cells and associated cytokines, inducing B-cell proliferation and differentiation to plasma cells which produce antibodies to the SARS-CoV-2's S-protein.
    - Cytotoxic T-cells interact with MHC-1 to produce CD8 cells that destroy host cells if infected with the given target (SARS-CoV-2) in the future, not the host cells processing the vaccine at that time.
- AstraZeneca - Oxford and Johnson and Johnson's Janssen
    - Uses Chimpanzee adenovirus encapsulating viral DNA expressing the S-protein of SARS-CoV-2 and introducing it to viral DNA into the host cell cytoplasm.
    - The host nucleus then utilizes enzymes to convert the delivered viral DNA component into RNA to produce ribosomes directed to develop proteins (translation) to express either MHC-1 or 2 proteins.

High-Yield Clinical Knowledge
- mRNA Vaccine Administration
    - Moderna vaccine is administered as an intramuscular injection (IM) of 0.5 mL once, followed by a second 0.5 mL dose separated by 28 days.
    - Pfizer-BioNTech vaccine is also an IM dose of 0.3 mL once, followed by a second 0.3 mL dose separated by 21 days.
        - The second dose should be administered within four or fewer days from the missed dose if the dosing interval is not completed according to the product information.

- No additional doses should be administered if the second dose is administered before the 4-day period.
- If a delay beyond the 4-day window occurs, the second dose may be administered up to 6 weeks after the first dose.
  - Currently, the CDC does not recommend restarting the vaccination series if the second dose is administered beyond this time frame.
- **DNA Vaccine Administration**
  - Johnson & Johnson's Janssen vaccine is an IM administration of a single 0.5 mL dose.
  - The AstraZeneca vaccine is administered as two 0.5 mL IM administrations, with the first and second doses separated by 28 to 84 days.
    - Some reports recommend a separation of 56 to 84 days between doses.
- **Conversion Between Vaccines**
  - mRNA vaccines (Moderna and Pfizer-BioNTech) are interchangeable if a patient begins one series and cannot complete that product due to shortages.
- **Acute Febrile Illnesses**
  - In patients with severe acute febrile illness, mRNA vaccine administration is not recommended.
  - There is no reason to withhold vaccination for patients with mild acute illnesses.
- **History of SARS-CoV-2 Infection**
  - mRNA SARS-CoV-2 vaccination appears safe among patients with current or prior history of SARS-CoV-2 infection but should be deferred until the acute illness resolves and isolation is no longer required.
  - It is not currently known the impact of the prior receipt of passive SARS-CoV-2 antibody therapy on vaccination.
- **Post-Exposure Prophylaxis**
  - SARS-CoV-2 mRNA vaccination is not recommended for post-exposure prophylaxis.
- **Pregnancy**
  - The safety of any SARS-CoV-2 vaccine in pregnancy is not fully known as pregnant patients were excluded from the investigational research.

High-Yield Core Evidence
- **COVE (Moderna)**
  - This was a multicenter, observer-blinded, placebo-controlled trial that randomized individuals at high risk of SARS-CoV-2 infection or its complications to receive either mRNA-1273 (Moderna vaccine) via two IM injections separated by 28 days or a matching placebo.
  - A total of 30,420 subjects were randomized equally to receive vaccine or placebo, with nearly all (96%) receiving both injections.
  - Among subjects receiving the vaccine, there was a significant reduction in the incidence of symptomatic SARS-CoV-2 infection, and efficacy was similar across key secondary analyses.
  - Furthermore, among subjects developing severe SARS-CoV-2 infection occurred 30 participants, all of which were in the placebo group.
  - Moderate, transient reactogenicity after vaccination occurred more frequently in the Moderna vaccine group, but serious adverse events were rare, and the incidence was similar in the two groups.
  - The authors concluded that the Moderna vaccine showed 94.1% efficacy at preventing Covid-19 illness, including severe disease. In addition, aside from transient local and systemic reactions, no safety concerns were identified. (N Engl J Med 2021; 384:403-416.)
- **Pfizer-BioNTech**
  - This is a publication of an ongoing multinational, placebo-controlled, observer-blinded, pivotal efficacy trial that randomized subjects 16 years or older to receive either placebo or the Pfizer-BioNTech vaccine.
  - This study included 43,548 subjects who underwent randomization and were equally divided into placebo or Pfizer-BioNTech vaccine groups.
  - There was a statistically significant reduction of SARS-CoV-2 infection among subjects receiving the Pfizer-BioNTech vaccine compared to placebo.
  - There was no change in efficacy across subgroups, including subgroups defined by age, sex, race, ethnicity, baseline body-mass index, and the presence of coexisting conditions.

- There were 10 cases of severe SARS-CoV-2 infection, with nine occurring in the placebo group and a single case in the Pfizer-BioNTech group.
- The incidence of serious adverse events was low and was similar in the vaccine and placebo groups.
- The authors concluded that the two-dose regimen of Pfizer-BioNTech vaccine conferred 95% protection against Covid-19 in persons 16 years of age or older. Safety over a median of 2 months was similar to that of other viral vaccines. (N Engl J Med. 2020 Dec 31;383(27):2603-2615.)

- **AstraZeneca-Oxford**
  - This was an interim analysis of four ongoing blinded, controlled trials that randomized patients in the UK, Brazil, and South Africa to receive either the AstraZeneca-Oxford vaccine administered as two injections or control (meningococcal group A, C, W, and Y conjugate vaccine or saline).
  - A subgroup in the AstraZeneca-Oxford group received two doses, but the first dose was a half dose as their first dose and a standard dose as their second dose.
  - The full dose AstraZeneca-Oxford group experienced a vaccine efficacy of 62.1%, compared to a 90.0% efficacy in the half- then full-dose group. Both of which were significantly better than placebo at preventing symptomatic SARS-CoV-2 infection.
  - Furthermore, fewer hospitalizations occurred in either vaccine group and a similar frequency of adverse events occurring between vaccine or placebo groups.
  - The authors concluded that the AstraZeneca-Oxford vaccine has an acceptable safety profile and is efficacious against symptomatic COVID-19 in this interim analysis of ongoing clinical trials. (Lancet. 2021 Jan 9;397(10269):99-111.)

High-Yield Fast-Fact

- **Operation Warp Speed**
  Operation Warp Speed was a public and privately funded endeavor to facilitate developing a SARS-CoV-2 vaccine that ultimately led to the currently available vaccine products.

HIGH-YIELD BOARD EXAM ESSENTIALS
- **CLASSIC AGENTS:** AstraZeneca Oxford, Johnson & Johnson's Janssen, Moderna, Pfizer-BioNTech
- **DRUG CLASS:** SARS-CoV-2 Vaccines
- **INDICATIONS:** SARS-CoV-2 infection prevention
- **MECHANISM:** mRNA vaccines - Consist of an mRNA fragment of the SARS-CoV-2 S-protein encapsulated in a carrier molecule to direct the host to mount an adaptive immune response based on the protein created from the RNA. DNA vaccines - Recombinant adenovirus vector expressing SARS-CoV-2 S-protein incapable of viral propagation but induces a host adaptive immune response.
- **SIDE EFFECTS:** Flu-like illness, injection site reactions, venous/arterial thrombosis (J&J)
- **CLINICAL PEARLS:** Novel vaccine technology provides genetic information to mount an adaptive immune response to several genetic targets that extend beyond infectious diseases and holds the potential for other genetic targets, including certain cancers.

SARS-CoV-2 Vaccines - Drug Class Review				
High-Yield Med Reviews				
Mechanism of Action: ***mRNA vaccines*** - *Consist of an mRNA fragment of the SARS-CoV-2 S-protein encapsulated in a carrier molecule to direct the host to mount an adaptive immune response based on the protein created from the RNA.* ***DNA vaccines*** - *Recombinant adenovirus vector expressing SARS-CoV-2 S-protein incapable of viral propagation but induces a host adaptive immune response.*				
Class Effects: *Myagia, body aches*				
Generic Name	**Brand Name**	**Vaccine Format**	**Notes**	

AstraZeneca Oxford	N/A	- SARS-CoV-2 infection	- **Dosing (Adult):**
			  — IM: 0.5 mL with the first and second doses separated by 28 to 84 days.
			 - **Dosing (Peds):** Limited
			 - **Contraindications:**
			  — Anaphylaxis to first dose
			  — Allergy to polyethylene glycol
			 - **Allergies:** No relevant concerns
			 - **Dosage Forms:** Intramuscular suspension	

Johnson & Jonson's Janssen	N/A	- SARS-CoV-2 infection	- **Dosing (Adult):**
			  — IM: 0.5 mL once
			 - **Dosing (Peds):**
			  — IM: 0.5 mL once
			 - **Contraindications:**
			  — Anaphylaxis to first dose
			  — Allergy to polyethylene glycol
			 - **Allergies:** No relevant concerns
			 - **Dosage Forms:** Intramuscular suspension	

Moderna	N/A	- SARS-CoV-2 infection	- **Dosing (Adult):**
			  — IM: 0.5 mL once, followed by a second 0.5 mL dose separated by 28 days.
			 - **Dosing (Peds):**
			  — IM: 0.5 mL once, followed by a second 0.5 mL dose separated by 28 days.
			 - **Contraindications:**
			  — Anaphylaxis to first dose
			  — Allergy to polyethylene glycol
			 - **Allergies:** No relevant concerns
			 - **Dosage Forms:** Intramuscular suspension	

Pfizer-BioNTech	N/A	- SARS-CoV-2 infection	- **Dosing (Adult):**
			  — IM: 0.3 mL once, followed by a second 0.3 mL dose separated by 21 days.
			 - **Dosing (Peds):**
			  — IM: 0.3 mL once, followed by a second 0.3 mL dose separated by 21 days.
			 - **Contraindications:**
			  — Anaphylaxis to first dose
			  — Allergy to polyethylene glycol
			 - **Allergies:** No relevant concerns
			 - **Dosage Forms:** Intramuscular suspension	

2025

A COMPREHENSIVE *RAPID REVIEW*

NAPLEX

Pharmacology & Drug Classes

Infectious Diseases

INFECTIOUS DISEASES – AMINOGLYCOSIDES

Drug Class
- **Aminoglycosides**
- **Agents:**
  - Acute Care
    - Amikacin
    - Gentamicin
    - Tobramycin
    - Neomycin
    - Plazomicin
    - Streptomycin
  - Chronic Care
    - Tobramycin

Main Indications or Uses
- **Acute Care**
  - Bacterial Endocarditis
  - Brucellosis (Streptomycin)
  - Endocarditis
  - Meningitis
  - Plague (Streptomycin)
  - Pneumonia
  - Sepsis
  - Tuberculosis (Streptomycin)
  - Tularemia (Streptomycin)
  - Urinary Tract Infections
- **Chronic Care**
  - Cystic fibrosis

> **Fast Facts**
>
> ✓ Neomycin can be used topically for simple skin infections. Due to its very poor oral bioavailability, it can also be used orally for surgical prophylaxis for colorectal surgery.
>
> ✓ Amikacin liposome can be given by nebulization for MAC whereas tobramycin nebulization can be used for Pseudomonas infections in cystic fibrosis.
>
> ✓ For emergency preparedness, gentamicin or streptomycin can be used as a 10-day course for the plague!

Mechanism of Action
- Aminoglycosides interrupt bacterial protein synthesis by binding to the 30S ribosomal subunit, ultimately leading to the accumulation of abnormal initiation complexes, resulting in bacterial cellular death.
  - Aminoglycosides also may interfere with bacterial protein synthesis by binding to polysomes, leading to premature termination of mRNA translation and incorrect amino acid insertion into bacterial polypeptide chains.
    - As a result, proteins that are subsequently produced are inserted into the cell membrane, disrupt permeability but allow for increased aminoglycoside transport.

Primary Net Benefit
- Concentration-dependent bactericidal activity with post-antibiotic effect after concentrations fall below minimum inhibitory concentration.
- Main Labs to Monitor:
  - Cultures from infected sites at baseline (blood, sputum, urine, CSF, etc.)
  - Serum creatinine, urine output
  - Therapeutic drug concentrations

High-Yield Basic Pharmacology
- **Penetration To 30S**
  - For aminoglycosides to exert their inhibitory effect on the 30S ribosomal subunit, they must first enter the bacterial cell via diffusion through the outer membrane and inner membranes.
    - Inner membrane aminoglycoside transport relies on a transmembrane electrical gradient, a rate-limited process that can also be blocked or inhibited by numerous factors, including low pH, divalent cations (calcium and magnesium), hyperosmolarity, and anaerobic environments.
- **Bacterial Resistance Mechanisms**
  - Aminoglycoside resistance is an emerging therapeutic obstacle as bacteria may develop resistance via numerous mechanisms.
    - Aminoglycoside resistance may develop due to inactivation by microbial enzymes, the antibiotic's ability to penetrate intracellularly, or low affinity of the drug for the bacterial ribosome.
- **Neuromuscular blockade**
  - Aminoglycosides have been independently associated with acute neuromuscular blockade and apnea, with a higher risk of paralysis in patients with a history of myasthenia gravis.
  - Patients receiving neuromuscular blocking agents (depolarizing and non-depolarizing agents) may have a prolonged time to recovery (up to 25% longer) if concomitantly receiving aminoglycosides.

High-Yield Clinical Knowledge
- **Ototoxicity**
  - Aminoglycosides may cause irreversible vestibular and cochlear toxicity.
  - These adverse effects are known to be related to high doses and/or high drug concentrations.
  - The ototoxicity from aminoglycosides differs from ototoxicity caused by loop diuretics (i.e., furosemide) as it is irreversible and causes bilateral high-frequency hearing loss and temporary vestibular dysfunction.
    - This results directly in the hair cells and neurons in the cochlea and the effect that shares similarities to the drug-drug interaction of aminoglycosides and neuromuscular blocking agents.
- **Nephrotoxicity**
  - Similar to ototoxicity, aminoglycosides may cause nephrotoxicity, which is associated with high doses, and/or high drug concentrations or concomitant nephrotoxic agents (i.e., NSAIDs).
  - Although nephrotoxicity can occur in up to 8-26% of patients receiving aminoglycosides, it is frequently reversible.
- **Traditional or Extended Interval Dosing**
  - Once-daily or extended interval dosing is the preferred dosing strategy for aminoglycosides.
  - The concentration-dependent antimicrobial effect of aminoglycosides permits maximal initial bacterial killing and relies on the postantibiotic effect to ensure optimal outcomes while maintaining, or even lowering, the risk of nephrotoxicity and ototoxicity.
- **Dosing Weight**
  - Careful consideration must take place of which weight to select when determining weight-based doses of aminoglycosides.
    - Low body weight (total body weight [TBW] less than ideal body weight [IBW]), use TBW
    - Obese patients with TBW more than 1.25 times IBW, use adjusted body weight formula = [0.4 × (TBW - IBW)] + IBW
- **Alternative Routes**
  - Aminoglycosides may be administered as topical skin and mucous membrane agents (neomycin), ophthalmic products (gentamicin, neomycin, and tobramycin), or as inhaled agents (amikacin, tobramycin).

- **Core spectrum**
    - Gram-Positive
        - Staphylococcus aureus, methicillin-sensitive only
    - Gram-Negative
        - Enterobacteriaceae
            - Escherichia coli
            - Klebsiella pneumoniae
            - Shigella species
            - Yersinia pestis
        - Enterobacter sp
        - Moraxella catarrhalis
        - Serratia species
        - Pseudomonas aeruginosa
- **Core Indications**
    - Aminoglycosides are rarely used independently for empiric therapy but should be used combined with a beta-lactam or vancomycin to treat proven severe or suspected bacterial infections.
    - Aminoglycosides' role in modern clinical practice is to expand the empiric spectrum of activity of the antimicrobial regimen, provide synergistic bacterial killing, and/or the prevention of the emergence of resistance to the individual agents.

HIGH-YIELD BOARD EXAM ESSENTIALS
- **CLASSIC AGENTS:** Amikacin, gentamicin, tobramycin, neomycin
- **DRUG CLASS:** Aminoglycosides
- **INDICATIONS:** Bacterial endocarditis, cystic fibrosis (CF), bacterial meningitis, pneumonia, sepsis, urinary tract infections
- **MECHANISM:** Inhibit bacterial protein synthesis at the 30S ribosomal subunit, resulting in bacterial death.
- **SIDE EFFECTS:** Nephrotoxicity, ototoxicity
- **CLINICAL PEARLS:**
    - No oral dosage formulations available for "systemic infections", but can be used for enteric purposes (e.g., surgical bowel prep)
    - All agents cover against Pseudomonas
    - Once-daily or extended interval dosing provides concentration-dependent antimicrobial effect of aminoglycosides that permits maximal initial bacterial killing and relies on the postantibiotic effect to ensure optimal outcomes while maintaining, or even lowering, the risk of nephrotoxicity and ototoxicity.
    - Tobramycin nebs used for CF patients pulmonary Pseudomonas infections

Table: Drug Class Summary

Aminoglycosides - Drug Class Review High-Yield Med Reviews			
Mechanism of Action: *Inhibit bacterial protein synthesis at the 30S ribosomal subunit, resulting in bacterial death.*			
Class Effects: *Concentration-dependent bactericidal activity with a post-antibiotic effect; Associated with nephrotoxicity and ototoxicity*			
Generic Name	**Brand Name**	**Main Indication(s) or Uses**	**Notes**
Amikacin	Amikin	<ul><li>Bacterial Endocarditis</li><li>Cystic fibrosis</li><li>Meningitis</li><li>Pneumonia</li><li>Sepsis</li><li>Urinary Tract Infections</li></ul>	<ul><li>**Dosing (Adult):**<ul><li>Extended interval dosing<ul><li>IV: 15 to 20 mg/kg/day</li></ul></li><li>Conventional dosing<ul><li>IV/IM: 5 to 7.5 mg/kg/dose q8h</li></ul></li></ul></li><li>**Dosing (Peds):**<ul><li>IV/IM: 15 to 30 mg/kg/*day* divided q8h</li><li>IV: 15 to 20 mg/kg/*dose* q24h</li></ul></li><li>**CYP450 Interactions:** None</li><li>**Renal or Hepatic Dose Adjustments:**<ul><li>GFR: < 20 mL/minute should not receive extended interval dosing</li><li>Conventional dosing<ul><li>GFR: 10 to 50 mL/minute q24-72 hours follow serum concentrations</li><li>GFR: < 10 mL/minute q48-72 follow serum concentrations.</li></ul></li></ul></li><li>**Dosage Forms:** IV solution</li></ul>
Gentamicin	Garamycin Gentak (ophthalmic)	<ul><li>Bacterial Endocarditis</li><li>Cystic fibrosis</li><li>Meningitis</li><li>Ocular infections</li><li>Pneumonia</li><li>Sepsis</li><li>Urinary Tract Infections</li></ul>	<ul><li>**Dosing (Adult):**<ul><li>Extended interval dosing<ul><li>IV: 15 to 20 mg/kg/day</li></ul></li><li>Conventional dosing<ul><li>IV/IM: 3 to 5 mg/kg/dose q8h</li></ul></li></ul></li><li>**Dosing (Peds):**<ul><li>IV/IM: 2 to 2.5 mg/kg/day divided q8h</li><li>IV: 3 to 5 mg/kg/dose q24h</li></ul></li><li>**CYP450 Interactions:** None</li><li>**Renal or Hepatic Dose Adjustments:**<ul><li>GFR: < 20 mL/minute should not receive extended interval dosing</li><li>Conventional dosing<ul><li>GFR: 10 to 50 mL/minute q12-72 hours follow serum concentrations</li><li>GFR: < 10 mL/minute q48-72 follow serum concentrations.</li></ul></li></ul></li><li>**Dosage Forms:** IV (solution), Ophthalmic (solution, ointment), Topical (cream, ointment)</li></ul>

Aminoglycosides - Drug Class Review
High-Yield Med Reviews

Generic Name	Brand Name	Main Indication(s) or Uses	Notes

Tobramycin	Nebcin
	
	Tobi
	(Inhalation)
	
	Tobrex
	(ophthalmic)
		• Bacterial Endocarditis
		• Cystic fibrosis
		• Meningitis
		• Ocular infections
		• Pneumonia
		• Sepsis
		• Urinary Tract Infections
			• **Dosing (Adult):**
			   – Extended interval dosing
			      – IV: 15 to 20 mg/kg/day
			   – Conventional dosing
			      – IV/IM: 5 to 7.5 mg/kg/dose q8h
			• **Dosing (Peds):**
			   – IV/IM: 15 to 30 mg/kg/day divided q8h
			   – IV: 15 to 20 mg/kg/dose q24
			• **CYP450 Interactions:** None
			• **Renal or Hepatic Dose Adjustments:**
			   – GFR < 20 mL/minute should not receive extended interval dosing
			   – Conventional dosing
			      – GFR: 10 to 50 mL/minute q12-72 hours follow serum concentrations
			      – GFR: < 10 mL/minute q48-72 follow serum concentrations.
			• **Dosage Forms:** IV (solution), Ophthalmic (solution, ointment), Topical (cream, ointment), Nebulization solution, Inhalation (capsule)

Neomycin	Mycifradin, Neosporin	• GI decontamination
		• Skin and soft tissue infections
			• **Dosing (Adult):**
			   – Oral: 1 g q6-8h
			   – Topically applied as instructed q4-6h
			• **Dosing (Peds):**
			   – Oral: 25 to 50 mg/kg/day divided in 4 doses; Maximum 12 g/day
			• **CYP450 Interactions:** None
			• **Renal or Hepatic Dose Adjustments:** None
			• **Dosage Forms:** Oral (tablet), topical, urologic irrigation

Plazomicin	Zemdri	• UTI (Complicated)	• **Dosing (Adult):** – 15 mg/kg IV once daily • **Dosing (Peds):** n/a • **CYP450 Interactions:** None • **Renal or Hepatic Dose Adjustments:** Reduce once CrCl < 60 mL/min to 10 mg/kg and to every 48 hrs once CrCl < 30 mL/min • **Dosage Forms:** Solution for IV injection

Streptomycin		• Brucellosis
		• Plague
		• Tuberculosis
		• Tularemia
			• **Dosing (Adult):**
			   – Brucellosis: 1 g IV once daily + doxycycline
			   – Other: 15 mg/kg IV once or twice a day
			• **Dosing (Peds):**
			   – IV/IM: 20-40 mg/kg/day in 2-4 divided doses
			• **CYP450 Interactions:** None
			• **Renal or Hepatic Dose Adjustments:**
			   – Reduce once CrCl < 50 mL/min
			• **Dosage Forms:** Solution for injection

INFECTIOUS DISEASE – AMINOPENICILLIN AND EXTENDED-SPECTRUM PENICILLIN

Drug Class
- Beta-Lactam Antibiotic → Aminopenicillin and Extended-Spectrum Penicillin
- Agents:
  - Acute Care
    - Amoxicillin
    - Amoxicillin/Clavulanic acid
    - Ampicillin
    - Ampicillin/Sulbactam
    - Durlobactam/Sulbactam
    - Piperacillin/tazobactam
  - Chronic Care
    - Amoxicillin
    - Amoxicillin/Clavulanic acid

> **Counseling Point**
> ✓ Counsel patients taking amoxicillin/clavulanic acid (Augmentin) that the development of diarrhea around the 3-4th day is normal and reversible once completing treatment.

Main Indications or Uses
- Acute Care
  - Bacteremia
  - Endocarditis
  - GI tract infections
  - GU tract infections (including UTI)
  - Meningitis
  - Respiratory tract infections (CAP)
  - Ventilator/Hospital Acquired Pneumonia
    - Durlobactam/sulbactam

> **Knowledge Integration**
> ✓ Remember, ampicillin is added to ceftriaxone or cefotaxime + vancomycin for empiric dosing in suspected bacterial meningitis in patients < 1 month old or > 50 years of age. If allergic to PCN, then consider TMP/SMX.

Mechanism of Action
- Inhibit the final step in bacterial cell wall synthesis by binding to specific penicillin-binding proteins in the bacterial cytoplasmic membrane.
  - Beta-lactams also prevent the transpeptidation reaction and cross-linking of linear peptidoglycan chain constituents of the cell wall and activate autolytic enzymes that cause lesions in the bacterial cell wall.
- Clavulanic acid and sulbactam are beta-lactamase inhibitor compounds that prevent hydrolysis by class A beta-lactamases.

Primary Net Benefit
- Bactericidal to susceptible pathogens, leading to microbiologic clearance of the affecting organisms.
- Main Labs to Monitor:
  - Cultures from infected sites at baseline (blood, sputum, urine, CSF, etc.)

High-Yield Basic Pharmacology
- **Absorption differences**
  - Amoxicillin and ampicillin are very similar in pharmacologic action, but only amoxicillin is commercially available as an oral preparation in the United States.
    - Peak plasma concentrations of amoxicillin are roughly 2.5 times higher than an equal dose of ampicillin administered orally.
- **Probenecid**
  - Probenecid significantly decreased the renal tubular secretion of many penicillins and is most often used with penicillin G; however, it can be combined with ampicillin to yield the same effect.
    - Probenecid can specifically improve penicillin and ampicillin concentration in the CSF.
- **Beta-lactamase Inhibitors**

- Clavulanic acid, sulbactam, and tazobactam are beta-lactamase inhibitors that are active against plasmid-encoded beta-lactamases but not active against beta-lactamases with AmpC chromosomal mutations frequently encountered in Pseudomonas, Citrobacter, and Enterobacter spp.

High-Yield Clinical Knowledge
- Aminopenicillins were developed to improve antimicrobial spectrum extending to gram-negative organisms, including Haemophilus influenza, Escherichia coli, and Proteus mirabilis.
- Ampicillin is often used in combination with a cephalosporin for acute bacterial meningitis empiric therapy.
    - The combination of two beta-lactam antibiotics is not a duplication of therapy since the ampicillin component is specifically targeting L. monocytogenes.
        - Ampicillin should be added to patients with suspected meningitis if they are younger than 2 years of age, older than 50 years of age, or otherwise immunocompromised.
- Many patients, approximately 10%, develop a nonpruritic, non-urticarial rash after exposure to aminopenicillins, and almost all patients taking amoxicillin while infected with Epstein-Barr virus develop a morbilliform rash.
    - These eruptions are not allergic and should not be listed as such inpatient charts as they are not associated with anaphylaxis on subsequent exposure. Instead, they should be documented as adverse events.
- **Core spectrum**
    - **Gram-Positive**
        - Staphylococcus species, methicillin-sensitive only
        - Streptococcus species
        - Enterococcus species
        - Listeria monocytogenes
    - **Gram-Negative**
        - Acinetobacter baumannii-calcoaceticus
            - Only Durlobactam/sulbactam
        - Escherichia coli
        - Klebsiella pneumoniae
        - Shigella species
        - Proteus mirabilis
        - Haemophilus influenzae
        - Enterobacter sp
        - Pseudomonas aeruginosa
            - Only piperacillin/tazobactam
    - Anaerobes (piperacillin/tazobactam)
- **Core Indications**
    - **Community-acquired pneumonia**
        - High-dose amoxicillin (1g q8h) or amoxicillin/clavulanate 875 mg twice daily, or ampicillin/sulbactam 3 g IV q6h in combination with azithromycin or doxycycline are recommended treatments for patients with CAP.
    - **Hospital-acquired pneumonia**
        - Piperacillin/tazobactam provides gram-negative coverage (of note, Pseudomonas aeruginosa and the Enterobacteriaceae) and increased anaerobic coverage.
        - Durlobactam/sulbactam is available for HAP and also VAP but should only be used for nosocomial infections from Acinetobacter baumannii-calcoaceticus.
    - **Intra-Abdominal infections**
        - Because of the good coverage of GI gram-negative pathogens and anaerobes found in GI flora, piperacillin/tazobactam is a first-line agent for many intra-abdominal infections.
    - **Bacterial meningitis**
        - Ampicillin is a drug of choice for meningitis caused by Listeria monocytogenes and Streptococcus agalactiae.
    - **Group B Streptococci colonization in pregnancy**

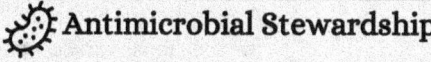

Antimicrobial Stewardship

✓ Only piperacillin / tazobactam (Zosyn) covers against Pseudomonas aeruginosa, not amoxicillin or ampicillin-based formulations.

✓ Amoxicillin is 1 of the top 10 drugs implicated in ED visits for adverse effects.

- Antepartum administration of ampicillin may be beneficial for prophylaxis against group B streptococcal infection in infants of mothers with birth canal colonization.
    - After administration of 2g IV to the mother, bactericidal concentrations of ampicillin are achieved in the amniotic fluid within 5 minutes.
- **Otitis Media**
    - Amoxicillin is the drug of choice for most cases of otitis media when antibiotics are indicated.
        - However, the dose is 40-45 mg/kg/dose twice a day to achieve proper penetration into the middle ear. Most max the dose at 2 g per dose.

High-Yield Fast-Facts
- **Oral Ampicillin**
    - For a localized GI tract Shigella infection, oral ampicillin has been favored for treatment because its lack of absorption is desirable.
- **Unasyn Dosing**
    - For the labeled 3 g vial of ampicillin/sulbactam, there is 2 g of ampicillin and 1 g of sulbactam, and for the 1.5 g dose vial, there is 1 g of ampicillin and 500 mg of sulbactam.
        - For weight-based dosing of ampicillin/sulbactam, the dose should be based on the ampicillin component.
- **Sulbactam for Acinetobacter**
    - The sulbactam component of ampicillin/sulbactam is uniquely active against the nosocomial pathogen Acinetobacter baumannii. That is to say, the reason for administration of ampicillin/sulbactam is strictly for the sulbactam component, as it is not commercially available alone in the United States.
- **Antimicrobial Stewardship (AS)**
    - Allergies should be investigated by providers or AS teams to determine if a true allergy occurred. Point-of-care skin testing and oral challenges can be performed in inpatient settings to determine tolerance, unless a non-IgE mediated allergic reaction is suspected. Only approximately 1% have true allergies.
        - Negative outcomes can occur from avoiding first-line antibiotics, including reduced efficacy and increased potential for adverse effects, resistance, and costs.
        - Amoxicillin is 1 of the top 10 drugs implicated in ED visits for adverse effects.

HIGH-YIELD BOARD EXAM ESSENTIALS
- **CLASSIC AGENTS:** Amoxicillin, amoxicillin/clavulanic acid, ampicillin, ampicillin/sulbactam, piperacillin/tazobactam
- **DRUG CLASS:** Aminopenicillin and extended-spectrum penicillin
- **INDICATIONS:** Bacteremia, endocarditis, GI tract infections, GU tract infections (e.g., UTI), meningitis, upper and lower respiratory tract infections (otitis media, sinusitis, strep pharyngitis pneumonia)
- **MECHANISM:** Inhibit the final step in bacterial cell wall synthesis by binding to specific penicillin-binding proteins in the bacterial cytoplasmic membrane.
- **SIDE EFFECTS:** Rash, diarrhea
- **CLINICAL PEARLS:**
    - These agents are renally eliminated, cause very little drug interactions, and are consider safe in pregnancy.
    - Many patients, approximately 10%, develop a nonpruritic, non-urticarial rash after exposure to aminopenicillins, and almost all patients taking amoxicillin while infected with Epstein-Barr virus (those with "mono") develop a morbilliform rash.
    - Only piperacillin/tazobactam in this group covers against Pseudomonas, none of the others. None of them cover against MRSA.
    - The dosing of amoxicillin is much higher for the treatment of otitis media than most people realize. The dose is 40-45 mg/kg/dose (most max the dose at 2 g/dose)

Table: Drug Class Summary

\multicolumn{4}{c}{**Aminopenicillin and Extended-Spectrum Penicillin - Drug Class Review**}
\multicolumn{4}{c}{High-Yield Med Reviews}

Aminopenicillin and Extended-Spectrum Penicillin - Drug Class Review
High-Yield Med Reviews

Mechanism of Action: *Inhibit the final step in bacterial cell wall synthesis by binding to specific penicillin-binding proteins in the bacterial cytoplasmic membrane.*

Class Effects: *Bactericidal to susceptible pathogens, leading to microbiologic clearance of the affecting organisms.*

Generic Name	Brand Name	Main Indication(s) or Uses	Notes
Amoxicillin	Moxatag	<ul><li>GI tract infections</li><li>GU tract infections</li><li>Respiratory tract infections</li><li>Urinary tract infection</li></ul>	<ul><li>**Dosing (Adult):**<ul><li>Oral: 250-875mg q8-12h</li></ul></li><li>**Dosing (Peds):**<ul><li>Oral: > 1 month and < 20 kg: 20-40 mg/kg/day in 3 divided doses</li></ul></li><li>**CYP450 Interactions:** None</li><li>**Renal or Hepatic Dose Adjustments:**<ul><li>GFR: 10 to 50 mL/minute: Decrease frequency to q12h</li><li>GFR: < 10 mL/minute: Decrease frequency to q12-24h.</li></ul></li><li>**Dosage Forms:** Oral (capsules, suspension, tablet)</li></ul>
Amoxicillin/ Clavulanic acid	Augmentin	<ul><li>GI tract infections</li><li>GU tract infections</li><li>Respiratory tract infections</li><li>Skin and soft tissue infections</li><li>Urinary tract infection</li></ul>	<ul><li>**Dosing (Adult):**<ul><li>Oral: 250-875mg q8-12h</li></ul></li><li>**Dosing (Peds):**<ul><li>Oral: > 1 month and < 20 kg: 20-40 mg/kg/day in 3 divided doses</li></ul></li><li>**CYP450 Interactions:** None</li><li>**Renal or Hepatic Dose Adjustments:**<ul><li>GFR: 10 to 50 mL/minute: Decrease frequency to q12h</li><li>GFR: < 10 mL/minute: Decrease frequency to q12-24h.</li></ul></li><li>**Dosage Forms:** Oral (capsules, extended-release capsule, suspension, tablet)</li></ul>
Ampicillin	Omnipen	<ul><li>Bacteremia</li><li>Endocarditis</li><li>GI tract infections</li><li>GU tract infections</li><li>Meningitis</li><li>Respiratory tract infections</li><li>Urinary tract infection</li></ul>	<ul><li>**Dosing (Adult):**<ul><li>IV: 1 to 2g IV q4h</li></ul></li><li>**Dosing (Peds):**<ul><li>IV/IM: 50 to 200 mg/kg/day in 4-6 divided doses</li></ul></li><li>**CYP450 Interactions:** None</li><li>**Renal or Hepatic Dose Adjustments:**<ul><li>GFR: 10 to 50 mL/minute: Decrease frequency to q6-12h</li><li>GFR: < 10 mL/minute: Decrease frequency to q8-24h.</li></ul></li><li>**Dosage Forms:** Oral (capsule, solution), IV/IM (solution)</li></ul>

| Aminopenicillin and Extended-Spectrum Penicillin - Drug Class Review ||||
| High-Yield Med Reviews ||||
Generic Name	Brand Name	Main Indication(s) or Uses	Notes
Ampicillin/ Sulbactam	Unasyn	<ul><li>Bacteremia</li><li>Endocarditis</li><li>GI tract infections</li><li>GU tract infections</li><li>Meningitis</li><li>Respiratory tract infections</li><li>Skin and soft tissue infections</li><li>Urinary tract infection</li></ul>	<ul><li>**Dosing (Adult):** – IV: 1.5 to 3g IV q6h</li><li>**Dosing (Peds):** – IV/IM of ampicillin 50 to 200 mg/kg/day in 4-6 divided doses</li><li>**CYP450 Interactions:** None</li><li>**Renal or Hepatic Dose Adjustments:** – GFR: 10 to 50 mL/minute: Decrease frequency to q6-12h – GFR: < 10 mL/minute: Decrease frequency to q8-24h.</li><li>**Dosage Forms:** IV (solution)</li></ul>
Durlobactam/ Sulbactam	Xacduro	<ul><li>Hospital Acquired Pneumonia</li><li>Ventilator Associated Pneumonia</li></ul>	<ul><li>**Dosing (Adult):** – IV: 1 g IV q6h x ~ 7 days</li><li>**Dosing (Peds):** – Not used</li><li>**CYP450 Interactions:** None</li><li>**Renal or Hepatic Dose Adjustments:** – GFR: 45 to 129 mL/minute: No adjustment – GFR: 30 to 44 mL/minute: 1 g every 8 hours – GFR: < 15 mL/minute: 1 g every 12 hrs</li><li>**Dosage Forms:** IV (solution)</li></ul>
Piperacillin/ Tazobactam	Zosyn	<ul><li>Bacteremia</li><li>Endocarditis</li><li>GI tract infections</li><li>GU tract infections</li><li>Respiratory tract infections</li><li>Skin and soft tissue infections</li><li>Urinary tract infection</li></ul>	<ul><li>**Dosing (Adult):** – IV: 3.375 to 4.5g IV q6h</li><li>**Dosing (Peds):** – IV of piperacillin 50 to 200 mg/kg/day in 4 divided doses</li><li>**CYP450 Interactions:** None</li><li>**Renal or Hepatic Dose Adjustments:** – GFR: 10 to 30 mL/minute: Decrease frequency to q12h – GFR: < 10 mL/minute: Reduce to q24h.</li><li>**Dosage Forms:** IV (solution)</li></ul>

INFECTIOUS DISEASE – ANTISTAPHYLOCOCCAL PENICILLINS

Drug Class
- Beta-Lactam Antibiotic → Antistaphylococcal Penicillins
- Agents:
  - Acute and Chronic Care
    - Dicloxacillin
    - Nafcillin

Main Indications or Uses
- Acute & Chronic Care
  - Endocarditis
  - Pneumonia
  - Bone and joint infections
  - Skin and soft tissue infections (from MSSA)

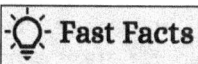

Fast Facts
- Since methicillin is no longer available, oxacillin is now used in the lab to determine if Staph. Aureus is sensitive or resistant. Thus MSSA / OSSA and MRSA / ORSA are interchangeable.

Mechanism of Action
- Inhibit the final step in bacterial cell wall synthesis by binding to specific penicillin-binding proteins in the bacterial cytoplasmic membrane.
  - Beta-lactams prevent the transpeptidation reaction and cross-linking of linear peptidoglycan chain constituents of the cell wall and activate autolytic enzymes that cause lesions in the bacterial cell wall.

Primary Net Benefit
- Bactericidal to susceptible pathogens, leading to microbiologic clearance of the affecting organisms.
- Main Labs to Monitor:
  - Cultures from infected sites at baseline (blood, sputum, urine, CSF, etc.)

High-Yield Basic Pharmacology
- **Penicillinase-Resistant**
  - Antistaphylococcal penicillins can also be referred to as penicillinase-resistant penicillins as they possess an additional side chain on the beta-lactam ring that protects it from acid hydrolysis by Staphylococcus species.
- **Gram-Positive Spectrum**
  - The antistaphylococcal penicillins have activity against most penicillinase-producing strains of Staphylococcus species and are less active against streptococcal species and enterococci.
  - These agents have no clinically relevant gram-negative activity or activity against Listeria monocytogenes.
- **Nafcillin Elimination**
  - Nafcillin is preferred in patients with renal impairment as it primarily undergoes biliary excretion.
  - Oxacillin and dicloxacillin are eliminated by both the biliary system and kidney.

High-Yield Clinical Knowledge
- **Nafcillin Vs. Oxacillin**
  - Nafcillin treatment is associated with higher rates of adverse events and treatment discontinuation than oxacillin among hospitalized adult patients. (Antimicrob Agents Chemother. 2016 Apr 22;60(5):3090-5.)
- **Nafcillin and CYP Interactions**
  - There is some evidence to suggest that nafcillin induces CYP3A4 and possibly CYP2C9, leading to clinically relevant drug interactions. (Br J Clin Pharmacol. 2003 Jun; 55(6): 588–590.)
- **Aminoglycoside Synergy**
  - In patients with endocarditis, the combination of aminoglycosides with nafcillin or oxacillin may provide a synergistic effect and an enhanced bactericidal effect, and a more rapid resolution of fever. (J Lab Clin Med 1976;88:118-124; Ann Intern Med 1982;97:496-503.)

- **Core spectrum**
  - Gram-Positive
    - Staphylococcus species, methicillin-sensitive only
    - Streptococcus species
- **Core indications**
  - Endocarditis, pneumonia, bone and joint infections, and skin and soft tissue infections caused by susceptible strains of methicillin-sensitive Staphylococci species.
  - **Endocarditis**
    - In patients with methicillin/oxacillin susceptible Staphylococci endocarditis (in the absence of prosthetic metal valves), an antistaphylococcal penicillin is preferred over vancomycin.
  - **Skin and Soft Tissue Infections and Bone and Joint Infections**
    - Nafcillin or oxacillin can be used for skin and soft tissue infections and bone and joint infections caused by Staphylococcal sp. sensitivity to methicillin/oxacillin.

High-Yield Fast-Fact
- **Methicillin or Oxacillin Resistant Staphylococcus Aureus?**
  - Methicillin is no longer available in the US with oxacillin taking its place in therapy.
    - Oxacillin resistant or sensitive Staphylococcus Aureus (ORSA or OSSA) would be a more accurate terminology compared to MSSA and MRSA.
- **Tissue Necrosis**
  - Nafcillin is associated with tissue necrosis if extravasation occurs during infusion. Since nafcillin is given as frequently as every 4 hours, or even as a continuous infusion, this may be a significant risk in patients.
- **Cloxacillin Availability**
  - Cloxacillin is frequently discussed in texts and primary literature; however, it is not available in the US.

HIGH-YIELD BOARD EXAM ESSENTIALS
- **CLASSIC AGENTS:** Dicloxacillin, nafcillin
- **DRUG CLASS:** Antistaphylococcal Penicillins
- **INDICATIONS:** Endocarditis, pneumonia, bone and joint infections, skin and soft tissue infections
- **MECHANISM:** Inhibit the final step in bacterial cell wall synthesis by binding to specific penicillin-binding proteins in the bacterial cytoplasmic membrane.
- **SIDE EFFECTS:** Hepatic injury (nafcillin), renal injury (dicloxacillin)
- **CLINICAL PEARLS:**
  - These agents do NOT cover against MRSA but do cover MSSA.
  - Nafcillin is associated with tissue necrosis if extravasation occurs during infusion. Since nafcillin is given as frequently as every 4 hours, or even as a continuous infusion, this may be a significant risk in patients.

Table: Drug Class Summary

Antistaphylococcal Penicillins - Drug Class Review High-Yield Med Reviews			
Mechanism of Action: *Inhibit the final step in bacterial cell wall synthesis by binding to specific penicillin-binding proteins in the bacterial cytoplasmic membrane.*			
Class Effects: *Bactericidal to mainly MSSA, but NOT MRSA.*			
Generic Name	**Brand Name**	**Indication(s) or Uses**	**Notes**

Dicloxacillin	Diclocil	<ul><li>Endocarditis</li><li>Pneumonia</li><li>Bone and joint infections</li><li>Skin and soft tissue infections</li></ul>	<ul><li>**Dosing (Adult):**
			  – Oral: 125 to 250 mg q6h</li><li>**Dosing (Peds):**
			  – Oral: 12.5 to 100 mg/kg/day divided in 4 doses</li><li>**CYP450 Interactions:** None</li><li>**Renal or Hepatic Dose Adjustments:** None</li><li>**Dosage Forms:** Oral (capsules)</li></ul>

Nafcillin	Nallpen, Unipen	<ul><li>Endocarditis</li><li>Pneumonia</li><li>Bone and joint infections</li><li>Skin and soft tissue infections</li></ul>	<ul><li>**Dosing (Adult):**
			  – IV: 1 to 2 g q4-6h</li><li>**Dosing (Peds):**
			  – IV: 50 to 200 mg/kg/day in 4-6 divided doses</li><li>**CYP450 Interactions:** Induces CYP3A4</li><li>**Renal or Hepatic Dose Adjustments:**
			  – Nafcillin: 50% dose reduction may be necessary for both renal and hepatic insufficiency.</li><li>**Dosage Forms:** IV (solution)</li></ul>

Oxacillin	Bactocil	<ul><li>Endocarditis</li><li>Pneumonia</li><li>Bone and joint infections</li><li>Skin and soft tissue infections</li></ul>	<ul><li>**Dosing (Adult):**
			  – IV: 1 to 2 g q4-6h</li><li>**Dosing (Peds):**
			  – IV: 50 to 200 mg/kg/day in 4-6 divided doses</li><li>**CYP450 Interactions:** None</li><li>**Renal or Hepatic Dose Adjustments:**
			  – GFR: < 10 mL/minute: Use lowest dose range initially.</li><li>**Dosage Forms:** IV (solution)</li></ul>

INFECTIOUS DISEASE – CARBAPENEMS

Drug Class
- Beta-Lactam Antibiotic → Carbapenems
- Agents:
    - Acute and Chronic Care
        - Doripenem
        - Ertapenem
        - Imipenem
            - Imipenem/Cilastatin/Relebactam
        - Meropenem
            - Meropenem/Vaborbactam

> **Fast Facts**
> ✓ Carbapenem antibiotics have a beta-lactam ring and while the cross-reactivity to those with penicillin allergy is very low, it is not zero.

Main Indications or Uses
- Acute & Chronic Care
    - Bacteremia (Sepsis)
    - Bone and joint infections
    - Gynecologic infections
    - Intra-abdominal infections
    - Pneumonia (Hospital and/or ventilator associated pneumonia)
    - Skin and soft tissue infection
    - Urinary tract infection (mainly pyelonephritis)

Mechanism of Action
- Inhibit the final step in bacterial cell wall synthesis by binding to specific penicillin-binding proteins in the bacterial cytoplasmic membrane.
    - Beta-lactams also prevent the transpeptidation reaction and cross-linking of linear peptidoglycan chain constituents of the cell wall as well as activate autolytic enzymes that cause lesions in the bacterial cell wall.

Primary Net Benefit
- Bactericidal to susceptible pathogens, including ESBL producing organisms and Pseudomonas (except ertapenem).
- Main Labs to Monitor:
    - Cultures from infected sites at baseline (blood, sputum, urine, CSF, etc.)

High-Yield Clinical Knowledge
- **Cilastatin And Renal Tubules**
    - Imipenem, although referred to independently in many resources, is always co-formulated with cilastatin.
    - Cilastatin prevents the inactivation of imipenem by renal tubule dehydropeptidases, thus limiting excessive elimination of the active imipenem component.
- **AmpC, ESBL, CRE**
    - Carbapenems can be used for susceptible ESBL positive organisms where other beta-lactams are not appropriate.
    - However, carbapenems may still be degraded by highly resistant organisms, including the emerging carbapenemase-producing gram-negative pathogens, which are referred to as carbapenem-resistant Enterobacteriaceae (CRE), and specific organisms referred to as Klebsiella producing carbapenemase (KPC).
- **Exception Ertapenem**
    - Ertapenem has a distinctly different spectrum of activity compared to other carbapenems. Notably, ertapenem does <u>NOT</u> cover Pseudomonas aeruginosa and Acinetobacter species.

High-Yield Basic Spectrum of Activity
- Carbapenem
    - Gram-Positive
        - Streptococcus
            - Streptococcus pneumoniae

- Streptococcus viridans
- Streptococcus groups A, B, C, G
- Staphylococcus aureus, methicillin-sensitive only
- Listeria monocytogenes
- **Gram-Negative**
    - Enterobacteriaceae (ESBL negative, CRE negative)
        - Escherichia coli
        - Klebsiella pneumoniae
        - Salmonella species
        - Shigella species
        - Yersinia pestis
    - Enterobacter sp (AmpC negative)
    - Moraxella catarrhalis
    - Serratia species
    - Providencia species
    - Morganella species
    - Citrobacter species
    - Aeromonas hydrophila
    - Pseudomonas aeruginosa
    - Neisseria gonorrhoeae
    - Neisseria meningitidis
- **Anaerobes**
    - Actinomyces
    - Bacteroides fragilis
    - Clostridium species
    - Fusobacterium necrophorum
    - Peptostreptococcus species
    - Prevotella melaninogenica

Antimicrobial Stewardship

- All of the carbapenems cover Pseudomonas aeruginosa except ertapenem.
- All of the carbapenems also cover against ESBL + organisms, but NOT CRE or KPC+ organisms. The exceptions are imipenem and meropenem formulations combined with a beta-lactamase inhibitor.

High-Yield Fast-Facts
- **Seizures Are Possible**
    - High doses, renal impairment, or a combination of the two may lead to excessive exposure to imipenem with the possibility of causing seizures.
        - The proposed mechanism is the carbapenem antagonist activity of the GABA-A receptor.
- **Penicillin Allergy**
    - Carbapenems are often used empirically in patients with a history of an allergic response to penicillin. However, many of these patients may be able to receive alternative (at times, more appropriate) beta-lactams after a thorough history of the offending allergy.
- **Extended infusion**
    - Most carbapenems are administered via extended infusions empirically in adult patients. While the prescribing information typically suggests an infusion rate of 30 minutes, extending the infusion to 3-4 hours capitalizes on the "Time over MIC" characteristics of carbapenem agents.

HIGH-YIELD BOARD EXAM ESSENTIALS
- **CLASSIC AGENTS:** Doripenem, ertapenem, imipenem, meropenem
- **DRUG CLASS:** Carbapenem
- **INDICATIONS:** Bacteremia, bone and joint infections, gynecologic infections, intra-abdominal infections, pneumonia (HAP & VAP), skin and soft tissue infection, urinary tract infection (pyelonephritis)
- **MECHANISM:** Inhibit the final step in bacterial cell wall synthesis by binding to specific penicillin-binding proteins in the bacterial cytoplasmic membrane.
- **SIDE EFFECTS:** Seizures (mainly at high-doses), hypersensitivity
- **CLINICAL PEARLS:** There is a small risk of cross-reaction with carbapenems in patients with reported penicillin allergy. While carbapenems are used in patients with PCN allergy, this does not negate close monitoring early on. Imipenem, although referred to independently in many resources, is always co-formulated with cilastatin. Cilastatin prevents the inactivation of imipenem by renal tubule dehydropeptidases, thus limiting excessive elimination of the active imipenem component. Ertapenem is the only agent in this class that does NOT cover against Pseudomonas.

Table: Drug Class Summary

	Carbapenem - Drug Class Review High-Yield Med Reviews		
Mechanism of Action: *Inhibit the final step in bacterial cell wall synthesis by binding to specific penicillin-binding proteins in the bacterial cytoplasmic membrane.*			
Class Effects: *Bactericidal, covers ESBL producing organisms and Pseudomonas (except ertapenem).*			
Generic Name	**Brand Name**	**Main Indication(s) or Uses**	**Notes**

Doripenem	Doribax	<ul><li>Intra-abdominal infections</li><li>Urinary tract infection</li></ul>	<ul><li>**Dosing (Adult):**
			  – IV: 500 mg IV q8h</li><li>**Dosing (Peds):** Not routinely used</li><li>**CYP450 Interactions:** None</li><li>**Renal or Hepatic Dose Adjustments:**
			  – GFR: 30 to 50 mL/minute: 250 mg q8h
			  – GFR: 11 to 29 mL/minute: 250 mg q12h
			  – GFR: < 11 mL/minutes: 250 mg q24h</li><li>**Dosage Forms:** IV (solution)</li></ul>

Ertapenem	Invanz	<ul><li>Intra-abdominal infections</li><li>Pelvic infection</li><li>Pneumonia</li><li>Skin and soft tissue infection</li><li>Surgical prophylaxis</li><li>Urinary tract infection</li></ul>	<ul><li>**Dosing (Adult):**
			  – IV: 1 g IV q24h</li><li>**Dosing (Peds):**
			  – IV: 15 mg/kg/dose twice daily
			  – Max 500 mg/dose</li><li>**CYP450 Interactions:** None</li><li>**Renal or Hepatic Dose Adjustments:**
			  – GFR: < 30 mL/minutes: 500 mg q24h</li><li>**Dosage Forms:** IV (solution)</li></ul>

Imipenem/ Cilastatin	Primaxin	<ul><li>Bacteremia</li><li>Bone and joint infections</li><li>Gynecologic infections</li><li>Intra-abdominal infections</li><li>Pneumonia</li><li>Skin and soft tissue infection</li><li>Urinary tract infection</li></ul>	<ul><li>**Dosing (Adult):**
			  – IV: 500 to 1000 mg q6h</li><li>**Dosing (Peds):**
			  – Oral: 20 to 100 mg/kg/day q6-12h</li><li>**CYP450 Interactions:** None</li><li>**Renal or Hepatic Dose Adjustments:**
			  – GFR: 60 to 90 mL/minute: 400 - 750 mg q6h
			  – GFR: 30 to 60 mL/minute: 300 - 500 mg q6h
			  – GFR: 15 and 30 mL/minute: 200 - 500 mg q6h
			  – GFR: < 15 mL/minute: Not recommended</li><li>**Dosage Forms:** IV (solution)</li></ul>

Infectious Diseases

Carbapenem - Drug Class Review
High-Yield Med Reviews

Generic Name	Brand Name	Main Indication(s) or Uses	Notes

Imipenem/ Cilastatin/ Relebactam	Recarbrio	- Intra-abdominal infections
		- Pneumonia
		- Urinary tract infection
		
		Note: Reserved for extensively resistant organisms
			- **Dosing (Adult):**
			  – IV: 1.25 g q6h
			- **Dosing (Peds):** Not routinely used
			- **CYP450 Interactions:** None
			- **Renal or Hepatic Dose Adjustments:**
			  – GFR: 60 to 90 mL/minute: 1g q6h
			  – GFR: 30 to 60 mL/minute: 750 mg q6h
			  – GFR: 15 and 30 mL/minute 500 q6h
			  – GFR: < 15 mL/minute: Not recommended
			- **Dosage Forms:** IV (solution)

Meropenem	Merrem	- Intra-abdominal infections
		- Bacterial meningitis
		- Skin and skin structure infection
			- **Dosing (Adult):**
			  – IV: 500 mg q6h or 1 to g q8h
			- **Dosing (Peds):**
			  – IV: 20 mg/kg/dose q8h
			    – Maximum 2g/dose
			- **CYP450 Interactions:** None
			- **Renal or Hepatic Dose Adjustments:**
			  – GFR: 25 to 50 mL/minute: 1-2g q12h
			  – GFR: 10 to 25 mL/minute: 500-1000 mg q12h
			  – GFR: < 15 mL/minute: 500-1000 mg q24h
			- **Dosage Forms:** IV (solution)

Meropenem/ Vaborbactam	Vabomere	- Urinary tract infection
		
		Note: Reserved for extensively resistant organisms
			- **Dosing (Adult):**
			  – IV: 4g q8h
			- **Dosing (Peds):**
			  – Oral: 20 to 100 mg/kg/day q6-12h
			- **CYP450 Interactions:** None
			- **Renal or Hepatic Dose Adjustments:**
			  – GFR: 30 to 49 mL/minute: 2g q8h
			  – GFR: 15 to 30 mL/minute: 2g q12h
			  – GFR: < 15 mL/minutes: 1 g q12h.
			- **Dosage Forms:** IV (solution)

INFECTIOUS DISEASE – CEPHALOSPORINS - 1st GENERATION

Drug Class
- Beta-Lactam Antibiotic → Cephalosporins – 1st Generation
- Agents:
  - Acute and Chronic Care
    - Cefadroxil
    - Cefazolin
    - Cephalexin

Main Indications or Uses
- Acute & Chronic Care
  - Bacteremia
  - Bone and joint infections
  - Endocarditis
  - GI Infection
  - Pharyngitis
  - Skin and soft tissue infections
  - Surgical prophylaxis
  - Urinary tract infections

> **Accelerate Your Knowledge**
>
> ✓ In trauma with any open fracture or penetrating injury requiring surgery, cefazolin is the drug of choice within the ER prior to going to surgery (for surgery prophylaxis).
>
> ✓ Cephalexin is not sufficient to cover for complicated UTIs (e.g., pyelonephritis) due to the lack of tissue penetration.

Mechanism of Action
- Inhibit the final step in bacterial cell wall synthesis by binding to specific penicillin-binding proteins in the bacterial cytoplasmic membrane.
  - Beta-lactams also prevent the transpeptidation reaction and cross-linking of linear peptidoglycan chain constituents of the cell wall as well as activate autolytic enzymes that cause lesions in the bacterial cell wall.

Primary Net Benefit
- Bactericidal to susceptible pathogens, leading to microbiologic clearance of the affecting organisms.
  - Does <u>NOT</u> cover against MRSA, Pseudomonas, ESBL or CRE organisms
- Main Labs to Monitor:
  - Cultures from infected sites at baseline (blood, sputum, urine, CSF etc.)

High-Yield Clinical Knowledge
- **First-Generation Uses**
  - Many oral first-generation cephalosporins are suitable for urinary tract infections and staphylococcal or streptococcal infections, including cellulitis or soft tissue abscess, but later generation agents should be selected for more serious systemic infections.
- **Culture & Sensitivity Interpretation**
  - Cefazolin is the only parenteral first-generation cephalosporin in the United States and is often listed on culture and sensitivity panels. For patients who may be eligible for oral first-generation cephalosporins, cefazolin susceptibility may be interpreted to cephalexin per CLSI.
- **Multiple Routes of Administration**
  - To ease administration, cefazolin may be administered with several different parenteral methods including intramuscular, intraosseous, intravenous infusion, or intravenous push.

High-Yield Basic Spectrum of Activity
- **First Generation Cephalosporins**
    - Gram-Positive
        - Streptococcus
            - Streptococcus pneumoniae
            - Streptococcus viridans
            - Streptococcus groups A, B, C, G
        - Staphylococcus aureus, methicillin-sensitive only
    - Gram-Negative
        - Enterobacteriaceae
            - Escherichia coli
            - Haemophilus influenzae
            - Klebsiella pneumoniae
            - Proteus mirabilis

> **Fast Facts**
> ✓ All cephalosporins are "bet-lactam" antibiotics due to their beta-lactam structures.
> ✓ 1st generation agents do NOT cover against MRSA, Pseudomonas or ESBLs.

High-Yield Fast-Facts
- **Cephalosporins and INR**
    - The cephalosporins that contain a methylthiotetrazole group such as cefotetan, and cefoperazone, are associated with prolonged prothrombin time, leading to clinically relevant bleeding in patients receiving warfarin.
- **Oldy Moldy**
    - Cephalosporin antibiotics were derived from the mold Acremonium, which was formerly known as Cephalosporium.
- **Cephalosporin Origin**
- Cephalosporins were first identified in 1945 by Giuseppe Brotzu from the University of Cagliari (Italy) when he isolated Cephalosporium acremonium

---

HIGH-YIELD BOARD EXAM ESSENTIALS
- **CLASSIC AGENTS:** Cefadroxil, cefazolin, cephalexin
- **DRUG CLASS:** Cephalosporins 1st generation
- **INDICATIONS:** Bacteremia, bone and joint infections, endocarditis, GI infection, pharyngitis, skin and soft tissue infections, surgical prophylaxis, urinary tract infections
- **MECHANISM:** Inhibit the final step in bacterial cell wall synthesis by binding to penicillin-binding proteins
- **SIDE EFFECTS:** Diarrhea, hypersensitivity, nausea
- **CLINICAL PEARLS:**
    - None of the agents in this class cover against MRSA, Pseudomonas, or ESBL producing organisms.
    - Many oral first-generation cephalosporins are suitable for uncomplicated:
        - Urinary tract infections (not pyelonephritis)
        - Staphylococcal or streptococcal infections, including cellulitis

Table: Drug Class Summary

\multicolumn{4}{c}{**Cephalosporins - 1st Generation - Drug Class Review**}

Cephalosporins - 1st Generation - Drug Class Review			
High-Yield Med Reviews			
Mechanism of Action: *Inhibit the final step in bacterial cell wall synthesis by binding to specific penicillin-binding proteins in the bacterial cytoplasmic membrane.*			
Class Effects: *Bactericidal to susceptible pathogens, but not MRSA, Pseudomonas, ESBL or CRE.*			
Generic Name	**Brand Name**	**Main Indication(s) or Uses**	**Notes**

Cefadroxil	Duricef	- Pharyngitis
		- Skin and soft tissue infections
		- Urinary tract infections
			- **Dosing (Adult):**
			  – Oral: 500 to 1000 mg q12-24h
			- **Dosing (Peds):**
			  – Oral: 30 mg/kg/day q12-24h
			- **CYP450 Interactions:** None
			- **Renal or Hepatic Dose Adjustments:**
			  – GFR: 25 to 50 mL/minute: 500 mg q12h
			  – GFR: 10 to 25 mL/minute: 500 mg q24h
			  – GFR: < 10 mL/minute: 500 mg q36h
			- **Dosage Forms:** Oral (capsules, suspension, tablet)

Cefazolin	Ancef	- Bacteremia
		- Bone and joint infections
		- Endocarditis
		- GI Infection
		- Pharyngitis
		- Skin and soft tissue infections
		- Surgical prophylaxis
		- Urinary tract infections
			- **Dosing (Adult):**
			  – IV/IO: 1 to 2 g IV q8h
			  – IM: 250 to 1500 mg q6-8h
			- **Dosing (Peds):**
			  – IV/IM: 25 to 150 mg/kg/day in q6 to 8h
			- **CYP450 Interactions:** None
			- **Renal or Hepatic Dose Adjustments:**
			  – GFR: 30 to 50 mL/minute: 1 to 2 g q8-12h
			  – GFR: 10 to 30 mL/minute: 500 mg q12h
			  – GFR: < 10 mL/minutes: 500 mg q24h
			- **Dosage Forms:** IV (solution)

Cephalexin	Keflex	- Bone and joint infections
		- Endocarditis
		- Otitis media
		- Skin and soft tissue infections
		- Urinary tract infections
			- **Dosing (Adult):**
			  – Oral: 250 to 1000 mg q12-24h
			- **Dosing (Peds):**
			  – Oral: 20 to 100 mg/kg/day q6-12h
			- **CYP450 Interactions:** None
			- **Renal or Hepatic Dose Adjustments:**
			  – GFR: 15 to 30 mL/minute: 250 to 500 mg q8-12h
			  – GFR: < 15 mL/minute: 250 to 500 mg q24h.
			- **Dosage Forms:** Oral (capsules, suspension, tablet)

INFECTIOUS DISEASE – CEPHALOSPORINS 2ND GENERATION

Drug Class
- Beta-Lactam Antibiotic → Cephalosporins - 2nd Generation
- Agents:
  - Acute and Chronic Care
    - Cefuroxime
    - Cefprozil
    - Cefoxitin
    - Cefotetan

Main Indications or Uses
- Acute & Chronic Care
  - Bacteremia
  - Bone and joint infections
  - Endocarditis
  - GI Infection
  - Pharyngitis
  - Pneumonia
  - Skin and soft tissue infections
  - Surgical prophylaxis
  - Urinary tract infections

> **Fast Facts**
> - All cephalosporins are "bet-lactam" antibiotics due to their beta-lactam structures.
> - Like 1st generation agents, the 2nd generation agents do NOT cover against MRSA, Pseudomonas or ESBLs.

Mechanism of Action
- Inhibit the final step in bacterial cell wall synthesis by binding to specific penicillin-binding proteins in the bacterial cytoplasmic membrane.
  - Beta-lactams also prevent the transpeptidation reaction and cross-linking of linear peptidoglycan chain constituents of the cell wall as well as activate autolytic enzymes that cause lesions in the bacterial cell wall.

Primary Net Benefit
- Bactericidal to susceptible pathogens, but not including MRSA, Pseudomonas, or ESBL+ organisms.
- Main Labs to Monitor:
  - Cultures from infected sites at baseline (blood, sputum, urine, CSF etc.)

High-Yield Core Knowledge
- **Cephamycin Sub-Category**
  - The second-generation cephalosporins possess an additional subclass known as cephamycins, including cefoxitin and cefotetan. The primary difference with these agents is their extended-spectrum including activity against anaerobes.
- **Perioperative Prophylaxis**
  - Cefoxitin and cefotetan are primarily utilized for perioperative prophylaxis in those undergoing intra-abdominal and gynecologic surgical procedures.
- **Extended Spectrum**
  - The oral second-generation cephalosporins extend their spectrum from first-generation agents by covering beta-lactamase-producing Haemophilus influenzae, and Moraxella catarrhalis and are useful to treat sinusitis, otitis, and lower respiratory tract infections.

High-Yield Basic Spectrum of Activity
- **Second Generation Cephalosporins**
  - Gram-Positive
    - Same as first-generation
  - Gram-Negative
    - Enterobacteriaceae
    - Moraxella catarrhalis
    - Serratia species (Cefotetan)
    - Providencia species (Cefotetan)
    - Morganella species (Cefotetan)
- Anaerobes
  - Clostridium species (not difficile)
  - Fusobacterium necrophorum
  - Peptostreptococcus species (Cefotetan)
  - Prevotella melaninogenica

High-Yield Fast-Facts
- **NMTT Side Chain**
  - Cephalosporins containing the NMTT sidechain (cefazolin, cefotetan) have been associated with a disulfiram-like reaction if combined with ethanol.
- **Beta-Lactamase Influence**
  - Cefuroxime may be more suitable for treatment of H. influenzae infections compared to cefazolin as a result of stability against the TEM beta-lactamase in ampicillin-resistant strains and beta-lactamase-producing Moraxella catarrhalis.
- **Third over Second-Generation**
  - Second generation cephalosporins have seen a decrease in their use, in place of either third-generation cephalosporins, or more narrow-spectrum first-generation agents.

HIGH-YIELD BOARD EXAM ESSENTIALS
- **CLASSIC AGENTS:** Cefuroxime, cefprozil, cefoxitin, cefotetan
- **DRUG CLASS:** Cephalosporins
- **INDICATIONS:** Bacteremia, bone and joint infections, endocarditis, GI infection, pharyngitis, skin and soft tissue infections, surgical prophylaxis, urinary tract infections
- **MECHANISM:** Inhibit the final step in bacterial cell wall synthesis by binding to specific penicillin-binding proteins in the bacterial cytoplasmic membrane.
- **SIDE EFFECTS:** Diarrhea, hypersensitivity, nausea
- **CLINICAL PEARLS:** Cephalosporins containing the NMTT sidechain (cefazolin, cefotetan) have been associated with a disulfiram-like reaction if combined with ethanol.

Table: Drug Class Summary

Cephalosporins - 2nd Generation - Drug Class Review
High-Yield Med Reviews

Mechanism of Action: *Inhibit the final step in bacterial cell wall synthesis by binding to specific penicillin-binding proteins in the bacterial cytoplasmic membrane.*

Class Effects: *Bactericidal to susceptible pathogens, but not including MRSA, Pseudomonas, or ESBL+ organisms.*

Generic Name	Brand Name	Main Indication(s) or Uses	Notes
Cefuroxime	Ceftin, Zinacef	<ul><li>Bone and joint infections</li><li>COPD exacerbation</li><li>Endocarditis</li><li>GI Infection</li><li>Lyme disease</li><li>Otitis media</li><li>Pharyngitis</li><li>Skin and soft tissue infections</li><li>Urinary tract infections</li></ul>	<ul><li>**Dosing (Adult):** − IM/IV: 1.5 g IV q8h − Oral: 250 to 500 mg q12-24h</li><li>**Dosing (Peds):** − Oral: 20 to 30 mg/kg/day q12-24h; Max: 500 mg/day − IM/IV: 100 to 200 mg/kg/day divided in 3-4 doses; Maximum 1500 mg/dose</li><li>**CYP450 Interactions:** None</li><li>**Renal or Hepatic Dose Adjustments:** − GFR: 10 to 30 mL/min: IV 750 - 1500 mg q12h; Oral 250 mg q12h or 500 mg q24h − GFR: < 10 mL/min: IV 750 - 1500 mg q24h; Oral 250 mg q24h or 500 mg q36h</li><li>**Dosage Forms:** Oral (caps, susp, tablet), IV (solution)</li></ul>
Cefprozil	Cefzil	<ul><li>COPD exacerbation</li><li>Otitis media</li><li>Pharyngitis</li></ul>	<ul><li>**Dosing (Adult):** − Oral: 250 to 500 mg q12-24h</li><li>**Dosing (Peds):** − Oral: 7.5 to 20 mg/kg/dose once to twice daily; Maximum 500 mg/dose</li><li>**CYP450 Interactions:** None</li><li>**Renal or Hepatic Dose Adjustments:** − GFR: < 30 mL/minute: reduce dose by 50%</li><li>**Dosage Forms:** Oral (suspension, tablet)</li></ul>
Cefoxitin	Mefoxin	<ul><li>Bacteremia</li><li>Bone and joint infections</li><li>GI/GYN Infection</li><li>Skin and soft tissue infections</li><li>Urinary tract infections</li></ul>	<ul><li>**Dosing (Adult):** − IV: 1 to 2 g IV q6-8h</li><li>**Dosing (Peds):** − Oral: 20 to 100 mg/kg/day q6-12h</li><li>**CYP450 Interactions:** None</li><li>**Renal or Hepatic Dose Adjustments:** − GFR: 30 to 50 mL/min: 1 - 2 g q8-12h − GFR: 10 to 29 mL/min: 1 - 2 g q12-24h − GFR: 5 to 9 mL/min: 500-1000 mg q12-24h</li><li>**Dosage Forms:** IV (solution)</li></ul>
Cefotetan	Cefotan	<ul><li>Bone and joint infections</li><li>GYN infections</li><li>Pneumonia</li><li>Skin and soft tissue infections</li><li>Surgical prophylaxis</li><li>Urinary tract infections</li></ul>	<ul><li>**Dosing (Adult):** IM/IV: 1 to 3 q12h</li><li>**Dosing (Peds):** IM/IV: 30 mg/kg/dose q12h</li><li>**CYP450 Interactions:** None</li><li>**Renal or Hepatic Dose Adjustments:** − GFR: 10 to 30 mL/min: Adjust frequency to q24h or reduce dose by 50% − GFR: < 10 mL/min: Adjust frequency to q48h or reduce dose by 25%</li><li>**Dosage Forms:** IV (solution)</li></ul>

INFECTIOUS DISEASES – CEPHALOSPORINS - 3RD GENERATION

Drug Class
- Beta-Lactam Antibiotic → Cephalosporins – 3rd Generation
- Agents:
  - Acute and Chronic Care
    - 3rd Generation
      - Cefotaxime
      - Ceftriaxone
      - Cefdinir
      - Cefixime
      - Cefpodoxime
      - Ceftazidime and Ceftazidime/avibactam

> **Antimicrobial Stewardship**
> ✓ Ceftazidime + avibactam (Avycaz) is, and should be, reserved for only multi-drug resistant infections as part of good antimicrobial stewardship.

Main Indications or Uses
- Acute & Chronic Care
  - Bacteremia
  - Bone and joint infections
  - Endocarditis
  - Intra-abdominal infections
  - Pharyngitis
  - Pneumonia
  - Skin and soft tissue infections
  - Surgical prophylaxis
  - Urinary tract infection

Mechanism of Action
- Inhibit the final step in bacterial cell wall synthesis by binding to specific penicillin-binding proteins in the bacterial cytoplasmic membrane.
  - Beta-lactams also prevent the transpeptidation reaction and cross-linking of linear peptidoglycan chain constituents of the cell wall as well as activate autolytic enzymes that cause lesions in the bacterial cell wall.

Primary Net Benefit
- Bactericidal to susceptible pathogens with increased gram-negative coverage and CNS penetration compared to the 1st and 2nd generation agents.
- Main Labs to Monitor:
  - Cultures from infected sites at baseline (blood, sputum, urine, CSF etc.)
  - C. diff stool antigen if starts to develop abdominal pain, diarrhea, and fever

High-Yield Clinical Knowledge
- **Ceftriaxone renal adjustment**
  - In patients with renal impairment, ceftriaxone does not require dose adjustment as it has mixed hepatic and renal elimination with approximately 50% recovered from the urine, and the remainder is eliminated by biliary excretion.
- **Cefotaxime neonatal meningitis**
  - Cefotaxime must be used in neonates in place of ceftriaxone, as it is contraindicated in this population due to its ability to displace bilirubin from albumin binding sites, causing a higher free bilirubin serum concentration with subsequent accumulation of bilirubin in the tissues.
- **Ceftazidime and Aztreonam**
  - Structurally, ceftazidime and aztreonam are nearly identical, except for the absence of a beta-lactam ring and accompanying side chains in the case of aztreonam.
    - As a result, their spectrum (including Pseudomonas aeruginosa), and pharmacokinetics are similar.

- In patients with a reported Type 1 allergy to ceftazidime, aztreonam should not be used because the likelihood of cross-reactivity is high given the identical R-1 side chains which are often the contributing antigenic component of the structure.
- **Ceftazidime and avibactam**
    - As cephalosporins generally have poor performance an activity against ESBL- and KPC-producing Enterobacteriaceae and AmpC β-lactamase-overexpressing Pseudomonas, but the addition of avibactam with ceftazidime extends the spectrum to include these pathogens.
        - Allows for use in hospital-acquired and ventilator-associated pneumonia (HAP & VAP) due to resistant organisms to other agents.
- **Intravitreal Route**
    - Ceftazidime can be used for endophthalmitis, but its route of administration should be intravitreal injections.

High-Yield Basic Spectrum of Activity
- **Third Generation Cephalosporins**
    - Gram-Positive
        - Same as second-generation; but no MRSA
    - Gram-Negative
        - Same as the second generation
        - Enterobacter sp (AmpC negative)
        - Citrobacter species
        - Aeromonas hydrophila
        - Yersinia enterocolitica
        - Pasteurella multocida
        - Pseudomonas aeruginosa (ceftazidime only)
        - Neisseria gonorrhoeae & N. meningitidis (ceftriaxone)
    - Anaerobes
        - Similar to the second generation
        - Actinomyces

Fast Facts
✓ Cefixime can be used for gonococcal STD infections when ceftriaxone not available or feasible.

✓ Lidocaine 1% can be used to reconstitute ceftriaxone for IM injection to reduce pain.

Counseling Point
✓ Cefdinir + oral iron supplements can cause maroon-colored stools → warn patients!

HIGH-YIELD BOARD EXAM ESSENTIALS
- **CLASSIC AGENTS:** Cefotaxime, ceftriaxone, cefdinir, cefixime, cefpodoxime, ceftazidime
- **DRUG CLASS:** 3rd Generation - Cephalosporins
- **INDICATIONS:** Bacteremia, bone and joint infections, endocarditis, GI infection, pharyngitis, skin and soft tissue infections, surgical prophylaxis, urinary tract infections
- **MECHANISM:** Inhibit the final step in bacterial cell wall synthesis by binding to specific penicillin-binding proteins in the bacterial cytoplasmic membrane.
- **SIDE EFFECTS:** Diarrhea (greater risk of C. diff), nausea, hypersensitivity reactions
- **CLINICAL PEARLS:**
    - In patients with renal impairment, ceftriaxone does not require dose adjustment as it has mixed hepatic and renal elimination with approximately 50% recovered from the urine, and the remainder is eliminated by biliary excretion.
    - No coverage against MRSA
    - Ceftazidime is the only agent to cover Pseudomonas
    - Ceftazidime + avibactam is reserved for drug resistant cases (ESBL, CRE, Amp-C, KPC + bacteria)

Table: Drug Class Summary

Cephalosporins - 3rd Generation - Drug Class Review High-Yield Med Reviews			
Mechanism of Action: *Inhibit the final step in bacterial cell wall synthesis by binding to specific penicillin-binding proteins in the bacterial cytoplasmic membrane.*			
Class Effects: *Bactericidal to susceptible pathogens with increased penetration into the CNS and gram negative coverage, including Pseudomonas (with ceftazidime only); risk of C. difficile infections.*			
Generic Name	**Brand Name**	**Main Indication(s) or Uses**	**Notes**
Cefotaxime	Claforan	<ul><li>Bacteremia</li><li>Bone and joint infections</li><li>CNS infections</li><li>GI Infection</li><li>Pharyngitis</li><li>Skin and soft tissue infections</li><li>Surgical prophylaxis</li><li>Urinary tract infections</li></ul>	<ul><li>**Dosing (Adult):** − IV: 1 to 2 g IV q6-8hours</li><li>**Dosing (Peds):** − IM/IV: 150 to 300 mg/kg/day − Maximum 12 g/day</li><li>**CYP450 Interactions:** None</li><li>**Renal or Hepatic Dose Adjustments:** − GFR: < 10 mL/minute: Decrease dose by 50% or administer every 24 hours</li><li>**Dosage Forms:** IV (solution)</li></ul>
Ceftriaxone	Rocephin	<ul><li>Bacteremia</li><li>Bone and joint infections</li><li>CNS infections</li><li>GI Infection</li><li>Gonococcal infection</li><li>Pharyngitis</li><li>Pneumonia</li><li>Skin and soft tissue infections</li><li>Surgical prophylaxis</li><li>Urinary tract infections</li></ul>	<ul><li>**Dosing (Adult):** − IV: 1 to 2 g IV q12-24h − IM: 250 to 2000 mg once to q12-24hours</li><li>**Dosing (Peds):** − IV/IM: 50 to 100 mg/kg/day in q12 to 24h</li><li>**CYP450 Interactions:** None</li><li>**Renal or Hepatic Dose Adjustments:** − None</li><li>**Dosage Forms:** IV (solution)</li></ul>
Cefdinir	Omnicef	<ul><li>Otitis media</li><li>Pneumonia</li><li>Sinusitis</li><li>Skin and soft tissue infections</li><li>Urinary tract infections</li></ul>	<ul><li>**Dosing (Adult):** − Oral: 300 mg BID or 600 mg Daily</li><li>**Dosing (Peds):** − Oral: 14 mg/kg/day divided q12-24h − Maximum 600 mg/day</li><li>**CYP450 Interactions:** None</li><li>**Renal or Hepatic Dose Adjustments:** − GFR: < 30 mL/minute: 300 mg once daily</li><li>**Dosage Forms:** Oral (capsules, suspension)</li></ul>
Cefixime	Suprax	<ul><li>Gonococcal infection</li><li>Rhinosinusitis</li><li>Typhoid fever</li></ul>	<ul><li>**Dosing (Adult):** − Oral: 400 mg q12-24hours</li><li>**Dosing (Peds):** − Oral: 14 mg/kg/day divided q12-24h − Maximum 600 mg/day</li><li>**CYP450 Interactions:** None</li><li>**Renal or Hepatic Dose Adjustments:** − GFR: 21 to 59 mL/minute: 260 mg once daily − GFR: < 20 mL/minute: 172 to 200 mg once daily</li><li>**Dosage Forms:** Oral (capsules, suspension)</li></ul>

Cephalosporins - 3rd Generation - Drug Class Review			
High-Yield Med Reviews			
Generic Name	Brand Name	Main Indication(s) or Uses	Notes
Cefpodoxime	Vantin	<ul><li>COPD exacerbation</li><li>Otitis media</li><li>Pneumonia</li><li>Rhinosinusitis</li><li>Sinusitis</li><li>Skin and soft tissue infections</li><li>Urinary tract infections</li></ul>	<ul><li>**Dosing (Adult):** - Oral: 200 to 400 mg q12-24hours</li><li>**Dosing (Peds):** - Oral: 5 mg/kg/day divided q24h - Maximum 400 mg/day</li><li>**CYP450 Interactions:** None</li><li>**Renal or Hepatic Dose Adjustments:** - GFR: < 30 mL/minute: Administer q24h</li><li>**Dosage Forms:** Oral (capsules, suspension)</li></ul>
Ceftazidime (+ avibactam)	Fortaz (Avycaz)	<ul><li>Bacteremia</li><li>Bone and joint infections</li><li>CNS infections</li><li>GI Infection</li><li>Gonococcal infection</li><li>Pharyngitis</li><li>Pneumonia</li><li>Skin and soft tissue infections</li><li>Surgical prophylaxis</li><li>Urinary tract infections</li></ul>	<ul><li>**Dosing (Adult):** - IV: 1 to 2 g IV q8h</li><li>**Dosing (Peds):** - Oral: 14 mg/kg/day divided q12-24h - Maximum 600 mg/day</li><li>**CYP450 Interactions:** None</li><li>**Renal or Hepatic Dose Adjustments:** - GFR: 31 to 50 mL/minute: 1 to 2 g IV q12h - GFR: 16 to 30 mL/minute: 1 to 2 g IV q24h - GFR: < 15 mL/minutes: 500 to 1g IV q24h</li><li>**Dosage Forms:** IV (solution) - Ceftazidime + avibactam (Avycaz) – IV solution; usually restricted use</li></ul>

INFECTIOUS DISEASE – CEPHALOSPORINS FOURTH GENERATION & OTHER

Drug Class
- Beta-Lactam Antibiotic → 4th Generation Cephalosporins & Other
- Agents:
  - **Acute and Chronic Care**
    - Cefepime
  - **Other**
    - Ceftaroline
    - Ceftolozane / tazobactam

> **Antimicrobial Stewardship**
> ✓ Ceftaroline should be reserved for MRSA when other options are not available.
> ✓ Ceftolozane + tazobactam is, and should be, reserved for only multi-drug resistant infections, including Pseudomonas and ESBL+ organisms, as part of good antimicrobial stewardship.

Main Indications or Uses
- **Acute & Chronic Care**
  - Bacteremia
  - Bone and joint infections
  - Endocarditis
  - GI Infection
  - Pharyngitis
  - Pneumonia
  - Skin and soft tissue infections
  - Surgical prophylaxis
  - Urinary tract infections

Mechanism of Action
- Inhibit the final step in bacterial cell wall synthesis by binding to specific penicillin-binding proteins in the bacterial cytoplasmic membrane.
  - Beta-lactams also prevent the transpeptidation reaction and cross-linking of linear peptidoglycan chain constituents of the cell wall as well as activate autolytic enzymes that cause lesions in the bacterial cell wall.

Primary Overall Net Benefit
- Bactericidal to susceptible pathogens, leading to microbiologic clearance of the affecting organisms.
- Main Labs to Monitor:
  - Cultures from infected sites at baseline (blood, sputum, urine, CSF etc.)

High-Yield Clinical Knowledge
- **ESBL Resistance**
  - Cefepime was developed to be more resistant to hydrolysis by chromosomal beta-lactamases but is hydrolyzed by extended-spectrum beta-lactamases.
- **Intermittent Vs Extended Interval**
  - Dosing for cefepime has traditionally been intermittent small volume parenteral infusions over 30 to 60 minutes. Newer evidence has supported a shift to extended infusion (4 hour infusions) with adjusted interval (q8-12h) to take advantage of beta-lactam antimicrobial kill characteristics of time over MIC.
- **MRSA Coverage**
  - Ceftaroline is unique and has increased binding to penicillin-binding protein 2a, which mediates methicillin resistance in staphylococci, resulting in bactericidal activity against these strains. It has some in vitro activity against enterococci and a broad gram-negative spectrum similar to ceftriaxone.

High-Yield Basic Spectrum of Activity
- **Cefepime and ceftolozane/tazobactam**
    - Gram-Positive
        - Same as third-generation
    - Gram-Negative
        - Same as the third-generation, but also
            - Acinetobacter species
            - Pseudomonas aeruginosa
    - Anaerobes
        - Peptostreptococcus
- **Anti-MRSA (Ceftaroline)**
    - Gram-Positive
        - Similar to fourth-generation, but then
            - Methicillin-Resistant Staphylococcus aureus (MRSA)
            - Enterococcus faecalis
    - Gram-Negative
        - Similar to THIRD-generation cephalosporins
        - Note - no pseudomonas coverage

High-Yield Fast-Facts
- **Empiric Coverage**
    - Cefepime is widely used in acute care settings as an empiric antibiotic when pseudomonas coverage is necessary, including in patients with febrile neutropenia.
- **Fourth to Fifth Generation**
    - Ceftaroline can also be considered a fifth-generation cephalosporin as it can cover MRSA and emerging resistant strains including vancomycin-intermediate S. aureus (VISA), heteroresistant VISA (hVISA), and vancomycin-resistant S. aureus (VRSA).
- **Prodrug Ceftaroline**
    - In its dosage format, ceftaroline is actually a prodrug (ceftaroline fosamil) and activated after administration to ceftaroline (active).

HIGH-YIELD BOARD EXAM ESSENTIALS
- **CLASSIC AGENTS:** Cefepime, ceftaroline, ceftolozane/tazobactam
- **DRUG CLASS:** Cephalosporins
- **INDICATIONS:** Bacteremia, bone and joint infections, endocarditis, GI infection, pharyngitis, skin and soft tissue infections, surgical prophylaxis, urinary tract infections
- **MECHANISM:** Inhibit the final step in bacterial cell wall synthesis by binding to specific penicillin-binding proteins in the bacterial cytoplasmic membrane.
- **SIDE EFFECTS:** Diarrhea, hypersensitivity, nausea
- **CLINICAL PEARLS:**
    - Cefepime and ceftolozane both cover Pseudomonas, but not MRSA. Whereas, ceftaroline covers MRSA but not Pseudomonas.
    - Cefepime was developed to be more resistant to hydrolysis by chromosomal beta-lactamases but is hydrolyzed by extended-spectrum beta-lactamases.
    - Considered generally safe in pregnancy.

Table: Drug Class Summary

Cephalosporins - 4th Generation & Anti-MRSA - Drug Class Review
High-Yield Med Reviews

Mechanism of Action: *Inhibit the final step in bacterial cell wall synthesis by binding to specific penicillin-binding proteins in the bacterial cytoplasmic membrane.*

Class Effects: *Bactericidal to susceptible pathogens, leading to microbiologic clearance of the affecting organisms.*

Generic Name	Brand Name	Indication(s) or Uses	Notes

Cefepime	Maxipime	- Intra-abdominal infection
		- Neutropenic fever
		- Pneumonia
		- Skin and soft tissue infection
		- Urinary tract infection
			- **Dosing (Adult):**
			  – IV: 1 to 2 g every 8 to 12 hours
			- **Dosing (Peds):**
			  – IV: 50 mg/kg/dose every 12 hours
			    – Maximum 2 g/dose
			- **CYP450 Interactions:** None
			- **Renal or Hepatic Dose Adjustments:**
			  – Various recommendations, consult local guidelines
			  – GFR: 10 to 30 mL/minute: 500 to 1000 mg q12-24h; or 2000 mg q24h
			  – GFR: < 10 mL/minute: 250 to 1000 mg q24h
			- **Dosage Forms:** IV (solution)

Ceftaroline	Teflaro	- Pneumonia
		- Skin and soft tissue infection
			- **Dosing (Adult):**
			  – IV: 600 mg q12hours for 5 to 14 days
			- **Dosing (Peds):**
			  – IV: 8 to 15 mg/kg/dose every 8 hours.
			    – Maximum 600 mg/dose
			- **CYP450 Interactions:** None
			- **Renal or Hepatic Dose Adjustments:**
			  – GFR: 30 to 50 mL/minute: 400 mg q12h
			  – GFR: 15 to 30 mL/minute: 300 mg q12h
			  – GFR: < 15 mL/minute or ESRD: 200 mg q12h
			- **Dosage Forms:** IV (solution)

Ceftolozane + Tazobactam	Zerbaxa	- Intra-abdominal infections
		- Pneumonia (Hospital Acquired or Ventilator Associated
		- UTI (Complicated)
		
		Note: Reserved only for multidrug resistant infections
			- **Dosing (Adult):**
			  – IV: 1.5 to 3 g every 8 hrs
			- **Dosing (Peds):** n/a
			- **CYP450 Interactions:** None
			- **Renal or Hepatic Dose Adjustments:**
			  – GFR: 30 to 50 mL/minute: 750 – 1.5 g q8h
			  – GFR: 15 to 30 mL/minute: 375 – 750 mg q8h
			  – GFR: < 15 mL/minute or ESRD: NR
			- **Dosage Forms:** IV (solution)

INFECTIOUS DISEASE – Monobactam

Drug Class
- Monobactam
- Agents:
  - Acute and Chronic Care
    - Aztreonam

Main Indications or Uses
- Acute & Chronic Care
  - Bacterial meningitis
  - Cystic Fibrosis (inhaled formulations)
  - Intra-abdominal infections
  - Osteomyelitis
  - Pneumonia
  - Surgical prophylaxis
  - Urinary tract infection

Mechanism of Action
- Inhibit the final step in bacterial cell wall synthesis by binding to specific penicillin-binding proteins in the bacterial cytoplasmic membrane.
  - Beta-lactams also prevent the transpeptidation reaction and cross-linking of linear peptidoglycan chain constituents of the cell wall as well as activate autolytic enzymes that cause lesions in the bacterial cell wall.

> **Knowledge Integration**
>
> ✓ An easy way to remember spectrum of coverage → "MONObactam only cover one type of bacteria, which can be "negative". This class only covers against gram-negative organisms.
>
> ✓ The inhaled formulation for nebulization is used for cystic fibrosis due to their risk of having Pseudomonas aeruginosa in the lung.
>
> ✓ While it can be used for the treatment of intra-abdominal infections and pneumonia, it is typically used only then a true penicillin allergy exists.

Primary Net Benefit
- Bactericidal to susceptible gram-negative pathogens (including Pseudomonas); BUT NO gram-positive coverage.
- Main Labs to Monitor:
  - Cultures from infected sites at baseline (blood, sputum, urine, CSF etc.)

High-Yield Clinical Knowledge
- **Penicillin-Allergic Patients**
  - Aztreonam is frequently used as an alternative agent in patients with penicillin-allergies, however, it is critical to ensure that the original allergy is not related to ceftazidime.
  - Cross-reactivity to aztreonam is likely in the case of ceftazidime allergy as these two agents share structural similarities, notably identical R1 sidechains (the antigenic component of the beta-lactam or monobactam structure).
- **Neonatal Risk**
  - Aztreonam should be avoided in neonates, infants, and young children as the risk of hepatotoxicity is higher compared to other populations.
- **Resistance Exists**
  - Aztreonam exclusively covers gram-negative pathogens but is still susceptible to hydrolysis by AmpC beta-lactamases and extended-spectrum beta-lactamases.

High-Yield Basic Spectrum of Activity
- Aztreonam
    - **Gram-Positive**
        - No coverage
    - **Gram-Negative**
        - Enterobacteriaceae (ESBL-neg, CRE-neg)
            - Escherichia coli
            - Klebsiella pneumoniae
            - Salmonella species
            - Shigella species
            - Yersinia pestis
        - Enterobacter sp (AmpC negative)
        - Moraxella catarrhalis
        - Serratia species
        - Providencia species
        - Morganella species
        - meningitidis
        - Citrobacter species
        - Aeromonas hydrophila
        - Pseudomonas aeruginosa
        - Neisseria gonorrhea
        - Neisseria
    - **Anaerobes**
        - No coverage

> **Antimicrobial Stewardship**
> ✓ Aztreonam covers against Pseudomonas but not MRSA. It should be reserved for cases when penicillin cannot be used. The exception could be ceftazidime which share similar structural characteristics as aztreonam.

High-Yield Fast-Facts
- **Inhaled Aztreonam**
    - Aztreonam can be administered via nebulization and is available under the brand name Cayston. It should be noted, the generic IV formulation can also be compounded for nebulization.
- **Pipeline combination with Avibactam**
    - There is the development of new combinations of aztreonam and avibactam to extend its use to certain pathogens that would otherwise be resistant.
- **Rare Events**
    - Aztreonam has been rarely associated with elevations in liver enzymes (AST, ALT), eosinophilia, and thrombocytopenia.

HIGH-YIELD BOARD EXAM ESSENTIALS
- **CLASSIC AGENTS:** Aztreonam
- **DRUG CLASS:** Monobactam
- **INDICATIONS:** Bacterial meningitis, osteomyelitis, surgical prophylaxis
- **MECHANISM:** Inhibit the final step in bacterial cell wall synthesis by binding to specific penicillin-binding proteins in the bacterial cytoplasmic membrane.
- **SIDE EFFECTS:** Elevations in liver enzymes, eosinophilia, thrombocytopenia
- **CLINICAL PEARLS:**
    - The dosage formulation marketed as Cayston is administered by nebulization and indicated for cystic fibrosis.
    - Aztreonam covers against Pseudomonas but not MRSA.
    - Cross-reactivity to aztreonam is likely in the case of ceftazidime allergy as these two agents share structural similarities, notably identical R1 sidechains (the antigenic component of the beta-lactam or monobactam structure).

Table: Drug Class Summary

Monobactam - Drug Class Review **High-Yield Med Reviews**			
Mechanism of Action: *Inhibit the final step in bacterial cell wall synthesis by binding to specific penicillin-binding proteins in the bacterial cytoplasmic membrane.*			
Class Effects: Bactericidal to susceptible gram-negative pathogens (including Pseudomonas); *BUT NO* gram-positive coverage.			
Generic Name	**Brand Name**	**Indication(s) or Uses**	**Notes**
Aztreonam	Azactam Cayston *(For cystic fibrosis only)*	<ul><li>Bacterial meningitis</li><li>Intra-abdominal infections</li><li>Osteomyelitis</li><li>Pneumonia</li><li>Surgical prophylaxis</li><li>Cystic fibrosis (Inhalation only; Cayston)</li></ul>	<ul><li>**Dosing (Adult):**<ul><li>IV/IM: 1 to 2 g q6-8h</li><li>Neb: 75 mg TID (at least 4 hrs apart) x 28 days. Give pre-treatment bronchodilator before each dose.</li></ul></li><li>**Dosing (Peds):**<ul><li>Oral: 30 mg/kg/day q12-24h</li></ul></li><li>**CYP450 Interactions:** None</li><li>**Renal or Hepatic Dose Adjustments:**<ul><li>GFR 10 to 30 mL/minute: 500 to 1000 mg q6-8h</li><li>GFR < 10 mL/minute: 250 to 500 mg q6-8h</li></ul></li><li>**Dosage Forms:** IV (solution), inhalation (via nebulization)</li></ul>

INFECTIOUS DISEASE – NATURAL PENICILLIN

Drug Class
- Beta-Lactam Antibiotic → Natural penicillin
- Agents:
    - Acute Care
        - Penicillin G Aqueous
        - Penicillin G Benzathine
        - Penicillin G Procaine
    - Chronic Care
        - Penicillin V Potassium

Main Indications or Uses
- Acute Care
    - Botulism
    - Diphtheria
    - Endocarditis
    - Meningitis
    - Pharyngitis (Group A Strep)
    - Syphilis
    - Streptococcus (group B), maternal prophylaxis
    - Tetanus (Clostridium tetani infection)

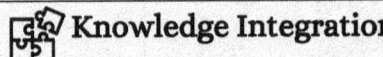

Dosing Pearl
- Penicillin B benzathine is to be only administered by IM injection (NOT IV) and has a duration of 1-4 weeks long after a single-injection allowing for a single-dose treatment for some conditions.

Knowledge Integration
- Treponema pallidum is a gram-negative bacteria known to cause syphilis and is still very susceptible to penicillin.

Mechanism of Action
- Inhibit the final step in bacterial cell wall synthesis by binding to specific penicillin-binding proteins in the bacterial cytoplasmic membrane.
    - Beta-lactams also prevent the transpeptidation reaction and cross-linking of linear peptidoglycan chain constituents of the cell wall as well as activate autolytic enzymes that cause lesions in the bacterial cell wall.

Primary Net Benefit
- Bactericidal to susceptible pathogens, leading to microbiologic clearance of the affecting organisms.
- Main Labs to Monitor:
    - Cultures from infected sites at baseline (blood, sputum, urine, CSF etc.)

High-Yield Basic Pharmacology
- Absorption differences
    - Amoxicillin and ampicillin are very similar in pharmacologic action, but only amoxicillin is commercially available as an oral preparation in the United States.
        - Peak plasma concentrations of amoxicillin are roughly 2.5 times higher than an equal dose of ampicillin administered orally.
- Probenecid
    - Probenecid significantly decreased the renal tubular secretion of many penicillins and is most often used with penicillin G; however, it can be combined with ampicillin to yield the same effect.
        - Probenecid can specifically improve penicillin and ampicillin concentration in the CSF.

High-Yield Clinical Knowledge
- Jarisch-Herxheimer Reaction
    - This reaction manifests as fever, chills, diaphoresis, tachycardia, hyperventilation, flushing, and myalgias, typically occurring within 2 hours of administration of penicillin G for treatment of syphilis.
    - The Jarisch-Herxheimer reaction typically persists for about 1 day and it can be treated with aspirin or prednisone.

- Other spirochetal infections such as leptospirosis, and Lyme disease, may also produce Jarisch-Herxheimer reactions after administration of penicillin G
    - It occurs in up to 50% of patients with primary syphilis being treated with penicillin G, and up to 75% in patients with secondary syphilis.
- **Penicillin Allergy**
    - Many patients with a penicillin allergy, report their exposure to be from penicillin VK, and typically complain of a rash. While this may be a relevant hypersensitivity, many beta-lactam alternatives can be selected that possess a dissimilar R-1 side chain, the structural element primarily responsible for type-1 hypersensitivity.

High-Yield Spectrum of Coverage
- **Core spectrum**
    - **Gram-Positive**
        - Staphylococcus species methicillin-sensitive only
        - Streptococcus species
        - Enterococcus species
        - Listeria monocytogenes
    - **Gram-Negative**
        - Escherichia coli
        - Klebsiella pneumoniae
        - Shigella species
        - Proteus mirabilis
        - Neisseria meningitides
        - Pasteurella multocida
        - Treponema pallidum
- **Core indications**
    - **Acute exacerbation of chronic bronchitis, epiglottitis, meningitis, pharyngitis, otitis media urinary tract infection (particularly Enterococcus spp infection), sinusitis.**
        - S. pneumoniae, S. pyogenes, H. influenzae.
    - **Group B Streptococci colonization in pregnancy**
        - Antepartum administration of ampicillin may be beneficial for prophylaxis against group B streptococcal infection in infants of mothers with birth canal colonization.
            - After administration of 2g IV to the mother, bactericidal concentrations of ampicillin are achieved in the amniotic fluid within 5 minutes.

High-Yield Fast-Facts
- **Units, not milligrams**
    - The unit of measure of the penicillin G dosage forms are 'units' where one unit is a concentration of drug that produces a given size zone of growth inhibition around an Oxford strain of Staphylococcus aureus.
- **The "Natural" Penicillins**
    - The natural penicillin agents are produced from the fermentation of Penicillium chrysogenum.

HIGH-YIELD BOARD EXAM ESSENTIALS
- **CLASSIC AGENTS:** Penicillin G (aqueous, benzathine, procaine); penicillin V potassium
- **DRUG CLASS:** Natural penicillin
- **INDICATIONS:** Botulism, diphtheria, endocarditis, meningitis, pharyngitis (group A strep), syphilis, Streptococcus (group B), Tetanus (Clostridium tetani infection)
- **MECHANISM:** Inhibit bacterial cell wall synthesis by binding to specific penicillin-binding proteins
- **SIDE EFFECTS:** Acute hypersensitivity, nausea, vomiting, diarrhea
- **CLINICAL PEARLS:** The unit of measure of the penicillin G dosage forms are 'units' where one unit is a concentration of drug that produces a given size zone of growth inhibition around an Oxford strain of Staphylococcus aureus.

Table: Drug Class Summary

\multicolumn{4}{c}{**Natural Penicillin - Drug Class Review**}
\multicolumn{4}{c}{High-Yield Med Reviews}
\multicolumn{4}{l}{**Mechanism of Action:** *Inhibit bacterial cell wall synthesis by binding to specific penicillin-binding proteins.*}
\multicolumn{4}{l}{**Class Effects:** *Bactericidal to susceptible pathogens, leading to microbiologic clearance of the affecting organisms.*}
Generic Name	**Brand Name**	**Main Indication(s) or Uses**	**Notes**
Penicillin G Aqueous	Pfizerpen	<ul><li>Botulism</li><li>Diphtheria</li><li>Endocarditis</li><li>Meningitis</li><li>Syphilis</li><li>Streptococcus (group B), maternal prophylaxis</li><li>Tetanus (Clostridium tetani infection)</li></ul>	<ul><li>Dosing (Adult): − IV: 4-6 million units q4h</li><li>Dosing (Peds): − IV: 20,000 to 65,000 units/kg IV q6-12h</li><li>CYP450 Interactions: None</li><li>Renal or Hepatic Dose Adjustments: − GFR 10 to 50 mL/minute: Reduce q6-8h − GFR < 10 mL/minute: Reduce dosing to q12h.</li><li>Dosage Forms: IV solution</li></ul>
Penicillin G Benzathine	Bicillin LA	<ul><li>Syphilis</li><li>Streptococcal infection</li></ul>	<ul><li>Dosing (Adult): − IM: 1.2 to 2.4 million units once</li><li>Dosing (Peds): − < 27 kg, IM 300,000 to 600,000 units once</li><li>CYP450 Interactions: None</li><li>Renal or Hepatic Dose Adjustments: None</li><li>Dosage Forms: Intramuscular suspension</li></ul>
Penicillin G Procaine	Bicillin CR, Wycillin	<ul><li>Streptococcal infection</li></ul>	<ul><li>Dosing (Adult): − IM: 600,000 to 1.2 million units daily x 10d</li><li>Dosing (Peds): − IM: 25,000 to 50,000 units/kg/day</li><li>CYP450 Interactions: None</li><li>Renal or Hepatic Dose Adjustments: None</li><li>Dosage Forms: Intramuscular suspension</li></ul>
Penicillin V Potassium	Pen-VK	<ul><li>Streptococcal pharyngitis</li><li>Lyme disease</li></ul>	<ul><li>Dosing (Adult): − Oral: 250 to 500 mg q6-12h for 10-30 days</li><li>Dosing (Peds): − Oral: 15 to 62.5 mg/kg/day in 3-6 divided doses for 10-30 days</li><li>CYP450 Interactions: None</li><li>Renal or Hepatic Dose Adjustments: − GFR < 10 mL/minute - decrease frequency</li><li>Dosage Forms: IV (solution)</li></ul>

INFECTIOUS DISEASES – CHLORAMPHENICOL – MISC ANTIBIOTIC

Drug Class
- Chloramphenicol
- Agents:
    - Acute Care
        - Chloramphenicol

Main Indications or Uses
- Acute Care
    - Bacteremia
    - Cystic fibrosis exacerbations
    - Meningitis

Mechanism of Action
- Binds to the 50S subunit of bacterial ribosomes and inhibits protein synthesis by interfering with the formation of initiation complexes and with aminoacyl translocation reactions.

Primary Net Benefit
- Bacteriostatic protein-synthesis inhibitor with activity against susceptible strains of Gram-positive pathogens and gram-positive anaerobes, including Clostridoides species, but reserved for last line therapy due to life-threatening or fatal blood dyscrasias.
- Main Labs to Monitor:
    - Cultures from infected sites at baseline (blood, sputum, urine, CSF, etc.)
    - CBC

High-Yield Basic Pharmacology
- **Similar 50S Spectrum**
    - The spectrum of chloramphenicol activity is very similar to that of other 50S ribosomal subunit inhibitors such as macrolides and clindamycin.
        - The spectrum consists primarily of Gram-positive organisms but has activity against Haemophilus influenzae, Neisseria meningitides, and anaerobes, including Bacteroides species.
- **Cross Resistance**
    - Given the similar binding sites, when resistance occurs to one of these classes, it confers others' resistance.
        - Clindamycin is active against pathogens with different resistance mechanisms to macrolides, specifically those with a macrolide efflux pump.
- **Oxidative Phosphorylation**
    - Chloramphenicol acts as an inhibitor of oxidative phosphorylation by inhibiting cytochrome c oxidase and proton-translocating ATPase.
        - This results in oxidative stress, decreased cellular ATP production, generation of free-radicals island ultimately cell death.

High-Yield Clinical Knowledge
- **Oral No More**
    - The oral dosage form of chloramphenicol is no longer available in the United States, as the IV product is the only dosage form available.
- **Aplastic Anemia**
    - Chloramphenicol exhibits a dose-dependent reversible suppression of erythrocyte production in normal therapeutic doses and increases with prolonged therapy after 1–2 weeks.
    - However, irreversible aplastic anemia due to chloramphenicol is an idiosyncratic reaction unrelated to dose but can manifest more frequently with prolonged use.

- Salvage therapy for aplastic anemia may include bone marrow transplantation or immunosuppressive therapy.
- **Drug Interactions**
  - Clinically relevant drug interactions exist with chloramphenicol as it inhibits CYP 2C9, with clinically relevant interactions with phenytoin, rifampin, and warfarin.
- **Resistance**
  - Chloramphenicol resistance usually occurs via plasmid-encoded acetyltransferase, which inactivates the drug or decreased permeability of the drug into the bacterial cell or ribosomal mutation.
- **Severe Beta-Lactam Allergy**
  - Chloramphenicol can be used as an alternative to beta-lactams in patients with severe allergies and otherwise no alternative agents available.
    - A detailed history of the allergy is necessary to avoid suboptimal care, and consultation with experts to explore penicillin desensitization may be reasonable interventions to avoid chloramphenicol.
- **Gray Baby Syndrome**
  - Neonates do not possess sufficient hepatic conjugation capacity to metabolized chloramphenicol, which can lead to accumulation, toxicity, and "Gray Baby Syndrome."
    - Gray Baby Syndrome derives its name from the vasomotor collapse resulting in skin mottling ashen-gray discoloration of the skin.
      - The vasomotor collapse is preceded by abdominal distention, vomiting, hypothermia, cyanosis, and cardiovascular instability.
  - Dose reductions with a maximum of 25 mg/kg/day in this population are recommended, along with close monitoring.

High-Yield Core Spectrum
- **Core spectrum**
  - **Gram-Positive**
    - Enterococcus species
    - Streptococcus species
    - Staphylococcus aureus (including methicillin-resistant)
    - Listeria monocytogenes
  - **Gram-Negative**
    - Enterobacteriaceae
      - E. coli
      - K. pneumoniae
    - Haemophilus influenzae
    - Salmonella species
    - Shigella species
    - Vibrio cholerae
  - **Atypical**
    - Mycoplasma species
    - Chlamydia
  - **Anaerobes**
    - Bacteroides species
    - Clostridium (not difficile)
- **Core Indications**
  - Reserved for last line therapy of bacteremia, meningitis, or tickborne rickettsial diseases

High-Yield Fast-Fact
- **Adverse Candidiasis**
  - The use of chloramphenicol has been associated with oral or vaginal candidiasis because of the alteration of normal microbial flora.
- **Jarisch-Herxheimer**

- The Jarisch-Herxheimer reaction can occur after the administration of chloramphenicol to treat either syphilis, brucellosis, or typhoid fever.
- **Adult Gray Syndrome**
  - Adult patients are still at risk of a similar 'gray syndrome' but is unlikely to occur outside of an accidental or intentional overdose of chloramphenicol.

HIGH-YIELD BOARD EXAM ESSENTIALS
- **CLASSIC AGENTS:** Chloramphenicol
- **DRUG CLASS:** Chloramphenicol
- **INDICATIONS:** Bacteremia, cystic fibrosis exacerbations, meningitis
- **MECHANISM:** Binds to the 50S subunit of bacterial ribosomes and inhibits protein synthesis by interfering with the formation of initiation complexes and with aminoacyl translocation reactions.
- **SIDE EFFECTS:** Gray Baby Syndrome, Jarisch-Herxheimer reaction, aplastic anemia
- **CLINICAL PEARLS:** Chloramphenicol can be used as an alternative to beta-lactams in patients with severe allergies and otherwise no alternative agents available. A detailed history of the allergy is necessary to avoid suboptimal care, and consultation with experts to explore penicillin desensitization may be reasonable interventions to avoid chloramphenicol.

Table: Drug Class Summary

Chloramphenicol - Drug Class Review			
High-Yield Med Reviews			
Mechanism of Action: Binds to the 50S subunit of bacterial ribosomes and inhibits protein synthesis by interfering with the formation of initiation complexes and with aminoacyl translocation reactions.			
Class Effects: Bacteriostatic protein-synthesis inhibitor with activity against susceptible strains of Gram-positive pathogens and gram-positive anaerobes, including Clostridoides species, but reserved for last line therapy due to life-threatening blood dyscrasias.			
Generic Name	**Brand Name**	**Indication(s) or Uses**	**Notes**

Chloramphenicol	Chloromycetin Econochlor	• Bacteremia
		• Meningitis
		• Tickborne rickettsial diseases
			• **Dosing (Adult):**
			  – IV: 50 to 100 mg/kg/day in divided q6h
			  – Maximum 4 g/day
			• **Dosing (Peds):**
			  – IV: 12.5 to 25 mg/kg/dose q6h; Max: 4 g/day
			• **CYP450 Interactions:** None
			• **Renal or Hepatic Dose Adjustments:** None
			• **Dosage Forms:** IV (solution)

INFECTIOUS DISEASES – LINCOSAMIDES

Drug Class
- Lincosamides
- Agents:
  - Acute & Chronic Care
    - Clindamycin
    - Lincomycin (not used clinically anymore)

Main Indications or Uses
- Acute & Chronic Care
  - Gynecological infections
  - Intraabdominal infection
  - Osteomyelitis
  - Pneumonia
  - Skin and soft tissue infection

> **Counseling Point**
> ✓ Counsel patients to return or seek evaluation if they start to develop new onset diarrhea with 3 or more unformed stools per day, especially if with a fever due to the greater risk of C. diff infection.

Mechanism of Action
- Binds to the 50S subunit of bacterial ribosomes and inhibits protein synthesis by interfering with the formation of initiation complexes and with aminoacyl translocation reactions.

Primary Net Benefit
- Bacteriostatic protein-synthesis inhibitor with activity against susceptible strains of Gram-positive pathogens and gram-positive anaerobes, including Clostiroides species.
- Main Labs to Monitor:
  - Cultures from infected sites at baseline (blood, sputum, urine, CSF, etc.)

High-Yield Basic Pharmacology
- The spectrum of clindamycin activity is limited to Gram-positive organisms as Gram-negative aerobic bacteria possess an outer membrane that clindamycin cannot penetrate.
- Clindamycin has reliable and nearly complete absorption when administered orally, making it a reliable agent for patients who can appropriately take oral antimicrobials.
- The 50S ribosomal subunit is a target of several other antibiotic agents, including the macrolides and chloramphenicol.
  - Given the similar binding sites, when resistance occurs to one of these classes, it confers others' resistance.
    - Clindamycin is active against pathogens with different resistance mechanisms to macrolides, specifically those with a macrolide efflux pump.

High-Yield Clinical Knowledge
- **C. difficile**
  - Clindamycin is associated with a high incidence of diarrhea (up to 20%), leading to discontinuation in many cases.
    - Clindamycin also carries a risk of diarrhea and colitis due to C difficile.
- **Clindamycin Resistance Issues**
  - Clindamycin has unique mechanisms of resistance to bacteria that can also confer cross-resistance to macrolides.
    - Resistance may be due to a mutation of the ribosomal receptor, the alteration of the 50S binding site by methylase, or an enzymatic inactivation of clindamycin.

- **HIV Patients and Rash**
  - Although skin rash incidence is relatively low in the general population taking clindamycin, in patients with HIV infection, the incidence of skin reactions occurs in up to 10% of patients.
    - In rare circumstances, these reactions can be severe erythema multiforme or Stevens-Johnson syndrome.
- **Necrotizing Fasciitis**
  - Clindamycin can be used in combination with penicillin G to manage life-threatening skin infections, including necrotizing fasciitis.
    - Clindamycin may be used empirically, as its spectrum included Group A Streptococcus and Clostridioides perfringens or Clostridioides neoformans.
- **Pneumocystis Jiroveci**
  - Since many HIV patients cannot tolerate trimethoprim-sulfamethoxazole for moderate to moderately severe Pneumocystis jiroveci pneumonia, clindamycin with primaquine is an alternative therapy.
  - Clindamycin plus pyrimethamine and leucovorin may also be used for AIDS-related toxoplasmosis of the brain.
- **Dental Procedure Prophylaxis**
  - In patients with beta-lactam allergies, clindamycin should be used for prophylaxis of endocarditis in patients with specific valvular heart disease undergoing certain dental procedures.

High-Yield Core Spectrum of Coverage
- **Core spectrum**
  - Gram-Positive
    - Streptococcus species
    - Staphylococcus aureus
  - Anaerobes
    - Bacteroides species
    - Clostridium difficile
    - Clostridium (not difficile)
- **Core Indications**
  - Clindamycin is used as an oral or parenteral agent to manage skin and soft-tissue infections.
  - It can be combined with an aminoglycoside or cephalosporin to treat penetrating wounds of the abdomen and the gut.
    - Other specific GI/GU infections clindamycin has a role in include infections originating in the female genital tract such as septic abortion, pelvic abscesses, or pelvic inflammatory disease.

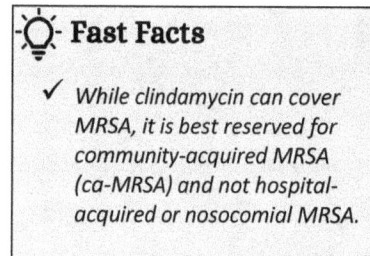

Fast Facts

✓ While clindamycin can cover MRSA, it is best reserved for community-acquired MRSA (ca-MRSA) and not hospital-acquired or nosocomial MRSA.

High-Yield Fast-Facts
- **D-Zone Test**
  - The double-disk diffusion method (D-zone test) is recommended for testing erythromycin-resistant and clindamycin-susceptible Group-B Streptococci.
- **Bite Wound Treatment**
  - For patients allergic to penicillin, clindamycin with sulfamethoxazole-trimethoprim is an appropriate combination for bite wound prophylaxis.
- **Lincosamides**
  - Clindamycin belongs to the lincosamide class of antibiotics, but since the removal of lincosamide from the US market, it is the only member of this class.

HIGH-YIELD BOARD EXAM ESSENTIALS
- **CLASSIC AGENTS:** Clindamycin
- **DRUG CLASS:** Lincosamide
- **INDICATIONS:** Gynecological infections, intraabdominal infection, osteomyelitis, pneumonia, Skin and soft tissue infection
- **MECHANISM:** Binds to the 50S subunit of bacterial ribosomes and inhibits protein synthesis by interfering with the formation of initiation complexes and with aminoacyl translocation reactions.
- **SIDE EFFECTS:** C. difficile, rash (HIV patients)
- **CLINICAL PEARLS:**
    - Can cover anaerobes and community-acquired MRSA
    - Must be administered 3 to 4 times per day → potential compliance issues
    - Pediatric patients → the suspension formulation for oral administration has a terrible taste → also compliance issue
    - Clindamycin is associated with a high incidence of diarrhea (up to 20%), leading to discontinuation in many cases
    - Common alternative to PCN allergic patients being treated for strep pharyngitis

Table: Drug Class Summary

Clindamycin - Drug Class Review High-Yield Med Reviews			
Mechanism of Action: *Binds to the 50S subunit of bacterial ribosomes and inhibits protein synthesis by interfering with the formation of initiation complexes and with aminoacyl translocation reactions.*			
Class Effects: Bacteriostatic protein-synthesis inhibitor against susceptible Gram-positive and gram-positive anaerobes.			
Generic Name	**Brand Name**	**Indication(s) or Uses**	**Notes**
Clindamycin	Cleocin	<ul><li>Gynecological infections</li><li>Intraabdominal infection</li><li>Osteomyelitis</li><li>Pneumonia</li><li>Skin and soft tissue infection</li></ul>	<ul><li>**Dosing (Adult):**<ul><li>IV/IM: 600 to 2700 mg/day divided q6-12h</li><li>Oral: 600 to 1800 mg/day divided q6-12h</li></ul></li><li>**Dosing (Peds):**<ul><li>IV/IM: 20 to 40 mg/kg/day divided q6-8h</li><li>Oral: 8 to 40 mg/kg/day divided q6-8h</li></ul></li><li>**CYP450 Interactions:**<ul><li>Substrate CYP3A4</li></ul></li><li>**Renal or Hepatic Dose Adjustments:** None</li><li>**Dosage Forms:** IV (solution), Oral (capsule, solution)</li></ul>

INFECTIOUS DISEASES – CYCLIC LIPOPETIDE

Drug Class
- Cyclic lipopeptide
- Agents:
    - Acute Care
        - Daptomycin

Main Indications or Uses
- Acute Care
    - Bacteremia
    - Skin and skin structure infection

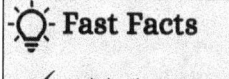

Fast Facts
✓ While daptomycin can penetrate the lung, it is inactivated by pulmonary surfactant and thus not useful for treating pneumonia.

Mechanism of Action
- Daptomycin binds to bacterial cytoplasmic membrane in a calcium-dependent manner, causing a rapid cellular loss of potassium, membrane depolarization, and bacterial cell death.

Primary Net Benefit
- A bactericidal agent with a spectrum of activity exclusive for Gram-positive aerobic, facultative, and anaerobic bacteria. Coverage includes MRSA.
- Main Labs to Monitor:
    - Cultures from infected sites at baseline (blood, sputum, urine, CSF, etc.)
    - Serum creatinine, urine output
    - Serum creatinine kinase, signs of myopathy

High-Yield Basic Pharmacology
- **Concentration Dependent**
    - Daptomycin demonstrates concentration-dependent (Cmax over MIC) bactericidal activity. As a result, some have used high doses (10-12 mg/kg) to improve the microbiologic cure.
- **Bactericidal Not Lytic**
    - The mechanism of daptomycin does not cause lysis of the bacterial cell but rather causes an inhibition of bacterial DNA, RNA, and protein synthesis resulting in cell death.

High-Yield Clinical Knowledge
- **Myopathy**
    - Myopathy is a common complaint with daptomycin therapy; however, this can progress to elevations in creatine phosphokinase levels, rhabdomyolysis, and renal failure in rare circumstances.
    - Patients currently taking statins.
- **Lung Penetration**
    - It is a common misconception that daptomycin does not penetrate lung tissue. In fact, daptomycin does penetrate lung tissue well; however, it is inactivated by pulmonary surfactant once it does.
- **Resistance**
    - Resistance to daptomycin occurs primarily via changes in bacterial cell surface charge that prevents daptomycin from binding to the cell wall.
        - Combination of daptomycin with beta-lactams may overcome resistance in scenarios where alternative therapies are not possible.
- **Outpatient IV Therapy**
    - In selected patients with susceptible infections, patients can be managed outpatient with home-health administration of daptomycin.
    - When home-health administered daptomycin is selected as therapy, it may be administered as an IV push over 2-5 minutes.
        - This can also be done in-patient when volume restriction is necessary or based on hospital protocol.

- **Antibiotic Lock**
  - In patients with chronic or long term IV catheters that become infected and removal/replacement is not possible, intra-catheter administration of daptomycin has been effective for salvaging the IV access.
    - The so-called "lock solution" is a concentrated daptomycin solution with or without heparin instilled into the lumen of the catheter and allowed to remain there for up to 72 hours.
- **Intraventricular**
  - For invasive CNS infections, rather than IV administration, daptomycin may be administered intraventricularly.
    - The intraventricular dose of daptomycin ranges from 2 to 5 mg daily and should be administered via a ventricular drain, with subsequent clamping of the drain for 15 to 60 minutes after administration.

High-Yield Core Spectrum of Coverage
- **Core spectrum**
  - Gram-Positive
    - Streptococcus species
      - Strep Group A, B, C, G
      - S pneumoniae
    - Enterococcus species
    - Staphylococcus aureus, methicillin-sensitive & -resistant (MSSA & MRSA)
    - Listeria monocytogenes
- **Core Indications**
  - Daptomycin is a narrow-spectrum antibiotic reserved for select infections caused by Gram-positive aerobic, facultative, and anaerobic bacteria.

High-Yield Fast-Facts
- **Expensive and Highly Used**
  - Daptomycin is a relatively expensive antibiotic and, at one point, one of the top 10 drug expenditures in hospitals within the United States.
- **Mount Ararat**
  - Daptomycin was discovered after observation of it being produced from Streptomyces rosesporus, which was first isolated on Mount Ararat in Turkey.

HIGH-YIELD BOARD EXAM ESSENTIALS
- **CLASSIC AGENTS:** Daptomycin
- **DRUG CLASS:** Cyclic lipopeptide
- **INDICATIONS:** Bacteremia, skin and skin structure infection
- **MECHANISM:** Binds to bacterial cytoplasmic membrane in a calcium-dependent manner, causing a rapid cellular loss of potassium, membrane depolarization, and bacterial cell death.
- **SIDE EFFECTS:** Myopathy, renal injury
- **CLINICAL PEARLS:** It is a common misconception that daptomycin does not penetrate lung tissue. In fact, daptomycin does penetrate lung tissue well; however, it is inactivated by pulmonary surfactant once it does.

Table: Drug Class Summary

| | Daptomycin - Drug Class Review
High-Yield Med Reviews |
|---|

Mechanism of Action: *Binds to the bacterial cytoplasmic membrane, causing a rapid cellular loss of potassium, membrane depolarization, and bacterial cell death.*			
Class Effects: A bactericidal agent with a spectrum of activity exclusive for Gram-positive aerobic, facultative, and anaerobic bacteria. Includes coverage against MRSA.			
Generic Name	**Brand Name**	**Indication(s) or Uses**	**Notes**
Daptomycin	Cubicin	<ul><li>Bacteremia</li><li>Skin and soft tissue infection</li></ul>	<ul><li>**Dosing (Adult):**<ul><li>IV: 4 to 12 mg/kg q24h</li></ul></li><li>**Dosing (Peds):**<ul><li>IV: 4 to 12 mg/kg q24h</li></ul></li><li>**CYP450 Interactions:** text</li><li>**Renal or Hepatic Dose Adjustments:**<ul><li>GFR: < 30 mL/minute: 4 to 6 mg/kg q48h</li></ul></li><li>**Dosage Forms:** IV (solution)</li></ul>

INFECTIOUS DISEASES – FLUOROQUINOLONES

Drug Class
- Fluoroquinolones
- Agents:
    - Acute Care
        - Besifloxacin
        - Ciprofloxacin
        - Delafloxacin
        - Levofloxacin
    - Chronic Care
        - Ciprofloxacin
        - Delafloxacin
        - Levofloxacin
        - Moxifloxacin
        - Norfloxacin
        - Ofloxacin

> 💬 **Counseling Point**
> ✓ Counsel patients to avoid taking any fluoroquinolone with 2 hours of a divalent or trivalent cations (e.g., calcium)

> 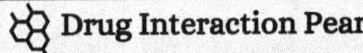 **Drug Interaction Pearl**
> ✓ Ciprofloxacin is one of the few well-known inhibitors of CYP1A2 for which theophylline is a major substrate.

Main Indications or Uses
- Acute & Chronic Care
    - Bacterial conjunctivitis (ophthalmic formulations)
    - Bone and joint infections
    - Infectious diarrhea
    - Intra-abdominal infections
    - Pneumonia
    - Skin and skin structure infections
    - Typhoid fever
    - Urinary tract infections

Mechanism of Action
- In Gram-Negative bacteria, fluoroquinolones inhibit DNA gyrase, causing bacterial DNA supercoiling and inhibiting bacterial growth.
- In Gram-Positive bacteria, fluoroquinolones inhibit topoisomerase IV, preventing separation of interlinked DNA strands from bacterial replication.

Primary Net Benefit
- Fluoroquinolones are broad-spectrum antimicrobial agents with good tissue penetration, distribution (including intracellularly), and pharmacokinetics that support once or twice daily dosing, however, are associated with increased resistance and adverse events that limit their use.
- Main Labs to Monitor:
    - Cultures (if applicable)
    - For ongoing therapy: CBC, blood glucose, signs and symptoms of tendinopathy; if diarrhea + fever develop consider stool antigen for C. diff.

High-Yield Basic Pharmacology
- **Peak to MIC**
    - Fluoroquinolones are bactericidal with concentration-dependent bacterial killing effects (i.e., peak:MIC effects).
        - For patients requiring renal dose adjustment, the peak:MIC effect should be maintained by preserving the dose (where possible) but prolonging the dosing interval.
    - These agents also possess a three to six-hour post-antibiotic effect on specific pathogens (staphylococci, Enterobacteriaceae, and pseudomonas aeruginosa).
- **Oral absorption**

- Fluoroquinolones have excellent oral bioavailability which facilitates IV to oral dosing conversion.
  - For levofloxacin and ofloxacin, oral bioavailability is 99%, and moxifloxacin oral bioavailability is 86%.
- **Hepatic metabolism**
  - Moxifloxacin is extensively hepatically metabolized, with ciprofloxacin and norfloxacin undergoing partial hepatic metabolism.
    - These agents generally undergo hepatic glucuronidation and sulfation (non-CYP oxidation metabolism) but can have inhibitory effects on CYP oxidation pathways.
      - Ciprofloxacin inhibits CYP1A2 and CYP3A4.

High-Yield Clinical Knowledge
- **Mechanism of resistance**
  - There are three primary mechanisms by which fluoroquinolones develop resistance:
    - Changes to the target sites of DNA gyrase and topoisomerase IV
    - Loss of bacterial outer membrane proteins, decreasing cell wall permeability
    - Mutations in the antibiotic efflux from the cell.
- **Common Adverse Events**
  - Connective Tissue Damage
    - Thought to be caused by oxidative damage and vascular ischemia
    - Most commonly causing tendinopathy of the Achilles tendon, presenting as either tendonitis or tendon rupture.
    - Pre-existing renal dysfunction and corticosteroid have been identified as possible risk factors.
    - Patients who engage in sports or frequent exercise should use caution when receiving fluoroquinolones.
  - Central Nervous System
    - Commonly manifests as dizziness, confusion, and headache but can also be associated with hallucinations, depression, psychotic reactions, and seizures.
    - Though to be caused by fluoroquinolone inhibition of GABA transmission.
  - Cardiovascular Toxicity
    - QT prolongation and arrhythmias including torsades de pointes.
    - Similar to other known QT-prolonging drugs, fluoroquinolones block the cardiac potassium rectifier channel.
    - The relative propensity for QT prolongation: moxifloxacin > levofloxacin = ciprofloxacin
- **Drug interactions**
  - Cations
    - All fluoroquinolones chelate with divalent cations (aluminum, calcium, iron, magnesium, and zinc).
      - Sucralfate can also decrease fluoroquinolone bioavailability up to 85%.
      - Fluoroquinolone doses should be spaced by four to six hours between administration of antacids or sucralfate.
  - Methylxanthines
    - Fluoroquinolones (primarily norfloxacin, ciprofloxacin, levofloxacin, and ofloxacin) can inhibit CYP1A2, and reduce the metabolism of theophylline or caffeine.
      - Patients receiving certain fluoroquinolones should be advised against excessive caffeine intake.
  - Tizanidine
    - The concomitant use of ciprofloxacin and tizanidine is contraindicated as ciprofloxacin inhibits the metabolism of tizanidine and can lead to a 10-fold increase in levels, and systemic toxicity including hypotension and seizures.
  - Warfarin
    - Ciprofloxacin and norfloxacin inhibit the metabolism of R-warfarin (CYP1A2 inhibition) and can lead to increased INR, bleeding, or both.
- **Ciprofloxacin and Streptococci**

- Ciprofloxacin is not reliably active against streptococcal species including Streptococcus Pyogenes, S. Pneumoniae, Streptococci Viridans group, and enterococcus species (aka group D streptococci).
- As a result, ciprofloxacin should not be empirically used for adult pneumonia, as it does not adequately cover this common pathogen.
  - In specific populations (i.e., children with cystic fibrosis), ciprofloxacin may be reasonable for pneumonia given its coverage of pseudomonas species, relative to other fluoroquinolones.
- **Futility for STD?**
  - The Center for Disease Control and Prevention (CDC) no longer recommends empiric use of fluoroquinolones for the treatment of gonococcal infections due to widespread resistance to these agents.
    - This pertains primarily to N. gonorrhea where there is a high level of resistance, however, for chlamydia, levofloxacin and ofloxacin have been able to achieve 90% cure rates with 7-day courses, and ciprofloxacin is effective in a 3-day course.
- **Pediatric use**
  - The use of fluoroquinolones has been discouraged in pediatric patients due to the possible higher risk of bone, cartilage, and connective tissue (tendinopathies) in this population.
    - However, emerging data from children with cystic fibrosis receiving ciprofloxacin is supporting a safer perspective on this drug class in pediatric populations.
      - So much so that the FDA has approved ciprofloxacin in patients as young as 1-year-old but emphasizes fluoroquinolones should not be used first-line in pediatric patients.

High-Yield Core Spectrum of Coverage
- **Gram-Positive**
  - Streptococcus
    - Streptococcus pneumoniae
    - Streptococcus viridans
    - Streptococcus groups A, B, C, G
  - Staphylococcus aureus, methicillin-sensitive only
    - Except delafloxacin (extends coverage to MRSA)
  - Listeria monocytogenes
- **Gram-Negative**
  - Enterobacteriaceae (ESBL negative, CRE negative)
    - Escherichia coli
    - Klebsiella pneumoniae
    - Salmonella species
    - Shigella species
    - Yersinia pestis
  - Enterobacter sp (AmpC negative)
  - Moraxella catarrhalis
  - Serratia species
  - Providencia species
  - Morganella species
  - Citrobacter species
  - Aeromonas hydrophila
  - Pseudomonas aeruginosa
  - Neisseria gonorrhoeae
  - Neisseria meningitidis
- **Atypical**
  - Legionella pneumophila
- **Anaerobes**
  - Actinomyces
  - Bacteroides fragilis
  - Clostridium species

> **Antimicrobial Stewardship**
>
> ✓ Delafloxacin should be reserved for pneumonia and/or skin infections due to MRSA.
>
> ✓ Fluoroquinolones in general should be limited unless necessary due to risk of C. diff and questionable benefit:risk ratio for many common infections.

- Fusobacterium necrophorum
- Peptostreptococcus species
- Prevotella melaninogenica

High-Yield Core Evidence
- **Levofloxacin Vs Imipenem-cilastatin For Nosocomial Pneumonia**
    - This was a multicenter, prospective, open-label trial in patients with nosocomial pneumonia who were randomized to receive either levofloxacin 750 mg IV q24h and then orally for 7 to 15 days or imipenem/cilastatin 500 mg to 1 g IV q6 to 8h, followed by oral ciprofloxacin 750 mg every 12 hours for 7 to 15 days.
    - There was no difference between therapies with regard to the primary outcome measure of the clinical response (cure, improvement, failure, or unable to evaluate) in microbiologically evaluable patients 3 to 15 days after the end of therapy.
    - For microbiological efficacy, there was no difference in the rates of eradication between therapies.
    - The authors concluded that levofloxacin was at least as effective and was as well tolerated as imipenem/cilastatin followed by ciprofloxacin in adult patients with nosocomial pneumonia, as demonstrated by comparable clinical and microbiologic success rates. (Clin Ther. 2003 Feb;25(2):485-506.)
- **Fluoroquinolone vs Cephalosporin for Acute Pyelonephritis**
    - This was a double-blind, multicenter trial, of adults with acute pyelonephritis who were randomized to receive norfloxacin or cefadroxil.
    - Norfloxacin was associated with a significantly higher rate of bacteriological cure when compared with cefadroxil, both at 3 to 10 days and up to eight weeks after cessation of treatment.
    - The clinical response during treatment did not differ between the two groups, but symptomatic recurrences at follow-up were more common in the cefadroxil group, and more adverse events were reported by patients receiving cefadroxil.
    - The authors concluded that a two-week course of norfloxacin was superior to a two-week course of cefadroxil for oral treatment of community-acquired acute pyelonephritis. (Eur J Clin Microbiol Infect Dis. 1990 May;9(5):317-23)

High-Yield Fast-Facts
- **Quinolone vs Fluoroquinolones**
    - This drug class can be referred to as quinolones or fluoroquinolones. However, all modern agents used in the USA are fluoroquinolones, with Nalidixic acid the only non-fluorinated quinolone, but it is no longer clinically used.
- **Anthrax**
    - Ciprofloxacin and levofloxacin are FDA approved for the prophylaxis of inhalational Bacillus anthracis infection.
        - In the event of an act of terrorism, these agents have been strategically stockpiled for use as post-exposure prophylaxis.
        - Ciprofloxacin is preferred for inhalational and cutaneous anthrax.
- **Tuberculosis**
    - While resistance rates preclude monotherapy, the fluoroquinolones levofloxacin and moxifloxacin are used for Mycobacterium tuberculosis infections in combination with other active antimicrobial agents.
- **Antimicrobial Stewardship**
    - FQs are commonly prescribed for uncomplicated UTIs (49%) when other antibiotics are preferred. This presents an opportunity to reduce use and resistance.
    - FQs can be utilized for ESBL-E complicated UTIs (1st-line) or CRE uncomplicated UTIs (1st-line), as well as ESBL-E uncomplicated UTIs (2nd-line), if susceptible.
    - Reducing FQ use has been associated with decreased Clostridioides difficile infections.
    - FQs have the highest admission rate after ED visits for adverse effects from antibiotics.

HIGH-YIELD BOARD EXAM ESSENTIALS
- **CLASSIC AGENTS:** Besifloxacin, ciprofloxacin, delafloxacin, levofloxacin, moxifloxacin, norfloxacin, ofloxacin
- **DRUG CLASS:** Fluoroquinolones
- **INDICATIONS:** Bacterial Conjunctivitis (ophthalmic formulations), Bone and joint infections, infectious diarrhea, intra-abdominal infections, pneumonia, skin and skin structure infections, typhoid fever, urinary tract infections
- **MECHANISM:** Inhibit DNA gyrase and topoisomerase IV, exerting a bactericidal effect on susceptible pathogens.
- **SIDE EFFECTS:** Connective Tissue Damage, QT prolongation, CNS toxicity (dizziness, confusion, headache, hallucinations, depression, psychotic reactions, and seizures)
- **CLINICAL PEARLS:**
    - Only ciprofloxacin and levofloxacin cover against Pseudomonas.
    - Only delafloxacin covered against MRSA.
    - Ciprofloxacin and norfloxacin inhibit the metabolism of R-warfarin (CYP1A2 inhibition) and can lead to increased INR, bleeding, or both.
    - Avoid administering di- and tri-valent cations at the same time as oral agents due to reduced absorption because of chelation.
    - Agents in this case are considered contraindicated in pregnancy and pediatric patients (except for unusual situations).

Table: Drug Class Summary

\multicolumn{4}{c}{**Fluoroquinolones - Drug Class Review**}
\multicolumn{4}{c}{High-Yield Med Reviews}
Mechanism of Action: Inhibit DNA gyrase and topoisomerase IV, exerting a bactericidal effect on susceptible pathogens.			
Class Effects: Bactericidal, peak to MIC dependent effect.			
Generic Name	**Brand Name**	**Main Indication(s) or Uses**	**Notes**
Besifloxacin	Besivance (ophthalmic)	• Bacterial Conjunctivitis	• **Dosing (Adult):** — Ocular: 1 gtt into affected eye TID x 7days • **Dosing (Peds):** — Ocular: 1 gtt into affected eye TID x 7days • **CYP450 Interactions:** n/a • **Renal or Hepatic Dose Adjustments:** n/a • **Dosage Forms:** Ophthalmic (suspension)
Ciprofloxacin	Cipro Ciloxan (ophthalmic) Cetraxal Otiprio (otic)	• Bacterial conjunctivitis • Bone and joint infections • Infectious diarrhea • Intra-abdominal infections • Otitis externa (otic form) • Pneumonia • Skin and skin structure infections • Typhoid fever • Urinary tract infections	• **Dosing (Adult):** — Oral: 100 to 750 mg BID to Daily — IV: 200 to 400 mg IV q12h — Ocular: varies by formulation for 5 days — Otic: bid x 7d or single dose (if 6% used) • **Dosing (Peds):** — Oral: 10 to 20 mg/kg/dose BID — Maximum 750 mg/dose — IV: 10 mg/kg/dose q8 to 12h • **CYP450 Interactions:** Inhibits CYP1A2, CYP3A4 • **Renal or Hepatic Dose Adjustments:** — GFR: < 30 mL/minute: oral maximum 500 mg q24h; IV 200 to 400 mg q24h • **Dosage Forms:** IV (solution), oral (tablet, suspension), ophthalmic (ointment & solution), otic (solution & suspension)
Delafloxacin	Baxdela	• Community-Acquired Pneumonia • Skin and Skin Structure Infection	• **Dosing (Adult):** — Oral: 450 mg po BID — IV: 300 mg BID • **Dosing (Peds):** n/a • **CYP450 Interactions:** None • **Renal or Hepatic Dose Adjustments:** Once CrCl < 15 mL/min • **Dosage Forms:** IV (solution), oral (tablet)

Fluoroquinolones - Drug Class Review
High-Yield Med Reviews

Generic Name	Brand Name	Main Indication(s) or Uses	Notes
Levofloxacin	Levaquin	<ul><li>Bacterial conjunctivitis</li><li>Bone and joint infections</li><li>Infectious diarrhea</li><li>Intra-abdominal infections</li><li>Pneumonia</li><li>Skin and skin structure infections</li><li>Urinary tract infections</li></ul>	<ul><li>**Dosing (Adult):** − Oral/IV: 250 to 750 mg Daily − Ocular: 1-2 gtt every 2-4 hrs x 7 days</li><li>**Dosing (Peds):** − Oral: 8 to 10 mg/kg/dose q12 to 24h − Maximum 750 mg/day</li><li>**CYP450 Interactions:** None</li><li>**Renal or Hepatic Dose Adjustments:** − GFR 20 - 50 mL/minute: max 500 mg q24h − GFR < 20 mL/minute: 250 mg q48h</li><li>**Dosage Forms:** IV (solution), oral (tablet), ophthalmic (solution)</li></ul>
Moxifloxacin	Avelox Vigamox (ophthalmic)	<ul><li>Bacterial conjunctivitis</li><li>Pneumonia</li></ul>	<ul><li>**Dosing (Adult):** − Oral/IV: 400 mg q24h − Ocular: 1 gtt into affected eye TID x 7d</li><li>**Dosing (Peds):** − Oral/IV: 4 to 5 mg/kg/dose q12h, maximum 200 mg/dose</li><li>**CYP450 Interactions:** None</li><li>**Renal or Hepatic Dose Adjustments:** None</li><li>**Dosage Forms:** IV (solution), oral (tablet), ophthalmic (solution)</li></ul>
Norfloxacin	Noroxin	<ul><li>Bone and joint infections</li><li>Infectious diarrhea</li><li>Intra-abdominal infections</li><li>Pneumonia</li><li>Skin and skin structure infections</li><li>Urinary tract infections</li></ul>	<ul><li>**Dosing (Adult):** − Oral/IV: 400 mg q12h</li><li>**Dosing (Peds):** − Not routinely used</li><li>**CYP450 Interactions:** None</li><li>**Renal or Hepatic Dose Adjustments:** − GFR < 30 mL/minute: 400 mg q24h</li><li>**Dosage Forms:** Oral (tablet)</li></ul>
Ofloxacin	Floxin Ocuflox (ophthalmic)	<ul><li>Bacterial conjunctivitis</li><li>Bone and joint infections</li><li>Corneal ulcer</li><li>Infectious diarrhea</li><li>Intra-abdominal infections</li><li>Pneumonia</li><li>Skin and skin structure infections</li><li>Urinary tract infections</li></ul>	<ul><li>**Dosing (Adult):** − Oral/IV: 200 to 400 mg q12h − Ocular: 1-2 gtt every 2-4 hrs x 2 days, then qid x 5 more days. If corneal ulcer more frequent (look up dosing)</li><li>**Dosing (Peds):** − Oral: 15 mg/kg/day divided q12h</li><li>**CYP450 Interactions:** None</li><li>**Renal or Hepatic Dose Adjustments:** − GFR: 20 to 50 mL/minute: maximum 200 to 400 mg q24h − GFR: < 20 mL/minute: 100 to 200 mg q24h</li><li>**Dosage Forms:** Oral (tablet), Ophthalmic (solution)</li></ul>

INFECTIOUS DISEASES – MISC ANTIBIOTICS

Drug Class
- Miscellaneous Antibiotics
- Agents:
  - Acute Care
    - Fosfomycin
    - Nitrofurantoin

Main Indications or Uses
- Acute Care
  - Uncomplicated urinary tract infections (i.e., cystitis)

> **Knowledge Integration**
> ✓ Neither of these agents are indicated for "complicated" UTIs, including pyelonephritis (a UTI involving the kidney) due to poor penetration into the kidney and insufficient data.

Mechanism of Action
- Nitrofurantoin
  - Converted by bacterial reductases to reactive intermediates, which react with bacterial ribosomal proteins causing inhibition of bacterial protein synthesis, aerobic energy metabolism, DNA, RNA, and cell wall synthesis.
- Fosfomycin
  - Inhibits the catalyzation of the initial step in bacterial cell wall synthesis by inactivating pyruvyl transferase.

Primary Net Benefit
- Bactericidal activity for Gram-positive and Gram-negative pathogens that commonly cause urinary tract infections.
- Main Labs to Monitor:
  - Cultures from infected sites at baseline (urine)

High-Yield Basic Pharmacology
- Macrobid Vs Macrodantin
  - Nitrofurantoin is formulated in two commonly used oral dosage forms, but the long-acting Macrobid, containing macrocrystalline nitrofurantoin, is preferred for treating urinary tract infections.
    - Clinical failure of treatment of UTI may occur with incorrect prescribing, despite supporting culture and sensitivity data.
- Resistance
  - Fosfomycin and nitrofurantoin have high barriers to resistance and lack acquired bacterial resistance, but should resistance occur, there is no cross-resistance between fosfomycin, nitrofurantoin, and other antimicrobial agents.
- Renal Insufficiency
  There are two major considerations of renal insufficiency when considering fosfomycin or nitrofurantoin:
    - In patients with renal failure, fosfomycin or nitrofurantoin urine levels are insufficient for antibacterial action but accumulate in the blood, causing systemic toxicities.
  - Nitrofurantoin is contraindicated in patients with significant renal insufficiency.
    - Still, there is currently a debate about the threshold as modern data suggest short-term nitrofurantoin treatment is reasonable in patients with creatinine clearance greater than 30 mL/minute.

High-Yield Clinical Knowledge
- Cystitis Treatment
  - Fosfomycin and nitrofurantoin are limited to treating lower urinary tract infections or cystitis in women due to lack of sufficient tissue penetration to upper urinary tract structures, including the ureters and kidneys.
- Adverse Events
  - Most patients tolerate fosfomycin or nitrofurantoin without complications.

- However, peripheral neuropathy and pulmonary toxicities may occur, especially when these agents are used for long periods of time or in patients with renal impairment.
- **Nitrofurantoin in Pregnancy**
  - There is controversy regarding nitrofurantoin's role since although it is not a teratogen, there have been cases with associations with congenital anomalies.
  - The greatest risk appears when nitrofurantoin is given to the mother close to delivery leading to a risk of hemolytic anemia in newborns.
  - It is currently recommended to avoid nitrofurantoin in pregnancy in the third trimester.

High-Yield Core Spectrum of Coverage
- **Core spectrum**
  - **Gram-Positive**
    - Streptococcus
      - Streptococcus pneumoniae
      - Streptococcus viridans
      - Streptococcus groups A, B, C, G
    - Staphylococcus aureus, methicillin-sensitive only
    - Enterococcus species
  - **Gram-Negative**
    - Enterobacteriaceae
      - Escherichia coli
      - Haemophilus influenzae
      - Klebsiella pneumoniae
      - Proteus mirabilis

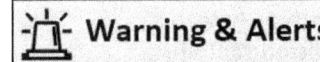

Warning & Alerts

✓ Avoid nitrofurantoin in patients with underlying G6PD deficiency due to risk of hemolysis leading to fatigue, SOB, jaundice, etc.

- **Core Indications**
  - Fosfomycin and nitrofurantoin are first-line agents for the treatment of cystitis in appropriately selected patients.

High-Yield Fast-Facts
- **Glucose-6-Phosphate**
  - Sensitivity testing for fosfomycin activity actually requires the supplementation of the media with glucose-6-phosphate. Interestingly, both fosfomycin and nitrofurantoin can cause hemolytic anemia can occur in patients with glucose-6-phosphate dehydrogenase deficiency.
- **Fosfomycin Oral**
  - In the US, fosfomycin is exclusively available as a powder (fosfomycin tromethamine) dissolved in water and taken orally.
- **Low Risk of C. difficile**
  - As a result of the narrow spectrum, there is a low risk of secondary C. difficile infection after treatment with either fosfomycin or nitrofurantoin.

Infectious Diseases

> ### HIGH-YIELD BOARD EXAM ESSENTIALS
> - **CLASSIC AGENTS:** Fosfomycin, nitrofurantoin
> - **DRUG CLASS:** Misc Antibiotics
> - **INDICATIONS:** Uncomplicated urinary tract infections (i.e., cystitis)
> - **MECHANISM:** Converted to reactive intermediates reacting with bacterial ribosomal proteins inhibiting bacterial protein synthesis, aerobic energy metabolism, DNA, RNA, and cell wall synthesis (nitrofurantoin); Inhibits the catalyzation of the initial step in bacterial cell wall synthesis by inactivating pyruvyl transferase (fosfomycin)
> - **SIDE EFFECTS:** Peripheral neuropathy and pulmonary toxicities
> - **CLINICAL PEARLS:**
>   - Nitrofurantoin is formulated in two commonly used oral dosage forms, but the long-acting Macrobid, containing macrocrystalline nitrofurantoin, is preferred for treating urinary tract infections and is easier to dose (twice a day; i.e., MacroBID).
>   - Fosfomycin is uniquely given as a single-dose.
>   - As a result of the narrow spectrum, there is a low risk of secondary C. difficile infection after treatment with either fosfomycin or nitrofurantoin.

Table: Drug Class Summary

Fosfomycin and Nitrofurantoin Drug Class Review			
High-Yield Med Reviews			
Mechanism of Action: *Nitrofurantoin: Converted to reactive intermediates reacting with bacterial ribosomal proteins inhibiting bacterial protein synthesis, aerobic energy metabolism, DNA, RNA, and cell wall synthesis. Fosfomycin: Inhibits the catalyzation of the initial step in bacterial cell wall synthesis by inactivating pyruvyl transferase.*			
Class Effects: *Bactericidal activity for Gram-positive and Gram-negative pathogens that commonly cause urinary tract infections.*			
Generic Name	**Brand Name**	**Indication(s) or Uses**	**Notes**

Fosfomycin	Monurol	- Urinary tract infection	- **Dosing (Adult):**
			  - Oral: 3 g once; Can be given as 3 g every other day for 3 doses
			- **Dosing (Peds):**
			  - Oral: 2 to 3 g once; Maximum 3 g/dose
			- **CYP450 Interactions:** None
			- **Renal or Hepatic Dose Adjustments:**
			  - GFR: 31 to 40 mL/min: Give 70% of daily dose
			  - GFR: 21 to 30 mL/min: Give 60% of daily dose
			  - GFR: 11 to 20 mL/min: Give 40% of daily dose
			  - GFR: < 10 mL/minute: Give 20% of daily dose
			- **Dosage Forms:** Oral (Packet)

Nitrofurantoin	Furadantin, Macrobid, Macrodantin	- Urinary tract infection	- **Dosing (Adult):**
			  - Oral: 100 mg q6-12h
			- **Dosing (Peds):**
			  - Oral: 12.5 to 100 mg q6h; Max: 100 mg/dose
			- **CYP450 Interactions:** None
			- **Renal or Hepatic Dose Adjustments:**
			  - GFR: < 60 mL/minute: Use contraindicated
			- **Dosage Forms:** Oral (capsule, suspension)

INFECTIOUS DISEASE – GLYCOPEPTIDES

Drug Class
- Glycopeptides
- Agents:
  - **Acute & Chronic Care**
    - Dalbavancin
    - Telavancin
    - Oritavancin
    - Vancomycin

Main Indications or Uses
- **Acute Care**
  - Bacteremia
  - Clostridoides difficile (vancomycin PO/PR only)
  - Endocarditis
  - Intra-abdominal infection
  - Meningitis
  - Osteomyelitis
  - Peritonitis
  - Pneumonia
  - Sepsis
  - Skin and soft tissue infections
  - Surgical prophylaxis
  - Urinary Tract Infections

> **Fast Facts**
> - Mainly used reserved for MRSA
> - Initial loading doses of vancomycin for serious infections is 20-25 mg/kg
> - Oral vancomycin has no use for systemic infections, but can treat the enteric infection, C. diff due to its poor oral bioavailability

> **Accelerate Your Knowledge**
> - There is a shift to using AUC:MIC ratios of vancomycin vs trough concentrations but is difficult to calculate for some places and thus both methods of assessment may still be seen clinically.

Mechanism of Action
- Inhibition of the polymerization or transglycosylase reaction, thus preventing bacterial cell wall synthesis in sensitive bacteria by binding with high affinity to the d-alanyl-d-alanine terminus of cell wall precursor units.

Primary Net Benefit
- Bactericidal for gram-positive bacteria (especially MRSA) and gram-positive anaerobes, including C. difficile.
- Main Labs to Monitor:
  - Cultures from infected sites at baseline (blood, sputum, urine, CSF etc.)
  - Renal function
  - Therapeutic drug concentrations (vancomycin)

High-Yield Basic Pharmacology
- **Telavancin and Oritavancin Mechanisms**
  - Similar to vancomycin, telavancin inhibits bacterial cell wall synthesis by binding to the D-ala-D-Ala terminus of peptidoglycan, but it also increases membrane permeability, disrupting the bacterial membrane potential.
  - Oritavancin similarly possesses the core mechanism of glycopeptides but also disrupts cell membrane permeability and inhibition of RNA synthesis in susceptible bacteria.
- **Bacterial Resistance Mechanisms**
  - Emerging vancomycin resistance, specifically, the Van A-type resistance among the Enterococcus species (E. faecium and faecalis), is caused by the expression of enzymes that modify cell wall precursors and substituting a terminal d-lactate for d-alanine, reducing affinity for vancomycin by 1000-fold.
  - Staphylococcus aureus resistance is associated with a heterogeneous phenotype, as well as plasmid gene transfer of Van A-type resistance from E. faecalis to MRSA.

- **Lipoglycopeptides Pro/Con**
    - Dalbavancin, oritavancin, and telavancin offer pharmacologic advancements from vancomycin but are limited by decreased activity against vancomycin-resistant enterococci, which shares the core mechanism of glycopeptides.
    - As a result of long half-lives, these agents can be administered at once weekly intervals or potentially as single-dose therapies.

High-Yield Clinical Knowledge
- **Clostridoides difficile**
    - Orally administered vancomycin is a key therapy for the treatment of C. difficile infections.
        - However, the oral dosage form must be used, which takes advantage of the minimal GI absorption, permitting high gut concentrations, and effective eradication of C. difficile.
            - The IV dosage form may be used orally.
- **Empiric Cornerstone**
    - Vancomycin is a key empiric antibiotic for many infections including bacteremia, cellulitis, endocarditis, meningitis, and pneumonia.
- **Therapeutic Drug Monitoring**
    - Therapeutic drug monitoring of the trough concentrations allows for titration of the empiric dose to achieve ideal concentrations between 15-20 mg/dL.
        - Updated recommendations have shifted the focus away from true trough concentrations, towards the assessment of the AUC of vancomycin, which better approximates therapeutic response.
- **Key Toxicities**
    - Acute renal injury is frequently encountered with therapeutic dosing of vancomycin.
        - Appropriate weight-based dosing, and therapeutic drug monitoring, as well as limiting concomitant nephrotoxins are interventions to reduce this risk.
    - "Redman" syndrome is an infusion rate-related histamine release eliciting flushing and red skin.
        - This is often listed as an allergy in patients charts but should be further clarified and documented as an adverse event to prevent future inappropriate antibiotic selection

High-Yield Core Spectrum of Coverage
- **Core spectrum**
    - Gram-Positive
        - Streptococcus species
            - Strep Group A, B, C, G
            - S pneumoniae
        - Enterococcus species
        - Staphylococcus aureus, methicillin-sensitive & -resistant (MSSA & MRSA)
        - Listeria monocytogenes
    - Anaerobes
        - Clostridoides difficile
- **Core Indications**
    - Vancomycin is a crucial component to numerous empiric antibiotic regimens, as previously outlined.
    - Dalbavancin, oritavancin, and telavancin have growing roles in the management of Skin and soft tissue infections, particularly in out-patient settings.

High-Yield Fast-Facts
- **Vancomycin Loading Dose**
    - Some experts have suggested administering a loading dose of 20-25 mg/kg once when initiating vancomycin therapy for serious infections.
        - Many institutions have adopted this practice and cap each dose at a maximum of 2 to 3 g.

- **Vancomycin Clinical Efficacy**
  - Vancomycin demonstrates clinical efficacy when the AUC:MIC ratio of ≥400 mg-h/L is achieved in treating staphylococcal infections.
    - There are emerging methods by which to calculate this target, however, the most widely used trough concentration is a surrogate for AUC:MIC.
- **Surgical Prophylaxis Alternative**
  - Vancomycin is an alternative agent for surgical prophylaxis in patients who have allergies to beta-lactams.

HIGH-YIELD BOARD EXAM ESSENTIALS
- **CLASSIC AGENTS:** Dalbavancin, telavancin, oritavancin, vancomycin
- **DRUG CLASS:** Glycopeptides
- **INDICATIONS:** Bacteremia, Clostridoides difficile (vancomycin PO/PR only), endocarditis, intra-abdominal infection, meningitis, osteomyelitis, peritonitis, pneumonia, sepsis, skin and soft tissue infections, surgical prophylaxis, urinary tract infections
- **MECHANISM:** Inhibition of the polymerization or transglycosylase reaction, thus preventing bacterial cell wall synthesis in sensitive bacteria by binding with high affinity to the d-alanyl-d-alanine terminus of cell wall precursor units.
- **SIDE EFFECTS:** Nephrotoxicity, infusion reaction (Redman syndrome)
- **CLINICAL PEARLS:**
  - Most commonly only used to cover against suspected or known MRSA
  - Infusion related reactions can be minimized with slowing the infusion, especially with large infusions
  - Initial loading doses (or empiric doses) for serious infections is usually 20-25 mg/kg up to 2-3 g per dose
  - Vancomycin demonstrates clinical efficacy when the AUC:MIC ratio of >400 mg-h/L is achieved in treating staphylococcal infections. There are emerging methods by which to calculate this target, however, the most widely used trough concentration is a surrogate for AUC:MIC.

Table: Drug Class Summary

	Glycopeptides - Drug Class Review High-Yield Med Reviews		
	**Mechanism of Action:** *Inhibition of the polymerization or transglycosylase reaction, thus preventing bacterial cell wall synthesis in sensitive bacteria by binding with high affinity to the d-alanyl-d-alanine terminus of cell wall precursor units.*		
	**Class Effects:** *Bactericidal for gram-positive bacteria and gram-positive anaerobes, including C. difficile.*		
Generic Name	**Brand Name**	**Main Indication(s) or Uses**	**Notes**

Dalbavancin	Dalvance	• Skin and soft tissue infections	• **Dosing (Adult):**
			  − IV: 1000 mg once, then 500 mg once in 7 days
			  − IV: 1500 mg once
			• **Dosing (Peds):**
			  − IV: 12 to 15 mg/kg once, then 6 to 7.5 mg/kg once in 7 days; Max 1000 mg/dose
			  − IV: 18 to 22.5 mg/kg once; Max 1500 mg/dose
			• **CYP450 Interactions:** None
			• **Renal or Hepatic Dose Adjustments:**
			  − GFR: < 30 mL/minute: IV 750 mg once, then 375 mg once in 7 days; or IV 1125 mg once
			• **Dosage Forms:** IV (solution)

Oritavancin	Orbactiv	• Skin and soft tissue infections	• **Dosing (Adult):** − IV: 1200 mg once • **Dosing (Peds):** Not routinely used • **CYP450 Interactions:** None • **Renal or Hepatic Dose Adjustments:** None • **Dosage Forms:** IV (solution)

Telavancin	Vibativ	• Pneumonia
		• Skin and soft tissue infections
			• **Dosing (Adult):**
			  − IV: 10 mg/kg q24h
			• **Dosing (Peds):**
			  − Not routinely used
			• **CYP450 Interactions:** None
			• **Renal or Hepatic Dose Adjustments:**
			  − GFR: 30 to 50 mL/minute: 7.5 mg/kg q24h
			  − GFR: 10 to 30 mL/minute: 10 mg/kg q48h
			  − GFR: < 10 mL/minute: Not recommended
			• **Dosage Forms:** IV (solution)

Vancomycin	Vancocin	• Bacteremia / Sepsis
		• Clostridoides difficile (PO/PR only)
		• Endocarditis
		• Intra-abdominal infection
		• Meningitis
		• Osteomyelitis
		• Peritonitis
		• Pneumonia
		• Skin & soft tissue infections
		• Surgical prophylaxis
		• Urinary Tract Infections
			• **Dosing (Adult):**
			  − Oral: 250 to 500 mg q6h
			  − IV: 10 to 20 mg/kg IV q12h (adjusted to renal function, body weight, indication)
			• **Dosing (Peds):**
			  − Oral: 10 mg/kg/dose q6h
			  − IV: 5 to 60 mg/kg/day divided q6-8h
			• **CYP450 Interactions:** None
			• **Renal or Hepatic Dose Adjustments:**
			  − Renal impairment: Therapeutic drug monitoring, adjusting dose to target concentration.
			• **Dosage Forms:** IV (solution), Oral (capsule)

INFECTIOUS DISEASE – MACROLIDES

Drug Class
- **Macrolides**
- **Agents:**
    - **Acute & Chronic Care**
        - Azithromycin
        - Clarithromycin
        - Erythromycin
        - Fidaxomicin

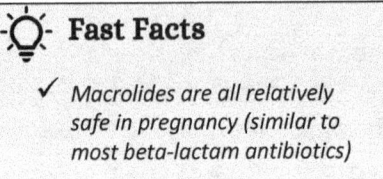

Main Indications or Uses
- **Acute & Chronic Care**
    - Pneumonia
    - Skin and soft tissue infections
    - Chlamydial infection
    - Helicobacter pylori infection
    - Mycobacterial infections

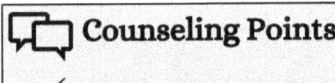

Mechanism of Action
- Inhibit susceptible bacterial protein synthesis by binding reversibly to 50S ribosomal RNA subunits preventing peptide chain elongation and causes peptidyl-transfer RNA to become dissociated from the ribosome.

Primary Net Benefit
- Bacteriostatic against susceptible pathogens (mainly gram-positive bacteria) and those that are primarily intracellular (e.g., atypical pathogens).
- Main Labs to Monitor:
    - Cultures from infected sites at baseline (blood, sputum, urine, CSF etc.)

High-Yield Basic Pharmacology
- **Erythromycin Base and GI Absorption**
    - The erythromycin base is destroyed in the acidic environment of the stomach and must be enteric-coated or formulated as an ester of the base (ie, ethyl succinate).
    - The prokinetic effect of erythromycin is not affected by the dosage form, including when administered parenterally.
- **Bacterial Resistance Mechanisms**
    - There are four general mechanisms by which otherwise susceptible bacteria may develop resistance to macrolide antibiotics:
        - Drug efflux via an active pump, ribosomal protection by the production of methylase enzymes, macrolide ring hydrolysis, or chromosomal mutations that alter a 50S ribosomal protein.
- **Fidaxomicin**
    - Fidaxomicin is minimally absorbed systemically, but achieves high fecal concentrations, making it a desirable agent for C. difficile infections.
    - According to the most recent IDSA guidelines, fidaxomicin may be considered first-line for treatment of C. difficile infection with or without oral vancomycin.

High-Yield Clinical Knowledge
- **Drug Interactions**
    - Erythromycin and clarithromycin are substrates and inhibitors of CYP3A4 leading to numerous clinically relevant drug interactions (notably, dronedarone, protease inhibitors, statins, budesonide, among others).
        - Azithromycin does not inhibit CYP3A4 at normal therapeutic dosing, but may at high concentrations.

- Chlamydia
  - Chlamydial infections can be treated with a single dose of azithromycin 1 g.
  - It is important that for sexually transmitted Chlamydial infections, the patient, and the patient's sexual partner must both receive treatment to avoid therapeutic failure, re-infection, or both.
- QT Prolongation
  - Erythromycin, clarithromycin, have been reported to cause cardiac arrhythmias, including QT prolongation with ventricular tachycardia.
  - Although azithromycin was believed to cause minimal QT prolongation, relative to other macrolides, a large database study observed that more patients receiving a macrolide (including azithromycin) developed cardiac arrhythmias compared to patients receiving fluoroquinolones. (N Engl J Med 2012; 366:1881-1890)

High-Yield Core Spectrum of Coverage
- Core spectrum
  - Gram-Positive
    - Streptococcus pneumoniae
    - Staphylococcus aureus, methicillin-sensitive
    - Listeria monocytogenes
  - Gram-Negative
    - Moraxella catarrhalis
    - Haemophilus influenzae
    - Legionella species
  - Atypical
    - Chlamydophila species
    - Mycoplasma pneumoniae
    - Mycobacterium avium
  - Anaerobes
    - Clostridium difficile (fidaxomicin only)
    - Clostridium (not difficile)

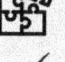 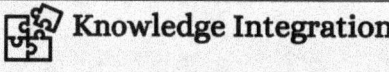

Knowledge Integration

✓ Clarithromycin (not the other macrolides) is the one used for managing H. pylori infections.

✓ Clarithromycin is also the preferred treatment for systemic infection from mycobacterium avium complex (MAC) disease, but azithromycin can be a substitute.

- Core Indications
  - Azithromycin is a key component for empiric management of community-acquired pneumonia and is the drug of choice for Chlamydial sexually transmitted infections.
  - Clarithromycin, in combination with a PPI/H2RA and/or antacid, is a core therapy for Helicobacter pylori infections.

High-Yield Fast-Facts
- Erythromycin GI Distress
  - Erythromycin is rarely used as an oral or IV antibiotic agent due to epigastric distress, which may be severe.
    - Erythromycin induces motilin receptors to stimulate GI motility but this can be a fortuitous effect for GI preparation to facilitate endoscopy/ esophagogastroduodenoscopy, particularly in patients with GI bleeds.
- Rare Effects
  - Macrolides are rarely associated with allergic reactions, however, they can manifest as fever, eosinophilia, and skin eruptions, which disappear shortly after therapy is stopped.
- Hepatotoxicity
  - Systemic use of erythromycin has been associated with cholestatic hepatitis, typically after 10-20 days of treatment.
  - Although the risk is much smaller with azithromycin and clarithromycin, they each still carry this warning.
- Antimicrobial Stewardship
  - Macrolides are most misused (25-35%) as first-line agents in adults.
  - Resistance is a significant problem for Streptococcus pneumoniae and group A Streptococcus.
    - Avoid macrolides for acute otitis media and sinusitis.
    - Use caution in Streptococcal pharyngitis.

HIGH-YIELD BOARD EXAM ESSENTIALS
- **CLASSIC AGENTS:** Azithromycin, clarithromycin, erythromycin, fidaxomicin
- **DRUG CLASS:** Macrolides
- **INDICATIONS:** Pneumonia, skin and soft tissue infections, chlamydial infection, helicobacter pylori infection, mycobacterial infections
- **MECHANISM:** Inhibit susceptible bacterial protein synthesis by binding reversibly to 50S ribosomal RNA subunits preventing peptide chain elongation and causes peptidyl-transfer RNA to become dissociated from the ribosome.
- **SIDE EFFECTS:** QT prolongation, hepatotoxicity, nausea/vomiting
- **CLINICAL PEARLS:**
    - Macrolide antibiotics have good intracellular penetration and coverage against intracellular organisms such as atypical bacteria.
    - Erythromycin and clarithromycin (but not azithromycin) are known strong inhibitors of CYP3A4 and cause drug-interactions.
    - Erythromycin, clarithromycin, have been reported to cause cardiac arrhythmias, including QT prolongation with ventricular tachycardia.
    - Erythromycin causes the most diarrhea due to its ability to stimulate bowel peristalsis.

Table: Drug Class Summary

Macrolides - Drug Class Review High-Yield Med Reviews			
Mechanism of Action: Inhibit susceptible bacterial protein synthesis by binding reversibly to 50S ribosomal.			
Class Effects: Bacteriostatic against susceptible pathogens (mainly gram-positive bacteria) and those that are primarily intracellular (e.g., atypical pathogens).			
Generic Name	Brand Name	Main Indication(s) or Uses	Notes

Azithromycin	Zithromax	<ul><li>Mycobacterium avium complex disease</li><li>Ophthalmic infections</li><li>Otitis media</li><li>Pneumonia</li><li>Scaling dermatoses</li><li>Strep pharyngitis</li></ul>	<ul><li>**Dosing (Adult):**
			  − Oral/IV: 250 to 500 mg daily</li><li>**Dosing (Peds):**
			  − Oral/IV: 5 to 10 mg/kg/day; Max 500 mg/dose</li><li>**CYP450 Interactions:**
			  − Substrate CYP3A4, inhibits P-gp</li><li>**Renal or Hepatic Dose Adjustments:** None</li><li>**Dosage Forms:** Oral (tablet, suspension), IV (solution), Ophthalmic (solution)</li></ul>

Clarithromycin	Biaxin	<ul><li>Mycobacterium avium complex disease</li><li>Helicobacter pylori infection</li><li>Rheumatic fever prophylaxis</li><li>Toxoplasma gondii encephalitis</li></ul>	<ul><li>**Dosing (Adult):**
			  − Oral: IR 500 mg q12h, or ER 1g q24h</li><li>**Dosing (Peds):**
			  − Oral: 15 mg/kg/day divided q12h; Max: 500 mg/dose</li><li>**CYP450 Interactions:**
			  − Substrate CYP3A4, inhibits CYP3A4, P-gp</li><li>**Renal or Hepatic Dose Adjustments:**
			  − GFR < 30 mL/minute reduce dose by 50%</li><li>**Dosage Forms:** Oral (tablet, suspension)</li></ul>

Erythromycin	Erythrocin	<ul><li>Oral dosage form: prokinetic agent for endoscopy/ esophagogastroduodenoscopy</li><li>Topical/Ophthalmic infections</li></ul>	<ul><li>**Dosing (Adult):**
			  − Oral (base): 250 to 500 mg q6-12h
			    − Maximum 4g/day
			  − Oral (EES): 400 to 800 q6-12h; Max: 4g/day
			  − IV: 15 to 20 mg/kg/day divided q6h; Max 4g/day</li><li>**Dosing (Peds):**
			  − Oral (base or EES): 30 to 50 mg/kg/day divided q6-12h; Maximum 4g/day
			  − IV: 15 to 20 mg/kg/day divided q6h; Max 4g/day</li><li>**CYP450 Interactions:**
			  − Substrate CYP2B6, CYP3A4. Inhibits CYP3A4, P-gp</li><li>**Renal or Hepatic Dose Adjustments:** None</li><li>**Dosage Forms:** Oral (capsule, tablet, suspension), IV (solution), Ophthalmic (ointment), Topical (gel, pad, solution)</li></ul>

Fidaxomicin	Dificid	<ul><li>Clostridoides difficile infection</li></ul>	<ul><li>**Dosing (Adult):**
			  − Oral: 200 mg BID for 10 days</li><li>**Dosing (Peds):**
			  − Oral: 16 mg/kg/dose BID x 10 days</li><li>**CYP450 Interactions:** Pgp substrate</li><li>**Renal or Hepatic Dose Adjustments:** None</li><li>**Dosage Forms:** Oral (tablet, suspension)</li></ul>

INFECTIOUS DISEASE – NITROIMIDAZOLE (METRONIDAZOLE, TINIDAZOLE)

Drug Class
- Metronidazole, Tinidazole
- Agents:
    - Acute Care
        - Metronidazole
        - Secnidazole
        - Tinidazole

Main Indications or Uses
- Acute Care (if relevant)
    - Amebiasis
    - Bacterial vaginosis
    - Clostridoides difficile (metronidazole)
    - Giardiasis
    - Trichomoniasis

> 💬 **Counseling Point**
>
> ✓ Warn to avoid drinking alcohol while taking metronidazole due to risk of disulfiram-like reaction.

Mechanism of Action
- Nitroimidazoles are reduced in susceptible pathogens producing an active metabolite taken up into bacterial DNA, forming unstable molecules, and disrupting DNA structure and replication.

Primary Overall Net Benefit
- Effective against most anaerobic bacteria plays a role in the treatment of Clostridoides difficile infections and some parasites.
- Main Labs to Monitor:
    - Main Labs to Monitor:
        - Cultures from infected sites at baseline (blood, sputum, urine, CSF, etc.)

High-Yield Basic Pharmacology
- **Renal Dose Adjustment**
    - Metronidazole is primarily eliminated in the urine to a large degree as unchanged drug or active metabolites (approximately 80%), yet renal dose adjustments are not routinely recommended.
    - There is a similar debate about dose adjustments' relevance in patients with severe hepatic impairment as the pharmacokinetics of metronidazole after a single dose are not altered in patients with cirrhosis.
        - Additional doses may require a 50% dose reduction.
- **Inhibits CYP2C9**
    - Metronidazole inhibits CYP2C9 and has clinically relevant drug interactions with warfarin, phenytoin, and phenobarbital.
        - With warfarin, metronidazole alters GI flora to increase warfarin absorption and inhibition of its metabolism by CYP2C9. Close monitoring of the INR is warranted.
- **Disulfiram Reaction**
    - Metronidazole is associated with a disulfiram-like effect in patients who are exposed to ethanol during therapy.
        - While this is relevant for knowledge on board examinations, its clinical relevance is questionable as the incidence of clinically relevant disulfiram reactions is extremely low.

High-Yield Clinical Knowledge
- **Helicobacter pylori Infection**
    - Metronidazole is a core element to combination therapy for H. pylori infections, including bismuth quad therapy (PPI/H2RA, bismuth, metronidazole, and tetracycline), concomitant therapy (PPI, amoxicillin, clarithromycin, and metronidazole), sequential therapy (PPI and amoxicillin for 5 days, then PPI, clarithromycin, and metronidazole for 5 days).
- **C. difficile Routes**

- Although metronidazole is no longer considered first-line therapy for C. difficile infections, it can be used in combination with oral vancomycin or fidaxomicin.
    - One advantage to metronidazole is that it can be administered orally or IV for this indication, and some propose higher colon penetration with the IV.
- **Metronidazole Pregnancy**
    - The controversy of metronidazole in pregnancy is dependent on the indication for use as it is contraindicated in the first trimester, but this specific to patients with trichomoniasis or bacterial vaginosis but acceptable for use during the second and third trimester.
    - For all other indications (C. difficile, intraabdominal infections, helicobacter infection, etc.), metronidazole is acceptable during pregnancy.
    - Despite conflicting recommendations, the available evidence suggests that metronidazole does not pose a significant risk of structural defects to the fetus.
        - The prescribing information of metronidazole from the manufacturer states For other indications, metronidazole can be used during pregnancy if there are no other alternatives with established safety profiles.

High-Yield Core Spectrum of Coverage
- **Core spectrum**
    - Anaerobes
        - Bacteroides fragilis
        - Clostridoides species (including C. difficile)
        - Fusobacterium necrophorum
        - Peptostreptococcus species
- **Core Indications**
    - Effective against most anaerobic bacteria plays a role in the treatment of Clostridoides difficile infections, Trichomoniasis, and some parasites.
    - Metronidazole is a crucial component in the combination therapy for H. pylori infections.

> **Drug Interaction Pearl**
> ✓ Metronidazole inhibits CYP2C9, which is the same pathway of metabolism for s-warfarin (the more potent isomer), thus increasing the risk for bleeding.

High-Yield Fast-Facts
- **Peripheral Neuropathy**
    - Metronidazole has been associated with the development of peripheral neuropathy with prolonged use, which can be seen during recurrent C. difficile infection treatment, or H. pylori treatment.
- **Possible Carcinogen**
    - Although the relevance in humans is questionable, metronidazole is considered carcinogenic by the U.S. National Toxicology Program, but this is based only on animal models and has also only been demonstrated to be mutagenic in bacterial cultures.
- **High Single Dose**
    - For the treatment of trichomoniasis, metronidazole is administered as a single 2000 mg dose orally. Although 4x the normal dose for other indications, this dose is well-tolerated and highly (greater than 90%) effective for treatment.

HIGH-YIELD BOARD EXAM ESSENTIALS
- **CLASSIC AGENTS:** Metronidazole, Tinidazole
- **DRUG CLASS:** Nitroimidazole
- **INDICATIONS:** Amebiasis, bacterial vaginosis, Clostridoides difficile, Giardiasis, Helicobacter pylori, trichomoniasis
- **MECHANISM:** Nitroimidazoles are reduced in susceptible pathogens producing an active metabolite taken up into bacterial DNA, forming unstable molecules, and disrupting DNA structure and replication.
- **SIDE EFFECTS:** Disulfiram reaction, peripheral neuropathy
- **CLINICAL PEARLS:** Metronidazole is known to inhibit CYP2C9 which can interact with warfarin and increase the risk of bleeding. Avoid alcohol when taking metronidazole due to a small risk in developing a "disulfiram-like reaction" (mainly nausea and vomiting). The controversy of metronidazole in pregnancy is dependent on the indication for use as it is contraindicated in the first trimester, but this specific to patients with trichomoniasis or bacterial vaginosis but acceptable for use during the second and third trimester.

Table: Drug Class Summary

| | Nitroimidazole - Drug Class Review
High-Yield Med Reviews |

	**Mechanism of Action:** *Reduced in susceptible pathogens to an active metabolite and taken up by bacterial DNA, forming unstable molecules and disrupting DNA structure and replication.*
	**Class Effects:** Bactericidal against anaerobic bacteria, including Clostridoides difficile, Trichomoniasis, as well as some parasites.
Generic Name	**Brand Name**	**Indication(s) or Uses**	**Notes**
Metronidazole	Flagyl	<ul><li>Amebiasis</li><li>Bacterial vaginosis</li><li>Clostridoides difficile</li><li>Giardiasis</li><li>Helicobacter pylori</li><li>Trichomoniasis</li></ul>	<ul><li>**Dosing (Adult):** – IV/Oral: 500 to 750 mg q8-12h</li><li>**Dosing (Peds):** – IV/Oral: 15 to 50 mg/kg/day divided q8h – Maximum 4 g/day</li><li>**CYP450 Interactions:** – Substrate of CYP2A6, inhibits CYP2C9</li><li>**Renal or Hepatic Dose Adjustments:** – Child-Pugh class C - reduce dose by 50%</li><li>**Dosage Forms:** IV (solution), Oral (capsule, tablet)</li></ul>
Secnidazole	Solosec	<ul><li>Bacterial Vaginosis</li><li>Trichomoniasis</li></ul>	<ul><li>**Dosing (Adult):** – Oral: 2 g as a single dose</li><li>**Dosing (Peds):** n/a</li><li>**CYP450 Interactions:** Unknown</li><li>**Renal or Hepatic Dose Adjustments:** None</li><li>**Dosage Forms:** Oral (packet)</li></ul>
Tinidazole	Tindamax	<ul><li>Amebiasis</li><li>Bacterial vaginosis</li><li>Clostridoides difficile</li><li>Giardiasis</li><li>Trichomoniasis</li></ul>	<ul><li>**Dosing (Adult):** – Oral: 2 g once daily</li><li>**Dosing (Peds):** – Oral: 50 mg/kg/day; Maximum 2 g/dose</li><li>**CYP450 Interactions:** Substrate CYP3A4</li><li>**Renal or Hepatic Dose Adjustments:** None</li><li>**Dosage Forms:** Oral (tablet)</li></ul>

INFECTIOUS DISEASE – OXAZOLIDINONES

Drug Class
- Oxazolidinones
- Agents:
  - Acute & Chronic Care
    - Linezolid
    - Tedizolid

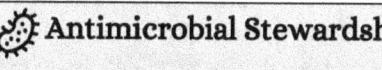

Antimicrobial Stewardship
✓ Should be reserved for patients with MRSA or VRE infections.

Main Indications or Uses
- Acute & Chronic Care (Labeled Indications)
  - Pneumonia
    - Linezolid
  - Skin and skin structure infections
    - Linezolid, tedizolid
  - Vancomycin-resistant Enterococcal infection
    - Linezolid

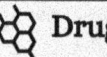

Drug Interaction Pearl
✓ Warning! Both agents can inhibit MAO and thus put patients at an increased risk for serotonin syndrome if used with certain drugs.

Mechanism of Action
- Binds to the 23S ribosomal RNA of the 50S subunit, stopping the formation of the ribosome complex responsible for protein synthesis, ultimately inhibiting bacterial protein synthesis.
  - Also, both agents can inhibit monoamine oxidase (MAO).

Primary Net Benefit
- Bacteriostatic against susceptible Gram-positive pathogens, including enterococci, staphylococci, and bactericidal against streptococci. Covers MRSA and VRE.
- Main Labs to Monitor:
  - Cultures from infected sites at baseline (blood, sputum, urine, CSF, etc.)
  - Muscle rigidity, hyperthermia, altered mental status (signs of serotonin syndrome, linezolid only)
  - Complete blood count (thrombocytopenia and risk of BMS)

High-Yield Basic Pharmacology
- **Unique Binding Site**
  - The unique 23S subunit binding site of linezolid results in no cross-resistance with other drug classes binding to the 50S subunit, such as clindamycin or macrolides.
- **Serotonin Syndrome**
  - Linezolid is a nonspecific inhibitor of monoamine oxidase (MAO), potentially leading to excess serotonin in patients concomitantly taking SSRI, SNRI, St. John's Wort, or ingesting excessive amounts of dietary tyramine.
- **IV to PO**
  - Both linezolid and tedizolid are well absorbed after oral administration and can be converted 1:1 from IV to oral (or vice versa).

High-Yield Clinical Knowledge
- **Mitochondrial toxicities**
  - Linezolid may directly inhibit intramitochondrial protein synthesis disrupting cellular energy production in tissues highly dependent on oxidative phosphorylation and leading to several clinically relevant adverse events: peripheral and optic neuropathy, lactic acidosis, and myelosuppression.
- **Myelosuppression**
  - Linezolid has been associated with myelosuppression (leukopenia, pancytopenia, and thrombocytopenia) and increases in incidence with prolonged therapy after 2 weeks of therapy.
    - Tedizolid also carries this risk, but this risk may be lower as clinical experience with this agent continues.

- **Vancomycin-Resistant Enterococci (VRE)**
    - The mechanism of resistance in enterococci and staphylococci results from specific point mutations of the 23S rRNA.
        - However, since most bacteria possess multiple copies of 23S rRNA genes, resistance to oxazolidinones to occur requires mutations in at least 2 copies.
- **Linezolid and Bacteremia**
    - Linezolid has excellent tissue penetration; however, blood concentrations are not adequate for reliable empiric management of bacteremia.
        - Exceptions that permit linezolid for bacteremia include VRE infections, or where alternatives otherwise do not exist.

High-Yield Core Spectrum of Coverage
- **Core spectrum**
    - Gram-Positive
        - Enterococci species (including vancomycin-resistant enterococci)
        - Staphylococcus aureus, methicillin-sensitive and methicillin-resistant
        - Streptococci species
        - Listeria monocytogenes
- **Core Indications**
    - Linezolid is a key agent for the management of vancomycin-resistant E. faecium infections.
    - As an IV form, it can be used as an alternative to vancomycin in healthcare-associated pneumonia or as an oral option to manage community-acquired pneumonia and skin and soft tissue infections.
    - These agents are oral options for the management of certain MRSA infections.

High-Yield Fast-Facts
- **Opioids and Serotonin Syndrome**
    - Specific opioids (fentanyl, tramadol, methadone) have been associated with serotonin syndrome and should be used cautiously combined with oxazolidinones.
- **VRE Alternatives**
    - Alternatives to oxazolidinones for VRE treatment include daptomycin, tigecycline, and possibly oritavancin.
- **Lactic Acidosis**
    - Lactic acidosis has been reported with linezolid with prolonged durations of use.
    - Potential lactic acidosis signs include patients with recurrent nausea and vomiting, acidosis, or low unexplained bicarbonate levels should be evaluated for linezolid-induced lactic acidosis.

HIGH-YIELD BOARD EXAM ESSENTIALS
- **CLASSIC AGENTS:** Linezolid, tedizolid
- **DRUG CLASS:** Oxazolidinones
- **INDICATIONS:** Pneumonia, skin and skin structure infections, vancomycin-resistant Enterococcal infection
- **MECHANISM:** Binds to the 23S RNS ribosomal RNA of the 50S subunit, inhibiting bacterial protein synthesis. Also inhibit MAO.
- **SIDE EFFECTS:** Serotonin syndrome, myelosuppression, peripheral and optic neuropathy, lactic acidosis
- **CLINICAL PEARLS:**
    - Both agents cover MRSA and are available in both oral and IV formulations at the same dose.
    - Both agents inhibit MAO and thus used with caution with SRI, SNRI, St. John's Wort, or ingesting excessive amounts of dietary tyramine.
    - Linezolid has excellent tissue penetration; however, blood concentrations are not adequate for reliable empiric management of bacteremia. Exceptions that permit linezolid for bacteremia include VRE infections, or where alternatives otherwise do not exist.

Table: Drug Class Summary

Oxazolidinones - Drug Class Review High-Yield Med Reviews			
Mechanism of Action: *Binds to the 23S RNS ribosomal RNA of the 50S subunit, inhibiting bacterial protein synthesis*			
Class Effects: *Both agents can inhibit MAO causing drug interactions. Bacteriostatic against susceptible Gram-positive pathogens, including enterococci, staphylococci, and bactericidal against streptococci; Covers MRSA and VRE.*			
Generic Name	**Brand Name**	**Indication(s) or Uses**	**Notes**

Linezolid	Zyvox	<ul><li>Pneumonia</li><li>Skin and skin structure infections</li><li>Vancomycin-resistant Enterococcal infection</li></ul>	<ul><li>**Dosing (Adult):**
			  – Oral/IV: 600 mg q12h</li><li>**Dosing (Peds):**
			  – Oral/IV: 10 mg/kg/dose q8h
			    – Maximum 600 mg/dose</li><li>**CYP450 Interactions:** None</li><li>**Renal or Hepatic Dose Adjustments:** None</li><li>**Dosage Forms:** Oral (tablet), IV (solution)</li></ul>

Tedizolid	Sivextro	<ul><li>Skin and skin structure infections</li></ul>	<ul><li>**Dosing (Adult):**
			  – Oral/IV: 200 mg daily</li><li>**Dosing (Peds):** Children 12 years and older
			  – Oral/IV: 200 mg daily</li><li>**CYP450 Interactions:** None</li><li>**Renal or Hepatic Dose Adjustments:** None</li><li>**Dosage Forms:** Oral (tablet), IV (solution)</li></ul>

ANTIMICROBIALS – POLYMYXINS

Drug Class
- **Polymyxins**
- **Agents:**
    - **Acute Care**
        - Polymyxin B
        - Colistimethate (may also be referred to as Colistin)

Main Indications or Uses
- **Acute Care**
    - Bacteremia
    - Meningitis
    - Pneumonia

> **Knowledge Integration**
> ✓ Due to the risk of nephrotoxicity and neurotoxicity from systemic drug exposure, giving polymyxin B via nebulization for pulmonary infections can help reduce some of the systemic drug exposure by topical administration.

Mechanism of Action
- Act as cationic detergents that interact strongly with phospholipids and disrupt bacterial cell membranes' structure, leading to bacterial cell lysis.

Primary Net Benefit
- Bactericidal, Gram-negative specific antimicrobials that have re-emerged to treat multi-drug resistant infections (including some cases of Pseudomonas aeruginosa and Acinetobacter spp), despite considerable toxicity.
- Main Labs to Monitor:
    - Cultures from infected sites at baseline (blood, sputum, urine, CSF, etc.)
    - Renal function (BUN, serum creatinine, urine output) due to risk of nephrotoxicity

High-Yield Basic Pharmacology
- **Polymyxins Binding Site**
    - Gram-negative bacteria sensitivity to the polymyxins is related to the phospholipids' content in the given bacterial cell wall.
        - The polymyxins' spectrum is limited to gram-negatives as their binding site to the lipopolysaccharide of the outer membrane of gram-negative bacteria inactivating it.
- **Resistance**
    - Resistance to polymyxins are acquired from bacterial exposure to polymyxins while on treatment has been documented and has become problematic among "*extensively* drug-resistant" Acinetobacter and Klebsiella.
- **Colistin**
    - Colistin is the active antimicrobial agent produced from the unstable compound colistin methane sulfonate both in vivo and in aqueous and biologic fluids ex vivo.

High-Yield Clinical Knowledge
- **Polymyxin B and Polymyxin E**
    - Although commonly referred to as colistin, it is otherwise known as polymyxin E.
    - It may be referred to as polymyxin E in the historical literature and is marketed either as colistimethate for intravenous administration or colistin base for topical use.
    - Polymyxin B itself not a single agent but is a mixture of polymyxins B1 and B2.
- **Nephrotoxicity**
    - The polymyxin agents are highly nephrotoxic, in a dose-dependent manner, and had fallen out of use due to this toxicity.
        - Their re-emergence into therapy is not because of increased safety but rather accepting the increased risk of renal injury to manage multi-drug resistant Gram-negative infections.

Infectious Diseases

- **Neurotoxicity**
    - Most commonly seen in patients with impaired renal function due to elevated drug levels.
        - Manifested as irritability, weakness, ataxia, and changes in vision
- **Pharmacokinetic Dosing**
    - As an alternative to fixed weight-based dosing, a pharmacokinetic model dosing has been proposed for colistin using the following calculation: maintenance dose = colistin steady-state target x [(1.50 x GFR)+ 30].
        - The suggested average target concentration of 2.5 mcg/mL (or 1.0 mcg/mL free-colistin).
- **Core spectrum**
    - Gram-Negative
        - Enterobacteriaceae (ESBL negative, CRE negative)
            - Escherichia coli
            - Klebsiella pneumoniae
        - Acinetobacter species
        - Pseudomonas aeruginosa
- **Core Indications**
    - Polymyxin B and colistin are used for nosocomial infections caused by multi-drug resistant pathogens or in select patients with cystic fibrosis.

High-Yield Fast-Facts

- **Return to Clinical Use**
    - The clinical use of colistin and polymyxin B had evaporated after the 1970s due to the early experience of nephrotoxicity and neurotoxicity.
    - Still, the rapid emergency of Gram-negative resistance to all other antibiotics since the early 2000s necessitated their resurgence.
- **Nebulization**
    - For certain pulmonary infections or cystic fibrosis, polymyxin B or colistin may be administered via nebulization rather than intravenously or as an adjunct to IV therapy.

HIGH-YIELD BOARD EXAM ESSENTIALS
- **CLASSIC AGENTS:** Polymyxin B, colistimethate
- **DRUG CLASS:** Polymyxins
- **INDICATIONS:** Bacteremia, meningitis, pneumonia
- **MECHANISM:** Act as cationic detergents that interact strongly with phospholipids and disrupt bacterial cell membranes' structure, leading to bacterial cell lysis.
- **SIDE EFFECTS:** Nephrotoxicity, neurotoxicity
- **CLINICAL PEARLS:** For certain pulmonary infections or cystic fibrosis, polymyxin B or colistin may be administered via nebulization rather than intravenously or as an adjunct to IV therapy.

Table: Drug Class Summary

Polymyxins - Drug Class Review High-Yield Med Reviews			
Mechanism of Action: *Act as cationic detergents that interact strongly with phospholipids and disrupt bacterial cell membranes' structure, leading to bacterial cell lysis.*			
Class Effects: *Bactericidal, Gram-negative specific antimicrobials that have re-emerged to treat multi-drug resistant infections (including some cases of Pseudomonas aeruginosa and Acinetobacter spp), despite considerable toxicity (nephrotoxicity and neurotoxicity).*			
Generic Name	**Brand Name**	**Indication(s) or Uses**	**Notes**

Colistimethate	Coly-Mycin M	• Bacteremia
		• Meningitis
		• Pneumonia
			• **Dosing (Adult):** Dosing based on colistin base activity (CBA)
			  − IV: 300 to 360 mg CBP/day divided q12h
			• **Dosing (Peds):**
			  − IV/IM: 2.5 to 5 mg CBA/kg/day divided q6-12h
			• **CYP450 Interactions:** text
			• **Renal or Hepatic Dose Adjustments:**
			  − Obese patients - dose based on adjusted body weight
			  − GFR 31 to 50 mL/minute: 183 to 250 mg CBA/day
			  − GFR 10 to 30 mL/minute: 150 to 183 mg CBA/day
			  − GFR < 10 mL/minute: 117 mg CBA/day
			• **Dosage Forms:** IV (solution)

Polymyxin B	Polytrim	• Bacteremia
		• Meningitis
		• Pneumonia
			• **Dosing (Adult):**
			  − IV: LD 20,000 to 25,000 units/kg, then 12,500 to 15,000 units/kg q12h
			• **Dosing (Peds):**
			  − IV: 25,000 to 30,000 units/kg/day divided q12h
			    − Maximum 2,000,000 units/kg per day
			• **CYP450 Interactions:** None
			• **Renal or Hepatic Dose Adjustments:** None
			• **Dosage Forms:** IV (solution)

INFECTIOUS DISEASE – QUINUPRISTIN-DALFOPRISTIN

Drug Class
- Streptogramin
- Agents:
    - Acute Care
        - Quinupristin/dalfopristin

Main Indications or Uses
- Acute Care
    - Bacteremia
    - Endocarditis
    - Meningitis
    - Skin and skin structure infections

> **Dosing Pearl**
> ✓ Best if administered diluted in 500 to 750 mL and given via a central line to avoid phlebitis (venous irritation usually experienced with a peripheral IV line.
> ✓ Give over at least 60 minutes as shorter durations are associated with infusion reactions.

Mechanism of Action
- Quinupristin and dalfopristin inhibit susceptible bacterial protein synthesis by binding reversibly to 50S ribosomal RNA subunits preventing peptide chain elongation and causes peptidyl-transfer RNA to become dissociated from the ribosome.
    - Dalfopristin possesses additional activity by enhancing quinupristin binding by binding to an adjacent location and resulting in a conformational change in the 50S ribosome.

Primary Net Benefit
- Bactericidal against gram-positive cocci and organisms responsible for atypical pathogens, and bacteriostatic against Enterococcus faecium (e.g., VRE).
- Main Labs to Monitor:
    - Cultures from infected sites at baseline (blood, sputum, urine, CSF, etc.)
    - Conjugated bilirubin due to risk of hyperbilirubinemia

High-Yield Basic Pharmacology
- **Early and Late Phase Inhibition**
    - The action of dalfopristin inhibits early-phase protein synthesis in bacterial cell production, whereas quinupristin inhibits late-phase inhibition of protein synthesis.
- **Interactions**
    - Quinupristin/dalfopristin is an inhibitor of CYP3A4 with clinically relevant drug interactions with warfarin, diazepam, quetiapine, simvastatin, and cyclosporine, to name a few.
- **VRE but Not Enterococcus faecalis**
    - Although quinupristin/dalfopristin is a key agent in the management of vancomycin-resistant enterococcus faecium, it is not effective against Enterococcus faecalis, as nearly all isolates are resistant to quinupristin/dalfopristin.

High-Yield Clinical Knowledge
- **Multi-Drug Resistant Pathogens**
    - As a result of other available agents that are better tolerated, the use of quinupristin/dalfopristin has been relegated to salvage therapy for complicated skin and skin structure infections caused by methicillin-susceptible strains of S. aureus or S. pyogenes or vancomycin-resistant strains of E. faecium.
- **Problematic Adverse Reactions**
    - Administration of quinupristin/dalfopristin is frequently associated with infusion reactions, including pain, inflammation in approximately half of all patients receiving this drug.
        - Administration via central IV access can reduce the incidence of infusion reactions and slow the rate of infusion.
    - Hyperbilirubinemia is also highly prevalent, occurring in up to 35% of patients.

High-Yield Core Spectrum of Coverage
- **Core spectrum**
  - **Gram-Positive**
    - Streptococcus species: Strep Group A, B, C, G and S pneumoniae
    - Enterococcus faecium (including vancomycin-resistant strains)
    - Staphylococcus aureus, methicillin-sensitive & -resistant (MSSA & MRSA)
    - Listeria monocytogenes
  - **Atypical:** Mycoplasma pneumoniae
  - **Anaerobes:** Prevotella melaninogenica
- **Core Indications**
  - The use of quinupristin/dalfopristin is limited to last-line therapy for MRSA and VRE.

High-Yield Fast-Fact
- **Combination Ratio**
  - Quinupristin/dalfopristin is formulated in a 30:70 ratio and work synergistically in their action on the 50S ribosome as described above.

HIGH-YIELD BOARD EXAM ESSENTIALS
- **CLASSIC AGENTS:** Quinupristin/Dalfopristin
- **DRUG CLASS:** Streptogramin
- **INDICATIONS:** Bacteremia, endocarditis, meningitis, skin and skin structure infections
- **MECHANISM:** Binds reversibly to 50S ribosomal RNA subunits inhibits susceptible bacterial protein synthesis
- **SIDE EFFECTS:** Infusion reactions, hyperbilirubinemia
- **CLINICAL PEARLS:** Covers against MRSA and VRE. Overall, IV infusions are hard to tolerate and as a result is not commonly used first line (note: give diluted in 500 mL via central line in most cases to avoid phlebitis and over at least 60 minutes to avoid infusion reactions). Quinupristin/dalfopristin is an inhibitor of CYP3A4 with clinically relevant drug interactions with warfarin, diazepam, quetiapine, simvastatin, and cyclosporine, to name a few.

Table: Drug Class Summary

Quinupristin-Dalfopristin - Drug Class Review High-Yield Med Reviews			
Generic Name	**Brand Name**	**Indication(s) or Uses**	**Notes**
Quinupristin-dalfopristin	Synercid	- Bacteremia - Endocarditis - Meningitis - Skin and skin structure infections	- **Dosing (Adult):** IV: 7.5 mg/kg q12h - **Dosing (Peds):** IV: 7.5 mg/kg q12h - **CYP450 Interactions:** Inhibits CYP3A4 - **Renal or Hepatic Dose Adjustments:** None - **Dosage Forms:** IV (solution)

INFECTIOUS DISEASE – SULFONAMIDES

Drug Class
- Sulfonamides
- Agents:
    - Acute & Chronic Care
        - Sulfacetamide
        - Sulfadiazine
        - Sulfamethoxazole/Trimethoprim

Main Indications or Uses
- Acute Care
    - Pneumocystis jiroveci (PJP) treatment
    - Toxoplasmosis
    - Skin and soft tissue infections
    - Urinary Tract Infections
- Chronic Care
    - Pneumocystis jiroveci (PJP) prophylaxis

> **Warnings or Alerts**
> - ✓ TMP/SMX should be avoid in the 1st & 3rd trimester of pregnancy but can be used in the 2nd trimester for UTIs.
> - ✓ TMP/SMX can significantly interfere with the metabolism of warfarin and increase the risk of bleeding. Consider not using TMP/SMX or reduce dose of warfarin on day 1.
> - ✓ Avoid use in patients with "sulfa" allergy due to risk of severe rash, including SJS.

Mechanism of Action
- Sulfonamides
    - Competitively inhibit dihydropteroate synthase, thus preventing the incorporation of para-aminobenzoic acid (PABA) into dihydropteroic acid and production of folic acid.
- Trimethoprim
    - Selective inhibition of bacterial dihydrofolic acid reductase prevents the conversion of dihydrofolic acid to tetrahydrofolic acid.

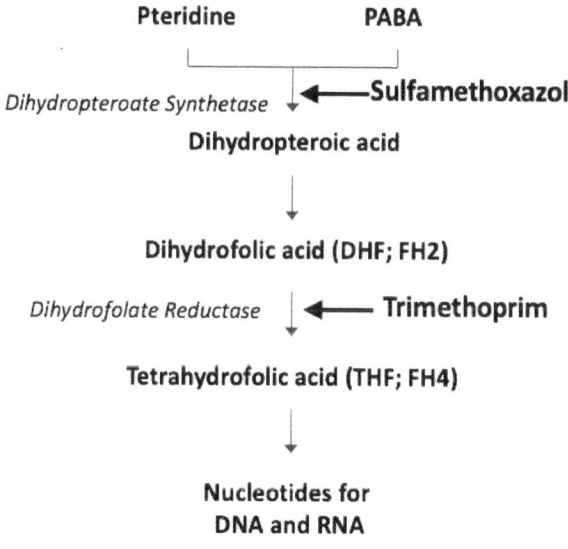

Primary Net Benefit

- Bacteriostatic as independent agents but can exert bactericidal in combination with other agents. Has some coverage against community-acquired MRSA (NOT nosocomial MRSA) and lacks strep coverage.
- Main Labs to Monitor:
    - Cultures from infected sites at baseline (blood, sputum, urine, CSF etc.)
    - Renal function (serum creatinine), K+ due to small risk of hyperkalemia

High-Yield Basic Pharmacology
- **Selective for Bacteria**
  - The action of sulfonamides on purine synthesis is selective for bacteria and does not affect mammalian purine synthesis.
    - Mammalian cells require preformed folic acid, cannot synthesize it, and are thus insensitive to drugs acting by this mechanism.
- **Bacterial Resistance Mechanisms**
  - There are three general mechanisms by which otherwise susceptible bacteria may develop resistance to sulfonamide antibiotics:
    - The decreased target site of action affinity (dihydropteroate synthase) for sulfonamides.
    - Active efflux from the bacterial cell or decreased penetration to the site of action.
    - Bacteria have developed an alternative metabolic pathway and/or increased production of PABA.
- **Trimethoprim Distribution**
  - Sulfamethoxazole/trimethoprim is considered a preferred agent for prostatitis, in part by the ability of trimethoprim to concentrate in the more acidic environment of the prostate relative to plasma.

High-Yield Clinical Knowledge
- **Pregnancy and UTIs**
  - Sulfamethoxazole/trimethoprim is generally contraindicated during the first and third trimester of pregnancy but for two different reasons.
    - First trimester it is contraindicated due to mechanistic concerns similar to methotrexate which could negatively impact dividing cells.
    - Third trimester it is contraindicated due to the potential risk of hemolysis in fetuses with undiagnosed or unknown G6PD deficiency which could lead to hyperbilirubinemia and risk of kernicterus (irreversible brain damage as a result of excess bilirubin generated from RBC breakdown.
- **Drug Interactions**
  - Sulfonamides have numerous drug interactions by inhibition of CYP2C9 with common medications including warfarin, sulfonylureas, and phenytoin.
  - Sulfonamides may also displace drugs bound to albumin, increasing free-fraction drug concentrations, and potentially causing toxicities or adverse events.
    - In patients taking warfarin and being started on sulfamethoxazole/trimethoprim, empiric dose reduction of warfarin by 10-20% with close follow up and/or monitoring of signs and symptoms of bleeding must occur.
  - Trimethoprim weakly inhibits CYP2C8 but can inhibit CYP2C9 and CYP3A4 at high concentrations.
- **Hypersensitivity**
  - Sulfonamides are associated with delayed onset hypersensitivity reactions which can range from morbilliform, urticarial, purpuric, and petechial rashes, to erythema multiforme, Stevens-Johnson syndrome, or toxic epidermal necrolysis.
  - The onset of these hypersensitivities can occur after the first week of therapy but may appear earlier in patients who have been previously sensitized.
    - Patients with HIV/AIDS have a markedly higher incidence of rashes with sulfonamide treatment which can influence therapeutic selection for PJP prophylaxis or treatment of opportunistic infections.
- **Hemolytic Anemia and G6PD Deficiency**
  - Acute hemolytic anemia may occur after administration of sulfonamide antibiotics, which can be related to an erythrocytic deficiency of G6PD activity.
  - Other hematologic effects can occur, albeit less frequently, including agranulocytosis, aplastic anemia, and thrombocytopenia.
    - Similar to the increased incidence of hypersensitivity in patients with HIV/AIDS taking sulfonamides, the incidence of hematologic toxicity is also higher in this population.

- **IV or Weight Based Dosing**
  - When dosing sulfamethoxazole/trimethoprim using a weight-based format, whether it is in an adult or pediatric patient, the trimethoprim component is used to calculate the appropriate dose.
    - Careful verification of the appropriate component should take place as well as confirming the dosage form, particularly if selecting the tablet format (single-strength "SS", or double-strength "DS").

High-Yield Core Spectrum of Coverage
- **Core spectrum**
  - Gram-Positive
    - Streptococcus pneumoniae
    - Staphylococcus aureus, methicillin-sensitive & -resistant (MSSA & MRSA)
    - Listeria monocytogenes
  - Gram-Negative
    - Escherichia coli
    - Haemophilus influenzae
    - Klebsiella pneumoniae
    - Proteus mirabilis
    - Burkholderia cepacia
    - Stenotrophomonas maltophilia
    - Yersinia enterocolitica
    - Francisella tularensis
    - Legionella sp
- **Core Indications**
  - Sulfonamide antibiotics were the first effective systemic antimicrobial agents for the prevention and cure of bacterial infections in humans.
  - However, because of resistance, toxicity, and the development of beta-lactams, sulfonamide antibiotics are rarely considered first-line agents in common infections.
    - Specific infections where they are still considered the first line:
      - Male UTI/Prostatitis
      - PJP infection treatment and prophylaxis
      - Toxoplasmosis
      - Oral treatment of MRSA skin infections (not strep)

High-Yield Fast-Facts
- **Adverse Effects**
  - Sulfamethoxazole/trimethoprim is 1 of the top 10 drugs implicated in ED visits for adverse effects.
- **Sulfonamide metabolism**
  - Sulfonamides are primarily metabolized in the liver, producing the major metabolite, N4-acetylated sulfonamide.
    - These metabolites possess no antibacterial activity but still has the toxic potential of the sulfonamide.
- **Silver Sulfadiazine**
  - Silver sulfadiazine is a topical product with limited antimicrobial activity.
    - Both the silver and sulfadiazine components possess antibacterial properties.
  - Although little silver is absorbed it must not be placed on the face and close to the eyes, as toxic silver deposits can occur in ophthalmologic tissues.
- **Nocardiosis**
  - Trimethoprim-sulfamethoxazole can be used for infections due to Nocardia spp, but for serious infections, it must be combined with a second agent, (amikacin, imipenem, or linezolid).

- **Hyperkalemia:**
  - Trimethoprim is structurally similar to the potassium sparing diuretic, amiloride.

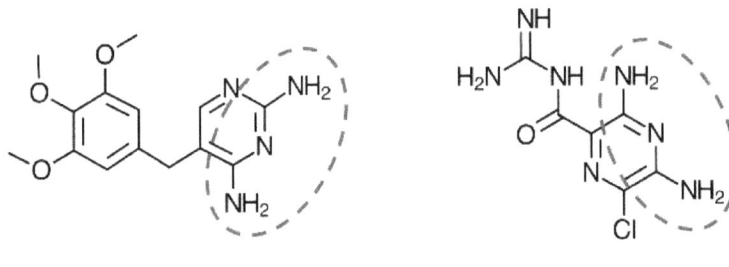

Trimethoprim   Amiloride

 HIGH-YIELD BOARD EXAM ESSENTIALS
- **CLASSIC AGENTS:** Sulfacetamide, sulfadiazine, sulfamethoxazole/trimethoprim
- **DRUG CLASS:** Sulfonamides
- **INDICATIONS:** PJP prophylaxis, toxoplasmosis, skin and soft tissue infections, urinary tract infections
- **MECHANISM:** Inhibit dihydropteroate synthase (sulfonamides). Inhibition of bacterial dihydrofolic acid reductase (trimethoprim)
- **SIDE EFFECTS:** Rash, hemolytic anemia, hepatic injury
- **CLINICAL PEARLS:**
  - Sulfonamides have numerous drug interactions by inhibition of CYP2C9 with common medications including warfarin, sulfonylureas, and phenytoin.
  - Sulfonamides may also displace drugs bound to albumin, increasing free-fraction drug concentrations, and potentially causing toxicities or adverse events.

Table: Drug Class Summary

Sulfonamides - Drug Class Review High-Yield Med Reviews			
Mechanism of Action: *Sulfonamides - Inhibit dihydropteroate synthase.* *Trimethoprim - Inhibition of bacterial dihydrofolic acid reductase*			
Class Effects: *Bacteriostatic as independent agents but can exert bactericidal in combination with other agents. Has some coverage against community-acquired MRSA (NOT nosocomial MRSA) and lacks strep coverage.*			
Generic Name	**Brand Name**	**Main Indication(s) or Uses**	**Notes**
Sulfacetamide	Bleph-10, Klaron, Ovace	<ul><li>Ophthalmic infections</li><li>Scaling dermatoses</li></ul>	<ul><li>**Dosing (Adult):**<ul><li>Ophthalmic application q2-4hours</li><li>Topical: apply to affected areas 1 to 3 times daily</li></ul></li><li>**Dosing (Peds):**<ul><li>Ophthalmic application q2-4hours</li><li>Topical: apply to affected areas 1 to 3 times daily</li></ul></li><li>**CYP450 Interactions:** None</li><li>**Renal or Hepatic Dose Adjustments:** None</li><li>**Dosage Forms:** Ophthalmic, Topical</li></ul>
Sulfadiazine	Lantrisul, Neotrizine, Sulfose, Terfonyl	<ul><li>Rheumatic fever prophylaxis</li><li>Toxoplasma gondii encephalitis</li></ul>	<ul><li>**Dosing (Adult):**<ul><li>Oral: 2 to 4 g/day in 3 to 6 divided doses</li></ul></li><li>**Dosing (Peds):**<ul><li>Oral: 25 to 50 mg/kg/dose q6-12h<ul><li>Maximum 6 g/day</li></ul></li></ul></li><li>**CYP450 Interactions:** Substrate CYP2C9, CYP2E1, CYP3A4</li><li>**Renal or Hepatic Dose Adjustments:** None</li><li>**Dosage Forms:** Oral (tablet)</li></ul>
Sulfamethoxazole / Trimethoprim	Bactrim	<ul><li>Toxoplasmosis</li><li>Skin and soft tissue infections</li><li>Urinary Tract Infections</li></ul>	<ul><li>**Dosing (Adult):**<ul><li>Oral: 1 to 2 SS or DS tablet q12-24h</li><li>IV: 8 to 20 mg/kg/day (trimethoprim) divided q6-12h</li></ul></li><li>**Dosing (Peds):**<ul><li>Oral: 5 to 12 mg/kg/day (trimethoprim) divided q12-24h</li><li>IV: 8 to 20 mg/kg/day (trimethoprim) divided q6-12h<ul><li>Maximum 320 mg/day of TMP</li></ul></li></ul></li><li>**CYP450 Interactions:** Substrate CYP2C9, CYP2E1, CYP3A4. Inhibits CYP2C9</li><li>**Renal or Hepatic Dose Adjustments:**<ul><li>GFR 15 to 30 mL/minute: Reduce dose by 50%</li><li>GFR < 15 mL/minute: reduce dose by 75%</li></ul></li><li>**Dosage Forms:** Oral (tablet, suspension), IV (solution)</li></ul>

INFECTIOUS DISEASE – TETRACYCLINES

Drug Class
- Tetracyclines
- Agents:
    - Acute & Chronic Care
        - Demeclocycline
        - Doxycycline
        - Eravacycline
        - Minocycline
        - Omadacycline
        - Sarecycline
        - Tetracycline
        - Tigecycline

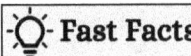 **Accelerate Your Knowledge**
- ✓ Tetracyclines are one of the treatments considered in emergency preparedness when exposure to biologic agents made to be weaponized has occurred (e.g., anthrax, plague).

Main Indications or Uses
- Acute & Chronic Care
    - Pneumonia
    - Rickettsial Infection
    - Plague
    - Brucellosis
    - Tularemia
    - Lyme disease
    - Bacillus anthracis (Anthrax)
    - Spirochetal infections
    - Skin and soft tissue infections
    - Urinary Tract Infections

Fast Facts
- ✓ Tigecycline is a derivative of minocycline and covers MRSA.

Mechanism of Action
- Bind to bacterial 30S ribosome, preventing access of tRNA to the acceptor site on the mRNA-ribosome complex ultimately inhibiting protein synthesis.

Primary Net Benefit
- Bacteriostatic antibiotics with activity against a wide range of aerobic and anaerobic gram-positive and gram-negative bacteria. Some agents extend coverage to MRSA.
- Main Labs to Monitor:
    - Cultures from infected sites at baseline (blood, sputum, urine, CSF etc.)

High-Yield Basic Pharmacology
- Bacterial cellular entry
    - Tetracyclines must enter the bacterial cell to exert their antimicrobial effect.
        - In gram-negative bacteria, this intracellular transport is accomplished by passive diffusion through channels formed by porins in the outer cell membrane and by active transport that pumps tetracyclines across the cytoplasmic membrane.
- Bacterial Resistance Mechanisms
    - There are three general mechanisms by which otherwise susceptible bacteria may develop resistance to tetracycline antibiotics including decreased antibiotic penetration into the ribosome or acquisition of an energy-dependent efflux pathway, displacement of the tetracycline from its target ribosomal site, and enzymatic inactivation.
- Cations
    - Concomitant oral administration of tetracyclines and di- or trivalent cations will impair absorption of both the antibiotic and the cation.
    - This interaction extends to food and dairy products high in di- and trivalent cations.

High-Yield Clinical Knowledge
- **Discoloration of Bony Structures and Teeth**
    - Tetracyclines may readily bind to calcium in newly formed bone or teeth in young children, or to fetal teeth if administered during pregnancy.
    - It must be noted, however, that the discoloration does not adversely affect bone function or growth, and the tooth discoloration is reversible.
        - Therefore, tetracyclines are not contraindicated in children but should be reserved for severe, potentially life-threatening infections, or when better alternatives are unavailable
- **Azithromycin Alternative**
    - For the treatment of community-acquired pneumonia, doxycycline may be used as an alternative to azithromycin for atypical pathogen coverage.
    - Doxycycline is now the preferred antibiotic compared to azithromycin for the treatment of sexually transmitted Chlamydial disease.
- **Photosensitivity**
    - Tetracyclines may cause photosensitivity in individuals exposed to sunlight during treatment.
    - Photosensitivity manifests in a range of symptoms from itching and burning sensations with mild erythemas, to erythematous plaques, blistering, lichenoid eruptions, and photoonycholysis.
- **Elevated ICP**
    - The tetracycline antibiotics have been historically linked on many board exams to causing idiopathic intracranial hypertension.

High-Yield Core Spectrum of Coverage
- **Core spectrum**
    - Gram-Positive
        - Streptococcus pneumoniae
        - Staphylococcus aureus, methicillin-sensitive & -resistant (MSSA & MRSA)
        - Listeria monocytogenes
    - Gram-Negative
        - Escherichia coli
        - Haemophilus influenzae
        - Klebsiella pneumoniae
        - Proteus mirabilis
        - Legionella sp
    - Atypical
        - Chlamydophila species
        - Mycoplasma pneumoniae
        - Rickettsia species
    - **Anaerobes**
        - Actinomyces
        - Bacteroides fragilis
        - Clostridium (not difficile)
        - Prevotella melaninogenica
        - Peptostreptococcus species
- **Core Indications**
    - Tetracyclines are commonly used as alternatives to azithromycin for empiric management of community-acquired pneumonia.
    - Tetracyclines also still play a role as first-line therapy for infections caused by rickettsiae, mycoplasmas, and chlamydiae.

High-Yield Fast-Facts
- **Demeclocycline for SIADH**
    - *Demeclocycline is rarely used as an antibacterial, but it has been used off-label in the treatment of inappropriate secretion of antidiuretic hormone because of its inhibition of antidiuretic hormone in the renal tubule*
- **Doxycycline dosage forms**
    - Doxycycline has numerous different salts including hyclate, monohydrate, and calcium salts. However, when consulting drug references, the doxycycline dose is almost always expressed as a doxycycline base.
- **Doxycycline Stockpile**
    - Doxycycline is a component of the US Strategic National Stockpile to be used for the prevention or treatment of anthrax exposures. For this indication, the dose is a conventional 100 mg q12h but should be taken for up to 60 days.

HIGH-YIELD BOARD EXAM ESSENTIALS
- **CLASSIC AGENTS:** Demeclocycline, doxycycline, eravacycline, minocycline, omadacycline, sarecycline, tetracycline, tigecycline
- **DRUG CLASS:** Tetracyclines
- **INDICATIONS:** Acne vulgaris, anthrax, Bartonella infection, Brucellosis, Lyme disease, pneumonia, Q-fever, Rocky Mountain Spotted Fever, sexually transmitted disease, skin and soft tissue infections, tularemia, urinary tract infections
- **MECHANISM:** Bind to bacterial 30S ribosome, preventing access of tRNA to the acceptor site on the mRNA-ribosome complex ultimately inhibiting protein synthesis.
- **SIDE EFFECTS:** Photosensitivity, bone/teeth discoloration
- **CLINICAL PEARLS:**
    - Tetracyclines may readily bind to calcium in newly formed bone or teeth in young children, or to fetal teeth if administered during pregnancy. It must be noted, however, that the discoloration does not adversely affect bone function or growth, and the tooth discoloration is reversible. Regardless, for board exams this is why they are generally contraindicated.
    - Due to the risk of chelation with di- or tri-valent cations, it is advised that dose of antibiotic be separated from cations by 2-4 hours to avoid decreases in bioavailability.
    - Tetracycline antibiotics (along with some of the aminoglycosides) are known to be used in various biological substances used in biological warfare. As such, these are treatments within emergency preparedness.

Table: Drug Class Summary

Tetracyclines - Drug Class Review High-Yield Med Reviews			
Mechanism of Action: *Bind to bacterial 30S ribosome, preventing access of tRNA to the acceptor site on the mRNA-ribosome complex ultimately inhibiting protein synthesis.*			
Class Effects: *Bacteriostatic antibiotics with activity against a wide range of aerobic and anaerobic gram-positive and gram-negative bacteria. Avoid in pregnancy and pediatric patients < 8 years of age.*			
Generic Name	**Brand Name**	**Main Indication(s) or Uses**	**Notes**
Demeclocycline	Declomycin, Declostatin, Ledermycin, Bioterciclin, Deganol, Deteclo	• SIADH	• **Dosing (Adult):** — Oral: 600 to 1200 mg/day • **Dosing (Peds > 8 yrs or age):** — Oral: 7 to 13 mg/kg/day q6-12h — Maximum 600 mg/day • **CYP450 Interactions:** None • **Renal or Hepatic Dose Adjustments:** None • **Dosage Forms:** Oral (tablet)
Doxycycline	Vibramycin	• Acne vulgaris • Anthrax • Bartonella infection • Brucellosis • Lyme disease • Pneumonia • Q-fever • Rocky Mountain Spotted Fever • Sexually transmitted disease • Skin and soft tissue infections • Tularemia • Urinary Tract Infections	• **Dosing (Adult):** — Oral/IV: 100 mg BID • **Dosing (Peds > 8 yrs of age):** — Oral/IV: 2.2 mg/kg/dose q12h — Maximum 100 mg/dose • **CYP450 Interactions:** None • **Renal or Hepatic Dose Adjustments:** None • **Dosage Forms:** Oral (capsule, tablet, suspension, syrup), IV (solution)
Eravacycline	Xerava	• Intra-abdominal infections	• **Dosing (Adult):** — IV: 1 mg/kg q12h • **Dosing (Peds):** — None • **CYP450 Interactions:** — Substrate CYP3A4 • **Renal or Hepatic Dose Adjustments:** — Child-Pugh class C, 1 mg/kg q12h x 1, then 1 mg/kg q24h • **Dosage Forms:** IV (solution)

Tetracyclines - Drug Class Review
High-Yield Med Reviews

Generic Name	Brand Name	Main Indication(s) or Uses	Notes

Minocycline	Minocin	- Acne vulgaris
		- Skin and soft tissue infections
		- Syphilis
			- **Dosing (Adult):**
			  - Oral/IV: 200 mg once, then 100 mg BID
			- **Dosing (Peds):**
			  - Oral/IV: 4mg/kg once, then 2 mg/kg/dose q12h
			    - Maximum 400 mg/day
			- **CYP450 Interactions:** None
			- **Renal or Hepatic Dose Adjustments:**
			  - GFR < 80 mL/minute maximum of 200 mg/day
			- **Dosage Forms:** Oral (capsule, tablet), IV (solution)

Omadacycline	Nuzyra	- Pneumonia
		- Skin and soft tissue infections
		- Tularemia
		- Urinary Tract Infections
			- **Dosing (Adult):**
			  - Oral: 300 mg daily
			  - IV: 200 mg once, then 100 mg daily
			- **Dosing (Peds):**
			  - Not routinely used
			- **CYP450 Interactions:** P-gp substrate
			- **Renal or Hepatic Dose Adjustments:** None
			- **Dosage Forms:** Oral (tablet), IV (solution)

Sarecycline	Seysara	- Acne vulgaris	- **Dosing (Adult):**
			  - Oral: 60 to 150 mg daily (weight based)
			    - 33 to 54 kg, 60 mg daily
			    - 55 to 84 kg, 100 mg daily
			    - 85 to 136 kg, 150 mg daily
			- **Dosing (Peds):**
			  - For children 9 and older, use weight-based dosing
			- **CYP450 Interactions:** None
			- **Renal or Hepatic Dose Adjustments:** None
			- **Dosage Forms:** Oral (tablet)

Tetracycline	Sumycin	- Acne vulgaris
		- Helicobacter pylori
		- Syphilis
		- Tularemia
		- Vibrio cholerae
			- **Dosing (Adult):**
			  - Oral: 250 to 500 mg q6-12h
			- **Dosing (Peds):**
			  - Oral/IV: 25 to 50 mg/kg/day divided q6h
			    - Maximum 250 to 500 mg/dose
			- **CYP450 Interactions:** Substrate of CYP 3A4
			- **Renal or Hepatic Dose Adjustments:**
			  - GFR 10 to 50 mL/minute - increase frequency to q8-12h)
			  - GFR < 10 mL/minute - increase frequency to q24h
			- **Dosage Forms:** Oral (capsule)

Tetracyclines - Drug Class Review
High-Yield Med Reviews

Generic Name	Brand Name	Main Indication(s) or Uses	Notes
Tigecycline	Tygacil	<ul><li>Pneumonia</li><li>Intraabdominal infections</li><li>Skin and soft tissue infections</li></ul>	<ul><li>**Dosing (Adult):** − IV: 100 mg once followed by 50 mg q12h</li><li>**Dosing (Peds):** − IV: 1.5 to 3mg/kg once then 1 to 2 mg/kg/dose q12h 　− Maximum 100 mg/dose (load) or 50 mg/dose (maintenance)</li><li>**CYP450 Interactions:** None</li><li>**Renal or Hepatic Dose Adjustments:** − Child-Pugh class C, 100 mg once then 25 mg q12h</li><li>**Dosage Forms:** IV (solution)</li></ul>

INFECTIOUS DISEASE – AMPHOTERICIN B

Drug Class
- **Amphotericin B**
- **Agents:**
    - **Acute & Chronic Care**
        - Amphotericin B (conventional)
        - Amphotericin B (lipid complex)
        - Amphotericin B (liposomal)

> 💉 **Dosing Pearl**
> ✓ Conventional amphotericin formulation is NOT interchangeable with lipid-based formulations and thus have different doses.

Main Indications or Uses
- **Acute Care**
    - Cryptococcal meningitis
    - Fungal infections
    - Leishmaniasis

Mechanism of Action
- Amphotericin B binds to fungal cell membrane ergosterol altering the membrane permeability and leading to leakage of cell components and subsequent fungal cell death.

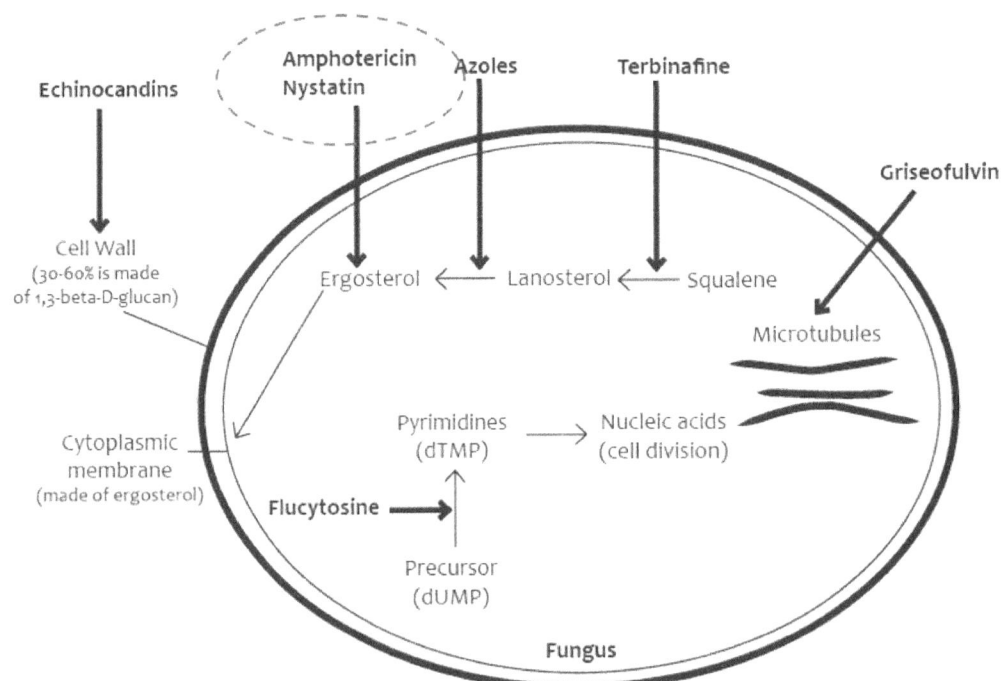

Primary Net Benefit
- Fungicidal agents are used for invasive fungal infections with the broadest spectrum of activity of available antifungal drugs, despite significant toxicity.
- Main Labs to Monitor:
    - Cultures from infected sites at baseline (blood, sputum, urine, CSF, etc.)
    - Renal function (serum creatinine, urine output), potential loss of electrolytes from kidneys (K+; Mg++)

High-Yield Basic Pharmacology
- **Lipid Delivery Vehicles**
    - Amphotericin B's two available formulations exist as lipid delivery vehicles (lipid complex and liposome), which reduce nephrotoxicity while preserving efficacy.

- When converting between conventional and lipid amphotericin B formulations, doses are not generalizable, and close attention should be made to avoid over/underdosing.
- **Lipid Physical Form**
  - The specific physical form of the lipid of amphotericin B can impact the volume of distribution and penetration into specific tissues such as the CNS or lung.
    - Amphotericin B (lipid complex) exists in a ribbon lipid formulation, which may increase penetration through the blood-brain barrier.
      - The spherical form of amphotericin (liposomal) may limit CNS penetration given the relatively larger spherical size and ability to pass the blood-brain barrier.
- **Conventional Dosing in Obesity**
  - For each amphotericin formulation, dosing in obesity follows different strategies:
    - Conventional amphotericin B should use adjusted body weight (IBW+[0.4(ABW-IBW)]
      - A maximum dosing weight of 100 kg has also been suggested.
    - Amphotericin B (liposomal or lipid complex) may use adjusted body weight, but a maximum dosing weight of 100 kg has also been suggested.

High-Yield Clinical Knowledge
- **Infusion-Related Reactions**
  - Amphotericin B infusion-related reactions are frequent and may manifest as fever, chills, muscle spasms, vomiting, headache, and hypotension.
  - Methods to limit these reactions include premedication with antipyretics, antihistamines, or corticosteroids and slowing the infusion rate or decreasing the dose.
- **Resistance**
  - Fungi may develop resistance to amphotericin B by altering its binding to the ergosterol site via decreased membrane ergosterol concentration or modifying the sterol target molecule.
- **Dose Adjustments**
  - No dose adjustments are recommended according to the prescribing information for patients with hepatic and/or renal impairment.
- **Cumulative Toxicity**
  - Although renal impairment may occur early in therapy, renal function may stabilize during therapy or progress to require dialysis.
    - The general mechanisms of nephrotoxicity include a reversible, pre-renal component, which is associated with decreased renal perfusion, and an irreversible, intrinsic renal tubular injury/renal tubular acidosis.

High-Yield Core Spectrum of Coverage
- **Core spectrum**
  - Candida albicans
  - Cryptococcus neoformans
  - Histoplasma capsulatum
  - Blastomyces dermatitidis
  - Coccidioides immitis
  - Aspergillus fumigatus
- **Core Indications**
  - Although a broad-spectrum antifungal, Amphotericin B has specific uses and indications because of the availability of safer alternatives for invasive fungal infections.
  - Cryptococcus meningitis, Leishmaniasis, and other resistant fungal infections are where amphotericin B is still widely used.

High-Yield Fast-Facts
- **Amphotericin A**
  - There once existed amphotericin A; however, it is not used clinically but was developed before the widespread use of amphotericin B.

- **Alternative Amphotericin B Routes**
  - Administration of amphotericin B may occur in other routes than just intravenously. These routes include topical ophthalmic administration, direct subconjunctival injections, bladder irrigation, or injection into joint spaces.
- **In-line IV Filter**
  - For the conventional amphotericin B, since it is insoluble in water and forms a colloid in water, a 0.5 micron or larger in-line filter should be used during infusion.
  - However, smaller filters (such as the commonly used 0.22-micron filter) will remove significant amounts of the drug and must be avoided.

HIGH-YIELD BOARD EXAM ESSENTIALS
- **CLASSIC AGENTS:** Amphotericin B (conventional, lipid complex, liposomal)
- **DRUG CLASS:** Antifungal
- **INDICATIONS:** Cryptococcal meningitis, fungal infections, leishmaniasis
- **MECHANISM:** Binds to fungal ergosterol leading to leakage of cell components and subsequent fungal cell death.
- **SIDE EFFECTS:** Acute kidney injury, infusion reactions (fever, chills, muscle spasms, vomiting, headache, and hypotension)
- **CLINICAL PEARLS:**
  - Although renal impairment may occur early in therapy, renal function may stabilize during therapy or progress to require dialysis. If the patient can tolerate, giving a small 250-500 mL bolus of fluid or using one of the non-conventional formulations of amphotericin B can facilitate removal from the kidneys and help reduce the risk.

Table: Drug Class Summary

	**Amphotericin B - Drug Class Review** High-Yield Med Reviews
	**Mechanism of Action:** *Binds to fungal ergosterol leading to leakage of cell components and subsequent fungal cell death.*
	**Class Effects:** *Fungicidal agents used for invasive fungal infections with the broadest spectrum of activity of available antifungal drugs, despite significant toxicity. Risk of nephrotoxicity especially with conventional amphotericin B.*
Generic Name	**Brand Name**	**Indication(s) or Uses**	**Notes**
Amphotericin B (conventional)	Fungizone IV	<ul><li>Fungal infections</li><li>Leishmaniasis</li></ul>	<ul><li>**Dosing (Adult):**<ul><li>IV: 0.3 to 1.5 mg/kg/day<ul><li>Typical range 0.3 to 0.7 mg/kg/day</li></ul></li></ul></li><li>**Dosing (Peds):**<ul><li>IV: 0.25 to 1 mg/kg/dose q24h</li></ul></li><li>**CYP450 Interactions:** None</li><li>**Renal or Hepatic Dose Adjustments:**<ul><li>Decrease dose by 50% or administer q48h if nephrotoxicity occurs.</li></ul></li><li>**Dosage Forms:** IV (solution)</li></ul>
Amphotericin B (lipid complex)	Abelcet	<ul><li>Cryptococcal meningitis</li><li>Fungal infections</li></ul>	<ul><li>**Dosing (Adult):**<ul><li>IV: 3 to 5 mg/kg/dose q24h</li></ul></li><li>**Dosing (Peds):**<ul><li>IV: 3 to 5 mg/kg/dose q24h</li></ul></li><li>**CYP450 Interactions:** None</li><li>**Renal or Hepatic Dose Adjustments:** None</li><li>**Dosage Forms:** IV (suspension)</li></ul>
Amphotericin B (liposomal)	AmBisome	<ul><li>Cryptococcal meningitis</li><li>Fungal infections</li></ul>	<ul><li>**Dosing (Adult):**<ul><li>IV: 3 to 6 mg/kg/dose q24h</li></ul></li><li>**Dosing (Peds):**<ul><li>IV: 3 to 6 mg/kg/dose q24h</li></ul></li><li>**CYP450 Interactions:** None</li><li>**Renal or Hepatic Dose Adjustments:** None</li><li>**Dosage Forms:** IV (suspension)</li></ul>

INFECTIOUS DISEASE – ANTIFUNGAL - AZOLE (SYSTEMIC TRIAZOLE)

Drug Class
- Systemic Azole Antifungal (Triazole)
- Agents:
    - Acute & Chronic Care
        - Fluconazole
        - Isavuconazole
        - Itraconazole
        - Posaconazole
        - Terconazole
        - Voriconazole

Main Indications or Uses
- Acute Care
    - Isavuconazole, Posaconazole, Voriconazole
        - Aspergillosis
        - Candidiasis
        - Mucormycosis
    - Itraconazole
        - Aspergillosis
        - Histoplasmosis
        - Mucormycosis
        - Onychomycosis
    - Terconazole
        - Vulvovaginal Candidiasis
    - Fluconazole
        - Blastomycosis
        - Candida intertrigo
        - Candidiasis (therapy or prophylaxis)
        - Coccidioidomycosis
        - Cryptococcosis
        - Tinea

Mechanism of Action
- Inhibit fungal CYP enzyme 14-α-sterol demethylase, which disrupts fungal ergosterol's biosynthesis, causing the accumulation of the toxic product 14α-methyl-3,6-diol, leading to fungal growth arrest.

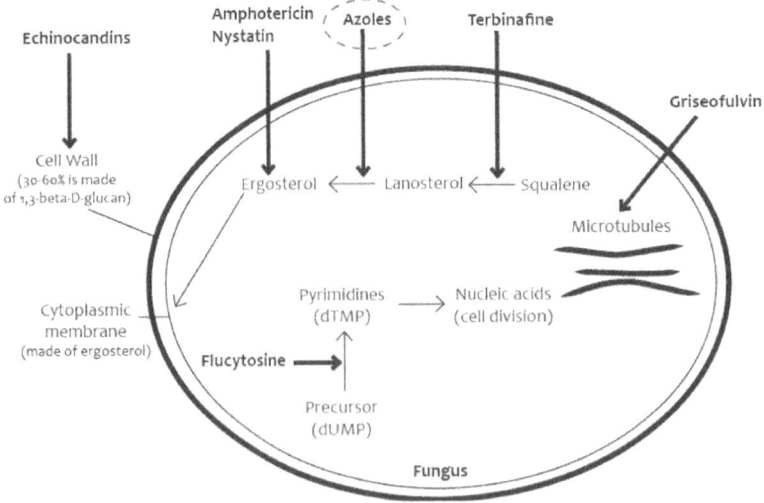

Infectious Diseases

Primary Net Benefit
- Broad-spectrum antifungal agents with limited adverse reactions but clinically relevant drug interactions.
- Main Labs to Monitor:
    - Cultures from infected sites at baseline (blood, sputum, urine, CSF, etc.)
    - Renal function (serum creatinine, urine output)
    - Liver enzyme and liver function tests

High-Yield Basic Pharmacology
- **Alternative MOAs**
    - In addition to their primary mechanism, Azole antifungal agents may disrupt phospholipid packing of acyl chains, impairing the function of membrane-bound enzyme systems and increasing the permeability of the fungal cell membrane.
- **Spectrum**
    - The azole antifungals are a broad-spectrum antifungal group with activity against Candida albicans, C. tropicalis, C. parapsilosis, C. neoformans, Blastomyces dermatitidis, Histoplasma capsulatum, Coccidioides spp., Paracoccidioides brasiliensis, and ringworm fungi.
        - Isavuconazole, posaconazole, and voriconazole are also active against Aspergillus species.
- **Resistance**
    - Resistance to azole antifungals is emerging among C. albicans isolates, with the primary mechanism of resistance being mutations of the gene encoding the azole target fungal binding site.
        - Other resistance mechanisms that have been described include increased azole export and decreased ergosterol content.

High-Yield Clinical Knowledge
- **Drug Interactions**
    - Although the azoles are well tolerated, there are numerous clinically relevant drug interactions as these agents are inhibitors of CYP2D6, 2C9, 2C19, 3A4, 3A5, AND 3A7.
    - The clinical effect of these interactions may be a) decreased azole antifungal effect (CYP inducers), b) increased azole exposure/toxicity (CYP inhibitors), or c) increased drug concentrations (CYP substrates).
        - Notable interactions include decreased elimination of carbamazepine, cyclosporine, digoxin, dofetilide, eplerenone, sulfonylureas, haloperidol, statins, methadone, midazolam, omeprazole, phenytoin, risperidone, HIV protease inhibitors, sildenafil, tacrolimus, and warfarin.
    - Fluconazole is associated with the fewest clinically relevant interactions as it has the least effect of all the azoles on hepatic CYP450 enzymes.
- **Itraconazole Acidic Absorption**
    - The absorption of itraconazole is dependent on gastric pH, with more acidic environments facilitating appropriate absorption.
    - Due to reduced bioavailability, clinical failure may occur when GI pH becomes more alkaline with PPI, H2RA, or antacid treatment.
    - There is also dosage form specific administration instructions:
        - Capsule and tablet absorption are best if taken with food.
        - The oral solution should be taken on an empty stomach.
            - To enhance absorption when coadministration of gastric pH increasing drugs is necessary, administration of itraconazole with cola may facilitate absorption.
- **Voriconazole Visual Disturbance**
    - A common adverse event (up to 30% of patients) that patients must be counseled regarding is the associated visual disturbances that include blurring and color vision changes or brightness.
        - These visual changes can occur immediately after a dose of voriconazole but typically resolve within 30 minutes.
- **Hepatotoxicity**
    - Azole antifungal agents have been associated with hepatotoxicity in rare circumstances.

High-Yield Core Spectrum of Coverage
- **Core spectrum**
  - Aspergillus fumigatus
  - Blastomyces dermatitidis
  - Candida species
  - Coccidioides immitis
  - Cryptococcus neoformans
  - Histoplasma capsulatum
  - Paracoccidioides brasiliensis
  - Scedosporium apiospermum
- **Core Indications**
  - It is a relatively non-toxic, broad-spectrum, including many Candida, C neoformans, the endemic mycoses, and dermatophytes.
  - Specific agents (itraconazole, posaconazole, isavuconazole, and voriconazole) possess antifungal activity against Aspergillus species.
  - Otherwise, well-tolerated but associated with clinically relevant drug interactions and rare incidence of clinical hepatitis.

High-Yield Fast-Facts
- **Hyperaldosteronism**
  - Posaconazole, once only available as an oral liquid but now as an oral capsule, is rarely associated with hyperaldosteronism, potentially leading to clinically relevant hypertension and hypokalemia.
- **QT Prolongation**
  - Some of the azole antifungal agents (posaconazole, voriconazole) can prolong the QTc interval or cause inhibition of the metabolism of other QTc prolonging drugs increasing the risk of Torsade de Pointes.
- **Fluconazole in Pregnancy**
  - According to many drug references, fluconazole should be avoided in pregnancy, with an increase in tetralogy of Fallot in babies born to mothers who received fluconazole.

HIGH-YIELD BOARD EXAM ESSENTIALS
- **CLASSIC AGENTS:** Fluconazole, isavuconazole, itraconazole, posaconazole, terconazole, voriconazole
- **DRUG CLASS:** Azole antifungals
- **INDICATIONS:** Fungal infections
- **MECHANISM:** Inhibit fungal CYP enzyme disrupting the biosynthesis of fungal ergosterol and fungal growth arrest.
- **SIDE EFFECTS:** Visual disturbance (voriconazole), QT prolongation (posaconazole, voriconazole), hepatotoxicity
- **CLINICAL PEARLS:**
  - Although the azoles are well tolerated, there are numerous clinically relevant drug interactions as these agents are inhibitors of CYP2D6, 2C9, 2C19, 3A4, 3A5, AND 3A7. The clinical effect of these interactions may be a) decreased azole antifungal effect (CYP inducers), b) increased azole exposure/toxicity (CYP inhibitors), or c) increased drug concentrations (CYP substrates).
  - Itraconazole capsules (not the solution) requires an acidic gastric environment for adequate absorption. Thus, avoid use of antacids while taking itraconazole capsules.

Table: Drug Class Summary

| \multicolumn{4}{c}{**Azole - Drug Class Review**} |
|||||

Azole - Drug Class Review			
High-Yield Med Reviews			
Mechanism of Action: *Inhibit fungal CYP enzyme disrupting fungal ergosterol biosynthesis and fungal growth arrest.*			
Class Effects: *Broad-spectrum antifungal agents with limited adverse reactions but clinically relevant drug interactions.*			
Generic Name	**Brand Name**	**Main Indication(s) or Uses**	**Notes**
Fluconazole	Diflucan	<ul><li>Blastomycosis</li><li>Candida intertrigo</li><li>Candidiasis (therapy or prophylaxis)</li><li>Coccidioidomycosis</li><li>Cryptococcosis</li><li>Tinea</li></ul>	<ul><li>**Dosing (Adult):**<ul><li>Oral: 50 to 200 mg q12-24h</li><li>IV: 100 to 800 mg q24h<ul><li>Extra info if needed</li></ul></li></ul></li><li>**Dosing (Peds):**<ul><li>IV/Oral: LD 6 to 12 mg/kg/dose, then 3 to 12 mg/kg/dose q24h</li><li>Maximum 600 mg/dose</li></ul></li><li>**CYP450 Interactions:** Inhibitor CYP2C9, CYP2C19, CYP3A4</li><li>**Renal or Hepatic Dose Adjustments:**<ul><li>GFR < 50 mL/minute: Reduce dose by 50%</li></ul></li><li>**Dosage Forms:** Oral (tablet, suspension), IV (solution)</li></ul>
Isavuconazole	Cresemba	<ul><li>Aspergillosis</li><li>Mucormycosis</li></ul>	<ul><li>**Dosing (Adult):**<ul><li>IV/Oral: 372 mg q8h x 6 doses, then 372 mg q24h</li></ul></li><li>**Dosing (Peds):** Not routinely used</li><li>**CYP450 Interactions:** Substrate and inhibits CYP3A4</li><li>**Renal or Hepatic Dose Adjustments:** None</li><li>**Dosage Forms:** IV (solution), Oral (capsule)</li></ul>
Itraconazole	Sporanox	<ul><li>Aspergillosis</li><li>Histoplasmosis</li><li>Mucormycosis</li><li>Onychomycosis</li></ul>	<ul><li>**Dosing (Adult):** Oral dosage forms not interchangeable<ul><li>Oral: (100 mg capsule or solution) 200 mg q8-12h</li><li>Oral: (65 mg capsule) 130 to 260 mg q24h</li></ul></li><li>**Dosing (Peds):**<ul><li>Oral: (solution) 2.5 to 5 mg/kg/dose twice daily</li><li>Maximum 400 mg/day</li></ul></li><li>**CYP450 Interactions:** Substrate and inhibits CYP3A4, P-gp</li><li>**Renal or Hepatic Dose Adjustments:** None</li><li>**Dosage Forms:** Oral (capsule, solution)</li></ul>

Azole - Drug Class Review High-Yield Med Reviews			
Generic Name	**Brand Name**	**Main Indication(s) or Uses**	**Notes**
Posaconazole	Noxafil	<ul><li>Aspergillosis</li><li>Candidiasis</li><li>Mucormycosis</li></ul>	<ul><li>**Dosing (Adult):**<ul><li>IV/Oral: tablet 300 mg q12h x 2 doses, then 300 mg q24h</li><li>Oral: suspension 200 mg q8h, or 400 mg q12h</li></ul></li><li>**Dosing (Peds):**<ul><li>Oral 4 to 7 mg/kg/dose q8-12h<ul><li>Maximum 400 mg/dose</li></ul></li></ul></li><li>**CYP450 Interactions:** Inhibits CYP3A4</li><li>**Renal or Hepatic Dose Adjustments:**<ul><li>IV form - GFR less than 50 mL/minute: avoid use (cyclodextrin accumulation)</li></ul></li><li>**Dosage Forms:** Oral (tablet, suspension), IV (solution)</li></ul>
Terconazole	Terazol, Zazole	<ul><li>Vulvovaginal candidiasis</li></ul>	<ul><li>**Dosing (Adult):**<ul><li>Intravaginal 1 applicatorful q24h for 3-7 days</li></ul></li><li>**Dosing (Peds):** Not routinely used</li><li>**CYP450 Interactions:** Topical dosage form - none (not absorbed systemically)</li><li>**Renal or Hepatic Dose Adjustments:** None</li><li>**Dosage Forms:** Topical (vaginal cream/suppository)</li></ul>
Voriconazole	Vfend	<ul><li>Aspergillosis</li><li>Candidiasis</li><li>Histoplasmosis</li><li>Mucormycosis</li><li>Onychomycosis</li></ul>	<ul><li>**Dosing (Adult):**<ul><li>Oral: 200 to 400 mg q12h</li><li>IV: 6 mg/kg q12h x 2 doses, then 4 mg/kg q12h</li></ul></li><li>**Dosing (Peds):**<ul><li>IV/Oral: 6 to 9 mg/kg/dose q12h<ul><li>Maximum 200 mg/dose</li></ul></li></ul></li><li>**CYP450 Interactions:** Substrate and inhibits CYP 2C9, 2C19, 3A4</li><li>**Renal or Hepatic Dose Adjustments:**<ul><li>Child-Pugh class A or B - Reduce maintenance dose by 50%</li></ul></li><li>**Dosage Forms:** IV (solution), Oral (tablet, solution)</li></ul>

INFECTIOUS DISEASE – AZOLE (TOPICAL IMIDAZOLES)

Drug Class
- Azole (Imidazole)
- Agents:
  - Acute & Chronic Care
    - Butoconazole
    - Clotrimazole
    - Econazole
    - Ketoconazole
    - Luliconazole
    - Miconazole
    - Oxiconazole
    - Sertaconazole
    - Sulconazole
    - Tioconazole

> **Fast Facts**
> ✓ Ketoconazole shampoo, cream, foam, and gel are uniquely indicated for seborrheic dermatitis.

Main Indications or Uses
- Acute Care
  - Topical treatment: Candida albicans, Malassezia furfur, tinea pedis, tinea cruris, and tinea corporis

Mechanism of Action
- Inhibit fungal CYP enzyme 14-α-sterol demethylase, which disrupts fungal ergosterol's biosynthesis, causing the accumulation of the toxic product 14α-methyl-3,6-diol, leading to fungal growth arrest.

Primary Net Benefit
- Broad-spectrum antifungal agents with limited adverse reactions limited to topical management of fungal infections.
- Main Labs to Monitor:
  - No routine monitoring

High-Yield Basic Pharmacology
- **Ketoconazole Oral Use**
  - Ketoconazole is rarely used orally as an antifungal agent but can still be used to manage Cushing syndrome.
    - Ketoconazole inhibits several steps in the synthesis of aldosterone, cortisol, and testosterone.
      - The inhibition of testosterone is linked to the characteristic adverse reaction of gynecomastia.
- **Oral Clotrimazole**
  - Clotrimazole is available as a product known as a troche (essentially a lozenge) that patients should be directed to allow to slowly dissolve in their mouth, which typically takes approximately 30 minutes.

High-Yield Clinical Knowledge
- **No Prescription Required**
  - Topical azole antifungals are widely available as over-the-counter products under various brand names of clotrimazole or miconazole.
- **Absorption of Topicals**
  - The topical azole antifungals can inhibit CYP450, but they are not systemically absorbed (with normal clinical use) and should not produce clinically relevant drug interactions.
- **Preferred Formulations**
  - Topical antifungal agents for cutaneous infections should be in the form of creams or solutions, as ointments are occlusive to the skin, worsening skin integrity.

- Although convenient, antifungal powders should be reserved for lesions of the feet, groin, and similar intertriginous areas.

High-Yield Core Spectrum of Coverage
- **Core spectrum**
  - Candida species
  - Dermatophytosis (ringworm)
  - Tinea versicolor, piedra, nigra
- **Core Indications**
  - Broad-spectrum, topical antifungal agents are otherwise well-tolerated but associated with local skin reactions.

High-Yield Fast-Fact
- **Pregnancy**
  - The topical antifungal agents are minimally absorbed but for use in pregnant patients.
  - However, rodent models have suggested teratogenicity, and no adverse effects on the human fetus have been attributed to the vaginal use of imidazoles or triazoles.
- **Partner Irritation**
  - During topical vaginal azole antifungal therapies, male sexual partners of the patient may experience mild penile irritation.
- **Look-Alike-Sound-Alike**
  - Although convenient for studying, the antifungal agents' generic names are very similar, prompting many to be considered high-risk for medication errors and employ tall-man lettering to highlight differences.
  - Another potential substitution error is with metronidazole, an antibiotic, but with a similar suffix to many azole antifungals.

HIGH-YIELD BOARD EXAM ESSENTIALS
- **CLASSIC AGENTS:** Butoconazole, clotrimazole, econazole ketoconazole, luliconazole, miconazole, oxiconazole, sertaconazole, sulconazole, tioconazole
- **DRUG CLASS:** Topical azole antifungal
- **INDICATIONS:** Topical treatment of Candida albicans, Malassezia furfur, tinea pedis, tinea cruris, and tinea corporis
- **MECHANISM:** Inhibit fungal CYP enzyme 14-alpha-sterol demethylase, which disrupts fungal ergosterol's biosynthesis, causing the accumulation of the toxic product 14-alpha-methyl-3,6-diol, leading to fungal growth arrest.
- **SIDE EFFECTS:** Skin irritation
- **CLINICAL PEARLS:** The topical azole antifungals can inhibit CYP450, but they are not systemically absorbed (with normal clinical use) and should not produce clinically relevant drug interactions.

Infectious Diseases

Table: Drug Class Summary

| | Azole Topical (Imidazole) - Drug Class Review
High-Yield Med Reviews |

Mechanism of Action: *Inhibit fungal CYP enzyme disrupting the biosynthesis of fungal ergosterol and fungal growth arrest.*

Class Effects: *Broad-spectrum antifungal agents with limited adverse reactions limited to topical management of fungal infections.*

Generic Name	Brand Name	Main Indication(s) or Uses	Notes
Butoconazole	Gynazole-1	• Vulvovaginal candidiasis	• **Dosing (Adult):** — Intravaginal 1 applicatorful (5 g) once • **Dosing (Peds):** Not routinely used • **CYP450 Interactions:** None (not absorbed systemically) • **Renal or Hepatic Dose Adjustments:** None • **Dosage Forms:** Vaginal cream
Clotrimazole	Alevazol, Clotrimazole 3 Day, Desenex, Gyne-Lotrimin 3, Lotrimin AF, Pro-Ex Antifungal	• Topical treatment of candidiasis, tinea pedis, tinea cruris, and tinea corporis	• **Dosing (Adult):** — Topical: to affected area twice daily • **Dosing (Peds):** — Topical: to affected area twice daily • **CYP450 Interactions:** None (not absorbed systemically) • **Renal or Hepatic Dose Adjustments:** None • **Dosage Forms:** Topical (cream, vaginal cream, ointment, solution)
Econazole	Econasil, Ecoza, Zolpak	• Topical treatment of candidiasis, tinea pedis, tinea cruris, and tinea corporis	• **Dosing (Adult):** — Topical: to affected area twice daily • **Dosing (Peds):** — Topical: to affected area twice daily • **CYP450 Interactions:** None (not absorbed systemically) • **Renal or Hepatic Dose Adjustments:** None • **Dosage Forms:** Topical (cream, foam, solution)
Ketoconazole	Extina, Ketodan, Nizoral, Xolegel	• Topical treatment of candidiasis, tinea pedis, tinea cruris, and tinea corporis	• **Dosing (Adult):** — Topical: application q12-24h • **Dosing (Peds):** — Topical: application q12-24h • **CYP450 Interactions:** Topical dosage form - none (not absorbed systemically) • **Renal or Hepatic Dose Adjustments:** None • **Dosage Forms:** Topical (cream, foam, gel, shampoo)

Azole Topical (Imidazole) - Drug Class Review High-Yield Med Reviews			
Generic Name	**Brand Name**	**Main Indication(s) or Uses**	**Notes**

Luliconazole	Luzu	- Topical treatment of tinea pedis, tinea cruris, and tinea corporis]	- **Dosing (Adult):**
			  − Topical: to affected area daily
			- **Dosing (Peds):**
			  − Topical: to affected area daily
			- **CYP450 Interactions:** Inhibits CYP2C9 (systemic absorption minimal)
			- **Renal or Hepatic Dose Adjustments:** None
			- **Dosage Forms:** Topica (cream)

Miconazole	Desenex Lotrimin AF Micaderm Micatin Vagistat	- Topical treatment of candidiasis, tinea pedis, tinea cruris, and tinea corporis	- **Dosing (Adult):**
			  − Topical: to affected area twice daily
			- **Dosing (Peds):**
			  − Topical: to affected area twice daily
			- **CYP450 Interactions:** Topical dosage form - none (not absorbed systemically)
			- **Renal or Hepatic Dose Adjustments:** None
			- **Dosage Forms:** Topica (aerosol, cream, vaginal cream, ointment, powder, solution, vaginal suppository)

Oxiconazole	Oxistat	- Topical treatment of tinea pedis, tinea cruris, and tinea corporis	- **Dosing (Adult):**
			  − Topical: to affected area q12-24h
			- **Dosing (Peds):**
			  − Topical: to affected area q12-24h
			- **CYP450 Interactions:** Topical dosage form - none (not absorbed systemically)
			- **Renal or Hepatic Dose Adjustments:** None
			- **Dosage Forms:** Topical (cream, lotion)

Sertaconazole	Ertaczo	- Topical treatment of tinea pedis, tinea cruris, and tinea corporis	- **Dosing (Adult):**
			  − Topical: to affected area q12h
			- **Dosing (Peds):**
			  − Topical: to affected area q12
			- **CYP450 Interactions:** Topical dosage form - none (not absorbed systemically)
			- **Renal or Hepatic Dose Adjustments:** None
			- **Dosage Forms:** Topical (cream)

Sulconazole	Exelderm	- Topical treatment of tinea pedis, tinea cruris, and tinea corporis	- **Dosing (Adult):** − Topical: to affected area q12-24h - **Dosing (Peds):** Not routinely used - **CYP450 Interactions:** Topical dosage form - none (not absorbed systemically) - **Renal or Hepatic Dose Adjustments:** None - **Dosage Forms:** Topical (cream, solution)

| Azole Topical (Imidazole) - Drug Class Review ||||
| High-Yield Med Reviews ||||
Generic Name	Brand Name	Main Indication(s) or Uses	Notes

Tioconazole	Vagistat-1	• Vulvovaginal candidiasis	• **Dosing (Adult):**
			  − Intravaginal 1 applicatorful q24h for 3-7 days
			• **Dosing (Peds):**
			  − Intravaginal 1 applicatorful q24h for 3-7 days
			• **CYP450 Interactions:** Topical dosage form - none (not absorbed systemically)
			• **Renal or Hepatic Dose Adjustments:** None
			• **Dosage Forms:** Topical (ointment)

INFECTIOUS DISEASE – ECHINOCANDIN

Drug Class
- Echinocandin
- Agents:
  - Acute Care
    - Anidulafungin
    - Caspofungin
    - Micafungin

> **Dosing Pearl**
> ✓ All echinocandins are administered by IV infusion. There are no oral dosage options.

Main Indications or Uses
- Acute Care
  - Disseminated and mucocutaneous Candidal infections
  - Febrile neutropenia

Mechanism of Action
- Inhibits the synthesis of 1,3-beta-D-glucan, disrupting fungal cell integrity and ultimately cell death.

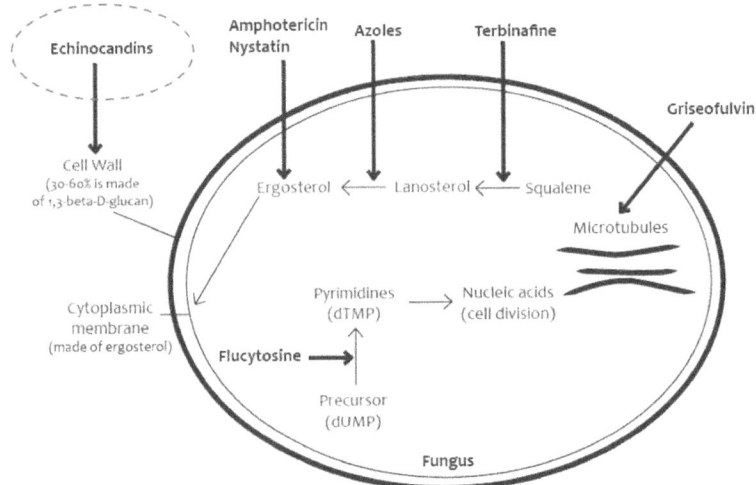

Primary Overall Net Benefit
- Fungicidal against Candida species, and fungistatic against Aspergillus species, plays a role in empiric therapy for febrile neutropenia.
- Main Labs to Monitor:
  - Cultures from infected sites at baseline (blood, sputum, urine, CSF, etc.)
  - Liver enzyme (AST/ALT, Alk Phos) and liver function (PT/INR, albumin, protein, bilirubin) tests

High-Yield Basic Pharmacology
- CNS Penetration
  - None of the echinocandins penetrate the CNS and thus do not play a role in managing CNS fungal infections.
- Resistance
  - Resistance to the echinocandins emerges from mutations that cause amino acid substitutions in the Fks subunits of glucan synthase.
- Fungal Specific
  - Unlike the azole antifungals, which target fungal CYP, which can overlap to human CYP inhibition (thus drug interactions), echinocandins are specific to fungal 1,3-beta-D-glucan, as mammalian cells do not require 1,3-beta-D-glucan.
  - Echinocandins exert the most potent antifungal effect in regions with active fungal cell growth.

High-Yield Clinical Knowledge
- **Febrile Neutropenia**
    - Antifungal treatment of febrile neutropenia is not typically started at the onset of illness, where broad-spectrum antibiotics play an essential role.
    - Echinocandins may be empirically started for febrile neutropenia if clinical improvement is not observed in patients on appropriate antimicrobial therapy for 4 to 7 days without other identified indications.
- **Use in Pregnancy**
    - All available echinocandins are contraindicated in pregnancy.
        - There have been no human studies, but in animal models, echinocandins have been observed to be embryotoxic, associated with incomplete ossification of the skull and torso, and increased risk of cervical ribs.
- **Dosing in Morbid Obesity**
    - Morbidly obese patients may have decreased exposure to echinocandins and require dose adjustments.
        - However, clear clinical guidance is lacking in this area.
    - For micafungin specifically, patients weighing over 115 kg should receive increased doses of micafungin of 200 mg.

High-Yield Core Spectrum of Coverage
- **Core spectrum**
    - Aspergillus fumigatus
    - Candida species
- **Core Indications**
    - Relatively non-toxic, Candida, C neoformans, the endemic mycoses, dermatophytes.

High-Yield Fast-Facts
- **Drug Interactions**
    - Caspofungin and micafungin are substrates of CYP 3A4 and may have clinically relevant cyclosporine interactions and other strong CYP3A4 inhibitors.
        - However, three clinical observational analyses have failed to observe clinically relevant hepatotoxicity with the combination of caspofungin and cyclosporine.
    - If patients are on inducers of CYP3A4 (carbamazepine, phenytoin, rifampin, isoniazid, etc.), the caspofungin dose should be increased to 70 mg daily.
- **Metabolism and Elimination**
    - Caspofungin and micafungin are both hepatically metabolized; however, anidulafungin is eliminated via chemical hydrolysis.

HIGH-YIELD BOARD EXAM ESSENTIALS
- **CLASSIC AGENTS:** Anidulafungin, caspofungin, micafungin
- **DRUG CLASS:** Echinocandin
- **INDICATIONS:** Disseminated and mucocutaneous Candidal infections, febrile neutropenia
- **MECHANISM:** Inhibits the synthesis of 1,3-beta-D-glucan disrupting fungal cell integrity, and ultimately cell death.
- **SIDE EFFECTS:** Peripheral edema, infusion reaction (chills, fever, phlebitis), liver enzyme elevation
- **CLINICAL PEARLS:** Caspofungin and micafungin are both hepatically metabolized; however, anidulafungin is eliminated via chemical hydrolysis.

Table: Drug Class Summary

Echinocandin - Drug Class Review High-Yield Med Reviews			
Mechanism of Action: *Inhibits the synthesis of 1,3-β-D-glucan, disrupting fungal cell integrity and ultimately cell death.*			
Class Effects: *Fungicidal against Candida species, fungistatic against Aspergillus species, and plays a role in empiric therapy for febrile neutropenia.*			
Generic Name	**Brand Name**	**Indication(s) or Uses**	**Notes**

Anidulafungin	Eraxis	• Candidemia
		• Esophageal Candidiasis
			• **Dosing (Adult):**
			  – IV: 200 mg x 1, then 100 mg q24h
			• **Dosing (Peds):**
			  – IV: 1.5 to 3 mg/kg/dose x 1, then 0.75 to 1.5 mg/kg/dose q24h
			    – Maximum 200 mg/dose (first dose); 100 mg/dose (subsequent doses)
			• **CYP450 Interactions:** None
			• **Renal or Hepatic Dose Adjustments:** None
			• **Dosage Forms:** IV (solution)

Caspofungin	Cancidas	• Aspergillosis
		• Candidemia
		• Esophageal Candidiasis
		• Neutropenic fever
			• **Dosing (Adult):**
			  – IV: 70 mg x 1, then 50 mg q24h
			    – IV: 150 mg q24h for endocarditis
			• **Dosing (Peds):**
			  – IV: 70 mg/m2/dose x 1, then 50 mg/m2 q24h
			• **CYP450 Interactions:** Inhibits CYP3A4
			• **Renal or Hepatic Dose Adjustments:**
			  – Child-Pugh class B or C: IV 70 mg x 1, then 35 mg q24h
			• **Dosage Forms:** IV (solution)

Micafungin	Mycamine	• Aspergillosis
		• Candidemia
		• Esophageal Candidiasis
		• Neutropenic fever
			• **Dosing (Adult):**
			  – IV: 100 to 150 mg IV q24h
			• **Dosing (Peds):**
			  – IV: 2 to 4 mg/kg/dose q24h
			    – Maximum 150 mg/dose
			• **CYP450 Interactions:** Inhibits CYP3A4
			• **Renal or Hepatic Dose Adjustments:** None
			• **Dosage Forms:** IV (solution)

INFECTIOUS DISEASE – FLUCYTOSINE

Drug Class
- Flucytosine
- Agents:
    - Acute Care
        - Flucytosine

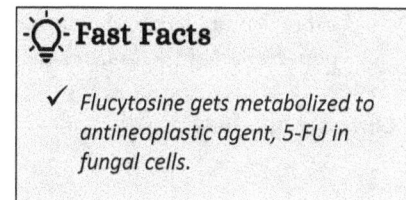

> **Fast Facts**
> ✓ Flucytosine gets metabolized to antineoplastic agent, 5-FU in fungal cells.

Main Indications or Uses
- Acute Care
    - Candida infections
    - Cryptococcus infections

Mechanism of Action
- Flucytosine inhibits susceptible fungal DNA and RNA synthesis after conversion to its active components, 5-fluorouracil (5-FU), 5-fluorodeoxyuridine monophosphate (FdUMP), and fluorouridine triphosphate (FUTP).

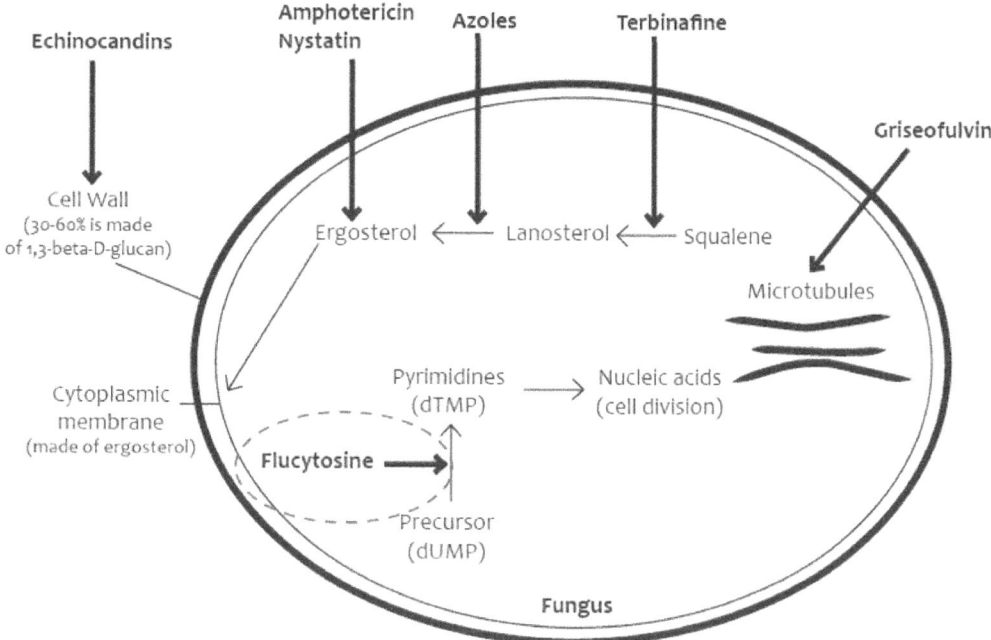

Primary Net Benefit
- Fungicidal agents are used for invasive fungal infections converted intracellularly to 5-FU.
- Main Labs to Monitor:
    - Cultures from infected sites at baseline (blood, sputum, urine, CSF, etc.)
    - Renal function (serum creatinine, urine output)
    - Liver enzyme (AST/ALT), liver function (INR/PT, albumin, total protein, bilirubin)

High-Yield Basic Pharmacology
- **Orally Administered**
    - Flucytosine is only available as an oral dosage form but is primarily used in cryptococcal meningitis, where patients may not take oral medications.
        - Thus, its administration frequently requires a nasogastric or orogastric tube and extemporaneous compounding from the oral capsule to an oral solution.

- **Fungal Specific**
  - The conversion of flucytosine to 5-FU is specific to fungal cells and does not occur in human cells, protecting them from toxicity.
    - However, intestinal flora can liberate 5-FU, permitting its absorption.
- **Amphotericin B Synergy**
  - When combined with amphotericin B, these agents demonstrate synergy, attributed to enhanced penetration of the flucytosine through amphotericin-damaged fungal cell membranes.

High-Yield Clinical Knowledge

- **Resistance**
  - Resistance to flucytosine occurs due to altered metabolism to its metabolites (5-FU, FdUMP, FUTP), which can happen in flucytosine monotherapy.
- **Therapeutic Drug Monitoring**
  - The normal therapeutic target range for flucytosine is 30 to 80 mcg/mL and should be taken on day 3 of therapy and after 2 hours from administration.
  - Concentrations above 100 mcg/mL should be avoided since the risk of bone marrow toxicity, and hepatotoxicity is higher with elevated concentrations.
- **Flucytosine to Fluconazole**
  - For cryptococcal meningitis treatment, high dose fluconazole has become an alternative to flucytosine in some clinical scenarios.

High-Yield Core Spectrum of Coverage
- **Core spectrum**
  - Candida infection
  - Cryptococcus neoformans
- **Core Indications**
  - Flucytosine is a narrow spectrum antifungal that has been limited in its use to cryptococcal meningitis and other invasive candida infections.

High-Yield Fast-Facts
- **Triple Therapy**
  - Although fluconazole may be used in place of flucytosine, it may also be used in combination along with amphotericin B as triple therapy for certain cryptococcal or candida infections.
- **Dosing Intervals**
  - Although fluconazole should be administered every 6 hours to reduce the risk of toxicity, this dosing interval should be maintained regardless of sleep - in other words, not q6h just during awake hours.

HIGH-YIELD BOARD EXAM ESSENTIALS
- **CLASSIC AGENTS:** Flucytosine
- **DRUG CLASS:** Antifungal
- **INDICATIONS:** Candida infections, Cryptococcus infections
- **MECHANISM:** Inhibits susceptible fungal DNA and RNA synthesis after conversion to its active components, 5-FU, FdUMP, and FUTP.
- **SIDE EFFECTS:** Nephrotoxicity, hepatotoxicity, bone marrow suppression
- **CLINICAL PEARLS:**
  - For cryptococcal meningitis treatment, high dose fluconazole has become an alternative to flucytosine in some clinical scenarios.
  - Monitor blood levels (> 100 mcg/mL is associated with BMS)

Table: Drug Class Summary

Flucytosine - Drug Class Review High-Yield Med Reviews			
Mechanism of Action: *Inhibits susceptible fungal DNA and RNA synthesis after conversion to 5-FU, FdUMP, and FUTP.*			
Class Effects: *Fungicidal agents used for invasive fungal infections converted intracellularly to 5-FU.*			
Generic Name	**Brand Name**	**Indication(s) or Uses**	**Notes**

Flucytosine	Ancobon	• Candida infections
		 • Cryptococcus infections
			• **Dosing (Adult):**
			   – Oral: 25 mg/kg/dose q6h
			     – Use IBW for obese patients
			 • **Dosing (Peds):**
			   – Oral: 25 mg/kg/dose q6h
			     – Extra info if needed
			 • **CYP450 Interactions:** None
			 • **Renal or Hepatic Dose Adjustments:**
			   – GFR 21 to 40 mL/min: 25 mg/kg/dose q12h
			   – GFR 11 to 20 mL/min: 25 mg/kg/dose q24h
			   – GFR < 10 mL/min: 25 mg/kg/dose q48h
			 • **Dosage Forms:** Oral (capsule)

INFECTIOUS DISEASE – OTHER ANTIFUNGALS

Drug Class
- Other Antifungal
- Agents:
  - Acute Care
    - Ciclopirox
    - Griseofulvin
    - Terbinafine
    - Maribavir
    - Naftifine
    - Nystatin

> 🚨 **Warning or Alert**
> ✓ Since griseofulvin binds to microtubules that are used for cell replication and division, its use is contraindicated in pregnancy.

Main Indications or Uses
- Acute Care
  - Topical treatment of tinea (pedis, corporis, cruris, versicolor), candidiasis
  - Onychomycosis
    - Ciclopirox
  - Oral candidiasis
    - Griseofulvin
  - Seborrheic dermatitis
    - Ciclopirox

> 💡 **Fast Facts**
> ✓ Since griseofulvin binds to keratin in new skin to prevent fungus infection of that tissue it can take up to 4 to 6 months to treat fungal infections of the finger or toenail.

Mechanism of Action
- Ciclopirox
  - Inhibits metal-dependent enzymes via chelation, causing degradation of peroxides within the fungal cell.
- Griseofulvin
  - Disrupts the assembly of the fungal mitotic spindle by inhibiting microtubule function, preventing fungal cell division.
- Maribavir
  - Inhibits protein kinase activity of CMV enzyme pUL97, inhibiting phosphorylation of proteins
- Naftifine, Terbinafine
  - Inhibits squalene-2,3-epoxidase, disrupting the synthesis of ergosterol in the fungal cell.
- Nystatin
  - Binds to fungal cell membrane ergosterol altering the membrane permeability leading to leakage of cell components and subsequent fungal cell death.

Primary Net Benefit
- Topical broad-spectrum antifungal therapy for infections where systemic agents are unnecessary or unwanted due to poor skin penetration.
- Griseofulvin and terbinafine are oral agents for tinea infections.
- Main Labs to Monitor:
  - No routine monitoring

High-Yield Basic Pharmacology
- Keratin Deposition
  - Griseofulvin has excellent penetration to keratin precursor cells, leading to prolonged antifungal effects.
    - As keratin cells differentiate, griseofulvin persists in keratin, leading to long-term resistance to fungal invasion, including new hair or nails.
  - Terbinafine exerts a similar effect on keratin; however, it is fungicidal, whereas griseofulvin is fungistatic.
- Distribution to Infection
  - Although orally administered, griseofulvin achieves good penetration to superficial sites of fungal infection due to the transfer of the drug via sweat and transepidermal fluid loss.

- **Amphotericin B and Nystatin**
  - Nystatin shares an identical mechanism of action to amphotericin B; however, it does not cause the same toxicities as nystatin is not absorbed systemically, even after oral administration.

High-Yield Clinical Knowledge
- **Barbiturates and Griseofulvin**
  - Coadministration of oral barbiturates (ex., phenobarbital, primidone, butalbital) decreases the absorption of griseofulvin by approximately 33% to 45%.
    - The mechanism is not related to CYP interactions, and the mechanism of this interaction remains unknown. Phenobarbital does not appear to increase griseofulvin metabolism but somehow impairs its absorption.
  - Griseofulvin is an inducer of CYP450 and should be used with caution in patients taking warfarin.
- **Non-CYP Ergosterol Inhibition**
  - Terbinafine inhibits ergosterol synthesis, a similar effect to azole antifungals, but terbinafine does not exert this effect through CYP450, as it inhibits the fungal enzyme squalene epoxidase.
  - Naftifine is an allylamine, similar to terbinafine but only used as a topical antifungal agent.
- **Oral Thrush**
  - Nystatin is an optimal agent for treating oral candidiasis or thrush in infants, as it is not absorbed systemically if swallowed.
    - Patients should be instructed to swish the drug around in the mouth and then swallow, but in neonates or infants, this can be difficult, if not impossible.
      - Caretakers should be instructed to paint nystatin suspension into the recesses of the mouth and avoid feeding for 5 to 10 minutes.

High-Yield Core Spectrum of Coverage
- **Core spectrum**
  - Candida species
  - Epidermophyton floccosum
  - Malassezia furfur
  - Trichophyton species
- **Core Indications**
  - Tinea pedis, corporis, cruris, versicolor, oral candidiasis or thrush.
  - Ringworm
  - Onychomycosis

High-Yield Fast-Facts
- **Palatability**
  - Oral nystatin is limited by its unpleasant taste, necessitating a therapeutic change to clotrimazole troches.
- **OTC vs. Rx**
  - Topical terbinafine is widely available as an OTC topical cream, but the alternative allylamine, naftifine, is only available as a prescription product.
- **Routes Not Interchangeable**
  - Topical antifungal products should not be substituted for oral, vaginal, or ocular use.

Table: Drug Class Summary

Other Antifungals - Drug Class Review High-Yield Med Reviews			
Mechanism of Action: *See each agent above.*			
Class Effects: *Topical broad-spectrum antifungal therapy for infections where systemic agents are unnecessary or unwanted due to poor skin penetration. Griseofulvin and terbinafine are oral agents for tinea infections.*			
Generic Name	**Brand Name**	**Main Indication(s) or Uses**	**Notes**
Ciclopirox	Ciclodan	<ul><li>Topical treatment of tinea (pedis, corporis, cruris, versicolor), candidiasis</li><li>Onychomycosis</li><li>Seborrheic dermatitis</li></ul>	<ul><li>**Dosing (Adult):** – Topical: application twice daily</li><li>**Dosing (Peds):** – Topical: application twice daily</li><li>**CYP450 Interactions:** None</li><li>**Renal or Hepatic Dose Adjustments:** None</li><li>**Dosage Forms:** Topical (cream, gel, shampoo, solution, suspension)</li></ul>

Griseofulvin	Gris-PEG	<ul><li>Systemic treatment of tinea pedis, corporis, cruris, capitis, and unguium</li></ul>	<ul><li>**Dosing (Adult):**
			– Oral: (ultramicrosize) 375 to 750 mg q24h
			– Oral: (microsize) 500 to 750 mg q24h</li><li>**Dosing (Peds):**
			– Oral: (ultramicrosize) 10 to 15 mg/kg/day
			   – Maximum 750 mg/day
			– Oral: (microsize) 20 to 25 mg/kg/day
			   – Maximum 1000 mg/day</li><li>**CYP450 Interactions:** None</li><li>**Renal or Hepatic Dose Adjustments:** Use contraindicated in hepatic failure</li><li>**Dosage Forms:** Oral (microsize suspension, ultramicrosize tablets)</li></ul>

Maribavir	Livtencity	<ul><li>CMV, refractory post-transplant</li></ul>	<ul><li>**Dosing (Adult):** – Oral 400 mg twice daily</li><li>**Dosing (Peds):** – Must be ≥ 12 years and ≥ 35 kg, oral 400 mg twice daily</li><li>**CYP450 Interactions:** Substrate CYP1A2, 3A4</li><li>**Renal or Hepatic Dose Adjustments:** Use contraindicated in hepatic failure</li><li>**Dosage Forms:** Oral (tablets)</li></ul>
Naftifine	Naftin	<ul><li>Topical treatment of tinea pedis, corporis, and cruris</li></ul>	<ul><li>**Dosing (Adult):** – Topical: to affected area twice daily</li><li>**Dosing (Peds):** – Topical: to affected area twice daily</li><li>**CYP450 Interactions:** None</li><li>**Renal or Hepatic Dose Adjustments:** None</li><li>**Dosage Forms:** Topical (cream, gel)</li></ul>

Other Antifungals - Drug Class Review
High-Yield Med Reviews

Generic Name	Brand Name	Main Indication(s) or Uses	Notes

Nystatin	Nystop	• Topical treatment of tinea (pedis, corporis, cruris, versicolor), candidiasis
		• Oral candidiasis
			• **Dosing (Adult):**
			  – Topical: to affected area twice daily
			  – Oral: 400,000 to 1,000,000 units q6-8h
			• **Dosing (Peds):**
			  – Topical: to affected area twice daily
			  – Oral: 200,000 to 600,000 units q6-8h
			• **CYP450 Interactions:** None
			• **Renal or Hepatic Dose Adjustments:** None
			• **Dosage Forms:** Oral (capsule, powder, suspension, tablet), topical (cream, ointment, powder)

Terbinafine	Lamisil	• Topical treatment of tinea (pedis, corporis, cruris, versicolor), candidiasis	• **Dosing (Adult):**
			  – Topical: to affected area once daily
			• **Dosing (Peds):**
			  – Topical: to affected area once daily
			• **CYP450 Interactions:** None
			• **Renal or Hepatic Dose Adjustments:** None
			• **Dosage Forms:** Topical (cream, gel, solution)

HIGH-YIELD BOARD EXAM ESSENTIALS
- **CLASSIC AGENTS:** Ciclopirox, griseofulvin, terbinafine, naftifine, nystatin
- **DRUG CLASS:** Antifungal
- **INDICATIONS:** Topical treatment of tinea (pedis, corporis, cruris, versicolor), onychomycosis (ciclopirox), oral candidiasis (griseofulvin), seborrheic dermatitis (ciclopirox).
- **MECHANISM:**
    - Ciclopirox - Inhibits metal-dependent enzymes via chelation, causing degradation of peroxides within the fungal cell
    - Griseofulvin - Disrupts the fungal mitotic spindle's assembly by inhibiting microtubule function, preventing fungal cell division
    - Naftifine and Terbinafine - Inhibits squalene-2,3-epoxidase, disrupting the synthesis of ergosterol in the fungal cell
    - Nystatin - Binds to fungal cell membrane ergosterol altering the membrane permeability leading to leakage of cell components and subsequent fungal cell death
- **SIDE EFFECTS:** Unpleasant taste, local irritation
- **CLINICAL PEARLS:**
    - Topical broad-spectrum antifungal therapy for infections where systemic agents are unnecessary or unwanted due to poor skin penetration.
    - Griseofulvin is contraindicated for use during pregnancy due to its ability to cross the placenta and bind to microtubules which can interfere with cellular replication and division.

INFECTIOUS DISEASE – ANTIMYCOBACTERIALS – GENERAL AGENTS

Drug Class
- Antimycobacterials
- Agents:
  - Acute & Chronic Care
    - Ethambutol
    - Pyrazinamide

Main Indications or Uses
- Acute & Chronic Care
  - Tuberculosis (Mycobacterium tuberculosis)

Mechanism of Action
- Ethambutol
  - It inhibits mycobacterial arabinosyl transferases, preventing the polymerization reaction of arabinoglycan from forming the mycobacterial cell wall.
- Pyrazinamide
  - Converted to pyrazinoic acid by mycobacterial pyrazinamide, disrupting the mycobacterial cell membrane metabolism and transport functions.

Primary Net Benefit
- First-line treatments for active tuberculosis are combined with isoniazid and rifamycins but carry risks of hepatotoxicity (pyrazinamide) and ophthalmic adverse events (ethambutol).
- Main Labs to Monitor:
  - Cultures from infected sites at baseline (sputum, CSF, etc.) and monthly (until two consecutive negative cultures reported
  - Liver enzyme (AST/ALT) and liver function (INR/PT, Albumin, Total Protein, Bilirubin) tests
  - Visual acuity, color vision (ethambutol, baseline, and periodically)

High-Yield Basic Pharmacology
- Central TB
  - In rare TB cases infecting the CNS, antimicrobial therapy with isoniazid and pyrazinamide achieve adequate CNS concentrations as they penetrate the blood-brain barrier readily.
  - Ethambutol and rifampin less readily penetrate the CNS, and alternative therapy, including fluoroquinolones, may be considered.
- Core Spectrum
  - Mycobacteria tuberculosis
  - Mycobacteria bovis
  - Mycobacterium kansasii

High-Yield Clinical Knowledge
- Hepatotoxicity
  - Pyrazinamide is associated with hepatotoxicity development, requiring baseline liver function tests when used in combination with rifampin or among patients with a history of liver disease.

- Ophthalmic Injury
  - Ethambutol has been associated with retrobulbar neuritis and is contraindicated among patients with optic neuritis.
  - Baseline visual acuity and color vision tests are required and should be monitored throughout ethambutol therapy.
    - Patients complaining of visual acuity changes or the loss of the ability to see green should prompt urgent ophthalmologic examination.

- Therapy with ethambutol may be delayed in children too young to undergo visual acuity and color vision assessments.
- **Pregnant Women**
  - To treat active TB in pregnant women, pyrazinamide should be avoided due to inadequate teratogenicity data.
    - However, there is growing data to support the safety of pyrazinamide in pregnancy.
- **Standard Regimen**
  - Pyrazinamide and ethambutol are combined with isoniazid and rifampin for two months as the standard initial regimen for TB, followed by an additional four months of isoniazid and rifampin.
  - Ethambutol can be discontinued if susceptibility to isoniazid, pyrazinamide, and rifampin is known.
  - Alternatively, therapy without pyrazinamide or ethambutol can be accomplished using isoniazid and rifampin for nine months.
- **Resistance**
  - Mycobacterial resistance to pyrazinamide develops due to impaired mycobacterial uptake or mutations in the pncA gene, which prevents the conversion to pyrazinoic acid.
  - Mutations in the mycobacterial embB gene or enhanced efflux pump activity are responsible for resistance to ethambutol.
  - Both pyrazinamide and ethambutol must always be combined with other antimycobacterial agents to avoid resistance.
- **Gout**
  - Pyrazinamide is associated with hyperuricemia as it reduces the renal clearance of uric acid by more than 80%.
    - Other common adverse events associated with pyrazinamide include GI distress and hepatotoxicity.
  - Ethambutol has also been associated with decreased renal elimination of uric acid and may contribute to gouty attacks.

High-Yield Core Evidence
- **Four Month Tuberculosis Regimen**
  - This was a noninferiority, open-label, controlled trial in adult patients with smear-positive, rifampin-sensitive, newly diagnosed pulmonary tuberculosis in five sub-Saharan African countries.
  - The subjects meeting inclusion criteria were randomized to a standard 6-month regimen that included ethambutol during the 2-month intensive phase was compared with a 4-month regimen in which gatifloxacin (400 mg per day) was substituted for ethambutol during the intensive phase and was continued, along with rifampin and isoniazid, during the continuation phase. T
  - There was no difference in the primary efficacy endpoint of an unfavorable outcome (treatment failure, recurrence, or death or study dropout during treatment) measured 24 months after the end of treatment, with a noninferiority margin of 6 percentage points, adjusted for country.
  - However, there was significant heterogeneity across countries, with differences in the rate of an unfavorable outcome, baseline cavitary status, and body-mass index.
  - The standard regimen, as compared with the 4-month regimen, was associated with a higher dropout rate during treatment and more treatment failures but fewer recurrences.
  - There was no evidence of increased risks of prolonging the QT interval or dysglycemia with the 4-month regimen.
  - The authors concluded that noninferiority of the 4-month regimen to the standard regimen concerning the primary efficacy endpoint was not shown. (N Engl J Med, 2014, 371:1588–1598.)

High-Yield Fast-Fact
- **Discovery**
  - Kushner and colleagues discovered pyrazinamide in 1952, and ethambutol was discovered at Lederle Laboratories in 1961.

HIGH-YIELD BOARD EXAM ESSENTIALS
- **CLASSIC AGENTS:** Ethambutol, pyrazinamide
- **DRUG CLASS:** Antimycobacterials
- **INDICATIONS:** Tuberculosis
- **MECHANISM:**
    - Ethambutol: Inhibits mycobacterial arabinosyl transferases, preventing the polymerization reaction of arabinoglycan used to form the mycobacterial cell wall.
    - Pyrazinamide: Converted to pyrazinoic acid by mycobacterial pyrazinamide, disrupting the mycobacterial cell membrane metabolism and transport functions
- **SIDE EFFECTS:** Hepatic injury, gout (pyrazinamide), retrobulbar neuritis (ethambutol)
- **CLINICAL PEARLS:**
    - Pyrazinamide and ethambutol are used in combination with isoniazid and rifampin for two months as the standard initial regimen for TB, followed by an additional four months of isoniazid and rifampin.
    - Ethambutol and pyrazinamide can both elevate uric acid levels and exacerbate gout.

Table: Drug Class Summary

Antimycobacterials - Drug Class Review High-Yield Med Reviews			
Mechanism of Action: *Ethambutol - Inhibits mycobacterial arabinosyl transferases, preventing the polymerization reaction of arabinoglycan used to form the mycobacterial cell wall.* *Pyrazinamide - Converted to pyrazinoic acid by mycobacterial pyrazinamide, disrupting the mycobacterial cell membrane metabolism and transport functions.*			
Class Effects: *First-line treatments for active tuberculosis used in combination with isoniazid and rifamycins but carries risks of hepatotoxicity (pyrazinamide) and ophthalmic adverse events (ethambutol)*			
Generic Name	**Brand Name**	**Main Indication(s) or Uses**	**Notes**

Ethambutol	Myambutol	- Tuberculosis	- **Dosing (Adult):**
			  - Oral: 800 to 1,600 mg daily
			  - Oral: 1,200 mg to 2,400 mg three times weekly DOT
			  - Oral: 2,000 to 4,000 mg twice weekly DOT
			- **Dosing (Peds):**
			  - Oral: 15 to 25 mg/kg/day or 5 times weekly DOT
			  - Oral: 50 mg/kg/dose two or three times weekly
			- **CYP450 Interactions:** None
			- **Renal or Hepatic Dose Adjustments:**
			  - GFR 10 to 50 mL/minute: q24-36h
			  - GFR < 10 mL/minute: q48h
			- **Dosage Forms:** Oral (tablet)

Pyrazinamide	Macrozide, Zinamide	- Tuberculosis	- **Dosing (Adult):**
			  - Oral: 1,000 to 2,000 mg daily
			  - Oral: 1,500 mg to 3,000 mg three times weekly DOT
			  - Oral: 2,000 to 4,000 mg twice weekly DOT
			- **Dosing (Peds):**
			  - Oral: 30 to 40 mg/kg/day or 5 times weekly DOT
			  - Oral: 50 mg/kg/dose two or three times weekly
			- **CYP450 Interactions:** None
			- **Renal or Hepatic Dose Adjustments:**
			  - GFR < 30 mL/minute: Three times weekly after dialysis
			- **Dosage Forms:** Oral (tablet)

INFECTIOUS DISEASE – ISONIAZID

Drug Class
- Isoniazid
- Agents:
  - Acute & Chronic Care
    - Isoniazid (INH)

> **Pharmacogenetics Tip**
> ✓ Slow-acetylators are at increased of INH induced hepatotoxicity and neuropathy.

Main Indications or Uses
- Acute & Chronic Care
  - Acute or latent tuberculosis (Mycobacterium tuberculosis)

Mechanism of Action
- Isoniazid is activated within the mycobacterium cell by KatG to its nicotinoyl radical, which reacts spontaneously with NAD+ inhibiting cell wall enzyme synthesis and inhibiting nucleic acid synthesis by reacting with NADP+.

Primary Net Benefit
- Bactericidal for actively growing Mycobacteria tuberculosis, with less effective activity against other Mycobacteria species.
- Main Labs to Monitor:
  - Cultures from infected sites at baseline (sputum, CSF, etc.) and monthly (until 2 consecutive negative cultures reported
  - Liver enzyme (AST/ALT) and liver function (INR/PT, Albumin, Total Protein, Bilirubin) tests due to risks of hepatotoxicity

High-Yield Basic Pharmacology
- **Collateral KatG Effects**
  - The activation of KatG by isoniazid has other effects, including superoxide production, hydrogen peroxide, nitric oxide radical, and alkyl hydroperoxides, contributing to isoniazid's mycobactericidal effects but also its toxicity.
- **Fast, Intermediate, or Slow Acetylators**
  - Phenotypic subgroups of isoniazid metabolism include fast, intermediate, or slow acetylators.
  - The patient's race can predict their phenotypic subtype with fast acetylation associated with Inuit and Japanese individuals.
    - It can be either heterozygous or homozygous expression of this autosomal dominant trait.
    - Scandinavians, Caucasians, and Jewish individuals are associated with slow acetylation.
- **Other Mycobacteria**
  - Isoniazid is most active against Mycobacterium tuberculosis but only has moderate activity against Mycobacterium bovis and Mycobacterium kansasii and poor activity in Mycobacterium Avium Complex.

High-Yield Clinical Knowledge
- **Pharmacodynamic Anti-Mycobacteria Action**
  - Similar to other antimicrobials, isoniazid's action on mycobacteria can be described as concentration-dependent, bactericidal (or mycobactericidal)
    - Isoniazid's actions can also exert peak concentration ratios over MIC or total exposure (area under the curve).
- **CYP2E1, Rifampin**
  - Isoniazid possesses alternative metabolism methods, including acetylation of isoniazid to acetyl isoniazid (by NAT2), either excreted by the kidney or further metabolized to acetyl hydrazine then oxidized by CYP2E1 to hepatotoxic metabolites.
  - In combination with rifampin for mycobacterium tuberculosis treatment, the risk of hepatotoxicity may be increased as it may induce CYP2E1 (in addition to the induction of 2E1 by isoniazid itself).
- **Pyridoxine Supplementation**

- Isoniazid is frequently administered with pyridoxine to limit neurological adverse events associated with its use.
    - Without pyridoxine, the risk of the hands and feet' peripheral neuropathies is approximately 2% but is much higher in patients who are slow acetylators, those with diabetes, or pre-existing anemia.
- **Resistance**
    - Mycobacterium resistance to isoniazid is primarily associated with a mutation in the heme-binding catalytic domain of KatG or deletion of KatG.
    - Other isoniazid resistance mechanisms include overexpression of the genes for InhA and mutations in the kasA and katG genes.
- **Neurological Adverse Events**
    - Isoniazid is frequently associated with an increased or recurrence of neurological disorders, including seizures in patients with pre-existing seizure disorders.
    - Other neurological adverse events include the development of optic atrophy, optic neuritis, dizziness, ataxia, paresthesias, and encephalopathy.
- **Isoniazid Overdose**
    - With isoniazid overdose, pyridoxine (vit B6) therapy can be potentially lifesaving.
    - Still, the dose is significantly higher than the dose used for peripheral neuropathy: 5 g administered IV and repeated every 5-10 minutes until seizures have stopped.
        - This often exhausts the total hospital pharmacy supply of pyridoxine.
- **Core Spectrum**
    - Mycobacteria tuberculosis
    - Mycobacteria bovis
    - Mycobacterium kansasii
- **Core Indications**
    - Acute or latent tuberculosis

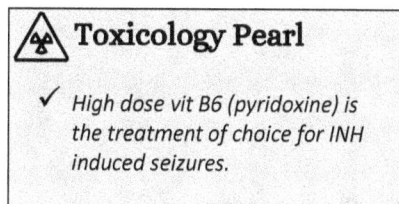

Toxicology Pearl

✓ High dose vit B6 (pyridoxine) is the treatment of choice for INH induced seizures.

High-Yield Core Evidence
- **Isoniazid DOT**
    - The difference in efficacy of directly observed therapy (DOT) for tuberculosis patients vs. self-administered therapy (SAT) in decreasing ADR, microbiologic failure, and relapse were analyzed using a meta-analysis of existing data.
    - A total of ten studies, five of which being prospective, randomized, and five being observational, were included (N=12,482)
    - There was no statistically significant difference between DOT versus SAT in the primary outcome of microbiologic failure rates for relapse or ADR.
    - In evidence-based medicine, the authors concluded that DOT was not significantly better than SAT in preventing microbiologic failure, relapse, or ADR. (Clin Infect Dis. 2013 Jul;57(1):21-31.)
- **Moxifloxacin or INH**
    - Moxifloxacin, active against Mycobacterium tuberculosis in vitro, maybe a safer alternative to isoniazid.
    - This randomized trial of adults with pulmonary TB compared moxifloxacin 400 mg plus isoniazid placebo or isoniazid 300 mg plus moxifloxacin placebo, administered 5 days/week for 8 weeks to rifampin, pyrazinamide, and ethambutol.
    - The primary outcome was negative sputum culture after 8 weeks of treatment.
    - 328 subjects were included in the primary efficacy analysis: 35 (11%) were HIV positive, 248 (76%) had cavitation on baseline chest radiograph, and 213 (65%) were enrolled at African sites.
    - There was no difference between moxifloxacin and isoniazid concerning the primary outcome.
    - The authors concluded that the substitution of moxifloxacin for isoniazid resulted in a small but statistically insignificant increase in Week-8 culture negativity. (Am J Respir Crit Care Med. 2009 Aug 1;180(3):273-80)

High-Yield Fast-Fact
- IN...H?
    - Isoniazid is commonly abbreviated INH; however, there is no H.
    - The H in the INH abbreviation refers to the alternative name of isoniazid, isonicotinic acid hydrazide.

HIGH-YIELD BOARD EXAM ESSENTIALS
- **CLASSIC AGENTS:** Isoniazid
- **DRUG CLASS:** Antitubercular agent
- **INDICATIONS:** Acute or latent tuberculosis
- **MECHANISM:** Activated in mycobacterium cells by KatG to a nicotinoyl radical inhibiting cell wall enzyme synthesis and inhibiting nucleic acid synthesis.
- **SIDE EFFECTS:** Seizures, optic atrophy, optic neuritis, dizziness, ataxia, paresthesias, and encephalopathy.
- **CLINICAL PEARLS:**
    - Isoniazid is frequently administered with pyridoxine to limit neurological adverse events associated with its use. Without pyridoxine, the risk of the hands and feet' peripheral neuropathies' risk is approximately 2% but is much higher in patients who are slow acetylators, those with diabetes, or pre-existing anemia.

Table: Drug Class Summary

Isoniazid - Drug Class Review </br> High-Yield Med Reviews			
Mechanism of Action: Activated in mycobacterium cells by KatG to a nicotinoyl radical inhibiting cell wall enzyme synthesis and inhibiting nucleic acid synthesis.			
Class Effects: Bactericidal for actively growing Mycobacteria tuberculosis, with less effective activity against other Mycobacteria species. Risk of hepatotoxicity and peripheral neuropathy.			
Generic Name	**Brand Name**	**Indication(s) or Uses**	**Notes**

Isoniazid		• Acute or latent tuberculosis	• **Dosing (Adult):**
			   – Oral/IM: 5 mg/kg or 300 mg q24h
			     – DOT: 15 mg/kg/dose or 900 mg, once-, twice-, or three-times-weekly
			 • **Dosing (Peds):**
			   – Oral/IM: 5 mg/kg q24h
			     – Maximum 300 mg/dose
			 • **CYP450 Interactions:**
			   – Inhibits CYP2C19, 3A4, 2D6. Induces CYP2E1
			 • **Renal or Hepatic Dose Adjustments:** None
			 • **Dosage Forms:** Oral (tablet, syrup), IM (solution)

INFECTIOUS DISEASE – RIFAMYCINS

Drug Class
- Rifamycins
- Agents:
    - Acute Care
        - Rifabutin
        - Rifampin
        - Rifamycin
        - Rifapentine
        - Rifaximin

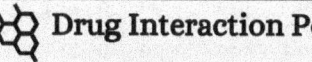

> **Drug Interaction Pearl**
> ✓ Rifampin is one of the most potent inducers of several CYP450 enzymes and can cause clinically relevant drug interactions.

Main Indications or Uses
- Acute Care
    - **Mycobacteria tuberculosis**
        - Rifabutin, Rifampin, Rifapentine
    - **Clostridoides difficile**
        - Rifaximin
    - **Traveler's diarrhea prophylaxis**
        - Rifamycin, Rifaximin
    - **Haemophilus influenzae meningitis prophylaxis**
        - Rifampin
    - **Hepatic encephalopathy**
        - Rifaximin
    - **Staphylococcal endocarditis or osteomyelitis**
        - Rifampin

Mechanism of Action
- Rifamycins bind to the beta subunit of bacterial DNA-dependent RNA polymerase, forming a stable drug-enzyme complex, inhibiting RNA synthesis.

Primary Net Benefit
- Bactericidal to mycobacteria, and other sensitive pathogens, particularly intracellular organisms and those sequestered in abscesses and lung cavities.
- Main Labs to Monitor:
    - Cultures from infected sites at baseline (sputum, CSF, etc.) and monthly (until 2 consecutive negative cultures reported
    - Liver enzyme (AST/ALT) and liver function (INR/PT, Albumin, Total Protein, Bilirubin) tests due to risk of hepatotoxicity

High-Yield Basic Pharmacology
- **With or Without Food**
    - Patients taking oral rifampin must be instructed to take it on an empty stomach as food decreases its peak concentration by 33%.
        - Since rifampin is concentration-dependent in its action, this may lead to clinical failure and/or resistance.
    - On the other hand, Rifapentine should be taken with food since the total exposure (AUC) is enhanced by 50%.
    - Food does not affect rifabutin absorption.
- **Resistance**
    - Mycobacterial resistance to rifamycins occurs due to a gene mutation in the bacterial DNA of the drug binding site.

- The vast majority (approximately 86% of resistant isolates) occur due to mutations at codons 526 and 531 of the rpoB gene.
- Efflux pumps have been identified as another resistance mechanism, occurring with a higher incidence in patients with AIDS and multi cavitary tuberculosis infections.
- **Rifaximin and Ammonia**
  - Rifaximin is used clinically to treat hepatic encephalopathy by eliminating bacteria that produce ammonia and other nitrogenous compounds.
    - Compared to lactulose, rifaximin may improve the successful resolution of encephalopathy and reduce the number of hospitalizations for hepatic encephalopathy while also being devoid of diarrhea, often caused by lactulose.

High-Yield Clinical Knowledge
- **CYP450 Inducer**
  - Rifamycins are inducers of CYP450 isoenzymes 1A2, 2C9, 2C19, 2E1, and 3A4, leading to numerous clinically relevant drug interactions.
    - Notable interactions include digoxin, prednisone, propranolol, phenytoin, sulfonylureas, warfarin, and zidovudine.
  - Not all rifamycins induce isoenzymes to the same degree.
    - Rifampin > Rifabutin > Rifapentine
    - Rifaximin and rifamycin are not absorbed to a clinically relevant degree to induce any CYP isoenzyme.
- **Red/Orange Discoloration**
  - Rifampin exerts a characteristic orange discoloration on urine, sweat, and tears.
  - However, cholestatic jaundice should be ruled out as a potential cause of skin discoloration.
- **Hepatotoxicity**
  - Systemically absorbed rifamycins may cause liver injury, hepatitis, and death.
  - Risk factors that increase the likelihood of hepatotoxicity include patients with preexisting chronic liver disease, alcoholism, old age, or concomitant hepatotoxic agents.
- **Biofilm Penetration**
  - Rifampin is not considered useful for monotherapy in susceptible isolates of S. aureus or coagulase-negative Staphylococci endocarditis. It must be used in combination with beta-lactam and/or vancomycin.
    - The use of rifampin is useful for this indication for its ability to penetrate biofilms established by these bacteria, preventing other antimicrobial agents from penetrating the bacterial colony.
- **High-dose rifampin**
  - Although isoniazid has been proposed to be given at once-, twice-, or thrice-weekly direct observed treatment, this strategy is not recommended with high dose rifampin due to increased incidence of intolerance.
  - Associated adverse events include flu-like syndrome (fever, chills, and myalgias), eosinophilia, interstitial nephritis, acute tubular necrosis, thrombocytopenia, hemolytic anemia, and shock.
    - Rare but serious events at any rifampin dose include thrombocytopenia and leukopenia.
- **Core Spectrum**
  - Mycobacteria tuberculosis, and non-tuberculosis Mycobacteria (bovis, kansasii, MAC)
  - Gram-positive
    - Streptococcus species
    - Staphylococcus aureus (including MRSA)
    - Listeria monocytogenes
  - Gram-Negative
    - Escherichia coli
    - Proteus species
    - Klebsiella species
    - Pseudomonas aeruginosa
    - Neisseria meningitidis
    - Haemophilus influenzae

High-Yield Core Evidence
- **Duration of Rifampin and Health System Costs**
    - This was a multicenter, randomized trial comparing latent tuberculosis treatment with isoniazid daily for 9 months or rifampin daily for 4 months. The primary objective was to compare the difference in health system costs between therapies.
    - Total health system cost per patient was significantly less with rifampin compared to isoniazid.
    - Furthermore, total costs related to managing adverse events with isoniazid were significantly higher than similar management costs due to rifampin.
        - The authors noted that the incremental cost-effectiveness analyses showed that 4RIF would be cost-saving and prevent more cases within 2 years if efficacy exceeded 74% and cost-saving if efficacy exceeded 65%.
    - The authors concluded that the rifampin 4-month regimen was significantly cheaper per patient completing treatment because of better completion and fewer adverse events. (Thorax. 2010 Jul;65(7):582-7.)
- **Rifaximin for Hepatic Encephalopathy**
    - This was a randomized, double-blind, placebo-controlled trial comparing rifaximin to placebo for recurrent hepatic encephalopathy resulting from chronic liver disease.
    - Rifaximin significantly reduced the risk of the primary outcome (time to the first breakthrough episode of hepatic encephalopathy) compared to placebo.
        - However, over 90% of patients received concomitant lactulose therapy.
    - The authors concluded that over a 6-month period, treatment with rifaximin maintained remission from hepatic encephalopathy more effectively than did placebo. (N Engl J Med. 2010 Mar 25;362(12):1071-81.)
- **Rifaximin for Clostridoides Difficile**
    - This was a randomized, double-blind, placebo-controlled pilot study to assess the rates of recurrent diarrhea in patients with Clostridoides difficile infection (CDI) given rifaximin versus placebo immediately after standard therapy.
    - Rifaximin therapy led to a significantly lower incidence of recurrent diarrhea than placebo.
    - The authors concluded that patients with CDI given a rifaximin chaser regimen experienced a decreased incidence of recurrent diarrhea than placebo. (J Antimicrob Chemother. 2011 Dec;66(12):2850-5.)

High-Yield Fast-Facts
- **Rifampicin**
    - Rifampin may be referred to as rifampicin, particularly in the literature outside the United States.
- **Rifaximin Absorption**
    - Rifaximin is not absorbed under normal clinical use; however, patients with severe hepatic impairment (Child-Pugh class C) may absorb sufficient concentrations to cause some degree of CYP3A4 induction.

HIGH-YIELD BOARD EXAM ESSENTIALS
- **CLASSIC AGENTS:** Rifabutin, rifampin, rifamycin, rifapentine, rifaximin
- **DRUG CLASS:** Rifamycin
- **INDICATIONS:** Mycobacteria tuberculosis (Rifabutin, Rifampin, Rifapentine), Clostridoides difficile (Rifaximin), Traveler's diarrhea prophylaxis (Rifamycin, Rifaximin), Haemophilus influenzae meningitis prophylaxis (Rifampin), Hepatic encephalopathy (Rifaximin), Staphylococcal endocarditis or osteomyelitis (Rifampin)
- **MECHANISM:** Rifamycins bind to the beta subunit of bacterial DNA-dependent RNA polymerase, forming a stable drug-enzyme complex, inhibiting RNA synthesis.
- **SIDE EFFECTS:** Orange discoloration to urine, sweat, and tears, hepatotoxicity
- **CLINICAL PEARLS:** Rifamycins are inducers of CYP450 isoenzymes 1A2, 2C9, 2C19, 2E1, and 3A4, leading to numerous clinically relevant drug interactions. Notable interactions include digoxin, prednisone, propranolol, phenytoin, sulfonylureas, warfarin, and zidovudine.

Table: Drug Class Summary

Rifamycins - Drug Class Review High-Yield Med Reviews			
Mechanism of Action: *Binds to the beta subunit of bacterial DNA-dependent RNA polymerase, inhibiting RNA synthesis.*			
Class Effects: *Bactericidal to mycobacteria, and other sensitive pathogens, particularly intracellular organisms and those sequestered in abscesses and lung cavities. Risk of hepatotoxicity and drug interactions are relevant.*			
Generic Name	**Brand Name**	**Main Indication(s) or Uses**	**Notes**
Rifabutin	Mycobutin	• Mycobacterium avium complex • Mycobacterium tuberculosis	• **Dosing (Adult):** – Oral: 5 mg/kg/dose q24h or 300 mg q24h • **Dosing (Peds):** – Oral: 5 to 20 mg/kg/dose q24h – Max 300 mg/dose • **CYP450 Interactions:** Substrate CYP1A2, 3A4; Induces CYP2C9, CYP3A4 • **Renal or Hepatic Dose Adjustments:** None • **Dosage Forms:** Oral (capsule)
Rifampin	Rifadin	• Mycobacterium tuberculosis • Meningococcal prophylaxis	• **Dosing (Adult):** – Oral/IV: 150 to 900 mg q24h – Numerous anti-TB regimens exist. • **Dosing (Peds):** – Oral/IV: 10 to 20 mg/kg/dose q12-24h – Maximum 900 mg/dose • **CYP450 Interactions:** Substrate Pgp; Induces CYP1A2, 2B6, 2C9, 2C19, 2C8, CYP3A4, Pgp • **Renal or Hepatic Dose Adjustments:** None • **Dosage Forms:** Oral (capsule), IV (solution)
Rifamycin	Aemcolo	• Traveler's diarrhea	• **Dosing (Adult):** – Oral: 388 mg BID x 3 days • **Dosing (Peds):** Not routinely used • **CYP450 Interactions:** Not systemically absorbed • **Renal or Hepatic Dose Adjustments:** None • **Dosage Forms:** Oral (tablet)
Rifapentine	Priftin	• Mycobacterium tuberculosis	• **Dosing (Adult):** – Oral: 600 mg BID • **Dosing (Peds):** Children 12 years and older – Oral: 600 mg BID • **CYP450 Interactions:** Induces CYP3A4 • **Renal or Hepatic Dose Adjustments:** None • **Dosage Forms:** Oral (tablet)
Rifaximin	Xifaxan	• Clostridoides difficile infection • Hepatic encephalopathy • Irritable bowel syndrome • Traveler's diarrhea	• **Dosing (Adult):** – Oral: 400 mg q8h or 550 mg q12h • **Dosing (Peds):** – Oral: 15 to 30 mg/kg/day divided q8h – Maximum 400 mg/dose • **CYP450 Interactions:** Not systemically absorbed • **Renal or Hepatic Dose Adjustments:** None • **Dosage Forms:** Oral (tablet)

INFECTIOUS DISEASE – CMV ANTIVIRALS

Drug Class
- **CMV Antivirals**
- **Agents:**
  - Acute & Chronic Care
    - Cidofovir
    - Foscarnet
    - Ganciclovir
    - Letermovir
    - Valganciclovir

Main Indications or Uses
- **Acute Care & Chronic Care**
  - Cytomegalovirus (CMV)

Mechanism of Action
- **Cidofovir, foscarnet, ganciclovir, valganciclovir**
  - Inhibit viral DNA synthesis by inhibiting viral DNA polymerases
- **Letermovir**
  - Interferes with viral DNA replication by inhibiting the DNA terminase complex responsible for DNA processing and packaging

Primary Net Benefit
- Provide treatment and/or prophylaxis for CMV and several other viral infections
- Main Labs to Monitor:
  - Serum creatinine, CBC, and platelet count at baseline and periodically during therapy

High-Yield Basic Pharmacology
- **Valganciclovir Metabolism and Absorption**
  - Valganciclovir is an orally bioavailable prodrug of ganciclovir.
    - Valganciclovir is rapidly converted to ganciclovir in the body by intestinal mucosal cells and hepatocytes.
    - The oral bioavailability of valganciclovir is 60% when administered with food, and high-fat meals further enhance absorption.
- **CMV Resistance**
  - CMV resistance to cidofovir, foscarnet, ganciclovir, and valganciclovir arises from mutations in the kinase, phosphotransferase, and/or DNA polymerase genes involved in viral replication.
    - The risk of resistance to ganciclovir and valganciclovir increases with the duration of therapy.
  - Resistance to letermovir is due to viral terminase complex genes involved in DNA packaging.

High-Yield Clinical Knowledge
- **Nephrotoxicity**
  - Cidofovir
    - Cidofovir has a Black Box Warning for nephrotoxicity.
    - The nephrotoxicity of cidofovir is related to its active tubular secretion in the kidney.
    - Nephrotoxicity can be minimized with the administration of probenecid and hydration before and following each cidofovir dose.
    - Probenecid competitively inhibits the organic anion transporter in the proximal tubule.
    - General dosing is probenecid 1 to 2 g and 1 liter of normal saline before and after the cidofovir infusion.
  - Foscarnet
    - Foscarnet has a Black Box Warning for renal impairment.

- Renal impairment may occur at any time during therapy, commonly during the second week of induction.
- Close monitoring of renal function is necessary, and dosage adjustments should be made for renal impairment.
- Ganciclovir and valganciclovir
  - There is an increased risk of nephrotoxicity in the elderly and with the use of concurrent nephrotoxic agents.

- **Myelosuppression**
  - Ganciclovir and valganciclovir
    - Myelosuppression is the dose-limiting adverse effect of ganciclovir and valganciclovir.
    - Neutropenia and thrombocytopenia are the most common effects.
      - Neutropenia is reversible upon discontinuation.
    - Myelosuppression usually develops within the first two weeks of treatment, and recovery occurs within three to seven days of discontinuation.
    - Use is not recommended with an absolute neutrophil count < 500 cells/mm^3, hemoglobin < 8 g/dL, or platelet count < 25,000 cells/mm^3.
  - Cidofovir
    - Neutropenia has been reported with cidofovir.

- **Carcinogenicity and Teratogenicity**
  - Cidofovir is carcinogenic and teratogenic and causes hypospermia in animals.
  - Ganciclovir and valganciclovir are carcinogenic and teratogenic and can impair fertility in humans.

- **Systemic and Intravitreal Administration**
  - CMV retinitis treatment with intravitreal injections should be given with concurrent systemic anti-CMV agents to prevent other end-organ diseases, including colitis, esophagitis, central nervous system disease, and pneumonitis

- **Treatment of Other CMV Infections**
  - CMV retinitis is the most common clinical manifestation of CMV infection.
  - Other manifestations include esophagitis, colitis, pneumonitis, and neurologic disease.
  - Esophagitis or colitis: IV ganciclovir followed by oral valganciclovir is the therapy of choice
  - Pneumonitis: ganciclovir or foscarnet is reasonable
    - Therapy for CMV pneumonitis has not been extensively studied.
  - Neurologic disease: both ganciclovir and foscarnet are recommended
    - Therapy for CMV neurologic disease has not been extensively studied.
    - Because patients with CMV neurologic disease have poor outcomes, experts recommend therapy initiation with both ganciclovir and foscarnet despite the risk of toxicities.

High-Yield Core Evidence
- **Prophylaxis In The Pre-modern Antiretroviral (ART) Era**
  - A prospective, randomized, double-blind, placebo-controlled study evaluated the efficacy and safety of oral ganciclovir in the prevention of CMV disease in people with acquired immunodeficiency syndrome (AIDS) and CD4+ lymphocyte counts less than 50 per cubic millimeter or less than 100 per cubic millimeter in those with a history of opportunistic infection.
  - Patients were randomized to receive either oral ganciclovir 1000 mg three times daily or a placebo.
  - The primary endpoint (development of CMV disease) occurred significantly less in the ganciclovir group than the placebo group, and there was no difference in mortality.
  - The authors concluded that prophylactic ganciclovir significantly reduces the risk of CMV disease in people with AIDS. (N Engl J Med. 1996 Jun 6;334:1491-7.)
  - In context, this study was before ART became widely available, and oral ganciclovir is no longer available in the United States.

- **Prophylaxis in The Modern ART Era**
  - A more recent prospective, randomized, double-blind, placebo-controlled study evaluated valganciclovir's efficacy in preventing CMV end-organ disease in people with AIDS and low CD4+ lymphocyte counts despite highly active antiretroviral therapy (HAART).
  - Patients were randomized to receive valganciclovir induction and maintenance doses (later amended to 900 mg daily when pharmacokinetic studies became available) or placebo.
  - The primary endpoint (time-to-CMV) and survival did not differ between the valganciclovir and placebo groups.
  - The authors concluded that prophylactic valganciclovir is not warranted for people with AIDS and low CD4+ lymphocyte counts who are receiving HAART given the low incidence of CMV end-organ disease and high all-cause mortality in the study population. (HIV Clin Trials. 2009 Sep 29;10(3):143-152.)
  - In context, the incidence of CMV has declined in the modern ART era, and primary prophylaxis is not recommended.

High-Yield Fast-Facts
- **Hazardous Agent**
  - Cidofovir is considered a hazardous agent by the National Institute for Occupational Safety and Health (NIOSH) due to its cytotoxic and mutagenic properties.
  - Appropriate precautions for preparing, receiving, handling, administration, and disposal should be taken.
    - Single gloves should be worn during receiving, unpacking, and placing in storage.
    - Double gloving, a gown, and closed system transfer devices are required during administration.
- **Once-Weekly Cidofovir Dosing**
  - Cidofovir has a half-life of about 2.6 hours.
  - The active metabolite of cidofovir, cidofovir diphosphate, has a half-life range of 24 to 87 hours, allowing for less frequent dosing.

HIGH-YIELD BOARD EXAM ESSENTIALS
- **CLASSIC AGENTS:** Cidofovir, foscarnet, ganciclovir, letermovir, valganciclovir
- **DRUG CLASS:** CMV antivirals
- **INDICATIONS:** CMV retinitis, HSV infection
- **MECHANISM:** Inhibit viral DNA synthesis by inhibiting viral DNA polymerases. Letermovir has a unique mechanism of inhibiting the CMV DNA terminase complex required for viral DNA processing and packaging.
- **SIDE EFFECTS:** Nephrotoxicity, hepatotoxicity, myelosuppression, teratogen
- **CLINICAL PEARLS:**
  - Valganciclovir is the prodrug of ganciclovir.
  - CMV retinitis treatment with intravitreal injections should be given with concurrent systemic anti-CMV agents to prevent other end-organ diseases, including colitis, esophagitis, central nervous system disease, and pneumonitis.

Table: Drug Class Summary

\multicolumn{4}{c}{**CMV Antivirals - Drug Class Review**}
\multicolumn{4}{c}{High-Yield Med Reviews}

Mechanism of Action: *Inhibit viral DNA synthesis by inhibiting viral DNA polymerases. Letermovir has a unique mechanism of inhibiting the CMV DNA terminase complex required for viral DNA processing and packaging.*

Class Effects: *Provide treatment and/or prophylaxis for CMV and several other viral infections. Cidofovir and foscarnet are reserved for resistant cases due to toxicity.*

Generic Name	Brand Name	Main Indication(s) or Uses	Notes

Cidofovir	N/A	- CMV retinitis treatment	- **Dosing (Adult):**
			  – IV: 5 mg/kg once weekly for 2 consecutive weeks, then 5 mg/kg once every 2 weeks (with concomitant probenecid)
			- **Dosing (Peds):**
			  – IV: 5 mg/kg once weekly for 2 consecutive weeks, then 3 to 5 mg/kg once every other week (with concomitant probenecid and IV hydration)
			- **CYP450 Interactions:** None
			- **Renal or Hepatic Dose Adjustments:**
			  – SCr increase by 0.3 to 0.4 mg/dL reduce dose to 30 mg/kg
			  – SCr increase by ≥ 0.5 mg/dL or development of ≥ 3+ proteinuria discontinue therapy
			- **Dosage Forms:** IV (solution)

Foscarnet	Foscavir	- CMV retinitis treatment
		- Herpes simplex virus (HSV) treatment
			- **Dosing (Adult):**
			  – IV: 60 to 90 mg/kg every 8 to 12 hours for 14 to 21 days, then IV 90 to 120 mg/kg once daily
			  – Intravitreal: 2.4 mg for 1 to 4 doses over a period of 7 to 10 days
			- **Dosing (Peds):**
			  – IV: 120 to 180 mg/kg/day in divided doses every 8 or 12 hours for 7 to 42 days, then 90 mg/kg once daily
			  – Intravitreal: 2.4 mg injection for 1 to 4 doses over a period of 7 to 10 days
			- **CYP450 Interactions:** None
			- **Renal or Hepatic Dose Adjustments:**
			  – Renal dose adjustments required when CrCl < 1.4 mL/min/kg; refer to manufacturer labeling
			- **Dosage Forms:** IV (solution)

| CMV Antivirals - Drug Class Review ||||
| High-Yield Med Reviews ||||
Generic Name	Brand Name	Main Indication(s) or Uses	Notes
Ganciclovir	Cytovene	<ul><li>CMV retinitis treatment</li><li>CMV prophylaxis</li></ul>	<ul><li>**Dosing (Adult):**<ul><li>IV: 5 mg/kg every 12 hours for 14 to 21 days, then 5 mg/kg every once daily</li><li>Intravitreal 2 mg for 1 to 4 doses over a period of 7 to 10 days</li></ul></li><li>**Dosing (Peds):**<ul><li>IV: 5 to 7.5 mg/kg every 12 hours for 14 to 21 days, then 5 mg/kg once daily for 5 to 7 days per week</li></ul></li><li>**CYP450 Interactions:** None</li><li>**Renal or Hepatic Dose Adjustments:**<ul><li>Renal dose adjustments required when CrCl < 70 mL/minute; refer to manufacturer labeling</li></ul></li><li>**Dosage Forms:** IV (solution)</li></ul>
Letermovir	Prevymis	<ul><li>CMV prophylaxis in allogeneic hematopoietic stem cell transplant (HSCT)</li></ul>	<ul><li>**Dosing (Adult):**<ul><li>Oral/IV: 480 mg once daily between day 0 and day 28 post-HSCT through day 100</li></ul></li><li>**Dosing (Peds):** Not used</li><li>**CYP450 Interactions:** Substrate CYP2D6, CYP3A4, Pgp</li><li>**Renal or Hepatic Dose Adjustments:**<ul><li>Child-Pugh class C use not recommended</li></ul></li><li>**Dosage Forms:** Oral (tablet), IV (solution)</li></ul>
Valganciclovir	Valcyte	<ul><li>CMV retinitis treatment in patients with acquired immunodeficiency syndrome (AIDS)</li><li>CMV prophylaxis in solid organ transplant recipients</li></ul>	<ul><li>**Dosing (Adult):**<ul><li>Treatment: Oral 900 mg twice daily for 14 to 21 day, then 900 mg once daily</li><li>Prophylaxis: 900 mg once daily</li></ul></li><li>**Dosing (Peds):**<ul><li>Treatment: Oral 900 mg twice daily for 14 to 21 days, then 900 mg once daily</li><li>Prophylaxis: (7 x BSA x CrCl) once daily<ul><li>CrCl calculation using modified Schwartz formula</li><li>Maximum of 900 mg/day</li></ul></li></ul></li><li>**CYP450 Interaction:** None</li><li>**Renal or Hepatic Dose Adjustments:**<ul><li>Renal dose adjustments required when CrCl < 60 mL/minute; refer to manufacturer labeling</li></ul></li><li>**Dosage Forms:** Oral (tablet, solution)</li></ul>

INFECTIOUS DISEASES – COVID-19 – COVID ANTI-INFECTIVES

Drug Class
- COVID Drugs
- Agents:
    - Acute Care, Ambulatory
        - Bebtelovimab
        - Convalescent plasma
        - Molnupiravir
        - Nirmatrelvir/ritonavir
        - Tixagevimab/cilgavimab
    - Acute Care, Hospitalized
        - Baricitinib
        - Sarilumab
        - Tocilizumab
        - Tofacitinib
    - Acute Care, Ambulatory and Hospitalized
        - Remdesivir

Main Indications or Uses
- Acute Care
    - SARS-CoV-2 (COVID-19)

Mechanism of Action
- **Bebtelovimab, tixagevimab/cilgavimab:**
    - Inhibit cell attachment and entry by targeting the SARS-CoV-2 spike protein
- **Baricitinib, sarilumab, tocilizumab, tofacitinib:**
    - Inhibit cytokine-mediated inflammation by either inhibiting Janus kinase (JAK) (baricitinib, tofacitinib) or interleukin-6 (IL-6) (sarilumab, tocilizumab)
    - Baricitinib is also proposed to prevent viral endocytosis by inhibiting AP2-associated protein kinase (AAK) and cyclin G-associated kinase (GAK) membrane proteins
- **Molnupiravir, nirmatrelvir/ritonavir, remdesivir:**
    - Inhibit multiple viral processes, including replication, protease function, and RNA polymerase function
- **Convalescent plasma:**
    - Neutralizes SARS-CoV-2 by antibody delivery, induces antibody-dependent cellular cytotoxicity and phagocytosis, and modulates the inflammatory response among multiple proposed mechanisms

Primary Overall Net Benefit
- Provide treatment or prophylaxis for SARS-CoV-2 infection
- Main Labs to Monitor:
    - Serum creatinine, liver enzymes, CBC, signs/symptoms of infection

High-Yield Basic Pharmacology
- **Targeting the Spike Protein**
    - Bebtelovimab and tixagevimab/cilgavimab are monoclonal antibodies derived from B lymphocytes of patients recovering from SARS-CoV-2 infection.
    - These monoclonal antibodies target the SARS-CoV-2 spike (S) protein, a structural protein located on the viral envelope that binds to the host angiotensin-converting enzyme 2 (ACE2) protein and induces membrane fusion.
        - Tixagevimab and cilgavimab bind to two different sites on the S protein.
- **Resistance Mechanisms**
    - Multiple mutations in the spike protein have markedly reduced susceptibility to several SARS-CoV-2 therapies and increased viral transmissibility.
    - Some variants also have mutations associated with enhanced binding to ACE2.

- Key variants that have been identified include Alpha, Beta, Gamma, Delta, and Omicron.

High-Yield Core Knowledge
- **Emergency Use Authorization**
    - The United States Food and Drug Administration (FDA) issued Emergency Use Authorizations (EUAs) to allow the use of unapproved medications or unapproved uses of approved medications under certain conditions during the COVID-19 public health emergency.
    - Remdesivir was FDA-approved on October 22, 2020, for SARS-CoV-2 treatment in hospitalized patients, and as of January 21, 2022, FDA approval expanded to SARS-CoV-2 treatment in nonhospitalized patients.
    - EUA criteria must be met for the use of other SARS-CoV-2 therapies:
        - Bebtelovimab, nirmatrelvir/ritonavir
            - Age ≥ 12 years and weight ≥ 40 kg
            - Positive results of direct SARS-CoV-2 testing
            - At high risk for progression to severe COVID-19, including hospitalization or death
        - Tixagevimab/cilgavimab
            - Age ≥ 12 years and weight ≥ 40 kg
            - No known current or recent SARS-CoV-2 exposure
            - Have moderate to severe immunocompromise and inadequate vaccine response or inability to be vaccinated or mount adequate vaccine response
        - Molnupiravir
            - Age ≥ 18 years
            - Positive results of direct SARS-CoV-2 testing
            - At high risk for progression to severe COVID-19, including hospitalization or death
            - appropriate
        - Baricitinib, tocilizumab
            - Age ≥ 2 years
            - Require supplemental oxygen, non-invasive or invasive mechanical ventilation, or extracorporeal membrane oxygenation (ECMO)
            - Currently receiving systemic corticosteroids (tocilizumab only)
        - Convalescent plasma
            - Have an immunosuppressive disease or are receiving immunosuppressive treatment (not including immunosuppressive treatment administered specifically for SARS-CoV-2 treatment)
- **Safety Concerns**
    - **Fetal Toxicity**
        - Based on animal reproduction studies, molnupiravir may cause fetal harm in pregnant individuals.
        - Females of childbearing potential should use contraception for the duration of molnupiravir treatment and for four days after the last dose.
        - Sexually active males should use contraception for the duration of molnupiravir treatment and for three months after the last dose.
    - **Drug interactions**
        - Ritonavir acts as a pharmacokinetic enhancer of nirmatrelvir by inhibiting cytochrome P450 (CYP) 3A4 involved in the metabolism of nirmatrelvir and many other medications.
        - Thus, potential drug interactions between nirmatrelvir/ritonavir and the patient's current medications must be reviewed.
        - Dose adjustments, temporary cessation of medications, and/or additional monitoring may be needed during and after nirmatrelvir/ritonavir treatment.
        - Commonly prescribed medications in which nirmatrelvir/ritonavir should be avoided altogether include rivaroxaban and salmeterol.
    - **Hepatotoxicity**
        - Remdesivir, baricitinib, and tofacitinib may cause reversible increases in liver enzymes, especially in patients receiving concomitant hepatotoxic medications, without clinically significant effects.

- Sarilumab and tocilizumab are associated with increases in liver enzymes and should not be initiated in patients with alanine aminotransferase (ALT) or aspartate aminotransferase (AST) > 1.5 times the upper limit of normal (ULN).
  - **Black Box Warnings**
    - Tofacitinib, baricitinib, sarilumab, and tocilizumab have a black box warning for serious infections.
      - Include tuberculosis, invasive fungal infections, and other opportunistic infections
      - Infection risk increases with concomitant immunosuppressants such as corticosteroids.
    - Tofacitinib and baricitinib additionally have the following black box warnings:
      - Mortality and major adverse cardiovascular events
      - Malignancies
      - Thrombosis
        - Patients treated with tofacitinib for SARS-CoV-2 should be on at least a prophylactic dose anticoagulant.

High-Yield Clinical Knowledge
- **Selection of Therapy for Nonhospitalized Patients**
  - Pre-exposure prophylaxis: tixagevimab/cilgavimab
    - May be given ≥ 2 weeks following SARS-CoV-2 vaccination
  - Treatment:
    - Outpatient therapy is for patients with mild-to-moderate SARS-CoV-2 infection.
      - Mild infection: signs and symptoms of SARS-CoV-2 infection are present in the absence of shortness of breath, dyspnea, or abnormal chest imaging
      - Moderate infection: evidence of lower respiratory tract disease during clinical assessment or imaging, and oxygen saturation > 94% on room air
    - Treatment options based on symptom onset:
      - ≤ 5 days: nirmtrelvir/ritonavir, molnupiravir
      - ≤ 7 days: remdesivir, bebtelovimab
      - ≤ 8 days: convalescent plasma
      - > 8 days: supportive care
    - Preferred therapies (listed in order of preference): nirmatrelvir/ritonavir, remdesivir
    - Alternative therapies: bebtelovimab, molnupiravir, convalescent plasma
- **Selection of Therapy for Hospitalized Patients**
  - Convalescent plasma is not recommended in these patients.
  - Treatment selection for hospitalized patients depends on disease severity.
    - Mild-to-moderate infection:
      - Remdesivir: for patients requiring minimal supplemental oxygen (not mechanical ventilation or ECMO)
    - Severe infection: oxygen saturation ≤ 94% on room air, ratio of arterial partial pressure of oxygen to fraction of inspired oxygen (PaO2/FiO2) < 300 mm Hg, respiratory rate > 30 breaths/minute, or lung infiltrates > 50%
      - Remdesivir: for patients requiring minimal supplemental oxygen (not mechanical ventilation or ECMO)
        - Remdesivir or dexamethasone may be used alone or in combination.
      - Tofacitinib: for patients on room air, supplemental oxygen, or high-flow oxygen (not non-invasive or invasive ventilation)
        - Should not receive tocilizumab or sarilumab for SARS-CoV-2 treatment
      - Baricitinib or tocilizumab: for patients on dexamethasone with/without remdesivir who have rapidly increased oxygen needs and systemic inflammation
      - Tocilizumab with dexamethasone: for patients requiring mechanical ventilation or ECMO
        - Sarilumab: if tocilizumab is not available or feasible to use
  - Recommended timing of therapy
    - Remdesivir: as soon as possible after diagnosis, ≤ 72 hours of positive SARS-CoV-2 test

- Tofacitinib: ≤ 3 days of hospital admission
- Sarilumab: ≤ 3 days of hospital admission or ≤ 24 hours of ICU admission

High-Yield Core Evidence
- Nirmatrelvir/ritonavir and the EPIC trials
    - EPIC-HR was a phase 2/3, randomized, placebo-controlled trial that compared nirmatrelvir/ritonavir to placebo in unvaccinated, symptomatic COVID-19 patients with a high risk of disease progression. The study demonstrated statistically significant reductions in both hospitalizations (1% vs 6.7%, p<0.001) and 28-day mortality (0% vs 1.6%, p<0.001). Overall composite outcome of deaths and hospitalizations demonstrated an 89% reduction, an NNT 17 to prevent hospitalizations, and an NNT 62 to prevent death.
    - EPIC-SR was designed to evaluate nirmatrelvir/ritonavir versus placebo in vaccinated and unvaccinated patients with standard-risk for developing severe COVID-19. Unfortunately, the trial was terminated early due to low hospitalization or death rates in the standard-risk population.
- Molnupiravir and the MOVe trials
    - MOVe-OUT was a phase 3, double-blind, randomized, placebo-controlled trial that evaluated nonhospitalized patients initiated on molnupiravir within 5 days of COVID-19 symptom onset versus placebo. The primary endpoint of death or hospitalization for any cause at day 29 was lower in the molnupiravir group (7.3% vs. 14.1%, 95% CI, −5.9 to −0.1).
    - MOVe-IN was a phase 2/3, randomized, placebo-controlled, double-blind trial that evaluated hospitalized patients initiated on molnupiravir within 10 days of symptom onset versus placebo. Unfortunately, the study failed to demonstrate clinical benefit in this patient population.

High-Yield Fast-Fact
- **The Power of Thor's Hammer**
    - Thor's hammer, Mjölnir, inspired Molnupiravir's name.
- **Repurposed Medications**
    - There have been many attempts at repurposing medications for the treatment of COVID-19. Such examples include antimalarial agents (hydroxychloroquine, chloroquine), HIV protease inhibitors (lopinavir/ritonavir), and antiparasitic agents (ivermectin). Unfortunately, to date, none of these repurposed medications have demonstrated clinical benefit for the treatment of COVID-19.
    - The National Poison Data System had a 212% increase in reported ivermectin exposure cases between January and September 2021.

Table: Drug Class Summary

COVID Anti-Infectives - Drug Class Review High-Yield Med Reviews			
Mechanism of Action: *Inhibit multiple viral processes or modulate the inflammatory response*			
Class Effects: *Provide treatment or prophylaxis for SARS-CoV-2 infection*			
Generic Name	**Brand Name**	**Main Indication(s) or Uses**	**Notes**

Baricitinib	Olumiant	• COVID-19, severe	• **Dosing (Adult):** 4 mg PO daily x 14 days or until hospital discharge, whichever is first
			• **Dosing (Peds):** 2-4 mg PO daily x 14 days or until hospital discharge, whichever is first
			• **CYP450 Interactions:** None
			• **Renal or Hepatic Dose Adjustments:**
			  — eGFR 30-60 mL/min: 2 mg PO daily
			  — eGFR 15-30 mL/min: 1 mg PO daily
			  — eGFR < 15 mL/min: Use not recommended
			• **Dosage Forms:** Oral (tablet)

Bebtelovimab	N/A	• COVID-19, mild-to-moderate	• **Dosing (Adult):** 175 mg IV once
			  — Administer within 7 days of symptom onset
			  — Reserve use for those at high risk of progression to severe disease
			• **Dosing (Peds):** 175 mg IV once
			• **CYP450 Interactions:** None
			• **Renal or Hepatic Dose Adjustments:** None
			• **Dosage Forms:** IV (solution)

Convalescent plasma	N/A	• COVID-19	• **Dosing (Adult):** 1 unit (200-250 mL) IV once • **Dosing (Peds):** N/A • **CYP450 Interactions:** None • **Renal or Hepatic Dose Adjustments:** None • **Dosage Forms:** IV (plasma)
Molnupiravir	Lagevrio	• COVID-19, mild-to-moderate	• **Dosing (Adult):** 800 mg PO BID x 5 days — Administer within 5 days of symptom onset • **Dosing (Peds):** N/A • **CYP450 Interactions:** None • **Renal or Hepatic Dose Adjustments:** None • **Dosage Forms:** Oral (capsule)

Nirmatrelvir/ ritonavir	Paxlovid	• COVID-19, mild-to-moderate	• **Dosing (Adult):** Nirmatrelvir 300 mg/ritonavir 100 mg PO BID x 5 days
			  — Administer within 5 days of symptom onset
			• **Dosing (Peds):** Nirmatrelvir 300 mg/ritonavir 100 mg PO BID x 5 days
			• **CYP450 Interactions:** Substrate of CYP1A2, CYP2D6, CYP3A4; Inhibits CYP2D6, CYP3A4; Induces 1A2, 2B6, 2C19, 2C9
			• **Renal or Hepatic Dose Adjustments:**
			  — eGFR 30-60 mL/min: Nirmaltrelvir 150 mg/ritonavir 100 mg PO BID
			  — eGFR < 30 mL/min: Avoid use
			• **Dosage Forms:** Oral (tablet)

COVID Anti-Infectives - Drug Class Review
High-Yield Med Reviews

Generic Name	Brand Name	Main Indication(s) or Uses	Notes
Remdesivir	Veklury	• COVID-19	• **Dosing (Adult):** 100-200 mg IV daily x 3-10 days • **Dosing (Peds):** 2.5-5 mg/kg (up to 100-200 mg) IV daily x 3-10 days • **CYP450 Interactions:** Substrate of CYP2C8, CYP2D6, CYP3A4 • **Renal or Hepatic Dose Adjustments:** None • **Dosage Forms:** IV (solution)
Sarilumab	Kevzara	• COVID-19, severe	• **Dosing (Adult):** 400 mg IV once • **Dosing (Peds):** N/A • **CYP450 Interactions:** May modulate the expression and activity of CYP 450 enzymes • **Renal or Hepatic Dose Adjustments:** None • **Dosage Forms:** IV (solution)
Tixagevimab/ cilgavimab	Evusheld	• COVID-19, pre-exposure prophylaxis	• **Dosing (Adult):** Tixagevimab 300 mg/cilgavimab 300 mg IM once • **Dosing (Peds):** Tixagevimab 300 mg/cilgavimab 300 mg IM once • **CYP450 Interactions:** None • **Renal or Hepatic Dose Adjustments:** None • **Dosage Forms:** IM (solution)

Tocilizumab	Actemra	• COVID-19, severe	• **Dosing (Adult):** 8 mg/kg IV once
			   − May repeat dose once after ≥ 8 hours
			• **Dosing (Peds):** 8-12 mg/kg IV once
			   − May repeat dose once after ≥ 8 hours
			• **CYP450 Interactions:** May modulate the expression and activity of CYP 450 enzymes
			• **Renal or Hepatic Dose Adjustments:** None
			• **Dosage Forms:** IV (solution)

Tofacitinib	Xeljanz	• COVID-19, severe	• **Dosing (Adult):** 10 mg PO BID x 14 days or until hospital discharge, whichever is first
			• **Dosing (Peds):** N/A
			• **CYP450 Interactions:** None
			• **Renal or Hepatic Dose Adjustments:**
			   − Moderate to severe renal impairment or on hemodialysis: 5 mg PO BID
			   − Moderate hepatic impairment: 5 mg PO BID
			   − Severe hepatic impairment: Use not recommended
			• **Dosage Forms:** Oral (tablet)

INFECTIOUS DISEASE – HEPATITIS B ANTIVIRALS

Drug Class
- Hepatitis B Antivirals
- Agents:
    - Acute & Chronic Care
        - Adefovir dipivoxil
        - Entecavir
        - Lamivudine
        - Tenofovir disoproxil/Alafenamide

Main Indications or Uses
- Acute & Chronic Care
    - Hepatitis B (HBV)

Mechanism of Action
- Competitive inhibition of HBV DNA polymerase and reverse transcriptase, causing chain termination.

Primary Net Benefit
- Anti-HBV agents provide viral load suppression, although unable to establish a clinical cure.
- Main Labs to Monitor:
    - HBV DNA
    - HBeAg, anti-HBe, HBsAg
    - Liver enzymes (AST/ALT)
    - Liver function (INR/PT, albumin, protein, bilirubin)
    - Serum creatinine
    - CBC

High-Yield Basic Pharmacology
- Adefovir Prodrug
    - Adefovir dipivoxil is a prodrug of adefovir, an acyclic phosphonated adenine nucleotide analog.
- Nucleoside Vs. Nucleotide
    - All available agents in this class, except for tenofovir, are nucleosides that must be triphosphorylated to exert their activity.
    - Teno*fovir* is a nucleo*tide* monophosphate that must undergo two additional phosphorylations for its antiretroviral activity.
- Tenofovir Alafenamide Vs Disoproxil
    - Tenofovir is formulated as two separate prodrugs, alafenamide or disoproxil.
    - The alafenamide was developed to improve oral absorption substantially and is associated with a lower risk of renal toxicity and bone marrow toxicity.

High-Yield Clinical Knowledge
- Lamivudine and Tenofovir Dosing
    - Lamivudine and tenofovir disoproxil are used for HIV-1 and HIV-2 at 300 mg daily or 150 mg twice daily and 300 or 150 mg daily, respectively.
    - For hepatitis B, lamivudine can also be used, but at 100 mg twice daily.
        - To treat coinfection with HIV and HBV, the HIV dosing (300 mg or 150 mg BID dosing).
    - Tenofovir disoproxil for HBV is used at a dose of 300 or 100 mg daily, leading to virologic failure in HIV co-infected patients.
- Toxicities
    - Anti-HBV antivirals may adversely affect the DNA polymerase gamma of human mitochondria, resulting in mitochondrial toxicities, including myopathies, peripheral neuropathies, pancreatitis, anemias, and granulocytopenia.

- These agents are rarely associated with lactic acidosis and hepatic steatosis.
- **HIV and HBV Coinfection**
  - Of the anti-HBV agents, tenofovir and lamivudine have clinically relevant HIV antiretroviral activity.
  - In patients with HIV and HBV coinfection, exacerbations of HBV may occur if one of these agents is discontinued.
- **Resistance and Mutations**
  - The terminology for resistance describes the target amino acid, its position, and the amino acid that has been substituted.
    - For example, an M184V mutation where methionine is substituted for valine at position 184.
  - In patients with HIV coinfection, appropriate NRTI selection should reduce the likelihood of M184V variant resistance, as observed with entecavir therapy.
- **Serum Creatinine Changes**
  - Adefovir is associated with a reversible increase in serum creatinine that is not a reflection of changes in renal function.
- **Pregnancy**
  - Adefovir should be avoided in pregnant patients as animal models have suggested this agent is embryotoxic and genotoxic.
  - Lamivudine may be suitable for therapy in pregnant patients as it has effectively prevented vertical transmission of HBV when given for the last four weeks of gestation.

High-Yield Core Evidence
- **Tenofovir Disoproxil to Alafenamide Conversion**
  - This was a multicentre, double-blind, phase 3 non-inferiority study that evaluated the efficacy and safety of tenofovir alafenamide in patients with HBV infection switching from tenofovir disoproxil fumarate who are virally suppressed.
  - Patients were randomized to receive either tenofovir alafenamide 25 mg once a day or continue tenofovir disoproxil fumarate 300 mg once a day.
  - Non-inferiority between the agents was established regarding the primary outcome of loss of virological control, defined as the proportion of patients who received at least one dose of the study drug with HBV DNA of at least 20 IU/mL at week 48.
  - Tenofovir alafenamide was associated with a significant increase in bone mineral density at the hip, and at the spine, and improved markers of bone turnover and tubular function at week 48
  - However, tenofovir alafenamide was associated with a significantly decreased but not clinically relevant decrease in creatinine clearance by Cockcroft-Gault relative to tenofovir disoproxil fumarate.
  - The authors concluded that these findings suggest that tenofovir alafenamide can be substituted for tenofovir disoproxil fumarate in patients with HBV infection for improved safety without losing efficacy. (Lancet Gastroenterol Hepatol. 2020 May;5(5):441-453.)

High-Yield Fast-Fact
- **Telbivudine**
  - As a result of the emergence of resistance and questionable efficacy compared to existing anti-HBV agents, telbivudine is no longer recommended for HBV treatment.

HIGH-YIELD BOARD EXAM ESSENTIALS
- **CLASSIC AGENTS:** Adefovir dipivoxil, entecavir, lamivudine, tenofovir disoproxil/alafenamide
- **DRUG CLASS:** Hepatitis B antivirals
- **INDICATIONS:** HBV infection
- **MECHANISM:** Competitive inhibition of HBV DNA polymerase and reverse transcriptase, causing chain termination.
- **SIDE EFFECTS:** Myopathies, peripheral neuropathies, pancreatitis, anemias, and granulocytopenia.
- **CLINICAL PEARLS:** Adefovir is associated with a reversible increase in serum creatinine that is not a reflection of changes in renal function.

Table: Drug Class Summary

Hepatitis B Antivirals - Drug Class Review High-Yield Med Reviews			
Mechanism of Action: *Competitive inhibition of HBV DNA polymerase and reverse transcriptase, causing chain termination.*			
Class Effects: *Anti-HBV agents provide viral load suppression, although unable to establish a clinical cure.*			
Generic Name	**Brand Name**	**Main Indication(s) or Uses**	**Notes**
Adefovir dipivoxil	Hepsera	• Hepatitis B	• **Dosing (Adult):** — Oral: 10 mg daily • **Dosing (Peds):** — Oral: 0.25 to 0.3 mg/kg/dose daily — Maximum 10 mg/dose • **CYP450 Interactions:** None • **Renal or Hepatic Dose Adjustments:** — GFR 30 to 49 mL/minute - 10 mg q48h — GFR 10 to 29 mL/minute - 10 mg q72h • **Dosage Forms:** Oral (tablet)
Entecavir	Baraclude	• Hepatitis B	• **Dosing (Adult):** — Oral: 0.5 to 1 mg daily • **Dosing (Peds):** — Oral: 0.15 to 1 mg daily • **CYP450 Interactions:** text • **Renal or Hepatic Dose Adjustments:** — GFR 30 to 49 mL/minute - 0.25 to 0.5 mg q48h — GFR 10 to 29 mL/minute - 0.15 to 0.3 mg q72h — GFR < 10 - 0.05 mg to 0.1 mg daily or normal dose every 7 days • **Dosage Forms:** Oral (solution, tablet)
Lamivudine	Epivir, Epivir HBV	• HIV • Hepatitis B	• **Dosing (Adult):** — HIV — Oral: 300 mg daily or 150 mg BID — HBV — Oral: 100 mg daily • **Dosing (Peds):** — Oral 30 to 150 mg BID • **CYP450 Interactions:** None • **Renal or Hepatic Dose Adjustments:** HIV indication — GFR 30 to 49 mL/minute - 150 mg daily — GFR 15 to 29 mL/minute - 150 mg x1 then 100 mg daily — GFR less than 15 mL/minute - 150 mg x1 then 50 mg daily — GFR < 5 - 50 mg, then 25 mg daily • **Dosage Forms:** Oral (solution, tablet)

Hepatitis B Antivirals - Drug Class Review
High-Yield Med Reviews

Generic Name	Brand Name	Main Indication(s) or Uses	Notes
Tenofovir alafenamide	Vemlidy	- Hepatitis B	- **Dosing (Adult):** 　- HIV 　　- Only available in combination with other ART (Biktarvy, Genvoya, Odefsey, Symtuza) 　- HBV 　　- Oral: 25 mg daily - **Dosing (Peds):** 　- Not routinely used - **CYP450 Interactions:** None - **Renal or Hepatic Dose Adjustments:** 　- GFR < 15 mL/minute - Not recommended 　- Child-Pugh class B or C - Not recommended - **Dosage Forms:** Oral (tablet)
Tenofovir disoproxil	Viread	- Hepatitis B - HIV	- **Dosing (Adult):** 　- HIV 　　- Oral: 300 mg daily or 150 mg BID 　- HBV 　　- Oral: 100 or 300 mg daily - **Dosing (Peds):** 　- Oral: 8 mg/kg/dose daily 　　- Maximum 300 mg/day - **CYP450 Interactions:** None - **Renal or Hepatic Dose Adjustments:** HIV indication 　- GFR 30 to 49 mL/minute - 300 mg q48h 　- GFR 10 to 29 mL/minute - 300 mg q72h 　- GFR < 10 mL/minute - Not recommended - **Dosage Forms:** Oral (solution, tablet)

INFECTIOUS DISEASE – HEPATITIS C ANTIVIRALS

Drug Class
- Hepatitis C Antivirals
- Agents:
- Chronic Care
    - Elbasvir and Grazoprevir
    - Glecaprevir and Pibrentasvir
    - Ombitasvir, Paritaprevir, and Ritonavir
    - Ombitasvir, Paritaprevir, Ritonavir, and Dasabuvir
    - Sofosbuvir
    - Sofosbuvir and Velpatasvir
    - Sofosbuvir and Ledipasvir
    - Sofosbuvir, Velpatasvir, and Voxilaprevir

> **Knowledge Integration**
> ✓ Most strains of HCV can now be treated with these oral antivirals and be cured after only 12 weeks of therapy. This is a huge benefit compared to older regimens that could take up to 1 year and not always result in cure.

Main Indications or Uses
- Chronic Care
    - Hepatitis C infection

Mechanism of Action
- **NS3/4A Inhibitor (Grazoprevir, Paritaprevir)**
    - Inhibition of the NS3/4A protease, responsible for cleaving the HCV polyprotein into the proteins that enable HCV RNA replication and virion assembly.
- **NS5A Inhibitors (Elbasvir, Ledipasvir, Ombitasvir, Velpatasvir)**
    - Inhibits nonstructural protein 5A (NS5A), an RNA-binding protein essential for HCV RNA replication, virion assembly, and modulation of host cells.
- **NS5B RNA Polymerase Inhibitors (Dasabuvir, Sofosbuvir)**
    - Bind to the catalytic site of nonstructural protein 5B (NS5B), inhibiting RNA replication by causing chain termination and increasing transcription errors.

Primary Net Benefit
- The direct-acting antivirals have transformed HCV treatment and are significantly better tolerated than alternatives (interferon products).
- Main Labs to Monitor:
    - HCV viral load
    - HCV genotype and subtype
    - CBC with differential
    - Serum creatinine
    - Liver function (INR/PT, albumin, protein, bilirubin)
    - Liver enzymes (AST/ALT, alk phos)

> **Warnings & Alerts**
> ✓ Use caution or avoid the coadministration of sofosbuvir and amiodarone due to the risk of symptomatic bradycardia.

High-Yield Basic Pharmacology
- **Ritonavir**
    - The HIV protease inhibitor ritonavir lacks HCV antiviral properties but acts as a pharmacokinetic boosting agent in the combination referred to as PrOD (paritaprevir, ritonavir, ombitasvir, and dasabuvir).
- **Notable Drug Interactions**
    - The combination of sofosbuvir and amiodarone should be avoided as numerous reports of symptomatic bradycardia have occurred due to this interaction.
        - This interaction's mechanism is unclear, as sofosbuvir is not a CYP 450 substrate, and a P-glycoprotein-related mechanism would increase sofosbuvir concentrations, not those of amiodarone.
    - The interaction with digoxin is more apparent as competition for P-glycoprotein leads to decreased elimination of digoxin and results in clinical toxicity.

- Digoxin should also be avoided among patients receiving velpatasvir due to p-glycoprotein inhibition.
- Velpatasvir should not be used with pravastatin or rosuvastatin, as the AUC may increase by 35% or 170%, respectively.

High-Yield Clinical Knowledge
- **PPI and H2RA Spacing**
  - Patients taking HCV antivirals with concomitant H2RA or PPI require specific administration spacing considerations to avoid clinically relevant decreases in drug absorption.
  - H2RAs should not exceed doses of famotidine 40 mg twice daily, or equivalent, and may be taken simultaneously as HCV antivirals or spaced by 12 hours.
  - PPIs should be administered 4 hours before velpatasvir administration.
- **P-glycoprotein and CYP3A4**
  - All of these agents are substrates of P-glycoprotein.
    - Therefore, they should not be combined with inducers of P-gp, including rifampin, phenytoin, phenobarbital, or St. John's wort which could result in therapeutic failure.
  - These agents are also substrates of a relatively newly described efflux transporter, breast cancer resistance protein (BCRP).
  - All agents, except for sofosbuvir, are substrates of CYP3A4 with numerous drug interactions that may impact drug efficacy outcomes.
- **Ribavirin Combination**
  - For HCV regimens containing sofosbuvir/velpatasvir in patients without cirrhosis but who have Y93 resistance identified, ribavirin can be added to avoid conversion to an alternative regimen.
  - Ribavirin may also be used with other HCV regimens, with increased sustained virologic response rates and different NS5A resistance-associated variants.
- **HIV Coinfection**
  - Coinfection of HCV and HIV is encountered in clinical practice, and specific considerations of drug interactions are necessary to maintain efficacy and ensure safety.
  - Sofosbuvir/velpatasvir may significantly increase tenofovir disoproxil fumarate concentrations, leading to dose-dependent toxicities, including renal injury.
  - Efavirenz and tipranavir/ritonavir are associated with significant reductions in velpatasvir concentrations, and these combinations are not recommended.
  - Numerous combinations lack clinically relevant interactions, including newer protease inhibitors (e.g., atazanavir, darunavir) and elvitegravir/cobicistat/emtricitabine/tenofovir alafenamide.
- **Resistance Associated Variants (RAV)**
  - The emergency of resistance to HCV antiviral agents is termed resistance-associated variants (RAV).
  - The clinical consequences of RAVs are specific to the clinical outcomes of HCV drug therapy. Therefore, they are dependent on patient treatment experience (treatment-naive vs. treatment-experienced), and the particular RAVs identified.
- **Hemolytic Anemia**
  - In regimens that include ribavirin for HCV treatment, ribavirin's addition comes with an increased risk of dose-dependent toxicities, primarily hemolytic anemia.
  - Hemolytic anemia occurs within the first two weeks of ribavirin treatment in 20% of patients.
  - Patients receiving ribavirin must be instructed to use two effective contraception forms by each sexual partner during treatment and six months after drug discontinuation.

High-Yield Core Evidence
- **FISSION and NEUTRINO**
  - This was a single publication of two phases 3 studies sharing a primary endpoint of a sustained virologic response at 12 weeks after therapy.
  - The first study was a single group, open-label study of patients with untreated HCV infection who received a 12-week regimen of sofosbuvir plus peginterferon alfa-2a and ribavirin patients with HCV genotype 1, 4, 5, or 6 (of whom 98% had genotype 1 or 4).
    - Sustained virologic response was reported in 90% of patients.

- The second was a noninferiority trial of HCV genotype 2 or 3 infections randomized to either sofosbuvir plus ribavirin for 12 weeks or peginterferon alfa-2a plus ribavirin for 24 weeks. In the two studies.
    - The sustained response was reported in a similar proportion of patients in the sofosbuvir–ribavirin group and the peginterferon–ribavirin group.
- Response rates in the sofosbuvir–ribavirin group were lower among patients with genotype 3 infection than those with genotype 2 infection.
- Fatigue, headache, nausea, and neutropenia were less common with sofosbuvir than with peginterferon.
- The authors concluded that sofosbuvir combined with peginterferon–ribavirin, patients with predominantly genotype 1 or 4 HCV infection had a rate of sustained virologic response of 90% at 12 weeks. In a noninferiority trial, patients with genotype 2 or 3 infections who received either sofosbuvir or peginterferon with ribavirin had nearly identical response rates (67%). In addition, adverse events were less frequent with sofosbuvir than with peginterferon. (N Engl J Med 2013; 368:1878-1887.)

- **ASTRAL-1**
    - This was a phase 3, double-blind, placebo-controlled study that randomized untreated and previously treated patients with chronic HCV genotype 1, 2, 4, 5, or 6 infections, including those with compensated cirrhosis to receive sofosbuvir plus velpatasvir in a once-daily, fixed-dose combination tablet or matching placebo for 12 weeks.
    - For the primary endpoint of a sustained virologic response at 12 weeks after the end of therapy, sofosbuvir–velpatasvir achieved a sustained virologic response of 99%, compared to zero patients receiving placebo.
    - However, two patients receiving sofosbuvir–velpatasvir, both with HCV genotype 1, had a virologic relapse.
    - The authors concluded that once-daily sofosbuvir–velpatasvir for 12 weeks provided high rates of sustained virologic response among previously treated and untreated patients infected with HCV genotypes 1, 2, 4, 5, or 6, including those with compensated cirrhosis. (N Engl J Med 2015; 373:2599-2607.)

HIGH-YIELD BOARD EXAM ESSENTIALS
- **CLASSIC AGENTS:** Dasabuvir, elbasvir, grazoprevir, ledipasvir, ombitasvir, paritaprevir, sofosbuvir, velpatasvir
- **DRUG CLASS:** Hepatitis C antivirals
- **INDICATIONS:** Chronic hepatitis C
- **MECHANISM:** NS3/4A Inhibitor (Grazoprevir, Paritaprevir). NS5A Inhibitors (Elbasvir, Ledipasvir, Ombitasvir, Velpatasvir). NS5B RNA Polymerase Inhibitors (Dasabuvir, Sofosbuvir)
- **SIDE EFFECTS:** Hepatotoxicity, hemolytic anemia (ribavirin combination)
- **CLINICAL PEARLS:** Most regimens can treat common strains of hepatitis C after 12 weeks of oral therapy. Patients taking HCV antivirals with concomitant H2RA or PPI require specific administration spacing considerations to avoid clinically relevant decreases in drug absorption.

Table: Drug Class Summary

Hepatitis C Antivirals - Drug Class Review			
High-Yield Med Reviews			
Mechanism of Action: See text for additional details on each agent..			
Class Effects: *The direct-acting antivirals have transformed HCV treatment and are significantly better tolerated than alternatives (interferon products).*			
Generic Name	**Brand Name**	**Main Indication(s) or Uses**	**Notes**

Elbasvir and Grazoprevir	Zepatier	• Chronic Hepatitis C	• **Dosing (Adult):**
			    – Oral: 1 tablet daily for 12 to 16 weeks
			 • **Dosing (Peds):**
			    – Not routinely used
			 • **CYP450 Interactions:** Substrate CYP3A4, P-gp
			 • **Renal or Hepatic Dose Adjustments:**
			    – Child-Pugh class B or C - contraindicated
			 • **Dosage Forms:** Oral (capsule)

Glecaprevir and Pibrentasvir	Maviret	• Chronic Hepatitis C	• **Dosing (Adult):**
			    – Oral: three tablets daily for 8 to 16 weeks
			 • **Dosing (Peds):**
			    – For children at least 45 kg or at least 12 years of age, use adult dosing
			 • **CYP450 Interactions:** Substrate CYP3A4, P-gp; Inhibits CYP1A2, 3A4, P-gp
			 • **Renal or Hepatic Dose Adjustments:**
			    – Child-Pugh class B or C - contraindicated
			 • **Dosage Forms:** Oral (tablet)

Ombitasvir, Paritaprevir, and Ritonavir	Technivie	• Chronic Hepatitis C	• **Dosing (Adult):**
			    – Oral: two tablets daily for 12 weeks
			 • **Dosing (Peds):**
			    – Not routinely used
			 • **CYP450 Interactions:** Substrate CYP2D6, 3A4, P-gp; Inhibits CYP3A4; Induces CYP1A2, 2C19
			 • **Renal or Hepatic Dose Adjustments:**
			    – Child-Pugh class B or C - contraindicated
			 • **Dosage Forms:** Oral (tablet)

Ombitasvir, Paritaprevir, Ritonavir, and Dasabuvir	Viekira	• Chronic Hepatitis C	• **Dosing (Adult):**
			    – Oral: two to three tablets daily for 12 to 24 weeks
			 • **Dosing (Peds):**
			    – Not routinely used
			 • **CYP450 Interactions:** Substrate CYP2C8, 2D6, 3A4, P-gp; Inhibits CYP3A4; Induces CYP1A2, 2C19
			
			 • **Renal or Hepatic Dose Adjustments:**
			    – Child-Pugh class B or C - contraindicated
			 • **Dosage Forms:** Oral (tablet)

Hepatitis C Antivirals - Drug Class Review
High-Yield Med Reviews

Generic Name	Brand Name	Main Indication(s) or Uses	Notes

Sofosbuvir	Sovaldi	- Chronic Hepatitis C	- **Dosing (Adult):**
			   — Oral: 400 mg daily for 12 to 16 weeks
			- **Dosing (Peds):**
			   — Oral: 150 to 400 mg daily for 12 to 24 weeks
			- **CYP450 Interactions:** Substrate P-gp
			- **Renal or Hepatic Dose Adjustments:**
			   — Child-Pugh class B or C - contraindicated
			- **Dosage Forms:** Oral (tablet)

Sofosbuvir and Velpatasvir	Epclusa	- Chronic Hepatitis C	- **Dosing (Adult):**
			   — Oral: one tablets daily for 12 to 24 weeks
			- **Dosing (Peds):**
			   — Oral: sofosbuvir 200-400 mg/velpatasvir 50-100 mg daily for 12 to 24 weeks
			- **CYP450 Interactions:** Substrate CYP2B6, 2C8, 3A4, P-gp
			- **Renal or Hepatic Dose Adjustments:**
			   — Child-Pugh class B or C - contraindicated
			- **Dosage Forms:** Oral (tablet)

Sofosbuvir and Ledipasvir	Harvoni	- Chronic Hepatitis C	- **Dosing (Adult):**
			   — Oral: sofosbuvir 400 mg/ledipasvir 90 mg daily for 12 to 24 weeks
			- **Dosing (Peds):**
			   — Oral: sofosbuvir 150-400 mg/ledipasvir 33.75-90 mg daily for 12 to 24 weeks
			- **CYP450 Interactions:** Substrate P-gp
			- **Renal or Hepatic Dose Adjustments:** None
			- **Dosage Forms:** Oral (pellets, tablet)

Sofosbuvir, Velpatasvir, and Voxilaprevir	Vosevi	- Chronic Hepatitis C	- **Dosing (Adult):**
			   — Oral: two tablets daily for 12 to 24 weeks
			- **Dosing (Peds):**
			   — Not routinely used
			- **CYP450 Interactions:** Substrate CYP2B6, 2C8, 3A4, P-gp
			- **Renal or Hepatic Dose Adjustments:**
			   — Child-Pugh class B or C - contraindicated
			- **Dosage Forms:** Oral (tablet)

INFECTIOUS DISEASE – HSV AND VZV ANTIVIRALS

Drug Class
- HSV and VZV Antiviral
- Agents:
    - Acute Care
        - Acyclovir
        - Docosanol (Topical)
        - Famciclovir
        - Penciclovir (Topical)
        - Trifluridine (Topical)
        - Valacyclovir

> **Dosing Pearl**
> ✓ Valacyclovir is the prodrug of acyclovir and allows for improved oral absorption thereby allowing for less frequent daily dosing to improve compliance.

Main Indications or Uses
- Acute Care
    - Herpes simplex virus (HSV)
    - Varicella-zoster virus (VZV)

Mechanism of Action
- **Acyclovir, famciclovir, penciclovir, trifluridine, valacyclovir**
    - Inhibit viral DNA synthesis by inhibiting viral DNA polymerases. This results in decreases in viral replication.
        - Acyclovir and valacyclovir can also be incorporated into viral DNA and terminate viral DNA synthesis.
        - Trifluridine also irreversibly inhibits thymidylate synthase involved in viral DNA synthesis.
- **Docosanol**
    - Prevents viral entry into the cell by inhibiting fusion between the plasma membrane and viral envelope.

Primary Net Benefit
- Provide acute treatment and/or suppression for HSV, VZV, and several other viral infections
- Main Labs to Monitor:
    - Serum creatinine, liver enzymes, CBC

High-Yield Basic Pharmacology
- **Prodrug Metabolism**
    - Valacyclovir to Acyclovir
        - Valacyclovir is rapidly converted to acyclovir by intestinal mucosal cells and hepatocytes.
        - The oral bioavailability of valacyclovir is 54 to 70% compared to 15 to 20% with acyclovir; bioavailability is unaffected by food.
    - Famciclovir to Penciclovir
        - Famciclovir is rapidly deacetylated and oxidized to penciclovir by first-pass metabolism.
        - The oral bioavailability of famciclovir is 70%
            - Food decreases the rate of absorption and peak concentration of penciclovir but does not affect bioavailability.
- **Resistance Mechanisms**
    - HSV and VZV resistance to acyclovir, famciclovir penciclovir, and valacyclovir arise from decreased thymidine kinase production, altered thymidine kinase, and/or altered DNA polymerase.
        - Thymidine kinase is a viral enzyme involved in several initial steps of acyclovir phosphorylation that subsequently allows acyclovir to inhibit viral DNA polymerase.
    - Strains that are resistant to acyclovir via decreased thymidine kinase production are also cross-resistant to famciclovir and penciclovir.
    - Trifluridine is effective against acyclovir-resistant strains, although resistance has been reported.

High-Yield Clinical Knowledge

- **Nephrotoxicity**
  - Acyclovir and valacyclovir cause reversible nephrotoxicity via crystalluria, interstitial nephritis (via immune reaction), and tubular necrosis (via accumulation of cytotoxic metabolite).
    - Acyclovir crystal formation is the most common cause of nephrotoxicity.
    - Nephrotoxicity can be prevented by avoiding rapid infusion and maintaining adequate hydration.
      - Acyclovir should be infused over at least 1 hour.
    - Risk factors include higher doses, rapid infusion, volume depletion, hypertension, diabetes, concurrent nephrotoxic agents, and obesity.
- **Neurotoxicity**
  - Acyclovir and valacyclovir may cause neurologic disturbances, including confusion, agitation, lethargy, hallucination, and impaired consciousness.
    - Neurotoxicity is dose-related and caused by cytotoxic metabolite accumulation.
    - Risk factors include higher doses (weight-based), renal impairment, and increased cerebrospinal fluid:albumin ratio.
- **Timing of Antiviral Initiation**
  - HSV and VZV antivirals should be initiated as soon as possible after symptom onset to be most effective.
  - Specific indications and optimal timing of antiviral initiation (listed below) are generally based on what has been included in clinical trials.
    - Herpes zoster (shingles)
      - Famciclovir and valacyclovir: within 72 hours of rash
    - Herpes labialis (cold sores)
      - Famciclovir and penciclovir initiation within 1 hour of symptom onset can reduce healing time by two days and 17 hours, respectively.
      - Docosanol initiation within 12 hours of symptom onset can reduce healing time by 18 hours.
    - Genital herpes
      - Valacyclovir: within 72 hours of the first diagnosis, within 24 hours of recurrent episodes
    - Varicella (chickenpox)
      - Acyclovir and valacyclovir: within 24 hours of rash
- **Duration of Therapy**
  - HSV
    - HSV-1 and HSV-2 infections are lifelong.
    - Genital herpes can be managed with either episodic therapy to shorten the duration of lesions or daily suppressive therapy to reduce the frequency of recurrences.
    - Acyclovir, valacyclovir, and famciclovir are effective options.
    - Episodic therapy should be provided for 7 to 10 days for initial episodes and 5 to 10 days for recurrent episodes.
    - Suppressive therapy may be continued indefinitely without lab monitoring.
      - The need for continued therapy should be reassessed annually.
  - VZV
    - The recommended duration of therapy for dermatomal lesions is 7 to 10 days.
      - Longer durations should be considered when lesions resolve slowly.
    - Acute retinal necrosis requires prolonged treatment over several months or more.
- **Selecting Topical, Intravenous, or Oral Therapy**
  - Topical antiviral therapy provides little clinical benefit for genital herpes and herpes zoster infections.
    - Systemic therapy is strongly recommended as first-line treatment.
  - Oral antiviral agents generally provide adequate systemic therapy.
    - Initial intravenous therapy may be indicated for severe mucocutaneous HSV infections, HSV complications (e.g., disseminated infection, pneumonitis, hepatitis, meningoencephalitis).
    - Intravenous agents should be used for 2 to 7 days or until regression of symptoms and can be transitioned to oral therapy to complete the total duration of therapy.

High-Yield Core Evidence
- **Comparative Efficacy Between Antiviral Agents**
  - Acyclovir, famciclovir, and valacyclovir appear equally effective in the treatment of genital herpes.
    - A multicenter, randomized, double-blind, placebo-controlled study evaluated the efficacy and safety of valacyclovir versus acyclovir in treating recurrent genital herpes infection and found no difference in healing time or adverse events. (Genitourin Med. 1997 Apr; 73(2):110-6.)
    - Another multicenter, randomized, double-blind, placebo-controlled study evaluated the efficacy and safety of famciclovir versus acyclovir in treating recurrent genital herpes infection and found no difference in healing time or adverse events. (Br J Dermatol. 2001 Apr; 144(4):818-24.)
  - Famciclovir, however, may be less effective for the suppression of viral shedding.
    - A set of two randomized, double-blind, placebo-controlled studies evaluated the clinical and biologic effects of famciclovir and valacyclovir in suppressive therapy for genital herpes.
    - Patients were randomized to receive either famciclovir 250 mg twice daily or valacyclovir 500 mg once daily.
    - The primary endpoint in the first study (proportion of patients who had a clinically confirmed recurrence) did not differ between the two groups, but the primary endpoint in the second study (proportion of days with HSV shedding detected) was higher in the famciclovir group.
    - The authors concluded that valacyclovir appears to be superior to famciclovir in suppressing genital herpes and viral shedding, warranting further comparative studies. (Sex Transm Dis. 2006 Sep; 33(9):529-33.)
  - Given the available evidence, current guidelines do not recommend one oral antiviral agent over another.

High-Yield Fast-Facts
- **Benzyl Alcohol Toxicity**
  - Some dosage forms of docosanol may contain benzyl alcohol preservative.
  - Large amounts of benzyl alcohol in neonates (≥ 99 mg/kg/day) have been associated with "gasping syndrome."
    - Symptoms include metabolic acidosis, gasping respirations, seizures, intracranial hemorrhage, hematologic abnormalities, skin breakdown, hepatic and renal failure, hypotension, bradycardia, and cardiovascular collapse.
  - The proposed mechanism of toxicity is that benzoate displaces bilirubin from protein binding sites.
  - Fatal toxicity has been associated with intravascular solutions containing benzyl alcohol.
- **Extravasation**
  - Intravenous acyclovir is an irritant at concentrations > 7 mg/mL.
  - Intradermal hyaluronidase may be considered for refractory extravasation.
    - Hyaluronidase degrades hyaluronic acid, thereby increasing tissue permeability and allowing for increased dispersion of the extravasated agent.
    Hyaluronidase has been used to treat extravasation of many other drugs, including amiodarone, aminophylline, calcium salts, dextrose, etoposide, phenytoin, taxanes, and vinca alkaloids.
- **Thrombotic Thrombocytopenic Purpura (TTP) and Hemolytic-Uremic Syndrome (HUS)**
  - Acyclovir and valacyclovir may cause thrombotic microangiopathy resulting in damage to the brain, kidney, liver, heart, and pancreas.

Table: Drug Class Summary

| \multicolumn{4}{c}{HSV and VZV Antivirals - Drug Class Review
High-Yield Med Reviews} |

Mechanism of Action: *Inhibit viral DNA synthesis by inhibiting DNA polymerases and thymidylate synthase and/or incorporating them into viral DNA. Docosanol prevents viral entry into the cell by inhibiting fusion between the plasma membrane and viral envelope.*

Class Effects: *Provide acute treatment and/or suppression for HSV, VZV, and several other viral infections*

Generic Name	Brand Name	Main Indication(s) or Uses	Notes

Acyclovir	Zovirax	- HSV treatment
		- Herpes zoster (shingles) treatment
		- Varicella (chickenpox) treatment
			- **Dosing (Adult):**
			  – IV: 5 to 10 mg/kg every 8 hours
			  – Oral: 200 mg to 800 mg 2 to 5 times daily
			- **Dosing (Peds):**
			  – IV: 5 to 20 mg/kg every 8 hours
			  – Oral:
			    – 20 mg/kg 2 to 4 times daily
			    – 300 mg/m^2 every 8 hours
			    – 200 to 800 mg 2 to 5 times daily
			- **CYP450 Interactions:** Inhibits CYP1A2 (weak)
			- **Renal or Hepatic Dose Adjustments:**
			  – Renal dose adjustments required when CrCl < 50 mL/min/1.73 m^2
			- **Dosage Forms:** Oral (capsule, tablet, suspension), IV (solution)

Docosanol	Abreva	- Cold sore/fever blister	- **Dosing (Adult):**
			  – Topical: application 5 times daily to affected area of face
			- **Dosing (Peds):**
			  – Same as adult dosing for children ≥ 12 years and adolescents
			- **CYP450 Interactions:** None
			- **Renal or Hepatic Dose Adjustments:** None
			- **Dosage Forms:** Topical (cream)

Famciclovir	Famvir	- HSV treatment and suppression
		- Herpes zoster (shingles) treatment
			- **Dosing (Adult):**
			  – Oral: 125 to 500 mg 2 to 3 times daily
			- **Dosing (Peds):**
			  – 250 to 1,000 mg 2 to 3 times daily
			- **CYP450 Interactions:** None
			- **Renal or Hepatic Dose Adjustments:**
			  – Renal dose adjustments required when CrCl < 40 or 60 mL/min depending on indication
			- **Dosage Forms:** Oral (tablet)

HSV and VZV Antivirals - Drug Class Review
High-Yield Med Reviews

Generic Name	Brand Name	Main Indication(s) or Uses	Notes
Penciclovir	Denavir	• Herpes labialis (cold sores) treatment	• **Dosing (Adult):** – Topical application every 2 hours during waking hours for 4 days • **Dosing (Peds):** [same as adult] – Same as adult dosing for children ≥ 12 years and adolescents • **CYP450 Interactions:** None • **Renal or Hepatic Dose Adjustments:** None • **Dosage Forms:** Topical (cream)
Trifluridine	Viroptic	• Herpes keratoconjunctivitis and keratitis treatment	• **Dosing (Adult):** – Ophthalmic 1 drop into affected eye(s) every 2 to 4 hours while awake – Maximum of 9 drops per day • **Dosing (Peds):** – Same as adult dosing for children ≥ 6 years and adolescents – Maximum of 9 drops per day • **CYP450 Interactions:** None • **Renal or Hepatic Dose Adjustments:** None • **Dosage Forms:** Ophthalmic (solution)
Valacyclovir	Valtrex	• HSV treatment and suppression • Herpes zoster (shingles) treatment	• **Dosing (Adult):** – Oral: 500 to 2,000 mg 1 to 3 times daily • **Dosing (Peds):** – Oral: – 20 mg/kg 1 to 2 times daily – Maximum of 1,000 mg per dose – 250 to 2,000 mg 1 to 3 times daily • **CYP450 Interactions:** Inhibits CYP1A2 (weak) • **Renal or Hepatic Dose Adjustments:** – Renal dose adjustments if CrCl < 50 mL/min • **Dosage Forms:** Oral (tablet)

HIGH-YIELD BOARD EXAM ESSENTIALS

- **CLASSIC AGENTS:** Acyclovir, docosanol (topical), famciclovir, penciclovir (topical), trifluridine (topical), valacyclovir
- **DRUG CLASS:** HSV and VZV Antiviral
- **INDICATIONS:** HSV, VZV
- **MECHANISM:** Inhibit viral DNA synthesis by inhibiting viral DNA polymerases (• Acyclovir, famciclovir, penciclovir, trifluridine, valacyclovir); Prevents viral entry into the cell by inhibiting fusion between the plasma membrane and viral envelope (docosanol).
- **SIDE EFFECTS:** Neurotoxicity, nephrotoxicity
- **CLINICAL PEARLS:**
  - Valacyclovir is the prodrug of acyclovir and has better oral bioavailability than acyclovir thereby allowing it to be given less frequently.
  - Acyclovir and valacyclovir cause reversible nephrotoxicity via crystalluria, interstitial nephritis (via immune reaction), and tubular necrosis (via accumulation of cytotoxic metabolite).
  - Acyclovir crystal formation is the most common cause of nephrotoxicity.

INFECTIOUS DISEASE – INFLUENZA ANTIVIRAL

Drug Class
- Influenza Antiviral
- Agents:
    - Acute Care
        - Amantadine
        - Baloxavir
        - Oseltamivir
        - Peramivir
        - Rimantadine
        - Zanamivir

> **Knowledge Integration**
>
> ✓ Per the CDC: Patients at increased for complications of flu include those 65 yrs. or older, women who are pregnant or postpartum within 2 weeks, living in nursing home, American and Alaska natives, BMI over 40, chronic medical conditions (e.g., HIV, DM, CKD, COPD) or those on immunosuppressive agents. Any of these patients should be considered for treatment if beyond 48 hours from the onset of symptoms.

Main Indications or Uses
- Acute Care
    - Influenza A and B
        - Baloxavir
    - Influenza A
        - Amantadine
        - Rimantadine

Mechanism of Action
- **Amantadine, Rimantadine**
    - Inhibit viral uncoating and/or viral assembly of the influenza A virus, specifically on the M2 protein, causing conformational changes in hemagglutinin transport and replication.
- **Baloxavir**
    - A selective inhibitor of influenza cap-dependent endonuclease interferes with viral RNA transcription and blocks virus replication.
- **Oseltamivir, Peramivir, Zanamivir**
    - A selective inhibitor of influenza A and B virus neuraminidase leads to viral aggregation at the cell surface and reduces respiratory viral spread.

Primary Net Benefit
- None of these agents cure influenza but rather reduce the duration of influenza symptoms and severity, at the cost of an offsetting increase in adverse events.
- Main Labs to Monitor:
    - Confirmation of influenza infection

High-Yield Basic Pharmacology
- **Baloxavir Dosing**
    - Benefiting from its 80-hour half-life, baloxavir is administered as a single oral dose for the treatment or prophylaxis of seasonal influenza.
- **Baloxavir Absorption**
    - Baloxavir is administered in a single oral dose, where absorption is critical to drug efficacy.
    - Polyvalent cation-containing products such as laxatives, antacids, calcium supplements, or dairy products must not be taken with baloxavir, and this combination is contraindicated.
    - Baloxavir concentrations decrease substantially with these combinations.
- **Zanamivir Bioavailability**
    - Despite a 5-15% bioavailability, zanamivir still achieves concentrations in the respiratory tract 1000x the MIC50 for influenza viruses.

High-Yield Clinical Knowledge

- **Neuropsychiatric Adverse Events**
  - Although rare, according to the prescribing information, prospective and retrospective evidence suggests a clinically relevant risk of neurotoxic and neuropsychiatric effects of amantadine, rimantadine, baloxavir, oseltamivir, and zanamivir.
    - Patients are at the highest risk of concomitantly taking antihistamines and psychotropic or anticholinergic drugs or with previous psychiatric disease.
- **Inhaled Zanamivir**
  - Zanamivir is only administered via inhalation and should be used with caution in patients with or without pre-existing reactive airway disease.
    - Although not contraindication, patients with reactive airway disease, asthma, or COPD have experienced fatal bronchospasm.
- **Peramivir and 2009 H1N1**
  - Peramivir was initially used during the 2009 H1N1 pandemic as the first intravenously administered neuraminidase inhibitor.
  - Although it's administered as a single IV infusion, it must still be administered as early as possible to reduce influenza sequelae severity and/or duration.
- **Amantadine or Rimantadine Use**
  - According to the CDC, either amantadine or rimantadine is no longer recommended for treatment or prophylaxis of influenza A due to high resistance rates.
- **Influenza Vaccine Timing**
  - Any anti-influenza antivirals may diminish the efficacy of live/attenuated influenza virus vaccine administration.
- **Flu Resistance**
  - Resistance to amantadine and rimantadine occurs readily due to a single mutation in the RNA sequence encoding for the M2 protein.
    - These resistant isolates can occur during treatment, particularly within 2 to 3 days after initiation of therapy.
  - Mutations cause resistance to zanamivir in the viral hemagglutinin or neuraminidase.
    - This resistance results in cross-resistance to other neuraminidase inhibitors.
- **Amantadine and Rimantadine Role**
  - Although they have a limited role in clinical practice, amantadine and rimantadine can be used for prophylaxis influenza A in high-risk patients in the outpatient space or as an agent for nosocomial influenza prophylaxis.
    - Their role is essential in scenarios where the influenza vaccine cannot be administered or is ineffective as in immunocompromised patients.

High-Yield Core Evidence

- **Meta-Analysis 2009 Update**
  - Update to the 2005 Cochrane analysis assessing the effects of neuraminidase inhibitors in preventing or alleviating influenza symptoms, the transmission of influenza, and complications in healthy adults, and estimate the frequency of adverse effects.
  - Regarding prophylaxis, there was no effect against influenza-like illness using neuraminidase inhibitors.
  - In treating symptomatic, confirmed influenza, oral oseltamivir or zanamivir did not reduce influenza-related lower respiratory tract complications.
  - The authors concluded that neuraminidase inhibitors have modest effectiveness against the symptoms of influenza in otherwise healthy adults. Still, the lack of good data has undermined previous findings for oseltamivir's prevention of complications from influenza. Independent randomized trials to resolve these uncertainties are needed. (BMJ. 2009 Dec 8;339:b5106.)

- **CAPSTONE-1**
  - This was one publication of two randomized, double-blind, controlled trials comparing oral baloxavir or placebo (study one) or oseltamivir (study two) in patients with acute uncomplicated influenza.
  - Compared to placebo, baloxavir was associated with a significant improvement in the primary efficacy endpoint of time to alleviate influenza symptoms in the intention-to-treat infected population.
  - However, when compared to oseltamivir, baloxavir had a similar time alleviating symptoms. Still, baloxavir was associated with greater viral load reductions 1 day after initiation of the regimen than placebo or oseltamivir.
  - The authors concluded that single-dose baloxavir was without evident safety concerns, was superior to placebo in alleviating influenza symptoms, and was superior to both oseltamivir and placebo in reducing the viral load 1 day after initiation the trial regimen in patients with uncomplicated influenza. (N Engl J Med 2018; 379:913-923.)

High-Yield Fast-Facts
- **Oseltamivir Controversy**
  - The Cochrane Collaborative conducted an intensive meta-analysis of oseltamivir, including attaining previously unpublished data, demonstrating an absence of net clinical benefit for its use for influenza treatment.
  - This occurred after the World Health Organization recommended stockpiling the drug for future influenza pandemics.
- **Amantadine Uses**
  - Although rarely used as an antiviral, amantadine is commonly used for neuropsychiatric indications, including drug-induced extrapyramidal symptoms, dyskinesias due to Parkinson's disease, or fatigue to Multiple Sclerosis.
- **Pregnancy**
  - Although the oral/inhaled/IV anti-influenza agents can be administered during pregnancy, the ideal intervention is to ensure immunization for influenza unless contraindicated.

HIGH-YIELD BOARD EXAM ESSENTIALS
- **CLASSIC AGENTS:** Amantadine, baloxavir, oseltamivir, peramivir, rimantadine, zanamivir
- **DRUG CLASS:** Influenza antivirals
- **INDICATIONS:** Influenza prophylaxis and treatment
- **MECHANISM:** Inhibit viral M2 protein, stopping viral transport and replication (amantadine, rimantadine); Inhibits influenza cap-dependent endonuclease, blocking viral replication (baloxavir); Inhibits influenza A and B virus neuraminidase, and reduced respiratory viral spread (oseltamivir, peramivir, zanamivir)
- **SIDE EFFECTS:** Neuropsychiatric effects (oseltamivir)
- **CLINICAL PEARLS:**
  - Amantadine and rimantadine only cover influenza A, NOT type B. The other agents cover both strains of influenza.
  - Zanamivir is only administered via inhalation and should be used with caution in patients with or without pre-existing reactive airway disease. Although not a contraindication, patients with reactive airway disease, asthma, or COPD have experienced fatal bronchospasm.
  - Baloxavir is a single-dose oral treatment whereas peramivir is a single dose IV treatment for flu.

Table: Drug Class Summary

\multicolumn{4}{c}{**Influenza Antiviral - Drug Class Review**}
\multicolumn{4}{l}{**Mechanism of Action:** *Amantadine, Rimantadine: Inhibit viral M2 protein, stopping viral transport and replication. Baloxavir: Inhibits influenza cap-dependent endonuclease, blocking viral replication. Oseltamivir, Peramivir, Zanamivir: Inhibits influenza A and B virus neuraminidase and reduces respiratory viral spread.* **Class Effects:** *Reduce the duration of influenza symptoms and severity at the cost of an offsetting increase in adverse events.*}
Generic Name	**Brand Name**	**Main Indication(s) or Uses**	**Notes**

Amantadine	Gocovri	- Influenza A prophylaxis and treatment (no longer recommended)	- **Dosing (Adult):**
			  - Oral: 100 to 200 mg q12-24h
			- **Dosing (Peds):**
			  - Oral: 5 mg/kg/day divided q12h
			    - Maximum 150 mg/day
			- **CYP450 Interactions:** Substrate CYP3A4, Pgp
			- **Renal or Hepatic Dose Adjustments:**
			  - GFR 30 to 59 mL/min - 200 mg x1 then 100 mg/day
			  - GFR 15 to 29 mL/min - 200 mg x1 then 100 mg q24h
			  - GFR < 15 mL/minute - contraindicated
			- **Dosage Forms:** Oral (capsule, tablet, syrup)

Baloxavir	Xofluza	- Influenza prophylaxis and treatment	- **Dosing (Adult):**
			  - Patients weight less than 80 kg
			    - Oral: 40 mg
			  - Patients weight 80 kg or greater
			    - Oral: 80 mg
			- **Dosing (Peds):**
			  - Patients weight less than 20 kg
			    - Oral: 2 mg/kg
			  - Patients weight 20 kg or greater
			    - use adult dosing
			- **CYP450 Interactions:** Substrate CYP3A4, Pgp
			- **Renal or Hepatic Dose Adjustments:** None
			- **Dosage Forms:** Oral (tablet)

Influenza Antiviral - Drug Class Review
High-Yield Med Reviews

Generic Name	Brand Name	Main Indication(s) or Uses	Notes

Oseltamivir	Tamiflu	- Influenza prophylaxis and treatment	- **Dosing (Adult):**
			  – Oral: 75 mg daily (prophylaxis) or BID (treatment)
			- **Dosing (Peds):**
			  – Oral: 3 to 3.5 mg/kg/dose q12-24h
			  – < 15 kg - Oral 30 mg q12-24h
			  – 15 to 23 kg - Oral 45 q12-24h
			  – 23 to 40 kg - Oral 60 mg q12-24h
			  – 40 kg or greater - Oral 75 mg q12-24H
			    – Treatment (q12h), prophylaxis (q24h)
			- **CYP450 Interactions:** None
			- **Renal or Hepatic Dose Adjustments:**
			  – GFR 30 to 60 mL/min - 30 mg q12-24h
			  – GFR 10 to 30 mL/min - 30 mg q24-48h
			  – GFR < 10 mL/min - not recommended
			- **Dosage Forms:** Oral (capsule, solution)

Peramivir	Rapivab	- Influenza treatment	- **Dosing (Adult):**
			  – I:V 600 mg once
			    – Can be used q24h for 5-10 days
			- **Dosing (Peds):**
			  – IV: 12 mg/kg once
			    – Maximum 600 mg/dose
			- **CYP450 Interactions:** None
			- **Renal or Hepatic Dose Adjustments:**
			  – GFR 31 to 49 mL/min - 150 to 200 mg
			  – GFR 10 to 29 mL/min - 100 mg
			  – GFR < 10 mL/min - 100 mg x1 then 15 mg q24h days 2-10
			- **Dosage Forms:** IV (solution)

Rimantadine	Flumadine	- Influenza A treatment or prophylaxis	- **Dosing (Adult):**
			  – Oral: 100 mg BID x 7 days
			- **Dosing (Peds):**
			  – Oral: 5 mg/kg/day
			    – Maximum 150 mg/day
			- **CYP450 Interactions:** None
			- **Renal or Hepatic Dose Adjustments:**
			  – GFR < 30 mL/min - 100 mg daily
			- **Dosage Forms:** Oral (tablet)

Zanamivir	Relenza Diskhaler	- Influenza treatment	- **Dosing (Adult):**
			  – Inhalation - two inhalations daily for 5 to 7 days
			- **Dosing (Peds):**
			  – Children 7 and older, use adult dosing
			- **CYP450 Interactions:** None
			- **Renal or Hepatic Dose Adjustments:** None
			- **Dosage Forms:** Aerosol powder

INFECTIOUS DISEASE – PALIVIZUMAB

Drug Class
- Palivizumab
- Agents:
    - Acute Care
        - Palivizumab

Main Indications or Uses
- Acute Care
    - Respiratory syncytial virus (RSV) prophylaxis

Mechanism of Action
- Prevents cell entry by inhibiting the viral fusion protein.

> **Dosing Pearl**
> ✓ Since palivizumab is a monoclonal antibody, it has a long half-life thereby allowing it to be administered by IM injection on a once-a-month basis for prevention of RSV in high-risk patients.

Primary Net Benefit
- Prevents RSV infection in high-risk pediatric patients, including those with a history of premature birth, bronchopulmonary dysplasia (BPD), and congenital heart disease (CHD).

High-Yield Basic Pharmacology
- Monoclonal Antibody
    - Palivizumab is a humanized monoclonal antibody derived from that of mice using recombinant DNA technology.
    - Mouse antibodies are produced by introducing the RSV antigen to the mouse's B lymphocytes.
- Resistance Mechanism
    - Resistant RSV strains with viral fusion protein mutations have been observed in vitro.
    - These mutations currently do not significantly impact the clinical efficacy of palivizumab.
- Adverse Reactions
    - Palivizumab is safe and tolerable with minimal adverse effects, including skin rash and fever.
    - Rare cases of severe thrombocytopenia and injection site reactions have been reported.

High-Yield Clinical Knowledge
- Indications
    - Palivizumab is indicated for pediatric patients:
        - With a history of premature birth (≤ 35 weeks gestational) and who are ≤ 6 months of age at the beginning of RSV season
        - With BPD that required medical treatment within the previous 6 months and who are ≤ 24 months of age at the beginning of RSV season
        - With hemodynamically significant CHD and who are ≤ 24 months of age at the beginning of RSV season
    - Palivizumab is also recommended for pediatric patients who are < 24 months of age and have:
        - Chronic lung disease (CLD) of prematurity
        - Congenital airway abnormality or neuromuscular disorder that decreases the ability to manage airway secretions
        - Cystic fibrosis
        - Immunocompromising conditions
        - Cardiac transplantation during RSV season
- Duration of Efficacy
    - Palivizumab achieves therapeutic concentrations two days after intramuscular administration.
    - The RSV season in the United States generally falls between November and March.
    - The five-dose regimen is intended to provide about 160 days of coverage during RSV season.
        - The first dose should be given just before the onset of RSV season.

- Subsequent doses accumulate to provide the highest coverage during the peak of RSV season in late December to mid-February.
- A three-dose regimen has been tested but did not provide adequate serum concentrations for seasonal coverage.

High-Yield Core Evidence
- **IMpact-RSV Trial**
  - A multicenter, randomized, double-blind, placebo-controlled trial evaluated the efficacy and safety of palivizumab prophylaxis in reducing the incidence of hospitalization due to RSV in high-risk children (prematurity or BPD).
  - Patients were randomized to receive 5 intramuscular injections of either palivizumab 15 mg/kg or an equivalent volume of placebo.
  - The primary endpoint (hospitalization with confirmed RSV infection) occurred significantly less in the palivizumab group than the placebo group, and there was no difference in adverse events.
  - The authors concluded that monthly intramuscular injections of palivizumab are safe and effective for preventing severe RSV infection in high-risk children. (Pediatrics. Sep 1998;102(3 Pt 1):531-7.)

High-Yield Fast-Fact
- **Intravenous Administration**
  - Palivizumab was initially studied as an intravenous injection but was later studied as an intramuscular injection for ease of administration.

HIGH-YIELD BOARD EXAM ESSENTIALS
- **CLASSIC AGENTS:** Palivizumab
- **DRUG CLASS:** Monoclonal antibody
- **INDICATIONS:** RSV prophylaxis
- **MECHANISM:** Prevents cell entry by inhibiting the viral fusion protein
- **SIDE EFFECTS:** Rash, fever, thrombocytopenia, injection site reactions
- **CLINICAL PEARLS:** Prevents RSV infection in high-risk pediatric patients, including those with a history of premature birth, BPD, and CHD.

Table: Drug Class Summary

Palivizumab - Drug Class Review High-Yield Med Reviews			
Mechanism of Action: *Prevents cell entry by inhibiting the viral fusion protein*			
Class Effects: *Prevents RSV infection in at-risk pediatric patients (i.e., histories of bronchopulmonary dysplasia (BPD) or with congenital heart disease (CHD))*			
Generic Name	**Brand Name**	**Indication(s) or Uses**	**Notes**

Palivizumab	Synagis	• Respiratory syncytial virus (RSV) prophylaxis	• **Dosing (Adult):** Not used
			• **Dosing (Peds):**
			  – IM: 15 mg/kg once monthly throughout RSV season
			    – Maximum 5 doses per season
			• **CYP450 Interactions:** None
			• **Renal or Hepatic Dose Adjustments:** None
			• **Dosage Forms:** IM (solution)

INFECTIOUS DISEASE – RIBAVIRIN

Drug Class
- Ribavirin
- Agents:
    - Acute Care
        - Ribavirin

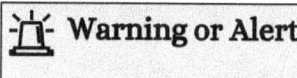

> **Warning or Alert**
> ✓ Ribavirin is BOTH embryotoxic and teratogenic while also being known to cause hemolytic anemia.

Main Indications or Uses
- Acute Care
    - Hepatitis C (HCV)

Mechanism of Action
- Interrupts viral RNA synthesis by inhibiting the production of guanosine triphosphate.

Primary Net Benefit
- Ribavirin was once a pivotal component of HCV treatment but has largely been replaced by direct-acting antiviral agents that may include ribavirin in select populations.
- Main Labs to Monitor:
    - HCV viral load
    - HCV genotype and subtype
    - CBC with differential
    - Serum Iron
    - Uric Acid
    - Liver function (INR/PT, albumin, protein, bilirubin)
    - Liver enzymes (AST/ALT, alk phos)
    - Pregnancy test

High-Yield Basic Pharmacology
- Spectrum
    - Ribavirin is effective for many DNA and RNA viruses, including influenza A and B, parainfluenza, respiratory syncytial viruses, hepatitis C, and HIV-1.

High-Yield Clinical Knowledge
- Teratogenicity
    - Ribavirin is embryotoxic and teratogenic.
    - Patients receiving ribavirin must be instructed to use two effective forms of contraception by each sexual partner during treatment and six months after drug discontinuation.
- Hemolytic Anemia
    - Although high-dose ribavirin is targeted for HCV treatment, this comes with an increased risk of dose-dependent toxicities, primarily hemolytic anemia.
    - Hemolytic anemia occurs within the first two weeks of ribavirin treatment in 20% of patients.
- Sofosbuvir Combination
    - For HCV regimens containing sofosbuvir/velpatasvir in patients without cirrhosis but who have Y93 resistance identified, ribavirin can be added to avoid conversion to an alternative regimen.
    - Ribavirin may also be used with sofosbuvir/ledipasvir.
- RSV Treatment
    - A nebulized form of ribavirin is available to treat severe respiratory syncytial virus (RSV) bronchiolitis or pneumonia in children.
    - Although the concerns for teratogenic and embryotoxic effects may not be relevant to the patient, they are concerns for healthcare workers exposed to the aerosolized ribavirin.
        - For these individuals at risk of ribavirin exposure, appropriate PPE is required.

- **Ribavirin and Didanosine**
  - The combination of ribavirin with didanosine should be avoided, as ribavirin increases the risk of didanosine-induced mitochondrial toxicity.
    - This occurs due to the ribavirin-induced formation of a triphosphorylated form of didanosine.

High-Yield Core Evidence
- **Sofosbuvir/Velpatasvir With and Without Ribavirin**
  - This was a phase 2 trial that randomized patients with genotype 3 HCV infection with compensated cirrhosis who lived in Spain to receive sofosbuvir/velpatasvir for 12 weeks or sofosbuvir/velpatasvir plus ribavirin for 12 weeks.
  - Patients randomized to sofosbuvir/velpatasvir plus ribavirin achieved a higher sustained virologic response 12 weeks after treatment (primary efficacy endpoint) than sofosbuvir/velpatasvir alone.
  - The most common adverse events included asthenia, headache, and insomnia in the sofosbuvir/velpatasvir plus ribavirin group.
  - The authors concluded that a high rate of patients with genotype 3 HCV infection and compensated cirrhosis achieved higher sustained virologic response 12 weeks after treatment. (Gastroenterology. 2018 Oct;155(4):1120-1127.e4.)
- **SOLAR-1**
  - This was a phase 2, open-label study, including two cohorts of patients with either cirrhosis and moderate or severe hepatic impairment who had not undergone liver transplantation or enrolled patients who had undergone liver transplantation: those without cirrhosis; those with cirrhosis, and mild, moderate, or severe hepatic impairment; and those with fibrosing cholestatic hepatitis.
  - Patients meeting inclusion criteria were randomized to receive either 12 or 24 weeks of a fixed-dose combination tablet containing sofosbuvir/ledipasvir, once daily, plus ribavirin.
  - Patients in the first cohort achieved sustained virologic response 12 weeks after treatment in 86%-89% of patients.
  - Among transplant recipients, sustained virologic response at 12 weeks after the end of treatment was achieved by 96%-98% of patients without cirrhosis or with compensated cirrhosis, by 85%-88% of patients with moderate hepatic impairment, by 60%-75% of patients with severe hepatic impairment, and by all six patients with fibrosing cholestatic hepatitis.
  - Response rates in the 12- and 24-week groups were similar.
  - The authors concluded that the combination of ledipasvir, sofosbuvir, and ribavirin for 12 weeks produced high rates of sustained virologic response at 12 weeks in patients with advanced liver disease and those with decompensated cirrhosis before and after liver transplantation. (Gastroenterology. 2015 Sep;149(3):649-59.)

High-Yield Fast-Fact
- **Sickle cell disease**
  - Ribavirin should be avoided in patients with sickle cell disease as it increases the risk of hemolytic anemia and sickle cell crisis.

HIGH-YIELD BOARD EXAM ESSENTIALS
- **CLASSIC AGENTS:** Ribavirin
- **DRUG CLASS:** Ribavirin
- **INDICATIONS:** Hepatitis C, RSV
- **MECHANISM:** Interrupts viral RNA synthesis by inhibiting the production of guanosine triphosphate.
- **SIDE EFFECTS:** Hemolytic anemia, teratogen, embryotoxic
- **CLINICAL PEARLS:**
  - Although high dose ribavirin is targeted for HCV treatment, this comes with an increased risk of dose-dependent toxicities, primarily hemolytic anemia.
  - Hemolytic anemia occurs within the first two weeks of ribavirin treatment in up to 20% of patients.

Table: Drug Class Summary

		Ribavirin - Drug Class Review High-Yield Med Reviews	
Mechanism of Action: *Interrupts viral RNA synthesis by inhibiting the production of guanosine triphosphate.*			
Class Effects: *Ribavirin was once a pivotal component of HCV treatment but has largely been replaced by direct-acting antiviral agents that may include ribavirin in select populations.*			
Generic Name	**Brand Name**	**Indication(s) or Uses**	**Notes**
Ribavirin	Copegus, Moderiba, Rebetol, Ribasphere, Virazole	<ul><li>Hepatitis C</li><li>Respiratory syncytial virus</li></ul>	<ul><li>**Dosing (Adult):**<ul><li>Oral: 1,000 to 1,200 mg in 2 divided doses</li><li>Inhalation - continuous nebulization 6 g over 12-18 hours OR intermittent 2 g over 2-4 hours q8h</li></ul></li><li>**Dosing (Peds):**<ul><li>Oral: 15 mg/kg/day in 2 divided doses<ul><li>Maximum 1,200 mg/dose</li></ul></li><li>Inhalation - continuous nebulization 6 g over 12-18 hours OR intermittent 2 g over 2-4 hours q8h</li></ul></li><li>**CYP450 Interactions:** None</li><li>**Renal or Hepatic Dose Adjustments:**<ul><li>GFR 50 mL/minute - contraindicated (Rebetol, Ribasphere capsules)</li><li>GFR 30 to 50 mL/minute - Alternate 200 mg/400 mg every other day (Copegus, Moderiba, Ribasphere tablets)</li><li>GFR < 30 mL/minute - 200 mg daily (Copegus, Moderiba, Ribasphere tablets)</li></ul></li><li>**Dosage Forms:** Oral (capsule, solution, tablet), Inhalation solution</li></ul>

HIV ANTIVIRALS – COMBINATION DOSAGE FORMS

Combination Dosage Forms - Drug Class Review
High-Yield Med Reviews

Mechanism of Action: *See drug class-specific reviews*

Class Effects: *Combination dosage forms allow for highly active antiretroviral therapeutic combinations while limiting pill burden on patients.*

Generic Name	Brand Name	Main Indication(s) or Uses	Notes

Efavirenz, emtricitabine, tenofovir disoproxil fumarate	Atripla	- HIV	- **Dosing (Adult):**
			  – Oral: 1 tablet daily
			- **Dosing (Peds):**
			  – For children at least 40 kg
			- **CYP450 Interactions:** see individual components
			- **Renal or Hepatic Dose Adjustments:**
			  – GFR < 50 mL/minute: not recommended
			  – Child-Pugh class C: not recommended
			- **Dosage Forms:** Oral (tablet)

Bictegravir, emtricitabine, and tenofovir alafenamide	Biktarvy	- HIV	- **Dosing (Adult):**
			  – Oral: 1 tablet daily
			- **Dosing (Peds):**
			  – For children at least 25 kg
			- **CYP450 Interactions:** see individual components
			- **Renal or Hepatic Dose Adjustments:**
			  – GFR < 30 mL/minute: not recommended
			  – Child-Pugh class C: not recommended
			- **Dosage Forms:** Oral (tablet)

Cabotegravir, relpivarine	Cabenuva	- HIV	- **Dosing (Adult):**
			  – IM: 600 mg / 900 mg (cabotegravir/rilpivirine) on last day of lead-in
			  – IM: 400 mg / 600 mg (cabotegravir/rilpivirine) once monthly
			- **Dosing (Peds):**
			  – Not routinely used
			- **CYP450 Interactions:** Substrate P-gp
			- **Renal or Hepatic Dose Adjustments:** None
			- **Dosage Forms:** SQ extended-release suspension

Lamivudine and tenofovir disoproxil fumarate	Cimduo, Temixys	- HIV	- **Dosing (Adult):**
			  – Oral: 1 tablet daily
			- **Dosing (Peds):**
			  – For children at least 35 kg
			- **CYP450 Interactions:** see individual components
			- **Renal or Hepatic Dose Adjustments:**
			  – GFR < 50 mL/minute - not recommended
			- **Dosage Forms:** Oral (tablet)

Lamivudine and zidovudine	Combivir	• HIV	• **Dosing (Adult):**
			    – Oral: 1 tablet twice daily
			• **Dosing (Peds):** Not routinely used
			• **CYP450 Interactions:** see individual components
			• **Renal or Hepatic Dose Adjustments:**
			    – ESRD: not recommended
			    – Child-Pugh class A, B or C: not used
			• **Dosage Forms:** Oral (tablet)

Emtricitabine, rilpivirine, tenofovir disoproxil fumarate	Complera	• HIV	• **Dosing (Adult):**
			    – Oral: 1 tablet daily
			• **Dosing (Peds):**
			    – For children at least 35 kg
			• **CYP450 Interactions:** see individual components
			• **Renal or Hepatic Dose Adjustments:**
			    – GFR < 50 mL/minute: not recommended
			• **Dosage Forms:** Oral (tablet)

Doravirine, lamivudine, and tenofovir diproxil fumarate	Delstrigo	• HIV	• **Dosing (Adult):**
			    – Oral: 1 tablet daily
			• **Dosing (Peds):**
			    – For children at least 35 kg
			• **CYP450 Interactions:** see individual components
			• **Renal or Hepatic Dose Adjustments:**
			    – GFR < 50 mL/minute: not recommended
			• **Dosage Forms:** Oral (tablet)

Emtricidabine and tenofovir alafenamide	Descovy	• HIV	• **Dosing (Adult):**
			    – Oral: 1 tablet daily
			• **Dosing (Peds):** For children at least 25 kg
			• **CYP450 Interactions:** see individual components
			• **Renal or Hepatic Dose Adjustments:**
			    – GFR < 30 mL/minute: not recommended
			    – Child-Pugh class C: not recommended
			• **Dosage Forms:** Oral (tablet)

Dolutegravir and lamivudine	Dovato	• HIV	• **Dosing (Adult):**
			    – Oral: 1 tablet daily
			• **Dosing (Peds):**
			    – For children at least 35 kg
			• **CYP450 Interactions:** see individual components
			• **Renal or Hepatic Dose Adjustments:**
			    – GFR < 50 mL/minute: not recommended
			    – Child-Pugh class C: not recommended
			• **Dosage Forms:** Oral (tablet)

Elvitegravir, cobicistat, emtricitabine, tenofovir alafenamide	Genvoya	• HIV	• **Dosing (Adult):**
			    – Oral: 1 tablet daily
			• **Dosing (Peds):** Not routinely used
			• **CYP450 Interactions:** see individual components
			• **Renal or Hepatic Dose Adjustments:**
			    – GFR < 50 mL/minute: not recommended
			    – Child-Pugh class C: not recommended
			• **Dosage Forms:** Oral (tablet)

Combination Dosage Forms - Drug Class Review
High-Yield Med Reviews

Generic Name	Brand Name	Main Indication(s) or Uses	Notes

Abacavir, lamivudine	Epzicom	- HIV	- **Dosing (Adult):**
			  − Oral: 1 tablet daily
			- **Dosing (Peds):**
			  − For children at least 25 kg
			- **CYP450 Interactions:** see individual components
			- **Renal or Hepatic Dose Adjustments:**
			  − GFR < 50 mL/minute: not recommended
			- **Dosage Forms:** Oral (tablet)

Atazanavir with cobicistat	Evotaz	- HIV	- **Dosing (Adult):**
			  − Oral: 1 tablet daily
			- **Dosing (Peds):**
			  − Not routinely used
			- **CYP450 Interactions:** see individual components
			- **Renal or Hepatic Dose Adjustments:**
			  − ESRD or hepatic impairment: not recommended
			- **Dosage Forms:** Oral (tablet)

Dolutegravir, rilpivirine	Juluca	- HIV	- **Dosing (Adult):**
			  − Oral: 1 tablet daily
			- **Dosing (Peds):**
			  − Not routinely used
			- **CYP450 Interactions:** see individual components
			- **Renal or Hepatic Dose Adjustments:**
			  − GFR < 30 mL/minute - not recommended
			  − Child-Pugh class C - not recommended
			- **Dosage Forms:** Oral (tablet)

Emtricitabine, rilpivirine, tenofovir alafenamide	Odefsey	- HIV	- **Dosing (Adult):**
			  − Oral: 1 tablet daily
			- **Dosing (Peds):**
			  − For children at least 35 kg
			- **CYP450 Interactions:** see individual components
			- **Renal or Hepatic Dose Adjustments:**
			  − GFR < 30 mL/minute: not recommended
			- **Dosage Forms:** Oral (tablet)

Darunavir and cobicistat	Prezcobix	- HIV	- **Dosing (Adult):**
			  − Oral: 1 tablet daily
			- **Dosing (Peds):**
			  − Not routinely used
			- **CYP450 Interactions:** see individual components
			- **Renal or Hepatic Dose Adjustments:**
			  − Child-Pugh class C: not recommended
			- **Dosage Forms:** Oral (tablet)

Combination Dosage Forms - Drug Class Review
High-Yield Med Reviews

Generic Name	Brand Name	Main Indication(s) or Uses	Notes

Elvitegravir, cobicistat, emtricitabine, tenofovir disoproxil fumarate	Stribild	- HIV	- **Dosing (Adult):**
			   − Oral: 1 tablet daily
			- **Dosing (Peds):**
			   − For children at least 35 kg
			- **CYP450 Interactions:** see individual components
			- **Renal or Hepatic Dose Adjustments:**
			   − GFR < 50 mL/minute: not recommended
			- **Dosage Forms:** Oral (tablet)

Efavirenz, lamivudine, tenofovir dioproxil fumarate	Symfi	- HIV	- **Dosing (Adult):**
			   − Oral 1 tablet daily
			- **Dosing (Peds):**
			   − For children at least 35 kg
			- **CYP450 Interactions:** see individual components
			- **Renal or Hepatic Dose Adjustments:**
			   − GFR 51 to 70 mL/minute: initial use not recommended
			   − GFR < 50 mL/minute: not recommended
			   − Child-Pugh class C: not recommended
			- **Dosage Forms:** Oral (tablet)

Darunavir, cobicistat, emtricitabine, tenofovir alafenamide	Symtuza	- HIV	- **Dosing (Adult):**
			   − Oral: 1 tablet daily
			- **Dosing (Peds):**
			   − Not routinely used
			- **CYP450 Interactions:** see individual components
			- **Renal or Hepatic Dose Adjustments:**
			   − GFR < 30 mL/minute: not recommended
			   − Child-Pugh class C: not recommended
			- **Dosage Forms:** Oral (tablet)

Abacavir, dolutegravir, lamivudine)	Triumeq	- HIV	- **Dosing (Adult):**
			   − Oral: 1 tablet daily
			- **Dosing (Peds):**
			   − For children at least 40 kg
			- **CYP450 Interactions:** see individual components
			- **Renal or Hepatic Dose Adjustments:**
			   − GFR < 50 mL/minute: not recommended
			   − Child-Pugh class C: contraindicated
			- **Dosage Forms:** Oral (tablet)

| \multicolumn{4}{c}{**Combination Dosage Forms - Drug Class Review**} |
|||| High-Yield Med Reviews |

Generic Name	Brand Name	Main Indication(s) or Uses	Notes

Abacavir, lamivudine, zidovudine	Trizivir	- HIV	- **Dosing (Adult):**
			  – Oral: 1 tablet twice daily
			- **Dosing (Peds):**
			  – For children at least 40 kg
			- **CYP450 Interactions:** see individual components
			- **Renal or Hepatic Dose Adjustments:**
			  – GFR < 50 mL/minute: not recommended
			  – Child-Pugh class C: contraindicated
			- **Dosage Forms:** Oral (tablet)

Emtricitabine and tenofovir disoproxil fumarate	Truvada	- HIV	- **Dosing (Adult):**
			  – Oral 1 tablet daily
			- **Dosing (Peds):**
			  – For children at least 35 kg
			- **CYP450 Interactions:** see individual components
			- **Renal or Hepatic Dose Adjustments:**
			  – GFR 30 to 49 mL/minute: q48h
			  – GFR < 30 mL/minute: not recommended
			- **Dosage Forms:** Oral (tablet)

HIV ANTIVIRALS – CYP450 Inhibitors

Drug Class
- CYP450 Inhibitors
- Agents:
  - Chronic Care
    - Cobicistat
    - Ritonavir (RTV)

Dosing Pearls

✓ The dose of ritonavir for "PI-boosting" or inhibition of CYP450 is a much lower dose that what is needed for antiviral efficacy.

Main Indications or Uses
- Chronic Care
  - Chronic Hepatitis C, genotype 1a or 1b
  - Chronic Hepatitis C, genotype 4
  - HIV

Mechanism of Action
- Cobicistat inhibits CYP3A* enzymes.
- Ritonavir is an HIV-1 protease inhibitor (PI) used clinically because of its inhibition of CYP450 enzymes.

Primary Net Benefit
- Improved exposure of protease inhibitor activity while limiting dose-related toxicities.
- Main Labs to Monitor:
  - Viral load (HIV, HCV)
  - CD4 count
  - Serum creatinine
  - Liver function (INR/PT, albumin, protein, bilirubin)
  - Liver enzymes (AST/ALT)

High-Yield Basic Pharmacology
- Relative CYP450 Inhibition
  - Ritonavir is classically a potent CYP3A4 inhibitor, but cobicistat exhibits more selective and characteristically stronger inhibition of CYP3A4.
- P-glycoprotein and Tenofovir
  - Tenofovir is a substrate of P-glycoprotein, inhibited by cobicistat and ritonavir, potentially leading to increased exposure and toxicities.

High-Yield Clinical Knowledge
- Serum Creatinine Changes
  - Cobicistat is associated with increased serum creatinine, causing a decreased calculation of GFR; however, this is not an actual change in renal function.
  - Cobicistat inhibits creatinine's renal tubular secretion, which leads to this calculated value, with no corresponding change in actual renal function.
- Drug Interactions
  - Cobicistat and ritonavir inhibit CYP450 isoenzymes and lead to numerous clinically relevant drug interactions.
    - Statins, calcium channel blockers, certain antiarrhythmics, inhaled corticosteroids, and estrogens are commonly administered medications with HIV or HCV regimens requiring close attention to appropriate agent selection and/or dose adjustments of changes in metabolism.
  - Other strong CYP3A4 or CYP2D6 inhibitors can decrease the metabolism of cobicistat, extending its pharmacokinetic actions.

- **HIV Activity**
  - Cobicistat has no intrinsic antiretroviral activity and is not considered an active drug when treating HIV.
  - Although a protease inhibitor, ritonavir has weak antiretroviral activity and dose-limiting toxicities and is not considered an active drug for HIV regimens.
- **Cobicistat Vs Ritonavir**
  - As cobicistat is inactive against HIV, it hypothetically reduces the likelihood of viral resistance to PIs.
  - Other advantages of cobicistat include specificity to CYP3A4 inhibition and the absence of lipid effects.
- **Combinations**
  - Although cobicistat is an independent dosage form, it's primarily used clinically in combination dosage forms with other antiretroviral medications.
  - This significantly reduces the pill burden of HIV patients and can help to improve compliance.

High-Yield Core Evidence
- **Cobicistat Vs Ritonavir**
  - This was a phase 3, non-inferiority study that enrolled treatment-naive patients with an HIV-1 RNA viral load of at least 5000 copies/mL and susceptibility to atazanavir, emtricitabine, and tenofovir, who were subsequently randomized to receive either elvitegravir/cobicistat/emtricitabine/tenofovir or atazanavir/ritonavir plus emtricitabine/tenofovir.
  - Elvitegravir/cobicistat/emtricitabine/tenofovir was non-inferior to the combination atazanavir/ritonavir plus emtricitabine/tenofovir in the HIV RNA viral load of 50 c/mL or less after 48 weeks.
  - Adverse events were reported with similar frequency and severity between the groups.
  - The combination of elvitegravir/cobicistat/emtricitabine/tenofovir was associated with fewer patients with abnormal liver function tests and lower median increases in fasting triglycerides.
  - There were small median increases in serum creatinine concentration with accompanying decreases in estimated glomerular filtration rate in both study groups by week two but stabilized by week eight and did not change up to week 48.
  - The authors concluded that the first integrase-inhibitor-based regimen would be given once daily and the only one formulated as a single tablet for initial HIV treatment. (Lancet. 2012 Jun 30;379(9835):2429-38.)
- **Cobicistat and PI Vs Efavirenz plus NRTI**
  - This was a phase 3, non-inferiority study that enrolled treatment-naive patients with an HIV-1 RNA viral load of at least 5000 copies/mL and susceptibility to atazanavir, emtricitabine, and tenofovir, who were subsequently randomized to receive either elvitegravir/cobicistat/emtricitabine/tenofovir or efavirenz plus emtricitabine/tenofovir.
  - Elvitegravir/cobicistat/emtricitabine/tenofovir was non-inferior to the combination of efavirenz plus emtricitabine/tenofovir concerning the primary endpoint of reduction in the HIV RNA viral load to less than 50 c/mL at week 48.
  - There was no difference between groups concerning the number of patients discontinuing drugs for adverse events.
  - However, serum creatinine concentration increased more by week 48 in the elvitegravir/cobicistat/emtricitabine/tenofovir group than in the group taking efavirenz plus emtricitabine/tenofovir.
  - The authors concluded elvitegravir/cobicistat/emtricitabine/tenofovir would be the only single-tablet, once-daily, integrase-inhibitor-based regimen for initial treatment of HIV infection. (Lancet. 2012 Jun 30;379(9835):2439-48.)

High-Yield Fast-Fact
- **Essential Medication**
  - Ritonavir is an essential medication according to the World Health Organization's List of Essential Medicines.

HIGH-YIELD BOARD EXAM ESSENTIALS
- **CLASSIC AGENTS:** Cobicistat, ritonavir
- **DRUG CLASS:** CYP450 Inhibitors
- **INDICATIONS:** HIV
- **MECHANISM:** Cobicistat inhibits CYP3A* enzymes. Ritonavir is an HIV-1 protease inhibitor but used clinically because of its inhibition of CYP450 enzymes.
- **SIDE EFFECTS:** Elevations in serum creatinine (cobicistat), hepatotoxicity (ritonavir)
- **CLINICAL PEARLS:** By definition, cobicistat and ritonavir inhibit CYP450 isoenzymes and lead to numerous clinically relevant drug interactions.

Table: Drug Class Summary

\multicolumn{4}{c}{**CYP450 Inhibitors - Drug Class Review**}
\multicolumn{4}{c}{High-Yield Med Reviews}
Mechanism of Action: *Cobicistat inhibits CYP3A* enzymes.* *Ritonavir is an HIV-1 protease inhibitor but used clinically because of its inhibition of CYP450 enzymes.*			
Class Effects: *Improved exposure of protease inhibitor activity while limiting dose-related toxicities.*			
Generic Name	**Brand Name**	**Main Indication(s) or Uses**	**Notes**

Atazanavir and cobicistat	Evotaz	- HIV	- **Dosing (Adult):**
			  – Oral: 1 tablet daily
			- **Dosing (Peds):**
			  – For children 35 kg and over: Oral 1 tablet daily
			- **CYP450 Interactions:** Substrate of CYP3A4; Inhibits CYP3A4
			- **Renal or Hepatic Dose Adjustments:**
			  – GFR < 70 mL/minute & tenofovir disoproxil fumarate - not recommended
			- **Dosage Forms:** Oral (tablet)

Cobicistat	Tybost	- HIV	- **Dosing (Adult):**
			  – Oral: 150 mg daily with atazanavir or darunavir
			- **Dosing (Peds):**
			  – For children 35 kg and over: Oral 150 mg daily
			- **CYP450 Interactions:** Substrate of CYP3A4; Inhibits CYP2D6, CYP3A4, P-gp
			- **Renal or Hepatic Dose Adjustments:**
			  – GFR < 70 mL/minute & tenofovir disoproxil fumarate: not recommended
			- **Dosage Forms:** Oral (tablet)

Darunavir, Cobicistat, Emtricitabine, and Tenofovir Alafenamide	Symtuza	- HIV	- **Dosing (Adult):**
			  – Oral: 1 tablet daily
			- **Dosing (Peds):**
			  – Not routinely used
			- **CYP450 Interactions:** Substrate of CYP3A4, P-gp; Inhibits CYP2D6, CYP3A4, P-gp
			- **Renal or Hepatic Dose Adjustments:**
			  – GFR < 30 mL/minute: not recommended
			  – Child-Pugh class C: not recommended
			- **Dosage Forms:** Oral (tablet)

CYP450 Inhibitors - Drug Class Review
High-Yield Med Reviews

Generic Name	Brand Name	Main Indication(s) or Uses	Notes
Elvitegravir, Cobicistat, Emtricitabine, and Tenofovir Alafenamide	Genvoya	- HIV	- **Dosing (Adult):** 　- One tablet daily - **Dosing (Peds):** 　- For children 25 kg and over - Oral 1 tablet daily - **CYP450 Interactions:** Substrate of CYP3A4; Inhibits CYP2D6, CYP3A4, P-gp - **Renal or Hepatic Dose Adjustments:** 　- GFR < 30 mL/minute: not recommended 　- Child-Pugh class C: not recommended - **Dosage Forms:** Oral (tablet)
Elvitegravir, Cobicistat, Emtricitabine, and Tenofovir Disoproxil Fumarate	Stribild	- HIV	- **Dosing (Adult):** 　- Oral: 1 tablet daily - **Dosing (Peds):** 　- For children 35 kg and over: Oral 1 tablet daily - **CYP450 Interactions:** Substrate of CYP3A4; Inhibits CYP2D6, CYP3A4, P-gp - **Renal or Hepatic Dose Adjustments:** 　- GFR < 70 mL/minute & tenofovir disoproxil fumarate: not recommended 　- Child-Pugh class C: not recommended - **Dosage Forms:** Oral (tablet)
Ombitasvir, Paritaprevir, and Ritonavir	Technivie	- Chronic Hepatitis C, genotype 4	- **Dosing (Adult):** 　- Oral: 2 tablets daily x 12 weeks with ribavirin - **Dosing (Peds):** 　- Not routinely used - **CYP450 Interactions:** Substrate of CYP2D6, CYP3A4, P-gp; Inhibits CYP3A4, P-gp; Induces CYP1A2, CYP2C19 - **Renal or Hepatic Dose Adjustments:** 　- Child-Pugh class C: contraindicated - **Dosage Forms:** Oral (tablet)
Ombitasvir, Paritaprevir, Ritonavir, and Dasabuvir	Viekira XR, Viekira Pak	- Chronic Hepatitis C, genotype 1a or 1b	- **Dosing (Adult):** 　- Oral: 2 to 3 tablets daily x 12 weeks with ribavirin - **Dosing (Peds):** 　- Not routinely used - **CYP450 Interactions:** Substrate of CYP2D6, CYP3A4, P-gp; Inhibits CYP3A4, P-gp; Induces CYP1A2, CYP2C19 - **Renal or Hepatic Dose Adjustments:** 　- Child-Pugh class C: contraindicated - **Dosage Forms:** Oral (tablet)

HIV ANTIVIRALS – ENTRY INHIBITORS

Drug Class
- Entry Inhibitors
- Agents:
    - Chronic Care
        - Ibalizumab
        - Enfuvirtide
        - Maraviroc

> **Dosing Pearls**
> ✓ Enfuvirtide must be reconstituted by the patient and injected subcutaneously twice a day. Once reconstituted, the solution for injection must be used within 24 hours.

Main Indications or Uses
- Chronic Care
    - HIV

Mechanism of Action
- Ibalizumab
    - Binds to the host CD4 receptor cell, blocking HIV from entering CD4 cells.
- Enfuvirtide
    - inhibits envelope fusion of HIV-1 with the target cell by binding to gp41 on the viral surface, stopping its fusion with the host cell.
- Maraviroc
    - Selectively binds to host CCR5 receptors, blocking HIV entry into CD4 cells.

Primary Net Benefit
- By blocking HIV entry into host CD4 cells, this group of agents provides novel antiretroviral mechanisms that can complement background therapy or salvage therapy when resistance limits regimen selection.
- Main Labs to Monitor:
    - CD4 count
    - HIV viral load
    - HIV genotype/phenotype
    - CCR5 tropism testing (Baseline for maraviroc)
    - Liver enzymes (AST/ALT)
    - Liver function (INR/PT, albumin, protein, bilirubin)

High-Yield Basic Pharmacology
- HIV Fusion
    - For HIV to enter human CD4 cells, it must attach to the host cell using its viral envelope glycoprotein complex.
    - This gp160 complex consists of gp120 and gp41, anchoring HIV to the host CD4 cell.
    - Chemokine receptor antagonists block gp120 (ibalizumab, maraviroc), whereas the fusion inhibitor enfuvirtide blocks gp41.
- CCR5 Vs. CXCR4
    - For maraviroc to be effective, the HIV isolates must be CCR5 expressing dominance.
    - HIV infection with CXCR-4 coreceptor dual or mixed tropism is present; maraviroc will not be effective.
    - Thus viral tropism assay susceptibility testing must occur before and during maraviroc therapy.
- Post-Attachment Interference
    - Ibalizumab binds to CD4 receptors, interfering with viral post-attachment activity necessary for viral entry into host cells.

Infectious Diseases

High-Yield Clinical Knowledge

- **Parenterally Administered**
  - Enfuvirtide is a twice-daily subcutaneous injection and the only parenteral antiretroviral for routine outpatient care.
  - Ibalizumab is also administered via infusion and is recommended for patients with multidrug-resistant HIV.
  - Cabotegravir plus rilpivirine is available as an injectable nanosuspension.
    - Zidovudine is also available in a parenteral dosage form but is not intended for routine outpatient care.
- **Injection Site Reactions**
  - Almost all patients taking enfuvirtide will experience injection site reactions.
  - These reactions are characterized by painful erythema and nodules at the injection site.
- **Hepatotoxicity Warning**
  - Like other antiretroviral agents, maraviroc has been associated with hepatotoxicity, necessitating baseline and periodic liver enzyme assessments.
    - The hepatotoxicity caused by maraviroc may be preceded by a systemic allergic response, which manifests as pruritic rash, eosinophilia, and elevated IgE.
- **Cardiovascular Disease**
  - The use of maraviroc has been associated with new or worsening myocardial ischemia or infarction and should be used with caution in patients at high cardiovascular disease risk.
- **Maraviroc Starting Doses**
  - As a result of its CYP3A4 metabolism, maraviroc is dosed based on the presence or absence of potent CYP3A4 inhibitors or inducers.
    - For patients starting maraviroc and who are currently taking CYP3A4 inhibitors, the starting dose of maraviroc is 150 mg BID.
    - For patients starting maraviroc while taking a CYP3A4 inducer, the starting dose is 600 mg BID.
    - A typical starting dose without a CYP3A4 inhibitor or inducer present is 300 mg BID.
- **Enfuvirtide Missed Doses**
  - Although enfuvirtide lacks cross-resistance to other antiretroviral classes, it has a low barrier to resistance as the viral mutation of the gp41 binding domain can occur.
  - As a result of a short half-life of approximately 4 hours, enfuvirtide must be administered twice daily.
  - If missed doses occur, there HIV viral mutation and resistance may occur.
- **Long Term CCR5 Antagonist**
  - Long-term use of maraviroc has been associated with increased susceptibility to flaviviruses, including West Nile virus and tick-borne encephalitis viruses.

High-Yield Core Evidence

- **TORO1**
  - This was a multicenter, open-label, phase 3 study.
  - Patients were randomized to enfuvirtide 90 mg SQ BID plus optimized background therapy or placebo plus optimized background therapy.
  - At the end of the 24-week study period, enfuvirtide therapy was associated with a significantly larger change in the plasma HIV-1 RNA level from baseline to week 24 compared to placebo.
  - Enfuvirtide was associated with a significantly larger mean increase in CD4 cell count compared to placebo-based therapy.
  - Injection site reactions were almost universal, with 98% of patients reporting at least one reaction, and more cases of pneumonia were observed in the enfuvirtide group.
  - The authors concluded that enfuvirtide to an optimized antiretroviral regimen provided significant antiretroviral and immunologic benefits through 24 weeks in patients who had previously received multiple antiretroviral drugs and had multidrug-resistant HIV-1 infection. (N Engl J Med 2003; 348:2175-2185.)

- **MOTIVATE 1 & 2 Studies**
  - This was a single publication of two studies which were both double-blind, placebo-controlled, phase 3 studies of patients with CCR5 HIV-1 only and who were randomized to either maraviroc once daily, maraviroc twice daily, or placebo, each with optimized background therapy (OBT) based on treatment history and drug-resistance testing.
  - In both studies, maraviroc led to a significant reduction in HIV-1 RNA from baseline compared to placebo.
  - Similarly, more patients receiving maraviroc once or twice daily had HIV-1 RNA levels of less than 50 copies per milliliter and a more significant improvement from baseline CD4 counts.
  - The authors concluded that maraviroc resulted in significantly greater suppression of HIV-1 and more significant increases in CD4 cell counts at 48 weeks in previously treated patients with CCR5 HIV-1 who were receiving OBT. (N Engl J Med 2008; 359:1429-1441.)
- **Ibalizumab for MDR HIV**
  - This was a single-group, open-label, phase 3 study that enrolled adult patients with multidrug-resistant (MDR) HIV-1 infection who were failing current antiretroviral therapy and had a viral load of 1000 c/mL or greater.
  - After a 7-day observation control period where patients continued their previous regimen, patients then received ibalizumab 2000 mg loading dose infusion, followed by 800 mg every 14 days combined with patient-specific background antiretroviral therapy for 25 weeks.
  - Compared to the baseline viral load, ibalizumab therapy significantly improved the proportion of patients with a 0.5 log10 decrease in viral load.
  - This effect was sustained through week 25, where patients receiving ibalizumab plus background ART had a mean decrease of 1.6 log10 c/mL from baseline, and 50% of patients achieved an undetectable viral load.
  - Twenty percent of patients experienced diarrhea, four patients died due to unrelated illnesses, and one patient experienced immune reconstitution inflammatory syndrome.
  - The authors concluded that ibalizumab had significant antiviral activity during a 25-week study. (N Engl J Med. 2018;379:645–654.)

High-Yield Fast-Fact
- **Exposure Prophylaxis**
  - Entry inhibitors present an option for HIV exposure prevention by preventing HIV viral entry into host cells rather than working on viral replication once already intracellularly.

HIGH-YIELD BOARD EXAM ESSENTIALS
- **CLASSIC AGENTS:** Ibalizumab, enfuvirtide, maraviroc
- **DRUG CLASS:** Entry inhibitors
- **INDICATIONS:** HIV
- **MECHANISM:** Ibalizumab - binds to the host CD4 receptor cell, blocking HIV from entering CD4 cells (ibalizumab); inhibits envelope fusion of HIV-1 with the target cell by binding to gp41 on the viral surface, stopping its fusion with the host cell (enfuvirtide); selectively binds to host CCR5 receptors, blocking HIV entry into CD4 cells (maraviroc).
- **SIDE EFFECTS:** Hepatotoxicity, new or worsening myocardial ischemia or infarction
- **CLINICAL PEARLS:** By blocking HIV entry into host CD4 cells, this group of agents provides novel antiretroviral mechanisms that can complement background therapy or for salvage therapy when resistance limits regimen selection.

Table: Drug Class Summary

Entry Inhibitor - Drug Class Review	
High-Yield Med Reviews	

Mechanism of Action:
Ibalizumab - binds to the host CD4 receptor cell, blocking HIV from entering CD4 cells.
Enfuvirtide - inhibits envelope fusion of HIV-1 with the target cell by binding to gp41 on the viral surface, stopping its fusion with the host cell.
Maraviroc - selectively binds to host CCR5 receptors, blocking HIV entry into CD4 cells.

Class Effects: By blocking HIV entry into host CD4 cells, this group of agents provides novel antiretroviral mechanisms that can complement background therapy or for salvage therapy when resistance limits regimen selection.

Generic Name	Brand Name	Main Indication(s) or Uses	Notes

Enfuvirtide	Fuzeon	- HIV	- **Dosing (Adult):**
			  - SQ: 90 mg BID
			- **Dosing (Peds):**
			  - SQ: 2 mg/kg/dose BID
			    - Maximum 90 mg/dose
			- **CYP450 Interactions:** None
			- **Renal or Hepatic Dose Adjustments:** None
			- **Dosage Forms:** Subcutaneous solution

Ibalizumab-uiyk	Trogarzo	- HIV	- **Dosing (Adult):**
			  - IV: 2,000 mg once, then 800 mg q14days
			- **Dosing (Peds):**
			  - Not routinely used
			- **CYP450 Interactions:** None
			- **Renal or Hepatic Dose Adjustments:** None
			- **Dosage Forms:** IV solution

Maraviroc	Selzentry	- HIV	- **Dosing (Adult):**
			  - Oral: 300 mg BID
			    - With CYP3A4 Inhibitors: 150 mg BID
			    - With CYP3A4 Inducers: 600 mg BID
			- **Dosing (Peds):**
			  - Weight above 30 kg: 300 mg BID
			    - With CYP3A4 Inhibitors: 50 to 150 mg BID
			    - With CYP3A4 Inducers: 600 mg BID
			- **CYP450 Interactions:** Substrate CYP3A4, P-gp
			- **Renal or Hepatic Dose Adjustments:** None
			- **Dosage Forms:** Oral (solution, tablet)

HIV ANTIVIRALS – INTEGRASE INHIBITORS

Drug Class
- Integrase Inhibitors
- Agents:
    - Chronic Care
        - Bictegravir
        - Cabotegravir
        - Dolutegravir
        - Elvitegravir
        - Raltegravir

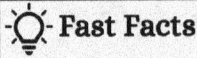

Fast Facts
- ✓ Integrase inhibitor based antiretroviral therapy (3-drug regimen) is now standard over protease inhibitor-based therapy due to better tolerability while maintaining good viral efficacy.

Main Indications or Uses
- Acute Care
    - Post-exposure prophylaxis
- Chronic Care
    - HIV

Mechanism of Action
- Inhibit integration of reverse-transcribed HIV DNA into host chromosomes.

Primary Net Benefit
- First-line antiretroviral agents with superior tolerability and safety profile.
- Main Labs to Monitor:
    - CD4 count
    - HIV viral load
    - HIV genotype/phenotype
    - Liver enzymes (AST/ALT)
    - Liver function (INR/PT, albumin, protein, bilirubin)

High-Yield Basic Pharmacology
- **Absorption and Cations**
    - Cation antacids (including aluminum, calcium, and magnesium) and iron products may interfere with the absorption of integrase inhibitors and must be separated by at least 2 hours before or 6 hours after cations.
- **Elvitegravir and Cobicistat**
    - Compared to the other integrase inhibitors, elvitegravir is primarily eliminated by CYP3A4, thus providing the opportunity for combination with "boosting" agents.
    - Although ritonavir could be used, cobicistat is the only boosting agent used routinely with elvitegravir.
- **Nanosuspension**
    - Cabotegravir is formulated as a nanosuspension with rilpivirine.
        - This combination follows a unique dosing schedule with an initial oral regimen followed by an intramuscular injection after the lead-in period with subsequent monthly injections after that.
        - Other parenteral antiretrovirals include enfuvirtide, ibalizumab, and zidovudine.

High-Yield Clinical Knowledge
- **HIV Resistance**
    - Integrase inhibitors, notably bictegravir and dolutegravir, protect a high genetic barrier to HIV resistance.
    - Although patients must be counseled not to miss or skip doses, should this occur, these agents with high genetic barriers to resistance are less likely to develop resistance.

- **OCT2 Interaction**
  - Metformin should be used cautiously with bictegravir and dolutegravir as it inhibits renal organic cation transporter (OCT2) and the multidrug and toxin extrusion transporter 1.
    - Dose and exposure-dependent effects of metformin may occur (lactic acidosis) with this combination.
  - Dofetilide is a substrate of OCT2, and its use is contraindicated with bictegravir and dolutegravir.
- **Serum Creatinine Changes**
  - Dolutegravir is associated with an increase in serum creatinine that does not represent a change in renal function.
    - This occurs due to competitive inhibition of tubular secretion of creatinine, with no actual impact on GFR.
  - Cobicistat has a similar effect on serum creatinine.
- **Well Tolerated**
  - Integrase inhibitors are well tolerated among patients with HIV, which is a welcome change from almost every other available antiretroviral class with numerous toxicities.
- **Dolutegravir and Pregnancy**
  - Dolutegravir should be avoided, if possible, in pregnant women as there has been an association with neural tube defects in infants.
    - With expert guidance, dolutegravir may be initiated or continued in women at least eight weeks from their last menstrual period.
- **Insomnia**
  - All integrase inhibitors are associated with insomnia.
  - Other neuropsychiatric effects associated with integrase inhibitors include depression and suicidality, particularly in preexisting psychiatric conditions.
- **Drug Interactions**
  - Most integrase inhibitors are glucuronidated but have some metabolism via CYP3A4.
  - Strong inducers, including carbamazepine, phenytoin, phenobarbital, and St. John's wort, may increase the elimination of integrase inhibitors, and coadministration should be avoided.

High-Yield Core Evidence
- **FLAIR Trial**
  - This was a multicenter, phase 3, randomized, open-label trial of adults with HIV-1 infection who had not previously received antiretroviral therapy.
  - Eligible patients underwent a 20-week run-in phase with daily oral dolutegravir, abacavir, and lamivudine,
  - Participants with an HIV viral load of less than 50 c/mL after 16 weeks were randomized to continue oral therapy or switch to oral cabotegravir plus rilpivirine for one month, followed by monthly injections of long-acting cabotegravir plus rilpivirine.
  - The combination of cabotegravir plus rilpivirine was non-inferior to dolutegravir, abacavir, and lamivudine concerning the primary outcome of HIV RNA less than 50 c/mL at week 48.
  - Almost all (99%) of patients receiving cabotegravir plus rilpivirine reported at least mild injection site reactions, but only four patients withdrew from the trial for this reason.
  - The authors concluded that cabotegravir plus rilpivirine was non-inferior to oral treatment with dolutegravir, abacavir, and lamivudine concerning maintaining HIV-1 suppression. (N Engl J Med 2020; 382:1124-1135.)

- **WAVES Trial**
  - This was a multicenter, active-controlled, double-blind, phase 3 clinical trial to assess the safety and efficacy of elvitegravir, cobicistat, emtricitabine, and tenofovir disoproxil fumarate compared with a boosted protease inhibitor regimen of ritonavir-boosted atazanavir with emtricitabine and tenofovir disoproxil fumarate.
  - Treatment-naive HIV-infected women with an estimated creatinine clearance of 70 mL/min were randomized to elvitegravir, cobicistat, emtricitabine, and tenofovir disoproxil fumarate or ritonavir-boosted atazanavir with emtricitabine and tenofovir disoproxil fumarate with matching placebos.
  - Elvitegravir, cobicistat, emtricitabine, and tenofovir disoproxil fumarate was non-inferior to ritonavir-boosted atazanavir with emtricitabine and tenofovir disoproxil fumarate at achieving HIV RNA viral load less than 50 c/mL at week 48.
  - No participant had a virological failure with resistance in the integrase inhibitor group than three participants in the protease inhibitor group.
  - The authors concluded that these findings recommend integrase inhibitor-based regimens in first-line antiretroviral therapy. (Lancet HIV. 2016 Sep;3(9):e410-e420.)

High-Yield Fast-Fact
- **Raltegravir and CK**
  - Although raltegravir contains a warning for elevated creatine phosphokinase, there has been no relationship between raltegravir or CK identified in post-market research.

HIGH-YIELD BOARD EXAM ESSENTIALS
- **CLASSIC AGENTS:** Bictegravir, cabotegravir, dolutegravir, elvitegravir, raltegravir
- **DRUG CLASS:** Integrase inhibitors
- **INDICATIONS:** HIV
- **MECHANISM:** Inhibit integration of reverse-transcribed HIV DNA into host chromosomes.
- **SIDE EFFECTS:** Insomnia, neural tube defects (dolutegravir)
- **CLINICAL PEARLS:** Metformin should be used cautiously with bictegravir and dolutegravir as it inhibits renal organic cation transporter (OCT2) and the multidrug and toxin extrusion transporter 1.

Table: Drug Class Summary

\multicolumn{4}{c}{**Integrase Inhibitors - Drug Class Review**}
\multicolumn{4}{c}{High-Yield Med Reviews}
\multicolumn{4}{l}{**Mechanism of Action:** *Inhibit integration of reverse-transcribed HIV DNA into host chromosomes.*}
\multicolumn{4}{l}{**Class Effects:** *First-line antiretroviral agents with superior tolerability and safety profile.*}
Generic Name	**Brand Name**	**Main Indication(s) or Uses**	**Notes**

Bictegravir	Biktarvy	• HIV	• **Dosing (Adult):**
			  – Oral: 1 tablet daily
			• **Dosing (Peds):**
			  – Limited to children at least 25 kg
			• **CYP450 Interactions:** Substrate CYP3A4
			• **Renal or Hepatic Dose Adjustments:**
			  – GFR < 30 mL/minute: Not recommended
			  – Child-Pugh class C: Not recommended
			• **Dosage Forms:** Oral (tablet)

Cabotegravir	Vocabria	• HIV	• **Dosing (Adult):**
			  – Oral: 30 mg daily with rilpivirine
			  – IM: 600 mg / 900 mg (cabotegravir/rilpivirine) on last day of lead-in
			  – IM: 400 mg / 600 mg (cabotegravir/rilpivirine) once monthly
			• **Dosing (Peds):**
			  – Not routinely used
			• **CYP450 Interactions:** Substrate P-gp
			• **Renal or Hepatic Dose Adjustments:** None
			• **Dosage Forms:** Oral (tablet), SQ extended-release suspension

Dolutegravir	Tivicay, Tivicay PD	• HIV	• **Dosing (Adult):**
			  – Oral: 50 mg once to twice daily
			• **Dosing (Peds):**
			  – Children 3 to < 14 kg
			    – Oral: 5 to 20 mg daily
			  – Children 14 kg and over
			    – Oral: 25 to 50 mg once to twice daily
			• **CYP450 Interactions:** Substrate CYP3A4, P-gp
			• **Renal or Hepatic Dose Adjustments:**
			  – Child-Pugh class C - Not recommended
			• **Dosage Forms:** Oral (Tablet)

Integrase Inhibitors - Drug Class Review
High-Yield Med Reviews

Generic Name	Brand Name	Main Indication(s) or Uses	Notes

Elvitegravir	Genvoya, Stribild	- HIV	- **Dosing (Adult):**
			   – Oral: 150 mg daily (in combination with cobicistat, emtricitabine, tenofovir disoproxil fumarate/tenofovir disproxil fumurate)
			- **Dosing (Peds):**
			   – Limited to children at least 25 kg
			- **CYP450 Interactions:** Substrate CYP3A4
			- **Renal or Hepatic Dose Adjustments:**
			   – Child-Pugh class C: Not recommended
			   – Genvoya
			      – GFR < 30 mL/minute: Not recommended
			   – Stribild
			      – GFR < 70 mL/minute: Initial use not recommended
			      – GFR < 50 mL/minute: continued use not recommended
			- **Dosage Forms:** Oral (Tablet)

Raltegravir	Isentress, Isentress HD	- HIV	- **Dosing (Adult):**
			   – Treatment naive
			      – Oral: 400 mg BID or 1,200 mg daily
			   – Treatment experience
			      – Oral 400 mg BID
			- **Dosing (Peds):**
			   – Oral suspension in children < 20 kg
			      – Oral: 6 mg/kg/dose twice daily
			         – Maximum 100 mg/dose
			   – Chewable tablets in children 11 kg and over
			      – Oral: 6 mg/kg/dose twice daily
			         – Maximum 300 mg/dose
			   – Film-coated tablets
			      – Limited to children at least 25 kg
			- **CYP450 Interactions:** None
			- **Renal or Hepatic Dose Adjustments:**
			   – Film-coated 600 mg tablet
			      – Child-Pugh class B or C: not recommended
			- **Dosage Forms:** Oral (chewable tablet, solution, tablet)

HIV ANTIVIRALS – NNRTI (NON-NUCLEOSIDE REVERSE TRANSCRIPTASE INHIBITORS)

Drug Class
- NNRTI
- Agents:
    - Chronic Care
        - Delavirdine
        - Doravirine
        - Efavirenz
        - Etravirine
        - Nevirapine
        - Rilpivirine

> **Fast Facts**
> ✓ Efavirenz can worsen underlying psychiatric disease and is contraindicated during pregnancy.
> ✓ Efavirenz can cause false positive test for marijuana on urine drug screen tests.

Main Indications or Uses
- Chronic Care
    - HIV

Mechanism of Action
- Bind directly to and inhibit HIV-1 reverse transcriptase, preventing RNA and DNA-dependent DNA polymerase activity.

Primary Net Benefit
- Antiretroviral agents with a long history of efficacy now include second-generation NNRTIs permitting once-daily dosing and improved adverse events.
- Main Labs to Monitor:
    - CD4 count
    - HIV viral load
    - HIV genotype/phenotype
    - Liver enzymes (AST/ALT)
    - Liver function (INR/PT, albumin, protein, bilirubin)

High-Yield Basic Pharmacology
- **NNRTI Vs. NRTI**
    - Unlike NRTIs, the NNRTIs do not compete with nucleoside triphosphates and do not require phosphorylation for their activity.
    - In other words, NNRTIs are not incorporated into viral DNA but prevent the movement of reverse transcriptase.
- **PPI Interaction**
    - The oral dosage form of rilpivirine should not be given with proton pump inhibitors as these agents reduce rilpivirine absorption.
        - However, when given intramuscularly, PPIs can be continued without rilpivirine.
- **CYP 450 Interactions**
    - As a class, NNRTIs are substrates for CYP3A4 and have mixed effects as either inducers, inhibitors, or mixed inhibitors/inducers.
    - Nevirapine induces CYP3A4, efavirenz, and etravirine both induce and inhibit CYP3A4, and delavirdine inhibits CYP3A4.
        - Delavirdine cannot be combined with fosamprenavir, but when combined with indinavir or saquinavir, it permits them to be administered on a twice-daily dosing schedule (rather than TID).
        - Efavirenz should not be combined with numerous other ARTs (doravirine and elvitegravir)
    - Uniquely, doravirine is a substrate of CYP 3A4 but neither induces nor inhibits its function.

High-Yield Clinical Knowledge
- **Class Adverse Events**
    - NNRTIs are commonly associated with GI intolerances and skin rashes.
    - Rashes can range from mild and self-limiting to toxic epidermal necrolysis.
        - Nevirapine initiation requires slow dose titration to minimize the risk of maculopapular rash.
    - Erythema multiforme, Stevens-Johnson syndrome, and toxic epidermal necrolysis are all immune-mediated epidermal conditions that differ based on clinical presentation:
        - Erythema multiforme affects less than 10% of total body surface area, most commonly involves hands and forearms, and presents with target lesions.
        - Stevens-Johnson syndrome also affects less than 10% of total body surface area but involves at least two mucosal sites.
        - Toxic epidermal necrolysis affects more than 30% of total body surface area, has an abrupt onset, and must be treated promptly.
    - Total serum cholesterol may increase with NNRTI therapy.
        - Efavirenz is associated with a 10-20% increase in total cholesterol.
- **Hepatic Injury**
    - Nevirapine should not be used in patients with CD4 counts above 250 cells/mL (women) or greater than 400 cells/mL (men) or patients with hepatitis B or C co-infection.
    - The characteristic rash associated with nevirapine initiation is closely related to hepatotoxicity, and the development of maculopapular rash should prompt liver enzyme and function assessment.
- **Efavirenz Timing**
    - As a result of its long half-life, efavirenz may be administered once daily but should be taken in the evening to avoid daytime hallucinations.
        - Other CNS effects of efavirenz include dizziness, insomnia, headache, depression, mania, and psychosis.
- **Genotypic Testing & Resistance**
    - Before initiation of NNRTI therapy, baseline genotypic testing is recommended.
    - Mutations can occur with single substitutions, which confer resistance across the medication class.
        - The nomenclature for resistance describes the target amino acid, its position, and the amino acid that has been substituted.
        - For example, a G190A mutation where glycine is substituted for alanine at position 190.
- **Parenterally Administered**
    - Cabotegravir plus rilpivirine is available as an injectable nanosuspension.
    - Other parenterally administered antiretroviral agents include:
        - Enfuvirtide is a twice-daily subcutaneous injection and the only parenteral antiretroviral for routine outpatient care.
        - Ibalizumab is also administered via infusion and is recommended for patients with multidrug-resistant HIV.
        - Zidovudine is also available in a parenteral dosage form but is not intended for routine outpatient care.
- **Efavirenz and Pregnancy**
    - Efavirenz may be avoided in pregnant women or in women planning to become pregnant due to neural tube defects.
    - However, as a result of this observation, but the absence of this effect in some literature, clinical guidance may permit it to be used with expert advice.
    - Dolutegravir has been associated with a similar effect of neural tube defects and should be avoided in the first four weeks from conception or six weeks from the last menstrual period.

High-Yield Core Evidence

- **ENCORE 1**
  - This was a multicenter, double-blind, randomized, non-inferiority study to compare the efficacy and safety of reduced-dose efavirenz with standard-dose efavirenz combined with tenofovir emtricitabine as first-line treatment for HIV infection.
  - Patients with HIV and viral loads above 1000 log10 copies/mL and CD4 counts between 50 to 500 cells/mL were randomized to either efavirenz 400 mg or 600 mg (both combined with tenofovir and emtricitabine).
  - Efavirenz 400 mg was non-inferior to 600 mg per day concerning the primary endpoint of the difference in proportions of participants with plasma HIV-RNA of less than 200 copies/mL at 48 weeks.
  - However, CD4 T-cell counts at week 48 were significantly higher for the 400 mg group than for the 600 mg group.
  - Furthermore, there were significantly more adverse events in the group receiving 600 mg/day, and considerably more patients stopped study drug treatment in the 600 mg/day group.
  - The authors concluded that lower dose efavirenz should be recommended for routine care. (Lancet, 2014, 383:1474–1482.)
- **Efavirenz and Pregnancy**
  - This systematic review and meta-analysis of efavirenz safety in HIV-infected pregnant women.
  - Of twenty-three studies included in this review, 21 reported the birth outcomes of 2026 live births among women exposed to efavirenz during the first trimester of pregnancy.
  - A pooled proportion of 1.63% of births was associated with congenital anomalies as reported, with only one neural tube defect observed.
  - There was no difference in overall congenital abnormality risk observed from twelve studies that reported birth outcomes of women exposed to efavirenz or non-efavirenz-containing regimens during the first-trimester pregnancy.
  - The incidence of neural tube defects was similar to the incidence in the general population.
  - The authors concluded that there is no evidence of an increased risk of overall or central nervous system congenital anomalies associated with first-trimester exposure to efavirenz, similar to previous systematic reviews. Still, continued birth outcomes prospective surveillance is warranted. (AIDS, 2014, 28(suppl 2): S123–S131.)

High-Yield Fast-Facts

- **Efavirenz Abuse**
  - Because of its hallucinogenic properties, some have smoked or inhaled efavirenz to achieve this effect.
- **QT Prolongation**
  - Rilpivirine has been associated with QT prolongation at high doses.

HIGH-YIELD BOARD EXAM ESSENTIALS
- **CLASSIC AGENTS:** Delavirdine, doravirine, efavirenz, etravirine, nevirapine, rilpivirine
- **DRUG CLASS:** NNRTI
- **INDICATIONS:** HIV
- **MECHANISM:** Bind directly to and inhibit HIV-1 reverse transcriptase, preventing RNA and DNA dependent DNA polymerase activity.
- **SIDE EFFECTS:** GI intolerance, rash (erythema multiforme, SJS/TEN), hepatotoxicity (nevirapine), neuropsychiatric effects (efavirenz)
- **CLINICAL PEARLS:** As a class, NNRTIs are substrates for CYP3A4 and have mixed effects as either inducer, inhibitors, or mixed inhibitors/inducers. Nevirapine induces CYP3A4, efavirenz, and etravirine both induce and inhibit CYP3A4, and delavirdine inhibits CYP3A4.

Table: Drug Class Summary

	**NNRTI - Drug Class Review** **High-Yield Med Reviews**
	**Mechanism of Action:** *Bind directly to and inhibit HIV-1 reverse transcriptase, preventing RNA and DNA-dependent DNA polymerase activity.*
	**Class Effects:** *Antiretroviral agents with a long history of efficacy now include second-generation NNRTIs permitting once-daily dosing and improved adverse events.*
Generic Name	**Brand Name**	**Main Indication(s) or Uses**	**Notes**

Delavirdine	Rescriptor	• HIV	• **Dosing (Adult):**
			  – Oral: 400 mg TID
			• **Dosing (Peds):**
			  – For children 16 years and older, use adult dosing.
			• **CYP450 Interactions:** Substrate CYP2D6, 3A4; Inhibits CYP3A4
			• **Renal or Hepatic Dose Adjustments:** None
			• **Dosage Forms:** Oral (tablet)

Doravirine	Pifeltro	• HIV	• **Dosing (Adult):**
			  – Oral: 100 mg daily
			• **Dosing (Peds):**
			  – Not routinely used
			• **CYP450 Interactions:** Substrate CYP3A4
			• **Renal or Hepatic Dose Adjustments:**
			  – GFR < 50 mL/minute: not recommended
			• **Dosage Forms:** Oral (tablet)

Efavirenz	Sustiva	• HIV	• **Dosing (Adult):**
			  – Oral: 600 mg daily
			  – Oral: 400 mg daily (when combined with tenofovir disoproxil fumarate and lamivudine)
			• **Dosing (Peds):**
			  – Children at least 3 months old and at least 3.5 kg
			    – Oral: 100 to 250 mg daily
			  – Children 3 years and older
			    – Oral: 200 to 600 mg daily
			• **CYP450 Interactions:** Substrate CYP2B6, 3A4; Induces CYP2B6, 2C19, 3A4
			• **Renal or Hepatic Dose Adjustments:**
			  – Child-Pugh class B or C: not recommended
			• **Dosage Forms:** Oral (capsule, tablet)

NNRTI - Drug Class Review
High-Yield Med Reviews

Generic Name	Brand Name	Main Indication(s) or Uses	Notes

Etravirine	Intelence	- HIV	- **Dosing (Adult):**
			    – Oral: 200 mg BID
			- **Dosing (Peds):**
			    – Children at least 10 kg and 2 years and older
			    – Oral: 100 to 200 mg BID
			- **CYP450 Interactions:** Substrate CYP2C19, 2C9, 3A4; Induces 3A4; Inhibits CYP2C19
			- **Renal or Hepatic Dose Adjustments:** None
			- **Dosage Forms:** Oral (tablet)

Nevirapine	Viramune, Viramune XR	- HIV	- **Dosing (Adult):**
			    – Oral: 200 mg daily x 14 days, then IR 200 mg BID, or ER 400 mg daily
			- **Dosing (Peds):**
			    – Oral: IR 120 to 200 mg/m2/dose daily x 14 days, then 120 to 200 mg/m2/dose BID
			    – Maximum 200 mg/dose
			    – Oral: ER 200 to 400 mg daily (after IR lead-in period)
			- **CYP450 Interactions:** Substrate CYP2B6, 2D6, 3A4; Induces CYP2B6
			- **Renal or Hepatic Dose Adjustments:**
			    – Child-Pugh class B or C: contraindicated
			- **Dosage Forms:** Oral (suspension, tablet)

Rilpivirine	Endurant	- HIV	- **Dosing (Adult):**
			    – Oral: 25 mg daily (with or without cabotegravir)
			    – IM: 600 mg / 900 mg (cabotegravir/rilpivirine) on last day of lead-in
			    – IM: 400 mg / 600 mg (cabotegravir/rilpivirine) once monthly
			- **Dosing (Peds):**
			    – Limited to children at least 25 kg
			- **CYP450 Interactions:** Substrate CYP3A4
			- **Renal or Hepatic Dose Adjustments:** None
			- **Dosage Forms:** Oral (tablet), SQ extended-release suspension

HIV ANTIVIRALS – NUCLEOTIDE/NUCLEOSIDE REVERSE TRANSCRIPTASE INHIBITORS (NRTI)

Drug Class
- NRTI
- Agents:
    - Chronic Care
        - Abacavir (ABC)
        - Didanosine (ddI)
        - Emtricitabine (FTC)
        - Lamivudine (3TC)
        - Stavudine (d4T)
        - Tenofovir alafenamide (TAF)
        - Tenofovir disoproxil (TDF)
        - Zalcitabine (DDC)
        - Zidovudine (AZT)

> **Pharmacogenetics Tip**
> ✓ Avoid abacavir in patients with the genetic polymorphism, HLA-B*5701 due to the risk of hypersensitivity reaction.

Main Indications or Uses
- Chronic Care
    - Hepatitis B
    - HIV

Mechanism of Action
- Inhibition of HIV reverse transcription into the emerging proviral DNA.

Primary Net Benefit
- A core component to highly-active antiretroviral regimens, but are associated with class toxicities including lactic acidosis, myopathies, peripheral neuropathies, pancreatitis, and bone marrow toxicities.
- Main Labs to Monitor:
    - CD4 count
    - HIV viral load
    - HIV genotype/phenotype
    - Liver enzymes (AST/ALT)
    - Liver function (INR/PT, albumin, protein, bilirubin)
    - Serum creatinine
    - CBC
    - HLA-B*5701 screening (abacavir)

High-Yield Basic Pharmacology
- **Nucleoside Vs. Nucleotide**
    - All available agents in this class, except for tenofovir, are nucleosides that must be triphosphorylated to exert their activity.
    - Tenofovir is a nucleotide monophosphate that must undergo two additional phosphorylations for its antiretroviral activity.
- **Reverse Transcriptase Inhibition**
    - After intracellular phosphorylation, nucleoside and nucleotide analogs inhibit HIV replication by competitive inhibition of native nucleotides and by eliminating elongation of nascent proviral DNA.
- **Antiviral Spectrum**
    - All agents in the NRTI class are active against susceptible HIV-1 and HIV-2.
    - Emtricitabine, lamivudine, and tenofovir can be used to treat hepatitis B.
    - Tenofovir is rarely used but can be used to treat herpes viruses.

High-Yield Clinical Knowledge
- **NRTI Toxicities**
  - NRTIs may adversely affect the DNA polymerase gamma of human mitochondria, resulting in mitochondrial toxicities including myopathies, peripheral neuropathies, pancreatitis, anemias, and granulocytopenia.
    - Zidovudine is associated with the highest risk of cytopenias and bone marrow toxicities.
  - Didanosine, stavudine, and zidovudine are associated with potentially fatal lactic acidosis and hepatic steatosis.
  - Emtricitabine, lamivudine, and tenofovir do not possess mitochondrial toxicities.
- **HLA-B*5701**
  - Before initiation of abacavir, patients must be screened for HLA-B*5701, as patients with positive HLA-B*5701 locus are at high risk of acute hypersensitivity syndrome.
- **Tenofovir Alafenamide Vs Disoproxil**
  - Tenofovir is formulated as two separate prodrugs, alafenamide or disoproxil.
  - The alafenamide was developed to improve oral absorption substantially and is associated with a lower risk of renal toxicity and bone marrow toxicity.
- **Renal Dose Adjustment**
  - All NRTIs, except for abacavir, require renal dose adjustments when the estimated GFR is less than 60 mL/minute or less than 50 mL/minute.
  - Abacavir is often preferred in patients with chronic kidney disease who have susceptible HIV and lack HLA-B*5701 positive screening.
- **Cross-Resistance**
  - NRTIs can be grouped by their amino acid analog backbone, which correlates with resistance and cross-resistance within this substructural class:
    - Abacavir is a guanosine analog.
    - Emtricitabine, lamivudine, and zalcitabine are cytidine.
    - For example, tenofovir and didanosine are adenosine analogs.
    - Stavudine and zidovudine are thymidine analogs.
  - The nomenclature for resistance describes the target amino acid, its position, and the amino acid that has been substituted.
    - For example, an M184V mutation where methionine is substituted for valine at position 184.
- **Combinations to Avoid**
  - The combination of stavudine and zidovudine, or lamivudine and zalcitabine, can cause mutual inhibition of their antiretroviral activity and thus should be avoided.
  - Peripheral neuropathies are more likely to occur with the combination of didanosine, stavudine, and zalcitabine.
- **Lamivudine Dosing**
  - Lamivudine is used for HIV-1 and HIV-2 at 300 mg daily or 150 mg twice daily.
  - For hepatitis B, lamivudine can also be used, but at 100 mg twice daily.
    - To treat coinfection with HIV and HBV, the HIV dosing (300 mg or 150 mg BID dosing).

High-Yield Core Evidence
- **SMART**
  - This was a multicenter, randomized clinical trial to assess early antiretroviral therapy in patients with HIV and CD4 cell counts of greater than 350 c/mcL (early intervention group) compared to episode use when CD4 cell counts decreased to less than 250 c/mcL until they rose to 350 c/mcL (episodic treatment group).
  - Early intervention patients had a significantly lower rate of development of any opportunistic infection or death from any cause.
  - When examined as individual endpoints, death from any cause, major cardiovascular, renal, or hepatic disease were significantly less likely to occur in patients in the early intervention group.
  - The authors concluded that early intervention with antiretroviral therapy significantly reduced the risk of opportunistic disease or death from any cause, mainly due to lowering the CD4+ cell count and increasing the viral load. (N Engl J Med. 2006 Nov 30;355(22):2283-96.)

- **INSIGHT START**
    - This was a multicenter, multinational, randomized clinical trial of the benefits and risks of initiating antiretroviral therapy in patients with asymptomatic HIV infection with a CD4 count of more than 350 cells/mL.
    - HIV-positive adults with CD4 above 500 c/mcL were randomized to receive either immediate antiretroviral treatment or deferred antiretroviral treatment until the CD4 count decreased to 350 c/mcL or an AIDS-defining illness occurred.
    - Midway through the study, subjects randomized to deferred treatment were offered immediate antiretroviral therapy, regardless of CD4 count.
    - Patients randomized to the immediate intervention group had a significantly lower risk of severe AIDS-related events, serious AIDS-related events, or death from any cause.
    - The authors concluded that antiretroviral therapy initiation in HIV-positive adults with a CD4 count of more than 500 c/mcL provided net benefits over starting such therapy in patients after the CD4 count had declined to 350 c/mcL. (N Engl J Med. 2015 Aug 27;373(9):795-807.)

High-Yield Fast-Fact
- **NNRTI Vs. NRTI**
    - Unlike NRTIs, the NNRTIs do not compete with nucleoside triphosphates and do not require phosphorylation for their activity.
    - In other words, NNRTIs are not incorporated into viral DNA but prevent the movement of reverse transcriptase.

HIGH-YIELD BOARD EXAM ESSENTIALS
- **CLASSIC AGENTS:** Abacavir (ABC), didanosine (ddI), emtricitabine (FTC), lamivudine (3TC), stavudine (d4T), tenofovir alafenamide (TAF), tenofovir disoproxil (TDF), zalcitabine (DDC), zidovudine (AZT)
- **DRUG CLASS:** NRTI
- **INDICATIONS:** HIV
- **MECHANISM:** Inhibition of HIV reverse transcription into the emerging proviral DNA.
- **SIDE EFFECTS:** Myopathies, peripheral neuropathies, pancreatitis, anemias, granulocytopenia; potentially fatal lactic acidosis and hepatic steatosis (didanosine, stavudine, zidovudine)
- **CLINICAL PEARLS:** Before initiation of abacavir, patients must be screened for the presence of HLA-B*5701, as patients with positive HLA-B*5701 locus are at high risk of acute hypersensitivity syndrome.

Table: Drug Class Summary

NRTI - Drug Class Review High-Yield Med Reviews			
Mechanism of Action: *Inhibition of HIV reverse transcription into the emerging proviral DNA.*			
Class Effects: *A core component to highly-active antiretroviral regimens but are associated with class toxicities including lactic acidosis, myopathies, peripheral neuropathies, pancreatitis, bone marrow toxicities.*			
Generic Name	**Brand Name**	**Main Indication(s) or Uses**	**Notes**

Abacavir	Ziagen	- HIV	- **Dosing (Adult):**
			   – Oral: 300 mg BID
			   – Oral: 600 mg daily with other antiretrovirals
			- **Dosing (Peds):**
			   – Oral: 8 mg/kg/dose BID
			      – Maximum 300 mg/dose
			   – Oral: 16 mg/kg/dose daily
			      – Maximum 600 mg/dose
			- **CYP450 Interactions:** None
			- **Renal or Hepatic Dose Adjustments:**
			   – Child-Pugh class A: 200 mg BID
			   – Child-Pugh class B or C: contraindicated
			- **Dosage Forms:** Oral (solution, tablet)

Didanosine	Videx	- HIV	- **Dosing (Adult):**
			   – Oral: 200 to 400 mg once daily
			   – Oral: 125 to 200 mg BID
			- **Dosing (Peds):**
			   – Oral: 50 to 100 mg/m2/dose q12h
			- **CYP450 Interactions:** None
			- **Renal or Hepatic Dose Adjustments:**
			   – GFR 30 to 59 mL/minute: reduce dose by 50%
			   – GFR 10 to 29 mL/minute: reduce dose by approximately 62.5%
			   – GFR < 10 mL/minute: reduce dose by approximately 75 %
			- **Dosage Forms:** Oral (capsule, solution)

NRTI - Drug Class Review
High-Yield Med Reviews

Generic Name	Brand Name	Main Indication(s) or Uses	Notes

Emtricitabine	Emtriva	- HIV	- **Dosing (Adult):**
			  - Oral: capsule 200 mg daily
			  - Oral: solution 240 mg daily
			- **Dosing (Peds):**
			  - Oral: solution 3 to 6 mg/kg/dose daily
			    - Maximum 240 mg/day
			  - For oral capsule use, must weigh more than 33 kg
			- **CYP450 Interactions:** None
			- **Renal or Hepatic Dose Adjustments:**
			  - GFR 30 to 49 mL/minute: Capsule 200 mg q48h, solution 120 mg q24h
			  - GFR 15 to 29 mL/minute: Capsule 200 mg q72h, solution 80 mg q24h
			  - GFR < 15 mL/minute: Capsule 200 mg q96h, solution 60 mg q24h
			- **Dosage Forms:** Oral (capsule, solution)

Lamivudine	Epivir, Epivir HBV	- HIV
		- Hepatitis B
			- **Dosing (Adult):**
			  - HIV
			    - Oral: 300 mg daily or 150 mg BID
			  - HBV
			    - Oral: 100 mg daily
			- **Dosing (Peds):**
			  - Oral: 30 to 150 mg BID
			- **CYP450 Interactions:** None
			- **Renal or Hepatic Dose Adjustments:** HIV indication
			  - GFR 30 to 49 mL/minute: 150 mg daily
			  - GFR 15 to 29 mL/minute: 150 mg x1 then 100 mg daily
			  - GFR < 15 mL/minute: 150 mg x1 then 50 mg daily
			  - GFR < 5 - 50 mg, then 25 mg daily
			- **Dosage Forms:** Oral (solution, tablet)

Stavudine	Zerit	- HIV	- **Dosing (Adult):**
			  - Oral: 30 to 40 mg q12h
			- **Dosing (Peds):**
			  - Oral: 1 mg/kg/dose q12h
			    - Maximum 30 mg/dose
			- **CYP450 Interactions:** None
			- **Renal or Hepatic Dose Adjustments:**
			  - GFR 26 to 50 mL/minute: 15 or 20 mg q12h
			  - GFR 10 to 25 mL/minute: 15 or 20 mg q24h
			- **Dosage Forms:** Oral (capsule, solution)

| \multicolumn{4}{c}{**NRTI - Drug Class Review**} |
| \multicolumn{4}{c}{High-Yield Med Reviews} |
Generic Name	Brand Name	Main Indication(s) or Uses	Notes

Tenofovir alafenamide	Vemlidy	- Hepatitis B	- **Dosing (Adult):**
			  – HIV
			    – Only available in combination with other ART (Biktarvy, Genvoya, Odefsey, Symtuza)
			  – HBV
			    – Oral: 25 mg daily
			- **Dosing (Peds):**
			  – Not routinely used
			- **CYP450 Interactions:** None
			- **Renal or Hepatic Dose Adjustments:**
			  – GFR < 15 mL/minute - Not recommended
			  – Child-Pugh class B or C - Not recommended
			- **Dosage Forms:** Oral (tablet)

Tenofovir disoproxil	Viread	- Hepatitis B
		- HIV
			- **Dosing (Adult):**
			  – HIV
			    – Oral: 300 mg daily or 150 mg BID
			  – HBV
			    – Oral: 100 or 300 mg daily
			- **Dosing (Peds):**
			  – Oral 8 mg/kg/dose daily
			    – Maximum 300 mg/day
			- **CYP450 Interactions:** None
			- **Renal or Hepatic Dose Adjustments:** HIV indication
			  – GFR 30 to 49 mL/minute: 300 mg q48h
			  – GFR 10 to 29 mL/minute: 300 mg q72h
			  – GFR < 10 mL/minute: Not recommended
			- **Dosage Forms:** Oral (solution, tablet)

Zalcitabine	Hivid	- HIV	- **Dosing (Adult):**
			  – Oral: 0.75 mg q8h
			- **Dosing (Peds):**
			  – Not routinely used
			- **CYP450 Interactions:** None
			- **Renal or Hepatic Dose Adjustments:**
			  – GFR 10 to 40 mL/minute: 0.75 mg q12h
			  – GFR < 10 mL/minute: 0.75 mg q24h
			- **Dosage Forms:** Oral (tablet)

| \multicolumn{4}{c}{**NRTI - Drug Class Review**} |
| \multicolumn{4}{c}{High-Yield Med Reviews} |

Generic Name	Brand Name	Main Indication(s) or Uses	Notes

Zidovudine	Retrovir	- HIV	- **Dosing (Adult):**
			    - IV: 2 mg/kg loading dose, then 1 mg/kg/hour
			    - Oral: 300 mg BID
			- **Dosing (Peds):**
			    - Oral: 9 to 12 mg/kg/dose
			        - Maximum 300 mg BID
			    - IV: 120 mg/m2/dose q4-6h
			        - Maximum 160 mg/dose
			- **CYP450 Interactions:** None
			- **Renal or Hepatic Dose Adjustments:**
			    - GFR < 15 mL/minute: Oral: 100 mg TID or 300 mg daily
			- **Dosage Forms:** Oral (capsule, solution, tablet), IV solution

HIV ANTIVIRALS – PROTEASE INHIBITOR

Drug Class
- Protease Inhibitor
- Agents:
    - Chronic Care
        - Atazanavir
        - Darunavir
        - Fosamprenavir
        - Indinavir
        - Lopinavir
        - Nelfinavir
        - Ritonavir
        - Saquinavir
        - Tipranavir

> **Fast Facts**
>
> ✓ Lopinavir/ritonavir solution contains 42% ethanol and also has methanol and propylene glycol.
>
> ✓ All protease inhibitors can inhibit CYP450 3A4
>
> ✓ All protease inhibitors can cause elevations in blood glucose and triglycerides, but atazanavir is the least likely to cause this.

Main Indications or Uses
- Chronic Care
    - HIV

Mechanism of Action
- Inhibit the processing of HIV viral proteins, forming immature, non-functional proteins incapable of infecting other cells.

Primary Net Benefit
- Lopinavir and ritonavir were among the first antiretrovirals associated with high pill burden and poor tolerability, but new protease inhibitors improved efficacy and safety, permitting long-term use.
- Main Labs to Monitor:
    - CD4 count
    - HIV viral load
    - HIV genotype/phenotype
    - Liver enzymes (AST/ALT)
    - Liver function (INR/PT, albumin, protein, bilirubin)
    - Lipid panel

High-Yield Basic Pharmacology
- **Pharmacokinetic "Boosting"**
    - Protease inhibitors can benefit from their common hepatic oxidation pathway by causing a pharmacokinetically predictable inhibition of their metabolism using the CYP3A4 inhibitors cobicistat or ritonavir.
    - When ritonavir is used as a boosting agent, it must not be included in "active" antiretroviral agents.
        - Nelfinavir is the only protease inhibitor not pharmacokinetically boosted by ritonavir.
    - Cobicistat does not possess the antiretroviral activity and is only used as a pharmacokinetic boosting agent.
- **PPI Interaction**
    - Many protease inhibitors require acidic environments for adequate absorption and thus cannot be combined with proton pump inhibitors.
        - A combination of indinavir and ritonavir can permit indinavir administration with food.
    - PPI use must be avoided with atazanavir, fosamprenavir, indinavir, and nelfinavir.

High-Yield Clinical Knowledge

- **Protease Inhibitor Class Adverse Effects**
  - Protease inhibitors are frequently associated with GI intolerance (diarrhea), central fat redistribution (buffalo hump plus peripheral fat wasting), hyperglycemia (and diabetes), hyperlipidemia, PR and QT prolongation, and numerous drug-drug interactions via cytochrome oxidation inhibition.
- **Hyperbilirubinemia**
  - Atazanavir and indinavir are associated with increased unconjugated bilirubin, potentially causing jaundice.
  - In atazanavir therapy, scleral icterus is a surrogate for patient compliance with ART therapy and otherwise does not require drug adjustment or intervention.
  - Indinavir may also cause asymptomatic hyperbilirubinemia.
- **Oral Contraceptives**
  - Nelfinavir and ritonavir decrease oral contraceptives' concentration through induction of their hepatic metabolism (induce CYP1A2, 2B6).
- **Darunavir Rash**
  - Darunavir therapy is associated with approximately a 5% risk of rash, which can become severe due to its sulfonamide moiety.
  - Patients with a history of sulfa allergy may exhibit a higher likelihood of rash due to darunavir.
- **Ritonavir Solution**
  - The oral solution preparation of ritonavir contains ethanol and should be avoided in patients concomitantly taking metronidazole, disulfiram, NMTT side chain containing cephalosporins (cefazolin, cefotetan), or calcium carbamide.
    - A combination of ritonavir solution with amprenavir suspension should also be avoided as amprenavir suspension contains propylene glycol.
- **Indinavir Nephrolithiasis**
  - Indinavir is poorly soluble at pH above 7.5, such as in urine, which increases the risk of crystalluria and nephrolithiasis.
    - Patients must maintain adequate hydration (approximately 2,000 mL/day) to provide sufficiently dilute urine to prevent crystalluria.
  - Atazanavir has been observed to precipitate in urine, increasing the risk of kidney stones.

High-Yield Core Evidence

- **CASTLE**
  - This was a multicenter, open-label, noninferiority trial that randomized ART treatment-naive patients to receive atazanavir 300 mg plus ritonavir 100 mg once daily or lopinavir/ritonavir 400/100 mg twice daily with tenofovir/emtricitabine 300/200 mg once daily for 48 weeks.
  - There was no difference between groups concerning the primary endpoint of the proportion of patients with viral load less than 50 c/mL at week 48.
  - There was no difference in the mean increases from baseline in CD4 cell count or serious adverse events.
  - As anticipated, more jaundice was observed in the atazanavir/ritonavir group, but this group experienced significantly less diarrhea than lopinavir/ritonavir treated patients.
  - The authors concluded that in treatment-naive patients, atazanavir/ritonavir once-daily demonstrated similar antiviral efficacy to lopinavir/ritonavir twice-daily, with less gastrointestinal toxicity but with a higher rate of hyperbilirubinemia. (Lancet. 2008 Aug 23;372(9639):646-55.)

- **Cobicistat vs Ritonavir**
  - This was a multicenter, noninferiority study of treatment-naive patients with HIV viral load of 5000 c/mL or higher who were randomized to either elvitegravir, cobicistat, emtricitabine, and tenofovir disoproxil fumarate or ritonavir-boosted atazanavir plus co-formulated emtricitabine and tenofovir disoproxil fumarate.
  - Elvitegravir, cobicistat, emtricitabine, and tenofovir disoproxil fumarate was non-inferior to ritonavir-boosted atazanavir plus co-formulated emtricitabine and tenofovir disoproxil fumarate regarding the endpoint of HIV viral load of 50 c/mL or less at 48 weeks.
  - There was no significant difference between groups regarding safety and tolerability, but fewer patients in the elvitegravir-based therapy experienced abnormal results in liver function tests than did those receiving atazanavir-based treatment.
  - However, patients receiving atazanavir-based therapy had smaller increases in fasting triglycerides than elvitegravir-based treatment.
  - The authors concluded that elvitegravir-based therapy was non-inferior to atazanavir-based ART therapy and would be the first integrase-inhibitor-based regimen given once daily and the only one formulated as a single tablet for initial HIV treatment. (Lancet. 2012;379:2429–2438.)

High-Yield Fast-Fact
- **Indinavir Effects**
  - Indinavir therapy is associated with numerous dermatologic adverse events, including alopecia and ingrown toenails.

HIGH-YIELD BOARD EXAM ESSENTIALS
- **CLASSIC AGENTS:** Atazanavir, darunavir, fosamprenavir, indinavir, lopinavir, nelfinavir, ritonavir, saquinavir, tipranavir
- **DRUG CLASS:** Protease inhibitor
- **INDICATIONS:** HIV
- **MECHANISM:** Inhibit the processing of HIV viral proteins, forming immature, non-functional proteins incapable of infecting other cells.
- **SIDE EFFECTS:** GI intolerance (diarrhea), central fat redistribution (buffalo hump plus peripheral fat wasting), hyperglycemia (and diabetes), hyperlipidemia, PR and QT prolongation, and numerous drug-drug interactions via cytochrome oxidation inhibition.
- **CLINICAL PEARLS:** Atazanavir and indinavir are associated with an increase in unconjugated bilirubin, potentially causing jaundice due to inhibition of UGT1A1. In the course of atazanavir therapy, scleral icterus is a surrogate for patient compliance with ART therapy and otherwise does not require drug adjustment or intervention.

Table: Drug Class Summary

	Protease Inhibitor - Drug Class Review High-Yield Med Reviews
	**Mechanism of Action:** *Inhibit the processing of HIV viral proteins, forming immature, non-functional proteins incapable of infecting other cells.*
	**Class Effects:** *Lopinavir and ritonavir were among the first antiretrovirals associated with high pill burden and poor tolerability, but new protease inhibitors improved efficacy and safety, permitting long-term use.*
Generic Name	**Brand Name**	**Main Indication(s) or Uses**	**Notes**

Atazanavir	Reyataz, Evotaz (with cobicistat)	- HIV	- **Dosing (Adult):**
			  – Oral: 300 mg daily plus ritonavir or cobicistat
			  – Oral: 400 mg daily
			- **Dosing (Peds):**
			  – Boosted regimen in children 3 months or older
			    – Oral: 200 to 300 mg daily
			  – Unboosted regimen in children 3 months or older
			    – Oral: 520 to 620 mg/m2/daily
			- **CYP450 Interactions:** Substrate CYP3A4; Inhibits CYP3A4
			- **Renal or Hepatic Dose Adjustments:**
			  – ESRD - not recommended
			  – Child-Pugh class C: not recommended
			- **Dosage Forms:** Oral (capsule, packet)

Darunavir	Prezista	- HIV	- **Dosing (Adult):**
			  – Oral: 800 mg once daily plus ritonavir or cobicistat
			  – Oral: 600 mg twice daily plus ritonavir or cobicistat
			- **Dosing (Peds):**
			  – Oral: 20 mg/kg BID plus ritonavir
			  – Oral: 200 to 600 mg BID plus ritonavir
			- **CYP450 Interactions:** Substrate CYP3A4, P-gp; Inhibits CYP2D6, 3A4
			- **Renal or Hepatic Dose Adjustments:**
			  – Child-Pugh class C: not recommended
			- **Dosage Forms:** Oral (suspension, tablet)

| \multicolumn{4}{c}{**Protease Inhibitor - Drug Class Review**} |
| \multicolumn{4}{c}{High-Yield Med Reviews} |

Generic Name	Brand Name	Main Indication(s) or Uses	Notes

Fosamprenavir	Lexiva	• HIV	• **Dosing (Adult):**
			  − Oral: 1,400 mg BID
			  − Oral: 700 mg BID plus ritonavir BID
			• **Dosing (Peds):**
			  − Oral: 30 mg/kg/dose without ritonavir
			    − Maximum 1,400 mg/day
			  − Oral: 18 to 45 mg/kg/dose BID plus ritonavir 3 to 7 mg/kg BID
			• **CYP450 Interactions:** Substrate CYP2C9, 2D6, 3A4, P-gp; Inhibits CYP3A4
			• **Renal or Hepatic Dose Adjustments:**
			  − Child-Pugh class A: 700 mg BID without ritonavir or ritonavir once daily
			  − Child-Pugh class C: 700 mg BID without ritonavir or 450 mg BID with ritonavir once daily
			  − Child-Pugh class C: 350 mg BID without ritonavir or 300 mg BID with ritonavir once daily
			• **Dosage Forms:** Oral (suspension, tablet)

Indinavir	Crixivan	• HIV	• **Dosing (Adult):**
			  − Oral: 800 mg q8h
			  − Oral: 800 mg BID plus ritonavir 100 to 200 mg BID
			• **Dosing (Peds):**
			  − Oral: 400 mg/m2/dose q12h plus ritonavir
			• **CYP450 Interactions:** Substrate CYP2D6, 3A4, P-gp; Inhibits CYP3A4
			• **Renal or Hepatic Dose Adjustments:**
			  − Child-Pugh class A or B: 600 mg q8h without ritonavir
			  − Child-Pugh class C: not recommended
			• **Dosage Forms:** Oral (capsule)

Lopinavir	Kaletra (with ritonavir)	• HIV	• **Dosing (Adult):**
			  − Oral: 400 mg BID with ritonavir 100 mg BID
			  − Oral: 800 mg with ritonavir 200 mg daily
			• **Dosing (Peds):**
			  − Oral: 10 to 16 mg/kg/dose or 300 mg/m2/dose BID
			  − Oral
			• **CYP450 Interactions:** Substrate CYP1A2, 2B6, 2D6, 3A4, P-gp; Inhibits CYP2D6, 3A4
			• **Renal or Hepatic Dose Adjustments:**
			  − Child-Pugh class C - use with caution
			• **Dosage Forms:** Oral (solution, tablet)

Protease Inhibitor - Drug Class Review
High-Yield Med Reviews

Generic Name	Brand Name	Main Indication(s) or Uses	Notes
Nelfinavir	Viracept	• HIV	• **Dosing (Adult):** — Oral: 750 mg TID or 1,250 mg BID • **Dosing (Peds):** — Oral: 45 to 55 mg/kg/dose BID — Maximum 1,250 mg/dose — Oral: 25 to 35 mg/kg/dose TID — Maximum 750 mg/dose • **CYP450 Interactions:** Substrate CYP2C9, 2C19, 2D6, 3A4, P-gp; Inhibits CYP3A4; Induces CYP1A2, 2B6 • **Renal or Hepatic Dose Adjustments:** — Child-Pugh class C - not recommended • **Dosage Forms:** Oral (tablet)
Ritonavir	Norvir	• HIV	• **Dosing (Adult):** — Oral: 100 to 400 mg daily in 1-2 divided doses • **Dosing (Peds):** — Oral: 250 to 400 mg/m2/dose q12h • **CYP450 Interactions:** Substrate CYP1A2, 2B6, 2D6, 3A4, P-gp; Inhibits CYP2D6, 3A4; Induces CYP1A2, 2B6, 2C19, 2C9 • **Renal or Hepatic Dose Adjustments:** — Child-Pugh class C: not recommended • **Dosage Forms:** Oral (capsule, packet, solution, tablet)
Tipranavir	Aptivus	• HIV	• **Dosing (Adult):** — Oral: 500 mg BID with ritonavir 200 mg BID • **Dosing (Peds):** — Oral: 14 mg/kg/dose BID plus ritonavir 6 mg/kg/dose BID — Maximum 500 mg (tipranavir), 200 mg (ritonavir) • **CYP450 Interactions:** Substrate CYP3A4; Inhibits CYP2D6 • **Renal or Hepatic Dose Adjustments:** — Child-Pugh class C: contraindicated • **Dosage Forms:** Oral (capsule, packet)

2025

A COMPREHENSIVE *RAPID REVIEW*

NAPLEX

Pharmacology & Drug Classes

Musculoskeletal

BONE MINERAL HOMEOSTASIS – ANTI-FGF23 MABs

Drug Class
- Anti-FGF23 MABs
- Agents:
  - Chronic Care
    - Burosumab

Main Indications or Uses
- Chronic Care
  - Tumor-induced osteomalacia
  - X-linked Hypophosphatemia

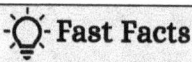

Fast Facts
- ✓ Burosumab is a fully human IgG1 monoclonal antibody and like all MABs, it is very specific to FGF23, cannot be administered by mouth, and has a long half-life allowing for a longer duration of time between shots.

Mechanism of Action
- Decreases renal phosphate excretion and 1,25(OH)2-D production by inhibition of FGF23.

Primary Net Benefit
- Burosumab is an orphan drug approved for X-linked hypophosphatemia, a rare autosomal dominant hypophosphatemia.
- Main Labs to Monitor:
  - Serum 25(OH)D
  - Serum phosphorus (baseline and q4weeks x 12 weeks)

High-Yield Basic Pharmacology
- Reverses Pathophysiology
  - In patients with FGF23-related genetic diseases, burosumab reverses the inhibition of renal uptake of phosphate and promotes 1,25(OH)2D production.

High-Yield Clinical Knowledge
- Use with Oral Phosphate or Vitamin D
  - In patients with vitamin D-dependent rickets, supplementation with standard doses of vitamin D, in combination with phosphate supplementation and calcitriol, are typically considered first-line interventions.
    - However, prolonged treatment can lead to secondary hyperparathyroidism.
  - Patients diagnosed with XLH who are started on burosumab cannot receive concomitant oral phosphate or active vitamin D analogs.
- Injection Site Reactions
  - Burosumab is typically administered via subcutaneous injection every 2 weeks and is associated with a relatively high incidence of self-limiting local injection site reactions.
- X-linked hypophosphatemia
  - Hypophosphatemia leading to the manifestations of rickets in children or adults has been linked to increased biologically active FGF23, promoting phosphate wasting in the urine.
  - XLH occurs due to mutations in the gene encoding endopeptidase (PHEX protein).
- Autosomal dominant hypophosphatemia
  - This occurs due to FGF23 gene mutations that result in decreased proteolysis and stabilized FGF23.
- Tumor-Induced Osteomalacia
  - Burosumab is also indicated for tumor-induced osteomalacia, which is similar in pathophysiology to autosomal dominant hypophosphatemia, where tumors increase the expression of FGF23.

High-Yield Core Evidence

- **AXLES 1**
  - This was a double-blind, placebo-controlled, phase 3 trial that randomized patients with symptomatic X-linked hypophosphatemia (XLH) and hypophosphatemia and pain to either burosumab 1 mg/kg or placebo subcutaneously every 4 weeks.
  - Patients randomized to receive burosumab experience significant improvements in mean serum phosphate concentrations to above the lower limit of normal compared with placebo.
  - Burosumab treated patients also experienced a significantly reduced Western Ontario and the McMaster Universities Osteoarthritis Index stiffness subscale compared with placebo.
  - Patients with baseline active fractures were fully healed in significantly more patients randomized to burosumab compared to placebo at week 24.
  - There were no treatment-related serious adverse events or meaningful changes from baseline in serum or urine calcium, intact parathyroid hormone, or nephrocalcinosis.
  - The authors concluded that these data support the conclusion that burosumab is a novel therapeutic addressing an important medical need in adults with XLH. (Lancet. 2019 Jul 13;394(10193):120.)

- **XLH in Children**
  - This was a multicenter, active-controlled, open-label, phase 3 trial that randomized children meeting inclusion criteria with X-linked hypophosphatemia (XLH) between the ages of 1 to 12 years to receive either burosumab 0.8 mg/kg SQ q2weeks or conventional therapy prescribed by investigators.
  - Patients randomized to burosumab experienced a significantly greater improvement in the primary endpoint of change in rickets severity at week 40, assessed by the Radiographic Global Impression of Change global score.
  - However, significantly more patients receiving burosumab experienced treatment-emergent adverse events considered possibly, probably, or definitely related to treatment by the investigator, but there was no difference in the incidence of serious adverse events.
  - The authors concluded that significantly greater clinical improvements were shown in rickets severity, growth, and biochemistries among children with XLH treated with burosumab compared with those continuing conventional therapy. (Lancet. 2019 Jun 15;393(10189):2416-2427.)

High-Yield Fast-Fact

- **Breakthrough Designation**
  - The FDA approved burosumab as an orphan breakthrough drug.
  - The FDA uses this designation to describe therapies exhibiting superior efficacy against serious diseases.

HIGH-YIELD BOARD EXAM ESSENTIALS

- **CLASSIC AGENTS:** Burosumab
- **DRUG CLASS:** Anti-FGF23 MAB
- **INDICATIONS:** Tumor-induced osteomalacia, X-linked Hypophosphatemia
- **MECHANISM:** Decreases renal phosphate excretion and 1,25(OH)2-D production by inhibition of FGF23
- **SIDE EFFECTS:** Injection site reaction, hypophosphatemia
- **CLINICAL PEARLS:** In patients with FGF23 related genetic diseases, burosumab reverses the inhibition of renal uptake of phosphate and promotes 1,25(OH)2D production.

Table: Drug Class Summary

	Anti-FGF23 MABs - Drug Class Review High-Yield Med Reviews
	**Mechanism of Action:** *Decreases renal phosphate excretion and 1,25(OH)2-D production by inhibition of FGF23*
	**Class Effects:** *Burosumab is an orphan drug approved for X-linked hypophosphatemia, a rare autosomal dominant hypophosphatemia.*
Generic Name	**Brand Name**	**Indication(s) or Uses**	**Notes**
Burosumab	Crysvita	<ul><li>Tumor-induced osteomalacia</li><li>X-linked Hypophosphatemia</li></ul>	<ul><li>**Dosing (Adult):**<ul><li>SQ: 0.5 to 1 mg/kg q4weeks, followed by serum phosphorus-guided dosing.<ul><li>Maximum 90 mg/dose</li></ul></li></ul></li><li>**Dosing (Peds):**<ul><li>SQ: 0.8 to 1 mg/kg/dose q2-4weeks, followed by serum phosphorus-guided dosing.<ul><li>Maximum 90 mg/dose</li></ul></li></ul></li><li>**CYP450 Interactions:** None</li><li>**Renal or Hepatic Dose Adjustments:**<ul><li>GFR < 30 mL/minute: Use contraindicated</li></ul></li><li>**Dosage Forms:** Subcutaneous solution</li></ul>

BONE MINERAL HOMEOSTASIS – BISPHOSPHONATES

Drug Class
- **Bisphosphonates**
- **Agents:**
    - Acute Care
        - Pamidronate
        - Zoledronic acid
    - **Chronic Care**
        - Alendronate
        - Ibandronate
        - Pamidronate
        - Risedronate
        - Zoledronic acid

Main Indications or Uses
- **Acute Care**
    - Hypercalcemia of malignancy
        - Pamidronate
        - Zoledronic acid
    - Multiple myeloma
        - Zoledronic acid
- **Chronic Care**
    - Osteolytic bone metastases/lesions
        - Pamidronate
        - Zoledronic acid
    - Osteoporosis or Paget disease
        - Alendronate
        - Ibandronate
        - Pamidronate
        - Risedronate
        - Zoledronic acid

> **Fast Facts**
>
> ✓ Unlike many of the other bisphosphonates, pamidronate is reserved for hypercalcemia of malignancy.
>
> ✓ The two options that can be given parenterally for the management of osteoporosis are ibandronate and zolendronic acid.
>
> ✓ All of these agents have a very low oral bioavailability.
>
> ✓ All of these agents have dosing reductions or restrictions once the CrCl is < 40 ml/min

Mechanism of Action
- Inhibit bone resorption by interfering with the activity of osteoclasts.

Primary Net Benefit
- Indirectly increase BMD and reduce the risk of hip, spine, and other fractures with potential for increasing atypical femur fractures
- Main Labs to Monitor:
    - Serum calcium (baseline, periodically)
    - Vitamin D (baseline, periodically)
    - SCr (baseline, periodically)
    - DEXA scan (baseline, based on patient and treatment but generally every 1-3 years), T-score

High-Yield Basic Pharmacology
- **Active Remodeling Sites**
    - Bisphosphonates concentrate in areas of bone that undergo active remodeling and remain in the bone until it is remodeled.

- **Oral Absorption**
  - All bisphosphonates are poorly absorbed from the intestines.
  - Alendronate and risedronate have bioavailabilities of < 1%.
  - Absorption can be further reduced if coadministered with divalent cations (calcium, magnesium), other antacids, or oral iron.
- **Elimination Characteristics**
  - Due to the large volume of distribution into bone and limited re-distribution out of bone, bisphosphonates undergo minimal hepatic elimination and are renally eliminated as unchanged molecules.
- **Elimination Half-Life**
  - The elimination half-life of these drugs is influenced by their distribution and elimination characteristics and is profoundly long.
  - The terminal half-life of bisphosphonates is approximately 11 *years*.

High-Yield Clinical Knowledge
- **Hypercalcemia of Malignancy**
  - In some patients with acute leukemias or those at risk of tumor lysis syndrome, IV bisphosphonates are a component of a cocktail to limit hypercalcemia associated with massive cell lysis.
  - Pamidronate and zoledronic acid are the only two bisphosphonates currently available in an IV dosage form and are used as single doses for hypercalcemia.
    - Ibandronate is also available as an IV formulation but is not used for hypercalcemia.
  - As their onset of action is hours to days, other interventions are critical, including IV volume replacement, diuresis, corticosteroids, calcitonin, and denosumab.
- **Esophageal Adverse Events**
  - Patients must be instructed to take oral bisphosphonates on an empty stomach with at least eight ounces of water and remain upright for 30 to 60 minutes.
    - Specific forms of risedronate, specifically the delayed-release preparation, may be taken 30 minutes after a morning meal.
  - This is to minimize GI adverse effects that range in severity from heartburn to esophageal irritation to GI ulceration, perforation, or rupture leading to critical GI bleeding.
- **Fractures and Osteonecrosis**
  - Bisphosphonates are associated with an increased risk of osteonecrosis of the jaw (rare) and an increased risk of stress fractures in the femoral shaft's lateral cortex (atypical fractures).
  - Because of these risks, limit bisphosphonate therapy to approximately 3-5 years (maybe less), as the risks begin to outweigh the benefits.
    - Bisphosphonates' benefits on BMD persist for 4-5 years and are sustained for longer periods of time even after discontinuation.
- **Renal Disease**
  - Patients with an estimated CrCl less than 30 to 35 mL/min (drug dependent) must not receive bisphosphonates.
- **Dosing Form and Frequency**
  - Bisphosphonates are available in dosage forms that allow daily, weekly, or yearly dosing.
  - Alendronate is available in oral daily or weekly dosage forms.
  - Ibandronate is available in an oral monthly or IV formulation given every 3 months.
  - Risedronate is available in an oral daily, weekly, or monthly formulation.
  - Pamidronate and zoledronic acid are only available as an IV infusion administered monthly (pamidronate) or every 1 to 2 years (zoledronic acid).

High-Yield Core Evidence
- **HORIZON-PFT**
    - This was a multicenter, double-blind, placebo-controlled trial that randomized postmenopausal women with osteoporosis to either an infusion of zoledronic acid 5 mg or placebo at baseline, 12 months, and 24 months and followed them for a total of 36 months.
    - Patients randomized to receive zoledronic acid infusions experienced a significant reduction in the risk of morphometric vertebral fracture and the risk of hip fracture during the 36-month study period compared to placebo.
    - Similarly, zoledronic acid significantly reduced the risk of nonvertebral fractures, clinical fractures, and clinical vertebral fractures compared to placebo and significantly improved BMD.
    - New atrial fibrillation was observed in significantly more patients who received zoledronic acid compared to placebo.
    - The authors concluded that a once-yearly infusion of zoledronic acid during a 3-year period significantly reduced the risk of vertebral, hip, and other fractures. (N Engl J Med. 2007 May 3;356(18):1809-22.)
- **Alendronate Cochrane Review and Meta-Analysis**
    - This was a systematic review and meta-analysis conducted to assess the efficacy of alendronate in the primary and secondary prevention of osteoporotic fractures in postmenopausal women.
    - Relevant randomized controlled trials published between 1966 to 2007 included postmenopausal women receiving at least one year of alendronate 10 mg for postmenopausal osteoporosis, which were compared to those receiving placebo and/or concurrent calcium/vitamin D.
    - The outcome was fracture incidence, where at least a 15% relative change was considered clinically significant.
    - A total of eleven trials representing 12,068 women were included in the review.
    - Alendronate was associated with a significant relative risk reduction for primary and secondary prevention of vertebral fractures.
    - Secondary prevention, but not primary prevention, with alendronate was associated with a relative risk reduction of nonvertebral fractures, hip fractures, and wrist fractures.
    - There were no significant adverse events in any included study, but observational data raise concerns regarding a potential risk for upper GI injury and, less commonly, osteonecrosis of the jaw.
    - The authors concluded that alendronate 10 mg/day demonstrated both clinically important and statistically significant reductions in vertebral, nonvertebral, hip, and wrist fractures as secondary prevention. No statistically significant results for primary prevention were evident and clinically meaningful, except for vertebral fractures. (Cochrane Database Syst Rev. 2008 Jan 23;(1): CD001155.)

High-Yield Fast-Fact
- **First-Generation**
    - First-generation bisphosphonates are no longer clinically used (clodronate, etidronate, and medronate).

HIGH-YIELD BOARD EXAM ESSENTIALS
- **CLASSIC AGENTS:** Alendronate, ibandronate, pamidronate, risedronate, zoledronic acid
- **DRUG CLASS:** Bisphosphonates
- **INDICATIONS:** Hypercalcemia of malignancy, multiple myeloma, osteolytic bone metastases/lesions, osteoporosis, or Paget disease
- **MECHANISM:** Inhibit bone resorption by interfering with the activity of osteoclasts.
- **SIDE EFFECTS:** Dyspepsia, GI ulceration, GI perforation, increased risk of atypical femur fractures
- **CLINICAL PEARLS:** Bisphosphonates have almost no oral absorption and thus must be given parenterally or on an empty stomach with water. Increase the risk of osteonecrosis of the jaw and femur stress fractures. Limit bisphosphonate therapy to approximately 3-5 years, as the risks begin to outweigh the benefits. Avoid with CrCl < 30-35 mL/min.

Table: Drug Class Summary

Bisphosphonates - Drug Class Review High-Yield Med Reviews			
Mechanism of Action: *Inhibit bone resorption by interfering with the activity of osteoclasts.*			
Class Effects: *Indirectly increase BMD, reduce the risk of hip, spine, and other fractures, increased risk of atypical femur fractures w/ long-term use, GI adverse effects, specific oral administration directions, avoid with CrCl < 30-35 mL/min*			
Generic Name	**Brand Name**	**Main Indication(s) or Uses**	**Notes**

Alendronate	Binosto Fosamax	• Osteoporosis
		• Paget disease
			• **Dosing (Adult):**
			  – Oral: 35 to 70 mg once weekly or 5 to 10 mg daily
			• **Dosing (Peds):**
			  – < 30 kg: 5 mg daily
			  – Between 30 and 40 kg: 5 to 10 mg daily
			  – Over 40 kg: 10 mg daily
			• **CYP450 Interactions:** None
			• **Renal or Hepatic Dose Adjustments:**
			  – CrCl < 35 mL/min: Not recommended
			• **Dosage Forms:** Oral (solution, tablet, effervescent tablet)

Ibandronate	Boniva	• Osteoporosis	• **Dosing (Adult):**
			  – IV: 2 to 6 mg over 1-2 hours q3-4weeks, up to 4 years
			  – Oral: 150 mg monthly
			• **Dosing (Peds):** N/A
			• **CYP450 Interactions:** None
			• **Renal or Hepatic Dose Adjustments:**
			  – CrCl < 30 mL/min: Not recommended
			• **Dosage Forms:** Oral (tablet), IV (solution)

Pamidronate	Areda	• Hypercalcemia of malignancy
		• Osteolytic bone metastases/lesions
		• Paget disease
			• **Dosing (Adult):**
			  – IV: 60 to 90 mg once or up to monthly
			• **Dosing (Peds):**
			  – IV: 0.25 to 2 mg/kg/dose, max 90 mg/dose
			• **CYP450 Interactions:** None
			• **Renal or Hepatic Dose Adjustments:**
			  – CrCl < 30 mL/min or SCr > 3 mg/dL: Not recommended (breast cancer, osteolytic bone metastases), reduce dose, or weigh risk/benefit
			• **Dosage Forms:** IV (solution)

Risedronate	Actonel Atelvia	• Osteoporosis
		• Paget disease
			• **Dosing (Adult):**
			  – Oral: 5 mg daily, 35 once weekly, or 150 mg once monthly
			• **Dosing (Peds):** N/A
			• **CYP450 Interactions:** None
			• **Renal or Hepatic Dose Adjustments:**
			  – CrCl < 30 mL/min: Not recommended
			• **Dosage Forms:** Oral (tablet)

Bisphosphonates - Drug Class Review
High-Yield Med Reviews

Generic Name	Brand Name	Main Indication(s) or Uses	Notes
Zoledronic acid	Reclast Zometa	<ul><li>Hypercalcemia of malignancy</li><li>Multiple myeloma</li><li>Osteolytic bone metastases/lesions</li><li>Osteoporosis</li><li>Paget disease</li></ul>	<ul><li>**Dosing (Adult):**<ul><li>IV: 4 mg q1-26weeks</li><li>IV: 5 mg q2years or as a single dose once</li></ul></li><li>**Dosing (Peds):**<ul><li>IV: 0.0125 to 0.05 mg/kg/dose, max 4 mg/dose</li></ul></li><li>**CYP450 Interactions:** None</li><li>**Renal or Hepatic Dose Adjustments:**<ul><li>CrCl < 35 mL/minute: Contraindicated</li></ul></li><li>**Dosage Forms:** IV (concentrate solution, solution)</li></ul>

BONE MINERAL HOMEOSTASIS – CALCIMIMETICS

Drug Class
- Calcimimetics
- Agents:
  - Chronic Care
    - Cinacalcet
    - Etelcalcetide

Main Indications or Uses
- Chronic Care
  - Hyperparathyroidism (primary and secondary)
  - Parathyroid carcinoma

Mechanism of Action
- Increase sensitivity for calcium-sensing receptor (CaSr) receptor for activation by extracellular calcium, leading to reduced parathyroid hormone secretion and serum calcium concentrations.

Primary Net Benefit
- Pharmacologic interventions for secondary hyperparathyroidism in patients on dialysis, additional indications for cinacalcet in the management of parathyroid carcinoma, and primary hyperparathyroidism where parathyroidectomy cannot be performed.
- Main Labs to Monitor:
  - Serum calcium, phosphorus, albumin (baseline, one week after initiation)

High-Yield Basic Pharmacology
- Corrected Calcium
  - Serum albumin must be followed to account for falsely low laboratory calcium in hypoalbuminemia.

High-Yield Clinical Knowledge
- Drug Interactions
  - Cinacalcet is a substrate of CYP1A2, 2D6, 3A4, and inhibits CYP2D6.
  - Numerous narrow therapeutic agents, including amitriptyline, flecainide, thioridazine, and vinblastine, are at risk of reduced elimination and toxicities combined with cinacalcet.
  - Etelcalcetide is not a substrate or inhibitor of CYP 450.
- Baseline Calcium
  - Cinacalcet and etelcalcetide cannot be started without first assessing a baseline serum calcium.
  - Serum calcium must be 8.4 mg/dL or above to safely initiate cinacalcet.
- Combination
  - Cinacalcet cannot be combined with etelcalcetide due to severe, life-threatening hypocalcemia.
  - When converting from cinacalcet to etelcalcetide, cinacalcet must be tapered off before initiation of etelcalcetide.
- Dose Titration
  - Cinacalcet must be started at a dose of 30 mg daily and titrated every 2 to 4 weeks to either a maximum of 180 mg/day or the goal PTH level is reached.
  - Etelcalcetide follows a simpler titration and is administered at the end of dialysis (three times weekly) as it is removed by dialysis.

High-Yield Core Evidence
- **Cinacalcet Vs Etelcalcetide**
    - This was a multicenter, double-blind, double-dummy clinical trial that randomized patients receiving hemodialysis with serum parathyroid hormone (PTH) concentrations above 500 pg/mL on active therapy to either oral cinacalcet daily and IV placebo three times weekly with dialysis or IV etelcalcetide three times weekly with dialysis and oral placebo daily.
    - Etecalcetide met both the noniferior margin and superiority margin compared to cinacalcet therapy concerning the primary efficacy outcome of a 30% reduction from baseline in mean predialysis PTH concentrations during weeks 20-27.
    - Furthermore, significantly more patients randomized to receive etelcalcetide than placebo achieved at least a 50% reduction in PTH.
    - The most common adverse effect was decreased blood calcium, which did not differ significantly between groups.
    - The authors concluded that among patients receiving hemodialysis with moderate to severe secondary hyperparathyroidism, etelcalcetide was not inferior to cinacalcet in reducing serum PTH concentrations over 26 weeks; it also met superiority criteria. (JAMA. 2017 Jan 10;317(2):156-164.)
- **EVOLVE**
    - This was a multicenter, multinational clinical trial of patients with moderate-to-severe secondary hyperparathyroidism undergoing hemodialysis who were randomized to receive either cinacalcet or placebo to assess the impact on the risk of death or nonfatal cardiovascular.
    - There was no difference between groups concerning the primary composite endpoint of time until death, myocardial infarction, hospitalization for unstable angina, heart failure, or a peripheral vascular event.
    - However, more patients receiving cinacalcet experienced hypocalcemia and gastrointestinal adverse events than placebo.
    - In an unadjusted intention-to-treat analysis, the authors concluded that cinacalcet did not significantly reduce the risk of death or major cardiovascular events in patients with moderate-to-severe secondary hyperparathyroidism who were undergoing dialysis. (N Engl J Med. 2012 Dec 27;367(26):2482-94.)

High-Yield Fast-Fact
- **Food Effect**
    - The bioavailability of cinacalcet is increased significantly when taken with food, and patients should always be educated to take cinacalcet with food.

HIGH-YIELD BOARD EXAM ESSENTIALS
- **CLASSIC AGENTS:** Cinacalcet, etelcalcetide
- **DRUG CLASS:** Calcimimetics
- **INDICATIONS:** Hyperparathyroidism (primary and secondary), parathyroid carcinoma
- **MECHANISM:** Increase sensitivity for CaSr receptor for activation by extracellular calcium, leading to reduced parathyroid hormone secretion and serum calcium concentrations
- **SIDE EFFECTS:** QT prolongation, GI bleed, hypocalcemia
- **CLINICAL PEARLS:**
    - Cinacalcet is a substrate of CYP1A2, 2D6, 3A4, and inhibits CYP2D6.
    - Numerous narrow therapeutic agents, including amitriptyline, flecainide, thioridazine, and vinblastine, are at risk of reduced elimination and toxicities combined with cinacalcet.

Table: Drug Class Summary

	Calcimimetics - Drug Class Review		
	High-Yield Med Reviews		
Mechanism of Action: *Increase sensitivity for calcium-sensing receptor (CaSr) receptor for activation by extracellular calcium, leading to reduced parathyroid hormone secretion and serum calcium concentrations.*			
Class Effects: *Pharmacologic interventions for secondary hyperparathyroidism in patients on dialysis and additional indications for cinacalcet in the management of parathyroid carcinoma and primary hyperparathyroidism where parathyroidectomy cannot be performed.*			
Generic Name	**Brand Name**	**Indication(s) or Uses**	**Notes**
Cinacalcet	Sensipar	<ul><li>Hyperparathyroidism (primary and secondary)</li><li>Parathyroid carcinoma</li></ul>	<ul><li>**Dosing (Adult):**<ul><li>Oral: 30 to 120 mg q6-24h</li></ul></li><li>**Dosing (Peds):**<ul><li>Oral: 0.2 mg/kg/dose daily titrated q4weeks to target intact parathyroid hormone 100-300 pg/mL<ul><li>Maximum 180 mg/day or 2.5 mg/kg/dose, whichever is lower</li></ul></li></ul></li><li>**CYP450 Interactions:** Substrate CYP1A2, 2D6, 3A4; Inhibits CYP2D6</li><li>**Renal or Hepatic Dose Adjustments:**<ul><li>Child-Pugh class B or C: Close monitoring</li></ul></li><li>**Dosage Forms:** Oral (tablet)</li></ul>
Etelcalcetide	Parsabiv	<ul><li>Hyperparathyroidism (secondary)</li></ul>	<ul><li>**Dosing (Adult):**<ul><li>IV: 5 mg IV three times per week<ul><li>Adjusted up to 15 mg three times weekly</li></ul></li></ul></li><li>**Dosing (Peds):**<ul><li>Not routinely used</li></ul></li><li>**CYP450 Interactions:** None</li><li>**Renal or Hepatic Dose Adjustments:** None</li><li>**Dosage Forms:** IV (solution)</li></ul>

BONE MINERAL HOMEOSTASIS – CALCITONIN

Drug Class
- Calcitonin
- Agents:
  - Acute & Chronic Care
    - Calcitonin

Main Indications or Uses
- Acute & Chronic Care
  - Hypercalcemia
  - Osteogenesis imperfecta
  - Osteoporosis
  - Paget disease

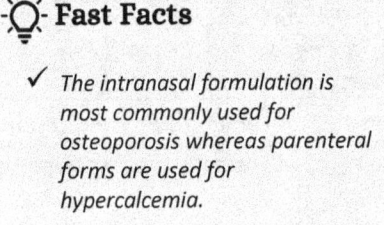

Fast Facts

✓ The intranasal formulation is most commonly used for osteoporosis whereas parenteral forms are used for hypercalcemia.

Mechanism of Action
- It inhibits osteoclast resorption and reduces renal calcium and phosphate (as well as sodium, potassium, and magnesium) reabsorption.

Primary Net Benefit
- Lowers serum calcium and phosphate through actions on both the bone and kidneys.
- Main Labs to Monitor:
  - Serum calcium
  - Serum 25(OH)D
  - Serum total alkaline phosphatase at 6 and 12 weeks, periodically thereafter.

High-Yield Basic Pharmacology
- Endogenous Calcitonin
  - Calcitonin is normally secreted by the thyroid gland, specifically from the parafollicular cells.
  - It consists of a single-chain peptide with 32 amino acids, with specific attention to the disulfide bond between positions 1 and 7, necessary for its biologic activity.
- British Medical Research Council
  - Although calcitonin is a relatively small single-chain peptide, it can be present in heterogeneous forms and sizes.
  - As a result of this heterogeneity, calcitonin's activity is compared to a standard maintained by the British Medical Research Council, which expresses calcitonin activity in MRC units.
- Salmon Calcitonin
  - Salmon calcitonin, the commonly used product, has a much longer half-life of 50 minutes than human calcitonin (half-life of 10 minutes).

High-Yield Clinical Knowledge
- Osteoporosis
  - The current role of calcitonin for postmenopausal osteoporosis is limited and reserved for salvage therapy.
    - Compared to other therapies, calcitonin only reduces the risk of vertebral fractures.
- Intranasal Formulation
  - Calcitonin is only available in an IV formulation or an intranasal formulation.
  - Patients report low satisfaction and do not prefer intranasal administration, but it has a limited role in the short-term relief of vertebral fracture pain.
- Hypercalcemia
  - Calcitonin is a component of drug therapy for acute hypercalcemia and can help reduce calcium concentrations within 24 to 48 hours.
    - Either the IV form or the intranasal form can be used.

- **Tachyphylaxis**
  - Salmon calcitonin is associated with developing antibodies, leading to tachyphylaxis with use beyond four months.

High-Yield Core Evidence
- **Postmenopausal Osteoporosis Meta-Analysis**
  - This was a meta-analysis of the effect of calcitonin on bone density and fractures in postmenopausal women.
  - A total of 30 studies that randomized women to calcitonin or placebo or calcium and/or vitamin D and measured bone density or fracture incidence for at least one year were included.
  - Calcitonin was associated with a reduced risk of vertebral fractures compared to placebo or calcium supplementation.
  - There was no benefit observed for nonvertebral fractures, lumbar spine bone density, or femoral neck density.
  - The authors concluded that calcitonin likely increases bone density in postmenopausal women predominantly at the lumbar spine and forearm for weekly doses of greater than 250 IU. However, the actual effect may be smaller than the pooled estimate. In addition, calcitonin likely reduces the risk of vertebral fracture; its impact on nonvertebral fracture remains uncertain. (Endocr Rev. 2002 Aug;23(4):540-51.)

High-Yield Fast-Fact
- **Salmon Sperm**
  - Salmon calcitonin is derived from the sperm of salmon.

HIGH-YIELD BOARD EXAM ESSENTIALS
- **CLASSIC AGENTS:** Calcitonin
- **DRUG CLASS:** Calcitonin
- **INDICATIONS:** Hypercalcemia, osteogenesis imperfecta, osteoporosis, Paget disease
- **MECHANISM:** It inhibits osteoclast resorption and reduces renal calcium and phosphate (as well as sodium, potassium, and magnesium) reabsorption.
- **SIDE EFFECTS:** Hypocalcemia, tachyphylaxis, allergy (cross sensitivity to Salmon allergy)
- **CLINICAL PEARLS:**
  - The IM or SQ (not intranasal) dosage formulation is used for hypercalcemia of malignancy after failure of IV fluids to reduce calcium.
  - The current role of intranasal calcitonin for postmenopausal osteoporosis is limited and reserved for salvage therapy. Compared to other therapies, calcitonin only reduces the risk of vertebral fractures.

Table: Drug Class Summary

Calcitonin - Drug Class Review High-Yield Med Reviews			
Mechanism of Action: *Inhibits osteoclast resorption and reduces renal calcium and phosphate (as well as sodium, potassium, and magnesium) reabsorption.*			
Class Effects: *Lowers serum calcium and phosphate through actions on both the bone and kidneys.*			
Generic Name	**Brand Name**	**Indication(s) or Uses**	**Notes**

Calcitonin	Miacalcin	- Hypercalcemia
		 - Osteogenesis imperfecta
		 - Osteoporosis
		 - Paget disease
			- **Dosing (Adult):**
			    – IM/SQ: 4 to 8 units/kg q12h
			    – IM/SQ: 100 units daily
			    – Intranasal 200 units in one nostril daily
			 - **Dosing (Peds):**
			    – IM/SQ: 2 units/kg/dose three times weekly
			 - **CYP450 Interactions:** None
			 - **Renal or Hepatic Dose Adjustments:** None
			 - **Dosage Forms:** Injection solution, Nasal solution

BONE MINERAL HOMEOSTASIS – CALCIUM SALTS

Drug Class
- Calcium Salts
- Agents:
    - Acute Care
        - Calcium chloride
        - Calcium gluconate
    - Chronic Care
        - Calcium acetate
        - Calcium carbonate
        - Calcium citrate
        - Calcium glubionate
        - Calcium lactate

Main Indications or Uses
- Acute Care
    - Cardiac arrest
    - Hyperkalemia
- Chronic Care
    - Antacid
    - Calcium supplementation
    - Hyperphosphatemia
    - Hypoparathyroidism
    - Hypocalcemia
    - Hypermagnesemia

> **Fast Facts**
> - The GI tract can only absorb up to 600 mg of elemental calcium per dose which is why most agents are given more than once-a-day.
> - In patients with lower albumin levels the corrected calcium = measured calcium (mg/dL) + 0.8 x [4.0 - albumin {g/dL}].
> - Calcium chloride has 3 times the amount of elemental calcium compared to calcium gluconate.
> - Patients with low calcium should have vitamin D levels checked and a 12-lead ECG to look for QT prolongation.

Mechanism of Action
- Calcium is an essential element necessary for a range of physiologic functions, including neuromuscular activity, endocrine regulation, coagulation, bone metabolism, and cardiac conduction.

Primary Net Benefit
- Calcium is the most abundant mineral in the body, required for normal functioning, but less than 1% of the total body calcium is located outside the bone.
- Main Labs to Monitor:
    - Serum calcium, magnesium, phosphorus, albumin

High-Yield Basic Pharmacology
- Calcium Distribution
    - The vast majority (about 99%) of the body's calcium stores are located in the bone.
    - Factors affecting calcium concentrations include the parathyroid hormone, phosphorus, vitamin D, and calcitonin.
- Albumin Bound
    - When calcium is located in the extracellular fluid, it is primarily bound to albumin, and only ionized/free calcium is physiologically active.
- Elemental Calcium Content
    - The available calcium salts have varied concentrations of elemental calcium, and knowledge of this essential calcium is necessary to select the appropriate dose for a given indication.
    - Of the oral calcium products, calcium carbonate contains the most elemental calcium (40%), with acetate, citrate, lactate, glubionate, and gluconate containing 23%, 21-24%, 13%, 9%, and 9%, respectively.
    - Calcium chloride contains approximately 27% elemental calcium (1 g = 10.5 mEq)

High-Yield Clinical Knowledge
- **Serum Calcium Correction**
  - In patients with hypoalbuminemia (albumin less than 4.0), a corrected serum calcium calculation must account for free or active calcium concentration changes.
  - Corrected calcium = measured calcium (mg/dL) + 0.8 x [4.0 - albumin {g/dL}].
    - This calculation must be correlated clinically as hypocalcemia may exist in the critically ill, despite normal albumin.
- **Dietary Requirements**
  - Most healthy adults require between 1,000 to 1,200 mg of calcium daily, which should be combined with
    - The elemental calcium in calcium salts must be considered when determining the daily intake of calcium since the GI tract can only absorb up to 600 mg of elemental calcium per dose. This is why it is normally dosed twice a day.
- **GI Complaints**
  - The most common adverse event with oral calcium intake is bloating and constipation, but selecting an alternative calcium salt may alleviate these effects.
  - Calcium carbonate is associated with the highest likelihood of constipation.
- **Drug-Induced Hypocalcemia**
  - Numerous medications may chelate calcium or increase renal elimination, lowering serum levels.
    - Furosemide (and other loop diuretics) increase calcium elimination, while sodium phosphate, EDTA, and foscarnet are common chelation causes.
  - Agents used for osteoporosis or parathyroid disease can also decrease serum calcium.
    - Calcitonin, cinacalcet, bisphosphonates, and denosumab.
  - Aminoglycosides are a rare cause of hypocalcemia as a secondary effect due to their hypomagnesemia effects.
- **Blood Administration**
  - Blood product administration can also cause hypocalcemia; citrate is used as a preservative.
    - Patients receiving massive transfusion protocols must receive calcium gluconate or calcium chloride and blood product administration.
- **Cardiac and Neural Conduction**
  - The physiologic functions of calcium are numerous, and knowledge of these actions informs multiple agents' pharmacology.
  - Skeletal muscle and cardiac/smooth muscles contain L-type calcium channels.
  - T-type calcium channels are located in cardiac pacemaker cells and are a component of neural conduction.
  - N-type, P-type, and R-type calcium channels exist in the CNS and peripheral nervous system.

High-Yield Core Evidence
- **Calcium Supplementation in Post-Menopausal Women**
  - This was a double-blind, placebo-controlled trial that randomized postmenopausal women to receive either calcium carbonate, calcium citrate malate, or placebo for two years.
  - There was no significant effect of calcium supplementation as assessed by bone loss from the spine in women who had undergone menopause five or fewer years earlier.
  - However, in the group of postmenopausal women who were postmenopausal for six years or more, calcium supplementation was associated with a significantly lower rate of bone loss compared to placebo.
  - Calcium citrate malate prevented bone loss during the two years of the study, explicitly slowing the rate of bone loss in the femoral neck, radius, and spine.
  - Calcium carbonate maintained bone density at the femoral neck and the radius only.
  - The authors concluded that healthy older postmenopausal women with a daily calcium intake of less than 400 mg could significantly reduce bone loss by increasing their calcium intake to 800 mg per day. In addition, at the dose we tested, supplementation with calcium citrate malate was more effective than supplementation with calcium carbonate. (N Engl J Med 1990; 323:878-883.)

- **Calcium Supplementation in Men**
  - This was a single-center, double-blind trial that randomized men who were at least 40 years of age to supplementation with calcium 600 mg/day or 1,200 mg/day or placebo to examine their effects on bone mineral density (BMD).
  - Calcium 1,200 mg/day, but not at a 600 mg/day dose, supplementation significantly increased BMD compared to placebo.
  - This observed effect was not affected by either patient's age or dietary calcium intake; however, there were calcium dose-dependent effects on parathyroid hormone levels, alkaline phosphatase, and procollagen type 1N-terminal peptide in the group receiving calcium 1,200 mg/day.
  - There was no difference between groups concerning adverse events, including tooth loss, constipation, and cramp, but calcium was associated with fewer falls but more vascular events compared to placebo.
  - The authors concluded that calcium, 1200 mg/day has effects on BMD in men compared with those found in postmenopausal women, but a 600 mg/day dosage is ineffective for treating BMD. (Arch Intern Med. 2008;168(20):2276-2282.)

High-Yield Fast-Fact
- **Fluoride Exposure**
  - Calcium chloride or calcium gluconate can be used topically to treat hydrofluoric acid burns.
- **Thiazides and Lithium**
  - Thiazide diuretics and lithium can cause an increased renal tubular reabsorption of calcium.

HIGH-YIELD BOARD EXAM ESSENTIALS
- **CLASSIC AGENTS:** Calcium chloride, calcium gluconate, calcium acetate, calcium carbonate, calcium citrate, calcium glubionate, calcium lactate
- **DRUG CLASS:** Calcium salts
- **INDICATIONS:** Antacid, cardiac arrest, calcium supplementation, hyperphosphatemia, hypoparathyroidism, hypocalcemia, hypermagnesemia
- **MECHANISM:** Calcium is an essential element necessary for a range of physiologic functions, including neuromuscular activity, endocrine regulation, coagulation, bone metabolism, and cardiac conduction.
- **SIDE EFFECTS:** Bloating, constipation
- **CLINICAL PEARLS:**
  - Calcium chloride has 3 times the amount of elemental calcium and should mainly be given by central line (or IO in cardiac arrest) whereas calcium gluconate has less elemental Ca can be given by peripheral IV.
  - In patients with hypoalbuminemia (albumin less than 4.0), a corrected serum calcium calculation must account for changes in free or active calcium concentrations. Corrected calcium = measured calcium (mg/dL) + 0.8 x [4.0 - albumin {g/dL}].

Table: Drug Class Summary

| | Calcium Salts - Drug Class Review
High-Yield Med Reviews |

Mechanism of Action: *Calcium is an essential element necessary for a range of physiologic functions, including neuromuscular activity, endocrine regulation, coagulation, bone metabolism, and cardiac conduction.*

Class Effects: *Calcium is the most abundant mineral in the body, required for normal functioning, but less than 1% of the total body calcium is located outside the bone.*

Generic Name	Brand Name	Main Indication(s) or Uses	Notes
Calcium acetate	Calphron Eliphos PhosLo Phoslyra	• Hyperphosphatemia	• **Dosing (Adult):** — Oral: 1,334 to 2,668 mg qmeal • **Dosing (Peds):** — Oral: 667 to 1,000 mg qmeal • **CYP450 Interactions:** None • **Renal or Hepatic Dose Adjustments:** None • **Dosage Forms:** Oral (capsule, solution, tablet)
Calcium carbonate	Antacid Cal-Carb Caltrate Florical Maalox Oysco Tums	• Antacid • Calcium supplementation • Hyperphosphatemia • Hypoparathyroidism	• **Dosing (Adult):** — Oral: 500 to 8,000 mg per day — Maximum for CKD 2,000 mg/day • **Dosing (Peds):** — Oral: 375 to 7,500 mg/day — Maximum for CKD 2,000 mg/day • **CYP450 Interactions:** None • **Renal or Hepatic Dose Adjustments:** None • **Dosage Forms:** Oral (capsule, powder, suspension, tablet)
Calcium chloride	Calciject	• Cardiac arrest • Hyperkalemia • Hypocalcemia • Hypermagnesemia	• **Dosing (Adult):** — IV: 20 mg/kg, maximum 1 to 2 g/dose q10-20minutes • **Dosing (Peds):** — IV: 20 mg/kg, maximum 1 g/dose q10-20minutes — IV: 0.5 to 2 mEq/kg/day • **CYP450 Interactions:** None • **Renal or Hepatic Dose Adjustments:** None • **Dosage Forms:** IV (solution)
Calcium citrate	Calcitrate	• Hypoparathyroidism	• **Dosing (Adult):** — Oral: 200 to 1,000 mg q8-12h • **Dosing (Peds):** — Oral: (elemental calcium) 45 to 65 mg/kg/day in 4 divided doses • **CYP450 Interactions:** None • **Renal or Hepatic Dose Adjustments:** None • **Dosage Forms:** Oral (tablet)

Calcium Salts - Drug Class Review
High-Yield Med Reviews

Generic Name	Brand Name	Main Indication(s) or Uses	Notes
Calcium glubionate	Calcionate	- Dietary supplement	- **Dosing (Adult):** 　− Oral: 345 mg q6-8h - **Dosing (Peds):** 　− Oral: 115 to 345 mg q4-8h 　　− Extra info if needed - **CYP450 Interactions:** None - **Renal or Hepatic Dose Adjustments:** None - **Dosage Forms:** Oral (syrup)
Calcium gluconate	Cal-Glu	- Cardiac arrest - Hyperkalemia - Hypocalcemia - Hypermagnesemia	- **Dosing (Adult):** 　− IV: 60 mg/kg q10-20minutes as needed or 60 to 120 mg/kg/hour infusion 　− IV: 1,500 to 3,000 mg IV over 2-5 minutes 　− IV: 1,000 to 4,000 mg over 2-4 hours 　− Oral: 500 to 4,000 mg/day - **Dosing (Peds):** 　− IV: 0.5 to 4 mEq/kg/day (TPN) 　− IV: 60 mg/kg (maximum 3,000 mg/dose) q10-20minutes as needed 　− Oral: 500 mg/kg/day divided in 4 doses (maximum 1,000 mg/dose) - **CYP450 Interactions:** None - **Renal or Hepatic Dose Adjustments:** None - **Dosage Forms:** IV (solution), Oral (capsule, tablet)
Calcium lactate	Cal-Lac	- Dietary supplementation	- **Dosing (Adult):** 　− Oral: 252 mg daily - **Dosing (Peds):** 　− Oral: (elemental calcium) 45 to 65 mg/kg/day in 4 divided doses - **CYP450 Interactions:** None - **Renal or Hepatic Dose Adjustments:** None - **Dosage Forms:** Oral (capsule, tablet)

BONE MINERAL HOMEOSTASIS – PARATHYROID HORMONE ANALOGS

Drug Class
- Parathyroid Hormone Analogs
- Agents:
    - Chronic Care
        - Abaloparatide
        - Parathyroid Hormone
        - Teriparatide

Main Indications or Uses
- Chronic Care
    - Hypoparathyroidism (parathyroid hormone)
    - Osteoporosis (abaloparatide, teriparatide)

Mechanism of Action
- Mimic the effects of endogenous parathyroid hormone (PTH), causing an anabolic effect and increasing bone formation. All have slightly different mechanisms.
- Parathyroid hormone: replaces endogenous parathyroid hormone to increase serum calcium concentrations by increasing renal tubular calcium reabsorption, intestinal calcium absorption, and osteoblast activity.
    - Intermittent exposure to PTH stimulates osteoblast activity more than osteoclast activity. Chronic, excessive PTH will promote bone turnover through stimulation of osteoclasts.

> **Fast Facts**
>
> ✓ Parathyroid hormone analogs are all administered parenterally and may cause orthostatic hypotension. Advise the patient to be sitting with dose administration.
>
> ✓ Abaloparatide, teriparatide, and PTH are associated with a high incidence of hypercalcemia (3.4-6.4%), leading to toxic effects of digoxin.

Primary Net Benefit
- **Hypoparathyroidism (parathyroid hormone):** replace PTH to improve hypocalcemia and other associated changes.
- **Osteoporosis (abaloparatide, teriparatide):** alternative therapies that reduce the risk of osteoporotic fractures.
- Main Labs to Monitor:
    - Serum calcium (all)
        - Parathyroid hormone: check within 3-7 days of initiation or dose changes)
    - BMD (osteoporosis)

High-Yield Basic Pharmacology
- **Abaloparatide Is a Synthetic PTHrP Analog**
    - As a synthetic analog of parathyroid hormone-related protein (PTHrP) that agonizes PTH1 receptors, abaloparatide exerts a PTH mimicking effect and an increased anabolic effect to increase bone mass.
- **Recombinant PTH**
    - Teriparatide is a recombinant PTH consisting of the first 34 amino acid sequence in endogenous human PTH.
- **Drug Interactions**
    - Clinically relevant pharmacodynamic interactions exist. Abaloparatide, teriparatide, and PTH are associated with a high incidence of hypercalcemia (3.4-6.4%), leading to toxic effects of digoxin.
    - Alendronate likely diminishes the effect of parathyroid hormone since it diminishes bone resorption and should be avoided in combination.

High-Yield Clinical Knowledge
- **Discontinuation Effect**
    - The parathyroid hormone analogs must be continued to reduce the risk of vertebral and nonvertebral fractures in postmenopausal women.
        - Alternative antiresorptive therapy should be started if discontinued to maintain a reduced fracture risk.
- **Osteosarcoma Risk**

- Teriparatide and abaloparatide therapy is limited to 2 years of cumulative treatment to reduce the risk of osteosarcoma.
- **Orthostatic Hypotension**
  - Parathyroid hormone analogs are all administered parenterally and may cause orthostatic hypotension after administration.
    - Patients should be educated to administer several of their first doses while sitting or lying down until their patient-specific response is known.
- **Comorbidity Cautions**
  - Parathyroid hormone analogs should not be used in patients with Paget disease, bone metabolism diseases, or elevated calcium or alkaline phosphatase levels.
- **Combination Therapy**
  - Combination therapy with teriparatide and bisphosphonates provides no additional benefit for bone health and may be associated with diminished BMD benefits compared to either monotherapy.
  - Combination with denosumab shows a synergistic effect on BMD that may help high-risk patients.
- **Severe Hypercalcemia or Hypocalcemia**
  - PTH may cause severe hypercalcemia, especially when initiating or making dose adjustments.
  - PTH may cause severe hypocalcemia, especially when doses are missed or withheld. May increase vitamin D and/or calcium supplements (or restart) if therapy interruption is needed to prevent hypocalcemia.

High-Yield Core Evidence

- **Pharmacologic Interventions to Prevent Fractures - Systematic Review**
  - This was a systematic review of clinical trials, observational studies, and other systematic reviews of pharmacologic treatments used to prevent fractures in adults at risk.
  - From 315 articles included, the authors noted high-quality evidence that bisphosphonates, denosumab, and teriparatide reduce fractures compared with placebo.
  - Specific relative risk reductions were observed for vertebral fractures and nonvertebral fractures with all bisphosphonates, denosumab, and teriparatide, but raloxifene only reduced vertebral fractures.
  - However, atypical subtrochanteric femur fractures were increased with long-term bisphosphonate use.
  - Gastrointestinal side effects, hot flashes, thromboembolic events, and infections varied among drugs.
  - Concluded that good-quality evidence supports several medications to improve BMD in osteoporosis and reduce hip and vertebral fracture risk, while bisphosphonates increased the risk of atypical femur fractures. (Ann Intern Med. 2014 Nov 18;161(10):711-23.)
- **ACTIVE Study**
  - A multicenter, placebo-controlled trial of postmenopausal women with BMD T-scores of between -2.5 to -5.0 at the lumbar spine or femoral neck and radiologic evidence of at least 2 mild or at least 1 moderate lumbar or thoracic vertebral fracture or a history of low-trauma nonvertebral fracture within the past 5 years who randomized to receive abaloparatide 80 mcg, open-label teriparatide 20 mcg, or placebo.
  - Abaloparatide and teriparatide significantly reduced the risk of the primary endpoint of the percentage of participants with a new vertebral fracture.
  - Abaloparatide significantly lowered the estimated event rate for nonvertebral fracture and was associated with significant improvements in BMD compared to placebo.
  - Hypercalcemia was lower with abaloparatide than teriparatide.
  - Concluded that abaloparatide reduced the risk of new vertebral and nonvertebral fractures compared to placebo among postmenopausal women with osteoporosis. (JAMA 2016 Aug 16;316(7):722-33.)

High-Yield Fast-Facts

- **Fracture Repair**
  - Teriparatide has been used to aid in the repair of fractures and for the treatment of fracture nonunions.
  - Professional athletes have used teriparatide off-label for this and to speed recovery from fractures.

HIGH-YIELD BOARD EXAM ESSENTIALS

- **CLASSIC AGENTS:** Abaloparatide, parathyroid hormone, teriparatide
- **DRUG CLASS:** Parathyroid hormone analogs
- **INDICATIONS:** Hypoparathyroidism, osteoporosis
- **MECHANISM:** Mimic the effects of endogenous parathyroid hormone (PTH), causing an anabolic effect and increasing bone resorption.
- **SIDE EFFECTS:** Orthostatic hypotension, hypercalcemia, osteosarcoma
- **CLINICAL PEARLS:**
    - Start antiresorptive therapy if discontinued to retain reduced fracture risk.
    - Combination therapy with bisphosphonates is not recommended.
    - Abaloparatide and teriparatide cause hypercalcemia which can lead to toxic effects with digoxin.

Table: Drug Class Summary

Parathyroid Hormone Analogs - Drug Class Review			
High-Yield Med Reviews			
Mechanism of Action: Mimic the effects of endogenous parathyroid hormone (PTH), causing an anabolic effect and increasing bone formation.			
Class Effects: Alternate therapies for osteoporosis that reduce the risk of vertebra but not hip fractures.			
Generic Name	**Brand Name**	**Indication(s) or Uses**	**Notes**
Abaloparatide	Tymlos	- Osteoporosis	- **Dosing (Adult):** − SQ: 80 mcg once daily - **Dosing (Peds):** N/A - **CYP450 Interactions:** None - **Renal or Hepatic Dose Adjustments:** None - **Dosage Forms:** SC pen-injector

Parathyroid Hormone	Natpara	- Hypoparathyroidism	- **Dosing (Adult):**
			    − SQ: 25 to 100 mcg once daily
			    − Adjust dose based on calcium
			- **Dosing (Peds):** N/A
			- **CYP450 Interactions:** None
			- **Renal or Hepatic Dose Adjustments:** None
			- **Dosage Forms:** SC cartridge

Teriparatide	Forteo	- Osteoporosis	- **Dosing (Adult):** − SQ: 20 mcg once daily - **Dosing (Peds):** N/A - **CYP450 Interactions:** None - **Renal or Hepatic Dose Adjustments:** None - **Dosage Forms:** SC pen-injector

BONE MINERAL HOMEOSTASIS – RANKL INHIBITOR

Drug Class
- RANKL Inhibitor
- Agents:
    - Acute & Chronic Care
        - Denosumab

Main Indications or Uses
- Acute Care
    - Hypercalcemia of malignancy
- Chronic Care
    - Bone metastases from solid tumors
    - Giant cell tumor of bone
    - Multiple myeloma
    - Osteoporosis

> **Fast Facts**
>
> ✓ Denosumab is a human monoclonal antibody (MAB) that binds to and inhibits RANKL.
>
> ✓ Like the bisphosphonates, denosumab impacts bone turn over and can cause osteonecrosis of the jaw.

Mechanism of Action
- Human monoclonal antibody (MAB) that binds to and inhibits RANKL from binding to the RANK receptor, preventing the activity and maturation of osteoclasts.

Primary Net Benefit
- Potential first-line option for osteoporosis in men and women who are at a high risk of fracture to decrease the risk of vertebral, hip, and nonvertebral fractures.
- Main Labs to Monitor:
    - Serum calcium, magnesium, and phosphorus (baseline and 14 days after administration [Prolia] and within the first weeks [Xgeva])
    - BMD screening every 1-3 years (osteoporosis patients)
    - HBV screening (cancer patients)

High-Yield Basic Pharmacology
- **Rapid Onset**
    - The onset of action is relatively rapid (85% reduction in bone resorption markers at 3 days) with a peak effect after ten days and maximum reductions at 1 month, despite its infrequent administration.
- **Duration of Therapy**
    - Denosumab has been studied for use in patients for a duration of 10 years.
    - Denosumab offers a long-term treatment strategy compared to other agents like bisphosphonates that are limited to 5 years of cumulative therapy.

High-Yield Clinical Knowledge
- **Hypocalcemia**
    - Serum calcium (corrected) levels must be above the lower limit of normal before starting denosumab since denosumab may cause severe, life-threatening hypocalcemia.
    - Risk factors for severe hypocalcemia include pre-existing hypocalcemia, inadequate or absent calcium supplementation, or renal impairment.
        - Hypoparathyroidism, parathyroid or thyroid surgery, malabsorptive states, or other drugs or conditions predisposing to hypocalcemia should also be considered with caution.
- **Fractures and Osteonecrosis**
    - Denosumab carries warnings for atypical femoral fractures and osteonecrosis of the jaw like bisphosphonates, but there is limited high-quality evidence suggesting an unacceptable risk.
- **Hypercalcemia of Malignancy**
    - In some patients with acute leukemias or those at risk of tumor lysis syndrome, denosumab can be used in combination therapy to treat hypercalcemia.

- Management of hypercalcemia also includes IV volume replacement, diuresis, corticosteroids, calcitonin, and IV bisphosphonates (pamidronate, zoledronic acid).
- **Glucocorticoid-Induced Osteoporosis**
  - Denosumab is indicated to increase BMD and prevent fractures in patients receiving high-dose or chronic glucocorticoids that develop secondary osteoporosis.
  - This includes men with nonmetastatic prostate cancer who are taking androgen-deprivation therapy as a means to increase bone mass and women receiving an adjuvant aromatase inhibitor for breast cancer.
- **Dental Procedures**
  - Recommend undergoing major dental procedures before denosumab initiation if possible.
- **Oncology Supportive Care**
  - Denosumab may be used in treating numerous oncologic disorders, including bone metastases from solid tumors, giant cell tumor of bone, or multiple myeloma.
  - The dose and frequency of denosumab are different for these indications.
    - Denosumab 120 mg SC every 4 weeks (additional 120 mg on days 8 and 15 during initiation)

High-Yield Core Evidence
- **FREEDOM**
  - This was a multicenter, double-blind, placebo-controlled trial of postmenopausal women who had a BMD T score between -2.5 and -4.0 at the lumbar spine or total hip and were randomized to receive either denosumab 60 mg SC q6months or placebo for 36 months.
  - Denosumab significantly reduced the risk of the primary outcome of new radiographic vertebral fractures compared to placebo (68% relative risk reduction) and also significantly reduced the risk of nonvertebral fractures.
  - Safety outcomes were similar, including new cancer, infection, CVD, delayed fracture healing, or hypocalcemia. No cases of osteonecrosis of the jaw or administration reactions occurred.
  - Concluded denosumab given SC twice yearly for 36 months was associated with reductions in vertebral, nonvertebral, and hip fractures in women with osteoporosis. (NEJM 2009 Aug 20;361(8):756-65.)
- **Denosumab Safety Meta-Analysis**
  - This was a meta-analysis of denosumab's safety in postmenopausal women with osteoporosis or low BMD compared with bisphosphonates or placebo.
  - Pooled data from the clinical trials included revealed no significant difference between denosumab, bisphosphonates, or placebo concerning the outcome of any adverse events, serious adverse events, cancer, or death.
  - Denosumab was associated with a potentially increased risk of serious adverse events related to infection and reduction in nonvertebral fractures compared to bisphosphonates or placebo (confidence intervals included 1).
    - There was no difference between denosumab and bisphosphonates concerning serious adverse events related to infections or reduction in nonvertebral fractures in a subgroup analysis.
  - Concluded that denosumab treatment decreased the risk of nonvertebral fracture but increased the risk of serious adverse events related to infection compared to placebo in postmenopausal women with osteoporosis or low BMD, but there was no difference compared to bisphosphonates. (Int J Clin Exp Pathol. 2014 Apr 15;7(5):2113-22.)

High-Yield Fast-Fact
- **SC Administration**
  - If patients are not comfortable or otherwise unable to administer denosumab, pharmacists in some states can administer denosumab to patients.

HIGH-YIELD BOARD EXAM ESSENTIALS
- **CLASSIC AGENTS:** Denosumab
- **DRUG CLASS:** RANKL inhibitor
- **INDICATIONS:** Bone metastases from solid tumors, giant cell tumor of bone, hypercalcemia of malignancy, multiple myeloma, osteoporosis
- **MECHANISM:** Human monoclonal antibody (MAB) that binds to and inhibits the ability of RANKL from binding to the RANK receptor, preventing the activity and maturation of osteoclasts.
- **SIDE EFFECTS:** Hypocalcemia, bone fractures, osteonecrosis of the jaw
- **CLINICAL PEARLS:**
  - Before starting denosumab, serum calcium (corrected) levels must be above the lower limit of normal, as denosumab may cause severe, life-threatening hypocalcemia.
  - Denosumab reduces markers of bone resorption within 3 days and return to normal within 12 months of treatment discontinuation.

Table: Drug Class Summary

RANKL Inhibitor - Drug Class Review High-Yield Med Reviews				
Mechanism of Action: Binds to and inhibits the ability of RANKL from binding to the RANK receptor, preventing the activity and maturation of osteoclasts.				
Class Effects: Used as first-line agent in osteoporosis for men and women who are at high risk of fracture to decrease risk of vertebral, hip, and nonvertebral fractures.				
Generic Name	**Brand Name**	**Main Indication(s) or Uses**	**Notes**	
Denosumab	Xgeva	<ul><li>Bone metastases from solid tumors</li><li>Giant cell tumor of bone</li><li>Hypercalcemia of malignancy</li><li>Multiple myeloma</li></ul>	<ul><li>**Dosing (Adult):**<ul><li>SQ: 120 mg q4weeks<ul><li>First month: administer additional 120 mg on days 8 and 15</li></ul></li></ul></li><li>**Dosing (Peds):**<ul><li>Adolescents over 45 kg: use adult dosing</li></ul></li><li>**CYP450 Interactions:** None</li><li>**Renal or Hepatic Dose Adjustments:** None</li><li>**Dosage Forms:** SC solution</li></ul>	
Denosumab	Prolia	<ul><li>Osteoporosis</li></ul>	<ul><li>**Dosing (Adult):**<ul><li>SQ: 60 mg q6months</li></ul></li><li>**Dosing (Peds):**<ul><li>Not routinely used</li></ul></li><li>**CYP450 Interactions:** None</li><li>**Renal or Hepatic Dose Adjustments:** None</li><li>**Dosage Forms:** SC prefilled syringe</li></ul>	

BONE MINERAL HOMEOSTASIS – SCLEROSTIN INHIBITOR

Drug Class
- Sclerostin Inhibitor
- Agents:
  - Chronic Care
    - Romosozumab

Main Indications or Uses
- Chronic Care
  - Osteoporosis treatment

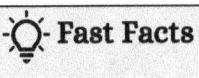

> **Fast Facts**
> ✓ The ending of the drug name, "-zumab" indicates that it is a humanized monoclonal antibody MAB) vs. "-umab" without the "z" indicates a fully human MAB.

Mechanism of Action
- A humanized monoclonal antibody that binds to sclerostin, which is a regulatory factor that inhibits Wnt/Betacatenin signaling pathway that manages bone growth, thereby increasing bone formation (primary effect) and reducing bone resorption.

Primary Net Benefit
- Significantly reduces the risk of fracture in postmenopausal women at high risk of fractures compared to alendronate alone.
- Main Labs to Monitor:
  - Serum calcium, phosphorus, vitamin D (initiation, then periodically)
  - BMD (baseline, then in 6-12 months)

High-Yield Basic Pharmacology
- Anabolic Agent
  - Romosozumab is considered an anabolic agent but works primarily by binding sclerostin, promoting Wnt signaling mediated gene transcription and increased osteoblast formation, differentiation, and bone matrix growth.
- Antibodies
  - Up to 20% of patients may develop antibodies to romosozumab; however, these have not been associated with neutralizing activity and do not impact efficacy or safety.

High-Yield Clinical Knowledge
- Cardiovascular Risk
  - Romosozumab was associated with a higher risk of CV events, as observed in the ARCH and BRIDGE trial.
    - There were observations of increased CV events in the FRAME trial that compared romosozumab to placebo.
  - Romosozumab is contraindicated in patients who have had a stroke or MI within the past year.
- Osteonecrosis of The Jaw
  - May increase the risk of osteonecrosis of the jaw, like bisphosphonates.
- Limited Treatment
  - Romosozumab is currently limited to 12 months of treatment based on the FDA indication.
- Adverse Events
  - Other relevant adverse events associated with romosozumab include hypocalcemia, an increased risk of femoral fractures, and off-target TNF-alfa mediated aggravation of arthritis.

High-Yield Core Evidence
- **FRAME**
  - This was a multicenter, double-blind, placebo-controlled trial of postmenopausal women with a T score of -2.5 to -3.5 at the total hip or femoral neck who were randomized to receive either romosozumab 210 mg SQ or placebo SQ monthly for 12 months, with each group then receiving denosumab 60 mg q6months for two doses. Total follow-up was 24 months.
  - At 12 months, there was a statistically significant reduction in the incidence of new vertebral fractures and new clinical fractures associated with romosozumab compared to placebo.
  - However, there was no difference in the incidence of new non-vertebral fractures at 12 months.
  - At the 24-month follow-up, the incidence of new vertebral fractures remained significantly lower among patients randomized to romosozumab than placebo.
  - There was no difference concerning adverse events between treatment groups.
  - The authors concluded that in postmenopausal women with osteoporosis, romosozumab was associated with a lower risk of vertebral fractures than placebo at 12 months and, after the transition to denosumab, at 24 months. The lower risk of clinical fracture that was seen with romosozumab was evident at one year. (NEJM 2016;375(16):1532-1543.)
- **ARCH**
  - This was a multicenter, double-blind trial of postmenopausal women with osteoporosis and a fragility fracture who were randomized to either romosozumab 210 mg SQ monthly or alendronate 70 mg once weekly for 12 months, with each group then receiving open-label alendronate 70 mg once weekly for an additional 12 months for a total follow-up of 24 months.
  - Patients who received romosozumab followed by alendronate experienced a significantly lower incidence in the primary outcome of new vertebral fracture at 24 months and the cumulative incidence of clinical fracture compared to the alendronate group.
  - New non-vertebral fractures, new hip fractures, and new clinical fractures occurred in significantly fewer patients randomized to receive romosozumab.
  - Patients randomized to romosozumab experienced more positively adjudicated severe CV adverse events than with alendronate, but the incidence in other safety endpoints was similar.
  - The authors concluded that in postmenopausal women with osteoporosis who were at high risk for fracture, romosozumab treatment for 12 months followed by alendronate resulted in a significantly lower fracture risk than alendronate alone. (NEJM 2017;377(15):1417-1427.)

High-Yield Fast-Fact
- **Wnt Pathway**
  - As a result of the impact of romosozumab, other Wnt pathway compounds are under investigation to treat various diseases.

HIGH-YIELD BOARD EXAM ESSENTIALS
- **CLASSIC AGENTS:** Romosozumab
- **DRUG CLASS:** Sclerostin Inhibitor
- **INDICATIONS:** Osteoporosis
- **MECHANISM:** A humanized monoclonal antibody that binds to sclerostin, thereby increasing bone formation and reducing bone resorption through the Wnt/Betacatenin pathway.
- **SIDE EFFECTS:** Increased risk of CV events, osteonecrosis of the jaw, hypocalcemia, increased risk of fractures
- **CLINICAL PEARLS:** According to the FDA-approved indication, romosozumab is currently limited to a one-year (or 12 months) treatment course.

Table: Drug Class Summary

| Sclerostin Inhibitor - Drug Class Review ||||
High-Yield Med Reviews			
Mechanism of Action: *A humanized monoclonal antibody binds to sclerostin, increasing bone formation and reducing bone resorption through the Wnt/Betacatenin pathway*			
Class Effects: *Reduces the risk of fracture in postmenopausal women with osteoporosis at high risk of fracture, potential increased CV risk, ONJ, hypocalcemia, increased fracture risk*			
Generic Name	**Brand Name**	**Indication(s) or Uses**	**Notes**
Romosozumab	Evenity	• Osteoporosis	• **Dosing (Adult):** – SQ: 210 mg as two 105 mg injections once monthly for 12 months • **Dosing (Peds):** N/A • **CYP450 Interactions:** None • **Renal or Hepatic Dose Adjustments:** None • **Dosage Forms:** SC prefilled syringe

BONE MINERAL HOMEOSTASIS – SELECTIVE ESTROGEN RECEPTOR MODULATORS

Drug Class
- Selective Estrogen Receptor Modulators
- Agents:
    - Chronic Care
        - Clomiphene
        - Bazedoxifene
        - Ospemifene
        - Raloxifene

Main Indications or Uses
- Chronic Care
    - Breast cancer risk reduction in postmenopausal females
    - Dyspareunia
    - Osteoporosis
    - Ovulation induction
    - Vasomotor symptoms associated with menopause
    - Vaginal dryness

> **Fast Facts**
> ✓ A SERM means that the molecule "selectively" act like an agonist on one tissue receptor but then act like an antagonist to another tissue receptor.
>
> ✓ Out of the SERMs, clomiphene is the main agent used to stimulate ovulation for the purpose of increasing changes of getting pregnant.

Mechanism of Action
- Competitive and partial agonist inhibitor (mixed agonist/antagonist effects) of estradiol at the estrogen receptor

Primary Net Benefit
- SERMs are used in breast cancer prevention in high-risk postmenopausal women and postmenopausal women with vasomotor symptoms also requiring osteoporosis prevention.
- Clomiphene is used to improve ovulation in women desiring pregnancy.
- Ospemifene is used to improve vaginal dryness with menopause.
- Main Labs to Monitor:
    - Estrogen
    - CBC
    - Serum calcium
    - Liver function (INR/PT, albumin, total protein, bilirubin)
    - Lipid profile
    - DEXA scan
    - Pregnancy test

High-Yield Basic Pharmacology
- Raloxifene Selectivity
    - Raloxifene is a mixed estrogen agonist/antagonist that has selective activity on lipids and bone but not on the endometrium or breast tissue.
- Clomiphene
    - Clomiphene is related to the SERMs as it is a partial agonist of estrogen receptors.

High-Yield Clinical Knowledge
- Lipid Effects and Thrombosis
    - Raloxifene decreases total cholesterol, LDL, and LPA but does not affect HDL or triglycerides.
    - Despite this CV benefit, raloxifene is associated with a significantly increased risk of DVT/PE.
- Cancer Risk Reduction
    - Raloxifene has been associated with a significant reduction in estrogen-receptor-positive breast cancer.
- Endometrial Cancer Risk
    - Bazedoxifene/estrogen may increase the risk of endometrial cancer in patients with a uterus because the estrogen component may reduce endometrial hyperplasia, which may predispose to endometrial cancer.

- **Hot Flashes**
  - Patients taking SERMs frequently experience flushing, hot flashes, nausea, and vomiting.
  - Bazedoxifene/estrogen does not cause flushing with the estrogen component.
- **Ovulation Stimulation**
  - Clomiphene is primarily used in women wishing to become pregnant by blocking the hypothalamus inhibitory feedback of estrogen and stimulating ovulation.
  - Clomiphene may result in multiple pregnancies in approximately 10% of cases.
  - Ovary enlargement is a common adverse effect of clomiphene.
- **Osteoporosis**
  - Raloxifene is an alternative in the management of osteoporosis for patients with menopausal symptoms as it reduces the rate of bone loss and may increase bone mass in the spine.
- **Pregnancy**
  - For SERM therapy, patients of childbearing potential must have a negative pregnancy test before the initiation of treatment.

High-Yield Core Evidence
- **RUTH**
  - This was a multicenter, double-blind, parallel-group, controlled trial of postmenopausal women with coronary heart disease (CHD) or those who had multiple CVD risk factors who were randomized to receive either raloxifene 60 mg daily or placebo and were followed for a median of 5.6 years.
  - There was no significant difference in the incidence of coronary events, including death from CV causes, MI, or hospitalization for ACS, but raloxifene significantly reduced the risk of invasive breast cancer.
  - Although there was no significant difference in death rates from any cause or total stroke according to group assignment, raloxifene was associated with an increased risk of fatal stroke and VTE.
  - Patients randomized to raloxifene experienced a reduced risk of vertebral fractures.
  - The authors concluded that raloxifene did not significantly affect the risk of CVD; however, raloxifene's benefits in reducing the risk of invasive breast cancer and vertebral fracture should be weighed against the increased risks of VTE and fatal stroke. (N Engl J Med. 2006 Jul 13;355(2):125-37.)
- **STAR P-2**
  - This was a multicenter, double-blind, parallel-group, controlled trial of postmenopausal women with an increased 5-year break cancer risk who were randomized to receive either raloxifene or tamoxifen to assess their impact on the risk of developing invasive breast cancer and other disease outcomes.
  - There was no difference between groups concerning the incidence of invasive breast cancer, uterine cancer, other invasive cancers, bone fractures, ischemic heart disease, stroke, or death, but tamoxifen significantly reduced the incidence of noninvasive breast cancer,
  - Conversely, raloxifene was associated with a significantly lower incidence of thrombotic events, fewer cataracts, and cataract surgeries.
  - The authors concluded that raloxifene is as effective as tamoxifen in reducing invasive breast cancer risk and has a lower risk of thromboembolic events and cataracts but a nonstatistically significant higher risk of noninvasive breast cancer. (JAMA. 2006 Dec 27;296(24):2926.)

High-Yield Fast-Fact
- **Clomiphene Visual Disturbances**
  - Clomiphene may increase the incidence of "afterimages" and hallucinations, which are self-limiting.
  - Activities such as driving are not recommended until the patient has a trial of clomiphene to know if these occur. Driving or similar activities are not recommended if patients experience visual disturbances.
- **SERMs and Estrogen Receptor Antagonists**
  - Tamoxifen and toremifene are SERMs and estrogen receptor antagonists that may be utilized in oncology for breast cancer treatment and risk reduction (tamoxifen only). Toremifene is not currently utilized.

HIGH-YIELD BOARD EXAM ESSENTIALS

- **CLASSIC AGENTS:** Clomiphene, bazedoxifene, ospemifene, raloxifene (also, tamoxifen and toremifene)
- **DRUG CLASS:** Selective estrogen receptor modulators
- **INDICATIONS:** Breast cancer risk reduction, dyspareunia, osteoporosis, ovulation induction, vasomotor symptoms associated with menopause, vaginal dryness
- **MECHANISM:** Competitive and partial agonist inhibitor (mixed agonist/antagonist effects) of estradiol at the estrogen receptor.
- **SIDE EFFECTS:** Increased risk of DVT/PE, visual disturbances, hot flashes
- **CLINICAL PEARLS:**
  - Raloxifene would be considered an alternative agent for osteoporosis in patients also experiencing postmenopausal symptoms.
  - Clomiphene can result in multiple pregnancies (10% cases).

Table: Drug Class Summary

Selective Estrogen Receptor Modulators - Drug Class Review High-Yield Med Reviews			
Mechanism of Action: *Competitive and partial agonist inhibitor (mixed agonist/antagonist effects) of estradiol at the estrogen receptor.*			
Class Effects: *Used in breast cancer prevention in high-risk postmenopausal women (raloxifene) or osteoporosis in postmenopausal women with symptoms (raloxifene, bazedoxifene/estrogen), increased VTE risk, hot flashes, multiple pregnancies (clomiphene)*			
Generic Name	**Brand Name**	**Main Indication(s) or Uses**	**Notes**

Clomiphene	Clomid
	Serophene
		• Ovulation induction	• **Dosing (Adult):**
			   – 50 mg daily x 5 days, followed by 100 mg x 5 days only if ovulation does not occur
			   – Max 100 mg/day for 5 doses up to 6 cycles
			• **Dosing (Peds):** N/A
			• **CYP450 Interactions:** None
			• **Renal or Hepatic Dose Adjustments:**
			   – Hepatic dysfunction: Contraindicated
			• **Dosage Forms:** Oral (tablet)

Bazedoxifene and Estrogens (conjugated, equine)	Duavee	• Osteoporosis
		• Vasomotor symptoms associated with menopause
			• **Dosing (Adult):**
			   – Oral: bazedoxifene/estrogens 20mg/0.45 mg
			• **Dosing (Peds):**
			   – Not routinely used
			• **CYP450 Interactions:** CYP1A2, 2A6, 2B6, 2C19, 2C9, 2D6, 2E1, 3A4 substrate; CYP1A2 inhibitor
			• **Renal or Hepatic Dose Adjustments:**
			   – Hepatic dysfunction: contraindicated
			• **Dosage Forms:** Oral (tablet)

Ospemifene	Osphena	• Dyspareunia
		• Vaginal dryness
			• **Dosing (Adult):**
			   – Oral: 60 mg daily
			• **Dosing (Peds):** N/A
			• **CYP450 Interactions:** CYP2C19, 2C9, 3A4 substrate
			• **Renal or Hepatic Dose Adjustments:**
			   – Child-Pugh class C: not recommended
			• **Dosage Forms:** Oral (tablet)

Raloxifene	Evista	• Osteoporosis
		• Risk reduction for invasive breast cancer in postmenopausal females
			• **Dosing (Adult):**
			   – Oral: 60 mg daily
			• **Dosing (Peds):** N/A
			• **CYP450 Interactions:** None
			• **Renal or Hepatic Dose Adjustments:**
			   – CrCl < 50 mL/minute: use with caution
			   – Hepatic dysfunction: use with caution
			• **Dosage Forms:** Oral (tablet)

BONE MINERAL HOMEOSTASIS – VITAMIN D ANALOGS

Drug Class
- Vitamin D Analogs
- Agents:
  - Chronic Care
    - Calcifediol
    - Calcipotriene
    - Calcitriol
    - Cholecalciferol
    - Doxercalciferol
    - Ergocalciferol
    - Paricalcitol

Main Indications or Uses
- Chronic Care
  - Hypoparathyroidism
    - Calcitriol
  - Plaque psoriasis
    - Calcipotriene
  - Osteoporosis
    - Ergocalciferol (cholecalciferol: off-label)
  - Secondary hyperparathyroidism
    - Calcifediol
    - Calcitriol
    - Doxercalciferol
    - Paricalcitol
  - Vitamin D deficiency
    - Ergocalciferol (cholecalciferol: off-label)

> **Fast Facts**
> - Calcitriol is the active form of vitamin D and thus does not require activation.
> - Active vitamin D requires the conversion of 7-dehydrocholesterol to cholecalciferol (aka Vitamin D) by sunlight. Cholecalciferol is then hydroxylated in the liver to form 25-OH-D and then converted to the active form, 1,25(OH)-D (calcitriol), in the kidneys.

Mechanism of Action
- Active forms of vitamin D that act on vitamin D receptors in the GI tract, stimulating intestinal calcium absorption and transport, with additional actions in the bone, renal tissue, and parathyroid glands.

Primary Net Benefit
- Vitamin D supports a range of physiologic functions and is also a fat-soluble vitamin that can result in toxicities.
- Main Labs to Monitor:
  - Serum calcium, phosphorus, vitamin D, magnesium
  - SCr, BUN, CrCl
  - PTH
  - Serum alkaline phosphatase

High-Yield Basic Pharmacology
- **Final Hydroxylation and CKD**
  - For the final conversion of calcitriol to active vitamin D in renal tissue, 1-alpha-hydroxylase activity is required.
  - However, with progressing CKD, the activity of 1-alpha-hydroxylase is gradually lost, leading to a decline in calcitriol activation.
- **Vitamin D and RANKL**
  - The active form of vitamin D can induce RANKL activity in osteoblasts, preventing osteoclasts' activity and maturation.

High-Yield Clinical Knowledge

- **Vitamin D2 or D3**
  - Plant-derived vitamin D2 and vitamin D3 are present in the typical American diet and supplemented through fortification of various foods.
    - Vitamin D2, or ergocalciferol, requires activation, whereas cholecalciferol is in the active vitamin D3 format.
    - Ergocalciferol is also less avidly bound to transport proteins, is not as well absorbed, and has a shorter half-life than cholecalciferol.
- **Active Vitamin D**
  - Patients with CKD cannot renally convert vitamin D to its active form of 1,25-hydroxyvitamin D (1,25(OH)D).
    - Without sufficient 1,25(OH)D, dysregulation of parathyroid hormone release allows for calcium excretion and diminished bone resorption.
- **Hypocalcemia Risk**
  - The synthetic analogs, doxercalciferol and paricalcitol, are used in place of calcitriol as they are less likely to cause hypercalcemia when lowering PTH.
    - For this reason, these agents may be preferred in clinical scenarios where calcium levels are high.
- **Plaque Psoriasis**
  - Calcipotriene is a topical synthetic vitamin D3 analog that is used for plaque psoriasis.
  - Calcitriol is also available in a topical preparation for use in plaque psoriasis and is similarly useful to calcipotriene.
- **Secondary Hyperparathyroidism**
  - Paricalcitol is a synthetic form of vitamin D2 that specifically reduces serum PTH levels without affecting serum calcium or phosphorus.
  - This advantage is of clinical use and importance in patients with CKD who are at risk of hyperphosphatemia and hypercalcemia.

High-Yield Core Evidence

- **VIOLET**
  - This was a single-center, double-blind, placebo-controlled trial of critically ill, vitamin D-deficient patients at high risk for death who were randomized within 12 hours of admission to the ICU to receive either a single enteral dose of vitamin D3 540,000 units or matched placebo.
  - There was no significant difference in the primary endpoint of 90-day all-cause and all-location mortality between treatment groups.
  - Baseline vitamin D levels were similar between groups, and patients receiving vitamin D3 had a significantly higher 25-hydroxyvitamin D level at three days, compared to patients who received placebo.
  - There was no significant difference between groups concerning safety or any secondary endpoint.
  - The authors concluded that early administration of high-dose enteral vitamin D3 did not provide an advantage over placebo concerning 90-day mortality or other nonfatal outcomes among critically ill, vitamin D-deficient patients. (NEJM 2019 Dec 26;381(26):2529-2540.)

High-Yield Fast-Fact

- **Sunshine**
  - Active vitamin D requires the conversion of 7-dehydrocholesterol to cholecalciferol (aka Vitamin D) by sunlight. Cholecalciferol is then hydroxylated in the liver to form 25-OH-D and then converted to 1,25(OH)-D (calcitriol) in the kidneys.
  - 40 units are equal to 1 mcg of vitamin D.

HIGH-YIELD BOARD EXAM ESSENTIALS

- **CLASSIC AGENTS:** Calcifediol, calcipotriene, calcitriol, cholecalciferol, doxercalciferol, ergocalciferol, paricalcitol
- **DRUG CLASS:** Vitamin D analogs
- **INDICATIONS:** Hypoparathyroidism (calcitriol), plaque psoriasis (calcipotriene), secondary hyperparathyroidism (calcifediol, calcitriol, doxercalciferol, paricalcitol), vitamin D deficiency, osteoporosis (ergocalciferol)
- **MECHANISM:** Active forms of vitamin D, acting on vitamin D receptors in the GI tract, stimulating intestinal calcium absorption and transport, with additional actions in the bone, renal tissue, and parathyroid glands.
- **SIDE EFFECTS:** Hypercalcemia, hyperphosphatemia, headache, polydipsia
- **CLINICAL PEARLS:**
    - Calcitriol is the active form of vitamin D and thus does not require activation.
    - The synthetic analogs, doxercalciferol and paricalcitol, are used in place of calcitriol as they are less likely to cause hypercalcemia when lowering PTH.
    - Cholecalciferol is used off-label but commonly for osteoporosis prevention and vitamin D deficiency.

Table: Drug Class Summary

Vitamin D - Drug Class Review High-Yield Med Reviews				
Mechanism of Action: Active forms of vitamin D, acting on vitamin D receptors in the GI tract, stimulating intestinal calcium absorption and transport, with additional actions in the bone, renal tissue, and parathyroid glands.				
Class Effects: Precursors or active vitamin D support for various physiologic functions, fat-soluble vitamin (potential overexposure and toxicity)				
Generic Name	**Brand Name**	**Main Indication(s) or Uses**	**Notes**	
Calcifediol	Rayaldee	- Secondary hyperparathyroidism	- **Dosing (Adult):** - Oral: 30 to 60 mcg at bedtime - **Dosing (Peds):** N/A - **CYP450 Interactions:** None - **Renal or Hepatic Dose Adjustments:** None - **Dosage Forms:** Oral (capsule)	

Calcipotriene	Calcitrene Dovonex Sorilux	- Plaque psoriasis	- **Dosing (Adult):**
			  - Topically applied to affected area once to twice daily
			- **Dosing (Peds):**
			  - Children ≥ 2 years: Topically applied to affected area once to twice daily
			- **CYP450 Interactions:** None
			- **Renal or Hepatic Dose Adjustments:** None
			- **Dosage Forms:** Topical (cream, foam, ointment, solution)	

Calcitriol	Rocaltrol	- Hypocalcemia in hypoparathyroidism
		- Secondary hyperparathyroidism in CKD
			- **Dosing (Adult):**
			  - Oral: 0.25 to 2 mcg/day
			  - IV: 0.5 to 4 mcg three times weekly
			- **Dosing (Peds):**
			  - Oral: 0.05 to 2 mcg daily, adjusted to corrected calcium, phosphorus, and iPTH levels
			- **CYP450 Interactions:** CYP3A4 substrate
			- **Renal or Hepatic Dose Adjustments:** None
			- **Dosage Forms:** Oral (capsule, solution), IV (solution)	

Cholecalciferol	Aqueous Vitamin D D-Vi-Sol D3 Vitamin Decara Dialyvite, various others	- Hypoparathyroidism
		- Osteoporosis
		- Vitamin D deficiency
			- **Dosing (Adult):**
			  - Oral: 800 to 7,000 units/day
			    - Alternative: 50,000 units weekly
			- **Dosing (Peds):**
			  - Oral: 400 to 10,000 units/day
			    - Up to 50,000 units weekly
			- **CYP450 Interactions:** None
			- **Renal or Hepatic Dose Adjustments:** None
			- **Dosage Forms:** Oral (capsule, liquid, sublingual, tablet)	

\multicolumn{4}{c}{**Vitamin D - Drug Class Review**}
\multicolumn{4}{c}{High-Yield Med Reviews}
Generic Name	**Brand Name**	**Main Indication(s) or Uses**	**Notes**

Doxercalciferol	Hectorol	• Secondary hyperparathyroidism	• **Dosing (Adult):**
			  – Not on dialysis
			    – Oral: 1 mcg daily
			  – On dialysis
			    – Oral: 10 to 20 mcg 3 times weekly
			    – IV: 4 to 6 mcg 3 times weekly
			• **Dosing (Peds):**
			  – Not routinely used
			• **CYP450 Interactions:** None
			• **Renal or Hepatic Dose Adjustments:** None
			• **Dosage Forms:** Oral (capsule), IV (solution)

Ergocalciferol	Calcidol
	Drisdol
	Ergocal
		• Osteoporosis
		• Vitamin D deficiency
			• **Dosing (Adult):**
			  – Oral: 800 to 7,000 units/day
			    – Alternative: 50,000 units weekly
			• **Dosing (Peds):**
			  – Oral: 400 to 10,000 units/day
			    – Up to 50,000 units weekly
			• **CYP450 Interactions:** None
			• **Renal or Hepatic Dose Adjustments:** None
			• **Dosage Forms:** Oral (capsule, liquid, tablet)

Paricalcitol	Zemplar	• Secondary hyperparathyroidism	• **Dosing (Adult):**
			  – On dialysis
			    – IV: 0.04 to 0.1 mcg/kg with dialysis, adjusted to iPTH level
			      – Max 0.24 mg/kg/day
			    – Oral: dose based on iPTH level divided by 80
			  – Predialysis
			    – Oral: 1 - 2 mcg daily or 2 - 4 mcg 3 times weekly
			• **Dosing (Peds):**
			  – Children between 10 to 16 years
			    – Oral: dose based on iPTH level divided by 120
			    – IV through HD access: 0.04 to 0.08 mcg/kg/dose
			  – Predialysis
			    – Oral: 1 - 2 mcg daily or 2 - 4 mcg three times weekly
			• **CYP450 Interactions:** CYP3A4 substrate
			• **Renal or Hepatic Dose Adjustments:** None
			• **Dosage Forms:** Oral (capsule), IV (solution)

2025

A COMPREHENSIVE *RAPID REVIEW*

NAPLEX

Pharmacology & Drug Classes

Neurology

NEUROLOGY – ALZHEIMER'S AGENTS

Drug Class
- Alzheimer's Pharmacotherapy
- Agents:
  - Chronic Care
    - Donepezil
    - Galantamine
    - Memantine
    - Rivastigmine

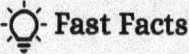

Fast Facts
- ✓ Donepezil is the most common agent used in this class for Alzheimer's disease due to its easy dose titration, once-a-day administration, tolerability, and indication for all levels of severity.
- ✓ GI side effects (N/V) are the most common complication to the use of these drugs.

Main Indications or Uses
- Chronic Care
  - Alzheimer dementia

Mechanism of Action
- Donepezil, Galantamine, Rivastigmine
  - Inhibitors of acetylcholinesterase, counteracting the loss of cholinergic neurons in Alzheimer's disease.
- Memantine
  - Noncompetitive inhibitor of NMDA receptor.

Primary Net Benefit
- Slow the cognitive dysfunction of patients with Alzheimer's disease, with significant safety improvement compared with the tacrine's historical use.
- Main Labs to Monitor:
  - No routine lab monitoring

High-Yield Basic Pharmacology
- Acetylcholinesterase Inhibition
  - The method of acetylcholinesterase inhibition differs between these agents:
    - Donepezil is a reversible, noncompetitive inhibitor of central acetylcholinesterase.
    - Galantamine is selective, competitive, reversible acetylcholinesterase inhibition that also improves acetylcholine interaction at nicotinic receptors in the CNS.
    - Rivastigmine is a reversible inhibitor of acetylcholinesterase as well as butyrylcholinesterase.
  - Despite these variances by which acetylcholinesterase inhibition occurs, the clinical relevance is unknown.
- Acetylcholinesterase Class
  - Rivastigmine belongs to the N-methylcarbamate class of cholinergic agents, including physostigmine, pyridostigmine, neostigmine, and some insecticides.
  - Donepezil and galantamine belong to the non-carbamate reversible anticholinergic class, including edrophonium and tacrine.
- NMDA Action
  - Memantine is a noncompetitive inhibitor of the NMDA glutamate receptor, blocking magnesium binding to its intra-pore active site.

High-Yield Clinical Knowledge
- Disease-Modifying
  - Currently, available pharmacotherapy for Alzheimer's does not modify the disease process but rather diminishes symptoms related to cognitive decline and the rate of cognitive decline.
  - However, some experts argue that pharmacotherapy combined with non-pharmacotherapy interventions possesses a disease-modifying effect of sustained cognitive decline reduction.
- Combination Therapy
  - The combination of donepezil with memantine has been shown to slow the rate of cognitive and functional decline in patients with Alzheimer's disease compared to monotherapy or no treatment.

- **Drug Interactions**
  - Trimethoprim (part of sulfamethoxazole/trimethoprim aka Bactrim) may increase the risk of memantine's adverse effects, namely myoclonus and delirium.
    - The proposed mechanism is competition for renal elimination via active tubular secretion.
  - In elderly patients with frequent UTIs, careful selection of antimicrobials should limit the risk of drug interactions.
- **Donepezil Dose**
  - The dosing of donepezil includes a 23 mg preparation, differing from the other 5 and 10 mg strengths.
  - There is a small improvement in cognitive function to the additional odd-numbered dosage form, which is counterbalanced by GI-related adverse effects.
- **Neurodegenerative Diseases**
  - Donepezil, galantamine, memantine, and rivastigmine can also be used for other neurodegenerative diseases where cholinergic effects play a role, including patients with Lewy bodies and vascular dementia.
- **Withdrawal**
  - If drug therapy changes or discontinuation occur, there is a risk of an acute withdrawal syndrome that manifests as a combination of worsening cognitive decline or excessive acetylcholinesterase effect (anticholinergic effect).

High-Yield Core Evidence
- **Memantine Study Group**
  - This was a multicenter, double-blind, placebo-controlled trial that randomized patients with moderate to severe Alzheimer's disease to receive either memantine or placebo.
  - Patients randomized to receive memantine had a significant improvement in the primary outcome of the change in Severe Impairment Battery and a modified Alzheimer Disease Cooperative Study-Activities of Daily Living Inventory (ADCS-ADL19).
  - Patients randomized to memantine also had significant improvements in all other secondary measures.
  - Adverse events and treatment discontinuations were similar between groups.
  - The authors concluded that patients with moderate to severe Alzheimer's disease receiving stable doses of donepezil and memantine resulted in significantly better outcomes than placebo on measures of cognition, activities of daily living, global outcome, and behavior and were well tolerated. (JAMA. 2004 Jan 21;291(3):317-24.)
- **CATIE-AD**
  - This double-blind, placebo-controlled trial randomized patients with psychosis, aggression, and agitation associated with Alzheimer's disease to receive either olanzapine, quetiapine, risperidone, or placebo.
  - Compared with placebo, the atypical antipsychotics olanzapine, quetiapine, and risperidone failed to improve outcomes related to Alzheimer's disease and psychosis, aggression, or agitation compared to placebo.
  - However, the median time to the discontinuation of treatment due to a lack of efficacy favored olanzapine and risperidone compared with quetiapine or placebo.
  - The time to the discontinuation of treatment due to adverse events or intolerability favored placebo.
  - The authors concluded that adverse effects offset advantages in the efficacy of atypical antipsychotic drugs for the treatment of psychosis, aggression, or agitation in patients with Alzheimer's disease. (N Engl J Med. 2006 Oct 12;355(15):1525-38.)

High-Yield Fast-Facts
- **NaMenDA**
  - The brand name of memantine reflects its mechanism of action, NMDA competitive inhibition.
- **Physostigmine Alternatives**
  - Donepezil, galantamine, or rivastigmine are possible alternatives to physostigmine in patients who are experiencing anticholinergic delirium.

HIGH-YIELD BOARD EXAM ESSENTIALS
- **CLASSIC AGENTS:** Donepezil, galantamine, memantine, rivastigmine
- **DRUG CLASS:** Alzheimer's pharmacotherapy
- **INDICATIONS:** Alzheimer's dementia
- **MECHANISM:** Inhibitors of acetylcholinesterase, counteracting the loss of cholinergic neurons in Alzheimer's disease (donepezil, galantamine, rivastigmine); noncompetitive inhibitor of NMDA receptor (memantine)
- **SIDE EFFECTS:** Diarrhea, insomnia, nausea.
- **CLINICAL PEARLS:**
    - Currently, available pharmacotherapy for Alzheimer's does not modify the disease process but rather diminishes symptoms related to cognitive decline and the rate of cognitive decline. However, some experts argue that pharmacotherapy combined with non-pharmacotherapy interventions possesses a disease-modifying effect of a sustained cognitive decline reduction.
    - Donepezil owns the majority of the market for its most inclusive indications for all severity levels, once-a-day administration, easy dosing titration, and tolerability profile.

Table: Drug Class Summary

Alzheimer's Pharmacotherapy - Drug Class Review High-Yield Med Reviews			
Mechanism of Action: *Inhibitors of acetylcholinesterase, counteracting the loss of cholinergic neurons in Alzheimer's disease.*			
Class Effects: *Slow the cognitive dysfunction of patients with Alzheimer's disease, with significant safety improvement compared with the tacrine's historical use.*			
Generic Name	**Brand Name**	**Main Indication(s) or Uses**	**Notes**
Donepezil	Aricept	• Alzheimer disease	• **Dosing (Adult):** — Oral: 5 to 23 mg daily • **Dosing (Peds):** Not routinely used • **CYP450 Interactions:** Substrate of CYP2D6, 3A4 • **Renal or Hepatic Dose Adjustments:** None • **Dosage Forms:** Oral (tablet, disintegrating tablet)
Galantamine	Razadyne	• Alzheimer disease	• **Dosing (Adult):** — Oral: IR 4 to 24 mg q12h — Oral: ER 8 to 24 mg daily • **Dosing (Peds):** Not routinely used • **CYP450 Interactions:** Substrate of CYP2D6, 3A4 • **Renal or Hepatic Dose Adjustments:** — GFR 9 to 59 mL/minute OR Child-Pugh class B: Maximum 16 mg/day — GFR < 9 mL/minute OR Child-Pugh class C: Not recommended • **Dosage Forms:** Oral (capsule, solution, tablet)
Memantine	Namenda	• Alzheimer disease	• **Dosing (Adult):** — Oral: 5 to 28 mg/day • **Dosing (Peds):** — Not routinely used • **CYP450 Interactions:** None • **Renal or Hepatic Dose Adjustments:** — GFR 5 to 29 mL/minute: Maximum 5 mg q12h IR, or 14 mg/day ER — GFR < 5 or Child-Pugh class C: Not recommended • **Dosage Forms:** Oral (capsule, solution, tablet)
Rivastigmine	Exelon	• Alzheimer disease	• **Dosing (Adult):** — Oral: 1.5 to 6 mg q12h — Transdermal patch 4.6 to 13.3 mg q24h • **Dosing (Peds):** — Not routinely used • **CYP450 Interactions:** None • **Renal or Hepatic Dose Adjustments:** — Child-Pugh class A or B: Maximum dose of 1.5 mg oral daily, or 4.6 mg daily transdermal — Child-Pugh class C: Not recommended • **Dosage Forms:** Oral (capsule), Transdermal patch

ANALGESICS – LOCAL ANESTHETICS

Drug Class
- Local Anesthetics
- Agents:
  - **Acute Care**
    - Articaine
    - Benzocaine
    - Bupivacaine
    - Chloroprocaine
    - Cocaine
    - Dibucaine
    - Lidocaine
    - Mepivacaine
    - Prilocaine
    - Proparacaine
    - Ropivacaine
    - Tetracaine

Main Indications or Uses
- **Acute Care**
  - Dental anesthesia
  - Topical anesthesia
  - Local anesthesia
  - Regional anesthesia

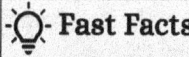 **Fast Facts**

✓ Lidocaine should not be given at doses exceeding 4.5 mg/kg (or 7 mg/kg if used with epinephrine) for local anesthetic purposes due to the risk CNS and cardiac toxicity.

Mechanism of Action
- Reversible inhibition of voltage-gated sodium channels causes a failure to initiate and propagate action potentials.
  - Analgesic properties are attributed to inhibiting axonal transmission of nerve impulses caused by pain or temperature.

Primary Net Benefit
- At normal therapeutic doses, local anesthetics provide isolated pain relief without affecting mental status, respiratory rate, heart rate, or blood pressure.
- Main Labs to Monitor:
  - No routine monitoring

High-Yield Basic Pharmacology
- **Amide or Ester**
  - Local anesthetics can be grouped into two structural classes: amino amides or esters.
  - Amino esters typically have one "i" in their drug name and are mostly all metabolized by plasma cholinesterase to a toxic metabolite para-aminobenzoic acid (PABA).
    - Patients with altered plasma cholinesterase function, hepatic impairment, or decreased hepatic blood flow are at risk of ester toxicity.
  - Patients with allergies to esters are likely to have cross-sensitivity to other ester anesthetics.
    - However, patients with ester allergies can safely receive amino amide anesthetics.
- **Epinephrine coformulation**
  - Many local anesthetics are co-formulated with dilute epinephrine (either 1:100,000 or 1:200,000), intended to limit bleeding, increase the anesthetic effect duration, and further limit systemic exposure to the drug.
    - These co-formulated products must not be administered IV and can only be administered for local infiltration.
- **Lidocaine Metabolites**
  - When used for cardiac indications, lidocaine can be given as a continuous infusion and monitored therapeutically using lidocaine plasma levels.
  - One of the toxic metabolites of lidocaine, monoethylglycinexylidide (MEGX), should also be monitored alongside lidocaine.
    - Glycinexylidide (GX) and MEGX are thought to cause seizures.

- **Benzocaine and Methemoglobin**
  - Benzocaine is metabolized to the toxic oxidizing metabolites phenylhydroxylamine and nitrobenzene.
    - Oxidation
  - Standard doses of benzocaine have been associated with clinically relevant methemoglobinemia.
  - Increased risk of methemoglobin exists when local anesthetics are administered in excessive doses or a breakdown of mucosal barriers to systemic absorption.
- **Maximum doses**
  - Local anesthetics should be dosed with the awareness of a maximum dose for each agent.
  - Lidocaine should not be given at doses exceeding 4.5 mg/kg for local anesthetic purposes.
    - When co-formulated with epinephrine, this maximum dose increases to 7 mg/kg.
  - Bupivacaine doses should not exceed 2.5 mg/kg, but epinephrine can be given at doses up to 3 mg/kg.
  - Mepivacaine's maximum dose is 5 mg/kg, but it can be given up to 7 mg/kg when co-formulated with epinephrine.
  - Ropivacaine has a maximum dose of 3 mg/kg.
- **Cardiac and Central Effects**
  - Local anesthetics may cause cardiac or central nervous system adverse events.
  - The local anesthetics are sodium channel blockers; they can act on cardiac tissue as antiarrhythmics or cause arrhythmias.
    - Lidocaine is classified as a Vaughn Williams 1B antiarrhythmic.
    - Bupivacaine is also thought to affect mitochondrial function, limiting cardiac cellular energy production from carbohydrates and precipitating cardiac arrest.
  - Seizures are also observed from excessive exposure to local anesthetics, which can often be preceded by tinnitus.

High-Yield Clinical Knowledge
- **EMLA or LMX Creams**
  - Topical admixtures of local anesthetics known as EMLA cream (lidocaine/prilocaine) or LMX (lidocaine) can be used for an outpatient application.
  - EMLA cream is used with caution as the incidence of methemoglobin is higher due to the combination of lidocaine and prilocaine.
- **Cocaine as An Anesthetics**
  - Cocaine is still available as a 4% solution for topical anesthesia and local vasoconstriction in patients with epistaxis.
    - Its use is controversial given the risk of adverse cardiac effects due to coronary vasoconstriction and the availability of alternative therapies that are similarly effective.
- **Intralipid Reversal**
  - In patients who experience adverse cardiac events associated with local anesthetic administration (including cardiac arrest), intravenous lipid emulsion 20% should be administered as a bolus of 1.5 mg/kg.
  - Intravenous intralipid is believed to shift cardiac cellular metabolism to lipolysis and fatty acid oxidation as an ATP source, as the local anesthetics impair carnitine-dependent mitochondrial lipid transportation.
    - Lipid emulsion is also thought to create a lipophilic compartment where the local anesthetic can distribute into or away from cardiac binding sites.
    - The lipid may also independently activate sodium channels, overcoming sodium channel blockade caused by local anesthetics.

High-Yield Core Evidence
- **Local Anesthetics for Neuropathic Pain**
    - This systematic review and meta-analysis of randomized controlled trials examined the efficacy and safety of systemically administered local anesthetics compared with placebo or active drugs.
    - The authors included 19 studies in the meta-analysis portion of the publication and 27 trials in the systematic review.
    - Specifically, regarding neuropathic pain, lidocaine and mexiletine were superior to placebo but similarly effective compared to amantadine, amitriptyline, gabapentin, and morphine.
    - These agents were associated with more drowsiness, fatigue, nausea, and dizziness than placebo or active controls.
    - The authors concluded that lidocaine and mexiletine produced no significant adverse events in controlled clinical trials. Furthermore, they were superior to placebo to relieve neuropathic pain and were as useful as other analgesics used for this condition. (Anesth Analg. 2005 Dec;101(6):1738-49.)

High-Yield Fast-Facts
- **Methylene Blue**
    - If methemoglobinemia occurs due to local anesthetics, methylene blue should be considered.
    - However, methylene blue itself can induce methemoglobin.
- **Liposomal Bupivacaine**
    - Bupivacaine is available as a liposomal encapsulation that permits sustained release of bupivacaine, extending its local anesthesia duration.

HIGH-YIELD BOARD EXAM ESSENTIALS
- **CLASSIC AGENTS:** Benzocaine, bupivacaine, lidocaine, proparacaine, tetracaine
- **DRUG CLASS:** Local anesthetics
- **INDICATIONS:** Local (bupivacaine, lidocaine) & Topical analgesia (benzocaine, proparacaine, tetracaine)
- **MECHANISM:** Inhibit nerve impulses for pain by blocking Na+ channels in nerve axons
- **SIDE EFFECTS:** At high doses cardiac and seizures. Benzocaine spray can cause methemoglobinemia.
- **CLINICAL PEARLS:**
    - Amino esters typically have one "i" in their drug name and amides have two "i"s.
    - Max dose of lidocaine WITHOUT epi is 4.5 mg/kg, but WITH epi is 7 mg/kg.

Table: Drug Class Summary

Local Anesthetics - Drug Class Review
High-Yield Med Reviews

Mechanism of Action: *Reversible inhibition of voltage-gated sodium channels causing a failure to initiate and propagate action potentials*

Class Effects: *Local anesthetics provide isolated pain relief without affecting mental status, respiratory rate, heart rate, or blood pressure at normal therapeutic doses.*

Generic Name	Brand Name	Main Indication(s) or Uses	Notes

Articaine and Epinephrine	Articadent
	Orabloc
	Septocaine
	Zorcaine
		- Dental anesthesia	- **Dosing (Adult):**
			   – Infiltrate: 20 to 204 mg (max 7 mg/kg)
			- **Dosing (Peds):**
			   – Infiltrate: 20 to 204 mg (max 7 mg/kg)
			- **CYP450 Interactions:** None
			- **Renal or Hepatic Dose Adjustments:** None
			- **Dosage Forms:** Injection solution

Benzocaine	Anacaine
	Anbesol
	Cepacol
	HurriCaine
		- Topical anesthesia
		- Poison ivy/sumac
			- **Dosing (Adult):**
			   – Topically applied to affected area up to 4 times daily
			   – Lozenge - allow to dissolve slowly in the mouth every 2 hours as needed
			- **Dosing (Peds):**
			   – Topically applied to affected area up to 4 times daily
			   – Lozenge - allow to dissolve slowly in the mouth every 2 hours as needed
			- **CYP450 Interactions:** None
			- **Renal or Hepatic Dose Adjustments:** None
			- **Dosage Forms:** Topical (aerosol, gel, liquid, lozenge, ointment, solution, stick, strip, swab)

Benzocaine, Butamben, and Tetracaine	Cetacaine	- Topical anesthesia	- **Dosing (Adult):**
			   – Topically spray for less than 1 second
			   – Gel/liquid: 200 mg applied topically
			- **Dosing (Peds):**
			   – Not recommended
			- **CYP450 Interactions:** None
			- **Renal or Hepatic Dose Adjustments:** None
			- **Dosage Forms:** Topical (aerosol, gel, liquid)

Local Anesthetics - Drug Class Review
High-Yield Med Reviews

Generic Name	Brand Name	Main Indication(s) or Uses	Notes
Bupivacaine	Marcaine Sensorcaine	<ul><li>Local anesthesia</li><li>Regional anesthesia</li></ul>	<ul><li>**Dosing (Adult):**<ul><li>Infiltration: 5 to 50 mL once<ul><li>Available as 0.25%, 0.5%, or 0.75%</li><li>Maximum 400 mg/24 hours</li></ul></li></ul></li><li>**Dosing (Peds):**<ul><li>Infiltration: 0.3 to 0.6 mL/kg<ul><li>Maximum volume of 20 mL/dose</li><li>Maximum dose 3 mg/kg or 200 mg, whichever is less</li></ul></li></ul></li><li>**CYP450 Interactions:** SubCYP1A2, 2C19, 2D, 3A4</li><li>**Renal or Hepatic Dose Adjustments:** None</li><li>**Dosage Forms:** Implant, Solution for injection</li></ul>
Bupivacaine and epinephrine	Marcaine E Sensorcaine/epinephrine	<ul><li>Local anesthesia</li></ul>	<ul><li>**Dosing (Adult):**<ul><li>Infiltration: 2 to 50 mL once<ul><li>Available as 0.25%, 0.5%, or 0.75%</li><li>Maximum 400 mg/24 hours</li></ul></li></ul></li><li>**Dosing (Peds):**<ul><li>See adult dosing</li></ul></li><li>**CYP450 Interactions:** SubCYP1A2, 2C19, 2D, 3A4</li><li>**Renal or Hepatic Dose Adjustments:** None</li><li>**Dosage Forms:** Solution for injection</li></ul>
Bupivacaine (liposomal)	Exparel	<ul><li>Local anesthesia</li><li>Regional anesthesia</li></ul>	<ul><li>**Dosing (Adult):**<ul><li>Infiltration: 7 to 30 mL</li></ul></li><li>**Dosing (Peds):**<ul><li>Not routinely used</li></ul></li><li>**CYP450 Interactions:** Sub CYP1A2, 2C19, 3A4</li><li>**Renal or Hepatic Dose Adjustments:** None</li><li>**Dosage Forms:** Suspension for injection</li></ul>
Chloroprocaine	Clorotekal Nesacaine	<ul><li>Local anesthesia</li></ul>	<ul><li>**Dosing (Adult):**<ul><li>Infiltration: 0.5 to 10 mL once<ul><li>Max dose 800 mg</li></ul></li></ul></li><li>**Dosing (Peds):**<ul><li>Infiltration: 0.5 to 10 mL once<ul><li>Max dose 11 mg/kg</li></ul></li></ul></li><li>**CYP450 Interactions:** None</li><li>**Renal or Hepatic Dose Adjustments:** None</li><li>**Dosage Forms:** Solution for injection</li></ul>

Local Anesthetics - Drug Class Review
High-Yield Med Reviews

Generic Name	Brand Name	Main Indication(s) or Uses	Notes

Cocaine	Goprelto, Numbrino	• Local anesthesia	• **Dosing (Adult):**
			  – Insert 2 cocaine solution cottonoid pledgets in each affected nostril for up to 20 minutes
			    – Max 4 pledgets, 160 mg or 3 mg/kg
			• **Dosing (Peds):**
			  – Insert 2 cocaine solution cottonoid pledgets in each affected nostril for up to 20 minutes
			    – Max 2 pledgets, or 3 mg/kg
			• **CYP450 Interactions:** Substrate CYP3A4
			• **Renal or Hepatic Dose Adjustments:** None
			• **Dosage Forms:** Topical (solution)

Dibucaine	Nupercainal	• Topical anesthesia	• **Dosing (Adult):**
			  – Apply to affected area up to 4 times daily
			• **Dosing (Peds):**
			  – Apply to affected area up to 4 times daily
			• **CYP450 Interactions:** None
			• **Renal or Hepatic Dose Adjustments:** None
			• **Dosage Forms:** Ointment

Lidocaine	Xylocaine	• Topical anesthesia
		• Local anesthesia
		• Regional anesthesia
			• **Dosing (Adult):**
			  – Infiltration: 2 to 50 mL
			    – Max 4.5 mg/kg/dose
			  – IV 1.5 mg/kg or 100 mg once
			    – Max 3 mg/kg
			  – IV infusion 1 to 4 mg/minute
			• **Dosing (Peds):**
			  – Infiltration 2 to 50 mL
			    – Max 4.5 mg/kg/dose
			  – IV 1.5 mg/kg or 100 mg once
			    – Max 3 mg/kg
			  – IV infusion 1 to 4 mg/minute
			• **CYP450 Interactions:** Sub CYP1A2, 2A6, 2B6, 2C9, 3A4
			• **Renal or Hepatic Dose Adjustments:**
			  – GFR < 30 mL/min or hepatic impairment: lower maintenance infusion dose
			• **Dosage Forms:** Solution for injection, Topical (aerosol, gel, liquid, ointment)

| \multicolumn{4}{|c|}{**Local Anesthetics - Drug Class Review**} |

| **Local Anesthetics - Drug Class Review** ||||
| *High-Yield Med Reviews* ||||
Generic Name	**Brand Name**	**Main Indication(s) or Uses**	**Notes**
Lidocaine with epinephrine	Xylocaine with epinephrine	• Local anesthesia	• **Dosing (Adult):** — Infiltration 1 to 5 mL/dose (max 7 mg/kg) • **Dosing (Peds):** — Infiltration 1 to 5 mL/dose (max 7 mg/kg) • **CYP450 Interactions:** Substrate CYP1A2, 2A6, 2B6, 2C9, 3A4 • **Renal or Hepatic Dose Adjustments:** — GFR < 30 mL/minute or hepatic impairment: lower maintenance dose • **Dosage Forms:** Solution for injection
Mepivacaine	Carbocaine Polocaine	• Local anesthesia • Regional anesthesia	• **Dosing (Adult):** — Infiltration: 5 to 40 mL — Max 400 mg, or 500 mg with epinephrine • **Dosing (Peds):** — Infiltration: 5 to 6 mg/kg — Max dose: 270 mg • **CYP450 Interactions:** None • **Renal or Hepatic Dose Adjustments:** None • **Dosage Forms:** Solution for injection
Prilocaine	Citanest Plain Dental	• Dental anesthesia	• **Dosing (Adult):** — Infiltration of 400 mg or 6 mg/kg — Max dose: 400 mg • **Dosing (Peds):** — Infiltration: 1 mL of 4% solution for single tooth procedures • **CYP450 Interactions:** None • **Renal or Hepatic Dose Adjustments:** None • **Dosage Forms:** Solution for injection
Proparacaine	Alcaine	• Topical anesthesia	• **Dosing (Adult):** — Ophthalmic: 1 to 2 drops per eye every 5 to 10 minutes for up to 7 doses • **Dosing (Peds):** — Ophthalmic: 1 to 2 drops per eye every 5 to 10 minutes for up to 7 doses • **CYP450 Interactions:** None • **Renal or Hepatic Dose Adjustments:** None • **Dosage Forms:** Ophthalmic solution

Local Anesthetics - Drug Class Review High-Yield Med Reviews			
Generic Name	**Brand Name**	**Main Indication(s) or Uses**	**Notes**

Ropivacaine	Naropin	- Local anesthesia
		- Regional anesthesia
			- **Dosing (Adult):**
			  – Infiltration: 5 to 50 mL
			    – Maximum 3 mg/kg
			    – Available as 0.5%, 0.75%, 1%
			- **Dosing (Peds):**
			  – Infiltration: 0.5 to 50 mL
			    – Maximum 3 mg/kg
			    – Available as 0.5%, 0.75%, 1%
			- **CYP450 Interactions:** Sub CYP1A2, 2B6, 2D6, 3A4
			- **Renal or Hepatic Dose Adjustments:** None
			- **Dosage Forms:** Solution for injection

Tetracaine	Altacaine
	Tetcaine
		- Topical anesthesia	- **Dosing (Adult):**
			  – Ophthalmic instill 1 to 2 drops in the affected eye as needed q3-5minutes up to 3 doses
			- **Dosing (Peds):**
			  – Ophthalmic instill 1 to 2 drops in the affected eye prn q3-5min up to 3 doses
			- **CYP450 Interactions:** None
			- **Renal or Hepatic Dose Adjustments:** None
			- **Dosage Forms:** Ophthalmic solution

ANALGESICS – NON-OPIOID - ACETAMINOPHEN

Drug Class
- Non-Opioid Analgesic
- Agents:
  - Acetaminophen (multi-dosage formulations available to guide each scenario)

Main Indications or Uses
- Acute & Chronic Care
  - Fever
  - Pain (mild to moderate pain; as monotherapy or adjunct)

> **Fast Facts**
> ✓ Patients who have taken more than 3,000 or 4,000 mg for several days are at risk of acetaminophen toxicity.
>
> ✓ Unlike NSAIDs, acetaminophen does not have antiinflammatory effects.

Mechanism of Action
- Acts as a central indirect inhibitor of COX-2 enzymes, decreasing PGE_2 synthesis by selectively inhibiting prostaglandin synthesis when prostaglandin and arachidonic acid concentrations are low.

Primary Net Benefit
- OTC, analgesic, and antipyretics are commonly used and also present alone or in combination with various products.
- Main Labs to Monitor:
  - No routine monitoring
  - Acetaminophen level if concerned for toxicity (normal range 10 to 20 mcg/mL)

High-Yield Clinical Pharmacology
- **Central COX-2 Effects**
  - Acetaminophen possesses numerous actions that contribute to its analgesic and antipyretic effects.
    - Indirectly inhibits prostaglandin production by reducing heme on the peroxidase portion of prostaglandin H_2.
  - Its prostaglandin synthesis inhibition occurs where prostaglandin synthesis and arachidonic acid are low.
    - Macrophages and platelets are present when arachidonic acid and prostaglandin synthesis are high; therefore, acetaminophen is minimally affected during normal therapeutic uses.
    - Conversely, the CNS where peroxide tone (a.k.a., arachidonic acid synthesis) is low.
- **Therapeutic Range**
  - The analgesic and antipyretic effects of acetaminophen are dose-dependent in nature.
  - Analgesic activity occurs at a serum acetaminophen concentration of approximately 10 mcg/mL, whereas antipyretic effects occur at higher levels closer to 18 mcg/mL.
- **Metabolism**
  - Acetaminophen normally undergoes hepatic glucuronidation and sulfation at normal therapeutic doses.
  - If glucuronidation or sulfation capacity is exceeded, either in overdose or hepatic dysfunction, the acetaminophen oxidation pathway is induced where CYP2E1 metabolizes the drug.
    - CYP2E1 metabolism of acetaminophen yields a toxic metabolite, N-acetyl-p-benzoquinone imine (NAPQI), which is then complexed with glutathione and safely eliminated.
    - When glutathione capacity is exceeded, NAPQI can accumulate, causing hepatic centrilobular necrosis and hepatic failure.

- **Maximum Dose**
    - Acetaminophen has maximum dose differences depending on whether the drug is used on a prescription or nonprescription (over-the-counter) basis.
    - For OTC use of acetaminophen, the maximum daily dose is 3,000 mg/day.
    - For prescription use of acetaminophen, the maximum daily dose is 4,000 mg/day.
        - Close attention must be paid to combination products that contain acetaminophen, as the omission of this quantity from the daily dose calculation will lead to overdosing.
- **N-Acetylcysteine**
    - A weight-based dose of 150 mg/kg or greater than 12,000 mg ingested over a single 4-hour period is considered a toxic dose.
    - If acetaminophen toxicity is suspected, a four-hour post-ingestion level should be drawn and plotted on the Rumack-Matthew Nomogram.
        - An acetaminophen level greater than 150 mcg/mL at 4 hours warrants N-acetylcysteine therapy.
- **Delayed Peak**
    - Acetaminophen is rapidly absorbed after oral administration within 2 hours, but peak plasma concentrations occur approximately 4 hours after ingestion.
        - For acetaminophen level screening in possible or confirmed overdose, a 4-hour level is recommended to account for this delay.
- **TRPV Pathway**
    - Acetaminophen's analgesic effects are also mediated by a collection of pathways, including cannabinoid, opioid, serotonergic, and transient receptor potential vanilloid cation channel subfamily V (TRPV) receptors.
        - TRPV receptors are also involved in the sensation of heat, as in from capsaicin.
- **Repeated Supratherapeutic Ingestions (RSTI)**
    - Patients who have taken more than 3,000 or 4,000 mg for several days are at risk of acetaminophen toxicity.
    - Acetaminophen level testing is of questionable use in this scenario as the Rumack-Matthew nomogram is not valid in this population, but AST/ALT screening should take place.
        - For AST levels above 2-times the upper limit of normal should be treated with N-acetylcysteine.
- **Renal and Metabolic Effects**
    - After a massive overdose, considered doses greater than 300 mg/kg, acetaminophen has been associated with nephrotoxic effects and anion-gap metabolic acidosis.

- While N-acetylcysteine should be used as a component of treatment, hemodialysis should be considered.

High-Yield Core Evidence
- **HEAT Trial**
    - This was a randomized trial of critically ill patients with fever and known or suspected infection who received either acetaminophen 1,000 mg IV or placebo every 6 hours until ICU discharge, resolution of fever, cessation of antimicrobial therapy, or death.
    - There was no significant difference between acetaminophen IV and placebo concerning the primary outcome of ICU-free days (days alive and free from the need for intensive care) from randomization to day 28.
    - There was also no difference in 90-day mortality between treatment groups.
    - The authors concluded that early administration of acetaminophen to treat fever due to probable infection did not affect the number of ICU-free days. (N Engl J Med. 2015 Dec 3;373(23):2215-24.)
- **Acetaminophen for Pain and Osteoarthritis**
    - This was a systematic review and meta-analysis of randomized controlled trials comparing the efficacy and safety of acetaminophen with placebo for spinal pain (neck or low back pain) and osteoarthritis of the hip or knee.
    - Of the evidence considered high-quality, acetaminophen did not demonstrate effectiveness in reducing pain intensity and disability or improving quality of life in the short term in people with low back pain.
    - Conversely, acetaminophen did provide significant, yet not clinically important, pain relief among patients with hip or knee osteoarthritis.
    - Adverse events were similar between acetaminophen and placebo.
    - The authors concluded that acetaminophen is ineffective in treating low back pain and provides minimal short-term benefit for people with osteoarthritis. (BMJ. 2015;350:h1225.)

High-Yield Fast-Facts
- **Paracetamol**
    - In other parts of the world, acetaminophen is known as paracetamol.
- **Non-Linear Elimination**
    - Although the common graphic representation of the Rumack-Matthew nomogram appears linear, it is actually a log-linear graph, representing the non-linear elimination of acetaminophen.
- **Antipyretic Effects**
    - Antipyresis from acetaminophen is a result of its inhibition of endogenous pyrogens at the hypothalamic thermoregulatory center.

HIGH-YIELD BOARD EXAM ESSENTIALS
- **CLASSIC AGENTS:** Acetaminophen (Tylenol)
- **DRUG CLASS:** Non-opioid analgesic
- **INDICATIONS:** Fever, Pain
- **MECHANISM:** Antipyresis is a result of its inhibition of endogenous pyrogens (i.e., prostaglandins) at the hypothalamic thermoregulatory center.
- **SIDE EFFECTS:** None unless toxicity occurs from doses exceeding 4,000 mg/d from NAPQI formation.
- **CLINICAL PEARL(S):** No antiinflammatory effects like NSAIDS. Safe in pregnancy. No major drug interactions.

Table: Drug Class Summary

Acetaminophen - Drug Class Review High-Yield Med Reviews			
Mechanism of Action: *Central indirect inhibitor of COX-2, selectively decreasing PGE_2 synthesis when prostaglandin and arachidonic acid concentrations are low.*			
Class Effects: • Over the counter, analgesic (but no antiinflammatory) effects, and antipyretic are commonly used and present alone or in combination in a variety of different products. Safe in pregnancy. No major drug interactions. • Toxic single dose: 200 mg/kg. Toxicity risk: liver damage from metabolite NAPQI. Per Rumack-Matthew Nomogram the first drug level check is at 4 hours (if time of overdose is known).			

Generic Name	Brand Name	Indication(s) or Uses	Notes

Acetaminophen	Ofirmev, Tylenol	• Fever
		 • Pain
			• **Dosing (Adult):**
			  – Oral: 325 to 1000 mg q4-6hours, maximum 3,000 mg/day (OTC) or 4,000 mg/day (Rx)
			  – IV: 12.5 mg/kg or 650 mg q4-6hours, maximum 75 mg/kg/day or 4,000 mg/day
			  – Rectal: 325 to 650 mg q4-6h, maximum 3,900 mg/day
			 • **Dosing (Peds):**
			  – Oral: 10 to 15 mg/kg/dose q4-6hours, maximum 75 mg/kg/day or 4,000 mg/day
			  – IV: 12.5 mg/kg q4-6hours, maximum 75 mg/kg/day or 4,000 mg/day
			  – Rectal: 10 to 15 mg/kg/dose q4-6hours, maximum 75 mg/kg/day or 3,900 mg/day
			 • **CYP450 Interactions:** Substrate mainly CYP2E1, but also 1A2, 2A6, 2C9, 2D6, 2E1, 3A4
			 • **Renal or Hepatic Dose Adjustments:**
			  – Child-Pugh class B or C: maximum 3,000 mg/day
			 • **Dosage Forms:** Oral (capsule, elixir, liquid, powder, solution, suspension, syrup, tablet), IV (solution; Ofirmev)

ANALGESICS – NONOPIOID - NSAIDs

Drug Class
- NSAIDs
- Agents:
  - Acute Care
    - Celecoxib
    - Diclofenac
    - Diflunisal
    - Etodolac
    - Fenoprofen
    - Flurbiprofen
    - Ibuprofen
    - Indomethacin
    - Ketoprofen
    - Ketorolac
    - Meclofenamate
    - Mefenamic acid
    - Meloxicam
    - Nabumetone
    - Naproxen
    - Oxaprozin
    - Piroxicam
    - Sulindac

Main Indications or Uses
- Acute Care
  - Analgesia
  - Antipyresis
    - Diclofenac
  - Closure of patent ductus arteriosus (infants only)
    - Indomethacin
  - Dysmenorrhea
  - Ischemic stroke or transient ischemic attack
- Chronic Care
  - Anti-inflammatory
  - Cardiovascular disease primary and secondary prevention

> **Fast Facts**
> - NSAIDs have both antipyretic and antiinflammatory effects.
> - NSAIDs do not provide any CV protection like aspirin.
> - NSAID induced ulceration is partially influenced by each NSAID's COX 1:COX2 ratio. Those that are more COX2 selective have less GI side effects.
> - NSAIDs can increase the risk of bleeding, worsen BP, worsen HF, and reduce renal function.

Mechanism of Action
- Inhibit the conversion of arachidonic acid to prostaglandins by inhibiting COX-1 and/or COX-2 either reversibly (NSAIDs).
  - NSAIDs differ in the degree of inhibition of COX1:COX2. NSAIDs that have more inhibition of COX-2 over COX-1 are thought to be "COX-2 selective" (e.g., celecoxib, etodolac, meloxicam) and thus cause less gastritis and/or risk of bleeding.
  - NSAIDs are unlike aspirin which has irreversible inhibition of preferentially COX-1.

Primary Overall Net Benefit
- NSAIDs produce dose-dependent analgesia, anti-inflammatory, and antiplatelet effects, which are devoid of CNS effects but are associated with GI bleeding, adverse cardiac effects (other than aspirin), and may be nephrotoxic.
- Main Labs to Monitor:
  - No routine lab monitoring

High-Yield Core Pharmacology
- Prostaglandin Products
  - NSAID inhibition of cyclooxygenase decreases the production of prostaglandins, thromboxane, and prostacyclin.
    - Prostaglandin H2 typically produces prostacyclin, Prostaglandin D, E, and F, and thromboxanes.
  - Thromboxanes stimulate platelet aggregation and decrease renal blood flow.
    - Thus, inhibition of thromboxane (typically TXA2) by NSAIDs decreases platelet aggregation and may augment renal blood flow.
  - Prostaglandin inhibition may also produce vasoconstriction and bronchoconstriction.

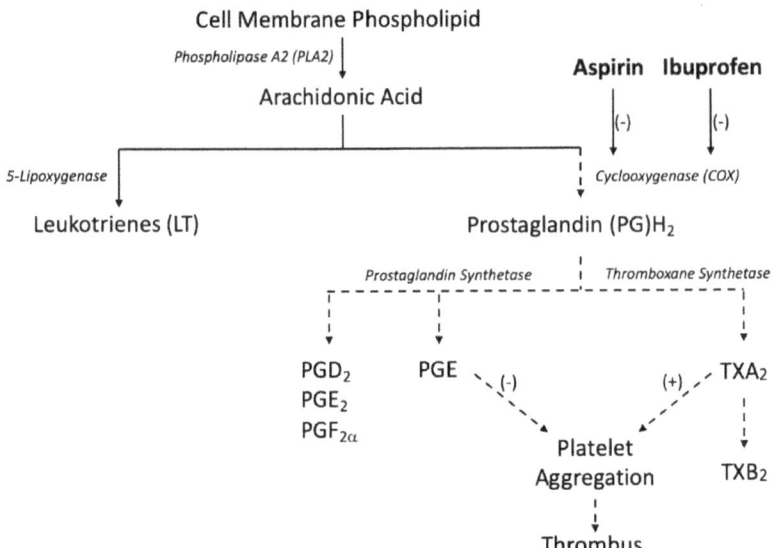

- **Central Vs. Peripheral Prostaglandin Inhibition**
    - The anti-inflammatory properties of NSAIDs are attributed to their inhibition of peripherally located prostaglandins.
    - The analgesic properties of NSAIDs are a result of inhibition of prostaglandins located in the CNS.
- **Analgesic Properties**
    - Upon tissue injury and the accompanying inflammation contributing pain is caused by the release of prostaglandins by cytokines such as bradykinin.
    - Local or systemic inhibition of COX, and prostaglandins, by salicylates contribute to analgesia which may be combined with other pain management strategies.
- **Cardiovascular Risk**
    - Inhibition of COX-2 by NSAIDs produces an inhibition of endothelial-derived prostacyclin I2 and lack of potent TXA2 inhibitory effect on platelets, leading to an increased risk of cardiovascular adverse events.
    - COX-2 selective inhibitors were originally developed to reduce the risk of GI and cardiac adverse events, but rofecoxib and valdecoxib were removed from the market due to their association with increased cardiac events.
        - Celecoxib remains in the market but carries a black boxed warning concerning this cardiovascular risk.
    - Aspirin is the exception to this class effect, as it has a net clinical benefit in reducing cardiovascular morbidity and mortality.
- **GI Bleeds**
    - Inhibition of COX-1 by NSAIDs prevents the production of PGE2 and PGI2, which leads to a decline in the production of the protective mucous lining in the GI mucosal lining, exposing the underlying tissue to gastric acid.
        - Normal coagulation may be impaired due to NSAIDs due to their inhibition of TXA2 and direct cytotoxic and irritating effects.
    - The most common ulcers formed by NSAIDs are located in the duodenum.
- **Kidney Injury**
    - Renal perfusion and glomerular filtration rate are partially regulated by COX-1 and PGI2, PGE2, and PGD2.
    - Inhibition of COX-1 can decrease renal blood flow and counteract renal hemodynamics by causing increased sodium reabsorption and decreased renin synthesis.
        - This can lead to increased plasma volume which could cause an increase in BP and heart failure exacerbation in patients with underlying HFrEF.

High-Yield Clinical Knowledge
- **Selective Vs. Non-Selective NSAIDs**
  - Selective COX-2 inhibitors (celecoxib, etodolac, meloxicam) maintain the anti-inflammatory properties of non-selective COX inhibition, potentially reducing the risk of GI and kidney adverse effects, as well as modification of platelet function.
    - However, prostacyclin synthesis is inhibited, which still may cause adverse cardiovascular effects.
    - COX-2 inhibitors have also been historically controversial as rofecoxib was removed from the market as it was associated with an increased risk of cardiovascular events.
- **Closing Patent Ductus Arteriosus**
  - Ibuprofen and indomethacin can be used intravenously in preterm infants for the closure of patent ductus arteriosus.
    - Other parenteral NSAIDs include ketorolac and meloxicam, although these are only used in adult patients.
- **NSAIDs in Pregnancy**
  - The use of NSAIDs during pregnancy is associated with premature closure of the ductus arteriosus which impairs fetal circulation in utero.
    - This was observed among patients who were given indomethacin for the purposes of terminating preterm labor.

High-Yield Core Evidence
- **PRECISION**
  - This was a multicenter, double-blind, noninferiority trial of patients taking NSAIDs for osteoarthritis or rheumatoid arthritis who were at an increased cardiovascular risk subsequently randomized to receive celecoxib, ibuprofen, or naproxen.
  - Among both the intent-to-treat population and per-protocol analysis, celecoxib, ibuprofen, and naproxen were non-inferior concerning the primary composite outcome of cardiovascular death, nonfatal myocardial infarction, or nonfatal stroke.
  - However, celecoxib was associated with significantly fewer gastrointestinal events compared to naproxen or ibuprofen.
  - Celecoxib was also associated with fewer renal events than ibuprofen but was not significantly lower with celecoxib than with naproxen.
  - Of note, the doses used in this trial were reflective of therapeutic dosing for arthritis (approximate mean daily doses of celecoxib 210 mg, naproxen 850, ibuprofen 2100).
  - Furthermore, a large portion of patients (68.8%) stopped taking study drugs during the study period, as well as 27.4% were lost to follow up.
  - The authors concluded that at moderate doses, celecoxib was found to be non-inferior to ibuprofen or naproxen concerning cardiovascular safety. (N Engl J Med. 2016 Dec 29;375(26):2519-29.)
- **Ketorolac Dose Response**
  - This was a single-center, double-blind, parallel-group trial that compared the efficacy of 3 doses of intravenous ketorolac (10, 15, and 30 mg) in patients aged 18 to 65 years and presenting to the ED with moderate to severe acute pain.
  - Thirty minutes after administering IV ketorolac, there was no significant difference between groups concerning the primary outcome of pain reduction at 30 minutes.
  - Analgesia, as demonstrated by the change in pain score of changes from 10 mg (7.7 to 5.1), 15 mg (7.5 to 5.0), and 30 mg (7.8 to 4.8), were similar between groups.
  - The authors did not disclose any serious adverse events.
  - The authors concluded that ketorolac has similar analgesic efficacy at intravenous doses of 10, 15, and 30 mg, showing that intravenous ketorolac administered at the analgesic ceiling dose (10 mg) provided effective pain relief ED patients with moderate to severe pain without increased adverse effects. (Ann Emerg Med. 2017 Aug;70(2):177-184.)

High-Yield Fast-Facts
- **Indomethacin Indications**
  - Indomethacin may be particularly useful in gouty arthritis as it may reduce neutrophil migration but comes with a relatively high risk of GI bleeding.
- **NSAIDs and Methotrexate**
  - Although patients with Rheumatoid Arthritis may take both, NSAIDs may increase the serum levels of methotrexate, potentially leading to toxicity.
  - NSAIDs are believed to decrease the renal excretion of methotrexate by inhibiting its renal transport and a decreased renal perfusion.
- **Adverse Events**
  - In addition to GI, renal, and cardiovascular adverse events, NSAIDs may also cause hematologic adverse events (thrombocytopenia, neutropenia, aplastic anemia), hepatic dysfunction, drug-induced asthma, and drug-induced rashes.

HIGH-YIELD BOARD EXAM ESSENTIALS
- **CLASSIC AGENTS:** Ibuprofen, Ketorolac, Meloxicam, Naproxen
- **DRUG CLASS:** Non-opioid analgesic NSAID
- **INDICATIONS:** Fever, Pain, Inflammation, Closure of patent ductus arteriosus (indomethacin only; infants)
- **MECHANISM:** Inhibition of COX decreases the production of not just prostaglandins but also thromboxane and prostacyclin that regulate inflammation and platelet activation.
- **SIDE EFFECTS:** Gastritis, nausea, bleeding, renal effects (AKI, ATN, Interstitial nephritis), increase risk of CVD.
- **CLINICAL PEARLS:**
  - Avoid in pregnancy.
  - Drug interactions with ACE inhibitors/ARBs, other anticoagulants, antiplatelet agents, and lithium, methotrexate.

Table: Drug Class Summary

NSAIDs - Drug Class Review				
High-Yield Med Reviews				
Mechanism of Action: *Inhibit the conversion of arachidonic acid to prostaglandins by inhibition of COX-1 and/or COX-2 either reversibly (NSAIDs) or irreversibly (aspirin).*				
Class Effects: *NSAIDs produce dose-dependent analgesia, anti-inflammatory, and antiplatelet effects, which are devoid of CNS effects but are associated with GI bleeding, adverse cardiac effects (other than aspirin), and may be nephrotoxic.*				
Generic Name	**Brand Name**	**Main Indication(s) or Uses**	**Notes**
Aspirin	Bayer Aspirin	<ul><li>Analgesia</li><li>Antipyresis</li><li>Anti-inflammatory</li><li>Cardiovascular disease primary and secondary prevention</li><li>Ischemic stroke or transient ischemic attack</li></ul>	<ul><li>**Dosing (Adult):**<ul><li>Oral: 81 to 1000 mg q4-24h</li><li>Rectal: 300 to 600 mg q4-24h</li></ul></li><li>**Dosing (Peds):**<ul><li>Oral: 1 to 15 mg/kg/dose q4-6h<ul><li>Maximum 4000 mg/day or 100 mg/kg/day, whichever is less</li></ul></li></ul></li><li>**CYP450 Interactions:** Substrate of CYP2C9</li><li>**Renal or Hepatic Dose Adjustments:**<ul><li>None</li></ul></li><li>**Dosage Forms:** Oral (caplet, capsule, suppository, tablet chewable, tablet delayed release, tablet enteric coated)</li></ul>
Celecoxib	Celebrex	<ul><li>Analgesia</li></ul>	<ul><li>**Dosing (Adult):**<ul><li>Oral: 100 to 200 mg q12-24h<ul><li>Maximum 400 mg/day</li></ul></li></ul></li><li>**Dosing (Peds):**<ul><li>Oral: 50 to 100 mg q12h</li></ul></li><li>**CYP450 Interactions:** Substrate CYP2C9, 3A4; Inhibits CYP2D6</li><li>**Renal or Hepatic Dose Adjustments:**<ul><li>GFR < 30 mL/minute: Avoid use</li><li>Child-Pugh class B: Reduce dose by 50%</li><li>Child-Pugh class C: Avoid the use</li></ul></li><li>**Dosage Forms:** Oral (capsule)</li></ul>
Diclofenac	Cambia Cataflam Zipsor Zorvolex	<ul><li>Analgesia</li><li>Dysmenorrhea</li></ul>	<ul><li>**Dosing (Adult):**<ul><li>Oral: 25 to 75 mg q8-12h</li><li>IV: 37.5 mg q6h as needed, maximum 150 mg/day</li></ul></li><li>**Dosing (Peds):**<ul><li>Not routinely used</li></ul></li><li>**CYP450 Interactions:** Substrate CYP1A2, 2B6, 2C19, 2C9, 2D6, 3A4; Inhibits UGT 1A6</li><li>**Renal or Hepatic Dose Adjustments:**<ul><li>GFR < 30 mL/minute: Avoid use</li><li>Child-Pugh class B or C: Avoid use</li></ul></li><li>**Dosage Forms:** Oral (capsule, packet, solution, tablet)</li></ul>

| NSAIDs - Drug Class Review || ||
| High-Yield Med Reviews || ||
Generic Name	Brand Name	Main Indication(s) or Uses	Notes

Diflunisal	Dolobid	• Analgesia	• **Dosing (Adult):**
			  – Oral: 250 to 750 mg q12h
			    – Maximum 1,500 mg/day
			• **Dosing (Peds):**
			  – Oral: 250 to 750 mg q12h
			    – Maximum 1,500 mg/day
			• **CYP450 Interactions:** None
			• **Renal or Hepatic Dose Adjustments:**
			  – GFR < 50 mL/minute: reduce dose by 50%
			• **Dosage Forms:** Oral (tablet)

Etodolac	Lodine	• Acute pain
		• Arthritis
			• **Dosing (Adult):**
			  – Oral: 200 to 400 mg q6-12h
			    – Maximum 1,000 mg/day
			• **Dosing (Peds):**
			  – Oral: 7.5 to 10 mg/kg/dose q12h
			    – Maximum 1,000 mg/day
			• **CYP450 Interactions:** None
			• **Renal or Hepatic Dose Adjustments:**
			  – GFR < 37 mL/minute: Avoid use
			• **Dosage Forms:** Oral (capsule, tablet)

Fenoprofen	Fenortho
	Nalfon
		• Analgesia
		• Arthritis
			• **Dosing (Adult):**
			  – Oral: 400 to 600 mg q6-8h
			    – Maximum 3,200 mg/day
			• **Dosing (Peds):** Not routinely used
			• **CYP450 Interactions:** None
			• **Renal or Hepatic Dose Adjustments:** None
			• **Dosage Forms:** Oral (capsule, tablet)

Flurbiprofen		• Arthritis	• **Dosing (Adult):** – Oral: 50 to 100 mg q6-12h • **Dosing (Peds):** Not routinely used • **CYP450 Interactions:** Substrate CYP2C9 • **Renal or Hepatic Dose Adjustments:** None • **Dosage Forms:** Oral (tablet)

| | | NSAIDs - Drug Class Review |||
		High-Yield Med Reviews		
Generic Name	Brand Name	Main Indication(s) or Uses	Notes

Ibuprofen	Caldolor
	Motrin
		• Analgesia
		• Antipyresis
		• Anti-inflammatory
			• **Dosing (Adult):**
			  – Oral: 200 to 800 mg q6-8h
			    – Max: 3,200 mg/day
			  – IV: 200 to 800 mg q4-6h PRN pain
			    – Maximum 2,400 mg/day
			• **Dosing (Peds):**
			  – Oral: 4 to 10 mg/kg/dose q6-8h
			    – Maximum 400 mg/dose
			  – IV: 10 mg/kg/dose q4-6 hours PRN pain
			    – Maximum: 2,400 mg/day
			• **CYP450 Interactions:** Substrate CYP2C9/19
			• **Renal or Hepatic Dose Adjustments:**
			  – GFR < 30 mL/minute: not recommended
			• **Dosage Forms:** IV (solution), oral (capsule, kit, suspension, tablet)

Indomethacin	Indocin
	Tivorbex
		• Analgesia
		• Antipyresis
		• Anti-inflammatory
		• Closure of patent ductus arteriosus (infants only)
			• **Dosing (Adult):**
			  – Oral/Rectal: 20 to 75 mg q12-24h
			    – Maximum 150 mg/day
			• **Dosing (Peds):**
			  – Oral/Rectal: 1 to 2 mg/kg/day divided q6-12h
			    – Maximum 4 mg/kg/day or 200 mg/day, whichever is less
			  – IV: 0.2 mg/kg then 0.1 to 0.25 mg/kg for 2 doses
			• **CYP450 Interactions:** Substrate CYP2C19, 2C9
			• **Renal or Hepatic Dose Adjustments:**
			  – GFR < 30 mL/minute: Avoid use
			• **Dosage Forms:** Oral (capsule, suppository, suspension), IV (solution)

Ketoprofen	Anafen
	Ketoprofen
		• Analgesia
		• Anti-inflammatory
			• **Dosing (Adult):**
			  – Oral: 25 to 100 mg q6-12h
			    Maximum 300 mg/day
			• **Dosing (Peds):** Not routinely used
			• **CYP450 Interactions:** text
			• **Renal or Hepatic Dose Adjustments:**
			  – GFR < 30 mL/minute: Avoid use
			• **Dosage Forms:** Oral (capsule)

NSAIDs - Drug Class Review
High-Yield Med Reviews

Generic Name	Brand Name	Main Indication(s) or Uses	Notes
Ketorolac	Toradol	<ul><li>Analgesia</li><li>Anti-inflammatory</li></ul>	<ul><li>**Dosing (Adult):**<ul><li>Oral: 10 mg q4-6h as needed for pain<ul><li>Maximum 40 mg/day for 5 days</li></ul></li><li>IV: 15 to 30 mg once q6h as needed for pain<ul><li>Maximum 120 mg/day for 5 days</li></ul></li><li>IM: 30 to 60 mg once q6h PRN pain<ul><li>Maximum 120 mg/day for 5 days</li></ul></li></ul></li><li>**Dosing (Peds):**<ul><li>IV: 0.5 mg/kg/dose q6-8h<ul><li>Maximum 30 mg/dose for 5 days</li></ul></li><li>Oral: 1 mg/kg/dose q4-6h<ul><li>Maximum 10 mg/dose for 5 days</li></ul></li></ul></li><li>**CYP450 Interactions:** None</li><li>**Renal or Hepatic Dose Adjustments:**<ul><li>GFR 10 to 50 mL/min: reduce dose 50%</li><li>GFR < 10 mL/minute: avoid use</li></ul></li><li>**Dosage Forms:** Oral (tablet), IV (solution)</li></ul>
Meclofenamate	Meclomen	<ul><li>Analgesia</li><li>Anti-inflammatory</li><li>Primary dysmenorrhea</li></ul>	<ul><li>**Dosing (Adult):**<ul><li>Oral 50 mg to 100 mg q4-6h<ul><li>Maximum 400 mg/day</li></ul></li></ul></li><li>**Dosing (Peds):** Not routinely used</li><li>**CYP450 Interactions:** None</li><li>**Renal or Hepatic Dose Adjustments:**<ul><li>GFR < 30 mL/minute – Avoid use</li></ul></li><li>**Dosage Forms:** Oral (capsule)</li></ul>
Mefenamic acid	Ponstel	<ul><li>Analgesia</li><li>Anti-inflammatory</li><li>Primary dysmenorrhea</li></ul>	<ul><li>**Dosing (Adult):**<ul><li>Oral: 500 mg once, then 250 mg q6h for 3 days</li></ul></li><li>**Dosing (Peds):**<ul><li>Not routinely used</li></ul></li><li>**CYP450 Interactions:** Substrate of CYP2C9</li><li>**Renal or Hepatic Dose Adjustments:**<ul><li>GFR < 30 mL/minute: Avoid use</li></ul></li><li>**Dosage Forms:** Oral (capsule)</li></ul>
Meloxicam	Anjeso Mobic Vivlodex	<ul><li>Analgesia</li><li>Antipyresis</li><li>Anti-inflammatory</li></ul>	<ul><li>**Dosing (Adult):**<ul><li>Oral: 5 to 15 once daily</li><li>IV: 30 mg daily</li></ul></li><li>**Dosing (Peds):**<ul><li>Oral: 0.125 mg/kg daily<ul><li>Maximum 7.5 mg/day</li></ul></li></ul></li><li>**CYP450 Interactions:** Substrate CYP2C9, 3A4</li><li>**Renal or Hepatic Dose Adjustments:**<ul><li>GFR < 30 mL/minute: Avoid use</li><li>Child-Pugh class C: Avoid use</li></ul></li><li>**Dosage Forms:** Oral (capsule, tablet), IV (solution)</li></ul>

| NSAIDs - Drug Class Review ||||
| High-Yield Med Reviews ||||
Generic Name	Brand Name	Main Indication(s) or Uses	Notes

Nabumetone	Relafen	• Analgesia	• **Dosing (Adult):**
			  – Oral: 1,000 to 2,000 mg daily
			• **Dosing (Peds):**
			  – Not routinely used
			• **CYP450 Interactions:** None
			• **Renal or Hepatic Dose Adjustments:**
			  – GFR 30 to 49 mL/minute: maximum 1,500 mg/day
			  – GFR < 30 mL/minute: maximum 1,000 mg/day
			• **Dosage Forms:** Oral (tablet)

Naproxen	Aleve
	Naprosyn
		• Analgesia
		• Antipyresis
		• Anti-inflammatory
			• **Dosing (Adult):**
			  – Oral: 250 to 1,000 mg q12-24h
			    – Maximum 1,500 mg/day
			• **Dosing (Peds):**
			  – Oral: 5 to 10 mg/kg/dose q12h
			    – Maximum 1,000 mg/day
			• **CYP450 Interactions:** Substrate CYP1A2, 2C9
			• **Renal or Hepatic Dose Adjustments:**
			  – GFR < 30 mL/minute: Avoid use
			• **Dosage Forms:** Oral (capsule, suspension, tablet)

Oxaprozin	Daypro	• Analgesia	• **Dosing (Adult):**
			  – Oral: 1,200 mg daily
			    – Maximum 1,800 mg/day or 26 mg/kg/day, whichever is less
			• **Dosing (Peds):**
			  – Oral: 10 to 20 mg/kg/dose
			    – Maximum 1,200 mg/day
			• **CYP450 Interactions:** None
			• **Renal or Hepatic Dose Adjustments:**
			  – GFR < 30 mL/minute: Avoid use
			• **Dosage Forms:** Oral (tablet)

Piroxicam	Feldene	• Analgesia	• **Dosing (Adult):**
			  – Oral: 20 mg daily
			• **Dosing (Peds):**
			  – Oral: 0.2 to 0.4 mg/kg/day
			    – Maximum 20 mg/day
			• **CYP450 Interactions:** Substrate CYP2C9
			• **Renal or Hepatic Dose Adjustments:**
			  – GFR < 30 mL/minute: Avoid use
			• **Dosage Forms:** Oral (capsule)

| NSAIDs - Drug Class Review || ||
| High-Yield Med Reviews || ||
Generic Name	Brand Name	Main Indication(s) or Uses	Notes

Sulindac	Clinoril
	Sulin
		▪ Analgesia
		▪ Anti-inflammatory
			▪ **Dosing (Adult):**
			   − Oral: 150 to 200 mg q12h for 7 to 14 days
			▪ **Dosing (Peds):**
			   − Oral: 2 to 6 mg/kg/day divided q12h
			      − Maximum 400 mg/day
			▪ **CYP450 Interactions:** None
			▪ **Renal or Hepatic Dose Adjustments:**
			   − GFR < 30 mL/minute: Avoid use
			▪ **Dosage Forms:** Oral (tablet)

ANALGESICS – SALICYLATES

Drug Class
- Salicylates
- Agents:
    - Acute Care
        - Aspirin
        - Choline Magnesium Trisalicylate
        - Methyl salicylate
        - Salsalate
        - Trolamine
    - Chronic Care
        - Aspirin

Main Indications or Uses
- Acute Care
    - Analgesia
        - Aspirin
        - Choline Magnesium Trisalicylate
        - Methyl salicylate
        - Trolamine
    - Antipyresis
        - Aspirin
    - Myocardial infarction
        - Aspirin
- Chronic Care
    - Antiinflammatory
        - Aspirin
    - Ischemic cardiac disease
        - Aspirin
    - Ischemic stroke or transient ischemic attack
        - Aspirin
    - Kawasaki disease
        - Aspirin
    - Rheumatic fever
        - Aspirin

> **Fast Facts**
>
> ✓ Unlike NSAIDs, aspirin causes an irreversible inhibition of COX-1 and does provide protection in the secondary prevention of CVD (but not primary prevention)
>
> ✓ High-dose aspirin is normally not given to pediatric patients due to the risk of Rye syndrome. The exception to this rule is with Kawasaki disease.
>
> ✓ Overdoses on aspirin can be life threatening and cause a mixed acid base disturbance where the patient initially develops a respiratory alkalosis followed by a metabolic acidosis.

Mechanism of Action
- Irreversible inhibition of cyclooxygenase 1 and 2 (COX-1, COX-2) decreasing prostaglandin precursors, inhibition of thromboxane A2.

Primary Net Benefit
- Salicylates are not routinely used for analgesic properties where better-tolerated alternatives exist, but aspirin is widely used for cardiovascular benefits.
- Main Labs to Monitor:
    - No routine monitoring

High-Yield Basic Pharmacology
- **Non-Acetylated Salicylates**
    - The non-acetylated salicylates, including choline magnesium trisalicylate, methyl salicylate, salsalate, and trolamine, possess antiinflammatory properties but lack any antiplatelet properties.
        - Their use is limited but may be options in patients with asthma with sensitivity to aspirin for antiinflammatory indications.

- **Antiinflammatory Effects**
  - Salicylates provide antiinflammatory effects through the direct inhibition of neutrophils.
- **Salicylic Acid Esters**
  - Two types of salicylic acid esters exist: phenolic esters like aspirin and carboxylic acid esters, including methyl salicylate.
  - These agents' actions are ultimately similar, given they're all converted to salicylic acid after absorption.
- **Irreversible Inhibition**
  - Aspirin is an irreversible inhibitor of platelet COX, producing platelet activity inhibition for the duration of the platelet's life (approximately 8 to 10 days).
  - NSAIDs other than aspirin inhibit platelet activity reversibly, typically for the duration of the given drugs' duration of analgesic effect.

High-Yield Clinical Knowledge
- **Analgesic Properties**
  - Upon tissue injury and the accompanying inflammation contributing pain is caused by the release of prostaglandins by cytokines such as bradykinin.
  - Local or systemic COX inhibition and prostaglandins by salicylates contribute to analgesia, combined with other pain management strategies.
- **Antipyresis**
  - The physiologic process by which fever is produced is mediated by inflammatory cytokines (IL-1, IL-6, TNF-alpha), which increase the synthesis of prostaglandin E2, triggering the hypothalamic response to elevate the body temperature set point.
  - Inhibition of prostaglandins using salicylates can contribute to an antipyretic of salicylates.
  - The antipyretic dose range of aspirin is much higher than that for cardiovascular indications, 324 to 1,000 mg by mouth q4-6h.
    - The maximum daily dose for adults is 4 g.
- **Antiplatelet Effects**
  - The covalent modification of COX-1 and COX-2 by aspirin leads to irreversible platelet function for the duration of the platelet's life as these cells are not capable of independently generating COX-1.
- **GI Bleeds**
  - Inhibition of COX-1 by salicylates prevents PGE2 and PGI2 production, which leads to a decline in the production of the protective mucous lining in the GI mucosal lining, exposing the underlying tissue to gastric acid.
  - As aspirin possesses a potent antiplatelet effect, normal coagulation may be impaired due to its inhibition of TXA2 and direct cytotoxic and irritating effects.
  - The most common ulcers formed by NSAIDs are located in the duodenum.
- **Aspirin in Pediatrics**
  - High doses of aspirin may be given to children with Kawasaki disease in combination with IV immune globulin.
    - Kawasaki disease is a vasculitis syndrome that may lead to heart disease in children, including coronary artery dilation and coronary aneurysms.
  - This is an essential distinction from over-the-counter aspirin use in children for analgesia and antipyresis recovering from chickenpox or influenza, which may develop Reye syndrome.
- **Niacin Flushing**
  - Patients who take high-dose niacin for cholesterol modulating effects can experience intense facial flushing due to the release of prostaglandin D2.
  - This prostaglandin-mediated flushing reaction can be blunted with concomitant aspirin use.
- **Hypersensitivity and Cross-Reactivity**
  - Patients who report an allergy to aspirin or NSAIDs may experience cross-sensitivity to other NSAIDs or aspirin.
  - Aspirin is contraindicated in patients with a history of hypersensitivity to NSAIDs.
    - In some clinical scenarios where aspirin is still necessary, desensitization protocols permit aspirin's safe use, but these must occur in an acute-care setting.

High-Yield Core Evidence
- **ISIS-2**
  - This was a multicenter, double-blinded, two-by-two factorial, placebo-controlled trial that randomized patients with an acute MI within 24 hours of symptom onset to one of four treatment groups: streptokinase, aspirin, aspirin plus streptokinase, or placebo.
  - Compared to placebo, all intervention treatment arms significantly reduced the risk of vascular mortality at five weeks.
    - Examining the individual treatment arms, aspirin reduced 5-week vascular mortality by 20%, streptokinase reduced this same measure by 23%, and the combination of aspirin and streptokinase reduced the same outcome by 40%.
  - Aspirin use was also associated with significantly reduced non-fatal reinfarction and nonfatal stroke and did not increase clinically significant bleeding risk.
  - The authors concluded that aspirin and streptokinase are practicable interventions that have demonstrated safety and efficacy in an MI population, and when widely used, can reduce excess mortality. (The Lancet. 1988. 332(8607):349-360.)

High-Yield Fast-Facts
- **Resistance**
  - Genetic variants of COX can lead to alternative pathways and ultimately clinical failure of aspirin, referred to as aspirin resistance.
- **Salicylate Toxicity**
  - Salicylate overdose is a potentially life-threatening toxicity that can be fatal within hours of a massive overdose.
  - This mechanism involves the uncoupling of oxidative phosphorylation and the inability to form ATP from glucose.

HIGH-YIELD BOARD EXAM ESSENTIALS
- **CLASSIC AGENTS:** Aspirin, choline magnesium trisalicylate, methyl salicylate, salsalate, trolamine
- **DRUG CLASS:** Salicylate
- **INDICATIONS:** Analgesic, antiinflammatory, antipyretic, ischemic cardiac disease, ischemic stroke or transient ischemic attack, Kawasaki disease, myocardial infarction, rheumatic fever
- **MECHANISM:** Irreversible inhibition of cyclooxygenase 1 and 2 (COX-1, COX-2) decreasing prostaglandin precursors, inhibition of thromboxane A2.
- **SIDE EFFECTS:** Dyspepsia, GI bleed, rash
- **CLINICAL PEARLS:** High doses of aspirin may be given to children with Kawasaki disease in combination with IV immune globulin. Kawasaki disease is a vasculitis syndrome that may lead to heart disease in children, including coronary artery dilation and coronary aneurysms.

Table: Drug Class Summary

Salicylates - Drug Class Review High-Yield Med Reviews			
Mechanism of Action: Irreversible inhibition of cyclooxygenase 1 and 2 (COX-1, COX-2) decreasing prostaglandin precursors, inhibition of thromboxane A2.			
Class Effects: Salicylates are not routinely used for analgesic properties where better-tolerated alternatives exist, but aspirin is widely used for cardiovascular benefits.			
Generic Name	**Brand Name**	**Main Indication(s) or Uses**	**Notes**
Aspirin	Bayer Aspirin	<ul><li>Analgesic</li><li>Antiinflammatory</li><li>Antipyretic</li><li>Ischemic cardiac disease</li><li>Ischemic stroke or transient ischemic attack</li><li>Kawasaki disease</li><li>Myocardial infarction</li><li>Rhematic fever</li></ul>	<ul><li>Dosing (Adult):<ul><li>Oral: 81 to 325 mg daily</li><li>Oral: 325 to 1,000 mg q4-6h, maximum 4,000 mg/day</li><li>Rectal: 300 to 600 mg/day</li></ul></li><li>Dosing (Peds):<ul><li>Oral/Rectal: 10 to 15 mg/kg/dose q4-6h<ul><li>Maximum 90 mg/kg/day or 4,000 mg/day</li></ul></li></ul></li><li>CYP450 Interactions: None</li><li>Renal or Hepatic Dose Adjustments:<ul><li>Severe hepatic disease: Avoid use</li></ul></li><li>Dosage Forms: Oral (caplet, capsule, tablet), Rectal (suppository)</li></ul>
Choline Magnesium Trisalicylate	Trilisate	<ul><li>Analgesia</li></ul>	<ul><li>Dosing (Adult):<ul><li>Oral: 1,500 to 3,000 mg q8-24h</li></ul></li><li>Dosing (Peds):<ul><li>Oral: 25 mg/kg/dose q12h</li></ul></li><li>CYP450 Interactions: None</li><li>Renal or Hepatic Dose Adjustments: None</li><li>Dosage Forms: Oral (Liquid)</li></ul>
Magnesium Salicylate	Doans Pills	<ul><li>Analgesia</li></ul>	<ul><li>Dosing (Adult):<ul><li>Oral: 1 - 2 tablet q4-6h as needed for pain</li></ul></li><li>Dosing (Peds):<ul><li>Not routinely used</li></ul></li><li>CYP450 Interactions: None</li><li>Renal or Hepatic Dose Adjustments: None</li><li>Dosage Forms: Oral (tablet)</li></ul>
Methyl salicylate	BenGay Icy Hot Salonpas Thera-Gesic	<ul><li>Analgesia</li></ul>	<ul><li>Dosing (Adult):<ul><li>Topically apply to affected area q6-8h as needed</li><li>Topical patch applied to affected area q6-8h as needed</li></ul></li><li>Dosing (Peds):<ul><li>Not routinely used</li></ul></li><li>CYP450 Interactions: None</li><li>Renal or Hepatic Dose Adjustments: None</li><li>Dosage Forms: Topical (balm, cream, foam, spray, stick)</li></ul>

| \multicolumn{4}{c}{**Salicylates - Drug Class Review**} |

Generic Name	Brand Name	Main Indication(s) or Uses	Notes

Salsalate	N/A	- Analgesia	- **Dosing (Adult):**
			  – Oral: 1 g q8h
			- **Dosing (Peds):**
			  – Not routinely used
			- **CYP450 Interactions:** None
			- **Renal or Hepatic Dose Adjustments:** None
			- **Dosage Forms:** Oral (tablet)

Trolamine	Arthricream
	Asper-flex
	Myoflex
		- Analgesia	- **Dosing (Adult):**
			  – Topically apply to affected area q6-8h as needed
			- **Dosing (Peds):**
			  – Topically apply to affected area q6-8h as needed
			- **CYP450 Interactions:** None
			- **Renal or Hepatic Dose Adjustments:** None
			- **Dosage Forms:** Topical (cream, lotion)

Salicylates - Drug Class Review — High-Yield Med Reviews

ANALGESICS – SKELETAL MUSCLE RELAXANTS

Drug Class
- **Skeletal Muscle Relaxants**
- **Agents:**
    - **Acute & Chronic Care**
        - AbobotulinumtoxinA
        - Baclofen
        - Carisoprodol
        - Chlorzoxazone
        - Cyclobenzaprine
        - Dantrolene
        - IncobotulinumtoxinA
        - Metaxalone
        - Methocarbamol
        - Meprobamate
        - OnabotulinumtoxinA A
        - Orphenadrine
        - PrabotulinumtoxinA
        - RimabotulinumtoxinB
        - Riluzole
        - Tizanidine

Main Indications or Uses
- **Acute & Chronic Care**
    - Amyotrophic lateral sclerosis (ALS)
        - Riluzole
    - Axillary hyperhidrosis
        - OnabotulinumtoxinA
    - Blepharospasm
        - IncobotulinumtoxinA
    - Cervical dystonia
        - AbobotulinumtoxinA
        - OnabotulinumtoxinA
        - RimabotulinumtoxinB
    - Chronic migraine
        - OnabotulinumtoxinA
    - Glabellar lines
        - PrabotulinumtoxinA
    - Malignant hyperthermia
        - Dantrolene
    - Neurogenic detrusor overactivity
        - OnabotulinumtoxinA
    - Overactive bladder
        - OnabotulinumtoxinA
    - Skeletal muscle relaxant
    - Urinary incontinence
        - OnabotulinumtoxinA

Mechanism of Action
- **Baclofen**
    - GABA-B agonist acts at the spinal cord level to inhibit transmission of reflexes resulting in skeletal muscle relaxation.

- **Botulinum toxin type A & B**
  - Inhibits synaptic exocytosis through clipping of vesicle fusion proteins in the presynaptic nerve terminal
- **Carisoprodol/Meprobamate**
  - Inhibits NMDA receptors and directly opens GABA-A receptors, similar to barbiturates.
- **Chlorzoxazone**
  - GABA-A and GABA-B agonists, as well as voltage-gated calcium channel antagonists.
- **Cyclobenzaprine**
  - Structurally similar to tricyclic antidepressants, producing antimuscarinic effects and skeletal muscle relaxation.
- **Dantrolene**
  - Ryanodine calcium channel receptor blocker, preventing increases in myoplasmic calcium and inhibition.
- **Metaxalone & Methocarbamol**
  - Inhibitions acetylcholinesterase, producing anticholinergic effects at the spinal cord level and within the CNS.
- **Orphenadrine**
  - Central and spinal antimuscarinic effects, producing analgesia and skeletal muscle relaxation.
- **Riluzole**
  - Inhibits the release of glutamate and inactivates voltage-dependent sodium channels.
- **Tizanidine**
  - Spinal alpha-2 receptor agonist.

Primary Net Benefit
- Skeletal muscle relaxants provide relief of muscle spasms and can be combined with other analgesics but can be associated with an anticholinergic adverse event of particular concern in the elderly.
- Main Labs to Monitor:
  - No routine laboratory monitoring

High-Yield Basic Pharmacology
- **GABA-B**
  - GABA-B receptors are G-protein-coupled receptors distinct from the GABA-A receptors, which are chloride ligand-gated receptors.
  - Furthermore, GABA-B receptors may be either presynaptic or postsynaptic and are located throughout the CNS and PNS.
- **Tricyclic Structures**
  - Some skeletal muscle relaxants, namely cyclobenzaprine, share a core tricyclic structure that confers many similar effects, including cardiac (QRS prolongation) and CNS toxicity (seizures).
- **Diphenhydramine**
  - Orphenadrine is the O-methyl analog of diphenhydramine and possesses many of the same central sedative effects but lacks peripheral antihistamine effects.

High-Yield Clinical Knowledge
- **Baclofen Toxicity and Withdrawal**
  - Baclofen in supratherapeutic doses can produce profound CNS depression, seizures, and respiratory depression in the setting of an overdose or baclofen infusion pump dysfunction.
  - Conversely, baclofen withdrawal presents similarly with altered mental status and seizures.
  - Patients on chronic baclofen therapy, particularly those who receive it through an implanted infusion device, must be educated on the signs and symptoms of baclofen toxicity or withdrawal.
- **Tizanidine and CYP1A2**
  - Concomitant use of tizanidine with either ciprofloxacin or fluvoxamine is contraindicated as a result of the risk of significant tizanidine toxicity from CYP1A2 inhibition.
- **Abuse Potential**
  - Carisoprodol and meprobamate are schedule IV drugs, as they pose a significant abuse potential risk due to their sedating properties.

- Although sedative properties are concerning, so too is acute or abrupt discontinuation of chronic therapy, which can precipitate an acute withdrawal syndrome consisting of anxiety, tremors, muscle spasms, insomnia, and hallucinations.
  - Although other agents in this group also carry an abuse potential, no other agents are currently scheduled controlled substances.
- **Dantrolene Use**
  - Oral dantrolene is used to manage chronic spasticity in patients with spinal cord injuries, cerebral palsy, multiple sclerosis, or previous stroke.
  - Parenteral dantrolene is reserved for use in malignant hyperthermia cases, which is most often encountered as a result of anesthetic gases or succinylcholine.
  - Anesthetic gases in some patients are associated with unregulated calcium release from the sarcoplasmic reticulum, causing a potentially fatal cascade of excessive muscle contraction, ATP depletion, oxidative stress, and hyperthermia.
  - The ryanodine calcium channel is specifically identified in the pathophysiologic course of malignant hyperthermia.
    - Its inhibition by dantrolene can be helpful in conjunction with invasive cooling, benzodiazepines, and supportive care.
- **Botulinum Toxin**
  - OnabotulinumtoxinA, the pharmacological product of botulinum toxin, is derived from Clostridium botulinum.
  - Toxin A inhibits the presynaptic calcium-dependent release of acetylcholine, causing muscle inactivation until new fibrils grow and new junctions are formed.
  - Other botulinum toxin products include abobotulinumtoxinA, incobotulinumtoxinA, prabotulinumtoxinA, and rimabotulinumtoxinB.
    - Toxin B cleaves synaptic VAMPs, preventing docking and fusion of the synaptic vesicle to the presynaptic membrane, thus preventing neurotransmitter release.

High-Yield Core Evidence
- **Low Back Pain Treatment - Orphenadrine or Methocarbamol**
  - This was a double-blind, parallel-group, comparative-effectiveness study that randomized patients with acute low back pain to a one-week course of naproxen plus placebo or naproxen plus either orphenadrine or methocarbamol.
  - There was no difference between treatment groups concerning the primary outcome of improving the Roland-Morris Disability Questionnaire between ED discharge and one week later.
  - However, fewer adverse events were reported in the orphenadrine group than the placebo or methocarbamol groups.
  - The authors concluded that among ED patients with acute, nontraumatic, nonradicular low back pain, combining naproxen with either orphenadrine or methocarbamol did not improve functional outcomes naproxen plus placebo. (Ann Emerg Med. 2018 Mar;71(3):348-356.e5.)
- **Low Back Pain Treatment - Baclofen, Metaxalone, Or Tizanidine**
  - This was a double-blind, parallel-group, comparative-effectiveness study that randomized patients with acute low back pain to a 1-week course of ibuprofen plus placebo versus ibuprofen plus a skeletal muscle relaxant (either baclofen, metaxalone, or tizanidine).
  - There was no difference between treatment groups concerning the primary outcome of improvement on the Roland-Morris Disability Questionnaire between ED discharge and one week later.
  - The authors concluded that the addition of baclofen, metaxalone, or tizanidine to ibuprofen does not appear to improve functioning or pain any more than placebo plus ibuprofen by one week after an ED visit for acute low back pain. (Ann Emerg Med. 2019 Oct;74(4):512-520.)

High-Yield Fast-Facts
- **Dantrolene and Phenytoin**
  - Dantrolene is a derivative of phenytoin but does not share the same pharmacology.
- **OTC Formulations**
  - When co-formulated with acetaminophen, methocarbamol is available over the counter in Canada, but all dosage forms in the US are prescription-only agents.

HIGH-YIELD BOARD EXAM ESSENTIALS
- **CLASSIC AGENTS:** AbobotulinumtoxinA, baclofen, carisoprodol, chlorzoxazone, cyclobenzaprine, dantrolene
- incobotulinumtoxinA, metaxalone, methocarbamol, meprobamate, onabotulinumtoxinA, orphenadrine, prabotulinumtoxinA, rimabotulinumtoxinB, riluzole, tizanidine
- **DRUG CLASS:** Skeletal Muscle Relaxants
- **INDICATIONS:** Anxiety, blepharospasm, cervical dystonia, malignant hyperthermia,
- **MECHANISM:**
  - Baclofen - GABA-B agonist; Onabotulinumtoxin A & B - Inhibits synaptic exocytosis of acetylcholine
  - Carisoprodol/Meprobamate - Inhibits NMDA receptors and directly opens GABA-A receptors
  - Chlorzoxazone - GABA-A and GABA-B agonists
  - Cyclobenzaprine - Antimuscarinic effects and skeletal muscle relaxation
  - Dantrolene - Ryanodine calcium channel receptor blocker
  - Metaxalone & Methocarbamol - Inhibits acetylcholinesterase
  - Orphenadrine - Central and spinal antimuscarinic effects
  - Riluzole - Inhibits the release of glutamate and inactivates voltage-dependent sodium channels
  - Tizanidine - Spinal alpha-2 receptor agonist.
- **SIDE EFFECTS:** Abuse potential, CNS depression, seizures, and respiratory depression.
- **CLINICAL PEARLS:** Concomitant use of tizanidine with either ciprofloxacin or fluvoxamine is contraindicated as a result of the risk of significant tizanidine toxicity from CYP1A2 inhibition.

Table: Drug Class Summary

Skeletal Muscle Relaxants - Drug Class Review
High-Yield Med Reviews

Mechanism of Action:
Baclofen - GABA-B agonist
Onabotulinumtoxin A & B - Inhibits synaptic exocytosis of acetylcholine.
Carisoprodol/Meprobamate - Inhibits NMDA receptors and directly opens GABA-A receptors.
Chlorzoxazone - GABA-A and GABA-B agonists.
Cyclobenzaprine - Antimuscarinic effects and skeletal muscle relaxation.
Dantrolene - Ryanodine calcium channel receptor blocker.
Metaxalone & Methocarbamol - Inhibitions acetylcholinesterase.
Orphenadrine - Central and spinal antimuscarinic effects
Riluzole - Inhibits the release of glutamate and inactivates voltage-dependent sodium channels.
Tizanidine - Spinal alpha-2 receptor agonist.

Class Effects: Skeletal muscle relaxants provide relief of muscle spasms and can be combined with other analgesics but can be associated with an anticholinergic adverse event of particular concern in the elderly.

Generic Name	Brand Name	Main Indication(s) or Uses	Notes

Abobotulinumtoxin A	Dysport	- Cervical dystonia
		- Skeletal muscle relaxant
			- **Dosing (Adult):**
			   – IM: 100 to 1,000 units divided among affected areas
			- **Dosing (Peds):**
			   – Not routinely used
			- **CYP450 Interactions:** None
			- **Renal or Hepatic Dose Adjustments:** None
			- **Dosage Forms:** IV (solution)

Baclofen	Gablofen
	Lioresal
	Ozobax
		- Skeletal muscle relaxant	- **Dosing (Adult):**
			   – Oral: 5 to 10 mg TID, maximum 120 mg/day
			   – Intrathecal: 50 mcg test dose followed by incremental doses to determine maintenance dose range.
			- **Dosing (Peds):**
			   – Oral: 2.5 to 10 mg TID, maximum 60 mg/day
			   – Intrathecal: 25 mcg test dose followed by incremental doses to determine maintenance dose range.
			- **CYP450 Interactions:** None
			- **Renal or Hepatic Dose Adjustments:**
			   – GFR 50 to 80 mL/minute: 5 mg q12h
			   – GFR 30 to 50 mL/minute: 2.5 mg q8h
			   – GFR < 30 mL/minute: avoid use
			- **Dosage Forms:** Oral (solution, tablet), Intrathecal solution

Skeletal Muscle Relaxants - Drug Class Review
High-Yield Med Reviews

Generic Name	Brand Name	Main Indication(s) or Uses	Notes
Carisoprodol	Soma, Vanadom	• Skeletal muscle relaxant	• **Dosing (Adult):** – Oral: 250 to 350 mg TID, maximum 3 weeks • **Dosing (Peds):** – Oral: 250 to 350 mg TID, maximum 3 weeks – Maximum 1,400 mg/day • **CYP450 Interactions:** Substrate CYP2C19 • **Renal or Hepatic Dose Adjustments:** None • **Dosage Forms:** Oral (tablet)
Chlorzoxazone	Lorzone, Parafon Forte	• Skeletal muscle relaxant	• **Dosing (Adult):** – Oral: 250 to 750 mg q6-8h • **Dosing (Peds):** – Oral: 20 mg/kg/day in 3-4 divided doses – Maximum 750 mg/dose • **CYP450 Interactions:** Substrate CYP1A2, 2A6, 2D6, 2E1, 3A4; Inhibits CYP3A4 • **Renal or Hepatic Dose Adjustments:** None • **Dosage Forms:** Oral (tablet)
Cyclobenzaprine	Amrix, Fexmid, Flexeril	• Skeletal muscle relaxant	• **Dosing (Adult):** – Oral: 5 to 15 mg q8-24h • **Dosing (Peds):** – Oral: 5 to 10 mg q8h • **CYP450 Interactions:** Substrate CYP1A2, 2D6, 3A4 • **Renal or Hepatic Dose Adjustments:** – Child-Pugh class B or C: use not recommended • **Dosage Forms:** Oral (tablet)
Dantrolene	Dantrium, Revonto, Ryanodex	• Skeletal muscle relaxant • Malignant hyperthermia	• **Dosing (Adult):** – Oral: 25 to 100 mg q8-24h – Maximum 400 mg/day – IV: 2.5 mg/kg once followed by 1 mg/kg as needed to a maximum of 10 mg/kg • **Dosing (Peds):** – Oral: 4 to 8 mg/kg/day in 3 to 4 divided doses – IV: 2.5 mg/kg once followed by 1 mg/kg as needed to a maximum of 10 mg/kg • **CYP450 Interactions:** Substrate CYP3A4 • **Renal or Hepatic Dose Adjustments:** None • **Dosage Forms:** Oral (capsule), IV (solution, suspension)

		Skeletal Muscle Relaxants - Drug Class Review High-Yield Med Reviews	
Generic Name	**Brand Name**	**Main Indication(s) or Uses**	**Notes**

Incobotulinumtoxin A	Xeomin	• Blepharospasm
		• Skeletal muscle relaxant
			• **Dosing (Adult):**
			  – IM: 25 to 100 units divided among affected areas
			• **Dosing (Peds):**
			  – IM: 4 to 22.5 units to the parotid or submandibular gland
			  – IM: 0.5 to 3 units/kg divided among affected areas
			    – Maximum 50 units/dose
			• **CYP450 Interactions:** None
			• **Renal or Hepatic Dose Adjustments:** None
			• **Dosage Forms:** IV (solution)

Meprobamate	N/A	• Anxiety	• **Dosing (Adult):**
			  – Oral: 1,200 to 1,600 mg/day in 3-4 divided doses
			    – Maximum 2,400 mg/day
			• **Dosing (Peds):**
			  – Oral: 200 to 600 mg/day in 2-3 divided doses
			• **CYP450 Interactions:** None
			• **Renal or Hepatic Dose Adjustments:**
			  – GFR 10 to 50 mL/minute: q9-12h
			  – GFR < 10 mL/minute: q12-18h
			• **Dosage Forms:** Oral (tablet)

Metaxalone	Skelaxin	• Skeletal muscle relaxant	• **Dosing (Adult):**
			  – Oral: 400 to 800 mg q6-8h
			• **Dosing (Peds):**
			  – Oral: 400 to 800 mg q6-8h
			• **CYP450 Interactions:** Substrate CYP1A2, C19, 2C8, 2C9, 2D6, 2E1, 3A4
			• **Renal or Hepatic Dose Adjustments:** None
			• **Dosage Forms:** Oral (tablet)

Methocarbamol	Robaxin	• Skeletal muscle relaxant	• **Dosing (Adult):**
			  – Oral 1.5 g q6-8h for 3 days
			  – IM/IV 1 g q8h prn for muscle spasm
			• **Dosing (Peds):**
			  – Oral: 1.5 g q6-8h for 3 days
			  – IM/IV: 15 mg/kg/dose q6-8h prn for muscle spasm
			• **CYP450 Interactions:** None
			• **Renal or Hepatic Dose Adjustments:** None
			• **Dosage Forms:** Oral (tablet), IV (solution)

Skeletal Muscle Relaxants - Drug Class Review
High-Yield Med Reviews

Generic Name	Brand Name	Main Indication(s) or Uses	Notes
OnabotulinumtoxinA	Botox	<ul><li>Axillary hyperhidrosis</li><li>Cervical dystonia</li><li>Chronic migraine</li><li>Neurogenic detrusor overactivity</li><li>Overactive bladder</li><li>Skeletal muscle relaxant</li><li>Urinary incontinence</li></ul>	<ul><li>**Dosing (Adult):** − IM: 5 to 75 units (total dose) − Maximum 400 units/3 months or cumulative dose of 6 units/kg</li><li>**Dosing (Peds):** − Not routinely used</li><li>**CYP450 Interactions:** None</li><li>**Renal or Hepatic Dose Adjustments:** None</li><li>**Dosage Forms:** IV (solution)</li></ul>
Orphenadrine	Norflex	<ul><li>Skeletal muscle relaxant</li></ul>	<ul><li>**Dosing (Adult):** − Oral: 100 mg BID − IM/IV: 60 mg q12h</li><li>**Dosing (Peds):** − Not routinely used</li><li>**CYP450 Interactions:** Substrate CYP1A2, 2B6, 2D6, 3A4</li><li>**Renal or Hepatic Dose Adjustments:** None</li><li>**Dosage Forms:** Oral (tablet), IV (solution)</li></ul>
PrabotulinumtoxinA	Nuceiva	<ul><li>Glabellar lines</li></ul>	<ul><li>**Dosing (Adult):** − IM: 4 units to up to 5 sites, or total dose of 20 units q3months</li><li>**Dosing (Peds):** − Not routinely used</li><li>**CYP450 Interactions:** None</li><li>**Renal or Hepatic Dose Adjustments:** None</li><li>**Dosage Forms:** IV (solution)</li></ul>
Riluzole	Rilutek Tiglutik	<ul><li>Amyotrophic lateral sclerosis (ALS)</li></ul>	<ul><li>**Dosing (Adult):** − Oral: 50 mg BID</li><li>**Dosing (Peds):** − Not routinely used</li><li>**CYP450 Interactions:** Substrate CYP1A2</li><li>**Renal or Hepatic Dose Adjustments:** None</li><li>**Dosage Forms:** Oral (suspension, tablet)</li></ul>
RimabotulinumtoxinB	Myobloc	<ul><li>Cervical dystonia</li></ul>	<ul><li>**Dosing (Adult):** − IM: 2,00 to 5,000 units divided to affected areas</li><li>**Dosing (Peds):** − Not routinely used</li><li>**CYP450 Interactions:** None</li><li>**Renal or Hepatic Dose Adjustments:** None</li><li>**Dosage Forms:** IV (solution)</li></ul>

Skeletal Muscle Relaxants - Drug Class Review			
High-Yield Med Reviews			
Generic Name	**Brand Name**	**Main Indication(s) or Uses**	**Notes**

Tizanidine	Zanaflex	- Skeletal muscle relaxant	- **Dosing (Adult):**
			  - Oral: 2 to 4 mg q6-12h
			    - Maximum 24 mg/day
			- **Dosing (Peds):**
			  - Oral: 1 to 4 mg at bedtime
			- **CYP450 Interactions:** Substrate CYP1A2
			- **Renal or Hepatic Dose Adjustments:**
			  - GFR < 25 mL/minute: Reduce dose by 50%
			- **Dosage Forms:** Oral (capsule, tablet)

ANALGESICS – OPIOIDS – LONG-ACTING

Drug Class
- Opioid Analgesics, Long-Acting
- Agents:
    - Acute & Chronic Care
        - Diphenoxylate
        - Fentanyl (buccal tablets, lozenges, sublingual spray, transdermal)
        - Levorphanol
        - Loperamide
        - Methadone
        - Morphine (sustained-release)
        - Oxycodone (extended-release)
        - Tapentadol
        - Tramadol

Main Indications or Uses
- Acute Care
    - Analgesia
- Chronic Care
    - Opioid use disorder

Mechanism of Action
- Opioid receptor agonists blunt the perception and response to pain by inhibiting ascending pain pathways.

> **Fast Facts**
> ✓ Methadone has more drug interactions associated with its use than most opioids. It also has a long half-life and can cause dose-dependent increases in the QT interval.

Primary Overall Net Benefit
- Long-acting opioid agonists are a component of chronic pain management but are associated with opioid dependence, which can lead to the need for methadone, a key element in treating opioid use disorder.
- Main Labs to Monitor:
    - No routine laboratory monitoring

High-Yield Basic Pharmacology
- Methadone
    - Methadone is a racemic mixture of R- and S-methadone.
    - S-methadone is a substrate of CYP3A4 and 2D6 and associated with the QT-prolonging effects of methadone.
        - R-methadone is available in Europe, which is devoid of QT-prolonging effects.
- Absorption Changes
    - Extended-release preparations of oxymorphone should not be taken with high-fat meals, as the drug's absorption can significantly increase, potentially leading to opioid toxicity.
- Other Neurotransmitter Effects
    - In addition to its opioid agonist effects, levorphanol is also an NMDA receptor agonist, which may potentiate seizures.

High-Yield Core Knowledge
- Methadone QT and Hepatic Oxidation
    - Methadone is associated with dose-dependent prolongation of the QT interval.
    - It is also a major substrate of CYP 3A4 and 2B6 and a minor substrate of CYP 2C19, 2C9, and 2D6.
    - Numerous drug interactions may increase the risk of respiratory depression and QT-prolonging effects.

- **Diphenoxylate and Loperamide**
  - Diphenoxylate and loperamide are over-the-counter opioids that are structurally similar to meperidine.
  - These agents are not absorbed systemically and used for self-care of diarrhea.
  - Diphenoxylate is co-formulated with atropine to deter abuse, as massive doses of it or loperamide may overcome P-glycoprotein in the gut, which produces sufficient systemic levels to cause CNS opioid effects.
    - Alternatively, co-ingestion with a P-glycoprotein inhibitor, such as clarithromycin, colchicine, diltiazem, erythromycin, omeprazole, or duloxetine, can also produce a systemic opioid agonist effect at standard dosing of diphenoxylate or loperamide.
- **Opioid Cross-Reactivity**
  - Patients who report allergies to opioids may have cross-reactivity to other similar opioid structural classes but may safely take opioids in different structural classes.
  - For example, patients with reported allergies to the phenanthrenes (codeine, morphine, heroin, hydrocodone, oxycodone) should not receive any agent within this class.
    - However, cross-reactivity risk is lower in distinct structural classes such as the phenylpiperidines (fentanyl, meperidine).
  - Opioid cross-reactivity may also refer to laboratory detection of opioids or opiates.
    - Like allergies, opioids with structural similarities (for example, morphine and oxycodone) may result in cross-reactivity on opioid screening assays.

High-Yield Clinical Knowledge
- **Tapentadol and Tramadol Seizures**
  - Seizures at regular doses or supratherapeutic doses have been observed with tapentadol and tramadol use.
  - These seizures should not be managed with naloxone as it has been associated with worsening seizures.
  - Benzodiazepines should be considered first-line agents for the management of drug-induced seizures.
- **Diminished Analgesic Effects**
  - Conversely to precipitating withdrawal, patients taking mixed opioid receptor agents may experience diminished responses to opioid analgesics, commonly in the post-surgical environment.
  - In these situations, patients may receive repeated doses, or high doses, to achieve analgesia; however, respiratory depression may be unaffected by this effect and can occur without other opioid-like products.
- **Fentanyl Transdermal Disposal**
  - Patients must be counseled on appropriate disposal of used fentanyl patches, as these patches, although therapeutically no longer beneficial, still contain significant quantities of fentanyl.
  - Surreptitious removal of the remaining fentanyl reservoir is a common method of acquisition of illicit fentanyl.
    - Once removed from the patch, this fentanyl can be smoked or injected.
  - Used patches must be folded with the adhesive ends together, disposed of in a biohazard container, and returned to the patient's pharmacy.
  - Like the transdermal disposal, fentanyl buccal tablets, lozenges, sublingual spray, or other dosage forms that are not used must also be disposed of properly to avoid diversion.

High-Yield Core Evidence
- **Methadone Maintenance Dose**
  - This was a single-center, double-blind clinical trial that compared the relative clinical efficacy of moderate (40 to 50 mg) vs. high-dose (80 to 100 mg) methadone in treating opioid dependence.
  - Patients randomized to the high-dose methadone regimen experienced significantly lower opioid-positive urine sample rates than patients in the moderate group.
  - These differences persisted during withdrawal from methadone, but there was no significant difference between dose groups in treatment retention during the long-term follow-up portion of the study.
  - Although numerically higher (19 vs. 11), there was no difference in the proportion of patients completing detoxification.
  - The authors concluded that both moderate- and high-dose methadone treatment decreased illicit opioid use during methadone maintenance and detoxification. (JAMA. 1999 Mar 17;281(11):1000-5.)

- **Chronic Tramadol Use**
  - This was an observational study of administrative claims data among opioid-naive patients undergoing elective surgery.
  - The study cohort consisted of 357,884 patients who filled a discharge prescription for one or more opioids (most commonly hydrocodone or oxycodone) associated with one of 20 included operations.
  - In this population, the authors observed an unadjusted risk of prolonged opioid use after surgery was 7.1% with other opioid use, 1.0% with ongoing opioid use.
  - Compared with other short-acting opioids, tramadol was associated with a significant (6%) increase in the risk of other opioid use relative to people receiving other short-acting opioids and an almost 50% increase in the adjusted risk of continued opioids use.
  - The authors concluded that patients receiving tramadol alone after surgery had similar to somewhat higher risks of prolonged opioid use than those receiving other short-acting opioids. (BMJ. 2019 May 14;365:l1849.)

High-Yield Fast-Facts
- **Kratom Use**
  - Kratom is an extract from the plant *Mitragyna speciosa* that exhibits partial mu-opioid receptor agonist effects.
- **Neonatal Abstinence Syndrome**
  - Methadone or morphine is used to treat neonatal abstinence syndrome in neonates born to mothers who are chronically taking therapeutic opioids or illicit use of opioids.
- **Precipitating Acute Withdrawal**
  - Administration of an opioid agonist combined with a partial agonist or mixed agonist/antagonists (buprenorphine, butorphanol, nalbuphine, or pentazocine) may precipitate acute opioid withdrawal.

HIGH-YIELD BOARD EXAM ESSENTIALS
- **CLASSIC AGENTS:** Diphenoxylate, fentanyl, levorphanol, loperamide, methadone, morphine, oxycodone, tapentadol, tramadol
- **DRUG CLASS:** Opioid Analgesics, Long-Acting
- **INDICATIONS:** Analgesia, opioid-use disorder
- **MECHANISM:** Opioid receptor agonists blunt the perception and response to pain by inhibiting ascending pain pathways.
- **SIDE EFFECTS:** Constipation, altered mental status, respiratory depression, euphoria, abuse potential, QT prolongation (methadone)
- **CLINICAL PEARLS:**
  - Diphenoxylate and loperamide are over-the-counter opioids that are structurally similar to meperidine.
  - These agents are not absorbed systemically and used for self-care of diarrhea.

Table: Drug Class Summary

\multicolumn{4}{c}{**Opioid Analgesics, Long-Acting - Drug Class Review**}

Opioid Analgesics, Long-Acting - Drug Class Review
High-Yield Med Reviews

Mechanism of Action: *Opioid receptor agonists blunt the perception and response to pain by inhibiting ascending pain pathways.*

Class Effects: *Long-acting opioid agonists are a component of chronic pain management but are associated with opioid dependence, which can lead to the need for methadone, a key element in treating opioid use disorder.*

Generic Name	Brand Name	Main Indication(s) or Uses	Notes

Diphenoxylate and Atropine	Lomotil	- Diarrhea	- **Dosing (Adult):**
			  – Oral: 5 mg 4 times daily until control achieved; Maximum 20 mg/day
			- **Dosing (Peds):**
			  – Oral: 1.5 to 5 mL (2.5mg/5mL) 4 times daily until control achieved
			- **CYP450 Interactions:** None
			- **Renal or Hepatic Dose Adjustments:** None
			- **Dosage Forms:** Oral (liquid, tablet)

Fentanyl (buccal tablets, lozenges, sublingual spray, transdermal)	Actiq, Duragesic, Lazanda, Subsys	- Analgesia	- **Dosing (Adult):**
			  – Transmucosal lozenge 200 mcg over 15 min for 2 doses
			  – Buccal tablet 100 mcg followed by 100 mcg 30 minutes later, maximum 2 doses
			  – Sublingual spray/tablet 100 mcg followed by 100 mcg 30 minutes later, max 2 doses
			- **Dosing (Peds):**
			  – Intranasal 1.5 mcg/kg/dose
			    – Maximum 100 mcg/dose
			- **CYP450 Interactions:** Substrate CYP3A4
			- **Renal or Hepatic Dose Adjustments:**
			  – Transdermal patch
			    – GFR 10 to 50 mL/minute: Reduce dose by 25%
			    – GFR < 10 mL/minute: Reduce dose by 50%
			    – Child-Pugh class C: Not recommended
			- **Dosage Forms:** Oral (liquid, lozenge, tablet), Nasal solution, Transdermal patch

Levorphanol	Dromoran	- Analgesia	- **Dosing (Adult):**
			  – Oral: 1 to 4 mg q6-8h
			- **Dosing (Peds):**
			  – Not routinely used
			- **CYP450 Interactions:** None
			- **Renal or Hepatic Dose Adjustments:** None
			- **Dosage Forms:** Oral (tablet)

Opioid Analgesics, Long-Acting - Drug Class Review
High-Yield Med Reviews

Generic Name	Brand Name	Main Indication(s) or Uses	Notes

Loperamide	Diamode
	Imodium A-D
		• Diarrhea	• **Dosing (Adult):**
			  – Oral: 4 mg followed by 2 mg after each loose stool
			    – Maximum 16 mg/day
			• **Dosing (Peds):**
			  – Oral: 1 to 4 mg with the first loose stool followed by 1 to 2 mg after each loose stool
			    – Maximum dose by age
			      – Age 2-5; 3 mg/day
			      – Age 6-8; 4 mg/day
			      – Age 9-11; 6 mg/day
			• **CYP450 Interactions:** Substrate CYP2B6, 2C8, 2D6, 3A4, P-gp
			• **Renal or Hepatic Dose Adjustments:** None
			• **Dosage Forms:** Oral (capsule, liquid, suspension, tablet)

Methadone	Dolophine	• Analgesia
		• Opioid use disorder
			• **Dosing (Adult):**
			  – Oral: 10 to 100 mg daily (opioid use disorder)
			  – Oral: 2.5 to 10 mg q8-12h (analgesia)
			• **Dosing (Peds):**
			  – IV/SQ: 0.025 mg/kg/dose 4-8h
			  – Oral: 0.025 to 0.2 mg/kg/dose q4-8h
			• **CYP450 Interactions:** Substrate CYP2B6, 2C19, 2C9, 2D6, 3A4, P-gp; Inhibits CYP2D6
			• **Renal or Hepatic Dose Adjustments:** None
			• **Dosage Forms:** Oral (concentrate, tablet), IV (solution)

Morphine (sustained-release)	Duramorph
	Infumorph
	MS Contin
		• Analgesia	• **Dosing (Adult):**
			  – Oral: ER administer total oral morphine daily dose in two divided doses
			• **Dosing (Peds):**
			  – Oral: ER 0.3 to 0.6 mg/kg/dose q12h
			• **CYP450 Interactions:** Substrate of P-gp
			• **Renal or Hepatic Dose Adjustments:**
			  – GFR 30 - 60 mL/min: Reduce dose by 50%
			  – GFR 15 - 30 mL/min: Reduce dose by 75%
			  – GFR < 15 mL/minute: Not recommended
			• **Dosage Forms:** Oral (capsule, solution, tablet), Suppository, IV solution

| Opioid Analgesics, Long-Acting - Drug Class Review ||||
| High-Yield Med Reviews ||||
Generic Name	Brand Name	Main Indication(s) or Uses	Notes

Oxycodone (With or without acetaminophen)	<u>Without acetaminophen</u>
	Oxycontin
	
	<u>With acetaminophen</u>
	Percocet
		• Analgesia	• **Dosing (Adult):**
			  — Oral: ER 10 to 20 mg q12-24h
			• **Dosing (Peds):**
			  — Oral: IR 0.1 to 0.2 mg/kg/dose q4-6h
			  — Maximum 10 mg/dose
			• **CYP450 Interactions:** Substrate CYP2C6, CYP3A4
			• **Renal or Hepatic Dose Adjustments:**
			  — GFR < 30 mL/minute: Reduce dose by 50%
			  — Child-Pugh class C: Reduce dose by 50%
			• **Dosage Forms:** Oral (capsule, tablet)

Tapentadol	Nucynta	• Analgesia	• **Dosing (Adult):**
			  — Oral: IR 50 to 100 mg q4-6h
			    — Maximum 600 mg/day
			  — Oral: ER 50 to 250 mg q12h
			• **Dosing (Peds):**
			  — Not routinely used
			• **CYP450 Interactions:** text
			• **Renal or Hepatic Dose Adjustments:**
			  — GFR < 30 mL/minute: use not recommended
			  — Child-Pugh class B: IR start q8h; ER start q24h
			  — Child-Pugh class C: Not recommended
			• **Dosage Forms:** Oral (tablet immediate release, extended-release)

Tramadol	Ultram	• Analgesia	• **Dosing (Adult):**
			  — Oral: IR 50 to 100 mg q4-6h
			    — Maximum 400 mg/day
			  — Oral: ER 100 - 300 mg daily
			• **Dosing (Peds):**
			  — Extra info if needed
			    — Extra info if needed
			• **CYP450 Interactions:** text
			• **Renal or Hepatic Dose Adjustments:**
			  — GFR < 30 mL/minute: IR q12h; ER use not recommended
			  — Child-Pugh class C: Not recommended
			• **Dosage Forms:** Oral (tablet immediate release, extended-release)

ANALGESICS – OPIOID ANALGESICS, SHORT-ACTING

Drug Class
- **Opioid Analgesics, Short-Acting**
- **Agents:**
    - **Acute Care**
        - Alfentanil
        - Codeine
        - Dihydrocodeine
        - Fentanyl
        - Heroin
        - Hydrocodone
        - Hydromorphone
        - Meperidine
        - Morphine
        - Oxycodone
        - Oxymorphone
        - Remifentanil
        - Sufentanil

> **Fast Facts**
> - Codeine must be metabolized via CYP2D6 to form morphine sulfate.
> - Hydrocodone must be metabolized via CYP2D6 to form hydromorphone.
> - Morphine sulfate given by IV push or infusion causes the most histamine release which leads to itching and reductions in blood pressure.
> - Tylenol with codeine has a C-III designation, but codeine by itself has a C-II designation.

Main Indications or Uses
- **Acute Care**
    - Analgesia
    - Sedation

Mechanism of Action
- Opioid receptor agonists blunt the perception and response to pain by inhibiting ascending pain pathways.

Primary Net Benefit
- Rapid-acting analgesics have been a cornerstone of pain management, but the benefits must be balanced with the risk of dependence or abuse.
- Main Labs to Monitor:
    - No routine monitoring

High-Yield Basic Pharmacology
- **Mu Receptors**
    - Opioid agonist effects on the mu-1 receptors located in the CNS are the primary therapeutic target of opioids for analgesia.
        - Central mu-1 receptors are also partially responsible for the euphoric effects associated with opioid use.
    - Mu-2 receptors are also located in the CNS, but when stimulated, they cause a diminished sensitivity if the medullary chemoreceptors to hypercapnia, which decreases the ventilatory response to hypoxia.
        - An alternative nomenclature of opioid receptors has been proposed, which would rename mu receptors OP3 receptors.
- **Kappa Receptors**
    - Activation of kappa opioid receptors is associated with spinal analgesia and diuresis from inhibition of antidiuretic hormone release.
        - Kappa opioid receptor activation is not associated with respiratory depression or constipation.
        - This led to the development of pentazocine and nalbuphine.
    - Kappa agonist effects are also responsible for miosis.
        - Kappa-1 agonist effects produce spinal analgesia.
        - Kappa-2 agonism induces psychotomimesis.
            - Common agonists of kappa-2 include pentazocine and salvinorin A.

- Kappa-3 stimulation produces supraspinal analgesic effects.
- An alternative nomenclature of opioid receptors has been proposed, which would rename kappa receptors OP2 receptors.
- **Delta Receptors**
  - Delta opioid receptors are primary targets of endogenous opioid ligands.
  - An alternative nomenclature of opioid receptors has been proposed, which would rename delta receptors OP1 receptors.
    - Nociception receptors have also been identified as receptors to endogenous opioid ligands and have been proposed to be classified as OP4 receptors.

High-Yield Clinical Knowledge
- **Opioid-Induced Constipation**
  - Constipation associated with opioid use is mediated by mu-2 receptor stimulation in the intestinal wall.
  - Bowel regimens including fiber, stool softeners, and laxatives should be considered in patients taking opioid agonists.
    - Oral naloxone doses between 2 and 6 mg can be administered to help relieve opioid-induced constipation.
    - Doses of oral naloxone above 6 mg should be avoided to reduce the risk of sufficient systemic absorption to produce acute opioid withdrawal.
- **Histamine Release**
  - Parenteral administration of some opioids induces mast cell-mediated histamine release, producing pruritus.
  - Meperidine and morphine are most likely to cause clinically relevant histamine release, whereas fentanyl is least likely associated with histamine release.
- **Respiratory Depression**
  - Opioid agonists who act on mu-2 receptors are associated with a dose-dependent decrease in the hypercapnia's ventilatory response.
  - Respiratory depression observed due to opioids is more closely related to decreased tidal volume and not necessarily respiratory rate.
- **Opioid Hyperalgesia**
  - The phenomena of opioid hyperalgesia is an increased innate response to pain after exposure to opioid agents.
    - This can be confused with opioid tolerance as patients may require higher doses to achieve an appropriate analgesic response.
  - Opioid hyperalgesia was first observed in patients in methadone maintenance programs but has been contemporarily described in surgical and critical care populations.
- **Fentanyl Rigid Chest Syndrome**
  - The rapid administration of fentanyl, mainly when doses are above 300 mcg, can produce an intercostal muscle spasm and a "rigid chest syndrome."
    - This intercostal muscle spasm impairs respiratory accommodation and reduces spontaneous ventilation.
  - This is thought to be a non-opioid receptor effect caused by dopamine receptor antagonist effects in the basal ganglia but can be reversed with naloxone.
- **Codeine In Pediatrics**
  - The use of codeine in children under the age of 18 is discouraged as they are at higher risk of clinically relevant opioid toxicity in the setting of undiagnosed CYP2D6 polymorphisms.
  - As codeine is a prodrug, which is metabolized by CYP2D6 to morphine and by CYP3A4 to norcodeine.
    - In patients with polymorphism leading to CYP2D6 overexpression, patients may unpredictably produce significant quantities of morphine.
- **Meperidine Neurotoxicity**
  - Meperidine is an opioid agonist as well as a presynaptic serotonin reuptake inhibitor.
  - In patients with concomitant serotonergic agents, the use of meperidine carries a risk of serotonin syndrome characterized by muscle rigidity, hyperthermia, and altered mental status.

- Meperidine's active metabolite, normeperidine, is also neurotoxic and potentially induces delirium, tremor, myoclonus, and seizures.

High-Yield Core Evidence
- **SPACE Trial**
  - This pragmatic trial randomized patients recruited from Veterans Affairs primary care clinics to compare opioid vs. nonopioid medications over 12 months on pain-related function, pain intensity, and adverse effects.
  - Chronic pain diagnoses among eligible patients included moderate to severe chronic back pain or hip or knee osteoarthritis pain despite analgesic use.
  - Analgesic therapy, whether opioid or nonopioid, followed a treat-to-target strategy aiming for improved pain and function and included a stepwise process in an escalation of analgesic therapy.
  - There was no significant difference in the primary outcome of pain-related function over 12 months and the main secondary outcome of pain intensity according to the BPI severity scale.
  - However, the patient reported pain intensity was significantly better in the nonopioid group over 12 months than in the opioid group.
  - Furthermore, there was a higher incidence of adverse medication-related symptoms in the opioid group over 12 months.
  - The authors concluded that treatment with opioids was not superior to treatment with non-opioid medications for improving pain-related function over 12 months. (JAMA. 2018 Mar 6;319(9):872-882.)
- **Analgosedation With Fentanyl**
  - This was a retrospective, observational study that examined the efficacy and safety of analgosedation with fentanyl versus traditional sedation with propofol in critically ill patients receiving mechanical ventilation.
  - There was no difference in the median duration of mechanical ventilation and median ICU length of stay between patients receiving propofol and fentanyl infusions.
  - More patients receiving propofol required rescue opioids compared with patients receiving fentanyl.
  - However, there was no difference in the rate of intensive care unit delirium was noted between groups.
  - The authors concluded that analgosedation with fentanyl appears to be a safe and effective strategy to facilitate mechanical ventilation. (Pharmacotherapy. 2014 Jun;34(6):643-7.)

High-Yield Fast-Facts
- **Runner's High**
  - The physiologic basis for the euphoria experienced after running or intense exercise has been observed to be reversed by naloxone and thought to result from endogenous opioid release.
- **Opioid Vs. Opiate**
  - Opiates refer to natural opium derivatives (codeine, heroin, morphine, hydromorphone), whereas opioids are synthetic derivatives of opiates (fentanyl, methadone).
- **Heroin and Cocaine**
  - The combination of heroin and cocaine, known as a speedball, causes competition for their shared metabolic pathway via plasma cholinesterase and liver carboxylesterases.
  - The result is an increased physiologic response to one or both of these agents.

HIGH-YIELD BOARD EXAM ESSENTIALS
- **CLASSIC AGENTS:** Alfentanil, codeine, dihydrocodeine, fentanyl, heroin, hydrocodone, hydromorphone, meperidine, morphine, oxycodone, oxymorphone, remifentanil, sufentanil
- **DRUG CLASS:** Opioid analgesics, short-acting
- **INDICATIONS:** Analgesia
- **MECHANISM:** Opioid receptor agonists blunt the perception and response to pain through inhibition of ascending pain pathways
- **SIDE EFFECTS:** Constipation, rash, flushing, erythema, respiratory depression, hypotension
- **CLINICAL PEARLS:** Constipation associated with opioid use is mediated by mu-2 receptor stimulation in the intestinal wall. Bowel regimens including fiber, stool softeners, and laxatives should be considered in patients taking opioid agonists.

Table: Drug Class Summary

Opioid Analgesics, Short-Acting - Drug Class Review High-Yield Med Reviews			
Mechanism of Action: *Opioid receptor agonists blunt the perception and response to pain by inhibiting ascending pain pathways.*			
Class Effects: *Rapid-acting analgesics have been a cornerstone of pain management, but the benefits must be balanced with dependence or abuse risk.*			
Generic Name	**Brand Name**	**Main Indication(s) or Uses**	**Notes**
Alfentanil	Alfenta	<ul><li>Analgesia</li><li>Anesthesia</li></ul>	<ul><li>**Dosing (Adult):**<ul><li>IV: induction 8 to 235 mg/kg</li><li>IV: maintenance 0.5 to 1.5 mcg/kg/min</li></ul></li><li>**Dosing (Peds):**<ul><li>IV: induction 8 to 235 mg/kg</li><li>IV: maintenance 0.5 to 1.5 mcg/kg/min</li></ul></li><li>**CYP450 Interactions:** Substrate CYP3A4</li><li>**Renal or Hepatic Dose Adjustments:** None</li><li>**Dosage Forms:** IV (solution)</li></ul>
Codeine	N/A	<ul><li>Analgesia</li><li>Cough</li></ul>	<ul><li>**Dosing (Adult):**<ul><li>IM/SQ: 30 to 60 mg q4o6h as needed for pain</li><li>Oral: 15 to 60 mg q4h as needed for pain<ul><li>Extra info if needed</li></ul></li></ul></li><li>**Dosing (Peds):**<ul><li>Use with caution<ul><li>Oral: 0.5 to 1 mg/kg/dose q4-6h</li></ul></li></ul></li><li>**CYP450 Interactions:** Substrate CYP2D6, 3A4</li><li>**Renal or Hepatic Dose Adjustments:**<ul><li>GFR 10 to 50 mL/minute: Reduce dose by 25%</li><li>GFR < 10 mL/minute: Reduce dose by 50%</li></ul></li><li>**Dosage Forms:** Oral (tablet)</li></ul>
Dihydrocodeine-Aspirin-Caffeine	Synalgos-DC	<ul><li>Analgesia</li></ul>	<ul><li>**Dosing (Adult):**<ul><li>Oral: two capsules q4h as needed for pain</li></ul></li><li>**Dosing (Peds):** [same as adult]<ul><li>Extra info if needed<ul><li>Extra info if needed</li></ul></li></ul></li><li>**CYP450 Interactions:** Substrate CYP 2D6, 3A4</li><li>**Renal or Hepatic Dose Adjustments:**<ul><li>GFR < 10 mL/minute: Not recommended</li><li>Child-Pugh class C: Not recommended</li></ul></li><li>**Dosage Forms:** Oral (capsule)</li></ul>

| \multicolumn{4}{c}{**Opioid Analgesics, Short-Acting - Drug Class Review**} |
| | | | |

		Opioid Analgesics, Short-Acting - Drug Class Review High-Yield Med Reviews	
Generic Name	**Brand Name**	**Main Indication(s) or Uses**	**Notes**

Fentanyl	Actiq, Duragesic, Lazanda, Subsys	• Analgesia	• **Dosing (Adult):**
			– IV loading 1 to 2 mcg/kg
			– IV: 0.35 to 0.5 mcg/kg q30-60min or 25 to 200 mcg/hour
			– IM: 50 to 100 mcg q1-2hours
			– Intranasal: 100 mcg once
			– Transmucosal lozenge 200 mcg over 15 min for 2 doses
			– Buccal tablet 100 mcg followed by 100 mcg 30 minutes later, maximum 2 doses
			– Sublingual spray/tablet 100 mcg followed by 100 mcg 30 minutes later, maximum 2 doses
			• **Dosing (Peds):**
			– IV loading 1 to 2 mcg/kg
			– IV/IM: 0.35 to 0.5 mcg/kg q30-60min
			– Intranasal: 1.5 mcg/kg/dose
			   – Maximum 100 mcg/dose
			• **CYP450 Interactions:** Substrate CYP3A4
			• **Renal or Hepatic Dose Adjustments:**
			– Transdermal patch
			   – GFR 10 to 50 mL/minute: Reduce dose by 25%
			   – GFR < 10 mL/minute: Reduce dose by 50%
			   – Child-Pugh class C: Not recommended
			• **Dosage Forms:** IV (solution), Oral (liquid, lozenge, tablet), Nasal solution, Transdermal patch

Hydrocodone (With or without acetaminophen)	<u>With Acetaminophen</u> Lorcet, Lortab, Norco, Vicodin, Xodol <u>Without Acetaminophen</u> Hysingla ER Zohydro	• Analgesia	• **Dosing (Adult):** – Oral: IR 5 to 10 mg q4-6h as needed for pain – Oral: ER 10 to 20 mg q12-24h • **Dosing (Peds):** – Oral: IR 0.1 to 0.2 mg/kg/dose q4-6h – Maximum 10 mg/dose • **CYP450 Interactions:** Substrate CYP2C6, CYP3A4 • **Renal or Hepatic Dose Adjustments:** – GFR < 30 mL/minute: Reduce dose by 50% – Child-Pugh class C: Reduce dose by 50% • **Dosage Forms:** Oral (capsule, tablet)

\multicolumn{4}{c}{**Opioid Analgesics, Short-Acting - Drug Class Review**}

Generic Name	Brand Name	Main Indication(s) or Uses	Notes

Hydromorphone	Dilaudid
	Exalgo
		- Analgesia	- **Dosing (Adult):**
			  – Oral: 2.5 to 10 mg q4-6h as needed for pain
			  – IV: 0.2 to 1 mg q2-3h as needed for pain
			  – IM/SQ: 1 to 2 mg q2-3h as needed for pain
			- **Dosing (Peds):**
			  – Oral: 0.03 to 0.06 mg q4-6h as needed for pain
			  – IV: 0.015 mg/kg/dose q2-3h as needed for pain
			  – IM/SQ: 0.8 to 1 mg q2-3h as needed for pain
			- **CYP450 Interactions:** None
			- **Renal or Hepatic Dose Adjustments:**
			  – GFR 30 to 60 mL/minute: Reduce dose by 50%
			  – GFR < 30 mL/minute: Reduce dose by 75%
			  – Child-Pugh class C: Not recommended
			- **Dosage Forms:** Oral (liquid, tablet), Suppository, IV (solution)

Meperidine	Demerol	- Analgesia	- **Dosing (Adult):**
			  – IM/SQ: 12.5 to 150 mg q3-4h
			    – Extra info if needed
			- **Dosing (Peds):**
			  – IM/IV/SQ: 0.2 to 1 mg/kg/dose q2-3hours
			  – Oral: 0.5 to 4 mg/kg/dose q3-4h
			- **CYP450 Interactions:** None
			- **Renal or Hepatic Dose Adjustments:**
			  – GFR < 30 mL/minute: not recommended
			  – Child-Pugh class B or C: not recommended
			- **Dosage Forms:** Oral (tablet, solution), IV (solution)

| \multicolumn{4}{c}{**Opioid Analgesics, Short-Acting - Drug Class Review**} |

Generic Name	Brand Name	Main Indication(s) or Uses	Notes

Morphine	Duramorph
	Infumorph
	MS Contin
		- Analgesia	- **Dosing (Adult):**
			  − Oral IR/Rectal: 10 to 30 mg q4h as needed for pain
			  − IV: 0.01 mg/kg or 1 to 4 mg q1-4 hours
			  − SQ: 2 to 5 mg q3-4h as needed for pain
			- **Dosing (Peds):**
			  − IM/IV/SQ: 0.05 to 0.2 mg/kg/dose
			  − Infusion: 0.01 to 0.04 mg/kg/hour
			  − Oral: IR 0.2 to 0.5 mg/kg/dose q3-4h as needed for pain
			- **CYP450 Interactions:** Substrate of P-gp
			- **Renal or Hepatic Dose Adjustments:**
			  − GFR 30 to 60 mL/minute: Reduce dose by 50%
			  − GFR 15 to 30 mL/minute: Reduce dose by 75%
			  − GFR < 15 mL/minute: Not recommended
			- **Dosage Forms:** Oral (capsule, solution, tablet), Suppository, IV solution

Oxycodone (With or without acetaminophen)	<u>Without acetaminophen</u>
	Oxycontin
	
	<u>With acetaminophen</u>
	Percocet
		- Analgesia	- **Dosing (Adult):**
			  − Oral: IR 5 to 15 mg q4-6h as needed for pain
			  − Oral: ER 10 to 20 mg q12-24h
			- **Dosing (Peds):**
			  − Oral: IR 0.1 to 0.2 mg/kg/dose q4-6h
			    − Maximum 10 mg/dose
			- **CYP450 Interactions:** Substrate CYP2C6, CYP3A4
			- **Renal or Hepatic Dose Adjustments:**
			  − GFR < 30 mL/minute: Reduce dose by 50%
			  − Child-Pugh class C: Reduce dose by 50%
			- **Dosage Forms:** Oral (capsule, tablet)

Oxymorphone	Opana	- Analgesia	- **Dosing (Adult):**
			  − IM/SQ: 1 to 1.5 mg q4-6h
			  − IV: 0.5 to 1 mg
			  − Oral: IR: 5 to 10 mg q4-6h as needed for pain
			  − Oral: ER: 5 mg q12h
			- **Dosing (Peds):**
			  − Not routinely used
			- **CYP450 Interactions:** text
			- **Renal or Hepatic Dose Adjustments:** text
			- **Dosage Forms:** Oral (tablet), IV solution

| Opioid Analgesics, Short-Acting - Drug Class Review ||||
| High-Yield Med Reviews ||||
Generic Name	Brand Name	Main Indication(s) or Uses	Notes
Remifentanil	Ultiva	<ul><li>Analgesia</li><li>Anesthesia</li></ul>	<ul><li>**Dosing (Adult):**<ul><li>IV: 0.25 to 2 mg/kg/minute</li></ul></li><li>**Dosing (Peds):**<ul><li>IV: 0.15 to 2 mg/kg/minute</li></ul></li><li>**CYP450 Interactions:** None</li><li>**Renal or Hepatic Dose Adjustments:** None</li><li>**Dosage Forms:** IV (solution)</li></ul>
Sufentanil	Dsuvia	<ul><li>Analgesia</li><li>Anesthesia</li></ul>	<ul><li>**Dosing (Adult):**<ul><li>SL: 30 mcg q1h as needed for pain, maximum 360 mg/day</li><li>IV: 1 to 2 mcg/kg initially followed by 10 to 25 mcg as needed, maximum 1 mcg/kg/hour</li></ul></li><li>**Dosing (Peds):**<ul><li>IV: 5 to 25 mcg/kg initially followed by 1 to 5 mcg/kg/dose up to 50 mcg/dose as needed</li></ul></li><li>**CYP450 Interactions:** Substrate CYP3A4</li><li>**Renal or Hepatic Dose Adjustments:** None</li><li>**Dosage Forms:** Oral (sublingual tablet), IV (solution)</li></ul>

NEUROLOGY – OPIOIDS – PARTIAL AGONISTS

Drug Class
- Opioid Partial Agonists
- Agents
    - Buprenorphine
    - Buprenorphine/naloxone
    - Butorphanol (short course therapy only for acute pain management)*
    - Nalbuphine (short course therapy only for acute pain management)*
    - Pentazocine (not available in US)*
    - Note: * The focus of this review is primarily buprenorphine therapy as butorphanol and nalbuphine are less frequently used and pentazocine is not available in the US. Drug shortages for nalbuphine for injection is fairly common making it less utilized.

Main Indications or Uses
- Opioid use disorder
- Acute and chronic pain

Mechanism of Action
- Buprenorphine binds with a high-affinity to mu opioid receptors within the CNS. It is a partial agonist lending to less dopamine release compared to a full opioid agonist as well as a ceiling analgesic effect.
- Combining naloxone, an opioid antagonist, with buprenorphine is theorized to prevent misuse as the bioavailability of naloxone is low when administered orally or sublingually.

Primary Overall Net Benefit
- Opioid use disorder remission, analgesia for acute and chronic pain relief
- Monitoring:
    - Liver function tests prior to initiation and every 6 to 12 months thereafter
    - Social and environmental screenings
    - Concomitant disease screenings: Hepatitis B, Hepatitis C, HIV, tuberculosis
    - Withdrawal screenings (opioid use disorder indication) at baseline and during induction until adequate dose is achieved
    - Pain screenings (pain indication) at baseline and routinely until adequate dose is achieved
    - Urine drug screening at baseline and at discretion of prescriber/program thereafter

High-Yield Basic Pharmacology
- **Buprenorphine**
    - Lipophilic
    - 25 to 50 times as potent as morphine
    - Poor oral absorption due to extensive first pass metabolism
    - Metabolism via CYP450 3A4 to norbuprenorphine (active metabolite)
    - Displaces endogenous and exogenous opioids from receptor
- **Naloxone**
    - Minimal systemic availability when administered orally or sublingually, fully available if administered via intravenous route.

High-Yield Core Clinical Knowledge
- **Abuse Risk**
    - Despite theoretical pharmaco-kinetics and -dynamics, post-marketing experience has shown that buprenorphine/naloxone is still an abusable product, although not as abusable as buprenorphine mono-products

- **Pharmacokinetic and Pharmacodynamic Considerations**
    - Even though there is a low bioavailability of naloxone when administered sublingually, buprenorphine/naloxone poses adverse reactions that are not always replicated with buprenorphine mono-products
    - When discontinuing a traditional full opioid agonist in favor of a buprenorphine-containing product, it is preferable to dose at a similar frequency (ie. oxycodone every 4 hours to buprenorphine every 4 hours) or select a sustained-release product such as the transdermal patch
    - At 50% mu opioid receptor occupancy (approximately 1 ng/mL plasma concentration) patients experience withdrawal symptoms. At 70% mu opioid receptor occupancy (approximately 2ng/mL plasma concentration) withdrawal symptoms are relieved and abstinence can be maintained. Pharmacokinetic studies show that buprenorphine extended release subcutaneous monthly injection has less variance between C_{max} and C_{min} compared to sublingual products.
- **Dental Warnings**
    - Buprenorphine sublingual dosage forms have been associated with dental problems, including tooth decay, cavities, oral infections, and tooth loss, even in patients with no history of dental problems.

High-Yield Core Evidence
- **Cochrane Review of Buprenorphine Use for Illicit Opioid Use**
    - A 2014 Cochrane Review of 31 trials found that in patients with heroin dependence, buprenorphine is superior to placebo in treatment retention and suppression of illicit opioid use (high doses) at doses of at least 2 mg daily and 16 mg daily, respectively.
    - In comparison to methadone, buprenorphine was found to be inferior in regard to treatment retention and non-inferior in regard to illicit opioid use.
    - Cochrane Database Syst Rev. 2014 Feb 6;(2):CD002207.
- **Transdermal Buprenorphine**
    - A meta-analysis of buprenorphine products to treat a variety of pain syndromes revealed transdermal dosage forms were consistently beneficial, while other routes of administration had mixed results.
    - Anesthesiology. 2014 May; 120(5): 1262–1274.

High-Yield Fast-Facts
- **Effect of Coercive Policies**
    - Coercive policies do not yield clinically meaningful results and should not be grounds for dismissal according to the American Society of Addiction Medicine. Examples may include dismissal from treatment program if patient does not attend group counseling or is actively using marijuana.
- **Duration of Buprenorphine Use**
    - There is no minimum or maximum recommended duration of buprenorphine therapy. As such, initiation of buprenorphine does not guarantee full remission from opioid use disorder and inevitable cessation of buprenorphine itself.

HIGH-YIELD BOARD EXAM ESSENTIALS
- **CLASSIC AGENTS:** Buprenorphine, nalbuphine, pentazocine
- **DRUG CLASS:** Opioid Analgesics, Partial agonists
- **INDICATIONS:** Analgesia, opioid-use disorder
- **MECHANISM:** Partial mu-opioid agonist lending to less dopamine release compared to a full opioid agonist as well as a ceiling analgesic effect
- **SIDE EFFECTS:** Constipation, altered mental status
- **CLINICAL PEARLS:**
    - Buprenorphine/naloxone combinations are not used for chronic pain management but opioid abuse disorder.

Table: Drug Class Summary

Opioid Partial Agonists Drug Class Review High-Yield Med Reviews			
Generic Name	Brand Name	Main Indication(s) or Uses	Notes
Mechanism of Action: *buprenorphine is a partial mu opioid agonist and naloxone is an opioid antagonist*			
Dosing: buprenorphine should be initiated 12-18 hours after last use of a short-acting opioid (ie. heroin or oxycodone) and 24-48 hours after last use of a long-acting opioid (i.e. methadone)			
Drug-Drug Interactions: CYP3A4 inducers, inhibitors and substrates; CNS depressants			
Class Effects: [add here if applicable or relevant; can be benefits +/- disadvantages worth noting]			

Buprenorphine sublingual tablet	Subutex	• Opioid use disorder	• **Dose:**
			  – 2-4 mg initially increasing by max of 4 mg every hour until withdrawal symptoms controlled, max total daily dose of 24mg
			• **Dosing (Peds) ≥16 years:**
			  – [same as adult]
			• Reduce initial dose by 50% in severe hepatic impairment

Buprenorphine buccal film	Belbuca	• Chronic pain	• **Dose:** – Minimum dose 75 mcg daily to maximum dose 900 mcg every 12 hours • **Dosing (Peds):** no recommendation • Reduce initial dose by 50% in severe hepatic impairment
Buprenorphine transdermal patch	Butrans	• Chronic pain	• **Dose:** – Change patch every 7 days; minimum dose 5 mcg/hour to maximum dose 20 mcg/hour • **Dosing (Peds) ≥18 years:** [same as adult] • Not studied in severe hepatic impairment
Buprenorphine subcutaneous implant	Probuphine	• Opioid use disorder	• **Dose:** – 4 implants inserted in inner arm for 6 months, can repeat one time in alternate arm • **Dosing (Peds):** no recommendation • Not recommended in moderate to severe hepatic impairment
Buprenorphine extended release subcutaneous injection	Sublocade	• Opioid use disorder	• **Dose:** – 300 mg every month for 2 months, then 100 mg every month thereafter • **Dosing (Peds):** no recommendation • Not recommended in moderate to severe hepatic impairment

| \multicolumn{4}{c}{**Opioid Partial Agonists Drug Class Review**} |

Generic Name	Brand Name	Main Indication(s) or Uses	Notes
Buprenorphine/naloxone sublingual film	Suboxone	▪ Opioid use disorder	▪ **Dose:** – 2 mg/0.5 mg titrating every 2 hours until withdrawal symptoms controlled, max total daily dose of 24 mg/6 mg ▪ **Dosing (Peds):** [same as adult] ▪ Renal or Hepatic Dose Adjustments: ▪ Not recommended in severe hepatic impairment
Buprenorphine/naloxone sublingual tablet	Zubsolv	▪ Opioid use disorder	▪ **Dose:** – 1.4 mg/0.36 mg titrating every 2 hours until withdrawal symptoms controlled, max total daily dose of 17.2 mg/4.2 mg ▪ **Dosing (Peds):** [same as adult] ▪ Not recommended in severe hepatic impairment
Buprenorphine/naloxone buccal film	Bunavail	▪ Opioid use disorder	▪ **Dose:** – 2.1 mg/0.3 mg titrating every 2 hours until withdrawal symptoms controlled, max total daily dose of 12.6 mg/2.1 mg ▪ **Dosing (Peds):** no recommendation ▪ Not recommended in severe hepatic impairment

High-Yield Med Reviews

NEUROLOGY – OPIOID ROTATION / CONVERSION

General Principles
- Rationale for the below approach to switching from one opioid to another:
    - Individual responses will vary and thus doses must be titrated
    - Cross-tolerance between agents is usually incomplete
    - Balance control of pain and side effects
    - Consider use of non-pharmacologic (e.g., transcutaneous nerve stimulation, PT, etc) and non-opioid (adjuvant analgesic therapies)

OPIOID ORAL MME DRUG CONVERSIONS

Opioid (mg/day)	MME Conversion Factor
Codeine	0.15
Fentanyl TD Patch	2.4 (per day)
	7.2 (per 3 days)
Hydrocodone	1
Methadone	3
0 – 20 mg	4
21 – 40 mg	8
41 – 60 mg	10
61 - 80 mg	12
Morphine	1
Oxycodone	1.5
Oxymorphone	3
Tapentadol	0.4
Tramadol	0.1

Note: MME is intended for analytic purposes only
MME = oral Morphine Milligram Equivalent
MME/day = Strength per Unit X (Number of Units per Days Supply) X MME Conversion Factor
Reference:
CDC Oral Morphine Equivalent Factors. August 2017

Steps in Opioid Rotation
- **Calculate equianalgesic dose**
    - Oral dosage forms are for non-long acting dosage forms
    - Except for fentanyl and methadone, decrease the equianalgesic dose by 25% to 50% then titrate based on breakthrough dose usage.
        - Some experts recommend adjusting down by 50% of the initial calculated equivalent dose due to variability in response
        - Consideration should also be given on genetic polymorphisms, liver and renal function, potential for drug interactions, presence of other comorbidities and/or medication usage.
    - Special Opioid Considerations:
        - Fentanyl TD: No dose change when switching to fentanyl transdermal patch
        - Methadone: Decrease initial calculated equianalgesic dose of methadone by 75-90% then titrate up to error on side of precaution given its long-duration of activity
    - If liver, renal or pulmonary co-morbidities present:
        - Consider further reductions in addition to those above

- **Rescue or PRN dosing**
  - 5-15% of total daily opioid dose in divided doses at appropriate intervals
- **Reassess pain, side effects and titrate at appropriate intervals**

Example Case

- 45-year-old male with metastatic lung cancer with progressively worsening pain despite scheduled high dose morphine of 120 mg by mouth every 8 hours and use of morphine 20 mg every 4 hours. A switch to oxycodone is being considered.
  - Note: the development of tolerance is common where patients can require high doses. This is also common in oncology patients. Every patient is different so keep that in mind.
- Total Daily Morphine Use:
  - 120 mg x 3 = 360 mg
  - 20 mg x 6 = 120 mg
  - Total = 480 mg
- Dose Equivalence:
  - (Oral) Morphine 30 mg = oxycodone 20 mg
  - Morphine 480 mg = Oxycodone 320 mg
- New Dose:
  - Oxycodone 320 mg divided in every 12 hours
    - No change = 320 mg/d
    - 25% reduction = 240 mg/d
    - 50% reduction = 160 mg/d
  - Oxycodone (Oxycontin) dosage forms available for chronic administration:
    - 10, 20, 30, 40, 60, 80 mg
    - No dose change:
      - 160 mg po every 12 hrs
    - Dose adjusted at 25%:
      - 80 mg every 8 hours …(or)… 120 mg every 12 hours
    - Dose adjusted at 50%:
      - 80 mg every 12 hrs
- Calculate breakthrough pain dose for immediate release oxycodone 320 mg total per day
  - 320 mg x 5% of total dose = 16 mg/dose
  - 320 mg x 10% of total dose = 32 mg/dose
  - 320 mg x 15% of total dose = 48 mg/dose
  - Dosage forms of oxycodone IR tablets available for clinical use:
    - 5, 10, 15, 20, 30 mg IR tablets
      - Pick the strength and dosage form that is closest to what you think will be the best breakthrough dose for pain control.
    - Example Option (assuming the estimated 32 mg/dose option was determined to be the best, then give oxycodone IR 30 mg every 4-6 hrs by mouth PRN pain.
      - Some may use a shorter interval such as every 2 hrs depending on clinical scenario.

ANALGESICS – OPIOID ANTAGONISTS

Drug Class
- **Opioid Antagonists**
- **Agents:**
  - Acute Care
    - Alvimopan
    - Naldemedine
    - Naloxegol
    - Naloxone
    - Naltrexone
    - Methylnaltrexone

Main Indications or Uses
- **Acute Care**
  - Alcohol use disorder
    - Naltrexone
  - Opioid overdose
    - Naloxone
  - Postoperative ileus
    - Alvimopan
- **Chronic Care**
  - Opioid-induced constipation or pruritus
    - Naldemedine
    - Naloxegol
    - Naloxone
    - Naltrexone
    - Methylnaltrexone

> ### Fast Facts
> ✓ Naloxone (Narcan) can be given by almost every route of administration to reverse opioid effects EXCEPT ORAL. It has no oral bioavailability.
>
> ✓ The peripheral acting opioid antagonists are used for the treatment of opioid-induced constipation without impacting the analgesics effects of opioids since they cannot cross the blood brain barrier due to structural modifications.

Mechanism of Action
- Competitive opioid receptor (including mu, kappa, and delta) antagonists.

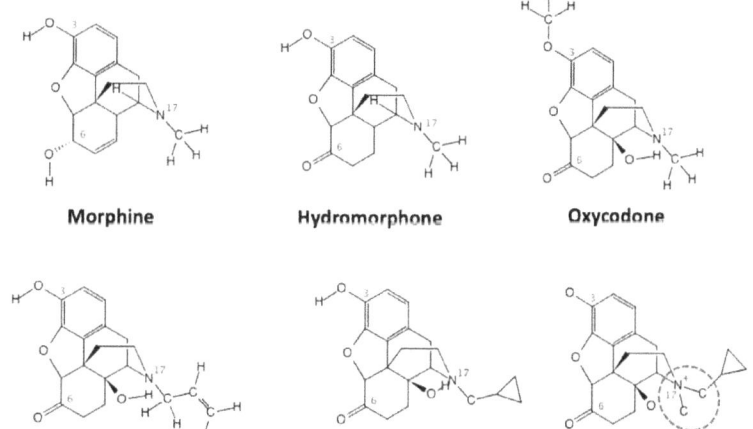

Naloxone works as a competitive antagonist.

Naltrexone (only one that is oral)

Methylnaltrexone (not work for apnea!!)

Primary Net Benefit
- Naloxone is a life-saving intervention in opioid intoxicated patients, but it and other opioid antagonists can be used for local opioid withdrawal effects, primarily constipation.
- Main Labs to Monitor:
  - No routine lab monitoring

High-Yield Basic Pharmacology
- **Oral Bioavailability**
    - At normal dose ranges, naloxone is minimally absorbed orally (bioavailability approximately 2%).
        - For acute opioid overdose, this route is not appropriate, and naloxone must be given parenterally or intranasally.
        - For opioid-induced constipation, oral administration of naloxone is possible, as it exerts a local effect on the GI.
    - Naltrexone, on the other hand, has a wide range of bioavailability due to first-pass metabolism between 5 and 60%.
    - Naloxegol is a pegylated derivative of naloxone, which increases oral bioavailability, and reduces penetration into the CNS.
- **Opioid Associated Effects**
    - Opioid receptor antagonists are intended to reverse the central respiratory depressive effects of opioid agonists.
    - Other opioid-related adverse effects include histamine release (morphine), QT prolongation due to methadone), and seizures related to tramadol or meperidine.

High-Yield Clinical Knowledge
- **Naloxone Dose-Response**
    - Low doses of naloxone (0.04 mg IV) are typically sufficient for most adult patients with opioid-related respiratory depression.
        - As opioids decrease the central respiratory response to hypoxia, this low dose of naloxone competitively inhibits opioid receptors in sufficient quantity to restore normal respiratory performance.
        - In opioid-naive patients, 1 mg of naloxone occupies 50% of available opioid receptors.
    - However, the duration of effect of most opioids (including heroin) is longer than naloxone; thus, the diminished response to hypoxia will return.
        - Additional doses of naloxone may be appropriate or as an infusion; however, airway, breathing, and ventilation support should also be utilized.
- **Bystander Naloxone Administration**
    - Naloxone distribution programs aim to provide opioid reversal via intranasal administration to lay individuals, bystanders, and medical professionals in non-acute care settings (such as pharmacies).
    - Patients, family members, and medical professionals should be educated on the role of naloxone and its administration and the importance of contacting 911 after administration.
- **Opioid-Induced Constipation**
    - Chronic opioid therapy decreases GI motility and frequently causes constipation.
    - Opioid antagonists, including those that act locally in the GI, can relieve constipation by causing a local opioid competitive inhibition without causing a systemic opioid withdrawal.
    - Methylnaltrexone is parenterally administered but does not cross the blood-brain barrier, thus causing peripheral opioid withdrawal and constipation relief.
        - Opioid antagonists are contraindicated in patients with bowel obstructions, as the risk of GI perforation is high in this setting.
    - Naldemedine and naloxegol are orally administered opioid antagonists that act locally on the GI to resolve constipation and are minimally absorbed.

- **Naloxone And ARDS**
    - Naloxone use for emergent reversal of opioid respiratory depression in opioid-dependent patients is at risk of secondary acute respiratory distress syndrome.
        - However, this is not proposed to be attributed directly to naloxone, but rather naloxone uncovers ARDS previously induced by the offending opioid.
- **Alvimopan And Recent Opioid Use**
    - Alvimopan is contraindicated in patients who have taken opioids for more than seven consecutive days.

- This is due to the risk of systemic opioid withdrawal, despite alvimopan being minimally absorbed.
- **Naltrexone for Alcohol Abstinence**
  - Naltrexone is available as an IM depot injection as adjunctive therapy in ethanol abstinence.
  - Opioid antagonism by naltrexone is proposed to inhibit central opioid-mediated ethanol craving, reduces ethanol intake and incidence of relapse.

High-Yield Core Evidence
- **Methylnaltrexone for Opioid-Induced Constipation**
  - This was a multicenter, double-blinded trial of patients who received opioids for two or more weeks and who had received stable doses of opioids and laxatives for three or more days without relief of opioid-induced constipation were randomized to either methylnaltrexone 0.15 mg/kg SQ or placebo every other day for two weeks.
  - Significantly more patients receiving methylnaltrexone achieved the coprimary outcomes of defecation within 4 hours after the first dose of the study drug and laxation within 4 hours after two or more of the first four doses.
  - Furthermore, the median time to laxation was significantly shorter in the methylnaltrexone group than in the placebo group.
  - The authors concluded that subcutaneous methylnaltrexone rapidly induced laxation in patients with advanced illness and opioid-induced constipation. Treatment did not appear to affect central analgesia or precipitate opioid withdrawal. (N Engl J Med 2008; 358:2332-2343.)
- **Pre-Hospital Intranasal Naloxone**
  - This was a prospective, nonrandomized trial of paramedics' intranasal (IN) naloxone (2 mg) administration patients with suspected opiate overdoses.
  - Patients included in this study received IN naloxone 2 mg immediately upon EMS contact, and after intravenous access was secured, a dose of naloxone 2 mg IV was administered.
  - This study included a total of 52 patients who were given naloxone, of which 43 (83%) appropriately responded to IN naloxone alone.
  - The authors concluded that IN naloxone is a novel alternative method for drug administration in high-risk patients in the prehospital setting with good overall effectiveness. (J Emerg Med. 2005 Oct;29(3):265-71.)

High-Yield Fast-Facts
- **Buprenorphine Binding Affinity**
  - Naloxone doses of 2 to 4 mg are the recommended dose for buprenorphine respiratory depression.
    - Patients on buprenorphine exhibit a bell-shaped dose-response to naloxone, with low (0.2-0.4 mg) and high (5-10mg) doses having little to no effect on the respiratory rate.
- **Acute Withdrawal**
  - It should be no surprise that naloxone administration induces opioid withdrawal where patients may become agitated and vomit.
  - Vomiting poses a risk of aspiration, mainly when naloxone can no longer overcome competition for opioid receptor sites.
- **Ultra-Rapid Withdrawal**
  - Although of questionable practice, some clinics sedate patients to permit rapid naloxone administration to precipitate opioid withdrawal at the beginning of an opioid abstinence treatment program.

HIGH-YIELD BOARD EXAM ESSENTIALS
- **CLASSIC AGENTS:** Alvimopan, naldemedine, naloxegol, naloxone, naltrexone, methylnaltrexone
- **DRUG CLASS:** Opioid antagonists
- **INDICATIONS:** Opioid-induced constipation, opioid overdose (naloxone), post-operative ileus
- **MECHANISM:** Competitive opioid receptor (including mu, kappa, and delta) antagonists.
- **SIDE EFFECTS:** Acute opioid withdrawal, diarrhea, ARDS
- **CLINICAL PEARLS:** Low doses of naloxone (0.04 mg IV) are typically sufficient for most adult patients with opioid-related respiratory depression.

Table: Drug Class Summary

\multicolumn{4}{c	}{**Opioid Antagonists - Drug Class Review**}
\multicolumn{4}{c	}{High-Yield Med Reviews}
\multicolumn{4}{l	}{**Mechanism of Action:** *Competitive opioid receptor (including mu, kappa, and delta) antagonists.*}
\multicolumn{4}{l	}{**Class Effects:** *Naloxone is a life-saving intervention in opioid intoxicated patients, but it and other opioid antagonists can be used for local opioid withdrawal effects, primarily constipation.*}
Generic Name	**Brand Name**	**Main Indication(s) or Uses**	**Notes**
Alvimopan	Entereg	• Postoperative ileus	• **Dosing (Adult):** – Oral: 12 mg 30 minutes to 5 hours before surgery, then 12 mg q12h for a maximum of 7 days • **Dosing (Peds):** – Not routinely used • **CYP450 Interactions:** None • **Renal or Hepatic Dose Adjustments:** – ESRD: Not recommended – Child-Pugh class C: Not recommended • **Dosage Forms:** Oral (capsule)
Naldemedine	Symproic	• Opioid-induced constipation	• **Dosing (Adult):** – Oral: 0.2 mg once daily • **Dosing (Peds):** – Not routinely used • **CYP450 Interactions:** Substrate CYP3A4, P-gp • **Renal or Hepatic Dose Adjustments:** – Child-Pugh class C - Not recommended • **Dosage Forms:** Oral (tablet)
Naloxegol	Movantik	• Opioid-induced constipation	• **Dosing (Adult):** – Oral: 12.5 to 25 mg daily • **Dosing (Peds):** – Not routinely used • **CYP450 Interactions:** Substrate CYP3A4, P-gp • **Renal or Hepatic Dose Adjustments:** – GFR < 60 mL/minute: initial dose of 12.5 mg – Child-Pugh class C: Not recommended • **Dosage Forms:** Oral (tablet)

Opioid Antagonists - Drug Class Review High-Yield Med Reviews			
Generic Name	**Brand Name**	**Main Indication(s) or Uses**	**Notes**

Naloxone	Narcan	- Opioid overdose
		- Opioid-induced constipation or pruritus
			- **Dosing (Adult):**
			  - IV/IM/SQ: 0.04 to 2 mg repeated as needed q2-3minutes
			  - Intranasal: 2 mg, repeated as needed q2-3minutes
			  - IV infusion: 0.25 to 3 mcg/kg/hour
			- **Dosing (Peds):**
			  - IV/IM/SQ: 0.04 to 2 mg repeated as needed q2-3minutes
			  - IV: 0.1 mg/kg/dose repeated as needed
			  - Intranasal: 2 mg, repeated as needed q2-3minutes
			  - IV infusion: 0.25 to 3 mcg/kg/hour
			- **CYP450 Interactions:** None
			- **Renal or Hepatic Dose Adjustments:** None
			- **Dosage Forms:** Nasal (liquid), IV (solution)

Naltrexone	Vivitrol	- Alcohol use disorder
		- Opioid use disorder
			- **Dosing (Adult):**
			  - Oral: 50 to 100 mg/day
			  - IM: 380 mg q4weeks
			- **Dosing (Peds):**
			  - Not routinely used
			- **CYP450 Interactions:** None
			- **Renal or Hepatic Dose Adjustments:** None
			- **Dosage Forms:** Oral (tablet), Suspension for intramuscular injection

Methylnaltrexone	Relistor	- Opioid-induced constipation	- **Dosing (Adult):**
			  - IM: 8 to 12 mg once
			  - IM: 0.15 mg/kg if less than 38 kg or greater than 114 kg
			  - Oral: 450 mg once daily
			- **Dosing (Peds):**
			  - Not routinely used
			- **CYP450 Interactions:** Substrate CYP2D6
			- **Renal or Hepatic Dose Adjustments:**
			  - GFR < 60 mL/minute: reduce dose by 50%
			- **Dosage Forms:** Solution for injection, Oral (Tablet)

NEUROLOGY – BRAIN CARBONIC ANHYDRASE INHIBITOR

Drug Class
- Brain Carbonic Anhydrase Inhibitor
- Agents:
    - **Acute Care**
        - Acetazolamide
    - **Chronic Care**
        - Acetazolamide
        - Topiramate
        - Zonisamide

> **Fast Facts**
> ✓ This class of drugs is known to increase the risk of hyperchloremic metabolic acidosis.
>
> ✓ Topiramate is most commonly used for migraine prevention and now is starting to get more use for weight management in obesity.

Main Indications or Uses
- **Acute Care**
    - Acute altitude/mountain sickness
        - Acetazolamide
- **Chronic Care**
    - Edema
        - Acetazolamide
    - Epilepsy
        - Acetazolamide
        - Topiramate (Partial seizures)
        - Zonisamide (Partial seizures)
    - Migraine Prevention
        - Topiramate

Mechanism of Action
- Carbonic anhydrase inhibitors at type II and type IV isoforms exist in the CNS, decreasing intracellular pH and causing a shift of potassium to the extracellular compartment, ultimately leading to hyperpolarization of cells and increasing seizure threshold.
- Additional antiepileptic effects have been attributed to inhibition of voltage-gated sodium channels, GABA-A agonist activity, and AMPA/kinate receptor inhibition.

Primary Net Benefit
- It can be used to treat specific epilepsies, but its benefits must be weighed against the adverse effects of carbonic anhydrase inhibition.
- Main Labs to Monitor:
    - Urine output, urine osmolarity daily
    - Serum electrolytes daily
    - Intraocular pressure every 30 to 60 minutes for acute angle-closure glaucoma

High-Yield Basic Pharmacology
- **Sulfonamide Derivatives**
    - There is a theoretical risk of cross-reactivity in patients with a history of sulfonamide hypersensitivity.
        - As a result of its sulfonamide structure, carbonic anhydrase inhibitors carry a risk of bone marrow depression, Stevens-Johnson Syndrome, and sulfonamide-like kidney injury.
    - Acetazolamide and methazolamide may cause a diversion of ammonia from urine into the systemic circulation, which can worsen existing hepatic encephalopathy.
- **Zonisamide**
    - In addition to the other actions in this class, zonisamide also inhibits T-type calcium channels, explaining its potential use in treating atypical absence seizures.
- **Glaucoma**
    - Carbonic anhydrase inhibitors are associated with acute myopia and acute closed-angle glaucoma.

High-Yield Clinical Knowledge

- **Hyperchloremic Metabolic Acidosis**
  - Carbonic anhydrase inhibitors block the excretion of hydrogen ions accumulating in the plasma.
    - In normal healthy kidneys, reabsorb bicarbonate and offsets the accumulation of hydrogen and ensuing acidosis.
    - With impaired renal function, high doses, or otherwise altered metabolic function, renal tubules' capacity to reabsorb bicarbonate is impaired, leading to an increasing acidosis.
      - The acidosis typically resolves upon discontinuation of the carbonic anhydrase inhibitor.
- **Topiramate Cognitive Impairment**
  - Patients taking topiramate may experience cognitive effects in a dose-dependent manner, including impaired expressive language function, impaired verbal memory, and slowed cognitive processing.
  - These cognition changes typically occur without changing mental status, without sedation, or mood changes.
    - Doses above 400 mg/day significantly increase adverse cognitive effects.
- **Topiramate and Oral Contraceptives**
  - Topiramate causes a dose-dependent induction of CYP3A4 metabolism of progestins, potentially decreasing the efficacy of birth control.
  - Substituting other contraceptive methods or changing to an ethinyl estradiol-based birth control with doses above 50 mcg/day may be reasonable.
- **Topiramate Paresthesias**
  - Therapeutic dosing of topiramate has been associated with paresthesias, occurring with more frequency early after initiation of treatment or at high doses.
  - Paresthesias may resolve spontaneously with continued treatment and without therapy modification.
- **Hyperthermia/Oligohydrosis**
  - Oligohydrosis may occur during topiramate therapy, causing hyperthermia, particularly during exposure to hot weather.
  - Exposure to hot weather, participating in strenuous exercise, or patients concomitantly taking carbonic anhydrase or anticholinergic agents.
- **Weight Loss**
  - Topiramate is used off-label for weight loss after observation from clinical trials consistently found this effect in patients receiving the drug.
    - Weight loss from topiramate is gradual, peaking at 12 to 18 months after the initiation of treatment.
    - Additional benefits include improving lipid profiles, glucose control, and blood pressure improvement.

High-Yield Core Evidence

- **Topiramate for Migraine Prevention**
  - Objective To assess the efficacy and safety of topiramate for migraine prevention in a large controlled trial.
  - This was a double-blind, placebo-controlled study that randomized adult and pediatric outpatients with a 6-month history of migraine and 3 to 12 migraines a month but no more than 15 headache days a month to either topiramate (50, 100, or 200 mg/d) or placebo.
  - Patients randomized to receive topiramate had a significantly improved primary outcome of change from baseline in mean monthly migraine frequency.
  - The responder rate was significantly greater with topiramate at all doses compared with placebo.
  - However, reductions in migraine days were significant for only the 100 mg per day and 200 mg per day group.
  - Adverse events resulting in discontinuation in the topiramate groups included paresthesia, fatigue, and nausea.
  - The authors concluded that topiramate showed significant efficacy in migraine prevention within the first month of treatment, an effect maintained for the double-blind phase duration. (JAMA. 2004;291(8):965-973.)

- **HEAT Trial**
  - This was a prospective, double-blind, randomized, placebo-controlled trial comparing ibuprofen, acetazolamide, or placebo to prevent high-altitude headaches and acute mountain sickness in healthy western trekkers in Nepal Himalaya.
  - There was no difference between ibuprofen and acetazolamide concerning the primary outcome of high-altitude headaches and acute mountain sickness. Still, both agents were significantly more effective than placebo.
  - The authors concluded that ibuprofen and acetazolamide were similarly effective in preventing high-altitude headaches and acute mountain sickness. (Wilderness Environ Med. 2010 Sep;21(3):236-43.)

High-Yield Fast-Facts
- **Topical Carbonic Anhydrase Inhibition**
  - The ophthalmologic carbonic anhydrase inhibitors (brinzolamide and dorzolamide) are key components of glaucoma management.
- **Skin Reactions**
  - Topiramate and zonisamide are associated with the rare occurrence of Stevens-Johnson syndrome and toxic epidermal necrolysis.
- **Eating Disorders**
  - Topiramate and zonisamide should be used with caution in patients with eating disorders. These disorders may be acutely worsened or manifest in patients without such disorders.

HIGH-YIELD BOARD EXAM ESSENTIALS
- **CLASSIC AGENTS:** Acetazolamide, topiramate, zonisamide
- **DRUG CLASS:** Brain carbonic anhydrase inhibitor
- **INDICATIONS:** Acute altitude/mountain sickness, glaucoma/elevated intraocular pressure, edema, epilepsy, migraine prophylaxis, seizures
- **MECHANISM:** Decrease intracellular pH and cause hyperpolarization of cells, increasing seizure threshold.
- Inhibition of voltage-gated sodium channels, GABA-A agonist activity, and AMPA/kinate receptor inhibition.
- **SIDE EFFECTS:** Hyperchloremic metabolic acidosis, cognitive impairment, paresthesia, hyperthermia/oligohidrosis
- **CLINICAL PEARLS:**
  - Acetazolamide is also for the outpatient management of pseudotumor cerebri in some patients to reduce the pressures applied to the eye and optic nerve.
  - Topiramate causes a dose-dependent induction of CYP3A4 metabolism of progestins, potentially decreasing the efficacy of birth control. Substituting other contraceptive methods or changing to an ethinyl estradiol-based birth control with doses above 50 mcg/day may be reasonable.

Table: Drug Class Summary

Brain Carbonic Anhydrase Inhibitor - Drug Class Review			
High-Yield Med Reviews			
Mechanism of Action: Decrease intracellular pH and cause hyperpolarization of cells, increasing seizure threshold. Inhibition of voltage-gated sodium channels, GABA-A agonist activity, and AMPA/kinate receptor inhibition.			
Class Effects: Can be used to treat specific epilepsies, but their benefits must be weighed against adverse effects related to carbonic anhydrase inhibition.			
Generic Name	**Brand Name**	**Main Indication(s) or Uses**	**Notes**
Acetazolamide	Diamox	<ul><li>Acute altitude/mountain sickness</li><li>Glaucoma/Elevated intraocular pressure</li><li>Edema</li><li>Epilepsy</li></ul>	<ul><li>**Dosing (Adult):**<ul><li>Oral: 125 to 500 mg once to four times per day<ul><li>Maximum 30 mg/kg/day</li></ul></li><li>IV: 500 mg once</li></ul></li><li>**Dosing (Peds):**<ul><li>Oral: 2.5 to 30 mg/kg/dose q12h<ul><li>Maximum 1000 mg/day</li></ul></li></ul></li><li>**CYP450 Interactions:** None</li><li>**Renal or Hepatic Dose Adjustments:**<ul><li>Contraindicated in severe renal impairment</li><li>Contraindicated in patients with cirrhosis or marked liver disease</li></ul></li><li>**Dosage Forms:** IV solution, oral (extended-release capsule, immediate-release tablet)</li></ul>
Topiramate	Topamax	<ul><li>Migraine prophylaxis</li><li>Seizures</li></ul>	<ul><li>**Dosing (Adult):**<ul><li>Oral: 15 to 25 mg daily slowly titrating up to 100 to 400 mg/day</li></ul></li><li>**Dosing (Peds):**<ul><li>Oral: 0.5 to 20 mg/kg/day following slow titration<ul><li>Maximum 400 mg/day</li></ul></li></ul></li><li>**CYP450 Interactions:** Possible CYP3A4 induction</li><li>**Renal or Hepatic Dose Adjustments:**<ul><li>GFR < 70 mL/minute: reduce dose by 50%, slower titration</li></ul></li><li>**Dosage Forms:** Oral (capsule, extended-release, sprinkle, tablet)</li></ul>
Zonisamide	Zonegran	<ul><li>Focal seizures</li></ul>	<ul><li>**Dosing (Adult):**<ul><li>Oral: 25 mg/day slowly titrating up to 100 to 600 mg/day</li></ul></li><li>**Dosing (Peds):**<ul><li>Oral: 1 to 2 mg/kg/day slowly titrating up to 5 to 8 mg/kg/day<ul><li>Maximum 12 mg/kg/day</li></ul></li></ul></li><li>**CYP450 Interactions:** Substrate of CYP2C19, CYP3A4</li><li>**Renal or Hepatic Dose Adjustments:**<ul><li>GFR < 50 mL/minute: use not recommended</li></ul></li><li>**Dosage Forms:** Oral (capsule)</li></ul>

NEUROLOGY – GABA UPTAKE INHIBITORS AND GABA TRANSAMINASE INHIBITOR

Drug Class
- GABA Uptake Inhibitors and GABA Transaminase Inhibitor
- Agents:
    - **Chronic Care**
        - Tiagabine
        - Vigabatrin

Main Indications or Uses
- **Chronic Care**
    - Tiagabine
        - Focal seizures
    - Vigabatrin
        - Infantile spasms
        - Refractory complex partial seizures

Mechanism of Action
- Increase synaptic availability of GABA, decreasing neuronal excitation.

Primary Net Benefit
- Antiepileptic agents are reserved for refractory patients who are intolerant to other agents due to significant toxicity.
- Main Labs to Monitor:
    - Ophthalmologic examination every 3 to 6 months
    - Tiagabine: 0.02 to 0.2 mg/L

High-Yield Basic Pharmacology
- **Tiagabine**
    - Prevents uptake of GABA into neurons, increasing extracellular GABA via selective inhibition of the GABA transporter GAT-1.
- **Paradoxical GABA-A Inhibition**
    - Vigabatrin is a GABA analog that prevents GABA breakdown by inhibiting GABA transaminase.
    - However, it may lead to a paradoxical inhibition of synaptic GABA-A receptors and prolong the activation of extrasynaptic GABA-A receptors.

High-Yield Clinical Knowledge
- **Irreversible Vision Loss**
    - Vigabatrin is associated with irreversible vision loss, causing it to be reserved for patients intolerant or not responding to other treatments.
        - Vision loss can occur within weeks of starting or may not manifest for months to years after initiation.
- **Agitation and Psychosis**
    - Vigabatrin is associated with new-onset or worsening existing agitation, confusion, and psychosis.
    - Alternative antiepileptic agents should be sought in patients with a history of psychiatric illness.

- **Worsening Seizures**
    - Tiagabine can paradoxically worsen myoclonic seizures and risk causing nonconvulsive status epilepticus, including among patients without a history of epilepsy.
        - Myoclonic seizure activity may result from the activation of extrasynaptic GABA-A receptors by tiagabine.
    - Seizures caused by tiagabine or vigabatrin may respond to benzodiazepines, barbiturates or propofol.

- **Lennox-Gastaut Syndrome**
  - Vigabatrin may decrease seizures refractory to valproic acid in patients with Lennox-Gastaut syndrome.

High-Yield Core Evidence
- **Northern European Tiagabine Study Group**
  - This was a multicenter, double-blind, parallel-group, placebo-controlled trial that randomized adult patients with refractory partial seizures to tiagabine or placebo.
  - Patients receiving tiagabine saw a significant reduction in the median 4-weekly seizure rate for all partial seizures and simple partial seizures, including the proportion of patients with a decrease of 50% or more in all partial seizures tiagabine group than in the placebo group.
  - Tiagabine and placebo had similar incidences of asthenia, headache, and somnolence, but tiagabine had more dizziness than the placebo group.
  - The authors concluded that tiagabine is generally well tolerated and demonstrates efficacy for refractory partial seizures. (Epilepsy Res. 1998 Mar;30(1):31-40.)
- **Long Term Vigabatrin Study**
  - This observational study of 66 patients with refractory complex partial seizures and a favorable initial response to vigabatrin for 5 to 72 months.
  - Thirty-seven patients discontinued vigabatrin due to a benefit-to-risk evaluation, seizure breakthroughs, adverse events, other undisclosed adverse events, moved or lost, no longer eligible for the study, non-drug-related death, narcotic abuse, and patient request.
  - The authors concluded that vigabatrin had been proven sufficiently safe to resume clinical trials of vigabatrin in the United States and Canada. (Neurology. 1991 Mar;41(3):363-4.)

High-Yield Fast-Facts
- **Tiagabine and Valproic Acid**
  - Tiagabine may decrease therapeutic concentrations of valproic acid; however, it may not lead to clinically relevant changes in response to valproic acid.
- **Endogenous GHB**
  - Vigabatrin may lower excessive endogenous gamma-hydroxybutyrate (GHB) in patients with genetic GABA metabolism deficiencies.
  - There is no effect on GHB from exogenous sources.

HIGH-YIELD BOARD EXAM ESSENTIALS
- **CLASSIC AGENTS:** Tiagabine, vigabatrin
- **DRUG CLASS:** GABA uptake inhibitors and GABA transaminase inhibitor
- **INDICATIONS:** Focal seizures, infantile spasms, refractory complex partial seizures
- **MECHANISM:** Increase synaptic availability of GABA, decreasing neuronal excitation.
- **SIDE EFFECTS:** Agitation, irreversible vision loss, seizures, psychosis
- **CLINICAL PEARLS:** Tiagabine can paradoxically worsen myoclonic seizures and pose a risk of causing nonconvulsive status epilepticus, including among patients without a history of epilepsy. Myoclonic seizure activity may be a result of the activation of extrasynaptic GABA-A receptors by tiagabine.

Table: Drug Class Summary

GABA Uptake Inhibitors and GABA Transaminase Inhibitor - Drug Class Review High-Yield Med Reviews			
Mechanism of Action: *Increase synaptic availability of GABA, decreasing neuronal excitation.*			
Class Effects: *Antiepileptic agents are reserved for refractory patients intolerant to other agents due to significant toxicities.*			
Generic Name	**Brand Name**	**Indication(s) or Uses**	**Notes**
Tiagabine	Gabitril	• Focal seizures	• **Dosing (Adult):** – Oral: 4 mg daily titrating to 32 to 56 mg/day • **Dosing (Peds):** – Oral: 4 mg daily titrating to 32 mg/day – Maximum 32 mg/day • **CYP450 Interactions:** Substrate of CYP3A4 • **Renal or Hepatic Dose Adjustments:** None • **Dosage Forms:** Oral (tablet)
Vigabatrin	Sabril	• Infantile spasms • Refractory complex partial seizures	• **Dosing (Adult):** – Oral: 500 mg BID up to 1,500 mg BID • **Dosing (Peds):** – Oral: 25 mg/kg/dose q12h – Maximum 150 mg/kg/day • **CYP450 Interactions:** None • **Renal or Hepatic Dose Adjustments:** – GFR 50 to 80 mL/minute: decrease by 25% – GFR 30 to 50 mL/minute: decrease by 50% – GFR 10 to 30 mL/minute: decrease by 75% • **Dosage Forms:** Oral (packet, tablet)

NEUROLOGY – GABAPENTINOIDS (AKA ALPHA 2 DELTA LIGANDS)

Drug Class
- Gabapentinoids
- Agents:
  - Chronic Care
    - Gabapentin
    - Pregabalin

Main Indications or Uses
- Chronic Care
  - Pregabalin
    - Fibromyalgia
    - Focal seizures
    - Neuropathic pain
    - Postherpetic neuralgia
  - Gabapentin
    - Focal seizures
    - Postherpetic neuralgia

Fast Facts
✓ Gabapentin and pregabalin are most commonly used for neuropathic pain and/or fibromyalgia in clinical practice.

✓ Both agents need renal dose adjustment and can cause sedation especially in the elderly.

Mechanism of Action
- Binds to the alpha-2-delta-1 subunit of the N-type calcium channel, reducing the frequency of calcium fusion of synaptic vesicles to membranes, thereby reducing glutamate exocytosis.

Primary Net Benefit
- Gabapentin and pregabalin can treat focal seizures but are more routinely used to treat neuropathic pain and certain anxiety disorders.
- Main Labs to Monitor:
  - Renal function (before initiation)

High-Yield Basic Pharmacology
- Voltage-Gated Calcium Channels
  - T-type and L-type calcium channels are more conventionally known for cardiology.
    - Still, both may be relevant in neurology with T-type channels on dendrites of thalamic neurons and L-type on presynaptic neurons.
  - High-voltage calcium channels include N-, P/Q-, and R-type calcium channels.
- No GABA
  - Although their names may suggest it, neither gabapentin nor pregabalin functionally acts as GABA.
  - These agents are amino acid-like structures that were first synthesized as analogs of GABA but were not observed to have any GABA-related action.
- NMDA Receptors
  - Gabapentinoids have been proposed to inhibit the alpha-2-delta-1 receptor's ability to move presynaptic NMDA receptors to the cell surface and thus neuronal synapses.

High-Yield Clinical Knowledge
- Pregabalin CV
  - Pregabalin is a federally controlled substance in schedule V (or C-V), whereas gabapentin is not.
- Withdrawal
  - Abrupt discontinuation of gabapentin is not recommended as a clinical withdrawal syndrome has been observed.
  - Gabapentin withdrawal manifests as agitation, confusion, tachycardia, and seizures.
  - Withdrawal should be managed by re-starting and then tapering gabapentin, as benzodiazepines are ineffective.

- **Renal Dose Adjustment**
    - The primary elimination route of the gabapentinoids is renal, with dose adjustments beginning when GFR falls below 50-60 mL/minute.
- **Gabapentin Absorption**
    - Gabapentin displays a saturable oral absorption with decreasing absorption, thus penetrating the CNS as doses increase.
        - This absorption of gabapentin is dependent on L-amino acid transport located exclusively in the upper small intestine.
        - Pregabalin displays more consistent absorption, with no observed saturation as it is absorbed by mechanisms other than L-amino acid transport.
    - At doses of 900 mg/day, bioavailability is approximately 60%, falling to 33% at 3,600 mg/day.
- **TDM**
    - Gabapentin and pregabalin can be monitored using therapeutic drug monitoring of serum levels but are not routinely recommended due to these agents' large therapeutic window and safety.
        - Gabapentin therapeutic range of 2 to 20 mg/L.
        - Pregabalin therapeutic range of 2.8 to 8.3 mg/L.
- **Pregabalin Safety**
    - Pregabalin has been associated with cardiac adverse events, including third-degree atrioventricular block, QT prolongation, encephalopathy, and respiratory failure.
    - Like gabapentin, pregabalin can lead to peripheral edema, weight gain, and decompensated congestive heart failure.

High-Yield Core Evidence

- **Gabapentin Monotherapy Study Group**
    - This prospective, double-blind trial in patients with newly diagnosed partial epilepsy were randomized to one of three masked doses of gabapentin (300, 900, or 1,800 mg/day) or open-label carbamazepine (600 mg/day).
    - This study's primary outcome was the proportion of patients required to exit the study if they experienced an exit event, defined as three simple or complex partial seizures, one generalized tonic-clonic (GTC) seizure, or status epilepticus.
    - The time to an exit event was longer for patients on gabapentin, 900 mg/day or 1,800 mg/day, than for patients receiving 300 mg/day.
    - Rates of an exit event plus adverse event withdrawal rate were similar for carbamazepine and 1,800 mg/day gabapentin but was better for 900 mg/day gabapentin.
    - The authors concluded that gabapentin at 900 or 1,800 mg/day is effective and safe as monotherapy for newly diagnosed partial epilepsy patients. (Neurology, 1998, 51:1282–1288.)
- **Gabapentin In Partial Seizures**
    - This was a double-blind, placebo-controlled study of gabapentin as add-on therapy in patients with partial and secondarily generalized seizures.
    - Patients randomized to gabapentin 1,200 mg/day experienced a significant decrease in seizure frequency from baseline than the 900 mg/day dose.
    - The authors noted a correlation between a reduced seizure incidence and serum gabapentin concentrations over 2 μg/ml.
    - The authors concluded that gabapentin effectively treats partial epileptic seizures in a dosage-related manner. (Epilepsia, 1991, 32:539–542.

High-Yield Fast-Facts

- **Seizures in OD**
    - Gabapentin overdose has been associated with the development of seizures.
    - Other antiepileptic agents that cause seizures in overdose include carbamazepine, topiramate, valproic acid, and zonisamide.

> **HIGH-YIELD BOARD EXAM ESSENTIALS**
> - **CLASSIC AGENTS:** Gabapentin, pregabalin
> - **DRUG CLASS:** Gabapentinoids
> - **INDICATIONS:** Fibromyalgia, focal seizures, neuropathic pain, postherpetic neuralgia
> - **MECHANISM:** Binds to the alpha-2-delta-1 subunit of the N-type calcium channel, reducing the frequency of calcium fusion of synaptic vesicles to membranes, thereby reducing glutamate exocytosis.
> - **SIDE EFFECTS:** Altered mental status, headache, withdrawal
> - **CLINICAL PEARLS:** Gabapentin is more commonly used for neuropathy than as an adjunct for seizures. Gabapentin and pregabalin are both renally cleared and need to be adjusted especially once the CrCl < 60 ml/min. Pregabalin has been associated with cardiac adverse events, including third-degree atrioventricular block, QT prolongation, as well as encephalopathy, and respiratory failure.

Table: Drug Class Summary

Gabapentinoids - Drug Class Review				
High-Yield Med Reviews			
Mechanism of Action: *Binds to the alpha-2-delta-1 subunit of the N-type calcium channel, reducing the frequency of calcium fusion of synaptic vesicles to membranes and reducing glutamate exocytosis.*			
Class Effects: Can be used to treat focal seizures but more routinely used to treat neuropathic pain and certain anxiety disorders.			
Generic Name	**Brand Name**	**Indication(s) or Uses**	**Notes**

Gabapentin	Neurontin	• Focal seizures
		• Postherpetic neuralgia
			• **Dosing (Adult):**
			  − Oral: 100 to 300 mg q8-12h
			    − Up to 3,600 mg/day has been used
			• **Dosing (Peds):**
			  − Oral: 10 to 15 mg/kg/day divided into 3 doses
			    − Maximum 3,600 mg/day
			• **CYP450 Interactions:** None
			• **Renal or Hepatic Dose Adjustments:**
			  − GFR 30 to 49 mL/minute: Maximum 900 mg/day
			  − GFR 15 to 29 mL/minute: Maximum 600 mg/day
			  − GFR < 15 mL/minute: Maximum 300 mg/day
			• **Dosage Forms:** Oral (capsule, solution, tablet)

Pregabalin	Lyrica	• Fibromyalgia
		• Focal seizures
		• Neuropathic pain
		• Postherpetic neuralgia
			• **Dosing (Adult):**
			  − Oral: 75 to 150 mg q12-24h
			• **Dosing (Peds):**
			  − Oral: 2.5 to 3.5 mg/kg/day divided q8h
			    − Maximum 14 mg/kg/day
			• **CYP450 Interactions:** None
			• **Renal or Hepatic Dose Adjustments:**
			  − GFR 30 to 60 mL/minute: Maximum 300 mg/day
			  − GFR 15 to 29 mL/minute: Maximum 150 mg/day
			  − GFR < 15 mL/minute: Maximum 75 mg/day
			• **Dosage Forms:** Oral (capsule, solution, tablet)

NEUROLOGY – NMDA RECEPTOR ANTAGONIST

Drug Class
- NMDA Receptor Antagonist
- Agents:
  - Chronic Care
    - Felbamate

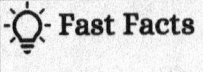

Fast Facts
- ✓ The overall use of felbamate is limited to rare forms of seizures due to risk of aplastic anemia and hepatic failure.

Main Indications or Uses
- Chronic Care
  - Focal seizures
  - Lennox-Gastaut syndrome

Mechanism of Action
- Selective use-dependent block of specific NMDA receptors and GABA-A activation independent of GABA.

Primary Net Benefit
- Limited role in focal seizure/Lennox-Gastaut seizure management due to toxicities, including aplastic anemia.
- Main Labs to Monitor:
  - Therapeutic range 30 to 100 mcg/mL
  - Monitor for early signs of aplastic anemia (reticulocyte counts and platelets, or symptoms of easy bruising, bleeding)
  - Liver enzymes (AST/ALT) and liver function (PT/INR, albumin, total protein, bilirubin)

High-Yield Basic Pharmacology
- GABA-A
  - In addition to its effects on the NMDA receptor, felbamate causes a weak inhibition of GABA-A receptors, similar to barbiturates.
  - Felbamate also possesses voltage-gated sodium channel blocking and calcium channel blocking properties.

High-Yield Clinical Knowledge
- Aplastic Anemia
  - Felbamate-related aplastic anemia was observed after FDA approval and through post-marketing research.
    - There is no evidence to suggest this is a dose-dependent effect.
  - Patients experiencing aplastic anemia had a history of allergies or toxicity to other antiepileptic drugs, a history of cytopenias, or a history of immune diseases.
- Hepatic Failure
  - Like aplastic anemia, felbamate-associated hepatic failure was noted first in post-marketing data, not in initial phase III research.
  - Patients with symptoms of jaundice, fatigue, and/or GI complaints should seek immediate medical care.
- Phenytoin
  - As a result of inhibition of CYP2C19, felbamate decreases the clearance of phenytoin, possibly leading to high therapeutic levels and potential toxicity.
- Valproic Acid
  - Valproic acid levels may increase in the presence of felbamate due to an inhibition of valproic acid beta-oxidation.
- Carbamazepine
  - Although felbamate may reduce carbamazepine levels, but increase 10,11-epoxide concentrations, potentially leading to neurotoxic sequelae.

High-Yield Core Evidence
- **Felbamate in Childhood Lennox-Gastaut**
  - This randomized study of patients with Lennox-Gastaut syndrome were randomized to felbamate or placebo after a run-in phase to assess the impact of felbamate on the frequency of refractory partial-onset seizures.
  - Patients randomized to receive felbamate had a significant decrease in the primary efficacy outcome of the total number of seizures counted during four hours of video recording heart failure total frequency of seizures.
  - Felbamate also significantly improved the global-evaluation scores than in the placebo group from day 49 to the end of the study.
  - There was no significant difference in adverse events between study groups.
  - The authors concluded that felbamate is beneficial in patients with Lennox-Gastaut syndrome. (N Engl J Med. 1993 Jan 7;328(1):29-33)
- **Felbamate for Partial Seizures**
  - This was a double-blind, placebo-controlled clinical that randomized patients with partial seizures and concomitantly taking either carbamazepine or phenytoin to receive felbamate or a placebo.
  - Patients randomized to felbamate had a significant reduction in the mean seizure frequency compared to placebo.
  - Felbamate was also significantly superior to placebo concerning percent seizure reduction and truncated percent seizure reduction.
  - The authors concluded that felbamate is safe and effective in treating medicated patients with severe refractory epilepsy. (Neurology. 1991 Nov;41(11):1785-9.)

High-Yield Fast-Fact
- **Felbamate and Meprobamate**
  - Felbamate is structurally related to meprobamate; however, there is no shared pharmacology or pharmacokinetics.

HIGH-YIELD BOARD EXAM ESSENTIALS
- **CLASSIC AGENTS:** Felbamate
- **DRUG CLASS:** NMDA receptor antagonist
- **INDICATIONS:** Focal seizures
- **MECHANISM:** Selective use-dependent block of certain NMDA receptors, and GABA-A activation independent of GABA.
- **SIDE EFFECTS:** Aplastic anemia, hepatic failure
- **CLINICAL PEARLS:** As a result of inhibition of CYP2C19, felbamate decreases the clearance of phenytoin, possibly leading to high therapeutic levels and potential toxicity.

Table: Drug Class Summary

NMDA Receptor Antagonist - Drug Class Review			
High-Yield Med Reviews			
Mechanism of Action: *Selective use-dependent block of certain NMDA receptors and GABA-A activation independent of GABA.*			
Class Effects: *Limited role in focal seizure/Lennox-Gastaut seizure management due to toxicities, including aplastic anemia.*			
Generic Name	**Brand Name**	**Indication(s) or Uses**	**Notes**

Felbamate	Felbatol	• Focal seizures	• **Dosing (Adult):**
			  – Oral: 1,200 mg/day divided q8-12h titrated up to 3,600 mg/day
			• **Dosing (Peds):**
			  – Oral: 15 mg/kg/day divided q8-12h titrated to maximum 45 mg/kg/day or 3,600 mg/day, whichever is less
			• **CYP450 Interactions:** Substrate of CYP 2E1, 3A4
			• **Renal or Hepatic Dose Adjustments:**
			  – GFR < 50 mL/minute: reduce dose by 50%
			• **Dosage Forms:** Oral (suspension, tablet)

NEUROLOGY – SODIUM CHANNEL BLOCKING DRUGS

Drug Class
- Sodium Channel Blocking Drugs
- Agents:
  - **Acute Care**
    - Phenytoin
    - Fosphenytoin
  - **Chronic Care**
    - Carbamazepine
    - Cenobamate
    - Eslicarbazepine
    - Lamotrigine
    - Oxcarbazepine
    - Phenytoin
    - Rufinamide
    - Topiramate
    - Valproic acid
    - Zonisamide

Main Indications or Uses
- **Acute Care**
  - Seizures
- **Chronic Care**
  - Absence seizures
    - Valproic acid
  - Bipolar disorder
    - Carbamazepine
    - Lamotrigine
    - Valproic acid
  - Lennox-Gastaut syndrome
    - Rufinamide
  - Seizures
    - Carbamazepine
    - Eslicarbazepine
    - Oxcarbazepine
    - Phenytoin/Fosphenytoin
    - Rufinamide
  - Focal seizures
    - Cenobamate
    - Lamotrigine
    - Valproic acid
  - Partial Seizures
    - Zonisamide
  - Migraine
    - Lamotrigine
    - Valproic acid

> **Fast Facts**
> - Valproic acid has several different indications where its use in clinical practice is still high despite drug level monitoring.
> - Valproic acid can uniquely cause hyperammonemia resulting in altered mental status.
> - Like Valproic Acid, Zonisamide has broad CNS effects with many actions on different receptors.

> **Dosing Pearls**
> - Fosphenytoin is the prodrug of phenytoin and can be given both IV or IM, but not by mouth whereas phenytoin can be given by mouth or IV.
> - The rate of IV infusion is 50 mg/min for phenytoin due to the presence of propylene glycol whereas fosphenytoin can be given at 150 mg/min because it does not have propylene glycol. Given either too fast can cause cardiac conduction problems and hypotension.
> - Both phenytoin and fosphenytoin follow first order elimination kinetics at standard doses but can covert to zero elimination kinetics at higher doses which can result in toxicity.

Mechanism of Action
- Inhibition of sodium channels by reducing their capacity for recovery from activation.

Primary Net Benefit
- The broad antiepileptic activity can be used acutely for seizures or status epilepticus.
- **Carbamazepine**
  - Carbamazepine is unique in that while it blocks voltage-sensitive sodium channels, it also inhibits the release of glutamate. Additionally, it has anticholinergic, antimanic, antineuralgic, antidepressant, and antiarrhythmic properties.
- **Cenobamate**
  - Inhibits voltage-gated sodium channels, and acts as a positive allosteric modulator of GABA-A ion channels.
- **Valproic Acid Actions**
  - Valproic acid has broad effects on the CNS and spinal cord neurons by reducing repetitive depolarizations.
  - The primary actions are attributed to valproic acid's voltage-gated sodium channel-blocking activity, inhibition of T-type calcium channels, stimulation of GABA synthesis, and inhibition of GABA degradation.
- **Zonisamide** (see voltage-gated calcium channel blockers)

- Inhibits T-type calcium channels, voltage-dependent sodium channels, and glutamate release. Also a weak inhibitor of carbonic anhydrase, and at lower doses than those used in epilepsy, it may inhibit MAO-B.

High-Yield Basic Pharmacology
- **Michaelis-Menten**
  - Michaelis-Menten pharmacokinetics (PK) describes the pk properties of phenytoin.
  - This pk model describes a process where phenytoin exhibits first-order (or linear) pharmacokinetics at low plasma concentrations, but as plasma levels increase, it shifts to non-linear kinetics.
  - There is wide patient-to-patient variability concerning the plasma level where this "switch" occurs, making phenytoin a medication requiring close therapeutic drug monitoring, particularly during initiation, dosing adjustments, or additions/subtraction of drugs interacting with phenytoin.
- **Phenytoin Binding Kinetics**
  - Numerous comorbidities or patient characteristics can alter phenytoin PK parameters, particularly distribution and protein binding.
    - Patients with renal failure, pregnant, neonates, or critical care patients may have altered phenytoin-binding kinetics.
- **Valproic Metabolism**
  - Valproic acid undergoes hepatic glucuronidation, and oxidation (beta-oxidation and omega-oxidation) occurring in the mitochondria, with possible toxic effects.
    - Initial valproic acid oxidation occurs in the mitochondrial matrix with passive diffusion of valproic acid across the mitochondrial membrane and eliminating valproic acid metabolites back out of the mitochondria using acetyl-CoA and carnitine as transporters.
      - This process sequesters CoA, preventing beta-oxidation of other fatty acids, potentially leading to hepatic steatosis.
      - If metabolized by carnitine, forming valproylcarnitine is normally renally eliminated. Still, it may inhibit L-carnitine's cellular uptake, leading to carnitine depletion and inducing omega-oxidation forming the hepatotoxic metabolite 4-en-valproate inhibition of the urea cycle leading to hyperammonemia.

High-Yield Clinical Knowledge
- **Bipolar Disorder**
  - Lamotrigine (bipolar depression), and valproic acid (bipolar mania), may be used for maintenance or treatment of bipolar mood disorders or used for migraine prophylaxis.
- **Dementia-associated agitation or aggression**
  - Valproate should not be used for this indication due to the increased risk of adverse effects and limited evidence for efficacy.
- **Many Names of Valproic Acid**
  - Valproic acid (VPA) may be referred to by many different names, including valproate, divalproex (a compound of sodium valproate and valproic acid).
- **Dosing, Dosage Forms, and/or Administration**
  - Notable toxicity related to dose titration (lamotrigine) or hyperammonemia (valproic acid).
  - **Carbamazepine**
    - Slowly titrated every 5 or more days based on tolerability, efficacy (control of seizures or mood), and therapeutic levels.
    - CYP 3A4 substrate and inducer that can impact its own metabolism and may require additional titration after 2-3 months of treatment if efficacy changes or levels decrease.
  - **Lamotrigine Titration**
    - Lamotrigine dose titration must follow a strict schedule with close monitoring of the patient for signs and symptoms of rash or hypersensitivity.
    - For patients who will be started on lamotrigine but are currently taking valproic acid, the initial dose titration should be slower, with a lower target maximum dose.
      - Starting with 25 mg every 48 hours for 2 weeks, then increasing to 25 mg every 24 hours for 2 weeks, after which doses can be increased by 25 to 50 mg/day every 1-2 weeks up to a maintenance dose of 100-150 mg/day divided into 2 doses.
  - **Valproate Dose Equivalencies**
    - Valproic acid 87 mg is equivalent to valproate sodium 100 mg.
    - Valproic acid 125 mg is equivalent to divalproex sodium 135 mg.
  - **Phenytoin IV Administration**
    - When phenytoin is administered intravenously, specific precautions must be taken to avoid phlebitis, tissue necrosis (purple-glove syndrome), vasodilation, and cardiac toxicity.
    - The maximum infusion rate for phenytoin is 50 mg/minute, but patients rarely tolerate rates greater than 20 mg/minute.
    - Phenytoin must be diluted in sodium chloride 0.9% and administered with an in-line filter.
    - Phenytoin should not be administered via intramuscular (IM) injection; however, fosphenytoin may be administered IM.

- The volume for a typical adult loading dose of fosphenytoin is around 10 mL, limiting IM sites to the gluteal tissue, though this is not ideal.
- **Fosphenytoin Administration**
  - Fosphenytoin may be administered at a rate of 150 mg/minute, diluted in either sodium chloride 0.9% or D5W, and does not require an in-line filter.
    - Fosphenytoin may still cause cardiac arrhythmias and has been associated with rate-dependent pruritus.
  - Although fosphenytoin can be administered three times faster than phenytoin, it has the same time to one activity due to the time required for dephosphorylation.
    - Fosphenytoin is dosed in "phenytoin-equivalents," which has the potential for confusion and dosing errors.
      - However, the clinical use of any dosing other than "phenytoin-equivalents" is infrequent.
- **Initiation Precautions**
  - Before initiating carbamazepine, eslicarbazepine, oxcarbazepine, or phenytoin, screening for the HLA-B*1502 allele is strongly recommended, particularly in patients of Asian or South Asian ancestry.
  - Patients with positive screening have a significantly higher risk of severe cutaneous adverse events, including DRESS (drug reactions with eosinophilia and systemic symptoms), Stevens-Johnson syndrome, or toxic epidermal necrolysis.
  - Hematological pretreatment testing should be conducted to evaluate for the risk of developing blood dyscrasias such as anemia or agranulocytosis before initiating carbamazepine.
- **Renal Dosing**
  - Oxcarbazepine should be initiated at 50% of the usual starting dose if eCrCl <30mL/min.
  - Topiramate dose reductions (50% decrease) for impaired renal function eCrCl < 70ml/min.

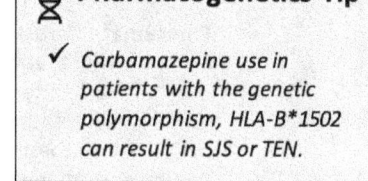

Pharmacogenetics Tip

✓ *Carbamazepine use in patients with the genetic polymorphism, HLA-B*1502 can result in SJS or TEN.*

- **Contraindications**
  - Carbamazepine: Bone marrow depression, MAO inhibitors within 14 days, use with nefazodone, or non-nucleoside reverse transcriptase inhibitors (NNRTIs) that are CYP3A4 substrates.
  - Topiramate ER is contraindicated with recent alcohol use (6 hours before and after dose) and in patients with metabolic acidosis who take metformin.
- **Boxed Warnings**
  - Carbamazepine: Skin reactions such as Stevens-Johnson and toxic epidermal necrolysis (HLA-B*1502), aplastic anemia, and agranulocytosis.
  - Phenytoin and fosphenytoin: Cardiovascular risk (arrhythmia, hypotension) with rapid infusion – do not exceed recommended infusion rates and closely monitor cardiac parameters. Reduction in dose or discontinuation may be necessary.
  - Lamotrigine: Serious skin rashes (Stevens-Johnson) which require medication discontinuation at the first sign of a rash and possible hospitalization.
  - Valproate has several boxed warnings.
    - Hepatoxicity for liver failure resulting in death.
    - Fetal risk due to the risk of major congenital malformations such as spina bifida. Should not be used in those of childbearing potential without contraception.
    - Pancreatitis that may occur with initiation or after several years of use.
    - Mitochondrial disease including DNA mutations of the mitochondrial DNA polymerase gamma (POLG) gene increases the risk of hepatoxicity.
- **Warnings**
  - Suicidal ideation, CNS depression.
  - Exercise caution in cardiac impairment, renal impairment, and hepatic impairment.
  - Caution in older adults who may be more sensitive to adverse effects.
- **Adverse Effects (AEs)**
  - CNS effects or CNS depression and suicidal ideation.
  - **Carbamazepine Adverse Effects and Toxicity**
    - Carbamazepine has a wide toxicity profile, ranging from teratogenic effects in pregnant patients to cardiac effects, respiratory failure, hepatoxicity, seizures, and anticholinergic toxicity.
    - Blood dyscrasias have occurred during normal carbamazepine therapeutic use, including leukocytosis, leukopenia, eosinophilia, thrombocytopenia, pancytopenia to agranulocytosis, aplastic anemia, and bone marrow depression.
    - Carbamazepine has been known to cause hyponatremia and inappropriate antidiuretic hormone (SIADH), occurring in 1 to 40% of patients throughout chronic therapy.
    - Other notable toxicities include QRS/QT prolongation, hypotension, nystagmus, diplopia, ataxia, dystonic reactions, choreoathetosis, and psychiatric effects such as confusion, agitation, or psychosis.
  - Oxcarbazepine has many similar AEs of carbamazepine: blood dyscrasias, hyponatremia, neuropsychiatric effects, and skin reactions.

- Phenytoin and Fosphenytoin: blood dyscrasias, cardiovascular effects, CNS effects, drowsiness, gingival hyperplasia (phen), hepatoxicity, hirsutism (phen), acne (phen), perineal itching (fos), and rash.
- Carbamazepine, phenytoin, and topiramate may cause or worsen sexual dysfunction.
- Lamotrigine has been associated with cases of aseptic meningitis, blood dyscrasias, immune activation or hemophagocytic lymphohistiocytosis (HLH), nausea, rash, edema, weight changes (gain or loss), GI symptoms, fatigue, and mood changes.
- Topiramate: metabolic acidosis, kidney stones, visual changes, and mood changes (mood disorder, depression) or psychiatric symptoms (anxiety, aggression).
  - **Topiramate Cognitive Impairment**
    - Patients taking topiramate may experience cognitive effects in a dose-dependent manner, but even at doses under 100 mg /day.
      - These effects may include impaired expressive language function, impaired verbal memory, and slowed cognitive processing.
      - These cognitive changes typically occur without changing mental status, without sedation, or notable mood changes.
      - Doses above 400 mg/day significantly increase adverse cognitive effects.
  - **Topiramate Paresthesias**
    - Therapeutic dosing of topiramate has been associated with paresthesias, occurring with more frequency early after initiation of treatment or at high doses.
    - Paresthesias may resolve spontaneously with continued treatment and without therapy modification.
    - Parathesis may also serve as an indication of therapeutic effectiveness.
  - **Topiramate Hyperthermia/Oligohidrosis**
    - Oligohidrosis may occur during topiramate therapy, causing hyperthermia, particularly during exposure to hot weather.
    - Exposure to hot weather, participating in strenuous exercise, or patients concomitantly taking carbonic anhydrase or anticholinergic agents.
  - **Topiramate Weight Loss**
    - Topiramate is used off-label for weight loss after observation from clinical trials consistently found this effect in patients receiving the drug.
      - Weight loss from topiramate is gradual, peaking at 12 to 18 months after the initiation of treatment.
      - Additional benefits include improving lipid profiles, glucose control, and blood pressure improvement.
      - It is used off-label for antipsychotic-induced weight gain, binge eating disorder, as well as alcohol use disorder.
      - Exacerbation and development of eating disorders such as anorexia and bulimia, have been reported in adolescents receiving topiramate for migraines or chronic headaches and in adults receiving topiramate for epilepsy.
  - **Valproic Acid Adverse Events (AEs)**
    - Valproic acid is associated with concentration-dependent toxicities inducing hypotension, hematological effects, respiratory depression, pancreatitis, encephalopathy, hepatotoxicity, and coma.
    - Associated with dose-dependent weight gain with doses at or above 1300 mg/day, so the lowest effective dose should be utilized. (Grosu C et al. J Clin Psychiatry 2024; 85(2):23m15008)
    - Byproducts of valproic acid metabolism, including ketoacids, carboxylic acid, and propionic acid, can cause anion-gap metabolic acidosis.
    - Chronic toxicities at normal therapeutic dosing include hepatic steatosis and hyperammonemia with encephalopathy.
    - **L-Carnitine**
      - L-carnitine is the treatment of choice for valproic acid hyperammonemia or hepatotoxicity and should be given in the IV dosage form as oral absorption is limited.
        - Oral L-carnitine can be an alternative in select patients with elevated ammonia levels, but the patients are otherwise asymptomatic.
- **Interactions - Drug, Supplement, Food, and/or Disease**
  - CYP Induction
    - Carbamazepine, eslicarbazepine, oxcarbazepine, phenytoin, and rufinamide are inducers of CYP 450 enzymes and contribute to numerous clinically significant drug interactions.
    - Carbamazepine is unique as it is an inducer of hepatic metabolism and an autoinducer - as it induces its metabolism.
      - As opposed to inhibition, hepatic induction occurs over time, and in the case of carbamazepine occurs over approximately 96 hours.
        - Dose adjustments should occur shortly after initiation and therapeutic drug monitoring of the parent carbamazepine and 10,11-epoxide metabolite concentration.
    - Carbamazepine: extensive drug-drug interactions, clozapine (enhanced myelosuppressive effects), hormonal contraceptives (decreased concentrations causing ineffectiveness), lamotrigine (enhanced toxic effects of lamotrigine), levetiracetam (enhanced toxic effects of carbamazepine), lurasidone

- (decreased concentrations), quetiapine (altered concentrations of both agents), rivaroxaban (decreased concentrations), thyroid medications (decreased concentrations), topiramate (decreased concentrations), valproate (altered concentrations of both agents).
- Oxcarbazepine has many similar drug-drug interactions as carbamazepine: clozapine, contraceptives, lamotrigine, levetiracetam, rivaroxaban, and valproate among others.
- Phenytoin can decrease the level of many antiepileptics, and many agents (anticoagulants, diltiazem, trimethoprim) can inhibit the metabolism of phenytoin, and phenytoin can decrease the effectiveness of contraceptives (oral, patch, ring, and implants).
- Lamotrigine:
  - Patients on lamotrigine inducers (carbamazepine, estrogens, phenytoin) may start at higher initial doses.
  - Increased risk of arrhythmias when combined with other sodium channel blockers
- Valproate: Diminished effects of apixaban and dabigatran; enhanced hepatotoxic effects when combined with cannabidiol; diminished concentration of valproate with carbapenems, carbamazepine, ethosuximide, ibuprofen; increased concentration of valproate with lithium; enhanced toxic effects of clozapine.
- **Oral Contraceptives**
  - Topiramate causes a dose-dependent induction of CYP3A4 metabolism of progestins, potentially decreasing the efficacy of birth control.
  - Substituting other contraceptive methods or changing to an ethinyl estradiol-based birth control with doses above 50 mcg/day may be reasonable.
  - Carbamazepine, oxcarbazepine, and rufinamide may reduce the efficacy of contraceptives.
  - Lamotrigine when combined with estrogen contraceptives may result in decreased efficacy of lamotrigine requiring larger doses of lamotrigine.
  - Valproate when combined with estrogen-containing products may result in decreased concentrations of valproate.
- **Monitoring**
  - Mood changes and suicidality.
  - CBC baseline and periodically every 2-4 weeks x 2 months, then every 3 to 6 months.
  - Thyroid function every 6-12 months with carbamazepine and valproate.
  - Renal function at baseline and periodically with carbamazepine and oxcarbazepine.
  - Serum sodium for agents associated with hyponatremia (e.g. carbamazepine, oxcarbazepine)
  - Liver enzymes (AST/ALT), liver function (albumin, protein, bilirubin, INR) at baseline and frequently.
    - Ammonia levels should be monitored with valproic acid if the patient experiences altered mental status.
    - Symptoms such as fatigue, facial edema, lethargy, weakness, vomiting, and anorexia should prompt liver evaluations for valproate.
  - Sodium bicarbonate at baseline and periodically, renal function with topiramate. Consider checking ammonia levels in those with lethargy, vomiting, or acute mental status changes.
  - HLA-B*1502 allele screening (carbamazepine, eslicarbazepine, oxcarbazepine, phenytoin).
  - Symptoms of pancreatitis with valproate (anorexia, abdominal pain, nausea, and vomiting).
  - Therapeutic drug monitoring should be balanced by significant dose-dependent and dose-independent toxicities.
    - Carbamazepine: 4 to 12 mg/L
    - Eslicarbazepine: 3 to 35 mg/L
    - Oxcarbazepine: 10 to 35 mg/L
    - Lamotrigine: 2 to 15 mg/L
    - Phenytoin
      - Total - 10 to 20 mg/L
      - Free - 1 to 2 mg/L
    - Rufinamide: 10 to 35 mg/L
    - Valproic acid: 50 to 100 mg/L
  - **Phenytoin Therapeutic Range & Toxicity**
    - Phenytoin has a narrow therapeutic range, and unique characteristics of toxicities occur when plasma levels exceed normal upper limits (total - 20 mg/L)
      - Nystagmus is one of the first signs of toxicity as phenytoin levels increase to between 20 and 30 mg/L.
      - If phenytoin levels rise to between 30 and 40 mg/L, cerebellar ataxia and dysequilibrium predominate where nystagmus may no longer be appreciated.
      - Confusion and altered mental status predominate with phenytoin levels between 40 to 50 mg/L.
      - As levels extend beyond 50 mg/L, patients may experience dystonias and depressed deep tendon reflexes.
        - It is currently controversial whether phenytoin toxicity can produce seizures in overdose/toxicity but is more likely attributed to the propylene glycol content of the IV phenytoin product.
      - Monitoring of free serum concentrations is recommended in severe renal dysfunction (eCrCl < 25ml/min)
  - **Free Vs. Total Phenytoin Levels**

- Depending on the standard laboratory configuration, phenytoin levels may be reported as total phenytoin levels or free phenytoin levels.
  - Total phenytoin levels should be considered in the context of albumin and corrected if albumin is less than 3.0 to 3.2 mg/dL using the Winter-Tozer equation.
  - Free phenytoin levels are not affected by protein binding fractions and may be more suitable if altered binding kinetics are suspected.
- **Patient Education**
  - Medications should be gradually tapered to discontinue, usually over months unless there is a serious adverse reaction.
  - Patients should be educated to report any mood changes, especially thoughts of self-harm or thoughts of death or dying whether the medication is being used for a psychiatric indication or not.
- **Pregnant Patients**
  - Avoiding phenytoin, carbamazepine, rufinamide, and topiramate during pregnancy is recommended, if possible, to reduce the risk of posterior cleft palate (carbamazepine, topiramate) and poor cognitive outcomes (phenytoin).
  - Monitoring of lamotrigine, levetiracetam, carbamazepine, oxcarbazepine, and phenytoin serum concentrations before (baseline control level) and during pregnancy should be considered if these agents are used to assist with dosing during pregnancy.
  - Patients should report mood changes or thoughts of harming themselves or ending their lives.
  - Valproic acid has indication-dependent use in patients who are pregnant.
    - Valproic acid is contraindicated in pregnant women since it is associated with neural tube defects in children born to mothers taking valproic acid during pregnancy.
      - Patients with bipolar disorder or seizures who are of childbearing age and are not currently taking valproic acid should not have the medication initiated if alternatives exist.
    - For patients with bipolar disorder or seizure disorders who are stable on chronic valproic acid therapy and become pregnant, a risk-benefit discussion must occur with providers to determine whether or not valproic acid should be continued.
    - It should not be used for the treatment of migraine during pregnancy as the benefit does not outweigh the risk.

High-Yield Core Evidence
- **Topiramate for Migraine Prevention**
  - Double-blind, placebo-controlled study that randomized adult and pediatric outpatients with a 6-month history of migraine and 3 to 12 migraines a month but no more than 15 headache days a month to either topiramate (50, 100, or 200 mg/d) or placebo to assess the efficacy and safety of topiramate.
  - Patients randomized to receive topiramate had a significantly improved primary outcome of change from baseline in mean monthly migraine frequency.
  - The responder rate was significantly greater with topiramate at all doses compared with placebo.
  - However, reductions in migraine days were significant for only the 100 mg per day and 200 mg per day group.
  - Adverse events resulting in discontinuation of topiramate included paresthesia, fatigue, and nausea.
  - The authors concluded that topiramate showed significant efficacy in migraine prevention within the first month of treatment, an effect maintained for the double-blind phase duration.
  - JAMA. 2004;291(8):965-973.
- **ESETT Trial** N Engl J Med. 2019 Nov 28;381(22):2103-2113
  - This was a blinded, adaptive trial that randomized adult and pediatric patients with convulsive status epilepticus unresponsive to benzodiazepines to one of three intravenous anticonvulsive agents; levetiracetam, fosphenytoin, or valproate.
  - There was no significant difference between treatment groups concerning the primary outcome of the absence of clinically evident seizures and improvement in consciousness level by 60 minutes after the start of drug infusion, without additional anticonvulsant medication.
  - More hypotension and intubation episodes occurred in the fosphenytoin group, and more deaths occurred in the levetiracetam group than in the other groups, but these differences were not significant.
  - The authors concluded that levetiracetam, fosphenytoin, and valproate led to seizure cessation and improved alertness by 60 minutes in approximately half the patients.
  - The three drugs were associated with similar incidences of adverse events.
- **Lamotrigine Vs. Valproic Acid Absence Seizures**
  - This open-label parallel-group trial randomized patients with a history of newly diagnosed children and adolescents with typical absence seizures to receive either lamotrigine or valproic acid.
  - Compared to lamotrigine, patients randomized to valproic acid had a significantly improved primary outcome at 1-month follow-up of seizure-free intervals, defined as lack of clinically observed seizures since the previous visit and lack of electroclinical seizures during ambulatory 24-h EEG testing and a video-EEG session with hyperventilation.
  - However, by the 3-month follow-up, treatment effects were similar between patients randomized to receive either lamotrigine or valproic acid.

- The authors concluded that either lamotrigine or valproic acid could be effective against absence seizures. However, valproic acid shows a much faster onset of action, at least in part because of its shorter titration schedule.
- Epilepsia. 2004;45(9):1049-1053.
- **Phenytoin TBI**
    - This landmark study examined the effectiveness of phenytoin compared to placebo in preventing post-traumatic seizures in patients with serious traumatic brain injuries.
    - Phenytoin was associated with a significant reduction in post-traumatic seizures from day 0 to day 7 compared to placebo.
    - However, after day 8 to the end of year 1, there was no significant difference in reducing post-traumatic seizures.
    - bThis lack of a late effect could not be attributed to differential mortality, low phenytoin levels, or treatment of some early seizures in patients assigned to the placebo group.
    - The authors concluded that phenytoin exerts a beneficial effect by reducing seizures only during the first week after a severe head injury.
    - N Engl J Med. 1990 Aug 23;323(8):497-502.

High-Yield Fast-Facts
- **Carbamazepine Alternatives**
    - Eslicarbazepine and oxcarbazepine are structurally and mechanistically related to carbamazepine but have improved safety and pharmacokinetic profile, as they are not autoinducer agents.
    - However, CYP induction is still an action of these agents.
- **Phenytoin Cardiology**
    - Phenytoin acts as a Vaughn Williams classification 1B antiarrhythmic and was once used for digoxin toxicity.
- **Carbamazepine TCA**
    - Carbamazepine structurally resembles a tricyclic antidepressant and shares many clinical and toxicological effects, namely cardiac sodium channel blockade and anticholinergic effects.
- **Skin Reactions**
    - Topiramate and carbamazepine are associated with the rare occurrence of Stevens-Johnson syndrome and toxic epidermal necrolysis.
- **Eating Disorders**
    - Topiramate should be used with caution in patients with eating disorders. These disorders may be acutely worsened or manifest in patients without such disorders.
- **Hemodialysis**
    - Severe valproic acid toxicity can be managed with hemodialysis, particularly when the levels are above 900 mg/L, requiring mechanical ventilation, pH less than 7.1, or coma.

HIGH-YIELD BOARD EXAM ESSENTIALS
- **CLASSIC AGENTS:** Carbamazepine, cenobamate, eslicarbazepine, fosphenytoin, lamotrigine, oxcarbazepine, phenytoin, rufinamide, topiramate, valproate.
- **DRUG CLASS:** Voltage-sensitive sodium channel antagonists (VSSCAs)
- **INDICATIONS:** Bipolar disorder, seizures, focal seizures, migraine.
- **MECHANISM:** Inhibition of sodium channels by reducing their capacity for recovery from activation.
- **SIDE EFFECTS:** Rash (lamotrigine), hepatotoxicity, dose-dependent toxicities (phenytoin), anticholinergic effects (carbamazepine), and suicidal ideation.
- **CLINICAL PEARLS:**
    - Before initiation of carbamazepine, eslicarbazepine, oxcarbazepine, or phenytoin, screening for HLA-B*1502 allele is strongly recommended, particularly in patients Asian or South Asian ancestry.
    - Lamotrigine dose titration must follow a strict schedule with close monitoring of the patient for severe hypersensitivity signs and symptoms. If patients who will be started on lamotrigine but are currently taking valproic acid, the initial dose titration should be slower, with a lower target maximum dose.
    - Avoid the use of phenytoin or fosphenytoin in a patient with TCA-induced seizure as it could worsen the seizure since both can inhibit sodium channels.
    - Fosphenytoin is the prodrug to phenytoin which can be given IM or IV whereas phenytoin should only be given IV or by mouth.
    - The administration rate of IV phenytoin is 50 mg/min due to the presence of propylene glycol whereas fosphenytoin is 150 mg/min and does NOT have propylene glycol.
    - Phenytoin initially exhibits first-order elimination kinetics, but at a certain dose it can convert to zero order elimination and result toxicity rapidly.
    - Topiramate causes a dose-dependent induction of CYP3A4 metabolism of progestins, potentially decreasing the efficacy of birth control. Substituting other contraceptive methods or changing to an ethinyl estradiol-based birth control with doses above 50 mcg/day may be reasonable.

Table: Drug Class Summary

Sodium Channel Blocking Drugs - Drug Class Review
High-Yield Med Reviews

Mechanism of Action: *Inhibition of sodium channels by reducing their capacity for recovery from activation. Topiramate with additional activity as GABA-A, and AMPA/kinate receptor inhibition, and weak carbonic anhydrase inhibition.*

Class Effects: Broad antiepileptic activity can be used acutely for seizures or status epilepticus and therapeutic drug monitoring but balanced by significant dose-dependent and dose-independent toxicities.

Generic Name	Brand Name	Main Indication(s)	Notes
Carbamazepine	Carbatrol Equetro Tegretol	• Bipolar disorder • Seizures	• **Dosing (Adult):** – Oral: 100 to 400 mg/day with gradual titrating ≤ 200 mg every ≥5 days – Maximum dose: 1.600 to 2 grams / day • **Dosing (Peds):** Not routinely used. • **CYP450 Interactions:** – Substrate of CYP2A6, CYP2B6, CYP2C19, CYP2E1, CYP3A4, UGT2B4, UGT2B7 • **Renal or Hepatic Dose Adjustments:** Child-Pugh class A or B maximum dose: 200 mg / day • **Dosage Forms:** Oral (capsule, suspension, tablet – chewable ER and IR)
Cenobamate	Xcopri	• Focal (partial onset) seizures	• **Dosing (Adult):** – Oral: 12.5 to 400 mg/day with gradual titrating weekly – Maximum dose: 400 mg / day • **Dosing (Peds):** – Oral: 10 to 20 mg/kg/day divided q6-8h, adjusted to therapeutic levels • **CYP450 Interactions:** Substrate of CYP2C8, 3A4; Induces CYP1A2, 2B6, 2C9, 3A4, P-gp. • **Renal or Hepatic Dose Adjustments:** Monitor 10,11-carbamazepine epoxide levels closely. • **Dosage Forms:** Oral (capsule, suspension, tablet – chewable ER and IR)
Eslicarbazepine	Aptiom	• Seizures	• **Dosing (Adult):** – Oral: 400 mg daily titrated to 1,600 mg daily • **Dosing (Peds):** – Oral: 200 mg/day titrated to weight-based maximum between 600 and 1,200 mg/day • **CYP450 Interactions:** Inhibits CYP2C19; Induces CYP3A4 • **Renal or Hepatic Dose Adjustments:** – GFR < 50 mL/minute: reduce initial dose by 50%, slow titration. • **Dosage Forms:** Oral (tablet)
Lamotrigine	Lamictal Subvenite	• Bipolar disorder • Focal seizures	• **Dosing (Adult):** Oral: 25 mg/day with slow titration to 100 to 200 mg/day target dose • **Dosing (Peds):** – Oral: 0.15 mg/kg/day with slow titration to target maintenance of 5.1 mg/kg/day – Maximum 5.1 mg/kg/day or 200 mg/day, whichever is less • **CYP450 Interactions:** None • **Renal or Hepatic Dose Adjustments:** – Child-Pugh class B or C without ascites: 25% reduction; with ascites: 50% reduction • **Dosage Forms:** Oral (kit, tablet, chewable tablet, orally disintegrating tablet)
Oxcarbazepine	Oxtellar Trileptal	• Seizures	• **Dosing (Adult):** Oral: 150 to 300 mg q12h, titrated to a maximum of 2,400 mg/day • **Dosing (Peds):** – Oral: 8 to 10 mg/kg/day, divided q12h – Maximum 2,400 mg/day • **CYP450 Interactions:** Induces CYP3A4 • **Renal/Hepatic Dose Adjustments:** GFR < 30 mL/minute: slower titration • **Dosage Forms:** Oral (suspension, tablet, XR tablet)

Sodium Channel Blocking Drugs - Drug Class Review
High-Yield Med Reviews

Generic Name	Brand Name	Main Indication(s) or Uses	Notes

Phenytoin	Dilantin
	Phenytek
		• Seizures
		• Status epilepticus
			• **Dosing (Adult):**
			  – IV: 15 to 20 mg/kg infused no faster than 50 mg/minute
			  – IV: maintenance 4 to 7 mg/kg/day, or 100 mg q8h
			  – Oral: 4 to 7 mg/kg/day divided q8h, or 100 mg q8h
			    – Target level 10 to 20 mg/L (total), or 1 to 2 mg/L (free)
			• **Dosing (Peds):**
			  – IV: 15 to 20 mg/kg infused no faster than 50 mg/minute
			  – IV: maintenance 4 to 7 mg/kg/day
			  – Oral: 4 to 7 mg/kg/day divided q8h
			    – Target level 10 to 20 mg/L (total), or 1 to 2 mg/L (free)
			• **CYP450 Interactions:** Substrate of CYP2C19, 2C9, 3A4; Induces CYP1A2, 2B6, 3A4, P-gp.
			• **Renal or Hepatic Dose Adjustments:**
			  – No empiric adjustments, follow drug levels.
			• **Dosage Forms:** Oral (suspension, tablet); As sodium salt: Oral (capsule), IV (solution)

Rufinamide	Banzel	• Lennox-Gastaut syndrome	• **Dosing (Adult):**
			  – Oral: 200 to 400 q12h, titrated to a maximum 1,600 mg/day
			• **Dosing (Peds):**
			  – Oral: 5 mg/kg/dose q12h, titrated to target of 22.5 mg/kg/dose q12h
			    – Maximum 1,600 mg/dose
			• **CYP450 Interactions:** Induces CYP3A4
			• **Renal or Hepatic Dose Adjustments:** None
			• **Dosage Forms:** Oral (suspension, tablet)

Topiramate	Topamax	• Migraine prophylaxis
		• Seizures
		• Other off-label uses (tremor, weight gain, alcohol use disorder, headaches, binge eating)
			• **Dosing (Adult):**
			  – Oral: 15 to 25 mg daily slowly titrating up to 100 to 400 mg/day
			• **Dosing (Peds):**
			  – Oral: 0.5 to 20 mg/kg/day following slow titration
			    – Maximum 400 mg/day
			• **CYP450 Interactions:** Possible CYP3A4 induction
			• **Renal or Hepatic Dose Adjustments:**
			  – GFR < 70 mL/minute: reduce dose by 50%, slower titration.
			• **Dosage Forms:** Oral (capsule, extended-release, sprinkle, tablet)

Valproic acid	Depacon
	Depakene
	Depakote
		• Bipolar disorder
		• Focal seizures
		• Migraine
			• **Dosing (Adult):**
			  – Oral: 10 to 60 mg/kg/day, adjusted to therapeutic levels
			  – IV: 20 to 40 mg/kg administered 10 mg/kg/minute, maximum dose of 3,000 mg
			• **Dosing (Peds):**
			  – Oral: 10 to 60 mg/kg/day, adjusted to therapeutic levels
			  – IV: 20 to 40 mg/kg administered 10 mg/kg/minute, maximum dose of 2,000 mg
			• **CYP450 Interactions:** Substrate of CYP2A6, 2B6, 2C19, 2C9, 2E1
			• **Renal or Hepatic Dose Adjustments:**
			  – Hepatic impairment: use not recommended.
			• **Dosage Forms:** Oral (capsule, solution, tablet), IV (solution)

NEUROLOGY – SV2A PROTEIN-LIGAND

Drug Class
- SV2A Protein-Ligand
- Agents:
  - Brivaracetam
  - Levetiracetam

Main Indications or Uses
- Acute Care
  - Seizures
    - Levetiracetam
  - Status epileptics
    - Levetiracetam
  - Traumatic brain injury, seizure prophylaxis
    - Levetiracetam
- Chronic Care
  - Partial onset seizures
    - Brivaracetam
    - Levetiracetam

> **Fast Facts**
> ✓ The dose of both agents is the same if given by mouth or by IV infusion making them easy to use and dose clinically.
>
> ✓ Levetiracetam is now used for status epilepticus as well as seizure prophylaxis for traumatic brain injury (TBI).

Mechanism of Action
- Selectively bind to the SV2A receptor in synaptic vesicles, reducing glutamate release during high-frequency activity.

Primary Net Benefit
- Broad antiepileptic activity with wide therapeutic window and relatively safe adverse event profile compared to other antiepileptic drugs.
- Main Labs to Monitor:
  - Brivaracetam
    - CBC
    - Liver function (PT/INR, albumin, total protein, bilirubin)
    - Liver enzymes (AST/ALT, alk.phos)
    - Serum creatinine

High-Yield Basic Pharmacology
- SV2A Role
  - SV2A is a synaptic vesicle essential to membrane proteins as it functions to recycle synaptic vesicles through vesicle endocytosis.
- N-Type Calcium Channels
  - Brivaracetam and levetiracetam also possess N-type calcium channel blocking properties, reducing calcium fusion of synaptic vesicles to membranes and reducing glutamate release.
- Bioavailability
  - The oral bioavailability of levetiracetam is approximately 100%, facilitating simple IV to the oral conversion of doses.

High-Yield Clinical Knowledge
- Adverse Events
  - Levetiracetam has a wide therapeutic range but may cause CNS depression and ataxia at high drug levels.
  - Agitation is a common adverse event in pediatric patients prescribed levetiracetam.
- Brivaracetam and Carbamazepine
  - Brivaracetam may decrease the elimination of 10,11-carbamazepine epoxide, the active metabolite of carbamazepine.

- The 10,11-carbamazepine epoxide is associated with neurologic toxicities and can be therapeutically monitored with a normal range of 1 to 10 mg/L.
- **Appropriate Levetiracetam Dosing**
    - Although conventional dosing of levetiracetam is typically between 500 to 1000 mg per dose, the recent ESETT, ConSEPT, and EcLiPSE trials used higher weight-based doses of 40 to 60 mg/kg per dose, with a maximum of 4,500 mg.
        - When considering the results suggesting similar effects to phenytoin, it's important to remember levetiracetam was studied at these doses, whereas phenytoin was used at doses more familiar to clinical practice.
- **Rapid IV Administration**
    - Levetiracetam may be administered via IV slow push, allowing for delivery of therapeutic dosing rapidly.
    - This contrasts with alternative agents used for acute seizures, such as phenytoin, which must be infused slowly over at a maximum rate of 50 mg/minute but rarely tolerated at rates above 20 mg/minute.

High-Yield Core Evidence
- **ConSEPT**
    - This was an open-label, multicenter trial that randomized children aged between 3 months and 16 years with convulsive status epilepticus that failed first-line benzodiazepine treatment to receive phenytoin 20 mg/kg or levetiracetam 40 mg/kg.
    - There was no significant difference between treatment groups concerning the primary outcome of the clinical cessation of seizure activity 5 min after completing the study drug's infusion.
    - The study authors concluded that levetiracetam is not superior to phenytoin for second-line pediatric convulsive status epilepticus. (Lancet. 2019 May 25;393(10186):2135-2145.)
- **EcLiPSE**
    - This was an open-label, multicenter trial that randomized children between the ages of 6 months to under 18 years with convulsive status epilepticus requiring second-line treatment to either levetiracetam 40 mg/kg over 5 min or phenytoin 20 mg/kg over at least 20 min.
    - There was no significant difference in the primary outcome of time from randomization to cessation of convulsive status epilepticus
    - The median time from randomization to the cessation of convulsive status epilepticus was similar.
    - The authors concluded that although levetiracetam was not significantly superior to phenytoin, the results, together with previously reported safety profiles and comparative ease of administration of levetiracetam, suggest it could be an appropriate alternative to phenytoin as the first-choice, second-line anticonvulsant in the treatment of pediatric convulsive status epilepticus. (Lancet. 2019 May 25;393(10186):2125-2134.)
- **Brivaracetam Combination Phase III Study**
    - This was a double-blind, placebo-controlled, multicenter study that randomized patients with uncontrolled partial-onset seizures despite ongoing treatment with 1-2 antiepileptic drugs to receive either brivaracetam 100 mg/day, brivaracetam 200mg/day, or placebo.
    - Both doses of brivaracetam significantly improved the co-primary efficacy outcomes of the percent reduction over placebo in 28-day adjusted partial-onset seizure frequency, and at least a 50% responder rate was based on percent reduction in partial-onset seizure frequency from baseline to the treatment period compared to placebo.
    - More patients receiving brivaracetam experienced adverse events leading to drug discontinuation compared with patients randomized to placebo.
    - The authors concluded that adjunctive brivaracetam at doses of 100 and 200 mg/day effectively reduced partial-onset seizures in adults without concomitant levetiracetam use and was well tolerated. (Epilepsia. 2015 Dec;56(12):1890-8.)

High-Yield Fast-Fact
- **Controlled Substance**
    - Unlike levetiracetam, which is not controlled, brivaracetam is a scheduled C-V medication.

HIGH-YIELD BOARD EXAM ESSENTIALS
- **CLASSIC AGENTS:** Brivaracetam, levetiracetam
- **DRUG CLASS:** SV2A Protein-Ligand
- **INDICATIONS:** Seizures, status epileptics
- **MECHANISM:** Selectively bind to the SV2A receptor in synaptic vesicles, reducing the release of glutamate during high-frequency activity.
- **SIDE EFFECTS:** Ataxia, CNS depression
- **CLINICAL PEARLS:**
    - Brivaracetam may decrease the elimination of 10,11-carbamazepine epoxide, the active metabolite of carbamazepine. The 10,11-carbamazepine epoxide is associated with neurologic toxicities and can be therapeutically monitored with a normal range of 1 to 10 mg/L.
    - The oral bioavailability of both agents is the same as IV (or close enough) to allow for easier dosing where the oral and IV dose are the same.
    - Levetiracetam needs to be renally dose adjusted.

Table: Drug Class Summary

SV2A Protein-Ligand - Drug Class Review			
High-Yield Med Reviews			
Mechanism of Action: *Selectively bind to the SV2A receptor in synaptic vesicles, reducing glutamate during high-frequency activity.*			
Class Effects: *Broad antiepileptic activity with wide therapeutic window and relatively safe adverse event profile compared to other antiepileptic drugs.*			
Generic Name	**Brand Name**	**Indication(s) or Uses**	**Notes**

Brivaracetam	Briviact	- Partial onset seizures	- **Dosing (Adult):**
			  - Oral/IV: 25 to 100 mg q12h
			- **Dosing (Peds):**
			  - Oral/IV: 0.5 to 1.25 mg/kg/dose q12h
			    - Maximum 5 mg/kg/day or 200 mg/day
			- **CYP450 Interactions:** Substrate CYP2C19
			- **Renal or Hepatic Dose Adjustments:**
			  - Child-Pugh class A, B, or C - Initial 25 mg q12h to maximum 75 mg q12h
			- **Dosage Forms:** Oral (solution, tablet), IV (solution)

Levetiracetam	Keppra	- Seizures
		- Status epileptics
			- **Dosing (Adult):**
			  - Oral/IV: 500 to 2,000 mg q12-24h
			  - IV: 60 mg/kg once, maximum 4,500 mg
			- **Dosing (Peds):**
			  - Oral/IV: 7 to 21 mg/kg/dose q12h
			    - Maximum 3,000 mg/day
			  - IV: 60 mg/kg once; Maximum 4,500 mg
			- **CYP450 Interactions:** None
			- **Renal or Hepatic Dose Adjustments:**
			  - GFR 30 to 50 mL/minute: 250 to 750 mg q12h
			  - GFR 15 to 30 mL/minute: 250 to 500 mg q12h
			  - < 15 mL/minute: 250 to 500 mg q24h
			- **Dosage Forms:** Oral (solution, tablet), IV (solution)

NEUROLOGY – VOLTAGE-GATED CALCIUM CHANNEL BLOCKERS

Drug Class
- Voltage-Gated Calcium Channel Blockers
- Agents:
  - Chronic Care
    - Ethosuximide
    - Zonisamide

Main Indications or Uses
- Chronic Care
  - Absence seizures
    - Ethosuximide
  - Focal/Partial Seizures
    - Zonisamide

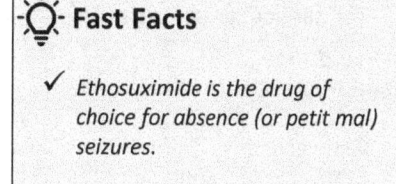

Fast Facts
- ✓ Ethosuximide is the drug of choice for absence (or petit mal) seizures.

Mechanism of Action
- Inhibition of voltage-gated T-type calcium channels, decreasing thalamic neuronal transmission.

Primary Net Benefit
- Antiepileptics with calcium channel blocking properties are useful for absence seizure treatment.

High-Yield Basic Pharmacology
- Zonisamide
  - Also inhibits voltage-dependent sodium channels, and glutamate release, and is a weak inhibitor of carbonic anhydrase.
    - At lower doses than those used in epilepsy, it may inhibit MAO-B and because of this has some data for use in Parkinson's disease though this is not a labeled indication.

High-Yield Clinical Knowledge
- Dosing, Dosage Forms, and/or Administration
  - Ethosuximide can be dosed once daily whereas zonisamide is administered once or twice daily.
  - Caution in renal and hepatic impairment as no dose adjustments exist in product labeling for ethosuximide, but the medicine has warnings related to possible hepatic and renal impairment.
  - Zonisamide should be avoided if eCrCl < 50 mL/min.
- Contraindications
  - Zonisamide in those with sulfonamide hypersensitivity because it is a sulfonamide drug, renal impairment (eCrCl < 50 mL/min).
- Warnings
  - CNS depression, skin reactions (including Stevens-Johnson Syndrome), hepatic impairment, renal impairment, and suicidal thoughts.
  - Ethosuximide: Blood dyscrasias, drug-induced immune thrombocytopenia, hypersensitivity (drug reaction with eosinophilia and systemic symptoms), and systemic lupus erythematosus.
  - Zonisamide: Encephalopathy, metabolic acidosis (weak carbonic anhydrase inhibitor), psychiatric symptoms (depression, psychosis, psychomotor slowing), skin reactions (toxic epidermal necrolysis), and in those with a sulfa allergy.
- Adverse Effects
  - **Ethosuximide:** Although the most common adverse events with ethosuximide therapy are GI complaints, there is a risk of CNS effects, including Parkinson-like symptoms, behavioral effects in patients with a history of psychiatric disorders, Stevens-Johnson syndrome, lupus erythematosus, and leukopenia, thrombocytopenia, pancytopenia, and aplastic anemia.
  - **Zonisamide:** Agranulocytosis, anorexia, sedation, dizziness, confusion, headache, renal stones, Stevens-Johnson syndrome, and toxic epidermal necrolysis.
  - **Skin Reactions:** Zonisamide and ethosuximide are associated with the rare occurrence of Stevens-Johnson syndrome and toxic epidermal necrolysis (zonisamide).
- Drug, Supplement, Food, and/or Disease Interactions
  - CNS depressants due to additive effects.
  - CYP 3A4 substrate so strong inducers may cause decreased levels of ethosuximide.
- Monitoring
  - Mood changes and suicidality at each appointment.
  - Liver enzymes (AST/ALT), and liver function (albumin, protein, bilirubin, INR) periodically.
  - CBC with differential at baseline and periodically.
  - Serum creatinine at baseline and periodically.
  - Therapeutic drug monitoring
    - Ethosuximide: 40 to 100 mcg/mL
    - Zonisamide: 10 to 40 mcg/mL
  - Ammonia level (encephalopathy) and serum bicarbonate with zonisamide.
- Patient Education

- It is important to be adherent with medications and appointments.
- Medications utilized in the treatment of seizures should be gradually tapered to be discontinued.
- Ethosuximide can be used in pregnancy (crosses placenta with birth defects reported) and lactation, if necessary, with close monitoring. If used baseline serum concentrations should be evaluated to target a patient-specific level during pregnancy.
- It is important to have blood monitoring with ethosuximide due to the risk of blood dyscrasias.
- Zonisamide: crosses the placenta, limited information in pregnancy; present in breast milk.

High-Yield Core Evidence
- **Childhood Absence Seizures**
  - This double-blind, controlled clinical trial randomized children with newly diagnosed childhood absence epilepsy to receive ethosuximide, valproic acid, or lamotrigine.
  - Ethosuximide and valproic acid had a similar frequency of freedom-from-failure rates (the primary outcome). Compared with lamotrigine, both ethosuximide and valproic acid had significantly better freedom rates from treatment failure after 16 weeks of therapy.
  - There were no differences between groups for discontinuation because of adverse events.
  - The authors concluded that ethosuximide and valproic acid are more effective than lamotrigine in the treatment of childhood absence epilepsy. Ethosuximide is associated with less adverse attention effects.
  - N Engl J Med. 2010;362(9):790-799.

High-Yield Fast-Facts
- **Eating Disorders**
  - Zonisamide should be used with caution in patients with eating disorders. It can be used off-label as a treatment for binge eating disorder. Disorders such as anorexia or bulimia may be acutely worsened or manifest in patients without such disorders.

 HIGH-YIELD BOARD EXAM ESSENTIALS
- **CLASSIC AGENTS:** Ethosuximide, zonisamide
- **DRUG CLASS:** Voltage-gated calcium channel blockers
- **INDICATIONS:** Absence seizures, focal seizures
- **MECHANISM:** Inhibition of voltage-gated T-type calcium channels, decreasing thalamic neuronal transmission.
- **SIDE EFFECTS:** CNS depression, pancreatitis, hepatotoxicity, skin reactions, and coma.
- **CLINICAL PEARLS:**
  - Caution with ethosuximide in renal and hepatic impairment as no dose adjustments exist in product labeling, but the medicine has warnings related to possible hepatic and renal impairment.
  - Zonisamide should be avoided if eCrCl < 50 mL/min.
  - Monitor closely and advise the patient to report any skin changes.

Table: Drug Class Summary

| Voltage-Gated Calcium Channel Blockers - Drug Class Review ||||
High-Yield Med Reviews			
Mechanism of Action: *Inhibition of voltage-gated T-type calcium channels, decreasing thalamic neuronal transmission.*			
Class Effects: *Antiepileptics with calcium channel blocking properties are useful for absence seizure treatment.*			
Generic Name	**Brand Name**	**Main Indication(s)**	**Notes**
Ethosuximide	Zarontin	• Absence seizures	• **Dosing (Adult):** Oral: 500 to 1,500 mg/day in divided doses • **Dosing (Peds):** Oral: 10 mg/kg/day divided q12h – Maximum 60 mg/kg/day or 2,000 mg/day • **CYP450 Interactions:** Substrate CYP3A4 • **Renal or Hepatic Dose Adjustments:** None recommended in product labeling • **Dosage Forms:** Oral (capsule, solution)
Zonisamide	Zonegran	• Focal seizures	• **Dosing (Adult):** Oral: 100 mg/day titrated to 600 mg/day in 100 mg increments every 7 days • **Dosing (Peds):** Oral: 1 to 2 mg/kg/day slowly titrating up to 5 to 8 mg/kg/day – Maximum 12 mg/kg/day • **CYP450 Interactions:** Substrate of CYP2C19, CYP3A4 • **Renal or Hepatic Dose Adjustments:** GFR < 50 mL/minute: use not recommended • **Dosage Forms:** Oral (capsule)

NEUROLOGY – ANTIMIGRAINE – CALCITONIN GENE-RELATED PEPTIDE RECEPTOR ANTAGONIST

Drug Class
- Calcitonin Gene-Related Peptide (CGRP) Receptor Antagonist
- Agents:
  - Acute & Chronic Care
    - Atogepant
    - Eptinezumab
    - Erenumab
    - Fremanezumab
    - Galcanezumab
    - Rimegepant
    - Ubrogepant
    - Zavegepant

> **Fast Facts**
> ✓ The dosage forms that can be given by mouth end with "-epant" and those that are parenterally administered end with "-mab".
>
> ✓ This drug class has increased in its use and options due to benefits in both the prevention and acute treatment of migraine headache.

Main Indications or Uses
- Acute Care
  - Migraine treatment (rimegepant, ubrogepant, zavegepant)
- Chronic Care
  - Migraine prophylaxis (atogepant, eptinezumab, erenumab, fremanezumab, galcanezumab)

Mechanism of Action
- **Eptinezumab, Erenumab, Galcanezumab, Fremanezumab**
  - Human monoclonal antibodies bind to and inhibit the CGRP receptor function.
- **Atogepant, Rimegepant, Ubrogepant, Zavegepant**
  - Small molecule antagonist of the CGRP receptor.

Primary Net Benefit
- Acute and chronic migraine pharmacotherapy that applies novel therapeutic targets and improves safety and efficacy compared to existing antimigraine therapeutics.
- Main Labs to Monitor:
  - No routine labs

High-Yield Basic Pharmacology
- **CGRP and Migraine**
  - CGRP is a neuropeptide with a strong association with migraine and cluster headaches.
  - CGRP levels are acutely elevated in the cerebral circulation during a migraine and decrease in response to triptans, dihydroergotamine, or onabotulinumtoxinA.
- **Umabs and Zumabs**
  - Of the CGRP-mab agents, erenumab is a fully human monoclonal antibody, whereas eptinezumab, galcanezumab, and fremanezumab are humanized murine or yeast antibodies.
- **Molecule Size**
  - The monoclonal antibodies are too large to cross the blood-brain barrier and exert antimigraine activity outside the CNS at the trigeminal nerve ending.
  - Conversely, the small molecule CGRP antagonists atogepant, rimegepant, ubrogepant, and zavegepant can work both within and outside the CNS.

High-Yield Clinical Knowledge
- **Combination Therapy**
  - The anti-CGRP agents are novel advances in migraine therapy that, in addition to an established efficacy, can be combined with other existing migraine pharmacotherapy, including triptans.
  - This offers multimodal pharmacotherapy intervention in patients with treatment-resistant migraines and avoids other drug therapies such as valproic acid, tricyclic antidepressants, or opioids.

- **Preventative Therapy**
    - Anti-CGRP pharmacotherapy is an alternative to topiramate for the prevention of episodic migraine.
    - Although there are no prospective head-to-head trials, anti-CGRP agents are associated with relatively mild adverse events, including upper respiratory tract infection and injection site pain.
        - Topiramate has been associated with anorexia, fatigue, memory problems, and paresthesias.
- **Safety**
    - Compared to existing antimigraine pharmacotherapy, the anti-CGRP agents do not risk serotonin syndrome, diminished sexual function and drive, or complicating existing coronary artery disease, angina, history of stroke, transient ischemic attack, or ischemic bowel disease.
- **Neutralizing Antibodies**
    - Neutralizing antibodies have been observed in 7 to 12% of patients exposed to eptinezumab, erenumab, or galcanezumab.
    - Fremanezumab is associated with a much lower incidence of neutralizing antibody development of 0.3 to 1.1%.
- **Administration**
    - Eptinezumab administration requires IV infusion, often taking place in a healthcare setting.
    - The remaining parenteral agents (erenumab, galcanezumab, fremanezumab) are all administered subcutaneously, which can be done by the patient, and on an every 1 to 3-month schedule.
    - Atogepant, rimegepant and ubrogepant are oral agents. Note the ending "-epant".
- **Every Other Day**
    - Oral rimegepant can be used to treat or prevent migraines but is taken on an every-other-day schedule, which may not be suitable for patients who may have difficulty with compliance.

High-Yield Core Evidence
- **LIBERTY**
    - This was a multicenter, double-blind, placebo-controlled trial of patients with a history of episodic migraine with or without aura for at least 12 months, had migraine for an average of 4-14 days per month during the three months before screening and had been treated unsuccessfully with between two and four preventive treatments.
    - Eligible patients were randomized to receive either erenumab 140 mg q4weeks or placebo q4weeks for 12 weeks.
    - Erenumab was associated with a significantly greater proportion of patients achieving a 50% or greater reduction in the mean number of monthly migraine days during weeks 9-12.
    - The tolerability and safety profiles of erenumab and placebo were similar, with injection site pain being the most commonly reported adverse event but similar between groups.
    - Compared with placebo, the authors concluded that erenumab was efficacious in patients with episodic migraine who previously did not respond to or tolerate between two and four previous migraine preventive treatments. (Lancet. 2018;392:2280-2287.)
- **Rimegepant Phase 2/3 Trial**
    - This was a multicenter, phase 2/3, double-blind, placebo-controlled trial that randomized adult patients with at least a one-year history of migraine.
    - After a 4-week observation period, they were randomized to either oral rimegepant 75 mg or matching placebo every other day for 12 weeks.
    - Patients randomized to rimegepant experienced a significantly fewer number of migraine days per month in the last four weeks of the double-blind treatment phase (weeks 9–12) compared to placebo.
    - A similar proportion of patients experienced adverse events, none of which were severe.
    - The authors concluded that taken every other day, rimegepant was adequate for the preventive treatment of migraine. Tolerability was similar to that of a placebo, and no severe or unexpected safety issues were noted. (Lancet. 2021;397:P51-60.)

High-Yield Fast-Fact
- **OnabotulinumtoxinA and CGRP**
    - OnabotulinumtoxinA has exhibited anti-CGRP properties in animal models by blocking necrotizing fasciitis due to S. pyogenes.

HIGH-YIELD BOARD EXAM ESSENTIALS
- **CLASSIC AGENTS:** Atogepant, eptinezumab, erenumab, fremanezumab, galcanezumab, rimegepant, ubrogepant
- **DRUG CLASS:** CGRP Receptor Antagonist
- **INDICATIONS:** Migraine treatment/prophylaxis
- **MECHANISM:** Human monoclonal antibodies bind to, and inhibit the CGRP receptor function (eptinezumab, erenumab, galcanezumab, fremanezumab); Small molecule antagonist of the CGRP receptor (atogepant, rimegepant, ubrogepant)
- **SIDE EFFECTS:** Neutralizing antibody formation
- **CLINICAL PEARLS:**
    - Compared to existing antimigraine pharmacotherapy, the anti-CGRP agents do not risk serotonin syndrome, diminished sexual function and drive, or complicating existing coronary artery disease, angina, history of stroke, transient ischemic attack, or ischemic bowel disease.
    - The agents ending with "-mab" are all biologic agents (i.e., monoclonal antibodies) that we require parenteral administration but have longer half-lives.

Table: Drug Class Summary

Calcitonin Gene-Related Peptide Receptor Antagonist - Drug Class Review High-Yield Med Reviews			
Mechanism of Action: Eptinezumab, Erenumab, Galcanezumab, Fremanezumab - Human monoclonal antibodies bind to, and inhibit the CGRP receptor function. Atogepant, Rimegepant, Ubrogepant, Zavegepant - Small molecule antagonist of the CGRP receptor.			
Class Effects: Acute and chronic migraine pharmacotherapy with novel therapeutic targets, improves safety and efficacy			
Generic Name	**Brand Name**	**Main Indication(s) or Uses**	**Notes**
Atogepant	Qulipta	• Migraine prophylaxis	• **Dosing (Adult):** — PO: 10, 30, or 60 mg daily • **Dosing (Peds):** — Not routinely used • **CYP450 Interactions:** None • **Renal or Hepatic Dose Adjustments:** — CrCl < 30 mL/min: 10 mg daily — Child-Pugh Class C: Not recommended • **Dosage Forms:** Oral (tablet)
Eptinezumab	Vyepti	• Migraine prophylaxis	• **Dosing (Adult):** — IV: 100 to 300 mg q3months • **Dosing (Peds):** — Not routinely used • **CYP450 Interactions:** None • **Renal or Hepatic Dose Adjustments:** None • **Dosage Forms:** IV (solution)
Erenumab	Aimovig	• Migraine prophylaxis	• **Dosing (Adult):** — SQ: 70 to 140 mg q1month • **Dosing (Peds):** — Not routinely used • **CYP450 Interactions:** None • **Renal or Hepatic Dose Adjustments:** None • **Dosage Forms:** Subcutaneous (solution)
Fremanezumab	Ajovy	• Migraine prophylaxis	• **Dosing (Adult):** — SQ: 225 or 675 mg q3months • **Dosing (Peds):** — Not routinely used • **CYP450 Interactions:** None • **Renal or Hepatic Dose Adjustments:** None • **Dosage Forms:** Subcutaneous (solution)
Galcanezumab	Emgality	• Migraine prophylaxis	• **Dosing (Adult):** — SQ: 120 to 300 mg q1months • **Dosing (Peds):** — Not routinely used • **CYP450 Interactions:** None • **Renal or Hepatic Dose Adjustments:** None • **Dosage Forms:** Subcutaneous (solution)

| Calcitonin Gene-Related Peptide Receptor Antagonist - Drug Class Review ||||
| High-Yield Med Reviews ||||
Generic Name	Brand Name	Main Indication(s) or Uses	Notes

Rimegepant	Nurtec	• Migraine prophylaxis	• **Dosing (Adult):**
			  – Oral: 75 mg every other day
			  – Oral: 75 mg once for migraine treatment
			• **Dosing (Peds):**
			  – Not routinely used
			• **CYP450 Interactions:** None
			• **Renal or Hepatic Dose Adjustments:**
			  – GFR < 15 mL/minute - Avoid use
			  – Child-Pugh class C - Avoid use
			• **Dosage Forms:** Oral (tablet disintegrating)

Ubrogepant	Ubrelvy	• Migraine prophylaxis	• **Dosing (Adult):**
			  – Oral: 50 to 100 mg x 1, may repeat once
			    – Maximum 200 mg/day
			• **Dosing (Peds):**
			  – Not routinely used
			• **CYP450 Interactions:** None
			• **Renal or Hepatic Dose Adjustments:**
			  – GFR < 15 to 29 mL/minute: Maximum 100 mg/day
			  – GFR < 15 mL/minute: Avoid use
			  – Child-Pugh class C: Maximum 100 mg/day
			• **Dosage Forms:** Oral (tablet)

Zavegepant	Zavzpret	• Acute, Severe Migraine Treatment	• **Dosing (Adult):**
			  – Intranasal: 1 spray (10 mg/spray) in 1 nostril x 1 dose
			    – Max dose: 1 spray per 24 hrs
			• **Dosing (Peds):**
			  – Not routinely used
			• **CYP450 Interactions:**
			  – Minor substrate: CYP2D6, 3A4, OATP1B1/1B3, P-gp
			• **Renal or Hepatic Dose Adjustments:**
			  – GFR < 30 mL/minute: Avoid use
			  – Child-Pugh class C: Avoid use
			• **Dosage Forms:** Intranasal Spray

NEUROLOGY – ANTIMIGRAINE AGENTS – SEROTONIN 5-HT1B/D RECEPTOR AGONISTS

Drug Class
- Antimigraine Agents
- Agents:
    - Acute
        - Almotriptan
        - Dihydroergotamine
        - Eletriptan
        - Ergotamine
        - Frovatriptan
        - Lasmiditan
        - Naratriptan
        - Rizatriptan
        - Sumatriptan
        - Zolmitriptan

> **Warnings & Alerts**
> ✓ This drug class should ONLY be used for the acute abortive treatment of migraine headache and limited to 1-2 doses to avoid the development of overuse headaches.
>
> ✓ Injectable options can sometimes cause chest pain (discomfort or pressure sensation).

Main Indications or Uses
- Acute Care
    - Migraine

Mechanism of Action
- Selective agonists of the 5HT-5HT-1D/1B (triptans) or non-selective 5HT-1D/1B agonists mediating cerebral vessel dilation, blocking the release of substance P and calcitonin gene-related peptide (CGRP) from the trigeminal nucleus caudalis).

Primary Net Benefit
- Compared to ergot derivatives, triptans evolved migraine care by maintaining abortive efficacy and improving safety.
- Main Labs to Monitor:
    - No routine monitoring

High-Yield Basic Pharmacology
- Natural Ergot Production
    - The fungus Claviceps purpurea that grows on grains like rye produces ergot, an alkaloid with partial agonist or antagonist effects on adrenergic, dopaminergic, and serotonergic receptors.
- Ergot Actions
    - The pharmacologic action of ergot alkaloids extends beyond 5HT-1B/1D agonist properties, as they interact with numerous serotonin receptors, including 1A, 1F, 2A, 2C, 3, and 4, in addition to dopamine and adrenergic receptors.
- Excess Serotonin Effects
    - In addition to the beneficial therapeutic effects, SSRIs increase serotonergic tone throughout the body, causing various, specifically gastrointestinal distress, early after initiation but resolving after one week of treatment.
        - The excess serotonergic activity has also been associated with diminished sexual function and drive.

High-Yield Clinical Knowledge
- Migraine Treatment
    - The triptans are effective in managing acute migraines and should not be used for the prevention of migraines.
        - Triptans must be administered as soon as possible after the onset of migraine signs and symptoms for maximum abortive efficacy.

- **Coronary Artery Disease**
  - All triptans are contraindicated in patients with coronary artery disease, angina, history of stroke, transient ischemic attack, or ischemic bowel disease.
  - Additional contraindications exist for specific triptans, including
    - Eletriptan, frovatriptan, and naratriptan are contraindicated in patients with peripheral vascular disease.
    - Eletriptan and naratriptan are contraindicated in patients with severe renal or hepatic impairment.
    - Patients with Wolff-Parkinson-White syndrome should not receive zolmitriptan.
- **Serotonin Syndrome**
  - Serotonin syndrome is the combination of a rapid onset of altered mental status, autonomic instability, hyperthermia, and hyperreflexia/myoclonus.
  - Triptans, dihydroergotamine, and ergotamine have been implicated in serotonin syndrome and other antidepressants, including MAO inhibitors, contribute to serotonin toxicity.
  - To reduce the likelihood of serotonin syndrome, most triptans may only be administered once or twice (depending on the agent) in 24 hours and cannot be combined with ergot derivatives.
  - Treatment of serotonin syndrome involves the management of hyperthermia through invasive or noninvasive cooling, skeletal muscle relaxation using benzodiazepines, and airway support.
    - Dantrolene and cyproheptadine have been suggested as adjuncts for managing serotonin syndrome but are of questionable patient-oriented benefit.
- **Ergotism**
  - Excessive ergot alkaloid use or administration may produce ergotism, characterized by the extremities' intense burning sensation, hemorrhagic vesiculation, gangrene, pruritus, formication, nausea, and vomiting.
  - Convulsive ergotism includes additional central effects such as headache, fixed miosis, hallucinations, delirium, cerebrovascular ischemia, and seizures.
  - Although excessive doses can cause ergotism, interactions with CYP3A4 inhibitors can also lead to ergotism.
- **Triptan Duration**
  - In many patients, the duration of the migraine is longer than the duration of effect for triptans.
  - All triptans except almotriptan and lasmiditan can be administered twice in acute migraine episodes.
    - Almotriptan and lasmiditan may only be administered once.

High-Yield Core Evidence
- **Subcutaneous Sumatriptan International Study Group**
  - This was a multicenter, double-blind, placebo-controlled, parallel-group clinical trial that randomized patients with migraine to receive either sumatriptan 6 mg SQ or 8 mg SQ or placebo and assessed associated migraine symptoms 30, 60, and 120 minutes after treatment.
  - Among patients who were not pain-free at 60 minutes, they were permitted to receive an additional administration of the study medication they were initially randomized to.
  - Patients randomized to either dose of sumatriptan achieved significant reductions in the severity of headache compared to placebo.
  - The response rates did not differ significantly among the sumatriptan regimens, and adverse events were minor and transient in all groups.
  - The authors concluded that a single 6-mg dose of sumatriptan given subcutaneously is a highly effective, rapid-acting, and well-tolerated treatment for migraine attacks. The administration of a second dose 60 minutes later to patients not responding well to an initial amount affords little additional benefit. (N Engl J Med 1991; 325:316-321.)

- **Headache Recurrence After ED Discharge**
    - This was a double-blind trial that randomized patients after initial treatment of primary headache in the ED with a recurrent primary headache to receive either naproxen 500 mg or sumatriptan 100 mg for headache recurrence after ED discharge.
    - Outcomes were assessed by telephone 48 hours after ED discharge.
    - There was no significant difference between groups concerning the primary endpoint of the between-group difference in change in pain intensity during the 2 hours after ingestion of either 500 mg naproxen or 100 mg sumatriptan.
    - Furthermore, findings were virtually identical among the migraine subset, and most patients rated their treatment satisfaction high, as they would want to take the same medication the next time.
    - Adverse effect profiles were also comparable.
    - The authors concluded that nearly three-quarters of patients reported headache recurrence within 48 hours of ED discharge, and naproxen 500 mg and sumatriptan 100 mg taken orally to relieve post-ED recurrent primary headache and migraine comparably. (Ann Emerg Med. 2010 Jul;56(1):7-17.)

High-Yield Fast-Fact
- **LSD**
    - Lysergic acid diethylamide, otherwise known as LSD, is an ergotamine alkaloid and a derivative of ergot.

HIGH-YIELD BOARD EXAM ESSENTIALS
- **CLASSIC AGENTS:** Almotriptan, dihydroergotamine, eletriptan, ergotamine, frovatriptan, lasmiditan, naratriptan, rizatriptan, sumatriptan, zolmitriptan
- **DRUG CLASS:** Antimigraine agents
- **INDICATIONS:** Migraine
- **MECHANISM:** Selective agonists of the 5HT-5HT-1D/1B (triptans) or non-selective 5HT-1D/1B agonists mediating cerebral vessel dilation, blocking the release of substance P and calcitonin gene-related peptide (CGRP) from the trigeminal nucleus caudalis).
- **SIDE EFFECTS:** Hypertension, ergotism, serotonin syndrome
- **CLINICAL PEARLS:**
    - The triptans are effective in managing acute migraines and should not be used for the prevention of migraines because they can worsen the frequency of migraines.
    - Triptans must be administered as soon as possible after the onset of migraine signs and symptoms for maximum abortive efficacy.
    - Injectable options can sometimes cause chest pain (discomfort or pressure sensation). Use with caution in patients with moderate to severe ischemic heart disease.

Table: Drug Class Summary

Antimigraine Agents - Drug Class Review High-Yield Med Reviews			
Mechanism of Action: *Selective agonists of the 5HT-5HT-1D/1B (triptans) or non-selective 5HT-1D/1B agonists mediating cerebral vessel dilation, blocking the release of substance P and calcitonin gene-related peptide (CGRP) from the trigeminal nucleus caudalis)*			
Class Effects: *Triptans evolved the care of migraine by maintaining abortive efficacy and improving safety compared to ergot derivatives.*			
Generic Name	**Brand Name**	**Main Indication(s) or Uses**	**Notes**

Almotriptan	Axert	• Migraine	• **Dosing (Adult):**
			  − Oral: 6.25 to 12.5 mg once
			    − Maximum 25 mg/day
			• **Dosing (Peds):**
			  − Oral: 6.25 to 12.5 mg once
			    − Maximum 25 mg/day
			• **CYP450 Interactions:** Substrate of CYP2D6, 3A4
			• **Renal or Hepatic Dose Adjustments:**
			  − GFR < 30 mL/minute: Max 12.5 mg/day
			• **Dosage Forms:** Oral (Tablet)

Dihydroergotamine	D.H.E, Migranal	• Migraine	• **Dosing (Adult):**
			  − IM/SQ: 1 mg at the first sign of headache then q1h as needed
			    − Maximum 3 mg/day or 6 mg/week
			  − IV: 1 mg at the first sign of headache then q1h as needed
			    − Maximum 2 mg/day or 6 mg/week
			  − Intranasal 1 spray per nostril once, repeat in 15 minutes for a total of 4 sprays.
			    − Maximum 6 sprays/24 hours or 8 sprays/week
			• **Dosing (Peds):**
			  − IV: 0.1 to 0.2 mg/dose q6h
			    − Maximum 8 doses per episodes
			• **CYP450 Interactions:** Substrate CYP3A4
			• **Renal or Hepatic Dose Adjustments:**
			  Severe renal or hepatic impairment: contraindicated
			• **Dosage Forms:** Injection solution, Nasal solution

Eletriptan	Relpax	• Migraine	• **Dosing (Adult):**
			  − Oral: 20 to 40 mg once, may repeat in 2 hours
			    − Maximum 80 mg/day
			• **Dosing (Peds):**
			  − Not routinely used
			• **CYP450 Interactions:** Substrate CYP3A4
			• **Renal or Hepatic Dose Adjustments:**
			  − Severe hepatic impairment - contraindicated
			• **Dosage Forms:** Oral (tablet)

Antimigraine Agents - Drug Class Review			
High-Yield Med Reviews			
Generic Name	**Brand Name**	**Main Indication(s) or Uses**	**Notes**
Ergotamine	Ergomar	▪ Migraine	▪ **Dosing (Adult):** – SL: 2 mg at first sign of migraine, then 2 mg q30minutes as needed – Maximum 6 mg/24 hours, 10 mg/week ▪ **Dosing (Peds):** – SL: 2 mg at first sign of migraine, then 2 mg q30minutes as needed – Maximum 6 mg/24 hours, 10 mg/week ▪ **CYP450 Interactions:** Substrate CYP3A4 ▪ **Renal or Hepatic Dose Adjustments:** – Severe renal or hepatic impairment - contraindicated ▪ **Dosage Forms:** Oral (sublingual tablet)
Frovatriptan	Frova	▪ Migraine	▪ **Dosing (Adult):** – Oral: 2.5 mg, may repeat after 2 hours – Maximum 7.5 mg/day ▪ **Dosing (Peds):** – Not routinely used ▪ **CYP450 Interactions:** Substrate CYP1A2 ▪ **Renal or Hepatic Dose Adjustments:** – Severe hepatic impairment: use with caution ▪ **Dosage Forms:** Oral (tablet)
Lasmiditan	Reyvow	▪ Migraine	▪ **Dosing (Adult):** – Oral: 50 to 200 mg once ▪ **Dosing (Peds):** – Not routinely used ▪ **CYP450 Interactions:** Substrate P-gp ▪ **Renal or Hepatic Dose Adjustments:** – Child-Pugh class C: not recommended ▪ **Dosage Forms:** Oral (tablet)
Naratriptan	Amerge	▪ Migraine	▪ **Dosing (Adult):** – Oral: 1 to 2.5 mg once, may repeat in 4 hours – Maximum 5 mg/24 hours ▪ **Dosing (Peds):** – Extra info if needed – Extra info if needed ▪ **CYP450 Interactions:** text ▪ **Renal or Hepatic Dose Adjustments:** – GFR < 15 mL/minute: contraindicated – Child-Pugh class C: contraindicated ▪ **Dosage Forms:** Oral (tablet)

Antimigraine Agents - Drug Class Review
High-Yield Med Reviews

Generic Name	Brand Name	Main Indication(s) or Uses	Notes

Rizatriptan	Maxalt	- Migraine	- **Dosing (Adult):**
			  – Oral: 5 to 10 mg once, may repeat in 2 hours
			    – Maximum 30 mg/24 hours
			- **Dosing (Peds):**
			  – Oral: 5 to 10 mg once
			- **CYP450 Interactions:** None
			- **Renal or Hepatic Dose Adjustments:** None
			- **Dosage Forms:** Oral (tablet)

Sumatriptan	Imitrex, Onzetra, Sumavel, Tosymra, Zembrace	- Cluster headache
		- Cyclic vomiting syndrome
		- Migraine
			- **Dosing (Adult):**
			  – Oral: 50 to 100 mg once, may repeat in 2 hours
			    – Maximum 100 mg/dose or 200 mg/24 hours
			  – SQ: 3 to 6 mg once
			    – Maximum 6 mg/dose or 12 mg/24 hours
			  – Nasal: 20 mg once in a single nostril contralateral to the side of headache
			    – Maximum 40 mg/24 hours
			- **Dosing (Peds):**
			  – Oral: 50 to 100 mg once, may repeat in 2 hours
			    – Maximum 100 mg/dose or 200 mg/24 hours
			  – SQ: 3 to 6 mg once
			    – Maximum 6 mg/dose or 12 mg/24 hours
			  – Nasal: 20 mg once in a single nostril contralateral to the side of headache
			    – Maximum 40 mg/24 hours
			- **CYP450 Interactions:** None
			- **Renal or Hepatic Dose Adjustments:**
			  – Severe hepatic impairment - use with caution
			- **Dosage Forms:** Oral (tablet), Nasal (powder, solution), subcutaneous solution

Antimigraine Agents - Drug Class Review High-Yield Med Reviews			
Generic Name	**Brand Name**	**Main Indication(s) or Uses**	**Notes**

Zolmitriptan	Zomig	- Migraine	- **Dosing (Adult):**
			   – Nasal: 2.5 to 10 mg at the onset of migraine
			   – Oral: 1.25 to 5 mg at the onset of migraine
			- **Dosing (Peds):**
			   – Nasal: 2.5 to 5 mg at the onset of migraine
			- **CYP450 Interactions:** Substrate CYP1A2
			- **Renal or Hepatic Dose Adjustments:**
			   – Child-Pugh class B or C: not recommended
			- **Dosage Forms:** Oral (tablet), Nasal (solution)

NEUROLOGY – BARBITURATES

Drug Class
- Barbiturates
- Agents:
    - Acute Care
        - Amobarbital
        - Methohexital
        - Phenobarbital
        - Pentobarbital
    - Chronic Care
        - Butalbital
        - Primidone

> **Fast Facts**
> - In patients with status epilepticus not responding to other standard treatments, phenobarbital or pentobarbital can be considered.
> - Primidone is metabolized to both phenobarbital and PEMA.

Main Indications or Uses
- Acute Care
    - Sedation
        - Amobarbital
        - Methohexital
        - Phenobarbital
        - Pentobarbital
    - Seizure treatment
        - Phenobarbital
        - Pentobarbital
    - Alcohol withdrawal
        - Phenobarbital
- Chronic Care
    - Headache/Migraine
        - Butalbital

Mechanism of Action
- Barbiturates bind to a specific barbiturate site on the GABA-A receptor, increasing the receptor's mean open time and intracellular influx of chloride.

Primary Net Benefit
- Dose-dependent CNS effects range from anxiolysis to sedation to coma and ultimately brain death at dosing extremes. Benzodiazepines have largely replaced use with improved safety and efficacy.
- Main Labs to Monitor:
    - Therapeutic drug monitoring
        - Phenobarbital
            - 5 to 20 mcg/mL
        - Pentobarbital
            - Sedation - 1 to 5 mcg/mL
            - Coma or intracranial pressure therapy - 30 to 40 mcg/mL

High-Yield Basic Pharmacology
- **Direct GABA-A Opening**
    - An important difference from benzodiazepines, barbiturates open GABA-A receptors independent of GABA.
    - This effect generally occurs at high concentrations and is coupled with other CNS inhibitory effects, including blocking AMPA/kainate receptors and inhibition of glutamate release.
- **Selective Antiepileptic Action**
    - Not all barbiturates possess antiepileptic properties at clinically used doses.

- Only those containing a 5-phenyl substituent (phenobarbital, pentobarbital) possess this action as conventionally used.
- **Hypnotic Dose Range**
  - As with other CNS effects, the hypnotic effects of barbiturates are dose-dependent in nature.
  - Generally, barbiturates extend the total sleep time, modify sleep stages, decrease the number of awakenings, and decrease REM sleep duration.
  - Tolerance also develops with repetitive use, where total sleep time can be cut in half after 2 weeks.
    - Conversely, rebound effects on sleep manifest as acute worsening of sleep parameters upon abrupt discontinuation.

High-Yield Clinical Knowledge
- **Tolerance, Abuse, and Dependence**
  - Barbiturates exhibit both pharmacokinetic and pharmacodynamic tolerance, each occurring at different time frames relative to drug therapy initiation.
  - The clinical implications of tolerance include narrowing the therapeutic index towards toxic ranges and cross-tolerance to other CNS depressant drugs.
    - Pharmacokinetic tolerance (equilibration of absorption, distribution, metabolism, and elimination) occurs rapidly after therapy initiation, achieving a peak within 3 to 7 days.
    - Pharmacodynamic tolerance to the euphoric, sedative and hypnotic effects occurs rapidly but develops over weeks to months.
- **CYP Inhibition-Induction**
  - Although barbiturates are known to cause induction of CYP 450 enzymes, acutely, they inhibit numerous CYP isoenzymes (1A2, 2C9, 2C19, 3A4), affecting both numerous medications and endogenous steroids.
  - With chronic administration, barbiturates cause numerous hepatic functions including CYP 450 oxidation (namely 1A2, 2C9, 2C19, 2E1, 3A4).
    - Just as with inhibition, induction of hepatic oxidation also increases the metabolism of numerous drugs and endogenous substances, including steroids, hormones, cholesterol, and vitamin K.
- **Respiratory Depression**
  - Barbiturates possess many respiratory depressant effects, including decreasing respiratory drive, hypoxic drive, chemoreceptor drive, and protective reflexes.
    - In the CNS, the respiratory drive is fully suppressed at three times normal anesthetic doses.
- **Cardiovascular System**
  - Barbiturates can cause vasodilation during rapid IV administration and decrease reflex responses via partial inhibition of ganglionic transmission.
    - Compensatory mechanisms are thus impaired, particularly in patients with heart failure, hypovolemic shock, and acute stroke (dependent on cerebral blood flow).

High-Yield Core Evidence
- **"The VA Study"**
  - This landmark clinical trial was a double-blind, multicenter trial that randomized patients with overt generalized status epilepticus or subtle status epilepticus to one of four intravenous regimens: diazepam followed by phenytoin, lorazepam, phenobarbital, and phenytoin.
  - Patients randomized to lorazepam experienced significantly superior successful treatment outcomes compared with phenytoin.
    - Treatment was considered successful when all motor and electroencephalographic seizure activity ceased within 20 minutes after the beginning of the drug infusion. There was no return of seizure activity during the next 40 minutes.
  - Overall, patients randomized to lorazepam, 64.9% experienced successful seizure control, those randomized to phenobarbital 58.2%, diazepam plus phenytoin 55.8%, and phenytoin 43.6%.
    - The intention-to-treat analysis discovered no significant differences among treatment groups, including patients with overt status epilepticus or those with subtle status epilepticus.
  - No differences were observed among the treatments concerning recurrence during the 12-hour study period, the incidence of adverse reactions, or the outcome at 30 days.

- The authors concluded that initial intravenous treatment for overt generalized convulsive status epilepticus, lorazepam is more effective than phenytoin. Although lorazepam is no more efficacious than phenobarbital or diazepam plus phenytoin, it is easier to use. (N Engl J Med. 1998;339(12):792.)
- **Status Epilepticus Treatment**
  - This was a non-blinded clinical trial of 36 consecutive patients with generalized convulsive status epilepticus randomized to receive either combination diazepam and phenytoin or phenobarbital.
  - Patients randomized to phenobarbital had a shorter cumulative convulsion time, median cumulative convulsion time, and response latency compared to the group receiving phenytoin and diazepam.
  - However, the frequencies of intubation, hypotension, and arrhythmias were similar in the two groups.
  - The authors concluded that the phenobarbital regimen is rapidly effective, comparable in safety, and enjoys certain practical advantages compared to the diazepam plus phenytoin regimen. (Neurology. 1988;38(2):202.)

High-Yield Fast-Facts
- **The Amytal Interview**
  - Amobarbital was once used to facilitate interviews of patients as a means of managing psychiatric disorders.
  - This therapy, popularized in the 1930s, was abandoned by the 1960s once evidence questioned its benefits.
  - Contemporary use of the Amytal interview has been considered, particularly with renewed interest in psilocybin and other psychotropic facilitated patient therapy interventions.
- **Thiopental in the US**
  - Thiopental is often described in textbooks and literature; however, it is not available in the United States.
- **Primidone (2-desoxyphenobarbital)**
  - Primidone is a prodrug releasing phenobarbital after metabolism.

HIGH-YIELD BOARD EXAM ESSENTIALS
- **CLASSIC AGENTS:** Amobarbital, butalbital, methohexital, phenobarbital, pentobarbital, primidone
- **DRUG CLASS:** Barbiturates
- **INDICATIONS:** Alcohol withdrawal treatment, headache/migraine, sedation, seizure treatment
- **MECHANISM:** Bind to a specific barbiturate site on the GABA-A receptor, increasing the mean open time of the receptor, thus increasing the influx of chloride intracellularly
- **SIDE EFFECTS:** Respiratory depression, altered mental status, hypotension, decreased cardiac output
- **CLINICAL PEARLS:** Although barbiturates are known to cause induction of CYP 450 enzymes, acutely, they inhibit numerous CYP isoenzymes (1A2, 2C9, 2C19, 3A4), affecting both numerous medications and endogenous steroids. With chronic administration, barbiturates cause numerous hepatic functions including CYP 450 oxidation (namely 1A2, 2C9, 2C19, 2E1, 3A4).

Table: Drug Class Summary

Barbiturates - Drug Class Review High-Yield Med Reviews			
Mechanism of Action: *Barbiturates bind to a specific barbiturate site on the GABA-A receptor, increasing the mean open time of the receptor, thus increasing the influx of chloride intracellularly.*			
Class Effects: *Dose-dependent CNS effects ranging from anxiolysis to sedation to coma and ultimately brain death at dosing extremes. Benzodiazepines have largely replaced use with improved safety and efficacy.*			
Generic Name	**Brand Name**	**Main Indication(s) or Uses**	**Notes**

Amobarbital	Amytal Sodium	• Sedative/hypnotic	• **Dosing (Adult):**]
			  – IM/IV: 30 to 200 mg q8-24h
			    – Maximum 1,000 mg/dose
			• **Dosing (Peds):**
			  – IM/IV: 2 to 3 mg/kg/dose
			    – Maximum 500 mg/dose
			• **CYP450 Interactions:** CYP Inducer
			• **Renal or Hepatic Dose Adjustments:** None
			• **Dosage Forms:** IV (solution)

Butalbital	Butisol (others in combination): Fioricet Fiornal Esgic	• Sedative/hypnotic
		• Tension headache
			• **Dosing (Adult):**
			  – Oral: 15 to 100 mg q6-24h
			• **Dosing (Peds):**
			  – Oral: 2 to 6 mg/kg/dose before surgery
			    – Maximum 100 mg/dose
			• **CYP450 Interactions:** CYP Inducer
			• **Renal or Hepatic Dose Adjustments:** None
			• **Dosage Forms:** Oral (capsule, tablet)

Methohexital	Brevital	• Anesthesia
		• Sedative/hypnotic
			• **Dosing (Adult):**
			  – IV: 0.5 to 1.5 mg/kg q2-5 minutes as needed
			• **Dosing (Peds):**
			  – IM: 6.6 to 25 mg/kg/dose
			    – Maximum 500 mg/dose
			  – IV: 0.5 to 2 mg/kg/dose
			    – Maximum 500 mg/dose
			• **CYP450 Interactions:** CYP Inducer
			• **Renal or Hepatic Dose Adjustments:** None
			• **Dosage Forms:** IV (solution)

Barbiturates - Drug Class Review
High-Yield Med Reviews

Generic Name	Brand Name	Main Indication(s) or Uses	Notes

Phenobarbital	Luminal	- Anesthesia
		- Sedative/hypnotic
		- Seizures
			- **Dosing (Adult):**
			  – Oral/IM/IV: 30 to 260 mg/kg q6-12h
			    – Maximum 400 mg/day
			  – IV: 15 to 20 mg/kg IV
			- **Dosing (Peds):**
			  – Oral: 2 to 5 mg/kg/dose
			    – Maximum 500 mg/dose
			  – IV: 10 to 20 mg/kg/dose
			    – Maximum 1000 mg/dose
			- **CYP450 Interactions:** CYP Inducer (CYP 1A2, 2A6, 2B6, 2C9, 3A4); Substrate of CYP2C19, 2C9, 2E1
			- **Renal or Hepatic Dose Adjustments:**
			  – GFR < 10 mL/minute: Decrease to q12-16 hours
			- **Dosage Forms:** Oral (elixir, tablet, solution), IV (solution)

Pentobarbital	Nembutal	- Anesthesia
		- Barbiturate coma
		- Sedative/hypnotic
			- **Dosing (Adult):**
			  – IM: 150 to 200 mg x1
			  – IV: bolus 5 to 15 mg/kg
			  – IV: infusion 0.5 to 5 mg/kg/hour
			- **Dosing (Peds):**
			  – IM: 2 to 6 mg/kg/dose
			    – Maximum 100 mg/dose
			  – IV: 1 to 15 mg/kg infusion
			    – Maximum 6 mg/kg or 100 mg/dose
			- **CYP450 Interactions:** CYP inducer
			- **Renal or Hepatic Dose Adjustments:** None
			- **Dosage Forms:** IV (solution)

Primidone	Mysoline	- Seizures
		- Essential tremor
			- **Dosing (Adult):**
			  – Oral: 100 to 1500 mg q6-24h
			- **Dosing (Peds):**
			  – Oral: 10 to 25 mg/kg/day divided q8-12h
			    – Maximum 500 mg/dose
			- **CYP450 Interactions:** CYP Inducer (CYP 1A2, 2A6, 2B6, 2C9, 3A4); Substrate of CYP2C19, 2C9, 2E1
			- **Renal or Hepatic Dose Adjustments:**
			  – GFR 10 to 50 mL/minute: Administer q12-24h
			  – GFR < 10 mL/minute: Administer q24h
			- **Dosage Forms:** Oral (tablet)

NEUROLOGY – BENZODIAZEPINES – Part 1

Drug Class
- **Benzodiazepines**
- **Agents:**
  - **Acute Care**
    - Diazepam
    - Lorazepam
    - Midazolam
    - Remimazolam
  - **Chronic Care**
    - Clobazam
    - Clorazepate

Main Indications or Uses
- **Acute Care**
  - Alcohol withdrawal
    - Diazepam
    - Lorazepam
  - Sedation
    - Diazepam
    - Lorazepam
    - Midazolam
    - Remimazolam
  - Seizures
    - Clorazepate
    - Diazepam
    - Lorazepam
    - Midazolam
  - Lennox-Gastaut syndrome
    - Clobazam
- **Chronic Care**
  - Anxiety disorders
    - Clorazepate
    - Diazepam
    - Lorazepam
  - Muscle spasms
    - Diazepam

Fast Facts

- As with all benzodiazepines, with chronic use patients can become physically dependent where they will need a taper to avoid risk of withdrawal seizures.

- Patients should be advised not to consume alcohol with benzodiazepines due to the additive risk of CNS depression.

- Prolonged IV infusions of lorazepam are commonly associated with the development of lactic acidosis. This is most commonly seen in patients in the ICU on a drip.

- Diazepam comes in a rectal suppository dosage formulation allowing caregivers to treat epileptic seizures at home.

- In status epilepticus, lorazepam is the initial drug of choice if an IV is present or midazolam by IM injection if no IV is present.

Mechanism of Action
- Benzodiazepines increase the frequency of GABA-A channel opening, potentiating GABAergic inhibition of neurotransmission.

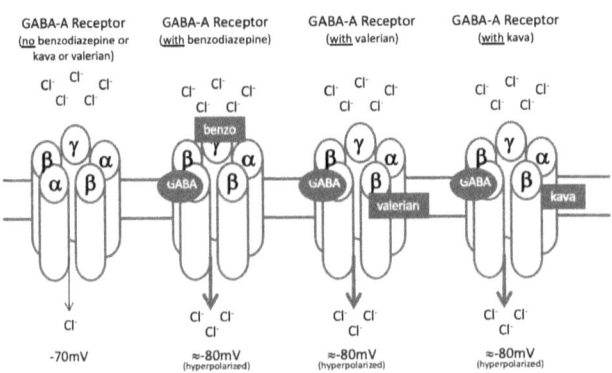

Primary Net Benefit
- Achieve CNS depressant activity related to barbiturates, but improved safety with sedative "ceiling" effect when used alone, and no direct negative cardiovascular or respiratory effects.
- Main Labs to Monitor:
  - No routine laboratory monitoring

High-Yield Basic Pharmacology
- **GABAergic Effects**
  - Benzodiazepines appear to increase GABAergic synaptic inhibition efficiency by binding to the alpha-1 subunit of GABA-A receptors containing a gamma-2 subunit.
- **GABA-A Receptor**
  - The GABA-A receptor most commonly contains a 5-subunit complex with alpha, beta, and gamma subunits.
  - The non-benzodiazepine sedative hypnotic "z-drugs" also bind to the alpha-1 subunit in a fashion similar to benzodiazepines.
- **Midazolam Physiologic Absorption**
  - Although a lipophilic drug, midazolam is in an aqueous solution buffered to a pH of approximately 3, which maintains the conformation of midazolam's structure in an "open ring" orientation. When exposed to a physiologic pH of 7.4, the benzodiazepine ring closes, allowing for midazolam to regain its lipophilic characteristics.
    - This preparation allows for safe and reliable IM administration of midazolam.
    - Although lorazepam and diazepam can be administered IM, their absorptions are not predictable due to their propylene glycol vehicles.

High-Yield Clinical Knowledge
- **Metabolism**
  - All benzodiazepines are metabolized hepatically but differ in hepatic metabolism, undergoing oxidation (phase 1) or glucuronidation (phase 2).
  - The "LOT" agents, lorazepam, oxazepam, and temazepam, are benzodiazepines that undergo glucuronidation.
  - Most other benzodiazepines (i.e., chlordiazepoxide, diazepam, midazolam, etc.) undergo hepatic oxidation by the CYP450 system.
    - Oxidation often produces metabolites that can accumulate with prolonged administration, leading to excessive sedation.

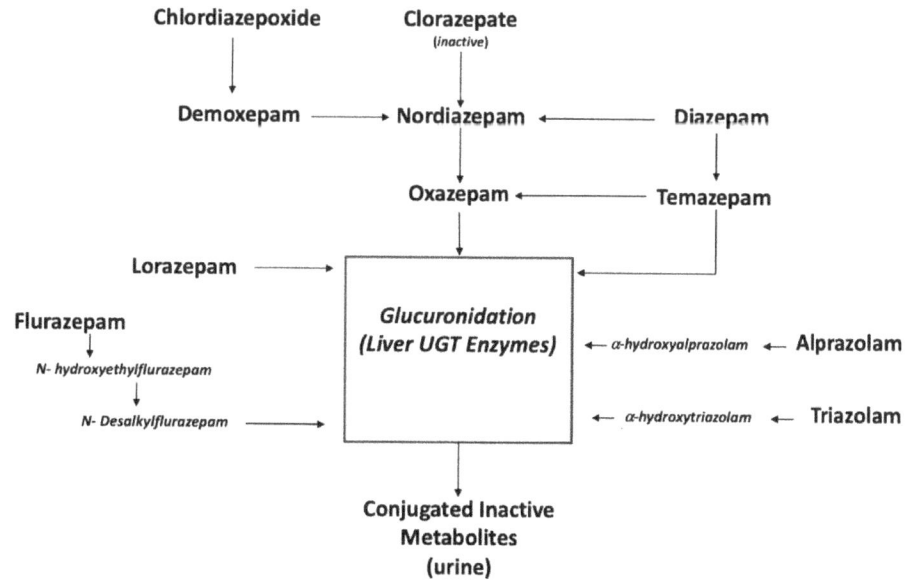

- **ICU Sedation**
  - Sedation of mechanically ventilated patients should be accomplished using propofol or dexmedetomidine, with benzodiazepines reserved for cases where either of the aforementioned agents cannot be used.
    - Benzodiazepine use for sedation of mechanically ventilated patients is associated with ICU delirium and the accumulation of metabolites (diazepam and midazolam), potentially prolonging mechanical ventilation.
  - If used, lorazepam is preferred over diazepam or midazolam as an agent for sedation of mechanically ventilated patients and should be administered using an intermittent push rather than continuous infusion.
- **Withdrawal**
  - As a result of chronic administration, followed by downregulation of GABA-A receptors, or GABA, abrupt discontinuation of benzodiazepines can cause a neurologic excitatory withdrawal syndrome, sharing many similarities with an alcohol withdrawal syndrome.
  - The management of benzodiazepine withdrawal involves providing appropriate doses of diazepam in a symptom-triggered fashion.
  - Benzodiazepine withdrawal is potentially fatal.
- **Anesthesia**
  - Beyond sedation and hypnosis, some benzodiazepines (diazepam, lorazepam, and midazolam) are used clinically to achieve anesthesia.
  - If used alone, respiratory depression is unlikely to occur, but if combined with other agents (opioids, anesthetic gases, propofol, etc.), clinically relevant respiratory depression may occur.
    - In patients who are otherwise not chronically taking benzodiazepines, flumazenil is routinely used to reverse respiratory depressant effects that may occur.
- **Anticonvulsant**
  - Diazepam, lorazepam, and midazolam are routinely used as an essential component for the acute management of seizures.
    - However, additional antiepileptic agents are necessary as this effect is short-lived with benzodiazepines.
  - Diazepam is the most lipophilic of the available agents used to treat seizures, permitting rapid entry to the CNS, and terminating seizures. However, this also leads to rapid redistribution of the CNS to other tissues, allowing for recurrent seizures.
    - However, diazepam is still used but is limited to outpatient use in the Dia-Stat rectal dosage form intended for parents/guardians to use on their dependents' seizure activity.
- **Flumazenil**
  - Flumazenil is a competitive antagonist of benzodiazepine binding to the GABA-A receptor, which can reverse unwanted effects of benzodiazepines, namely respiratory depression or excessive sedation.
  - In patients with chronic use of benzodiazepines, flumazenil may induce acute withdrawal. Still, given that the duration of action of flumazenil is much shorted than most offending benzodiazepines, this is a short-lived event.
    - Furthermore, acute withdrawal seizures can be treated using non-benzodiazepine agents, including propofol.
  - In benzodiazepine-naive patients, flumazenil is routinely used in the OR/PACU setting to speed the time to recovery from anesthesia.

High-Yield Core Evidence
- **Diazepam vs. Lorazepam vs. Placebo**
  - This randomized, double-blind trial compared IV diazepam, IV lorazepam, or placebo administered by paramedics to treat out-of-hospital status epilepticus.
  - Lorazepam was associated with a significant improvement in termination of status epilepticus on arrival at the emergency department compared with diazepam or placebo.
  - There was no difference in the rates of respiratory or circulatory complications after the study treatment was administered.

- The authors concluded that benzodiazepines are safe and effective when administered by paramedics for out-of-hospital status epilepticus in adults. Lorazepam is likely to be better therapy than diazepam. (N Engl J Med. 2001 Aug 30;345(9):631-7.)
- **RAMPART**
  - This was a double-blind, non-inferiority trial of adult and pediatric patients who were still seizing after paramedic arrival and initial treatment were randomized to receive either IM midazolam or IV lorazepam.
  - Patients randomized to receive IV lorazepam had an absence of seizures when of emergency department arrival compared to patients receiving IM midazolam.
  - Median times to active treatment were 1.2 minutes in the IM midazolam group and 4.8 minutes in the IV lorazepam group, corresponding median times from active treatment to cessation of convulsions of 3.3 minutes and 1.6 minutes.
  - There was no difference in the incidence of endotracheal intubation and recurrence of seizures.
  - The authors concluded that for subjects in status epilepticus, IM midazolam is at least as safe and effective as IV lorazepam for prehospital seizure cessation. (N Engl J Med. 2012 Feb 16;366(7):591-600.)

High-Yield Fast-Facts
- **Propylene Glycol Toxicity**
  - Prolonged infusions of lorazepam can lead to the accumulation of propylene glycol and the potential for developing a metabolic acidosis produced by this toxic alcohol.

- **GABA Antagonists**
  - Common GABA antagonists such as colchicine, clozapine, beta-lactams, and TCAs can potentially induce seizures at doses at or above therapeutic doses.

HIGH-YIELD BOARD EXAM ESSENTIALS
- **CLASSIC AGENTS:** Clobazam, clorazepate, diazepam, lorazepam, midazolam, remimazolam
- **DRUG CLASS:** Benzodiazepines
- **INDICATIONS:** Alcohol withdrawal, anxiety disorders, sedation, seizures, Lennox-Gastaut syndrome, muscle spasms
- **MECHANISM:** Increase the frequency of GABA-A channel opening, potentiating GABAergic inhibition of neurotransmission.
- **SIDE EFFECTS:** Altered mental status, withdrawal (abrupt discontinuation from chronic use)
- **CLINICAL PEARLS:**
  - Achieve CNS depressant activity related to barbiturates, but improved safety with sedative "ceiling" effect when used alone, and no direct negative cardiovascular or respiratory effects.
  - Avoid mixing with use of alcohol due to increase CNS depression.
  - Benzodiazepines are considered contraindicated in pregnancy.
  - Diazepam and lorazepam the drugs of choice in cocaine-induced MI and alcohol withdrawal.
  - Long infusions of lorazepam in the ICU can result in an anion gap metabolic acidosis due to conversion of propylene glycol to lactic acid.

Table: Drug Class Summary

Benzodiazepines - Drug Class Review			
High-Yield Med Reviews			
Mechanism of Action: Benzodiazepines increase the frequency of GABA-A channel opening, potentiating GABAergic inhibition of neurotransmission.			
Class Effects: Achieve CNS depressant activity related to barbiturates, but improved safety with sedative "ceiling" effect when used alone, and no direct negative cardiovascular or respiratory effects.			
Generic Name	**Brand Name**	**Main Indication(s) or Uses**	**Notes**

Clobazam	Onfi	• Lennox-Gastaut syndrome	• **Dosing (Adult):**
			  – Oral: 5 mg daily, up to 20 mg q12h
			• **Dosing (Peds):**
			  – 0.2 to 1 mg/kg/day divided q12h
			    – Maximum 40 mg/day
			• **CYP450 Interactions:** Substrate of CYP2B6, 2C19, 3A4, P-gp; Inhibits CYP2D6; Induces CYP3A4
			• **Renal or Hepatic Dose Adjustments:** None
			• **Dosage Forms:** Oral (film, suspension, tablet)

Clorazepate	Tranxene-T	• Alcohol withdrawal
		• Anxiety disorders
		• Seizures
			• **Dosing (Adult):**
			  – Oral: 30 mg/day in divided doses
			    – Maximum 90 mg/day
			• **Dosing (Peds):**
			  – Oral: 0.3 to 1 mg/kg/day divided q8-24h
			    – Maximum 90 mg/day
			• **CYP450 Interactions:** Substrate CYP3A4
			• **Renal or Hepatic Dose Adjustments:** None
			• **Dosage Forms:** Oral (tablet)

Diazepam	Diastat, Valium, Valtoco	• Alcohol withdrawal
		• Anxiety disorders
		• Muscle spasms
		• Sedation
		• Seizures
			• **Dosing (Adult):**
			  – IV/IN: 0.2 mg/kg as needed
			    – Maximum 20 mg/dose
			• **Dosing (Peds):**
			  – IV/IN: 0.2 mg/kg as needed
			    – Maximum 20 mg/dose
			  – Rectal: 0.2 to 0.5 mg/kg
			    – Maximum 20 mg/dose
			• **CYP450 Interactions:** Substrate CYP1A2, 2C19, 2C9, 3A4
			• **Renal or Hepatic Dose Adjustments:** None
			• **Dosage Forms:** Oral (concentrate, solution, tablet), Rectal (gel), IV (solution)

Benzodiazepines - Drug Class Review
High-Yield Med Reviews

Generic Name	Brand Name	Main Indication(s) or Uses	Notes

Lorazepam	Ativan	- Anxiety disorders
		- Sedation
		- Seizures
			- **Dosing (Adult):**
			  - IM/IV: 0.25 to 4 mg q3-5minutes to q3-6hours
			  - Oral: 0.5 to 2 mg q6-24hours
			- **Dosing (Peds):**
			  - Oral: 0.05 mg/kg/dose q4-8hours
			    - Maximum 2 mg/dose
			  - IV: 0.1 mg/kg up to 2 doses
			    - Maximum 5 mg/dose
			- **CYP450 Interactions:** None
			- **Renal or Hepatic Dose Adjustments:** None
			- **Dosage Forms:** Oral (concentrate, solution, tablet), IV (solution)

Midazolam	Versed	- Sedation
		- Seizures
			- **Dosing (Adult):**
			  - IN/IM/IV: 0.5 to 10 mg q3-5minutes
			  - IV: 0.05 to 2 mg/kg/hour infusion
			- **Dosing (Peds):**
			  - Oral/Rectal: 0.25 to 0.5 mg/kg/dose
			    - Maximum 10 mg/dose
			  - IN/IM/IV: 0.1 to 0.5 mg/kg/dose
			    - Maximum 10 mg/dose
			  - IV: infusion 0.05 to 2mg/kg/hour
			- **CYP450 Interactions:** Substrate CYP2B6, 3A4
			- **Renal or Hepatic Dose Adjustments:**
			  - No specific adjustments, but continuous administration will lead to the accumulation of midazolam and metabolites.
			- **Dosage Forms:** Oral (syrup), IV (solution)

Remimazolam	Byfavo	- Sedation	- **Dosing (Adult):** - IV: 1.25 to 5 mg as needed - **Dosing (Peds):** Not routinely used - **CYP450 Interactions:** None known - **Renal or Hepatic Dose Adjustments:** None - **Dosage Forms:** IV (solution)

NEUROLOGY – BENZODIAZEPINES – Part 2

Drug Class
- **Benzodiazepines**
- Agents:
  - **Acute Care**
    - Chlordiazepoxide
    - Oxazepam
  - **Chronic Care**
    - Alprazolam
    - Estazolam
    - Flurazepam
    - Quazepam
    - Temazepam
    - Triazolam

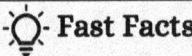

Fast Facts

✓ Benzodiazepines are the initial drug of choice in patients with alcohol withdrawal. At appropriate doses, they can prevent the patient from going into alcohol withdrawal seizures.

Main Indications or Uses
- **Acute Care**
  - Alcohol withdrawal
    - Chlordiazepoxide
    - Oxazepam
  - Chemotherapy nausea and vomiting
    - Alprazolam
- **Chronic Care**
  - Anxiety
    - Alprazolam
    - Chlordiazepoxide
    - Oxazepam
  - Insomnia
    - Estazolam
    - Flurazepam
    - Quazepam
    - Temazepam
    - Triazolam
  - Vertigo
    - Alprazolam

Mechanism of Action
- Benzodiazepines increase the frequency of GABA-A channel opening, potentiating GABAergic inhibition of neurotransmission.

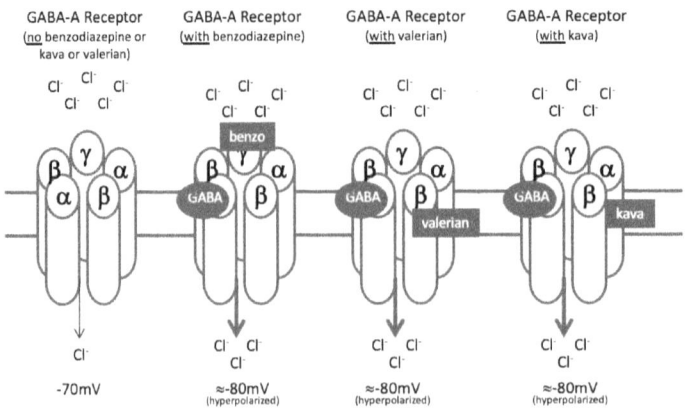

Primary Net Benefit
- Achieve CNS depressant activity related to barbiturates, but improved safety with sedative "ceiling" effect when used alone, and no direct negative cardiovascular or respiratory effects.
- Main Labs to Monitor:
    - No routine laboratory monitoring

High-Yield Basic Pharmacology
- **Chlordiazepoxide Metabolites**
    - CYP3A4 oxidizes chlordiazepoxide to numerous active metabolites, including nordiazepam and oxazepam.
    - For the management of alcohol withdrawal, this property is ideal. It permits self-titration and, when combined with symptom-triggered dosing (rather than a scheduled dose), allows for less drug to be used and fewer excessive sedation episodes.
- **GABAergic Effects**
    - Benzodiazepines appear to increase GABAergic synaptic inhibition efficiency by binding to the alpha-1 subunit of GABA-A receptors containing a gamma-2 subunit.
- **GABA-A Receptor**
    - The GABA-A receptor most commonly contains a 5-subunit complex with alpha, beta, and gamma subunits.
    - The non-benzodiazepine sedative hypnotic "z-drugs" also bind to the alpha-1 subunit in a fashion similar to benzodiazepines.

High-Yield Clinical Knowledge
- **Metabolism**
    - All benzodiazepines are metabolized hepatically but differ in hepatic metabolism, undergoing oxidation (phase 1) or glucuronidation (phase 2).
    - The "LOT" agents, lorazepam, oxazepam, and temazepam, are benzodiazepines that undergo glucuronidation.
    - Most other benzodiazepines (i.e., chlordiazepoxide, diazepam, midazolam, etc.) undergo hepatic oxidation by the CYP450 system.
        - Oxidation often produces metabolites that can accumulate with prolonged administration, leading to excessive sedation.
- **Tolerance**
    - Benzodiazepines use associated with development of a decreased clinical effect following continuous exposure.
        - Cross-tolerance can be a feature of this effect, including other sedative-hypnotics (barbiturates), non-benzodiazepine sleep aids (zolpidem), or ethanol.
    - Tolerance is thought to develop from the downregulation of GABA-A receptors as a counterregulatory response to excessive inhibition.
- **Withdrawal**
    - As a result of chronic administration, followed by downregulation of GABA-A receptors, or GABA, abrupt discontinuation of benzodiazepines can cause a neurologic excitatory withdrawal syndrome, sharing many similarities with an alcohol withdrawal syndrome.
    - The management of benzodiazepine withdrawal involves providing appropriate doses of diazepam in a symptom-triggered fashion.
    - Benzodiazepine withdrawal is potentially fatal.
- **Sedation**
    - As their class name implies, benzodiazepines exert dose-dependent anxiolytic effects, amnestic effects, and sedation as a member of the sedative-hypnotic group.
        - The amnestic effects produced by benzodiazepines are dose-dependent and are anterograde.
- **Hypnosis**
    - Hypnosis, or inducing sleep, can be achieved with doses above those used to achieve sedation with benzodiazepines.
    - Benzodiazepines decrease the onset of sleep, increase non-REM sleep duration, and reduce the duration of REM sleep and stage 4 non-REM sleep.

- **Cardiovascular and Renal Effects**
    - Although benzodiazepines do not cause adverse cardiovascular effects independently, clinically relevant cardiovascular events may occur if combined with other CNS depressants (including ethanol).
    - Furthermore, in patients who require positive pressure ventilation or have underlying sleep-related breathing disorders, benzodiazepines may lead to hypoxic events.

High-Yield Core Evidence
- **Symptom Triggered Vs. Fixed-Dose Oxazepam**
    - This was a prospective, double-blind trial of consecutive patients with alcohol dependence who were entering an alcohol treatment program randomized to receive oxazepam on a symptom-triggered schedule or oxazepam scheduled every 6 hours with additional as needed doses.
    - Patients randomized to the symptom-triggered arm received significantly less oxazepam (37.5 mg) than the scheduled or fixed-dose group (231.4 mg).
    - Furthermore, the treatment duration was significantly shorter in patients randomized to symptom-triggered therapy than fixed-dose groups (20.0 vs. 62.7 hours).
    - There were no differences in the measures of comfort between the 2 groups.
    - The authors concluded that symptom-triggered benzodiazepine treatment for alcohol withdrawal is safe, comfortable, and associated with decreased medication quantity and treatment duration. (Arch Intern Med. 2002 May 27;162(10):1117-21.)
- **Estazolam Vs. Flurazepam**
    - This was a double-blind, placebo-controlled, multicenter, 7-night study comparing estazolam to flurazepam in outpatients with insomnia.
    - There were no observed differences in the patients' subjective assessments in six sleep parameters.
    - However, patients who received estazolam 1 mg rated their sleep significantly better than did patients receiving placebo on all parameters except sleep latency.
    - The percentage of patients who reported any adverse events was similar between groups.
    - The authors concluded that estazolam 2 mg was found to be as effective a hypnotic as flurazepam 30 mg. Estazolam 1 mg is also effective in treating outpatients with insomnia, but to a lesser degree. (J Clin Pharmacol. 1991 Aug;31(8):747-50.)

High-Yield Fast-Facts
- **Glycine Receptors**
    - Glycine receptors are similar to GABA as they're voltage-gated chloride channels, but these receptors are a Cl- inhibitory receptor in the spinal cord.
    - Strychnine and tetanus toxin are glycine receptor inhibitors.
- **GABA-B Receptors**
    - GABA-B receptors differ from GABA-A in that they are typically ligand-gated channels and have their own agonists and antagonists.
    - Baclofen and gamma-hydroxybutyrate are GABA-B agonists.

HIGH-YIELD BOARD EXAM ESSENTIALS
- **CLASSIC AGENTS:** Alprazolam, chlordiazepoxide, oxazepam, estazolam, flurazepam, quazepam, temazepam, triazolam
- **DRUG CLASS:** Benzodiazepines
- **INDICATIONS:** Alcohol withdrawal, anxiety disorders, chemotherapy nausea and vomiting, insomnia, vertigo
- **MECHANISM:** Increase the frequency of GABA-A channel opening, potentiating GABAergic inhibition of neurotransmission.
- **SIDE EFFECTS:** Altered mental status, sedation, withdrawal (abrupt discontinuation from chronic use)
- **CLINICAL PEARLS:** All benzodiazepines are metabolized hepatically but differ in hepatic metabolism, undergoing either oxidation (phase 1) or glucuronidation (phase 2). The "LOT" agents, lorazepam, oxazepam, and temazepam, are benzodiazepines that undergo glucuronidation.

Table: Drug Class Summary

	**Benzodiazepines - Drug Class Review** **High-Yield Med Reviews**
	**Mechanism of Action:** *Benzodiazepines increase the frequency of GABA-A channel opening, potentiating GABAergic inhibition of neurotransmission.*
	**Class Effects:** *Achieve CNS depressant activity related to barbiturates, but improved safety with sedative "ceiling" effect when used alone, and no direct negative cardiovascular or respiratory effects.*
Generic Name	**Brand Name**	**Main Indication(s) or Uses**	**Notes**
Alprazolam	Xanax	<ul><li>Anxiety</li><li>Chemotherapy nausea and vomiting</li><li>Vertigo</li></ul>	<ul><li>**Dosing (Adult):**<ul><li>Oral: 0.25 to 1 mg q8-12h</li><li>Maximum 10 mg/day</li></ul></li><li>**Dosing (Peds):**<ul><li>0.005 to 0.02 mg/kg/dose q8h</li><li>Maximum 10 mg/day</li></ul></li><li>**CYP450 Interactions:** Substrate CYP3A4; Inhibits CYP3A4</li><li>**Renal or Hepatic Dose Adjustments:**<ul><li>Child-Pugh class C: 0.25 mg q8-12h</li></ul></li><li>**Dosage Forms:** Oral (concentrate, disintegrating tablet, tablet IR, tablet XR)</li></ul>
Chlordiazepoxide	Librium	<ul><li>Alcohol withdrawal</li><li>Anxiety</li></ul>	<ul><li>**Dosing (Adult):**<ul><li>Oral: 25 to 100 mg q6-24h</li></ul></li><li>**Dosing (Peds):**<ul><li>Oral: 5 to 10 mg q6-12h</li></ul></li><li>**CYP450 Interactions:** Substrate CYP3A4</li><li>**Renal or Hepatic Dose Adjustments:**<ul><li>GFR < 10 mL/minute: administer 50% of the dose</li></ul></li><li>**Dosage Forms:** Oral (capsule)</li></ul>
Estazolam	Prosom	<ul><li>Insomnia</li></ul>	<ul><li>**Dosing (Adult):**<ul><li>Oral 1 mg at bedtime</li></ul></li><li>**Dosing (Peds):** Not routinely used</li><li>**CYP450 Interactions:** Substrate CYP3A4</li><li>**Renal or Hepatic Dose Adjustments:** None</li><li>**Dosage Forms:** Oral (tablet)</li></ul>
Flurazepam	Som-Pam	<ul><li>Insomnia</li></ul>	<ul><li>**Dosing (Adult):**<ul><li>Oral: 15 to 30 mg at bedtime</li></ul></li><li>**Dosing (Peds):**<ul><li>Oral: 15 mg at bedtime</li></ul></li><li>**CYP450 Interactions:** Substrate CYP3A4</li><li>**Renal or Hepatic Dose Adjustments:** None</li><li>**Dosage Forms:** Oral (tablet)</li></ul>

Benzodiazepines - Drug Class Review
High-Yield Med Reviews

Generic Name	Brand Name	Main Indication(s) or Uses	Notes

Oxazepam	Oxpam	- Alcohol withdrawal
		- Anxiety
			- **Dosing (Adult):**
			  – Oral: 10 to 30 mg q6-24h
			- **Dosing (Peds):**
			  – Oral: 10 to 30 mg q6-24h
			- **CYP450 Interactions:** None
			- **Renal or Hepatic Dose Adjustments:** None
			- **Dosage Forms:** Oral (capsule)

Quazepam	Doral	- Insomnia	- **Dosing (Adult):** – Oral: 7.5 mg at bedtime - **Dosing (Peds):** Not routinely used - **CYP450 Interactions:** Substrate CYP3A4 - **Renal or Hepatic Dose Adjustments:** None - **Dosage Forms:** Oral (tablet)
Temazepam	Restoril	- Insomnia	- **Dosing (Adult):** – Oral: 7.5 to 30 mg at bedtime - **Dosing (Peds):** Not routinely used - **CYP450 Interactions:** Substrate CYP2B6, 2C19, 2C9, 3A4 - **Renal or Hepatic Dose Adjustments:** None - **Dosage Forms:** Oral (capsule)

Triazolam	Halcion	- Insomnia	- **Dosing (Adult):**
			  – Oral: 0.125 to 0.25 mg at bedtime
			- **Dosing (Peds):**
			  – Oral: 0.125 to 0.25 mg at bedtime
			- **CYP450 Interactions:** Substrate CYP3A4
			- **Renal or Hepatic Dose Adjustments:** None
			- **Dosage Forms:** Oral (tablet)

NEUROLOGY – CNS STIMULANTS

Drug Class
- Amphetamines
- Agents:
    - Chronic Care
        - Amphetamine
        - Armodafinil
        - Dexmethylphenidate
        - Dextroamphetamine
        - Lisdexamfetamine
        - Methamphetamine
        - Methylphenidate
        - Modafinil
        - Serdexmethylphenidate

> **Fast Facts**
> ✓ Stimulants are the drugs of choice for the management of ADD/ADHD.
>
> ✓ Lisdexamfetamine is a prodrug that can only be metabolized if taken by mouth which helps to prevent inappropriate use through other routes.

Main Indications or Uses
- Chronic Care
    - Attention-deficit/hyperactivity disorder (Amphetamine, dexmethylphenidate, lisdexamfetamine, methylphenidate)
    - Narcolepsy (Armodafinil, dextroamphetamine, methamphetamine, modafinil)
    - Obstructive sleep apnea (Armodafinil, modafinil)
    - Shift work sleep disorder (Armodafinil, modafinil)

Mechanism of Action
- **Amphetamines:**
    - Stimulate the release of biogenic amines, particularly dopamine, norepinephrine, and serotonin.
- **Methylphenidate:**
    - Inhibits the reuptake of biogenic amines, particularly dopamine, norepinephrine, and serotonin.
        - This is the same mechanism as cocaine!

Primary Net Benefit
- Stimulants are effective drug treatment options for attention-deficit/hyperactivity disorder (ADHD) and can be applied to other stimulant indications, including narcolepsy.
- Main Labs to Monitor:
    - Blood pressure, heart rate
    - Height, weight; growth charts

High-Yield Basic Pharmacology
- **Phenylethylamines**
    - Amphetamines are a broad class of compounds that share a phenylethylamine structure.
    - However, amphetamine itself refers explicitly to beta-phenylisopropylamine.
- **Amphetamines**
    - Amphetamines include compounds that are used for legitimate medical purposes, as well as illicit applications for use.
        - These chemicals and agents can range from methcathinone and MDMA (3,4-Methylenedioxymethamphetamine) with stimulant properties to N,N-Dimethyltryptamine (DMT) with potent hallucinogenic properties.
- **Structural Substitutions**
    - The development of alternative amphetamine products has, in part, been possible due to the detailed knowledge of its structural activity relationship and specific substitutions on its core structure.

- For example, substitutions on the alpha carbon permit resistance to oxidation by monoamine oxidase. In contrast, substituting the amino group for larger amino groups confers more beta-adrenergic effects.

High-Yield Clinical Knowledge
- **Psychiatric Adverse Events**
  - The FDA applied warnings to all ADHD and amphetamine stimulant medications regarding the increased risk of acute psychiatric adverse events, including psychosis, mood disturbances, and severe anxiety.
  - The MTA study (described below) found no statistically significant difference in the incidence of psychosis among children receiving stimulant medication for ADHD.
- **Height and Weight**
  - Amphetamine ADHD medications are strongly associated with growth deficits of approximately 1 to 1.4 cm/year and weight gain deficits of 3 kg in the first year of therapy.
  - However, long-term follow-up of patients taking amphetamines has revealed that patients generally achieve their predicted growth potential upon discontinuation.
- **Cardiac Events**
  - Stimulant medication is associated with a 3 to 10 beat per minute increase in heart rate and changes in systolic blood pressure of approximately 12 mmHg.
  - These changes are not associated with significant changes in cardiovascular events among children but may be relevant in adolescents and adults who continue taking these medications.
- **Dosage Forms**
  - As many of these agents are used in children, a wide range of formulations exist to enhance pharmacokinetics but also ease of administration and to encourage compliance.
  - Numerous products feature oral dosage forms, including immediate, delayed, and extended-release preparations and oral liquids or orally disintegrating tablets.
    - The disadvantage to immediate-release forms are a short duration of action, requiring multiple doses per day.
  - Methylphenidate is available as a transdermal patch, which may be used if oral administration is not suitable or other compliance issues have been identified.
- **Dependence, Tolerance, and Abuse**
  - With chronic use, patients may become psychologically dependent on amphetamines, but tolerance does develop to the anorexigenic effects of amphetamines and mood changes.
  - However, these agents have a high potential for abuse due to their stimulant, hallucinogenic, and adaptogenic properties.
- **Non-amphetamines**
  - Compared to amphetamines for treating ADHD, non-amphetamine stimulants such as atomoxetine, clonidine, and guanfacine, are not as effective but can be used adjunctively in selected patients.

High-Yield Core Evidence
- **The MTA Cooperative Group Study**
  - This was a long-term observational study of children with ADHD Combined Type, who were assigned to 14 months of medication management (titration followed by monthly visits); intensive behavioral treatment (parent, school, and child components, with therapist involvement, gradually reduced over time); the two combined; or standard community care (treatments by community providers).
  - All four groups showed sizable reductions in symptoms over time, with significant differences among them in degrees of change.
  - For most ADHD symptoms, children in the combined treatment and medication management groups showed significantly more significant improvement than those given intensive behavioral treatment and community care.
  - The authors concluded that medication management was superior to behavioral treatment and routine community care that included medication. (Arch Gen Psychiatry 1999 Dec;56(12):1073-86.)

- **ADHD Medication Meta-Analysis**
  - This was a meta-analysis of published and unpublished double-blind, randomized controlled trials comparing amphetamines (including lisdexamfetamine), atomoxetine, bupropion, clonidine, guanfacine, methylphenidate, and modafinil with each other or placebo.
  - A total of 133 double-blind, randomized controlled trials, 10 068 children and adolescents, and 8131 adults were included in the efficacy analysis.
  - For ADHD core symptoms rated by clinicians in children and adolescents closest to 12 weeks, all included drugs were superior to placebo.
  - However, only methylphenidate and modafinil were more efficacious than placebo, according to teacher-only evaluations.
  - In adults, amphetamines, methylphenidate, bupropion, and atomoxetine, but not modafinil, were better than placebo.
  - The authors concluded that this meta-analysis supports methylphenidate in children and adolescents, and amphetamines in adults, as preferred first-choice medications for the short-term treatment of ADHD. (Lancet Psych. 2018;5:727–738.)

High-Yield Fast-Fact
- **DMT Absorption**
  - DMT is not orally bioavailable, but when consumed with a MAO inhibitor and COMT inhibitor, it becomes enterally absorbed in the traditional central/south American drink Ayahuasca.

HIGH-YIELD BOARD EXAM ESSENTIALS
- **CLASSIC AGENTS:** Amphetamine, armodafinil, dexmethylphenidate, dextroamphetamine, lisdexamfetamine, methamphetamine, methylphenidate, modafinil
- **DRUG CLASS:** Amphetamines
- **INDICATIONS:** ADHD (amphetamine, dexmethylphenidate, lisdexamfetamine, methylphenidate), narcolepsy (armodafinil, dextroamphetamine, methamphetamine, modafinil), obstructive sleep apnea (armodafinil, modafinil), shift work sleep disorder (armodafinil, modafinil)
- **MECHANISM:** Stimulate the release of biogenic amines, particularly dopamine, norepinephrine, and serotonin.
- **SIDE EFFECTS:** Psychosis, mood disturbances, severe anxiety, tachycardia
- **CLINICAL PEARLS:**
  - Amphetamines (and derivatives) increase the release of norepinephrine (NE) and dopamine (DA) whereas methylphenidate agents inhibit the re-uptake of NE and DA.
  - Amphetamine ADHD medications are strongly associated with growth deficits of approximately 1 to 1.4 cm/year and weight gain deficits of 3 kg in the first year of therapy. However, long-term follow-up of patients taking amphetamines has revealed that patients generally achieve their predicted growth potential upon discontinuation.
  - Lisdexamfetamine is a pro-drug that must be taken by mouth to facilitate conversion to active form which can help prevent abuse if attempting to use it by another route of administration.

Table: Drug Class Summary

Amphetamines - Drug Class Review High-Yield Med Reviews			
Mechanism of Action: *Stimulate the release of biogenic amines, particularly dopamine, norepinephrine, and serotonin.*			
Class Effects: *Stimulants are effective drug treatment options for attention-deficit/hyperactivity disorder (ADHD) and can be applied to other stimulant indications including narcolepsy.*			
Generic Name	**Brand Name**	**Main Indication(s) or Uses**	**Notes**
Amphetamine	Adzenys, Dyanavel, Eveko	- Attention-deficit/hyperactivity disorder	- **Dosing (Adult):** 　− Oral: ER 12.5 to 30 mg daily 　− Oral: IR 10 to 60 mg daily - **Dosing (Peds):** 　− Oral: IR 2.5 to 40 mg/day in 1-2 divided doses 　− Oral: ER 3.1 to 18.8 mg daily - **CYP450 Interactions:** Substrate CYP2D6 - **Renal or Hepatic Dose Adjustments:** None - **Dosage Forms:** Oral (suspension, tablet, ODT)
Armodafinil	Nuvigil	- Narcolepsy - Obstructive sleep apnea - Shift-work disorder	- **Dosing (Adult):** 　− Oral: 150 to 250 mg daily - **Dosing (Peds):** 　− Not routinely used - **CYP450 Interactions:** Substrate CYP3A4; Inhibits CYP2C19; Induces CYP3A4 - **Renal or Hepatic Dose Adjustments:** 　− Child-Pugh class C: use reduced dose - **Dosage Forms:** Oral (tablet)
Dexmethylphenidate	Focalin	- Attention-deficit/hyperactivity disorder	- **Dosing (Adult):** 　− Oral: IR 2.5 to 10 mg BID 　− Oral: ER 10 to 40 mg daily - **Dosing (Peds):** 　− Oral: IR 2.5 to 10 mg BID 　− Oral: ER 10 to 40 mg daily - **CYP450 Interactions:** None - **Renal or Hepatic Dose Adjustments:** None - **Dosage Forms:** Oral (capsule, tablet)
Dextroamphetamine	Dexedrine, ProCentra, Zenzedi	- Narcolepsy	- **Dosing (Adult):** 　− Oral: IR/ER 10 to 60 mg daily - **Dosing (Peds):** 　− Oral: IR 2.5 to 40 mg daily divided q4-6h 　− Oral: ER 5 to 40 mg daily in 2 divided doses - **CYP450 Interactions:** Substrate CYP2D6 - **Renal or Hepatic Dose Adjustments:** None - **Dosage Forms:** Oral (capsule, solution, tablet)

\multicolumn{4}{c}{**Amphetamines - Drug Class Review**}
\multicolumn{4}{c}{High-Yield Med Reviews}
Generic Name	**Brand Name**	**Main Indication(s) or Uses**	**Notes**

Lisdexamfetamine	Vyvanse	- Attention-deficit/hyperactivity disorder	- **Dosing (Adult):**
			   – Oral: 30 to 70 mg daily
			- **Dosing (Peds):**
			   – Oral: 20 to 70 mg daily
			- **CYP450 Interactions:** Substrate CYP2D6
			- **Renal or Hepatic Dose Adjustments:**
			   – GFR 15 to 30 mL/minute: maximum 50 mg/day
			   – GFR < 15 mL/minute: maximum 30 mg/day
			- **Dosage Forms:** Oral (capsule, tablet)

Methamphetamine	Desoxyn	- Narcolepsy	- **Dosing (Adult):**
			   – Oral: 20 to 60 mg within 1 hour of awakening
			- **Dosing (Peds):**
			   – Oral: 5 to 25 mg daily
			- **CYP450 Interactions:** Substrate CYP2D6
			- **Renal or Hepatic Dose Adjustments:** None
			- **Dosage Forms:** Oral (tablet)

Methylphenidate	Adhansia, Aptensio, Concerta, Cotempla, Daytrana, Jornay, Metadate, Methylin, QuilliChew, Quillivant, Relexxii, Ritalin	- Attention-deficit/hyperactivity disorder	- **Dosing (Adult):**
			   – Oral: ER 10 to 100 mg/day
			   – Oral: SR 20 to 100 mg/day
			   – Oral: IR 10 to 60 mg/day in 2-3 divided doses
			   – Transdermal: 10 mg applied 2 hours before the effect is needed, and removed after 9 hours
			- **Dosing (Peds):**
			   – Oral: ER 10 to 100 mg/day
			   – Oral: SR 20 to 100 mg/day
			   – Oral: IR 2.5 to 60 mg/day in 2-3 divided doses
			   – Transdermal: 10 mg applied 2 hours before the effect is needed, and removed after 9 hours
			- **CYP450 Interactions:** None
			- **Renal or Hepatic Dose Adjustments:** None
			- **Dosage Forms:** Oral (capsule, solution, suspension, tablet), Transdermal patch

Amphetamines - Drug Class Review High-Yield Med Reviews			
Generic Name	**Brand Name**	**Main Indication(s) or Uses**	**Notes**

Modafinil	Provigil	- Narcolepsy
		- Obstructive sleep apnea
		- Shift-work disorder
			- **Dosing (Adult):**
			  - Oral: 100 to 400 mg daily
			- **Dosing (Peds):**
			  - Oral: 100 to 400 mg daily
			- **CYP450 Interactions:** Substrate CYP3A4; Inhibits CYP2C19; Induces CYP3A4
			- **Renal or Hepatic Dose Adjustments:**
			  - Child-Pugh class C: reduce dose by 50%
			- **Dosage Forms:** Oral (tablet)

Serdexmethyl-phenidate	Azstarys (with dexmethylphenidate	- Attention-deficit/hyperactivity disorder	- **Dosing (Adult):**
			  - Oral: 39.2 mg / 7.8 mg once daily
			    - Maximum 52.3 mg / 10.4 mg daily
			- **Dosing (Peds):**
			  - Children ≥ 6, same as adult dosing
			- **CYP450 Interactions:** None
			- **Renal or Hepatic Dose Adjustments:** None
			- **Dosage Forms:** Oral (capsule, solution, suspension, tablet), Transdermal patch

NEUROMUSCULAR BLOCKERS – DEPOLARIZING NEUROMUSCULAR BLOCKER

Drug Class
- Depolarizing Neuromuscular Blocker
- Agents:
  - Acute Care
    - Succinylcholine

Main Indications or Uses
- Acute Care
  - Neuromuscular blockade for endotracheal intubation, surgery, or mechanical ventilation

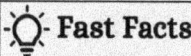

Fast Facts
- Succinylcholine is the only depolarizing neuromuscular blocker that manifests in fasciculations after administration and can also be given IM (if no IV available; IM is not preferred but can be used).

Mechanism of Action
- Binds to acetylcholine receptors of the motor endplate, causing an initial depolarization but causes a persistent effect resistant to acetylcholinesterase.

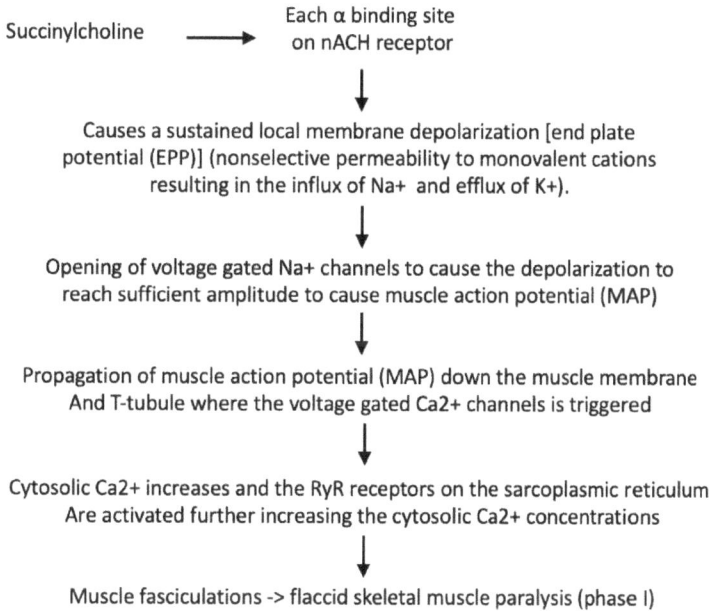

Primary Net Benefit
- Rapid onset and short duration of paralysis facilitating endotracheal intubation, but with potentially clinically relevant hyperkalemia and other neuromuscular adverse effects.
- Main Labs to Monitor:
  - Serum potassium

High-Yield Basic Pharmacology
- **Phase 1 to 2 Block**
  - With excessive doses or prolonged exposure, the initial depolarizing neuromuscular blockade of succinylcholine can transition to a phase 2 block that is competitive inhibition of acetylcholine.
- **Short Duration**
  - Succinylcholine is rapidly metabolized by butyrylcholinesterases, with a duration of action of approximately 10 minutes.
- **Dose-Dependent Effect**

- Neuromuscular blockers exert a dose-dependent effect on motor endplate function, ranging from muscle weakness to complete flaccid paralysis.

High-Yield Clinical Knowledge
- **Fasciculation**
  - Succinylcholine causes an initial depolarization before paralysis by nature of its mechanism.
  - The physical manifestation of this depolarization appears as fasciculations that are typically appreciated in the mandible.
    - To blunt fasciculations, small doses of non-depolarizing neuromuscular blockers (10% of a standard dose) can be administered shortly before succinylcholine.
    - The clinical role of this intervention is questionable and has mostly fallen out of favor.
- **Hyperkalemia**
  - Succinylcholine causes an increase in serum potassium, possibly due to its depolarizing action.
    - The magnitude of this increase can vary but is clinically estimated to be 0.5 mEq/L.
  - Patients with pre-existing renal disease are at increased risk of hyperkalemia due to succinylcholine.; however, the magnitude of these changes occurs within the normal range of pressures.
    - Furthermore, these studies were conducted in a neurosurgical population with existing intracranial pressure monitors, which is not consistent with the physiology of many emergency or critical care patients requiring intubation.
- **Prolonged Effect or Response**
  - Patients with a history of neuromuscular disease (ex., myasthenia gravis, multiple sclerosis, etc.) may have a prolonged and unpredictable paralysis duration.
- **Malignant hyperthermia**
  - Succinylcholine has been associated with malignant hyperthermia.
    - The proposed mechanism is via stimulation of ryanodine calcium channels of the sarcoplasmic reticulum leading to an uncontrolled calcium-dependent calcium release causing excessive muscle contraction, leading to energy depletion, generation of free radicals, and thermal energy.

High-Yield Core Evidence
- **Succinylcholine Vs. Rocuronium**
  - This Cochrane systematic review compared rocuronium to succinylcholine in their effect on creating intubating conditions suitable for rapid sequence intubation of the trachea.
  - The literature search included Cochrane Central Register of Controlled Trials, MEDLINE, and EMBASE for randomized controlled trials or controlled clinical trials that reported intubating conditions comparing rocuronium and succinylcholine for rapid or modified rapid sequence intubation.
  - The authors noted that succinylcholine was superior to rocuronium for achieving excellent intubating conditions and clinically acceptable intubation conditions.
  - However, there was a high incidence of detection bias amongst the trials coupled with significant heterogeneity; thus, the quality of evidence was moderate for these conclusions. (Anaesthesia. 2017 Jun;72(6):765-777.)
- **Pre-Hospital Succinylcholine Vs. Rocuronium**
  - This multicenter, single-blind, noninferiority trial randomized adult patients who needed out-of-hospital tracheal intubation to receive rocuronium 1.2 mg/kg or succinylcholine 1 mg/kg for rapid sequence intubation.
  - Patients receiving rocuronium experienced a higher rate of the primary outcome (intubation success rate on the first attempt), but this incidence did not meet the pre-defined noninferiority margin.
  - The most common intubation-related adverse events were hypoxemia and hypotension were similar between groups.
  - The authors concluded that compared with succinylcholine, rocuronium failed to demonstrate noninferiority in the first-attempt intubation success among patients undergoing endotracheal intubation in an out-of-hospital emergency setting. (JAMA. 2019;322(23):2303-2312.)

High-Yield Fast-Facts
- **Histamine Release**
    - Succinylcholine has been associated with mast-cell mediated histamine release, but this effect is not clinically relevant.
- **Dantrolene**
    - The treatment for malignant hyperthermia includes dantrolene, which is a ryanodine calcium channel blocker.

HIGH-YIELD BOARD EXAM ESSENTIALS
- **CLASSIC AGENTS:** Succinylcholine
- **DRUG CLASS:** Depolarizing neuromuscular blocker
- **INDICATIONS:** Neuromuscular blockade for endotracheal intubation, surgery, or mechanical ventilation
- **MECHANISM:** Binds to acetylcholine receptors of the motor endplate, causing an initial depolarization but causes a persistent effect resistant to acetylcholinesterase.
- **SIDE EFFECTS:** Hyperkalemia, rhabdomyolysis, malignant hyperthermia, fasciculations
- **CLINICAL PEARLS:**
    - The only neuromuscular blocker that you can use as IM injection although not preferred over IV.
    - Has a quick onset of action within 1 minute and short duration.
    - Patients with a history of neuromuscular disease (ex., myasthenia gravis, multiple sclerosis, etc.) may have a prolonged and unpredictable paralysis duration.
    - Traditionally avoided in patients with known hyperkalemia or at increased risk of hyperkalemia as the depolarizing effect can cause muscles to release intracellular potassium during muscle fasciculations.

Table: Drug Class Summary

Depolarizing Neuromuscular Blocker - Drug Class Review			
High-Yield Med Reviews			
Generic Name	Brand Name	Indication(s) or Uses	Notes

Succinylcholine	Anectine
	Quelicin
		• Neuromuscular blockade for endotracheal intubation, surgery, or mechanical ventilation	• Dosing (Adult):
			  – IV: 1.0 to 1.5 mg/kg
			  – IM: 3 to 4 mg/kg
			• Dosing (Peds):
			  – IV: 1.0 to 3 mg/kg
			  – IM: 4 to 5 mg/kg
			• CYP450 Interactions: None
			• Renal or Hepatic Dose Adjustments: None
			• Dosage Forms: IV (solution)

NEUROMUSCULAR BLOCKERS – NON-DEPOLARIZING NEUROMUSCULAR BLOCKER

Drug Class
- Non-Depolarizing Neuromuscular Blocker
- Agents:
    - Acute Care
        - Atracurium
        - Cisatracurium
        - Mivacurium
        - Pancuronium
        - Rocuronium
        - Vecuronium

> **Fast Facts**
> - Since these agents are "non-depolarizing" neuromuscular blockers they do NOT cause muscle fasciculations like succinylcholine.
> - Compared to succinylcholine they tend to have a slight delay in the onset of action but have a longer duration.

Main Indications or Uses
- Acute Care
    - Neuromuscular blockade for endotracheal intubation, surgery, or mechanical ventilation

Mechanism of Action
- Competitively inhibit acetylcholine at the skeletal muscle motor endplate.

Non-Depolarizing Agent
↓
Competitively antagonize acetylcholine
at the nACH (nicotinic) receptor
↓
Inhibit or block local membrane depolarization
[end plate potential (EPP)].
↓
Paralysis of skeletal muscle

Primary Net Benefit
- Produce a dose-dependent neuromuscular blockade without initial fasciculations or many other adverse events related to succinylcholine.
- Main Labs to Monitor:
    - Train-of-four

High-Yield Basic Pharmacology
- **Atracurium and Cisatracurium Metabolite**
    - Atracurium is metabolized to laudanosine, which can cross the blood-brain barrier and placental barrier leading to neuroexcitation without any neuromuscular blocking effects.
        - Laudanosine is a GABA antagonist and an antagonist of nicotinic acetylcholine receptors and opioid receptor antagonists.
    - Patients receiving prolonged infusions or liver disease, biliary obstruction, or renal impairment are at high risk of laudanosine accumulation.
- **Muscarinic Effects**
    - Pancuronium may cause dose-dependent and rate-dependent muscarinic effects, including tachycardia and hypertension.
        - This effect is caused by a parasympathetic response from activation of muscarinic receptors by pancuronium.

High-Yield Clinical Knowledge
- **Anaphylaxis**
  - Anaphylaxis may occur with a high incidence among patients receiving rocuronium that can be difficult to treat.
  - Although standard management of anaphylaxis should be a cornerstone of therapy, the reversal agent sugammadex can treat anaphylaxis due to rocuronium or vecuronium.
- **Limited Contraindications**
  - Compared with succinylcholine and its long list of contraindications and warnings, the non-depolarizing neuromuscular blockers have few contraindications.
    - These contraindications consist of a history of allergy or hypersensitivity to a neuromuscular blocker.
- **Persistent Weakness**
  - Non-depolarizing neuromuscular blockers that are administered as IV infusions for greater than 48 hours pose a risk of prolonged neuromuscular blockade even after discontinuation of the drug.
  - Risk factors for prolonged paralysis include patients with sepsis, ARDS, multiorgan failure, hyperglycemia, systemic corticosteroids, muscle injury, and thermal injury.
- **Pancuronium Adjustment**
  - Pancuronium is primarily renally excreted and requires dose adjustments for patients with impaired renal function.
  - Accumulation of pancuronium and its active metabolite, 3-desacetyl-pancuronium, can lead to prolonged paralysis even after drug discontinuation.
- **Reversal**
  - Non-depolarizing neuromuscular blocking agents can be reversed using one of two strategies: sugammadex or cholinergic competitive inhibition.
    - Sugammadex encapsulates rocuronium or vecuronium in a 1:1 ratio and prevents further binding to the nicotinic receptors.
    - Neostigmine or pyridostigmine inhibits plasma cholinesterase, increasing acetylcholine at the neuromuscular junction to overcome the competitive inhibition caused by paralytics.
- **Defasciculation**
  - To blunt the fasciculation response to succinylcholine, small (10% of normal doses) doses of non-depolarizing neuromuscular blockers can be administered before succinylcholine.

High-Yield Core Evidence
- **ACURASYS Trial**
  - This was a multicenter, double-blinded, placebo-controlled trial that randomized patients with early severe ARDS to either cisatracurium infusion or placebo for 48 hours.
  - Patients randomized to receive cisatracurium had improved 90-day survival and more ventilator-free days compared to patients receiving placebo.
  - This difference remained significant even after adjustment for both the baseline PaO2:FIO2 and plateau pressure and the Simplified Acute Physiology II score, as well as during the 28-day mortality analysis.
  - However, the crude 90-day mortality was not significantly different between groups.
  - The rate of ICU-acquired paresis did not differ significantly between the two groups.
  - The authors concluded that early administration of a neuromuscular blocking agent improved the adjusted 90-day survival for patients with severe ARDS and increased the time off the ventilator without increasing muscle weakness. (N Engl J Med. 2010 Sep 16;363(12):1107-16.)

- **ROSE Trial**
  - This was a multicenter clinical trial that randomized patients with moderate-to-severe ARDS to receive either cisatracurium 48-hour infusion with concomitant deep sedation or to a usual-care approach without routine neuromuscular blockade and with lighter sedation targets.
  - This study was stopped early due to futility after an interim analysis failed to show the benefit of cisatracurium infusion.
  - Of the patients enrolled, there was no difference in the primary outcome of in-hospital death from any cause at 90 days with a p=0.93.
  - While in the hospital, patients in the intervention group were less physically active and had more adverse cardiovascular events than patients in the control group.
  - The authors concluded that for patients with moderate-to-severe ARDS treated with a high PEEP strategy, there was no significant difference in mortality at 90 days between patients who received an early and continuous cisatracurium infusion and those who were treated with a usual-care approach with lighter sedation targets. (N Engl J Med 2019; 380:1997-2008.)

High-Yield Fast-Fact
- **Sugammadex Allergy**
  - Patients experiencing an allergic response to sugammadex should receive rocuronium, which forms a complex and interrupts antigenic activity of sugammadex itself.

HIGH-YIELD BOARD EXAM ESSENTIALS
- **CLASSIC AGENTS:** Atracurium, cisatracurium, mivacurium, pancuronium, rocuronium, vecuronium
- **DRUG CLASS:** Non-depolarizing neuromuscular blocker
- **INDICATIONS:** Neuromuscular blockade for endotracheal intubation, surgery, or mechanical ventilation
- **MECHANISM:** Competitively inhibit acetylcholine at the skeletal muscle motor endplate.
- **SIDE EFFECTS:** Anaphylaxis, persistent muscle weakness
- **CLINICAL PEARLS:**
  - Pancuronium is primarily renally excreted and requires dose adjustments for patients with impaired renal function. Accumulation of pancuronium and its active metabolite, 3-desacetyl-pancuronium, can lead to prolonged paralysis even after drug discontinuation.

Table: Drug Class Summary

\multicolumn{4}{c}{**Non-Depolarizing Neuromuscular Blocker - Drug Class Review**}
\multicolumn{4}{c}{High-Yield Med Reviews}
\multicolumn{4}{l}{**Mechanism of Action:** *Competitively inhibit acetylcholine at the skeletal muscle motor endplate.*}
\multicolumn{4}{l}{**Class Effects:** *Produce a dose-dependent neuromuscular blockade without initial fasciculations or many other adverse events related to succinylcholine.*}
Generic Name	Brand Name	Main Indication(s) or Uses	Notes

Atracurium	Tracrium	• Neuromuscular blockade for endotracheal intubation, surgery, or mechanical ventilation	• **Dosing (Adult):**
			  – IV: 0.4 to 0.5 mg bolus
			  – IV: infusion 4 to 20 mcg/kg/minute
			• **Dosing (Peds):**
			  – IV: 0.3 to 0.5 mg bolus
			  – IV infusion 4 to 20 mcg/kg/minute
			• **CYP450 Interactions:** None
			• **Renal or Hepatic Dose Adjustments:** None
			• **Dosage Forms:** IV (solution)

Cisatracurium	Nimbex	• Neuromuscular blockade for endotracheal intubation, surgery, or mechanical ventilation	• **Dosing (Adult):**
			  – IV: 0.1 to 0.2 mg/kg followed by 1 to 3 mcg/kg/minute
			• **Dosing (Peds):**
			  – IV: 0.1 to 0.2 mg/kg followed by 1 to 3 mcg/kg/minute
			• **CYP450 Interactions:** None
			• **Renal or Hepatic Dose Adjustments:** None
			• **Dosage Forms:** IV (solution)

Mivacurium	Mivacron	• Neuromuscular blockade for endotracheal intubation, surgery, or mechanical ventilation	• **Dosing (Adult):**
			  – IV: 0.15 to 0.25 mg/kg
			  – IV: 5 to 10 mcg/kg/minute
			• **Dosing (Peds):**
			  – IV: 0.15 to 0.25 mg/kg
			  – IV: 1 to 10 mcg/kg/minute
			• **CYP450 Interactions:** None
			• **Renal or Hepatic Dose Adjustments:**
			  – GFR < 30 mL/minute: maximum bolus 0.15 mg/kg, reduce infusion rates by 50%
			• **Dosage Forms:** IV (solution)

Non-Depolarizing Neuromuscular Blocker - Drug Class Review High-Yield Med Reviews			
Generic Name	**Brand Name**	**Main Indication(s) or Uses**	**Notes**

Pancuronium	Pavulon	• Neuromuscular blockade for endotracheal intubation, surgery, or mechanical ventilation	• **Dosing (Adult):**
			  – IV: 0.04 to 0.1 mg/kg
			  – IV: 0.8 to 2 mcg/kg/minute
			• **Dosing (Peds):**
			  – IV: 0.04 to 0.1 mg/kg
			  – IV: 0.8 to 2 mcg/kg/minute
			• **CYP450 Interactions:** None
			• **Renal or Hepatic Dose Adjustments:**
			  – GFR 10 to 50 mL/minute: Reduce by 50%
			  – GFR < 10 mL/minute: Avoid use
			  – Hepatic impairment: can have increased or decreased response
			• **Dosage Forms:** IV (solution)

Rocuronium	Zemuron	• Neuromuscular blockade for endotracheal intubation, surgery, or mechanical ventilation	• **Dosing (Adult):**
			  – IV: 0.6 to 1.2 mg/kg x 1
			  – IV: 8 to 12 mcg/kg/minute
			• **Dosing (Peds):**
			  – IV: 0.6 to 1.8 mg/kg x 1
			  – IV: 8 to 12 mcg/kg/minute
			• **CYP450 Interactions:** None
			• **Renal or Hepatic Dose Adjustments:**
			  – Hepatic impairment: no specific guidance, but may require higher doses
			• **Dosage Forms:** IV (solution)

Vecuronium	Norcuron	• Neuromuscular blockade for endotracheal intubation, surgery, or mechanical ventilation	• **Dosing (Adult):**
			  – IV: 0.08 to 0.1 mg/kg
			  – IV: 0.8 to 1.2 mcg/kg/minute
			• **Dosing (Peds):**
			  – IV: 0.08 to 0.1 mg/kg
			  – IV: 0.8 to 1.2 mcg/kg/minute
			• **CYP450 Interactions:** None
			• **Renal or Hepatic Dose Adjustments:** None
			• **Dosage Forms:** IV (solution)

NEUROMUSCULAR BLOCKERS – NEUROMUSCULAR BLOCKER REVERSAL

Drug Class
- Neuromuscular Blocker Reversal
- Agents:
    - Acute Care
        - Neostigmine
        - Pyridostigmine
        - Sugammadex

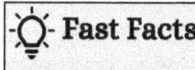

Fast Facts
- ✓ It is important to recognize that sugammadex does not reverse succinylcholine, but only rocuronium and vecuronium.

Main Indications or Uses
- Acute Care
    - Myasthenia gravis
    - Reversal of nondepolarizing neuromuscular
    - Reduction of secretions
    - Reversal of rocuronium or vecuronium

Mechanism of Action
- Neostigmine, Pyridostigmine
    - Inhibits acetylcholinesterase at the neuromuscular junction, thereby increasing acetylcholine.
- Sugammadex
    - Binds to steroid-based neuromuscular blockers (rocuronium, vecuronium), forming a 1:1 complex that prevents the neuromuscular blocker's binding to its nicotinic receptor site.

Primary Net Benefit
- Reversal agents for neuromuscular blocking agents improve recovery time from paralysis but are not associated with any patient-oriented benefits.
- Main Labs to Monitor:
    - No routine lab monitoring

High-Yield Basic Pharmacology
- Tertiary Vs. Quaternary Ammonium
    - Neostigmine and pyridostigmine are quaternary ammonium compounds and do not readily cross the blood-brain barrier at normal therapeutic doses.
        - Physostigmine, a similar cholinergic agent, is an example of a tertiary ammonium compound that does cross the blood-brain barrier causing a central cholinergic effect.
- Paralytic Encapsulation
    - Sugammadex is a modified cyclodextrin compound with a hydrophilic outer surface and a lipophilic central cavity that encapsulates both rocuronium and vecuronium.
    - This encapsulation creates a concentration gradient by which rocuronium or vecuronium leaves the neuromuscular junction for the plasma and then subsequently bound by sugammadex.

High-Yield Clinical Knowledge
- Killer B's
    - The administration of neostigmine or pyridostigmine carries a risk of bradycardia, bronchospasm, and bronchorrhea - otherwise known as the killer b's of cholinergic toxicity.
    - The coadministration of an antimuscarinic agent can manage these effects.
- Atropine Vs. Glycopyrrolate
    - To counterbalance the cholinergic effects (primarily bradycardia) of neostigmine or pyridostigmine, these agents are often administered with an anticholinergic agent, either atropine or glycopyrrolate.
    - Being a quaternary ammonium, glycopyrrolate does not cross the blood-brain barrier, thus does not possess central anticholinergic effects, causing confusion, delirium, or altered mental status.
- Dose-Dependent Time To Reversal

- Sugammadex exhibits a dose-dependent time to reversal paralysis, with the shortest time to reversal achieved using the 16 mg/kg dose.
- At a typical surgical reversal dose of 4 mg/kg, the median time to reach the train of four ratios of 0.9 is 2.4 minutes after rocuronium or 3.4 minutes for vecuronium compared to 49 minutes using neostigmine.
- **Sugammadex Allergy**
  - Some patients may experience an acute allergic reaction to sugammadex that can be treated by administering rocuronium or vecuronium.
  - The formation of the sugammadex-rocuronium/vecuronium complex, the reaction is halted.
- **Decreased Hormonal Contraceptive Effectiveness**
  - Sugammadex may bind with progesterone, decreasing its concentrations.
  - Thus, in women taking progesterone-based hormonal contraceptives, this birth control's effectiveness may be diminished for up to 7 days following sugammadex administration.

High-Yield Core Evidence
- **Sugammadex Vs Neostigmine**
  - This meta-analysis compared the efficacy and safety of sugammadex versus neostigmine in reversing neuromuscular blockade caused by nondepolarizing neuromuscular agents in adults.
  - The following databases were used in the authors' search: Cochrane Central Register of Controlled Trials, MEDLINE, Embase, www.controlled-trials.com, clinicaltrials.gov, and www.centerwatch.com.
  - The authors included relevant randomized controlled trials irrespective of publication status, date of publication, blinding status, outcomes published, or language.
  - A total of 41 studies (with 4206 participants) was included in this systematic review, with twelve trials eligible for meta-analysis of primary outcomes, and 28 trials were eligible for meta-analysis of secondary outcomes.
  - Sugammadex 2 mg/kg was 6.6 times faster than neostigmine at a dose of 0.05 mg/kg in reversing neuromuscular blockade from the second twitch to TOFR > 0.9.
  - Sugammadex 4 mg/kg was 16.8 times faster than neostigmine 0.07 mg/kg (2.9 vs 48.8 minutes) in reversing neuromuscular block from post-tetanic count 1 to 5 to TOFR > 0.9.
  - There were significantly fewer composite adverse events in the sugammadex group than the neostigmine group, specifically regarding the incidence of bradycardia, postoperative nausea and vomiting, and overall signs of postoperative residual paralysis.
  - The authors concluded that these results suggest that, compared with neostigmine, sugammadex can more rapidly reverse rocuronium-induced neuromuscular block regardless of the block's depth. With an NNT of 8 to avoid an adverse event, sugammadex appears to have a better safety profile than neostigmine. (Cochrane Database Syst Rev. 2017 Aug 14;8(8):CD012763.)

High-Yield Fast-Fact
- **Selective Reversal**
  - Sugammadex has no effect on the reversal of paralysis from atracurium, cisatracurium, or mivacurium.

HIGH-YIELD BOARD EXAM ESSENTIALS
- **CLASSIC AGENTS:** Neostigmine, pyridostigmine, sugammadex
- **DRUG CLASS:** Neuromuscular blocker reversal
- **INDICATIONS:** Reversal of nondepolarizing neuromuscular, reduction of secretions, myasthenia gravis
- **MECHANISM:** Inhibits acetylcholinesterase at the neuromuscular junction, thereby increasing acetylcholine (neostigmine, pyridostigmine); Binds to steroid-based neuromuscular blockers (rocuronium, vecuronium), forming a 1:1 complex that prevents the neuromuscular blocker's binding to its nicotinic receptor site (sugammadex)
- **SIDE EFFECTS:** Cholinergic effects (neostigmine, pyridostigmine), allergy/hypersensitivity (sugammadex)
- **CLINICAL PEARLS:** Sugammadex exhibits a dose-dependent time to reversal paralysis, with the shortest time to reversal achieved using the 16 mg/kg dose. At a typical surgical reversal dose of 4 mg/kg, the median time to reach the train of four ratios of 0.9 is 2.4 minutes after rocuronium or 3.4 minutes for vecuronium compared to 49 minutes using neostigmine.

Table: Drug Class Summary

Neuromuscular Blocker Reversal - Drug Class Review High-Yield Med Reviews			
Mechanism of Action: **Neostigmine, Pyridostigmine** - *Inhibits acetylcholinesterase at the neuromuscular junction, thereby increasing acetylcholine.* **Sugammadex** - *Binds to steroid-based neuromuscular blockers (rocuronium, vecuronium), forming a 1:1 complex that prevents the neuromuscular blocker's binding to its nicotinic receptor site.*			
Class Effects: *Reversal agents for neuromuscular blocking agents improve recovery time from paralysis but not associated with any patient-oriented benefits.*			
Generic Name	**Brand Name**	**Main Indication(s) or Uses**	**Notes**
Glycopyrrolate	Cuvposa	<ul><li>Reversal of nondepolarizing neuromuscular</li><li>Reduction of secretions</li></ul>	<ul><li>**Dosing (Adult):**<ul><li>IV: 0.2 mg for each 1 mg of neostigmine or 5 mg of pyridostigmine</li></ul></li><li>**Dosing (Peds):**<ul><li>IV: 0.2 mg for each 1 mg of neostigmine or 5 mg of pyridostigmine</li></ul></li><li>**CYP450 Interactions:** None</li><li>**Renal or Hepatic Dose Adjustments:** None</li><li>**Dosage Forms:** IV (solution), Oral (tablet)</li></ul>
Neostigmine	Bloxiverz	<ul><li>Myasthenia gravis</li><li>Reversal of nondepolarizing neuromuscular</li></ul>	<ul><li>**Dosing (Adult):**<ul><li>IV: 0.03 to 0.07 mg/kg</li><li>Maximum 5 mg</li></ul></li><li>**Dosing (Peds):**<ul><li>IV: 0.03 to 0.07 mg/kg</li><li>Maximum 5 mg</li></ul></li><li>**CYP450 Interactions:** None</li><li>**Renal or Hepatic Dose Adjustments:**<ul><li>GFR 10 to 50 mL/minute: Reduce dose by 50%</li><li>GFR < 10 mL/minute: Reduce dose by 75%</li></ul></li><li>**Dosage Forms:** IV (solution)</li></ul>
Pyridostigmine	Mestinon Regonol	<ul><li>Myasthenia gravis Reversal of nondepolarizing neuromuscular</li></ul>	<ul><li>**Dosing (Adult):**<ul><li>IV: 0.1 to 0.25 mg/kg</li></ul></li><li>**Dosing (Peds):**<ul><li>IV: 0.1 to 0.25 mg/kg</li></ul></li><li>**CYP450 Interactions:** None</li><li>**Renal or Hepatic Dose Adjustments:** None</li><li>**Dosage Forms:** IV (solution), Oral (tablet)</li></ul>
Sugammadex	Bridion	<ul><li>Reversal of rocuronium or vecuronium</li></ul>	<ul><li>**Dosing (Adult):**<ul><li>IV: 4 to 16 mg/kg once</li></ul></li><li>**Dosing (Peds):**<ul><li>IV: 2 mg/kg once</li></ul></li><li>**CYP450 Interactions:** None</li><li>**Renal or Hepatic Dose Adjustments:**<ul><li>GFR < 30 mL/minute: not recommended</li></ul></li><li>**Dosage Forms:** IV (solution)</li></ul>

NEUROLOGY – PARKINSONS AGENTS - ANTICHOLINERGICS

Drug Class
- Anticholinergics
- Agents:
  - Acute & Chronic Care
    - Benztropine
    - Procyclidine
    - Trihexyphenidyl

Main Indications or Uses
- Acute & Chronic Care
  - Drug-induced extrapyramidal symptoms
    - Benztropine
  - Parkinson disease
    - Benztropine
    - Procyclidine
    - Trihexyphenidyl

> **Knowledge Integration**
> ✓ Benztropine and diphenhydramine are the most common treatments of antipsychotic-induced dystonic reactions.
>
> ✓ This class has a limited use in Parkinson's disease due to the anticholinergic effects in this patient population.

Mechanism of Action
- Inhibits excess acetylcholine at muscarinic and nicotinic receptor sites, decreasing parasympathetic nervous system activity.

Primary Net Benefit
- Replaced mainly with safer alternatives, anticholinergic agents may reduce tremors and alleviate rigidity associated with Parkinson's diseases but lack bradykinetic effects.
- Main Labs to Monitor:
  - No routine lab monitoring

High-Yield Basic Pharmacology
- Anticholinergic Effect
  - The anticholinergic agents counteract diminished levels of dopamine by stimulating parasympathetic activity and relative hyperactivity of acetylcholine.
- Dopaminergic Pathway
  - The breakdown of dopaminergic neurons in the nigrostriatal pathway results in the depletion of dopamine related to Parkinson's disease.

High-Yield Clinical Knowledge
- Abrupt Discontinuation
  - Abrupt discontinuation of anticholinergic agents must be avoided as this may precipitate acute exacerbations of parkinsonisms.
  - Careful tapering of doses should take place if changes in the drug regimen are warranted.
- Elderly Patients
  - The use of anticholinergic drugs in elderly patients significantly increases their risk of falls and other adverse events that impact comorbidities such as dry mucus membranes, tachycardia, altered mental status, or orthostatic hypotension.
  - Since many patients with Parkinson's disease are elderly, the use of alternative agents (i.e., dopamine agonists) should be strongly considered to minimize these risks.
  - Furthermore, anticholinergic agents in this population have been associated with an increased incidence of dementia.
- Dopaminergic Agents Vs. Anticholinergic
  - Dopaminergic agents, such as bromocriptine or ropinirole, are similarly effective in managing Parkinson's tremor as the anticholinergic agents, without the risk of anticholinergic effects.

- **Blind As A Bat...**
  - Common adverse anticholinergic effects that lead to discontinuation include visual changes, confusion, constipation, xerostomia, altered mental status, hyperthermia/flushing, and urinary retention.

High-Yield Core Evidence
- **Benztropine Vs. Clozapine**
  - This was a double-blind crossover trial that randomized patients to clozapine or benztropine to treat tremor in Parkinson's disease.
  - There was no difference concerning the primary outcome of change in the tremor and the motor score of the United Parkinson's Disease Rating Scale.
  - Patients in each group experienced significant adverse events; however, there were no leukopenia cases related to clozapine therapy.
  - The study authors concluded that the atypical antipsychotic drug clozapine helps treat tremor in Parkinson's disease and should be considered when all other drug therapies fail. (Neurology. 1997 Apr;48(4):1077-81.)

High-Yield Fast-Facts
- **Acute Dystonic Reactions**
  - As an alternative to benzodiazepines, benztropine may be used to manage acute dystonic reactions secondary to antipsychotic drugs.
- **Abuse Potential**
  - Anticholinergic drugs possess an abuse potential via dopaminergic effects, which resemble similar results from sympathomimetic abuse.

HIGH-YIELD BOARD EXAM ESSENTIALS
- **CLASSIC AGENTS:** Benztropine, procyclidine, trihexyphenidyl
- **DRUG CLASS:** Anticholinergics
- **INDICATIONS:** Drug-induced extrapyramidal symptoms, Parkinson disease
- **MECHANISM:** Inhibits excess acetylcholine at muscarinic and nicotinic receptor sites, decreasing parasympathetic nervous system activity.
- **SIDE EFFECTS:** Dry mucus membranes, tachycardia, altered mental status, or orthostatic hypotension.
- **CLINICAL PEARLS:**
  - Abrupt discontinuation of anticholinergic agents must be avoided as this may precipitate acute exacerbations of parkinsonisms. Careful tapering of doses should take place if changes in the drug regimen are warranted.
  - Benztropine is a common treatment for acute dystonic reactions associated with antipsychotics.

Table: Drug Class Summary

\multicolumn{4}{c}{**Anticholinergics - Drug Class Review**}

Anticholinergics - Drug Class Review			
High-Yield Med Reviews			
Mechanism of Action: *Inhibits excess acetylcholine at muscarinic and nicotinic receptor sites, decreasing parasympathetic nervous system activity.*			
Class Effects: *Largely replaced with safer alternatives, anticholinergic agents may reduce tremor and alleviate rigidity associated with Parkinson's diseases but lack effects on bradykinesia.*			
Generic Name	**Brand Name**	**Indication(s) or Uses**	**Notes**
Benztropine	Cogentin	• Drug-induced extrapyramidal symptoms • Parkinson's disease	• **Dosing (Adult):** – IM/IV/Oral: 0.5 to 2 mg q8-12h – Maximum 6 mg/day • **Dosing (Peds):** – IM/IV/Oral: 0.02 to 0.05 mg/kg/dose q8-24h – Maximum 6 mg/day • **CYP450 Interactions:** Substrate of CYP2D6 • **Renal or Hepatic Dose Adjustments:** None • **Dosage Forms:** Oral (tablet), IV (solution)
Procyclidine	Kemadrin	• Parkinson's disease	• **Dosing (Adult):** – Oral: 2.5 mg three times daily after meals – Maximum 20 mg/day • **Dosing (Peds):** – Not routinely used • **CYP450 Interactions:** None • **Renal or Hepatic Dose Adjustments:** None • **Dosage Forms:** Oral (elixir, tablet)
Trihexyphenidyl	Artane, Parkin	• Drug-induced extrapyramidal symptoms • Parkinson's disease	• **Dosing (Adult):** – Oral: 1 mg/day titrated to 15 mg/day in 3-4 divided doses • **Dosing (Peds):** – Oral: 0.1 to 0.2 mg/kg/day divided in 2-3 doses – Maximum 2.6 mg/kg/day • **CYP450 Interactions:** None • **Renal or Hepatic Dose Adjustments:** None • **Dosage Forms:** Oral (tablet, solution)

NEUROLOGY – PARKINSONS AGENTS – CARBIDOPA/LEVODOPA

Drug Class
- Carbidopa/Levodopa
- Agents:
  - Chronic Care
    - Carbidopa/Levodopa
    - Carbidopa/Levodopa/Entacapone

Main Indications or Uses
- Chronic Care
  - Parkinson Disease

Mechanism of Action
- Levodopa
  - A precursor to dopamine that provides supplemental concentrations to the central nervous system.
- Carbidopa
  - Inhibits peripheral conversion of levodopa to dopamine.

> **Fast Facts**
> ✓ Carbidopa prevents the peripheral or systemic conversion of levodopa to dopamine thereby allowing the levodopa to be preferentially taken up in the CNS.
>
> ✓ This drug class does not prevent the progression of Parkinson's disease, but instead treats some of the symptoms for a period of about 5 years.

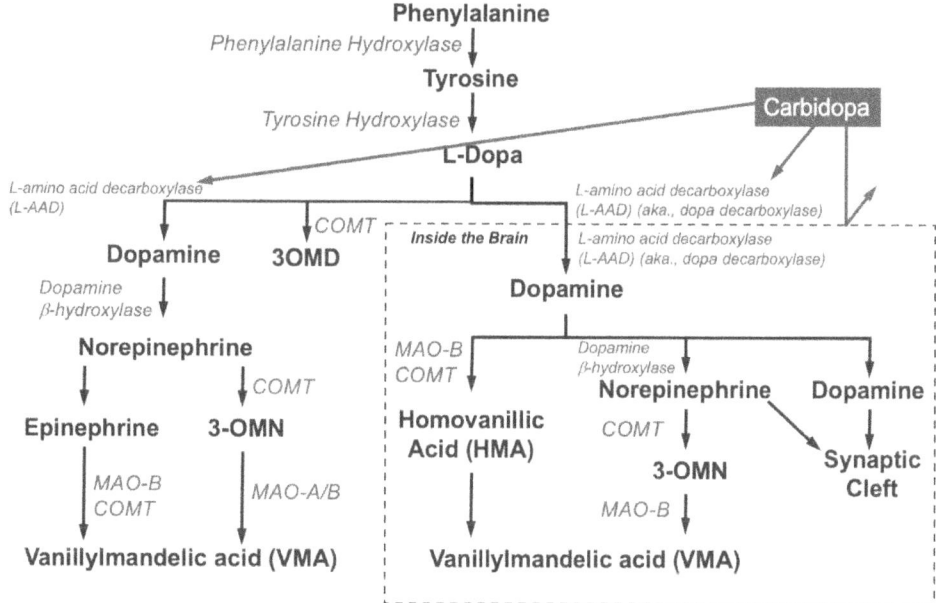

Primary Net Benefit
- Nearly all patients with Parkinson's disease will require carbidopa/levodopa and likely develop fluctuations and dyskinesias due to the drug combination.
- Main Labs to Monitor:
  - Liver function (INR, albumin, protein, bilirubin)
  - Serum creatinine
  - CBS
  - Blood pressure, orthostatic blood pressure
  - Intraocular pressure

High-Yield Basic Pharmacology
- **Carbidopa Rationale**

- Carbidopa reduces the premature conversion of levodopa to dopamine in the peripheral circulation by inhibiting dopa decarboxylase.
- Coformulation with levodopa reduces its daily dose by 75%, and the suppression of dopa decarboxylase typically requires a dose of 75 mg/day of carbidopa.
- **Alternative Metabolism**
    - As dopa decarboxylase is inhibited by carbidopa, peripheral metabolism may still occur by catechol-o-methyltransferase (COMT).
    - This secondary metabolic pathway can be inhibited using COMT inhibitors such as entacapone or tolcapone.
- **Continuous Administration**
    - Novel methods to reduce dose fluctuations of levodopa have employed a continuously administered solution of carbidopa-levodopa intraduodenally.
    - These drug delivery systems appear to reduce fluctuations in central dopamine concentrations and may reduce the development of dyskinesias.

High-Yield Clinical Knowledge
- **Dyskinesias**
    - The development of dyskinesias from levodopa is dose-dependent but generally occurs in upwards of 80% of patients after 10 years of continuous therapy.
        - The most common dyskinesias observed is choreoathetosis of the face and distal extremities.
        - Intraduodenal or intrajejunal continuous administration of carbidopa-levodopa has been suggested to reduce or slow the development of dyskinesias by reducing the chronic pulsatile stimulation of dopamine receptors leading to dopaminergic denervation.
- **Response Fluctuation Effects**
    - Long-term therapy with levodopa is associated with dyskinesias shortly after oral doses (peak effect) and an end of dose motor fluctuation termed "wearing-off effect."
        - These effects can manifest after inappropriately high dose initiation or long-term therapy as the approximate risk of developing these effects is 10% per year of levodopa therapy.
    - Substituting immediate-release for controlled-release formulations does not reduce the development of these movement disorders.
        - The addition of COMT inhibitors or MAO-B inhibitors may play a role and should be considered.
- **Numerous Formulations**
    - Combinations of carbidopa-levodopa are formulated as immediate-release, controlled-release, and extended-release preparations.
    - Doses are not interchangeable as bioavailabilities differ between these agents.
- **Fall Risk**
    - Patients with Parkinson's disease are at risk of falls due to the impaired gait or shuffling characteristic of walking.
    - Levodopa has been associated with the development of episodic akinesia of the lower extremities, which may place patients at a higher risk of falls.
        - This freezing phenomenon is worsened when patients encounter obstacles such as doorways, or corners, which are ubiquitous in healthcare facilities.
- **Acute On/Off Management**
    - After titration of levodopa and regimen modification with MAO-B inhibitors or COMT inhibitors, apomorphine has been used to manage acute off episodes.
- **Drug Holidays**
    - Extended periods where anti-Parkinson's medications are withheld, known as drug holidays, is a method to temporarily improve responsiveness to levodopa and alleviate some adverse events.
        - This does not reduce the on-off effect of levodopa chronic therapy.

High-Yield Core Evidence
- **Dyskinesia In Parkinson's Disease**
    - This was a prospective, double-blind trial that randomized patients with early Parkinson's disease to receive either ropinirole or levodopa over a period of five years, with supplementary doses of open-label levodopa permitted.

- At five years, the cumulative incidence of dyskinesias significantly favored patients randomized to receive ropinirole than those receiving levodopa.
- However, there was no significant difference between the two groups in the mean change in scores for daily living activities among those who completed the study.
- A similar proportion of patients in either group experienced adverse events that led to the study's early withdrawal.
- The authors concluded that early Parkinson's disease can be managed successfully for up to five years with a reduced risk of dyskinesia by initiating treatment with ropinirole alone and supplementing it with levodopa if necessary. (N Engl J Med. 2000 May 18;342(20):1484-91.)
- **Parkinson Study Group**
    - This was a double-blind, placebo-controlled trial that randomized patients with early Parkinson's disease who to receive either carbidopa-levodopa at a daily dose of 37.5 and 150 mg, 75 and 300 mg, or 150 and 600 mg, respectively, or a matching placebo for a period of 40 weeks, and then to undergo withdrawal of treatment for 2 weeks.
    - Patients randomized to placebo experienced a significantly worse change in scores on the Unified Parkinson's Disease Rating Scale (the primary outcome) between baseline and 42 weeks, compared to any carbidopa-levodopa dose.
    - There was no difference in the mean change between the total score on the UPDRS at baseline and at 42 weeks between carbidopa-levodopa groups.
    - However, patients receiving the highest levodopa dose had significantly more dyskinesia, hypertonia, infection, headache, and nausea than those receiving placebo.
    - The authors concluded that levodopa either slows Parkinson's disease progression or has a prolonged effect on the disease's symptoms. In contrast, the neuroimaging data suggest that levodopa accelerates the loss of nigrostriatal dopamine nerve terminals or that its pharmacologic effects modify the dopamine transporter. The potential long-term effects of levodopa on Parkinson's disease remain uncertain. (N Engl J Med. 2004 Dec 9;351(24):2498-508.)

High-Yield Fast-Facts
- **Glaucoma**
    - Levodopa should not be given to patients with acute angle-closure glaucoma but may be used in patients with chronic open-angle glaucoma if intraocular pressures are followed.
- **Psychiatric Disturbance**
    - Levodopa should not be used in patients with psychiatric history as it may exacerbate their disorder.
- **Melanoma**
    - Levodopa is a precursor of melanin and may induce malignant melanoma pathology.

HIGH-YIELD BOARD EXAM ESSENTIALS
- **CLASSIC AGENTS:** Carbidopa/levodopa, carbidopa/levodopa/entacapone
- **DRUG CLASS:** Anti-Parkinson's
- **INDICATIONS:** Parkinson disease, restless leg syndrome
- **MECHANISM:** Levodopa - Precursor to dopamine that providing supplemental concentrations to the central nervous system; Carbidopa - Inhibits peripheral conversion of levodopa to dopamine.
- **SIDE EFFECTS:** Dyskinesias, "wearing-off effect", GI side effects (constipation, nausea), orthostatic hypotension, psychosis (hallucinations)
- **CLINICAL PEARLS:** The development of dyskinesias from levodopa is dose-dependent but generally occurs in upwards of 80% of patients after 10 years of continuous therapy. Controlled and extended release formulations should not be used as initial therapy and are also not interchangeable on a dose to dose basis. Adjustments in dosing are necessary when switching between agents.

Table: Drug Class Summary

\multicolumn{4}{c}{**Carbidopa-Levodopa Drug Class Review**}

\multicolumn{4}{l}{**Carbidopa-Levodopa Drug Class Review** — High-Yield Med Reviews}
\multicolumn{4}{l}{**Mechanism of Action:** *Levodopa* - Precursor to dopamine that providing supplemental concentrations to the central nervous system. *Carbidopa* - Inhibits peripheral conversion of levodopa to dopamine.}
\multicolumn{4}{l}{**Class Effects:** *Nearly all patients with Parkinson's disease will require carbidopa/levodopa and likely develop fluctuations and dyskinesias due to the drug combination.*}
Generic Name	**Brand Name**	**Indication(s) or Uses**	**Notes**

Carbidopa-Levodopa	Duopa
	Rytary
	Sinemet
		• Parkinson disease
		• Restless leg syndrome
			• **Dosing (Adult):**
			  – IR/ODT: tablets carbidopa/levodopa 12.5 mg/50 mg BID to TID.
			    – Titrated by 1 tablet or up to 25 mg/100 mg every 1-2 days
			  – CR tablet: 50 mg/200 mg BID
			    – Titrated no faster than q3days to maximum levodopa dose of 2,400 mg/day
			  – ER: 23.75 mg/95 mg TID
			    – Titrated q3days to maximum levodopa dose of 2,450 mg/day
			• **Dosing (Peds):**
			  – Not routinely used
			• **CYP450 Interactions:** None
			• **Renal or Hepatic Dose Adjustments:** None
			• **Dosage Forms:** Oral (IR, CR, ER, ODT tablet, suspension)

Carbidopa-Levodopa-Entacapone	Stalevo	• Parkinson disease	• **Dosing (Adult):**
			  – Oral: initial dose is dependent on carbidopa/levodopa target
			    – All Stalevo products contain entacapone 200 mg
			• **Dosing (Peds):**
			  – Not routinely used
			• **CYP450 Interactions:** None
			• **Renal or Hepatic Dose Adjustments:**
			  – Severe hepatic impairment - avoid use
			• **Dosage Forms:** Oral (tablet)

NEUROLOGY – PARKINSON'S AGENTS – COMT INHIBITORS

Drug Class

- COMT Inhibitors
- Agents:
    - Chronic Care
        - Entacapone
        - Opicapone
        - Tolcapone

> **Fast Facts**
>
> ✓ Tolcapone is not preferred due to unclear clinical benefit but an increased risk of hepatotoxicity. Tolcapone has a BBW for this reason.

Main Indications or Uses

- Chronic Care
    - Parkinson disease

Mechanism of Action

- Inhibits catechol-O-methyltransferase (COMT), preventing premature metabolism of levodopa in the peripheral circulation.

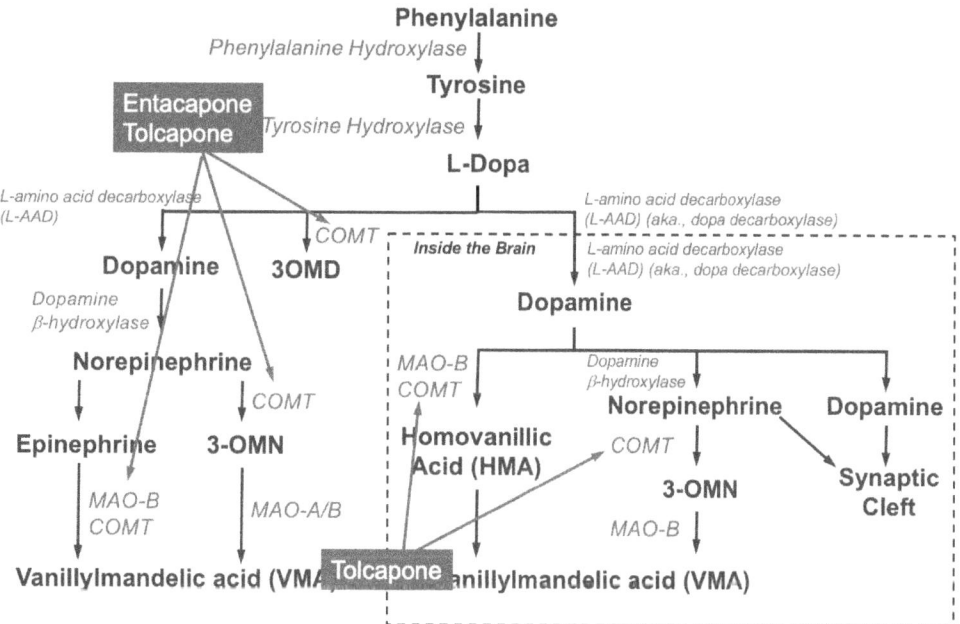

Primary Net Benefit

- COMT inhibitors can improve clinical response to levodopa/carbidopa therapy and reduce adverse events associated with excessive levodopa dosing.
- Main Labs to Monitor:
    - Hepatic function at baseline and periodically after that
    - Renal function at baseline and periodically thereafter

High-Yield Basic Pharmacology
- **3-OMD**
  - COMT directly increases plasma levels of 3-O-methyldopa (3-OMD), which competes with levodopa for transport in the intestine, or across the blood-brain-barrier.
  - Thus, inhibiting COM decreases 3-OMD, allowing better drug absorption and penetration into the CNS.
- **Half-Life Change**
  - The typical half-life of levodopa is 1 hour but extends to 1.5 hours with coadministration of carbidopa.
  - With a COMT inhibitor, the half-life of levodopa is extended further to 2 to 2.5 hours.

High-Yield Clinical Knowledge
- **COMT Addition**
  - A COMT inhibitor should be added to levodopa/carbidopa therapy once maximum daily doses are met or the need for frequent dosing throughout the day.
  - Alternatively to COMT inhibitors, MAO-B inhibitors such as rasagiline may be used.
- **No Monotherapy**
  - On their own, COMT inhibitors do not affect Parkinson's disease and must be used in conjunction with levodopa/carbidopa.
- **Hepatotoxicity**
  - Tolcapone, which can be administered less frequently than entacapone, is not preferred due to unclear clinical benefit but an increased risk of hepatotoxicity.
    - This effect is a black boxed warning for tolcapone.
- **Improved "on" Time**
  - COMT inhibitors, when added to levodopa/carbidopa therapy, improve the duration of therapeutic "on" time by approximately 1 to 2 hours per day.
- **Daily Doses**
  - Opicapone is a relative newcomer to the COMT inhibitor class and offers the advantage of once-daily dosing.
  - Although clinical experience is developing, there does not appear to be an excessive risk of hepatotoxicity.
- **Neuroleptic Malignant Syndrome**
  - If abrupt discontinuation of COMT inhibitors occurs for any reason, patients can experience acute and profound worsening of Parkinson's symptoms, including rigidity, altered mental status, and hyperthermia characteristic of NMS.
    - NMS can be life-threatening.

High-Yield Core Evidence
- **NOMECOMT Trial**
  - This was a 6-month, double-blind, placebo-controlled trial that assessed the effect and safety of entacapone as an adjunct to levodopa/carbidopa or placebo plus levodopa/carbidopa treatment in patients with Parkinson's disease with wearing-off motor fluctuations.
  - Patients receiving entacapone experiences significantly improved "on" time as observed in the patients' home diary recordings of "on" and "off" times and with Unified Parkinson's Disease Rating Scale scoring by the examiner.
  - Furthermore, patients taking entacapone saw significant reductions in their daily levodopa dose compared to placebo.
  - When entacapone was withheld, the observed benefits from levodopa was lost almost entirely.
  - The authors concluded that long-term entacapone treatment effectively prolonged the beneficial response to levodopa in parkinsonian patients with the wearing-off phenomenon. The improvement occurred irrespective of the reduction of the levodopa dose. (Neurology. 1998 Nov;51(5):1309-14.)

- **BIPARK-2 Trial**
  - This was a phase 3 international, multicenter, outpatient study that randomized patients with Parkinson's disease experiencing end-of-dose motor fluctuations to opicapone (25 or 50 mg/day) or a placebo an adjunct to optimized levodopa/carbidopa therapy.
  - Patients randomized to either dose of opicapone experienced a significantly improved change from baseline in absolute off-time vs. placebo based on patient diaries.
  - After an adjusted analysis of the treatment difference vs. placebo, the opicapone 50 mg dose was significant, but not for the opicapone 25 mg per day group.
  - The off-time reduction was sustained throughout the open-label phase.
  - The authors concluded that opicapone 50 mg daily was associated with a significant reduction in mean daily off-time in levodopa-treated patients with PD and motor fluctuations, and this effect is maintained for at least one year. Opicapone was safe and well-tolerated. (JAMA Neurol. 2017 Feb 1;74(2):197-206.)

High-Yield Fast-Fact
- **Newest Approval**
  - Opicapone was a recent addition to Parkinson's pharmacotherapy, being approved in 2020.

HIGH-YIELD BOARD EXAM ESSENTIALS
- **CLASSIC AGENTS:** Entacapone, opicapone, tolcapone
- **DRUG CLASS:** COMT inhibitor
- **INDICATIONS:** Parkinson disease
- **MECHANISM:** Inhibits catechol-O-methyltransferase (COMT), preventing levodopa's levodopa metabolism in the peripheral circulation.
- **SIDE EFFECTS:** Hepatotoxicity, NMS
- **CLINICAL PEARLS:** A COMT inhibitor should be added to levodopa/carbidopa therapy once maximum daily doses are met, or the need for frequent dosing throughout the day. Alternatively, to COMT inhibitors, MAO-B inhibitors such as rasagiline may be used.

Table: Drug Class Summary

	COMT Inhibitors - Drug Class Review High-Yield Med Reviews		
Mechanism of Action: *Inhibits catechol-O-methyltransferase (COMT), preventing levodopa's levodopa metabolism in the peripheral circulation.*			
Class Effects: *COMT inhibitors can improve clinical response to levodopa/carbidopa therapy and reduce adverse events associated with excessive levodopa dosing.*			
Generic Name	**Brand Name**	**Indication(s) or Uses**	**Notes**

Entacapone	Comtan	- Parkinson disease	- **Dosing (Adult):**
			  – Oral: 200 mg with each levodopa/carbidopa dose
			    – Maximum 1600 mg/day
			- **Dosing (Peds):**
			  – Not routinely used
			- **CYP450 Interactions:** None
			- **Renal or Hepatic Dose Adjustments:**
			  – Severe hepatic impairment: use with caution.
			- **Dosage Forms:** Oral (tablet)

Opicapone	Ongentys	- Parkinson disease	- **Dosing (Adult):**
			  – Oral: 50 mg daily at bedtime
			- **Dosing (Peds):**
			  – Not routinely used
			- **CYP450 Interactions:** Substrate of P-gp
			- **Renal or Hepatic Dose Adjustments:**
			  – Child-Pugh class B: 25 mg at bedtime
			  – Child-Pugh class C: avoid use
			- **Dosage Forms:** Oral (capsule)

Tolcapone	Tasmar	- Parkinson disease	- **Dosing (Adult):**
			  – Oral: 100 mg TID with levodopa/carbidopa
			- **Dosing (Peds):**
			  – Not routinely used
			- **CYP450 Interactions:** None
			- **Renal or Hepatic Dose Adjustments:**
			  – GFR < 25 mL/minute: use with caution
			- **Dosage Forms:** Oral (tablet)

NEUROLOGY – PARKINSON'S AGENTS – DOPAMINE AGONISTS

Drug Class
- Dopamine Agonists
- Agents:
    - Chronic Care
        - Amantadine
        - Apomorphine
        - Bromocriptine
        - Pramipexole
        - Ropinirole
        - Rotigotine

Main Indications or Uses
- Chronic Care
    - Diabetes mellitus, type 2
    - Hyperprolactinemia
    - Parkinson disease
    - Neuroleptic malignant syndrome
    - Restless leg syndrome

Mechanism of Action
- Amantadine
    - Enhances dopamine release from presynaptic terminals and inhibits NMDA receptors.
- Apomorphine and bromocriptine
    - Dopamine-2 (D2) receptor agonist, activating postsynaptic dopamine receptors in the tuberoinfundibular and nigrostriatal pathways.
- Pramipexole and ropinirole
    - Possess D2 agonist properties and D3 and D4 agonist effects stimulating dopaminergic activity in the striatum and substantia nigra.
- Rotigotine
    - D2 agonist effects stimulate dopaminergic activity in the striatum and substantia nigra.

Primary Net Benefit
- First-line agents for Parkinson's disease because of a lower incidence of response fluctuations and prolongs time to levodopa therapy, which spares some long-term adverse events, including dyskinesias.
- Main Labs to Monitor:
    - No routine lab monitoring

High-Yield Basic Pharmacology
- Ergot Vs. Non-ergot Agonist
    - The dopamine agonists can be grouped into either ergot derived agonists, such as bromocriptine, or non-ergot agonists such as apomorphine, pramipexole, ropinirole, and rotigotine.
    - Non-ergot agents provide similar efficacy with improved safety compared to bromocriptine.
- Apomorphine and Morphine
    - Apomorphine is a derivative of morphine but lacks analgesic or euphoric effects and is poorly bioavailable due to extensive first-pass metabolism.

High-Yield Clinical Knowledge
- Dopaminergic Vs. Levodopa
    - Dopamine agonists may provide a lower incidence of dopamine fluctuations to the CNS; their use is often limited by lower degrees of Parkinson-related symptom relief and more cognitive adverse events, fatigue, and edema.

- The use of dopamine agonists may be best as additive therapy to existing regimens with levodopa/carbidopa.
- **Adverse Events**
  - When initiating dopamine agonists, slow dose titration is required to avoid the onset of nausea and vomiting.
  - Patients may also develop compulsive behaviors, delusions, hallucinations, psychosis, and sudden unexpected sleep episodes.
- **Prior Psychiatric or Cardiac Disease**
  - Patients with a history of psychiatric illnesses, recent myocardial infarctions, or active peptic ulcers cannot receive dopamine agonists as they are contraindicated in these populations.
- **Withdrawal**
  - If dopamine agonists are to be discontinued, they must be slowly tapered off to avoid a withdrawal syndrome that manifests as anxiety, agitation, depression, panic attacks, fatigue, orthostatic hypotension, nausea and vomiting, diaphoresis, and drug cravings.
  - This withdrawal syndrome may be resistant to levodopa titration or other dopaminergic agents and can persist for months.
- **Erythromelalgia**
  - This is a unique syndrome associated with ergot derivatives, including bromocriptine, that manifests as painful, red, and swollen feet and/or hands that resolve after discontinuation of the offending drug.
- **Sleep Attacks**
  - Pramipexole or ropinirole have been associated with sleep attacks, which are more commonly observed if dopaminergic agents are abruptly stopped.
  - Should sleep attacks occur during pramipexole or ropinirole therapy, they should be discontinued.

High-Yield Core Evidence
- **Ropinirole Study Group**
  - This was a multicenter, blinded, placebo-controlled trial of patients with Parkinson's disease who were randomized to receive either ropinirole or placebo, each added to background levodopa/carbidopa therapy.
  - Patients randomized to receive ropinirole experienced a significant reduction of 20% or greater in both levodopa dose and in percent time spent "off" than placebo.
  - Adverse events and the incidence of patients discontinuing therapy for safety were similar between groups.
  - The authors concluded that ropinirole permits a reduction in L-dopa dose with enhanced clinical benefit for Parkinson's disease patients with motor fluctuations. (Neurology. 1998 Oct;51(4):1057-62.)
- **Parkinson Study Group**
  - This was a multicenter, parallel-group, double-blind trial that randomized patients with early Parkinson's disease to receive either pramipexole, 0.5 mg TID, with placebo or carbidopa/levodopa 25/100 mg TID, with placebo.
  - Patients randomized to pramipexole led to significantly less development of dyskinesias or on-off motor fluctuations than levodopa-based therapy.
  - Similarly, pramipexole was associated with a significant improvement in the Unified Parkinson's Disease Rating Scale; however, somnolence was significantly more common in the pramipexole group.
  - The authors concluded that fewer patients receiving initial treatment for Parkinson's disease with pramipexole developed dopaminergic motor complications than levodopa therapy. Despite supplementation with open-label levodopa in both groups, the levodopa-treated group had a more significant improvement in total UPDRS than the pramipexole group. (JAMA. 2000 Oct 18;284(15):1931-8.)

High-Yield Fast-Fact
- **Pergolide**
  - Pergolide is an ergot derivative that is no longer available in the United States due to its association with valvular heart disease development.

Table: Drug Class Summary

Dopamine Agonists - Drug Class Review High-Yield Med Reviews			
Mechanism of Action: *Amantadine - Enhances dopamine release.* *Apomorphine and bromocriptine - D2 agonist.* *Pramipexole and ropinirole - D2 agonist properties, but also has D3 and D4 agonist effects.* *Rotigotine - D2 agonist effects.*			
Class Effects: *First-line agents for Parkinson's disease because of a lower incidence of response fluctuations and prolongs time to levodopa therapy, which spares some long-term adverse events, including dyskinesias.*			
Generic Name	**Brand Name**	**Main Indication(s) or Uses**	**Notes**
Amantadine	Gocovri, Osmolex ER	<ul><li>Drug-induced parkinsonism</li><li>Parkinson disease</li></ul>	<ul><li>**Dosing (Adult):**<ul><li>Oral: 100 to 200 mg q12-24h</li></ul></li><li>**Dosing (Peds):**<ul><li>Oral: 5 mg/kg/day divided q12h<ul><li>Maximum 150 mg/day</li></ul></li></ul></li><li>**CYP450 Interactions:** Substrate CYP3A4, Pgp</li><li>**Renal or Hepatic Dose Adjustments:**<ul><li>GFR 30 to 59 mL/min: 200 mg x1 then 100 mg/day</li><li>GFR 15 to 29 mL/min: 200 mg x1 then 100 mg q24h</li><li>GFR < 15 mL/minute: contraindicated</li></ul></li><li>**Dosage Forms:** Oral (capsule, tablet, syrup)</li></ul>
Apomorphine	Apokyn, Kynmobi	<ul><li>Parkinson disease</li></ul>	<ul><li>**Dosing (Adult):**<ul><li>SL film 10 mg as needed by at most q2h<ul><li>Maximum 5 doses/day</li></ul></li><li>SQ: 2 to 6 mg as needed<ul><li>Maximum 20 mg/day</li></ul></li></ul></li><li>**Dosing (Peds):**<ul><li>Not routinely used</li></ul></li><li>**CYP450 Interactions:** Substrate of CYP1A2, CYP2C19, CYP3A4</li><li>**Renal or Hepatic Dose Adjustments:**<ul><li>GFR < 30 mL/minute - avoid use</li></ul></li><li>**Dosage Forms:** Sublingual film or kit</li></ul>
Bromocriptine	Cycloset, Parlodel	<ul><li>Diabetes mellitus, type 2</li><li>Hyperprolactinemia</li><li>Parkinson disease</li><li>Neuroleptic malignant syndrome</li></ul>	<ul><li>**Dosing (Adult):**<ul><li>Oral: 0.8 to 15 mg/day<ul><li>Up to 100 mg/day for Parkinsonism</li></ul></li></ul></li><li>**Dosing (Peds):**<ul><li>Oral: 0.8 to 15 mg/day</li></ul></li><li>**CYP450 Interactions:** Substrate CYP3A4</li><li>**Renal or Hepatic Dose Adjustments:** None</li><li>**Dosage Forms:** Oral (capsule, tablet)</li></ul>

Dopamine Agonists - Drug Class Review
High-Yield Med Reviews

Generic Name	Brand Name	Main Indication(s) or Uses	Notes

Pramipexole	Mirapex	- Parkinson disease
		- Restless leg syndrome
			- **Dosing (Adult):**
			  – Oral: 0.125 to 1.5 mg TID to QD
			- **Dosing (Peds):**
			  – Not routinely used
			- **CYP450 Interactions:** None
			- **Renal or Hepatic Dose Adjustments:**
			  – GFR 30 to 50 mL/minute: maximum 0.75 mg TID
			  – GFR 15 to 29 mL/minute: IR maximum 1.5 mg daily; ER not recommended
			  – GFR < 15: not recommended
			- **Dosage Forms:** Oral (tablet)

Ropinirole	Requip	- Parkinson disease
		- Restless leg syndrome
			- **Dosing (Adult):**
			  – Oral: IR 0.25 to 8 mg TID
			  – Oral: ER 2 to 24 mg daily
			- **Dosing (Peds):**
			  – Not routinely used
			- **CYP450 Interactions:** Substrate CYP1A2, 3A4
			- **Renal or Hepatic Dose Adjustments:**
			  – GFR < 30 mL/minute: use with caution
			- **Dosage Forms:** Oral (tablet)

Rotigotine	Neupro	- Parkinson disease
		- Restless leg syndrome
			- **Dosing (Adult):**
			  – Transdermal patch: 2 to 16 mg/24hour applied daily
			- **Dosing (Peds):**
			  – Not routinely used
			- **CYP450 Interactions:** None
			- **Renal or Hepatic Dose Adjustments:** None
			- **Dosage Forms:** Transdermal patch

HIGH-YIELD BOARD EXAM ESSENTIALS
- **CLASSIC AGENTS:** Amantadine, apomorphine, bromocriptine, pramipexole, ropinirole, rotigotine
- **DRUG CLASS:** Dopamine agonists
- **INDICATIONS:** Diabetes mellitus type 2, hyperprolactinemia, neuroleptic malignant syndrome, drug-induced parkinsonism, Parkinson disease
- **MECHANISM:** Enhances dopamine release (amantadine); D2 agonist (apomorphine and bromocriptine); D2 agonist properties, but also has D3 and D4 agonist effects (pramipexole and ropinirole); D2 agonist effects (rotigotine)
- **SIDE EFFECTS:** Compulsive behaviors, delusions, hallucinations, psychosis, and sudden unexpected sleep episodes
- **CLINICAL PEARLS:** Pramipexole or ropinirole have been associated with sleep attacks, which are more commonly observed if dopaminergic agents are abruptly stopped. Should sleep attacks occur during pramipexole or ropinirole therapy, they should be discontinued.

NEUROLOGY – PARKINSON'S AGENTS - MAO-B INHIBITORS

Drug Class
- MAO-B Inhibitors
- Agents:
  - Chronic Care
    - Rasagiline
    - Safinamide
    - Selegiline

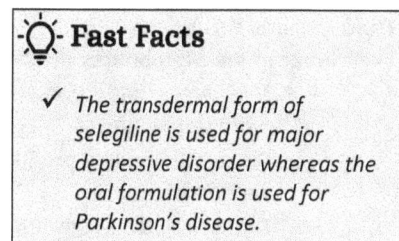

> **Fast Facts**
> ✓ The transdermal form of selegiline is used for major depressive disorder whereas the oral formulation is used for Parkinson's disease.

Main Indications or Uses
- Chronic Care
  - Depression
  - Parkinson disease

Mechanism of Action
- Inhibition of monoamine oxidase B prevents the metabolism of dopamine in the CNS.

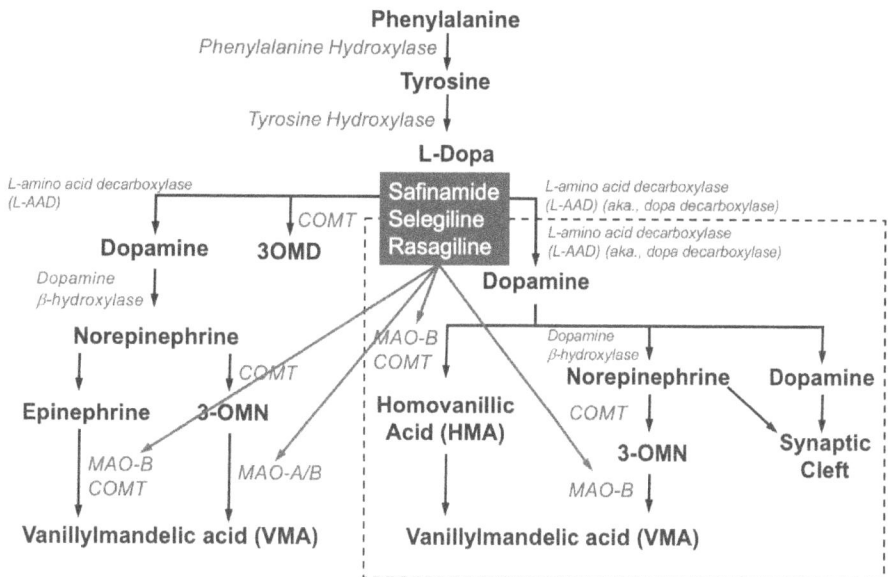

Primary Net Benefit
- MAO-B inhibition may slow Parkinson's disease progression and can be combined with levodopa to enhance its dose-response relationship.
- Main Labs to Monitor:
  - No routine lab monitoring

High-Yield Basic Pharmacology
- **Reversible Vs. Irreversible**
  - Rasagiline and selegiline are irreversible inhibitors of MAO-B, sometimes referred to as "suicide inhibition."
  - Safinamide reversibly inhibits MAO-B.
- **Glutamate Inhibition**
  - In addition to its selective MAO-B inhibition, safinamide also inhibits voltage-gated sodium channels inhibits the excitatory neurotransmitter glutamate.

- **MAO-A Vs. MAO-B**
  - MAO-A normally functions to metabolize monoamines, including norepinephrine, serotonin, and dopamine, in the CNS and outside the CNS.
  - MAO-B selectively functions to metabolize dopamine in the CNS but may also exist peripherally.

High-Yield Clinical Knowledge
- **Amphetamine Metabolites**
  - Selegiline undergoes hepatic first-pass metabolism, which produces amphetamine and methamphetamine.
  - These metabolites produce similar effects to their illicit counterparts, leading to insomnia, agitation, and hallucinations.
  - The orally disintegrating and transdermal dosage form of selegiline largely bypasses the first-pass circulation and can minimize the amount of amphetamine and methamphetamine produced.
- **Serotonin Syndrome**
  - Serotonin syndrome associated with MAO-B inhibitors is rare; however, it is still a hypothetical risk.
  - MAO-B inhibitors should not be used with tramadol, methadone, dextromethorphan, cyclobenzaprine, or St. John's wort.
    - The risk of serotonin syndrome with MAO-A inhibitors is substantially higher.
- **Neuroprotection Properties**
  - MAO-B inhibitors are postulated to provide disease-modifying benefits in Parkinson's disease as inhibition of this dopamine pathway diverts it to alternative routes (COMT), which do not produce free radicals.
- **Benefits and Risks**
  - The addition of selegiline may provide up to 1 hour of additional "on" time for patients wearing off phenomena.
  - Conversely, selegiline may increase a levodopa peak effect, further worsening dyskinesias or delusions associated with levodopa therapy.

High-Yield Core Evidence
- **ADAGIO Trial**
  - This was a multicenter, double-blind clinical trial in patients with untreated Parkinson's disease who were randomized to receive either an early start treatment of rasagiline for 72 weeks or a delayed-start treatment placebo for 36 weeks followed by rasagiline for 36 weeks.
  - Patients receiving the early start treatment with rasagiline experienced a significant improvement in all primary outcomes, including a smaller mean increase of the Unified Parkinson's Disease Rating Scale, assessed at three-time points.
  - All three endpoints were not met with rasagiline at a dose of 2 mg per day since the change in the UPDRS score between baseline and week 72 was not significantly different in the two groups.
  - The authors concluded that early treatment with rasagiline at a dose of 1 mg per day provided benefits consistent with a possible disease-modifying effect, but early treatment with rasagiline at a quantity of 2 mg per day did not. (N Engl J Med 2009; 361:1268-1278.)

High-Yield Fast-Fact
- **MPTP and Selegiline**
  - MPTP and its metabolite MPP+ are products of inappropriately synthesized illicit meperidine, which may lead to irreversible parkinsonism.
  - Selegiline may prevent or diminish the metabolism of MPTP to MPP+ and reduce its adverse neurologic sequelae.

Table: Drug Class Summary

\multicolumn{4}{c}{**MAO-B Inhibitors - Drug Class Review**}

MAO-B Inhibitors - Drug Class Review
High-Yield Med Reviews

Mechanism of Action: *Inhibition of monoamine oxidase B prevents the metabolism of dopamine in the CNS.*

Class Effects: *MAO-B inhibition may slow Parkinson's disease progression and can be combined with levodopa to enhance its dose-response relationship.*

Generic Name	Brand Name	Indication(s) or Uses	Notes

Rasagiline	Azilect	• Parkinson disease	• **Dosing (Adult):**
			  − Oral: 0.5 to 1 mg daily
			• **Dosing (Peds):**
			  − Not routinely used
			• **CYP450 Interactions:** Substrate CYP1A2
			• **Renal or Hepatic Dose Adjustments:**
			  − Child-Pugh Class C: Not recommended
			• **Dosage Forms:** Oral (tablet)

Safinamide	Xadago	• Parkinson disease	• **Dosing (Adult):**
			  − Oral: 50 to 100 mg daily
			• **Dosing (Peds):**
			  − Not routinely used
			• **CYP450 Interactions:** Substrate CYP3A4
			• **Renal or Hepatic Dose Adjustments:**
			  − Child-Pugh Class C: Not recommended
			• **Dosage Forms:** Oral (tablet)

Selegiline	Emsam
	Zelapar
		• Depression
		• Parkinson disease
			• **Dosing (Adult):**
			  − Oral: 1.25 to 5 mg BID
			  − Transdermal: 6 to 12 mg/24 hour patch
			• **Dosing (Peds):**
			  − Not routinely used
			• **CYP450 Interactions:** Substrate of CYP1A2, 2A6, 2B6, 2D6, 3A4
			• **Renal or Hepatic Dose Adjustments:**
			  − GFR < 30 mL/minute: Use not recommended
			  − Child-Pugh Class C: Not recommended
			• **Dosage Forms:** Oral (capsule, tablet), Transdermal patch

HIGH-YIELD BOARD EXAM ESSENTIALS
- **CLASSIC AGENTS:** Rasagiline, safinamide, selegiline
- **DRUG CLASS:** MAO-B Inhibitors
- **INDICATIONS:** Depression, Parkinson disease
- **MECHANISM:** Inhibition of monoamine oxidase B prevents the metabolism of dopamine in the CNS.
- **SIDE EFFECTS:** Hypertension, headache, serotonin syndrome
- **CLINICAL PEARLS:** MAO-B inhibitors are postulated to provide disease-modifying benefits in Parkinson's disease as inhibition of this dopamine pathway diverts it to alternative routes (COMT), which do not produce free radicals. The transdermal formulation of selegiline is indicated for major depressive disorder not Parkinson's disease.

NEUROLOGY – SEDATIVE HYPNOTICS - GENERAL

Drug Class
- **Melatonin, Ramelteon, Tasimelteon & Suvorexant**
- **Agents:**
  - Chronic Care
    - Melatonin
    - Ramelteon
    - Suvorexant
    - Tasimelteon

Main Indications or Uses
- **Chronic Care**
  - Insomnia (melatonin, ramelteon, suvorexant)
  - Non-24-hour sleep-wake disorder (Tasimelteon)

Mechanism of Action
- **Melatonin, Ramelteon, Tasimelteon**
  - Melatonin receptor agonists produce sleepiness and influence night-day circadian synchronization.
- **Suvorexant**
  - Orexin receptor antagonist, enhancing REM and non-REM sleep.

Primary Net Benefit
- Non-benzodiazepine sleep aids improve the sleep-wake cycle in patients and are an alternative to patients unable to take benzodiazepines.
- Main Labs to Monitor:
  - No routine monitoring

High-Yield Basic Pharmacology
- **Endogenous Melatonin**
  - Melatonin is usually produced in the pineal gland from the metabolism of serotonin.
  - The release of melatonin from the pineal gland follows a normal circadian rhythm and influences the sleep-wake behavior of humans.
- **Melatonin Receptors**
  - There have been three melatonin receptor subtypes identified: MT1, MT2, and MT3.
  - MT1 and MT2 receptors are typically located in the hypothalamus, influencing sleep-wake cycles.
    - MT1 activation causes sleepiness.
    - Stimulation of MT2 receptors influences light-dark synchronization.
    - The function of MT3 has not been fully described.
- **Orexin**
  - The lateral hypothalamus produces orexin, which has been linked to regulating sleep-wake cycles in humans.
  - Orexin pathway neurons promote wakefulness, but orexin activity inhibition influences the rapid eye movement (REM) phase of sleep and non-REM sleep.

High-Yield Clinical Knowledge
- **Jet Lag**
  - Melatonin is widely used as a food supplement for the treatment or prevention of jet lag.
  - When regularly taken at nighttime, melatonin can reduce subjective daytime fatigue while improving mood and faster recovery to regular sleep-wake cycles in a patient's home time zone.

- **Sleep Metric Improvement**
  - Suvorexant is an effective means to improve specific sleep metrics such as decreased time to persistent sleep and increased total sleep time.
  - Melatonin receptor agonists improve persistent sleep without other sleep architecture influences and are mainly devoid of withdrawal symptoms.
- **Drug Interactions**
  - Melatonin, ramelteon, and tasimelteon are metabolized by and may inhibit or induce CYP1A2, potentially leading to clinically relevant drug interactions with many antidepressants, including SSRIs, fluvoxamine, and ciprofloxacin.
  - Additive hypnotic effects can occur when any of these agents are combined with non-benzodiazepine "Z-drugs" such as zileuton.
  - Melatonin may independently decrease prothrombin time and may affect warfarin therapy.
  - As a CYP3A4 substrate, suvorexant is subject to numerous drug interactions from potent CYP3A4 inhibitors such as azole antifungals, macrolides, and non-dihydropyridine calcium channel blockers.
- **Reproductive Function**
  - Melatonin receptors have been identified in both female and male reproductive organs, raising speculative therapeutic targets.
  - In women, melatonin may be an adjunct to infertility treatment during in vitro fertilization and otherwise appears to be safe in pregnancy.
  - Melatonin may improve sperm function in men with poor sperm motility and early apoptosis.
- **Surgical Anxiolysis**
  - Melatonin may be similarly effective to midazolam in reducing preoperative anxiety among adult patients.
  - However, post-operative melatonin for anxiolysis is not as effective compared to other interventions, including benzodiazepines.
- **Abnormal Dreams**
  - Although ramelteon and tasimelteon are effective hypnotic agents, their use has increased the frequency and intensity of nightmares or abnormal dreams.
  - Other common adverse events include headache, dizziness, and fatigue.
- **Controlled Substance**
  - Suvorexant is a scheduled IV medication.
  - Conversely, melatonin is available over-the-counter, and ramelteon and tasimelteon are non-scheduled prescription agents.
- **Minimum 7 hours**
  - Suvorexant should be taken within thirty minutes before sleep, only if there are at least seven hours of projected sleep time before waking.
  - Increased daytime sleepiness, sudden onset of sleep, or worsening of depression and suicidal ideation are possible.

High-Yield Core Evidence
- **SET and RESET**
  - This was a publication of two consecutive trials, which were both multicentered, randomized, placebo-controlled, double-blinded trials in adult patients who were totally blind with a non-24-hour circadian period conducted in clinical research centers and sleep centers.
  - In the SET trial, patients were randomized to either tasimelteon 20 mg or placebo every 24 hours at a fixed time of 1 hour before target bedtime for 26 weeks.
  - Patients receiving tasimelteon in an open-label portion of SET but did not meet inclusion criteria had undergone re-randomization to have tasimelteon withdrawn among patients with a positive response to tasimelteon after a run-in period.
  - In SET, the primary endpoint was the proportion of entrained patients assessed in the intention-to-treat population.
    - Tasimelteon was associated with a significant improvement in circadian entrainment and clinical response compared to placebo.

- In RESET, the primary endpoint was the proportion of non-entrained patients assessed in the intention-to-treat population.
    - A significant improvement in circadian entrainment among patients who continued tasimelteon compared to patients who had tasimelteon withdrawn and continued a placebo.
- No deaths were reported in either study or discontinuation rates due to adverse events were comparable between the tasimelteon treatment courses.
- The authors concluded that once-daily tasimelteon could entrain blind people with non-24; however, continued tasimelteon treatment is necessary to maintain these improvements. (Lancet. 2015 Oct 31;386(10005):1754-64.)

High-Yield Fast-Fact
- **Agomelatine**
    - Agomelatine is an MT receptor agonist and 5HT2C antagonist in Europe but not currently licensed in the United States.

HIGH-YIELD BOARD EXAM ESSENTIALS
- **CLASSIC AGENTS:** Melatonin, ramelteon, suvorexant, tasimelteon
- **DRUG CLASS:** Hypnotic
- **INDICATIONS:** Insomnia
- **MECHANISM:** Melatonin receptor agonists produce sleepiness and influence night-day circadian synchronization (melatonin, ramelteon, tasimelteon); orexin receptor antagonist, enhancing REM and non-REM sleep (suvorexant).
- **SIDE EFFECTS:** Abnormal dreams, abuse potential, decreased PT (melatonin)
- **CLINICAL PEARLS:** Melatonin, ramelteon, and tasimelteon are metabolized by and may inhibit or induce CYP1A2, potentially leading to clinically relevant drug interactions with many antidepressants, including SSRIs, fluvoxamine, and ciprofloxacin.

Table: Drug Class Summary

\multicolumn{4}{c}{**Melatonin, Ramelteon, Tasimelteon & Suvorexant - Drug Class Review**}

Melatonin, Ramelteon, Tasimelteon & Suvorexant - Drug Class Review
High-Yield Med Reviews

Mechanism of Action:
Melatonin, Ramelteon, Tasimelteon - Melatonin receptor agonists produce sleepiness and influence night-day circadian synchronization.
Suvorexant - Orexin receptor antagonist, enhancing REM and non-REM sleep.

Class Effects: *Non-benzodiazepine sleep aids improve the sleep-wake cycle in patients and are an alternative to patients unable to take benzodiazepines.*

Generic Name	Brand Name	Main Indication(s) or Uses	Notes

Melatonin	Melatonin	- Insomnia	- **Dosing (Adult):**
			  - Oral: 0.3 to 20 mg before bedtime
			- **Dosing (Peds):**
			  - Use under direction of physicians 0.1 to 6 mg before bedtime
			- **CYP450 Interactions:** Substrate CYP1A2, 2B6, 2C19, 3A4
			- **Renal or Hepatic Dose Adjustments:**
			  - Severe renal or hepatic impairment: OTC not recommended
			- **Dosage Forms:** Oral (capsule, tablet

Ramelteon	Rozerem	- Insomnia	- **Dosing (Adult):**
			  - Oral: 8 mg within 30 minutes of bedtime
			- **Dosing (Peds):**
			  - Not routinely used
			- **CYP450 Interactions:** Substrate CYP1A2, 2C19, 3A4
			- **Renal or Hepatic Dose Adjustments:**
			  - Severe hepatic impairment: not recommended
			- **Dosage Forms:** Oral (tablet)

Suvorexant	Belsomra	- Insomnia	- **Dosing (Adult):**
			  - Oral: 10 to 20 mg 30 minutes before bedtime
			- **Dosing (Peds):**
			  - Oral: 5 to 20 mg at bedtime
			    - Maximum 20 mg/day
			- **CYP450 Interactions:** Substrate CYP2C19, 3A4
			- **Renal or Hepatic Dose Adjustments:**
			  - Severe hepatic impairment: not recommended
			- **Dosage Forms:** Oral (tablet)

| Melatonin, Ramelteon, Tasimelteon & Suvorexant - Drug Class Review ||||
| High-Yield Med Reviews ||||
Generic Name	Brand Name	Main Indication(s) or Uses	Notes

Tasimelteon	Hetlioz	- Non-24-hour sleep-wake disorder	- **Dosing (Adult):**
			  - Oral: 20 mg at the same time daily before bedtime
			- **Dosing (Peds):**
			  - Not routinely used
			- **CYP450 Interactions:** Substrate CYP1A2, 3A4
			- **Renal or Hepatic Dose Adjustments:**
			  - Severe hepatic impairment: not recommended
			- **Dosage Forms:** Oral (capsule)

NEUROLOGY – ETOMIDATE

Drug Class
- Etomidate

Main Indications or Uses
- Acute care
  - Anesthesia
  - Procedural sedation
  - Rapid sequence intubation

> **Fast Facts**
> - Etomidate is most commonly reserved for rapid sequence intubation and at appropriate doses generally does not cause hemodynamic instability.
> - Etomidate can cause drug-induced adrenal suppression though the clinical relevance is questionable.

Mechanism of Action
- Binds to the beta-2 subunit of the GABA-A receptor, which results in increased sensitivity of the GABAA receptor to GABA, enhancing the inhibitory neurotransmission and decreasing nervous system activity.

Primary Net Benefit
- Etomidate is a critical first-line sedation induction agent for patients undergoing emergent rapid sequence intubation.
- Main Labs to Monitor:
  - No routine labs

High-Yield Basic Pharmacology
- **Rapid Anesthesia**
  - Etomidate provides rapid onset anesthesia (< 30 seconds) but does not possess analgesic properties.
- **Propylene Glycol**
  - The propylene glycol content of etomidate is relatively high (35%) but does not carry a risk of toxic effects due to the single-dose therapy.
  - However, it may result in clinically relevant toxicity when co-administered with other propylene glycol-containing medications (including amiodarone, lorazepam, phenytoin).

High-Yield Clinical Knowledge
- **Adrenal Suppression**
  - Etomidate is known to cause adrenal insufficiency due to its dose-dependent inhibition of 11-beta-hydroxylase, resulting in the impaired conversion of cholesterol to cortisol.
    - However, there are no clinically relevant sequelae from this effect in single-dose therapy, which is the standard of care when utilizing etomidate.
    - Historical use of etomidate infusions as a post-procedural sedative is the basis for the clinically relevant adrenal insufficiency, resulting in patient deaths.
- **Seizure Effects**
  - Many resources cite etomidate as possibly activating seizure foci and its clinical use as an agent for inducing seizure activity on EEG.
  - However, there is clinical debate about whether this is an actual effect as etomidate also possesses antiepileptic properties.
- **Hemodynamic Effects**
  - Compared to other anesthetic induction agents (including barbiturates, propofol, and ketamine), etomidate does not produce hemodynamic changes, including blood pressure, heart rate, and respiratory rate.
  - This promotes the safety of single-dose usage of etomidate in the sedation of critically ill patients, combined with the low risk of clinically relevant adrenal suppression.

High-Yield Core Evidence
- **KETASED**
  - A multicenter, prospective, single-blind trial of patients requiring emergent intubation was prospectively randomized to receive either etomidate IV 0.3 mg/kg or ketamine IV 2 mg/kg for intubation.
  - There was no statistically significant difference between either ketamine or etomidate in the primary outcome of the maximum SOFA score during the first three days in the ICU.
  - No difference in the intubation difficulty score or adverse events between groups was observed; however, more patients receiving etomidate experienced laboratory evident adrenal insufficiency.
  - The authors concluded that ketamine is a safe and valuable alternative to etomidate for endotracheal intubation in critically ill patients and should be considered in those with sepsis. (Lancet. 2009 Jul 25;374(9686):293-300)
- **Etomidate Vs. Propofol**
  - Single-center, randomized, nonblinded prospective trial of adult patients undergoing procedural sedation with either propofol or etomidate for painful procedures in the ED.
  - No clinically significant difference was observed in procedure success rate, complications including subclinical and clinically relevant respiratory depression.
  - More myoclonus was noted etomidate recipients, but a lower risk of vasodilation.
  - The authors concluded that etomidate and propofol appear equally safe for ED procedural sedation; however, etomidate had a lower rate of procedural success and induced myoclonus in 20% of patients. (Ann Emerg Med. 2007 Jan;49(1):15-22.)

High-Yield Fast-Facts
- **Myoclonus**
  - The mechanism of etomidate-induced myoclonus is the activation of glycine receptors at the spinal cord level.

HIGH-YIELD BOARD EXAM ESSENTIALS
- **CLASSIC AGENTS:** Etomidate
- **DRUG CLASS:** Sedative-hypnotic
- **INDICATIONS:** Anesthesia, procedural sedation, rapid sequence intubation
- **MECHANISM:** GABA-A agonist
- **SIDE EFFECTS:** Myoclonus, adrenal suppression
- **CLINICAL PEARLS:** Adrenal suppression is not a clinical concern with single dose use

---

Table: Drug Class Summary

Etomidate - Drug Class Review High-Yield Med Reviews			
Mechanism of Action: *Binds to the beta-2 subunit of the GABA-A receptor, which results in increased sensitivity of the GABAA receptor to GABA, enhancing the inhibitory neurotransmission and decreasing nervous system activity.*			
Class Effects: *Etomidate is a first-line sedation induction agent for patients undergoing emergent intubation.*			
Generic Name	**Brand Name**	**Main Indication(s) or Uses**	**Notes**

Etomidate	Amidate	• Anesthesia
		• Procedural sedation
		• Rapid sequence intubation
			• **Dosing (Adult):**
			  – IV: 0.3 mg/kg
			• **Dosing (Peds):**
			  – IV: 0.3 mg/kg
			• **CYP450 Interactions:** None
			• **Renal or Hepatic Dose Adjustments:** None
			• **Dosage Forms:** IV solution

NEUROLOGY – PROPOFOL

Drug Class
- Propofol

Main Indications or Uses
- Acute care
  - General anesthesia
  - Mechanical ventilation sedation

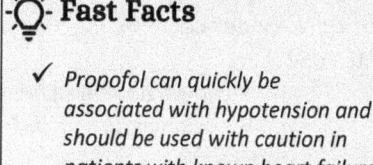

Fast Facts

✓ Propofol can quickly be associated with hypotension and should be used with caution in patients with known heart failure or CVD.

Mechanism of Action
- Postsynaptic GABA-A agonist, by binding to the beta-2 subunit of GABA-A, enhances nigral dopamine release from GABA-B receptors, an antagonist of NMDA receptors and partial agonist of dopamine-2 receptors.

Primary Net Benefit
- First-line anesthetic agent for sedation in mechanically ventilated patients plays a role in procedural sedation but is associated with the rate of administration hypotension and propofol infusion syndrome.
- Main Labs to Monitor:
  - Richmond Agitation–Sedation Scale (RASS)
  - Oxygen saturation
  - Blood pressure

High-Yield Basic Pharmacology
- **Free-Fatty Acid Metabolism**
  - Prolonged use of propofol is associated with reduced mitochondrial free-fatty acid metabolism and functional utilization, resulting in an imbalance of energy supply to these cells and myonecrosis.
- **White Liquid**
  - Propofol is a 10% emulsion solution (containing soybean oil, glycerol, and lecithin) that is white in color.
  - This fat-emulsion-based formulation is associated with numerous adverse events, including hypertriglyceridemia, anaphylactoid reaction, impaired macrophage function, and reduced platelet and coagulation factor function.

High-Yield Clinical Knowledge
- **Propofol Infusion Syndrome**
  - Prolonged propofol infusions are associated with a significant clinical syndrome known as propofol-infusion syndrome.
  - Propofol-infusion syndrome manifests as cardiac dysrhythmias (an early sign of right bundle branch block or ST-elevation), metabolic acidosis, and skeletal muscle injury.
  - Pediatric patients are at higher risk of propofol-infusion syndrome, often limiting the use of propofol in this age demographic.
    - Other risk factors include traumatic brain injury, concurrent glucocorticoids, inadequate carbohydrate intake, and mitochondrial myopathy that has not been diagnosed.
- **Antiseizure Effect**
  - Propofol is routinely used as a substitute for barbiturates in patients with status epilepticus mainly as it is regularly regarded as first-line sedative among these patients post endotracheal intubation.
  - Its reduction in cerebral blood flow, metabolic rate, and intracranial pressure control are advantages to propofol for this indication.
- **Profound Vasodilation**
  - Propofol is associated with arterial and venous vasodilation, resulting in cardiac function reduction (preload and afterload reduction) and acute hypotension.
  - This hypotension is dependent on high dose-range dosing (above 2 mg/kg bolus and 50 mcg/kg/minute infusion), rapid administration of the bolus, and identified patient risk factors, including elderly patients or patients with low intravascular volume.

- **Administration Pain**
  - Propofol administration is often associated with pain upon injection but prior administered opioids may manage this, administered with lidocaine or diluted propofol.

High-Yield Core Evidence
- **MENDS2**
  - Multicenter, double-blind, randomized trial of mechanically ventilated septic adult patients who received either dexmedetomidine IV 0.2 to 1.5 mcg/kg/hour or propofol 5 to 50 mcg/kg/minute for nurse-driven RASS target.
  - There was no difference between either agent regarding the primary endpoint of days alive without delirium or coma during the 14-day intervention.
  - The median dose of dexmedetomidine during the study was 0.27 mcg/kg/hour, compared to propofol's median dose of 10.21 mcg/kg/minute.
  - Furthermore, there was no difference between secondary endpoints, including ventilator-free days at 28 days, death at 90 days, or age-adjusted total score on the Telephone Interview for Cognitive Status questionnaire at 6 months.
  - The authors concluded that outcomes in patients who received dexmedetomidine did not differ from outcomes in those who received propofol. (N Engl J Med 2021; 384:1424-1436.)
- **The POKER Study**
  - This was a multicenter, double-blinded, randomized trial comparing ketofol (ketamine plus propofol in a 1:1 ratio) to propofol in patients undergoing procedure associated deep sedation.
  - The primary outcome was. Secondary outcomes included hypotension and patient satisfaction.
  - There was no significant difference in the primary outcome of the occurrence of a respiratory adverse event (desaturation, apnea, or hypoventilation) requiring an intervention by the sedating physician.
  - Propofol alone was more likely to result in hypotension than ketofol, but ketofol was associated with emergence delirium.
  - The authors concluded that although propofol resulted in more hypotension, the clinical relevance is questionable, and both agents are associated with high levels of patient satisfaction. (Ann Emerg Med. 2016 Nov;68(5):574-582.e1)

High-Yield Fast-Facts
- **Controlled Substance Controversy**
  - According to the FDA, propofol is not considered a controlled substance; however, many states and individual medical centers are tracking its use, administration, and disposal as if it were a controlled substance due to the risk of abuse.

HIGH-YIELD BOARD EXAM ESSENTIALS
- **CLASSIC AGENTS:** Propofol
- **DRUG CLASS:** Sedative-hypnotic
- **INDICATIONS:** General anesthesia, mechanical ventilation sedation
- **MECHANISM:** GABA-A agonist, NDMA antagonist
- **SIDE EFFECTS:** Hypotension, propofol infusion syndrome
- **CLINICAL PEARLS:** Dose and rate dependent vasodilation, but still considered first-line for mechanically ventilated ICU patients (alternative to dexmedetomidine).

Table: Drug Class Summary

	Propofol - Drug Class Review High-Yield Med Reviews
	**Mechanism of Action:** *Postsynaptic GABA-A agonist by binding to the beta-2 subunit of GABA-A, enhances nigral dopamine release from GABA-B receptors, an antagonist of NMDA receptors, and partial agonist of dopamine-2 receptors.*
	**Class Effects:** *First-line anesthetic agent for sedation in mechanically ventilated patients plays a role in procedural sedation but is associated with the rate of administration hypotension and propofol infusion syndrome.*
Generic Name	Brand Name	Main Indication(s) or Uses	Notes
Propofol	Diprivan	<ul><li>General anesthesia</li><li>Mechanical ventilation sedation</li></ul>	<ul><li>**Dosing (Adult):**<ul><li>IV bolus: 1-2 mg/kg followed by 5 to 50 mcg/kg/minute infusion titrated to target level of sedation (RASS score)</li><li>IV bolus: 0.5 to 2 mg/kg for procedural sedation</li></ul></li><li>**Dosing (Peds):**<ul><li>IV bolus: 1-2 mg/kg followed by 5 to 50 mcg/kg/minute infusion titrated to target level of sedation (RASS score)</li></ul></li><li>**CYP450 Interactions:** Substrate CYP 1A2, 2A6, 2B6, 2C19, 2C9, 2D6, 2E1, and 3A4</li><li>**Renal or Hepatic Dose Adjustments:** None</li><li>**Dosage Forms:** IV emulsion (either 10 mg/mL or 20 mg/mL)</li></ul>

2025

A COMPREHENSIVE *RAPID REVIEW*

NAPLEX
Pharmacology & Drug Classes

OB / GYN

OBSTETRICS & GYNECOLOGY – NON-ORAL CONTRACEPTIVES

Drug Class
- **Hormonal contraceptives**
  - Combined contraceptives
    - Ethinyl estradiol (EE) plus progestin
  - Progestin-only contraceptives
- **Non-hormonal contraceptive**

Main Indications or Uses
- Contraception
- Hot flashes
- Endometriosis
- Menstrual disorders (abnormal bleeding, menorrhagia, dysmenorrhea)

> **Fast Facts**
> ✓ Estrogen based therapy can reduce milk production if used in the post-partum setting.
>
> ✓ Estrogen can also increase the risk of clots especially in patients at increased risk of CVD and/or have a known hypercoagulable state.

Mechanism of Action
- **Synthetic estrogen**
  - Alters hypothalamic gonadotropin secretion of follicle-stimulating hormone and luteinizing hormone
- **Progestin (synthetic progesterone)**
  - Suppresses luteinizing hormone, thickens cervical mucus, the thin endometrial lining
- **Copper**
  - Prompts endometrium to release leukotrienes and prostaglandins, yielding a non-favorable environment for implantation

Primary Net Benefit
- Prevents ovulation, reducing the chance of conception
- Prevents/treats conditions associated with abnormal menstruation and hormonal imbalance
- Main Labs to Monitor:
  - Pregnancy status baseline
  - Blood pressure and weight baseline and annually after that
  - In relevant patient populations, glucose/HgbA1c, lipid panel, signs/symptoms of VTE
  - Menstrual changes (i.e., increased pain, blood volume)

High-Yield Basic Pharmacology
- **Mechanism and Metabolism**
  - Negative feedback on the hypothalamus disrupts the normal release of FSH and LH from the anterior pituitary
  - Thickening of cervical mucus
  - Ethinyl Estradiol
    - Hepatic metabolism via CYP3A4
      - Drug-drug interactions: antiretrovirals, anticonvulsants, antibiotics
    - Ethinyl estradiol is highly protein-bound
  - Etonogestrel, levonorgestrel, medroxyprogesterone, norelgestromin, segesterone acetate
    - Minor hepatic metabolism via CYP3A4

High-Yield Clinical Knowledge
- Additional contraception is *NOT* required following initiation of
  - Copper IUD
  - Progestin IUD (if within 7 days or menstruation start)
  - Progestin implant (if within 5 days of menstruation start)
  - Progestin injection (if within 7 days of menstruation start)

- Estrogen-containing versus progestin-only versus non-hormonal safety and efficacy should be considered when selecting a non—oral contraceptive agent for a woman
  - The most weight-offensive agents include the progestin injection followed by a progestin implant
  - The progestin injection has the longest return to fertility after discontinuation (up to 10 months)
  - Estrogen-free products are preferred in breastfeeding women
  - The non-hormonal IUD is associated with the most pain, dysmenorrhea, and menorrhagia
- **Product Selection Considerations**
  - Estrogen-containing products should be avoided/used cautiously in women:
    - With vascular disease history/risk factors (i.e., tobacco use) given, estrogen increases the risk of MI, stroke, and VTE
    - That are breastfeeding given estrogen decreases milk production
    - That are within 21 days post-partum high risk of VTE
    - A history of breast cancer given potential increased risk, especially with higher dose formulations
    - With migraines with aura given estrogen increases risk of exacerbations
    - With hepatic failure given estrogen increases risk of further hepatic damage
  - More than half of women with a hormonal IUD experience amenorrhea or oligomenorrhea after two years of use
  - Progestin injections have a maximum recommended duration of two years given loss of bone mineral density; however, difference in fracture frequency has not been demonstrated

High-Yield Core Evidence
- MMWR US Selected Practice Recommendations for Contraceptive Use, 2016
  - Long-Acting Reversible Contraceptives (LARC) such as intrauterine devices and implants are the most effective agents with typical usage compared to patient-administered preparations.
  - Perfect use and typical use efficacy differ with contraceptive injections, patches, and rings
  - MMWR Recomm Rep 2016;65(No. RR-4):1-66.
- LARC products likely have efficacy beyond current FDA-approved indications, as evidenced in the literature
  - Copper IUD up to 12 years (Contraception 2014;89:495-504)
  - Levonorgestrel IUD up to 7 years (Contraception 2016;93:498-506)
  - Etonogestrel implant up to 5 years (Human Reprod 2016;31:2491-8)

High-Yield Fast-Facts
- IUDs can be used in any non-pregnant woman if she is post-menarche, regardless of whether she has previously conceived/delivered

HIGH-YIELD BOARD EXAM ESSENTIALS
- **CLASSIC AGENTS:** Ethinyl estradiol (EE) +/- progestin
- **DRUG CLASS:** Non-oral Contraceptives
- **INDICATIONS:** Contraception, hot flashes, endometriosis
- **MECHANISM:** Suppression of follicle-stimulating hormone and luteinizing hormone prevent ovulation and decrease chance of conception (except for copper IUD).
- **SIDE EFFECTS:** Vaginal spotting or amenorrhea, DVT/PE, decreased milk production (estrogen)
- **CLINICAL PEARLS:** Avoid estrogen containing IUDs post-partum in patients who are breast-feeding as it can decrease milk production. Avoid estrogen containing agents in patients with known hypercoagulable disorders, CAD, or history of VTE due to the increase risk of forming clots.

Table: Drug Class Summary

| \multicolumn{4}{c}{**Non-Oral Contraceptives Drug Class Review**} |
| \multicolumn{4}{c}{**High-Yield Med Reviews**} |

Non-Oral Contraceptives Drug Class Review
High-Yield Med Reviews

Mechanism of Action: *Suppression of follicle-stimulating hormone and luteinizing hormone prevents ovulation and decreases the chance of conception (except for copper IUD)*

Pediatric Dosing: *Use after menarche; dose same as adult*

Generic Name	Brand Name	Main Indication(s) or Uses	Notes
Ethinyl estradiol + norelgestromin transdermal patch	Xulane (previously marketed as Ortho-Evra)	• Combined Hormonal Transdermal Contraceptive	• **Dosing (Adult):** apply 1 patch once weekly x 3 weeks, follow with a patch-free week • **CYP450 Interactions:** CYP3A4 inhibitors and inducers • **Renal or Hepatic Dose Adjustments:** contraindicated in hepatic impairment • If patch is inadvertently removed ≥48 hours, efficacy is compromised • Contraindicated in women with BMI ≥30 kg/m² due to increased risk of VTE; consider alternative contraceptive in women weighing >90 kg
Ethinyl estradiol + etonogestrel vaginal ring	EluRyng NuvaRing	• Combined Hormonal Vaginal Contraceptive	• **Dosing (Adult):** insert 1 ring vaginally continuously x 3 weeks, follow with a ring-free week – New ring inserted each cycle • **CYP450 Interactions:** CYP3A4 inhibitors and inducers • **Renal or Hepatic Dose Adjustments:** contraindicated in hepatic impairment • If ring is inadvertently removed > 3 hours, efficacy is compromised
Ethinyl estradiol + segesterone acetate vaginal ring	Annovera	• Combined Hormonal Vaginal Contraceptive	• **Dosing (Adult):** insert 1 ring vaginally continuously x 3 weeks, follow with a ring-free week – Each ring provides efficacy x 1 year • **CYP450 Interactions:** CYP3A4 inhibitors and inducers • **Renal or Hepatic Dose Adjustments:** contraindicated in hepatic impairment • If ring is inadvertently removed > 2 hours, efficacy is compromised

Medroxyprogesterone injection	Depo-Provera Depo-SubQ Provera 104 Provera	• Progestin Injection	• **Contraception Dosing (Adult):** injection every 3 months
			   – Intramuscular: 150 mg
			   – Subcutaneous: 104 mg
			• **CYP450 Interactions:** CYP3A4 inhibitors and inducers
			• **Renal or Hepatic Dose Adjustments:** contraindicated in hepatic impairment

| \multicolumn{4}{c}{**Non-Oral Contraceptives Drug Class Review**} |
| | | | **High-Yield Med Reviews** |

Generic Name	Brand Name	Main Indication(s) or Uses	Notes

Levonorgestrel intrauterine device (IUD)	Kyleena
	Liletta
	Mirena
	Skyla
		• Progestin IUD	• **Dosing (Adult):** inserted into uterine cavity
			  – Kyleena, Mirena: 5 years
			  – Liletta: 6 years
			  – Skyla: 3 years
			• **CYP450 Interactions:** CYP3A4 inhibitors and inducers
			• **Renal or Hepatic Dose Adjustments:** contraindicated in hepatic impairment

Etonogestrel implant	Nexplanon	• Progestin Implant	• **Dosing (Adult):** inserted into inner, upper arm – 3 years duration • **CYP450 Interactions:** none • **Renal or Hepatic Dose Adjustments:** contraindicated in hepatic failure • Consider an alternative contraceptive in women that weigh >130% of ideal body weight (possibly less effective)
Copper IUD	Paragard	• Non-hormonal IUD	• **Dosing (Adult):** inserted into uterine cavity – 10 years duration • **CYP450 Interactions:** none • **Renal or Hepatic Dose Adjustments:** none

OBSTETRICS & GYNECOLOGY – ORAL CONTRACEPTIVES

Drug Class
- **Oral Hormonal Contraceptives**
    - Combined oral contraceptives (COC)
        - Ethinyl estradiol (EE) plus progestin
    - Progestin-only pills (POP)

Main Indications or Uses
- Acne
- Contraception
- Hirsutism
- Endometriosis-induced pain
- Pre-menstrual dysphoric disorder
- Menstrual disorders (abnormal bleeding, menorrhagia, dysmenorrhea)

> **Fast Facts**
> ✓ In short, oral contraceptives attempt to trick the brain into thinking it is pregnant through a typical hormone feedback mechanism.
>
> ✓ The dose and degree of compliance with oral contraceptives directly influences its efficacy and ability to cause escape ovulations.

Mechanism of Action
- **Synthetic estrogen**
    - Alters hypothalamic gonadotropin secretion of follicle-stimulating hormone and luteinizing hormone
- **Progestin (synthetic progesterone)**
    - Suppresses luteinizing hormone, thickens cervical mucus, the thin endometrial lining

Primary Net Benefit
- Prevents ovulation, reducing the chance of conception
- Prevents/treats conditions associated with abnormal menstruation and hormonal imbalance
- Main Labs to Monitor:
    - Pregnancy status baseline
    - Blood pressure and weight baseline and annually after that
    - Serum potassium (specific formulations)
    - Signs/symptoms of venous thromboembolism (VTE)
    - In relevant patient populations, glucose/HgbA1c, lipid panel, signs/symptoms of depression

High-Yield Basic Pharmacology
- **Create Abbreviated / Short Title**
    - Negative feedback on the hypothalamus disrupts the normal release of FSH and LH from the anterior pituitary
    - **Ethinyl Estradiol**
        - Hepatic metabolism via CYP3A4
            - Drug-drug interactions: antiretrovirals, anticonvulsants, antibiotics
        - Ethinyl estradiol is highly protein-bound
    - **Drospirenone, norethindrone**
        - Minor hepatic metabolism via CYP3A4
    - POPs except for drospirenone have a short t ½ and necessitate daily administration of no more than a 3-hour variance

High-Yield Clinical Knowledge
- **Duration of Abstinence**
    - Women should use additional contraception measures or abstain from sexual intercourse until one week of therapy has been completed for the majority of oral contraception preparations
- **Missed Doses**
    - Missed doses should be managed according to the package insert of each specific preparation as there are numerous product-specific considerations.

- In general:
    - If one dose is missed, a patient can take two doses the following day and then resume the regular one dose daily schedule after that without compromising efficacy
    - If two or more doses are missed, a patient can take two doses for two days and then resume the one-dose daily schedule. Still, efficacy may be compromised by requiring additional contraception or abstinence for seven days. Emergency contraception may be considered in cases of two or more missed doses
- **Adverse Events**
    - Adverse effects such as bloating, irritability, and breakthrough bleeding often subside after three months of therapy
    - COCs or POPs are not associated with subsequent ability to conceive after discontinuation.
- **Oral Hormonal Contraction Considerations**
    - There is no difference in monophasic versus multiphasic efficacy or safety of monophasic versus multiphasic COCs. Extended-cycle preparations may be safer compared to standard 28-day pill preparations.
    - Women with hirsutism, acne, and oily skin should be prescribed COCs with low androgenic affinity.
    - The estrogen component of COCs increases the risk of VTE. However, breast cancer data is less affirmative, with low estrogen dose preparations hypothesized to carry little/no risk of breast cancer compared to higher estrogen dose preparations.
    - Contraindications/strong caution for COC use:
        - Breast cancer
        - Breastfeeding or within 21 days post-partum
        - Hepatic impairment
        - Active VTE or history of VTE increases the risk of VTE
        - Uncontrolled hypertension
        - Vascular disease, heart disease, cerebrovascular disease
        - Current tobacco use
        - Migraine with aura

High-Yield Core Evidence
- **MMWR US Selected Practice Recommendations for Contraceptive Use, 2016**
    - Efficacy is similar across COC and POP preparations with perfect use; however, efficacy with typical use, safety, affordability, and accessibility should be evaluated when determining contraceptive therapy. (MMWR Recomm Rep 2016;65(No. RR-4):1-66.)
- **Systematic Review**
    - A systematic review of contraceptive efficacy revealed that women taking COC preparations with shorter hormone-free intervals had lower rates of pregnancy and greater suppression of ovulation than preparations with 7-day hormone-free intervals. In addition, regarding missing doses, women on preparations with lower estrogen content (20 mcg) had greater follicular than women on practices with higher estrogen content (30 mcg) when doses were skipped. (Contraception 2013;87:685-700.)

High-Yield Fast-Fact
- **History of Hormonal Contraception**
    - Oral hormonal contraceptives have changed greatly since approval in the 1960s
        - Most notably, they have a fraction of the estrogen content as the initial preparations.
        - Less notably, there is even a chewable mint-flavored COC pill!
    - US History: Griswold v. Connecticut (1965) allowed all married women access to COCs and Eisenstadt v. Baird (1972) allowed all unmarried women access to COCs
    - Several states in the US allow pharmacists to prescribe COCs following guidance and required training per state boards of pharmacy

Table: Drug Class Summary

Oral Hormonal Contraceptives Drug Class Review High-Yield Med Reviews			
Mechanism of Action: *Suppression of follicle-stimulating hormone and luteinizing hormone prevents ovulation and decreases the chance of conception*			
Dosing: *EE < 35 mcg in women with pre-existing conditions that increase the risk of VTE, higher doses of EE can be considered with women with histories of non-adherence*			
Pediatric Dosing: *Use after menarche; dose same as an adult*			
CYP450 Interactions: *CYP3A4 inhibitors and inducers*			
Renal or Hepatic Dose Adjustments: *Contraindicated in hepatic failure*			
Generic Name	**Brand Name**	**Main Indication(s) or Uses**	**Notes**
EE + progestin (drospirenone, norethindrone acetate, levonorgestrel, desogestrel, ethynodiol diacetate)	Brand Name more than 50 branded preparations	▪ Monophasic COC	▪ **Dosing (Adult):** Same amount of EE:progestin in active pills − 4 or 7 hormone-free days per 28-day cycle ▪ **Additional Components:** ferrous fumarate, levomefolate calcium in select preparations
EE + progestin (desogestrel, norethindrone)	Brand Name Azurette Bekyree Kariva Kimidess Mircette Necon 10/11 Pimtrea Viorele Volnea	▪ Biphasic COC	▪ **Dosing (Adult):** two different EE:progestin ratios in active pills − 2 or 7 hormone-free days per 28 days cycle

Oral Hormonal Contraceptives Drug Class Review
High-Yield Med Reviews

Generic Name	Brand Name	Main Indication(s) or Uses	Notes

EE + progestin (norethindrone, desogestrel, norgestimate, levonorgestrel)	Brand Name Alyacen 7/7/7
	Aranelle
	Caziant
	Cesia
	Cyclessa
	Cyclafem 7/7/7
	Dasetta 7/7/7
	Enpresse
	Estrostep Fe
	Leena
	Levonest
	Ortho-Novum 7/7/7
	Ortho Tri-Cyclen
	Ortho Tri-Cyclen Lo
	Myzilra
	Necon 7/7/7
	Nortrel 7/7/7
	Tilia Fe
	Tri-Estarylla
	Tri-Legest Fe
	Tri-Linyah
	TriNessa
	Tri-Norinyl
	Tri-Previfem
	Tri-Sprintec
	Trivora
	Velivet
		▪ Triphasic COC	▪ **Dosing (Adult):** three different EE:progestin ratios in active pills
			   – 7 hormone-free days per 28 day cycle
			      – Extra info if needed

Estradiol valerate + dienogest	Natazia	▪ Four phasic COC	▪ **Dosing (Adult):** four different estradiol valerate:dienogest ratios in active pills – 2 hormone-free days per 28 day cycle

Ethinyl estradiol + norethindrone	Lo Loestrin Fe	▪ Multiphasic COC	▪ **Dosing (Adult):** EE + progestin day 1-24, EE day 25-26
			   – 2 hormone-free days per 28 day cycle
			      – Extra info if needed
			▪ **Additional Component:** ferrous fumarate day 27-28

EE + levonorgestrel	Amethyst
	Introvale
	Jolessa
	Quasense
	Seasonale
		▪ Extended cycle COC	▪ **Dosing (Adult):**
			   – EE + progestin x 365 days, no hormone-free interval
			   – EE + progestin x 84 days, 7 hormone-free days (4 times annually)

Oral Hormonal Contraceptives Drug Class Review
High-Yield Med Reviews

Generic Name	Brand Name	Main Indication(s) or Uses	Notes
EE + levonorgestrel	Amethia, Amethia Lo, Camrese, Camrese Lo, Jaimiess, Lo Jaimiess, LoSeasonique, Quartette, Seasonique	• Extended cycle multiphasic COC	• **Dosing (Adult):** EE + progestin x 84 − EE + progestin x 84 days, EE x 7 days − Four different EE:progestin ratios per 91 day cycle − No hormone-free interval
Drospirenone	Slynd	• POP	• **Dosing (Adult):** progestin day 1-24, 4 hormone-free days per 28 day cycle • **Missed doses:** only POP that has a 24-hour intake window
Norethindrone	Camila, Deblitane, Errin, Heather, Jencycla, Jolivette, Lyza, Nor-QD, Nora-BE, Norlyroc, Ortho Micronor, Sharobel	• POP	• **Dosing (Adult):** progestin x 365 days, no hormone-free interval

HIGH-YIELD BOARD EXAM ESSENTIALS
- **CLASSIC AGENTS:** Ethinyl estradiol (EE) +/- progestin
- **DRUG CLASS:** Oral Contraceptives
- **INDICATIONS:** Acne, contraception, hirsutism, hot flashes, endometriosis
- **MECHANISM:** Suppression of follicle-stimulating hormone and luteinizing hormone prevent ovulation and decrease chance of conception. They can also thicken cervical mucous to prevent sperm migration.
- **SIDE EFFECTS:** Vaginal spotting or amenorrhea, DVT/PE, decreased milk production (estrogen)
- **CLINICAL PEARLS:** Avoid estrogen containing IUDs post-partum in patients who are breast-feeding as it can decrease milk production. Avoid estrogen containing agents in patients with known hypercoagulable disorders, CAD, or history of VTE due to the increased risk of forming clots.

ENDOCRINE – GONADOTROPIN-RELEASING HORMONE AGONISTS AND ANTAGONIST

Drug Class
- Gonadotropin-Releasing Hormone Agonists and Antagonists
- Agents:
    - Chronic Care
        - Degarelix
        - Goserelin
        - Histrelin
        - Leuprolide
        - Nafarelin
        - Triptorelin

Main Indications or Uses
- Acute & Chronic Care
    - Breast cancer (Goserelin)
    - Central precocious puberty (Histrelin, leuprolide, nafarelin, triptorelin)
    - Controlled ovarian stimulation (Cetrorelix, ganirelix)
    - Endometriosis (Elagolix, goserelin, leuprolide, nafarelin)
    - Prostate cancer (Goserelin, histrelin, leuprolide, triptorelin)
    - Uterine leiomyomata (Leuprolide)

Mechanism of Action
- Gonadotropin-Releasing Hormone Agonists (Goserelin, histrelin, leuprolide, nafarelin, triptorelin)
    - Reversibly inhibiting follicle-stimulating hormone and luteinizing hormone secretion.
- Gonadotropin-Releasing Hormone Antagonist (Cetrorelix, degarelix, ganirelix, elagolix)
    - Reversibly inhibits GnRH receptors on the pituitary gland, reducing testosterone production.

Primary Net Benefit
- GnRH agonists are associated with an increased risk of cardiovascular death but with a lower risk of prostate cancer-specific mortality and all-cause mortality.
- Main Labs to Monitor:
    - Pregnancy (negative, before initiation)
    - Liver enzyme (AST/ALT, Alk Phos)
    - Liver function (PT/INR, albumin, protein, bilirubin)

High-Yield Basic Pharmacology
- Agonist vs Antagonist
    - Degarelix, a GnRH antagonist, can achieve a much more rapid therapeutic antiandrogenic effect in 7 days, compared to 28 days for other GnRH agonists.
- Pharmacologic Oophorectomy
    - The GnRH agonists mimic a reversible pharmacologic oophorectomy upon drug discontinuation and clearance.

High-Yield Clinical Knowledge
- Long Duration Dosage Forms
    - Many GnRH agonists are available in parenteral long-acting dosage forms, including leuprolide depot injection or leuprolide implant, triptorelin depot or implant, and goserelin acetate implant.
- Comparable Efficacy and Safety
    - The available evidence suggests no significant differences in either efficacy or toxicity among the GnRH agonists and orchiectomy.
    - Many experts consider the choice of pharmacologic intervention a patient-specific and patient-physician shared decision-making process.

- **Central precocious puberty**
    - Central precocious puberty is the onset of puberty before 7 or 8 years in girls or before 9 in boys.
    - Before GnRH agonist therapy, a test dose must be administered or have a positive gonadotropin response to GnRH.
- **Gonadotropic Flare**
    - Upon initiation of GnRH agonists, a short-lived gonadotropic flare occurs as long-term receptor downregulation develops.
    - Pain that may accompany this phase can be alleviated by the addition of combined hormonal contraceptives or progestin for up to three weeks.
- **Hypoestrogenic Effects**
    - GnRH agonists' common adverse effects relate to their hypoestrogenic effect but dissipate with long-term use beyond six months.
    - These effects include loss of bone mineral density and vasomotor symptoms.
- **Add-Back Therapy**
    - Add-back therapy of estrogens, progestin alone, and progestins plus bisphosphonates are commonly used in combination with GnRH agonists to minimize bone mineral density loss and relieve vasomotor symptoms.
        - Doses of estrogen must be low enough to avoid neutralizing the anti-estrogenic effects of GnRH agonist therapy.
- **GnRH Suppression in Women**
    - GnRH gonadal suppression with continuous use of GnRH agonists is a component of managing advanced breast cancer and ovarian cancer.

High-Yield Core Evidence
- **Diabetes and CVD Risk During GnRH Agonist Therapy**
    - This was a population-based cohort study of Medicare enrollees 66 years of age or older diagnosed with locoregional prostate cancer during the predefined observation period to determine whether androgen deprivation therapy is associated with an increased incidence of diabetes and cardiovascular disease.
    - The study investigators observed that GnRH agonist use was associated with an increased risk of incident diabetes, coronary heart disease, myocardial infarction, and sudden cardiac death.
    - Although men treated with orchiectomy were more likely to develop diabetes, they were less likely to develop coronary heart disease, myocardial infarction, or sudden cardiac death.
    - The authors concluded that GnRH agonist treatment for men with locoregional prostate cancer might increase the risk of incident diabetes and CV disease. (J Clin Oncol. 2006 Sep 20;24(27):4448-56.)
- **Androgen Deprivation Meta-Analysis**
    - This was a systematic review and meta-analysis of randomized trials to determine whether androgen deprivation therapy (ADT) causes excess cardiovascular deaths in men with prostate cancer.
    - The study authors included randomized clinical trials that included men with nonmetastatic disease, an intervention group with GnRH agonist-based ADT, a control group with no immediate ADT, complete information on cardiovascular deaths, and a median follow-up of more than one year.
    - This meta-analysis included eight randomized trials consisting of 4141 patients.
    - There was no significant difference observed concerning cardiovascular death in patients receiving ADT than control, and ADT was not associated with excess cardiovascular death in trials of less than six months and at least three years of ADT.
    - Data from eleven randomized trials associated ADT with lower prostate cancer-specific mortality, and lower all-cause mortality
    - The authors concluded that in a pooled analysis of randomized trials in unfavorable-risk prostate cancer, ADT use was not associated with an increased risk of cardiovascular death but was associated with a lower risk of prostate cancer-specific mortality and all-cause mortality. (JAMA. 2011 Dec 7;306(21):2359-66.)

High-Yield Fast-Fact
- **GnRH or LnRH**
    - The GnRH agonists are also sometimes referred to as luteinizing hormone-releasing hormone agonists.

Table: Drug Class Summary

\multicolumn{4}{c}{**Gonadotropin-Releasing Hormone Agonists and Antagonist - Drug Class Review**}

Gonadotropin-Releasing Hormone Agonists and Antagonist - Drug Class Review
High-Yield Med Reviews

Mechanism of Action:
GnRH Agonists - Reversibly inhibiting follicle-stimulating hormone and luteinizing hormone secretion.
GnRH Antagonist - Reversibly inhibits GnRH receptors on the pituitary gland, reducing the production of testosterone.

Class Effects: GnRH agonists are associated with an increased risk of cardiovascular death but are associated with a lower risk of prostate cancer-specific mortality and all-cause mortality.

Generic Name	Brand Name	Main Indication(s) or Uses	Notes
Cetrorelix	Cetrotide	• Controlled ovarian stimulation	• **Dosing (Adult):** — SQ: 0.25 mg of stimulation day 5 or 6 and continued daily until hCG administration • **Dosing (Peds):** — Not routinely used • **CYP450 Interactions:** None • **Renal or Hepatic Dose Adjustments:** — Severe renal impairment: contraindicated • **Dosage Forms:** SQ kit
Degarelix	Firmagon	• Prostate cancer	• **Dosing (Adult):** — SQ: 240 mg, then 80 mg q28days • **Dosing (Peds):** — Not routinely used • **CYP450 Interactions:** None • **Renal or Hepatic Dose Adjustments:** None • **Dosage Forms:** SQ solution
Ganirelix	Antagon	• Controlled ovarian stimulation	• **Dosing (Adult):** — SQ: 250 mcg on day 2 or 3 of the cycle, continued until hCG administration • **Dosing (Peds):** — Not routinely used • **CYP450 Interactions:** None • **Renal or Hepatic Dose Adjustments:** None • **Dosage Forms:** SQ kit
Elagolix	Orilissa	• Endometriosis	• **Dosing (Adult):** — Oral: 150 mg daily for a maximum of 24 months • **Dosing (Peds):** — Not routinely used • **CYP450 Interactions:** Substrate CYP3A4, P-gp; Inhibits CYP2C19, P-gp; Induces CYP3A4 • **Renal or Hepatic Dose Adjustments:** None • **Dosage Forms:** Oral (tablet)

Gonadotropin-Releasing Hormone Agonists and Antagonist - Drug Class Review
High-Yield Med Reviews

Generic Name	Brand Name	Main Indication(s) or Uses	Notes
Goserelin	Zoladex	<ul><li>Breast cancer</li><li>Endometriosis</li><li>Endometriosis</li><li>Prostate cancer</li></ul>	<ul><li>**Dosing (Adult):**<ul><li>SQ: (females) 3.6 mg q28days (duration indication dependent)</li><li>SQ: (males) 3.6 mg q28days or 10.8 mg q12weeks</li></ul></li><li>**Dosing (Peds):**<ul><li>Not routinely used</li></ul></li><li>**CYP450 Interactions:** None</li><li>**Renal or Hepatic Dose Adjustments:** None</li><li>**Dosage Forms:** SQ Implant</li></ul>
Histrelin	Supprelin LA, Vantas	<ul><li>Central precocious puberty</li><li>Prostate cancer</li></ul>	<ul><li>**Dosing (Adult):**<ul><li>SQ: 50 mg implant q12months</li></ul></li><li>**Dosing (Peds):**<ul><li>SQ: 50 mg implant q12months</li></ul></li><li>**CYP450 Interactions:** None</li><li>**Renal or Hepatic Dose Adjustments:** None</li><li>**Dosage Forms:** SQ kit</li></ul>
Leuprolide	Eligard, Fensolvi, Lupron	<ul><li>Central precocious puberty</li><li>Endometriosis</li><li>Prostate cancer</li><li>Uterine leiomyomata</li></ul>	<ul><li>**Dosing (Adult):**<ul><li>IM/SQ: (depot) 7.5 mg qmonth; 22.5 mg q12weeks; 30 mg q16weeks; 45 mg q24weeks</li><li>IM: 3.75 mg q1month for 6 months or 11.25 mg q3months for 6 months</li></ul></li><li>**Dosing (Peds):**<ul><li>IM: (depot) initial 7.5 to 15 mg qmonth, titrated by 3.75 mg q4weeks</li><li>SQ: 45 mg q6months</li><li>IM: 3.75 mg q1month for 6 months or 11.25 mg q3months for 6 months</li></ul></li><li>**CYP450 Interactions:** None</li><li>**Renal or Hepatic Dose Adjustments:** None</li><li>**Dosage Forms:** SQ kit, Injection kit</li></ul>
Nafarelin	Synarel	<ul><li>Central precocious puberty</li><li>Endometriosis</li></ul>	<ul><li>**Dosing (Adult):**<ul><li>Intranasal: 200 mcg (1 spray) in each nostril BID starting between days 2 and 4 of the menstrual cycle<ul><li>Up to 4 total sprays for no more than 6 months</li></ul></li></ul></li><li>**Dosing (Peds):**<ul><li>Intranasal: 400 mcg (2 sprays) per nostril BID<ul><li>Maximum 3 sprays TID (1,800 mcg/day)</li></ul></li></ul></li><li>**CYP450 Interactions:** None</li><li>**Renal or Hepatic Dose Adjustments:** None</li><li>**Dosage Forms:** Nasal solution</li></ul>

Gonadotropin-Releasing Hormone Agonists and Antagonist - Drug Class Review
High-Yield Med Reviews

Generic Name	Brand Name	Main Indication(s) or Uses	Notes

Triptorelin	Trelstar Mixject, Triptodur	- Central precocious puberty
		- Prostate cancer
			- **Dosing (Adult):**
			  – IM: 3.75 mg q4weeks or 11.25 mg q12weeks or 22.5 mg q24weeks
			- **Dosing (Peds):**
			  – IM: 22.5 mg q24weeks
			- **CYP450 Interactions:** None
			- **Renal or Hepatic Dose Adjustments:** None
			- **Dosage Forms:** IM suspension

HIGH-YIELD BOARD EXAM ESSENTIALS
- **CLASSIC AGENTS:** Degarelix, goserelin, histrelin, leuprolide, nafarelin, triptorelin
- **DRUG CLASS:** Gonadotropin-releasing hormone agonists and antagonist
- **INDICATIONS:** Breast cancer (goserelin), central precocious puberty (histrelin, leuprolide, nafarelin, triptorelin), controlled ovarian stimulation (cetrorelix, ganirelix), endometriosis (elagolix, goserelin, leuprolide, nafarelin), prostate cancer (goserelin, histrelin, leuprolide, triptorelin), uterine leiomyomata (leuprolide)
- **MECHANISM:** Reversibly inhibiting follicle-stimulating hormone and luteinizing hormone secretion (GnRH Agonists). Reversibly inhibits GnRH receptors on the pituitary gland, reducing the production of testosterone (GnRH Antagonist).
- **SIDE EFFECTS:** Gonadotropic flare, loss of bone mineral density and vasomotor symptoms.
- **CLINICAL PEARLS:** Upon initiation of GnRH agonists, a short-lived gonadotropic flare occurs as long-term

2025

A COMPREHENSIVE *RAPID REVIEW*

NAPLEX
Pharmacology & Drug Classes

Ophthalmology

OPHTHALMOLOGY – ALPHA AGONISTS

Drug Class
- Alpha Agonists
- Agents:
    - Acute & Chronic Care
        - Apraclonidine
        - Brimonidine

Main Indications or Uses
- Acute & Chronic Care
    - Elevated intraocular pressure

> **Fast Facts**
> ✓ Apraclonidine is a derivative of the alpha-2 agonist, clonidine.
>
> ✓ The goal is to reduce the IOP by about 20 - 30% from baseline.

Mechanism of Action
- Enhance normal and uveoscleral outflow of aqueous humor and decrease aqueous humor production.

Primary Net Benefit
- Considered second-line intraocular pressure (IOP) lowering agents for glaucoma.
- Main Labs to Monitor:
    - Intraocular pressure (baseline, at 4-6 weeks, then every 3-4 months)
    - Ophthalmic exam

High-Yield Basic Pharmacology
- Clonidine
    - Apraclonidine is a derivative of clonidine that is highly ionized at physiological pH, thus unable to cross the blood-brain barrier.
- Pre- and Postsynaptic Alpha-2
    - Apraclonidine and brimonidine possess both pre- and post-synaptic alpha-2 agonist properties.
    - Pre-synaptic agonist actions on the alpha-2 receptor reduce the quantity of sympathetic neurotransmitter release.
    - Post-synaptic alpha-2 agonist actions lead to a reduction in aqueous humor production.

High-Yield Clinical Knowledge
- Rebound Effects
    - The alpha-2 agonists are associated with vasoconstriction-vasodilation rebound effects that can cause eye redness.
    - This effect of brimonidine extends to its use as a topical skin agent to treat rosacea.
    - The red discoloration often responds to lowering the dose or conversion to an alternative agent.
- Children Younger Than 2
    - Apraclonidine and brimonidine are contraindicated in children younger than 2 because of the risk of CNS depression and apnea.
- Ophthalmic Drop Administration
    - Before administering any ophthalmic product, patients should be reminded to wash their hands and remove any contact lenses.
    - Most administrations should begin with 1 drop of solution in the affected eye.
    - No more than 1 drop should be administered at a time, and multiple drops should be separated by at least 1 minute since the aqueous chamber cannot hold the given volume.
    - If drops and ointments are given, the drop should be administered first, followed by the ointment.
- Monitoring Intraocular Pressure
    - Some patients with glaucoma may only affect individual eyes rather than a bilateral effect.
    - To monitor intraocular pressure changes throughout drug therapy, an initial pressure in the affected should be used as a baseline for monitoring rather than using the unaffected eye intraocular pressure.
    - This results from the possibility of ophthalmic agents applied to a single eye, affecting both eyes.

- **Intraocular Pressure Goals**
  - An acute reduction of 20 to 30% in the IOP is the initial goal of drug therapy, monitoring visual fields, and examination of the optic disk.
  - If goal pressures are not achieved with an initial agent, switching to a new agent rather than additional add-on agents is recommended.

High-Yield Core Evidence
- **Acute Primary Open-Angle Glaucoma Study**
  - This was a multicenter, prospective, double-blind trial that randomized patients with primary open-angle glaucoma to receive one of four treatments of either placebo, clonidine 0.125%, apraclonidine 1.0%, or brimonidine 0.2%.
  - The alpha-agonists clonidine, apraclonidine, and brimonidine significantly lowered IOP compared to placebo.
  - Clonidine therapy was associated with significant modifications of mean blood pressure, IOP, and visual field indices.
  - However, apraclonidine did not affect mean blood pressure, and there was no change in the analyzed parameters after brimonidine instillation.
  - The authors concluded that the lack of effects on the blood flow and the absence of vasomotor activity at the level of the posterior pole exhibited by brimonidine is related to its alpha-2 selectivity, as appears by comparing this compound with the other alpha-agonists available for the management of glaucoma. (Ophthalmologica. Jan-Feb 2003;217(1):39-44.)

High-Yield Fast-Fact
- **Oral Ingestion**
  - Oral ingestion of alpha-agonist ophthalmic products can produce profound diarrhea but may also lead to severe, life-threatening hemodynamic compromise similar to a massive clonidine overdose.
  - Ingestion of small amounts of ophthalmic products by a child is considered a medical emergency.

HIGH-YIELD BOARD EXAM ESSENTIALS
- **CLASSIC AGENTS:** Apraclonidine, brimonidine
- **DRUG CLASS:** Alpha agonists
- **INDICATIONS:** Elevated intraocular pressure
- **MECHANISM:** Enhance normal and uveoscleral outflow of aqueous humor and decrease the production of aqueous humor.
- **SIDE EFFECTS:** Rebound elevation in IOP, CNS depression, apnea
- **CLINICAL PEARLS:** Apraclonidine and brimonidine are contraindicated in children younger than 2 because of the risk of CNS depression and apnea.

Table: Drug Class Summary

Alpha Agonists - Drug Class Review High-Yield Med Reviews			
**Mechanism of Action:** *Enhance normal and uveoscleral outflow of aqueous humor and decrease the production of aqueous humor.*			
**Class Effects:** *Considered second line intraocular pressure (IOP) lowering agents.*			
Generic Name	**Brand Name**	**Indication(s) or Uses**	**Notes**
Apraclonidine	Iopidine	• Elevated intraocular pressure	• **Dosing (Adult):** — Ophthalmic: 1 to 2 drops into affected eye(s) 3 times daily • **Dosing (Peds):** — Not routinely used • **CYP450 Interactions:** None • **Renal or Hepatic Dose Adjustments:** None • **Dosage Forms:** Ophthalmic solution
Brimonidine	Alphagan P, Lumify	• Elevated intraocular pressure	• **Dosing (Adult):** — Ophthalmic: 1 drop into affected eye(s) q8-12h • **Dosing (Peds):** — Ophthalmic: 1 drop into affected eye(s) q8-12h • **CYP450 Interactions:** None • **Renal or Hepatic Dose Adjustments:** None • **Dosage Forms:** Ophthalmic solution

OPHTHALMOLOGY – ANTIGLAUCOMA – BETA ANTAGONISTS

Drug Class
- **Beta Antagonists**
- **Agents:**
    - Acute & Chronic Care
        - Betaxolol
        - Carteolol
        - Levobunolol
        - Metipranolol
        - Timolol

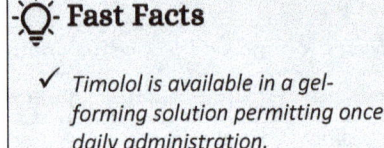

Fast Facts
- ✓ Timolol is available in a gel-forming solution permitting once-daily administration.

Main Indications or Uses
- **Acute & Chronic Care**
    - Elevated intraocular pressure

Mechanism of Action
- Beta-2 antagonists decrease intraocular pressure (IOP) and decreases aqueous humor production.

Primary Net Benefit
- Intraocular pressure (IOP) lowering agents with established safety and efficacy for ophthalmic care.
- Main Labs to Monitor:
    - Intraocular pressure (baseline, at 4-6 weeks, then every 3-4 months)
    - Ophthalmic exam
    - ECG, heart rate, and blood pressure at baseline and after any change in therapy.

High-Yield Basic Pharmacology
- **Beta-1 Selectivity**
    - The ophthalmic beta-antagonists are all non-selective beta-1 and beta-2 agents, except for betaxolol, a beta-1 selective antagonist.
    - The proposed benefit is a reduced likelihood of bronchospasm from systemically absorbed betaxolol.
- **ISA Activity**
    - Carteolol, while a non-selective beta-antagonist, also possesses intrinsic sympathomimetic activity.
    - This effect does not appear to impact its IOP lowering effect compared to other beta-antagonists.

High-Yield Clinical Knowledge
- **Alpha and Beta Effects**
    - Levobunolol is a mixed alpha and beta receptor antagonist that may have a specific benefit in controlling IOP after cataract surgery.
- **Timolol Formulations**
    - Although most ophthalmic beta-antagonists are administered multiple times daily, timolol is available in a gel-forming solution permitting once-daily administration.
- **Systemic Effects**
    - Ophthalmic beta-antagonists can be systemically absorbed and are expected to lead to common beta-antagonist adverse events, including bronchospasm, bradycardia, masking of sympathetic response to hypoglycemia, and sexual dysfunction.
        - Ophthalmic beta-antagonists should be used with caution in patients with reactive pulmonary disease, symptomatic bradycardia, heart failure, and diabetes.
    - Furthermore, patients already taking systemic beta-antagonists experience a lower IOP reduction from ophthalmic beta-antagonist therapy.

- **Monitoring Intraocular Pressure**
  - Some patients with glaucoma may only affect individual eyes rather than a bilateral effect.
  - To monitor intraocular pressure changes throughout drug therapy, an initial pressure in the affected should be used as a baseline for monitoring rather than using the unaffected eye intraocular pressure.
  - This results from the possibility of ophthalmic agents that are applied to a single eye, affecting both eyes.
- **Intraocular Pressure Goals**
  - An acute reduction of 20 to 30% in the IOP is the initial goal of drug therapy and monitoring visual fields and examination of the optic disk.
  - If goal pressures are not achieved with an initial agent, switching to a new agent is recommended rather than adding additional agents.
- **Ophthalmic Drop Administration**
  - Before administering any ophthalmic product, patients should be reminded to wash their hands and remove any contact lenses.
  - Most administrations should begin with 1 drop of solution in the affected eye.
  - No more than 1 drop should be administered at a time, and multiple drops should be separated by at least 1 minute since the aqueous chamber cannot hold the given volume.
  - If drops and ointments are to be given, the drop should be administered first, followed by the ointment.

High-Yield Core Evidence
- **United States Latanoprost Study Group**
  - This was a multicenter, double-blind, parallel-group study in patients with ocular hypertension or early primary open-angle glaucoma who were randomized to receive either latanoprost 0.005% daily or timolol 0.5 % twice daily for six months.
  - Patients receiving latanoprost experience a significantly superior reduction in IOP compared to timolol.
  - Heart rate was significantly lower among patients receiving timolol but not with latanoprost.
  - Compared to zero receiving timolol, patients in the latanoprost group experience iris color change.
  - No significant difference between treatment groups occurred in visual acuity, slit-lamp examination, blood pressure, and laboratory values.
  - The authors concluded that latanoprost has the potential to become a new first-line treatment for glaucoma. (Ophthalmology. 1996 Jan;103(1):138-47.)

High-Yield Fast-Fact
- **Hypoglycemic Masking**
  - Beta-antagonists diminish sympathetic-mediated responses to hypoglycemia (tachycardia, tremor, and hunger)
  - During the acute hypoglycemic stress response, sweating is not diminished as this response is mediated by nicotinic activation by acetylcholine.

HIGH-YIELD BOARD EXAM ESSENTIALS
- **CLASSIC AGENTS:** Betaxolol, carteolol, levobunolol, metipranolol, timolol
- **DRUG CLASS:** Beta antagonists
- **INDICATIONS:** Elevated intraocular pressure
- **MECHANISM:** Beta-2 antagonists decrease intraocular pressure (IOP) decreases aqueous humor production.
- **SIDE EFFECTS:** Eye discomfort, blurry vision, keratitis
- **CLINICAL PEARLS:** An acute reduction of 20 to 30% in the IOP is the initial goal of drug therapy, as well as monitoring visual fields and examination of the optic disk.

Table: Drug Class Summary

\multicolumn{4}{c}{**Beta Antagonists - Drug Class Review**}
\multicolumn{4}{c}{High-Yield Med Reviews}
\multicolumn{4}{l}{**Mechanism of Action:** *Beta-2 antagonists decrease intraocular pressure (IOP) decreases aqueous humor production.*}
\multicolumn{4}{l}{**Class Effects:** *Intraocular pressure (IOP) lowering agents with established safety and efficacy for ophthalmic care.*}
Generic Name	**Brand Name**	**Main Indication(s) or Uses**	**Notes**
Betaxolol	Betoptic-S	• Elevated intraocular pressure	• **Dosing (Adult):** 　– Ophthalmic: 1 to 2 drops into affected eye(s) q12h • **Dosing (Peds):** 　– Ophthalmic: 1 drop into affected eye(s) q12h • **CYP450 Interactions:** Substrate CYP1A2, 2D6 • **Renal or Hepatic Dose Adjustments:** None • **Dosage Forms:** Ophthalmic (solution, suspension)
Carteolol	Ocupress	• Elevated intraocular pressure	• **Dosing (Adult):** 　– Ophthalmic: 1 drops into affected eye(s) q12h • **Dosing (Peds):** 　– Not routinely used • **CYP450 Interactions:** Substrate CYP2D6 • **Renal or Hepatic Dose Adjustments:** None • **Dosage Forms:** Ophthalmic (solution)
Levobunolol	Betagan	• Elevated intraocular pressure	• **Dosing (Adult):** 　– Ophthalmic: 1 to 2 drops into affected eye(s) q24h • **Dosing (Peds):** 　– Not routinely used • **CYP450 Interactions:** None • **Renal or Hepatic Dose Adjustments:** None • **Dosage Forms:** Ophthalmic (solution)
Timolol	Betimol, Istalol, Timoptic	• Elevated intraocular pressure	• **Dosing (Adult):** 　– Ophthalmic: 1 drop into affected eye(s) q12h • **Dosing (Peds):** 　– Ophthalmic: 1 drop into affected eye(s) q12h • **CYP450 Interactions:** Substrate CYP2D6 • **Renal or Hepatic Dose Adjustments:** None • **Dosage Forms:** Ophthalmic (gel forming solution, solution)

OPHTHALMOLOGY – ANTIGLAUCOMA – CARBONIC ANHYDRASE INHIBITORS

Drug Class
- Carbonic Anhydrase Inhibitors
- Agents:
    - Acute & Chronic Care
        - Brinzolamide
        - Dorzolamide

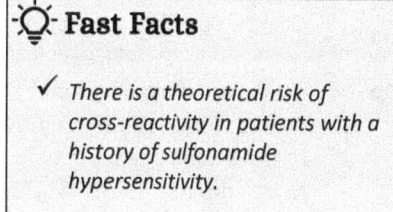

Fast Facts
- ✓ There is a theoretical risk of cross-reactivity in patients with a history of sulfonamide hypersensitivity.

Main Indications or Uses
- Acute & Chronic Care
    - Elevated intraocular pressure

Mechanism of Action
- Inhibit carbonic anhydrase causing a reduction in intraocular fluid transport from a reduction in the formation of bicarbonate.

Primary Net Benefit
- Reserved for second-line or combination therapy for the management of elevated intraocular pressure. Considerations of clinically relevant systemic absorption include patients with renal impairment.
- Main Labs to Monitor:
    - Intraocular pressure (baseline, at 4-6 weeks, then every 3-4 months)
    - Ophthalmic exam

High-Yield Basic Pharmacology
- Other Systemic Effects
    - Inhibition of carbonic anhydrase blunts the reabsorption of sodium bicarbonate, promoting diuresis.
    - Carbonic anhydrase is responsible for converting carbonic acid to carbon dioxide at the renal luminal membrane and rehydration of carbon dioxide to the carbonic acid in the cytoplasm.
    - By blocking these processes, carbonic anhydrase inhibitors promote a reduction of hydrogen secretion and increased renal excretion of sodium, potassium, bicarbonate, and water.

High-Yield Clinical Knowledge
- Systemic Vs. Topical Carbonic Anhydrase Inhibitors
    - The topical carbonic anhydrase inhibitors are primarily preferred to oral agents and reduce the incidence of fatigue, depression, paresthesias, and nephrolithiasis associated with the systemic route.
- Sulfonamide Derivatives
    - There is a theoretical risk of cross-reactivity in patients with a history of sulfonamide hypersensitivity.
    - As a result of its sulfonamide structure, carbonic anhydrase inhibitors carry a risk of bone marrow depression, Stevens-Johnson Syndrome, and sulfonamide-like kidney injury.
    - The ophthalmic carbonic anhydrase inhibitors are systemically absorbed and may pose a risk in patients with sulfonamide hypersensitivity.
- Renal Impairment
    - Unlike other topical ophthalmic agents, brinzolamide and dorzolamide should be avoided in patients with GFR less than 30 mL/minute as the risk of hyperchloremic acidosis is higher among this population.

- Systemic Carbonic Anhydrase Inhibition
    - The combination of systemic and topical carbonic anhydrase inhibitors is not recommended.
    - Although systemic CAIs reduce IOP by up to 40%, they should be reserved for third-line agents, as the frequency and severity of systemic adverse events limit their use.
        - These systemic effects range from fatigue, nausea, altered taste to depression, nephrolithiasis, increased uric acid, and blood dyscrasias.

- **Hyperchloremic Metabolic Acidosis**
  - Carbonic anhydrase inhibitors block the excretion of hydrogen ions accumulating in the plasma.
    - In normal healthy kidneys, reabsorb bicarbonate and offsets the accumulation of hydrogen and ensuing acidosis.
    - With impaired renal function, high doses, or otherwise altered metabolic function, renal tubules' capacity to reabsorb bicarbonate is impaired, leading to an increasing acidosis.
      - The acidosis typically resolves upon discontinuation of the carbonic anhydrase inhibitor.
- **Ophthalmic Drop Administration**
  - Before administering any ophthalmic product, patients should be reminded to wash their hands and remove contact lenses.
  - Most administrations should begin with 1 drop of solution in the affected eye.
  - No more than 1 drop should be administered at a time, and multiple drops should be separated by at least 1 minute since the aqueous chamber cannot hold the given volume.
  - If drops and ointments are to be given, the drop should be administered first, followed by the ointment.

High-Yield Core Evidence
- **Ocular Hypertension Treatment Study**
  - This multicenter clinical trial randomized patients with elevated IOP to either topical ocular hypotensive medication therapy or close observation to determine the safety and efficacy of topical ocular hypotensive medication in delaying or preventing the onset of primary open-angle glaucoma.
  - After the 60-month study period, there was a significant reduction in the cumulative probability of developing primary open-angle glaucoma among patients receiving ocular hypotensive medication compared to observation alone.
  - There was little evidence of increased systemic or ocular risk associated with the ocular hypotensive medication.
  - The authors concluded that topical ocular hypotensive medication effectively delayed or prevented the onset of primary open-angle glaucoma in individuals with elevated IOP. (Arch Ophthalmol. 2002 Jun;120(6):701-13.)

High-Yield Fast-Fact
- **Weight Loss**
  - The systemic carbonic anhydrase inhibitor topiramate is used off-label for weight loss after observation from clinical trials consistently found this effect in patients receiving the drug.

HIGH-YIELD BOARD EXAM ESSENTIALS
- **CLASSIC AGENTS:** Brinzolamide, dorzolamide
- **DRUG CLASS:** Carbonic anhydrase inhibitors
- **INDICATIONS:** Elevated intraocular pressure
- **MECHANISM:** Inhibit carbonic anhydrase, causing a reduction in intraocular fluid transport from a reduction in bicarbonate formation.
- **SIDE EFFECTS:** Very low risk for hyperchloremic acidosis, fatigue, depression, paresthesias, and nephrolithiasis when used topically.
- **CLINICAL PEARLS:** The topical carbonic anhydrase inhibitors are primarily preferred to oral agents and reduce the incidence of fatigue, depression, paresthesias, and nephrolithiasis associated with the systemic route.

Table: Drug Class Summary

Carbonic Anhydrase Inhibitors - Drug Class Review High-Yield Med Reviews			
Mechanism of Action: *Inhibit carbonic anhydrase, causing a reduction in intraocular fluid transport from a reduction in bicarbonate formation.*			
Class Effects: *Reserved for second line or combination therapy for the management of elevated intraocular pressure. Considerations of clinically relevant systemic absorption include patients with renal impairment.*			
Generic Name	**Brand Name**	**Indication(s) or Uses**	**Notes**

Brinzolamide	Azopt	• Elevated intraocular pressure	• **Dosing (Adult):**
			  – Ophthalmic: 1 drop into affected eye(s) q8h
			• **Dosing (Peds):**
			  – Not routinely used
			• **CYP450 Interactions:** Substrate CYP3A4
			• **Renal or Hepatic Dose Adjustments:**
			  – GFR < 30 mL/minute: use not recommended
			• **Dosage Forms:** Ophthalmic solution

Dorzolamide	Trusopt	• Elevated intraocular pressure	• **Dosing (Adult):**
			  – Ophthalmic: 1 drop into affected eye(s) q8h
			• **Dosing (Peds):**
			  – Ophthalmic: 1 drop into affected eye(s) q8h
			• **CYP450 Interactions:** Substrate CYP2C9, 3A4
			• **Renal or Hepatic Dose Adjustments:**
			  – GFR < 30 mL/minute: use not recommended
			• **Dosage Forms:** Ophthalmic solution

OPHTHALMOLOGY – CHOLINERGIC AGENTS

Drug Class
- Cholinergic Agents
- Agents:
  - Acute Care
    - Acetylcholine
    - Carbachol
    - Echothiophate iodide
    - Pilocarpine

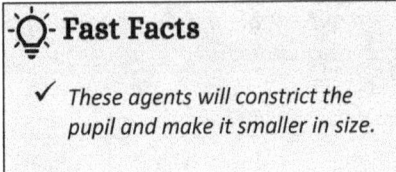

Fast Facts
- ✓ These agents will constrict the pupil and make it smaller in size.

Main Indications or Uses
- Acute Care
  - Accommodative esotropia (acetylcholine)
  - Elevated intraocular pressure (acetylcholine, carbachol, echothiophate iodide, pilocarpine)
  - Induce Miosis (acetylcholine, carbachol, pilocarpine)

Mechanism of Action
- Lower intraocular pressure (IOP) through ciliary muscle contraction, causing an opening of the trabecular meshwork and increasing aqueous humor trabecular outflow.

Primary Net Benefit
- Pilocarpine is the preferred cholinergic component of the combination treatment approach to primary open-angle glaucoma.
- Main Labs to Monitor:
  - Intraocular pressure

High-Yield Basic Pharmacology
- Pseudocholinesterase Vs Cholinesterase
  - Pseudocholinesterase is otherwise known as serum cholinesterase.
  - On the other hand, acetylcholinesterase is considered "true cholinesterase" and is located in erythrocytes, pulmonary tissue, spleen, and the CNS/PNS.

High-Yield Clinical Knowledge
- Cholinergic Ophthalmic Complications
  - Pilocarpine is associated with miosis and decreased vision in low light settings or among patients with central cataracts.
  - Other common adverse events associated with pilocarpine include headache, eyelid twitching, and conjunctival irritation.
- Systemic Cholinergic Effects
  - With continued use, cholinergic ophthalmic agents disrupt the blood-aqueous humor barrier and acutely worsen ophthalmic inflammatory conditions.
  - This can also lead to systemic cholinergic manifestations, including bradycardia, bronchospasm, bronchorrhea, diaphoresis, flushing, nausea/vomiting/diarrhea, urinary retention, and altered mental status.
  - As a result of a high likelihood of serious systemic cholinergic effects, the use of echothiophate is minimal.

- **Eyelid Closure**
  - After administering pilocarpine, patients may be instructed to close their eyes, which may improve clinical response and decrease pilocarpine administration frequency.
  - Eyelid closure has also been associated with reduced systemic adverse effects of echothiophate.
  - Patients should be instructed to gently close their eyes for 5 minutes following drug administration for optimal response.
  - The proposed mechanism is decreased nasolacrimal drainage and increased nasopharyngeal mucosal absorption of the drug.
- **Echothiophate and Cataracts**
  - The use of echothiophate is limited to selected patients with either aphakia or pseudophakia (without lenses or artificial lenses), as it is known to induce the formation of cataracts.
  - Echothiophate has also been associated with numerous adverse ophthalmic structural changes, including fibrinous iritis.
  - The hydrolysis of succinylcholine is slowed by echothiophate, which may significantly prolong paralysis and worsen the associated hyperkalemia.
- **Carbachol**
  - Carbachol is more resistant to cholinesterase hydrolysis than pilocarpine, providing a longer half-life.
  - While patients who do not adequately respond to pilocarpine can receive carbachol, it is associated with more systemic and ophthalmic adverse events.

High-Yield Core Evidence
- **Latanoprost Vs Pilocarpine/Timolol**
  - This prospective, cross-over trial randomized patients with primary open-angle glaucoma or ocular hypertension to receive either pilocarpine/timolol twice daily or latanoprost once daily in the evening with a placebo each morning.
  - According to the initial randomization, patients received eight weeks of treatment, then cross-over groups after eight weeks.
  - There was no statistical difference between treatments was observed at any individual time-point except at 10 hours, when the pilocarpine/timolol group demonstrated statistically, but not clinically, significantly decreased in IOP.
  - There were no statistical differences between groups in unsolicited systemic or ocular adverse events, but more patients receiving pilocarpine/timolol complained of mild blurred vision, stinging, and ocular pain.
  - The authors concluded that pilocarpine/timolol and latanoprost are efficacious in reducing diurnal IOP. (Acta Ophthalmol. 2008 Dec;86(8):860-5.)

High-Yield Fast-Fact
- **Pilocarpine Dose and Eye Color**
  - It has been observed that patients with darkly pigmented eyes require higher pilocarpine concentrations to elicit a reduction in IOP.

HIGH-YIELD BOARD EXAM ESSENTIALS
- **CLASSIC AGENTS:** Acetylcholine, carbachol, echothiophate iodide, pilocarpine
- **DRUG CLASS:** Cholinergic agents
- **INDICATIONS:** Accommodative esotropia, elevated intraocular pressure
- **MECHANISM:** Lower intraocular pressure (IOP) through ciliary muscle contraction, causing an opening of the trabecular meshwork and an increase in aqueous humor trabecular outflow.
- **SIDE EFFECTS:** Systemic cholinergic effects (lacrimation, urination, GI distress, altered mental status).
- **CLINICAL PEARLS:** Pilocarpine is associated with miosis and an associated decrease in vision in low light settings or among patients with central cataracts.

Table: Drug Class Summary

\multicolumn{4}{c}{**Cholinergic Agents - Drug Class Review**}
\multicolumn{4}{c}{High-Yield Med Reviews}
\multicolumn{4}{l}{**Mechanism of Action:** Lower intraocular pressure (IOP) through ciliary muscle contraction, causing an opening of the trabecular meshwork and increasing aqueous humor trabecular outflow.}
\multicolumn{4}{l}{**Class Effects:** Pilocarpine is the preferred cholinergic component of the combination treatment approach to primary open-angle glaucoma.}
Generic Name	Brand Name	Main Indication(s) or Uses	Notes
Acetylcholine	Michol-E	• Induce Miosis	• **Dosing (Adult):** — Intraocular: 0.5 to 2 mL to affected eye(s) • **Dosing (Peds):** — Intraocular: 0.5 to 2 mL to affected eye(s) • **CYP450 Interactions:** None • **Renal or Hepatic Dose Adjustments:** None • **Dosage Forms:** Ophthalmic solution
Carbachol	Miostat	• Elevated intraocular pressure • Induce Miosis	• **Dosing (Adult):** — Ophthalmic: 1 to 2 drops to affected eye(s) up to 3 times/day • **Dosing (Peds):** — Ophthalmic: 1 to 2 drops to affected eye(s) up to 3 times/day • **CYP450 Interactions:** None • **Renal or Hepatic Dose Adjustments:** None • **Dosage Forms:** Ophthalmic solution
Echothiophate iodide	Phospholine Iodide	• Accommodative esotropia • Elevated intraocular pressure	• **Dosing (Adult):** — Ophthalmic: 1 drop to affected eye(s) up to twice daily • **Dosing (Peds):** — Ophthalmic: 1 drop up to into both eyes at bedtime • **CYP450 Interactions:** None • **Renal or Hepatic Dose Adjustments:** None • **Dosage Forms:** Ophthalmic solution
Pilocarpine	Isopto Carpine	• Elevated intraocular pressure • Induce Miosis	• **Dosing (Adult):** — Ophthalmic: 1 drop to affected eye(s) up to 4 times/day • **Dosing (Peds):** — Ophthalmic: 1 drop to affected eye(s) up to 4 times/day • **CYP450 Interactions:** None • **Renal or Hepatic Dose Adjustments:** None • **Dosage Forms:** Ophthalmic solution

OPHTHALMOLOGY – OPHTHALMIC/NASAL – ANTIHISTAMINES

Drug Class
- Antihistamines (Nasal/Ophthalmic)
- Agents:
    - Acute & Chronic Care
        - Alcaftadine
        - Azelastine
        - Bepotastine
        - Cetirizine
        - Clemastine
        - Emedastine
        - Epinastine
        - Ketotifen
        - Olopatadine

Main Indications or Uses
- Chronic Care
    - Allergic conjunctivitis
    - Allergic rhinitis
    - Pruritus
    - Vasomotor rhinitis

> **Fast Facts**
> ✓ Numerous options available over-the-counter for patients to access.
>
> ✓ As with many eye drops, it is advised to remove any contact lens prior to administration and then wait 10 minutes before reinsertion.

Mechanism of Action
- Antihistamines (Alcaftadine, azelastine, bepotastine, cetirizine, clemastine, emedastine, epinastine, ketotifen, olopatadine)
    - Inverse agonists at H1 receptors compete with histamine for binding sites and stabilize the receptor's inactive state.
- Anticholinergic (Atropine, glycopyrrolate)
    - Competitive inhibitor of acetylcholine receptors

Primary Net Benefit
- Over-the-counter agents for managing common allergy-related complaints and acute care use of specific agents for numerous indications that are extensions of their central and peripheral antihistamine effect.
- Main Labs to Monitor:
    - No routine monitoring

High-Yield Basic Pharmacology
- Onset of Effect
    - Antihistamines are most effective when administered 1 to 2 hours before anticipated allergen exposure.
- Antihistamine
    - Commonly used antihistamines are inverse agonists of H1 receptors.
    - This distinction from H1 antagonists, which are competitive antagonists of histamine at the H1 receptor.

High-Yield Clinical Knowledge
- Contact Lens Insertion
    - Patients must be instructed to remove contact lenses before ophthalmic administration.
    - Patients should wait at least 10 minutes after administering ophthalmic antihistamines before inserting contact lenses.
- Multiple Ophthalmic Agent Administration
    - If the patient has more than one ophthalmic medication, they should be spaced at least five minutes.
- Oral Ingestion of Topical Products
    - Accidental ingestion may result in significant morbidity and mortality. Keep out of reach of children since there is no child protection cap after initial use.
- Symptomatic Management
    - These agents are ineffective at treating the underlying cause of ophthalmic redness, such as allergic conjunctivitis.

- Corticosteroids are more appropriate for addressing the underlying cause but are not always indicated as allergic conjunctivitis or rhinitis may be self-limiting.
- **Antihistamine Combinations**
    - Additive antihistamine effects and increased risk of adverse events can occur in patients taking over-the-counter topical antihistamines who may also be taking oral antihistamines.
- **Topical Dryness**
    - Azelastine topical nasal products have been associated with mucous membrane drying effects, headache, and decreased clinical response with long-term use.

High-Yield Core Evidence
- **Diphenhydramine Meta-Analysis**
    - This was a meta-analysis of diphenhydramine's sedating and performance-impairing effects relative to placebo and second-generation antihistamines.
    - The literature search included the MEDLINE database and included studies of patients with atopic disease and control subjects, were blinded and randomized clinical trials, objectively examined alertness and psychomotor performance, reported means and variances and were written in English.
    - The authors observed that of the analyzed literature, diphenhydramine impaired performance relative to placebo control and second-generation antihistamines, including acrivastine, astemizole, cetirizine, fexofenadine, loratadine, and terfenadine.
    - There was significant heterogeneity as the results were quite varied, the average sedating effect of diphenhydramine was modest.
    - In some instances, results of tests of performance in the diphenhydramine group showed less sedation than in the control or second-generation antihistamine groups.
    - Still, there was a statistically significant mild sedating effect caused by second-generation antihistamines in comparison with placebo.
    - The authors concluded that the absence of a consistent finding of diphenhydramine-induced sedation is surprising given that most studies have been designed to increase the probability of this outcome, including administering a 50-mg dose. (J Allergy Clin Immunol. 2003;111:770–776.)

High-Yield Fast-Fact
- **Atropine and Glycopyrrolate**
    - Although atropine and glycopyrrolate possess antihistamine effects, they are not used as OTC anticholinergics.

HIGH-YIELD BOARD EXAM ESSENTIALS
- **CLASSIC AGENTS:** Alcaftadine, azelastine, bepotastine, cetirizine, clemastine, emedastine, epinastine, ketotifen, olopatadine
- **DRUG CLASS:** Antihistamine
- **INDICATIONS:** Allergic conjunctivitis, allergic rhinitis, vasomotor rhinitis
- **MECHANISM:** Inverse agonists at H1 receptors that compete with histamine for binding sites and stabilizes the receptor's inactive state.
- **SIDE EFFECTS:** Dry mucous membranes, sedation
- **CLINICAL PEARLS:** Patients must be instructed to remove contact lenses before ophthalmic administration. Patients should wait at least 10 minutes after the administration of ophthalmic antihistamines before inserting contact lenses.

Table: Drug Class Summary

	Antihistamine (Nasal/Ophthalmic) - Drug Class Review High-Yield Med Reviews
	**Mechanism of Action:** Antihistamines - Inverse agonist at H1 receptors that compete with histamine for binding sites and stabilizes the receptor's inactive state. Anticholinergic - Competitive inhibitor of acetylcholine receptors
	**Class Effects:** Over-the-counter agents for managing common allergy-related complaints and acute care use of specific agents for numerous indications that are extensions of their central and peripheral antihistamine effect.
Generic Name	**Brand Name**	**Main Indication(s) or Uses**	**Notes**

Alcaftadine	Lastacaft	- Allergic conjunctivitis	- **Dosing (Adult):**
			  - Ophthalmic: 1 drop in each eye daily
			- **Dosing (Peds):**
			  - Ophthalmic: 1 drop in each eye daily
			- **CYP450 Interactions:** None
			- **Renal or Hepatic Dose Adjustments:** None
			- **Dosage Forms:** Ophthalmic solution

Atropine	Isopto Atropine	- Amblyopia
		- Mydriasis
			- **Dosing (Adult):**
			  - Ophthalmic: 1 drop in each eye 40 minutes prior to maximal dilation time
			  - Ophthalmic: apply a small amount in the conjunctival sac 1-2 times daily
			- **Dosing (Peds):**
			  - Ophthalmic: 1 drop in each eye 40 minutes prior to maximal dilation time
			- **CYP450 Interactions:** None
			- **Renal or Hepatic Dose Adjustments:** None
			- **Dosage Forms:** Ophthalmic (solution, ointment)

Azelastine	Astepro	- Allergic conjunctivitis
		- Allergic rhinitis
		- Vasomotor rhinitis
			- **Dosing (Adult):**
			  - Nasal: 1 to 2 sprays per nostril twice daily
			  - Ophthalmic: 1 drop in affected eye(s) twice daily
			- **Dosing (Peds):**
			  - Nasal: 1 to 2 sprays per nostril twice daily
			  - Ophthalmic: 1 drop in affected eye(s) twice daily
			- **CYP450 Interactions:** None
			- **Renal or Hepatic Dose Adjustments:** None
			- **Dosage Forms:** Ophthalmic solution, Nasal solution

Bepotastine	Bepreve	- Allergic conjunctivitis	- **Dosing (Adult):**
			  - Ophthalmic: 1 drop in affected eye(s) twice daily
			- **Dosing (Peds):**
			  - Ophthalmic: 1 drop in affected eye(s) twice daily
			- **CYP450 Interactions:** None
			- **Renal or Hepatic Dose Adjustments:** None
			- **Dosage Forms:** Ophthalmic solution

Antihistamine (Nasal/Ophthalmic) - Drug Class Review
High-Yield Med Reviews

Generic Name	Brand Name	Main Indication(s) or Uses	Notes

Cetirizine	Zyrtec, Zyrtec-D (with pseudoephedrine), Zerviate, Quzyttir	- Allergic rhinitis	- **Dosing (Adult):**
			  – Ophthalmic: 1 drop in affected eye(s) twice daily
			- **Dosing (Peds):**
			  – Ophthalmic: 1 drop in affected eye(s) twice daily
			- **CYP450 Interactions:** Substrate CYP3A4, P-gp
			- **Renal or Hepatic Dose Adjustments:**
			  – GFR 11 to 30 mL/minute: 5 mg daily
			  – GFR < 10 mL/minute: not recommended
			  – Child-Pugh class A, B or C: 5 mg daily
			- **Dosage Forms:** Oral (liquid, tablet), Ophthalmic solution, IV (solution)

Emedastine	Emadine	- Allergic conjunctivitis	- **Dosing (Adult):**
			  – Ophthalmic: 1 drop in affected eye(s) up to 4 times daily
			- **Dosing (Peds):**
			  – Ophthalmic: 1 drop in affected eye(s) up to 4 times daily
			- **CYP450 Interactions:** None
			- **Renal or Hepatic Dose Adjustments:** None
			- **Dosage Forms:** Ophthalmic solution

Epinastine	Elestat	- Allergic conjunctivitis	- **Dosing (Adult):**
			  – Ophthalmic: 1 drop in affected eye(s) twice daily
			- **Dosing (Peds):**
			  – Ophthalmic: 1 drop in affected eye(s) twice daily
			- **CYP450 Interactions:** None
			- **Renal or Hepatic Dose Adjustments:** None
			- **Dosage Forms:** Ophthalmic solution

Glycopyrrolate	Qbrexza	- Primary axillary hyperhidrosis	- **Dosing (Adult):**
			  – Topically apply to each underarm q24h
			- **Dosing (Peds):**
			  – Children over 9 years: Topically apply to each underarm q24h
			- **CYP450 Interactions:** None
			- **Renal or Hepatic Dose Adjustments:** None
			- **Dosage Forms:** Ophthalmic solution

Antihistamine (Nasal/Ophthalmic) - Drug Class Review High-Yield Med Reviews			
Generic Name	**Brand Name**	**Main Indication(s) or Uses**	**Notes**
Ketotifen	Zaditor	• Allergic conjunctivitis	• **Dosing (Adult):** – Ophthalmic: 1 drop in affected eye(s) twice daily • **Dosing (Peds):** – Ophthalmic: 1 drop in affected eye(s) twice daily • **CYP450 Interactions:** None • **Renal or Hepatic Dose Adjustments:** None • **Dosage Forms:** Ophthalmic solution
Olopatadine	Patanase, Pataday	• Allergic conjunctivitis • Allergic rhinitis	• **Dosing (Adult):** – Ophthalmic: 1 drop in affected eye(s) once to twice daily – Nasal: 2 sprays in each nostril BID • **Dosing (Peds):** – Ophthalmic: 1 drop in affected eye(s) once to twice daily – Nasal: 1 to 2 sprays in each nostril BID • **CYP450 Interactions:** None • **Renal or Hepatic Dose Adjustments:** None • **Dosage Forms:** Ophthalmic solution, Nasal solution

OPHTHALMOLOGY – GLUCOCORTICOIDS

Drug Class
- Glucocorticoids
- Agents:
  - **Acute & Chronic Care**
    - Dexamethasone
    - Difluprednate
    - Fluocinolone
    - Fluorometholone
    - Hydrocortisone
      - Hydrocortisone, Bacitracin, Neomycin, Polymyxin B
      - Hydrocortisone, Neomycin, Polymyxin B
    - Loteprednol
    - Prednisolone
    - Triamcinolone

> **Warnings & Alerts**
> ✓ Ophthalmic steroid use should never be used in patients with potential viral, fungal, or mycobacterial ocular infections as they can worsen the infection.

Main Indications or Uses
- **Acute & Chronic Care**
  - Inflammatory ocular conditions
    - Dexamethasone, fluorometholone, hydrocortisone, [hydrocortisone, bacitracin, neomycin, polymyxin b], [hydrocortisone, neomycin, polymyxin b], loteprednol, prednisolone, triamcinolone
  - Endogenous anterior uveitis
    - Difluprednate
  - Diabetic macular edema
    - Fluocinolone

Mechanism of Action
- Inhibit ophthalmic edema formation, capillary dilation, leukocyte migration, and scar formation.

Primary Net Benefit
- Ophthalmic glucocorticoids exert a wide range of effects from ocular allergies and external eye inflammation to anterior uveitis and intravitreal injections to treat diabetic retinopathy and cystoid macular edema.
- Main Labs to Monitor:
  - Intraocular pressure

High-Yield Basic Pharmacology
- **Implants/Injections**
  - Dexamethasone and fluocinolone are available as ophthalmic implants to treat noninfectious uveitis or macular edema.

High-Yield Clinical Knowledge
- **Cataracts**
  - The use of glucocorticoids is limited by developing posterior subcapsular cataracts that arise with long-term or high-dose therapy.
- **Secondary Open-Angle Glaucoma**
  - Ophthalmic glucocorticoids may also increase the risk of secondary open-angle glaucoma, high among patients with a positive family history of glaucoma.
  - Loteprednol carries the lowest risk of elevated IOP.
- **Eye Drop Administration**

- Nasolacrimal occlusion can reduce the systemic absorption of ophthalmic agents, including glucocorticoids.
- First, patients should be instructed to wash their hands, followed by gently pulling down the lower eyelid to form a pocket.
- Holding the drug bottle and bracing their hand with the side of their nose, the tip of the bottle should be placed close to the eye.
- With their head tilted back, place the prescribed number of drips in the eyelid pocket, then close their eye and immediately press their finger gently against the inside corner of the eye for 1 to 3 minutes.
- **Intraocular Pressure Measurement**
  - Tonometry is an intraocular pressure measurement and can be conducted with specialized devices known as tonometers.
  - Hand-held tonometers are often used in emergency departments, whereas larger tonometers are found elsewhere.

High-Yield Core Evidence
- **Optic Neuritis Treatment Trial**
  - This was a multicenter, prospective cohort study that randomized patients with acute optic neuritis to receive oral prednisone 1 mg/kg/day for 14 days, IV methylprednisolone 1 g /day for three days, followed by oral prednisone 1 mg/kg/day for 11 days, or oral placebo for 14 days.
  - Visual function assessed over a six-month follow-up period recovered significantly faster in the group receiving IV methylprednisolone than placebo.
  - Methylprednisolone was also associated with slightly better visual fields, contrast sensitivity, and color vision but not better visual acuity.
  - The outcome in the oral-prednisone group did not differ from that in the placebo group, but new episodes of optic neuritis in either eye were higher in the group receiving oral prednisone.
  - The authors concluded that intravenous methylprednisolone followed by oral prednisone speeds the recovery of visual loss due to optic neuritis and slightly better vision at six months. As prescribed in this study, oral prednisone alone is an ineffective treatment and increases the risk of new episodes of optic neuritis. (N Engl J Med. 1992 Feb 27;326(9):581-8.)

High-Yield Fast-Fact
- **Eye Drops in the Ear**
  - For some indications, ophthalmic products may be administered ophthalmically and tend to be both more widely available and less expensive than otic preparations of the same drug.
  - Otic products should never be administered ophthalmically.

HIGH-YIELD BOARD EXAM ESSENTIALS
- **CLASSIC AGENTS:** Dexamethasone, difluprednate, fluorometholone, hydrocortisone, loteprednol, prednisolone, triamcinolone
- **DRUG CLASS:** Glucocorticoids
- **INDICATIONS:** Inflammatory ocular conditions, endogenous anterior uveitis, diabetic macular edema
- **MECHANISM:** Inhibit ophthalmic edema formation, capillary dilation, leukocyte migration, and scar formation
- **SIDE EFFECTS:** Posterior subcapsular cataracts
- **CLINICAL PEARLS:** Ophthalmic glucocorticoids may also increase the risk of secondary open-angle glaucoma, with a high risk among patients with a positive family history of glaucoma. Ocular glucocorticoids should never be given to a patient with herpes keratitis unless an ophthalmologist is in involved and managing the patient.

Table: Drug Class Summary

Glucocorticoids - Drug Class Review			
High-Yield Med Reviews			
Mechanism of Action: *Inhibit ophthalmic edema formation, capillary dilation, leukocyte migration, and scar formation.*			
Class Effects: Ophthalmic glucocorticoids exert a wide range of effects from ocular allergies and external eye inflammation to anterior uveitis and intravitreal injections to treat diabetic retinopathy and cystoid macular edema.			
Generic Name	**Brand Name**	**Main Indication(s) or Uses**	**Notes**

Dexamethasone	Dextenza, Dexycu, Maxidex, Ozurdex	- Inflammatory ocular conditions	- **Dosing (Adult):**
			  - Ophthalmic: apply to inside of lower lid of affected eye(s) every 3 or 4 hours
			  - Ophthalmic: instill 1 to 2 drops to affected eye(s) q1hour during the day and every other hour at night
			  - Ophthalmic: instill 1 to 2 drops to affected eye(s) q4-6h
			- **Dosing (Peds):**
			  - Ophthalmic: instill 1 to 2 drops to affected eye(s) q1hour during the day and every other hour at night
			  - Ophthalmic: instill 1 to 2 drops to affected eye(s) q4-6h
			- **CYP450 Interactions:** None
			- **Renal or Hepatic Dose Adjustments:** None
			- **Dosage Forms:** Ophthalmic (ointment, solution, suspension)

Difluprednate	Durezol	- Endogenous anterior uveitis	- **Dosing (Adult):**
			  - Ophthalmic: instill 1 to 2 drops to affected eye(s) 4 times daily for 14 days, then taper
			- **Dosing (Peds):**
			  - Ophthalmic: instill 1 to 2 drops to affected eye(s) 4 times daily for 14 days, then taper
			- **CYP450 Interactions:** None
			- **Renal or Hepatic Dose Adjustments:** None
			- **Dosage Forms:** Ophthalmic emulsion

Fluocinolone	Iluvien, Retisert, Yutiq	- Diabetic macular edema	- **Dosing (Adult):**
			  - Intravitreal injected implant in affected eye for 30 to 36 months
			- **Dosing (Peds):**
			  - Children over 12 years, use adult dosing
			- **CYP450 Interactions:** None
			- **Renal or Hepatic Dose Adjustments:** None
			- **Dosage Forms:** Intravitreal implant

Glucocorticoids - Drug Class Review
High-Yield Med Reviews

Generic Name	Brand Name	Main Indication(s) or Uses	Notes

Fluorometholone	Flarex, FML, Forte	- Inflammatory ocular conditions	- **Dosing (Adult):**
			  - Ophthalmic: apply to inside of lower lid of affected eye(s) every 1 to 3 times daily
			  - Ophthalmic: instill 1 to 2 drops to affected eye(s) 2 to 4 times daily
			- **Dosing (Peds):**
			  - Ophthalmic: apply to inside of lower lid of affected eye(s) every 1 to 3 times daily
			  - Ophthalmic: instill 1 to 2 drops to affected eye(s) 2 to 4 times daily
			- **CYP450 Interactions:** None
			- **Renal or Hepatic Dose Adjustments:** None
			- **Dosage Forms:** Ophthalmic (ointment, suspension)

Hydrocortisone, Bacitracin, Neomycin, Polymyxin B	Neo-Polycin HC	- Inflammatory ocular conditions	- **Dosing (Adult):**
			  - Ophthalmic: apply to inside of lower lid of affected eye(s) every 3 or 4 hours
			- **Dosing (Peds):**
			  - Ophthalmic: apply to inside of lower lid of affected eye(s) every 3 or 4 hours
			- **CYP450 Interactions:** None
			- **Renal or Hepatic Dose Adjustments:** None
			- **Dosage Forms:** Ophthalmic ointment

Hydrocortisone, Neomycin, Polymyxin B	Brand Name (if available)	- Inflammatory ocular conditions	- **Dosing (Adult):**
			  - Ophthalmic: apply to inside of lower lid of affected eye(s) every 3 or 4 hours
			- **Dosing (Peds):**
			  - Ophthalmic: apply to inside of lower lid of affected eye(s) every 3 or 4 hours
			- **CYP450 Interactions:** None
			- **Renal or Hepatic Dose Adjustments:** None
			- **Dosage Forms:** Ophthalmic ointment

Loteprednol	Alrex, Eysuvis, Inveltys, Lotemax	- Inflammatory ocular conditions	- **Dosing (Adult):**
			  - Ophthalmic: instill 1 to 2 drops to affected eye(s) 4 times daily
			  - Ophthalmic: apply ½ inch ribbon to inside of lower lid of affected eye(s) 4 times daily
			- **Dosing (Peds):**
			  - Ophthalmic: instill 1 to 2 drops to affected eye(s) 4 times daily
			- **CYP450 Interactions:** None
			- **Renal or Hepatic Dose Adjustments:** None
			- **Dosage Forms:** Ophthalmic (gel, ointment, suspension)

Glucocorticoids - Drug Class Review
High-Yield Med Reviews

Generic Name	Brand Name	Main Indication(s) or Uses	Notes

Prednisolone	Omnipred, Pred Forte, Pred Mild	• Inflammatory ocular conditions	• **Dosing (Adult):**
			  − Ophthalmic: instill 1 to 2 drops to affected eye(s) 2 to 4 times daily
			• **Dosing (Peds):**
			  − Ophthalmic: instill 1 to 2 drops to affected eye(s) 2 to 4 times daily
			• **CYP450 Interactions:** None
			• **Renal or Hepatic Dose Adjustments:** None
			• **Dosage Forms:** Ophthalmic ointment

Triamcinolone	Triesence	• Inflammatory ocular conditions	• **Dosing (Adult):**
			  − Intravitreal: 1 to 4 mg once
			• **Dosing (Peds):**
			  − Intravitreal: 1 to 4 mg once
			• **CYP450 Interactions:** None
			• **Renal or Hepatic Dose Adjustments:** None
			• **Dosage Forms:** Ophthalmic suspension

OPHTHALMOLOGY – IMIDAZOLINE (NASAL/OPHTHALMIC)

Drug Class
- Imidazoline (Nasal/Ophthalmic)
- Agents:
    - **Acute & Chronic Care**
        - Naphazoline
        - Oxymetazoline
        - Tetrahydrozoline

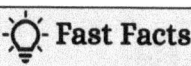 **Fast Facts**
- Naphazoline is a common agent available over-the-counter as Naphcon-A or Visine for ophthalmic use.

Main Indications or Uses
- **Chronic Care**
    - Allergic conjunctivitis
    - Allergic rhinitis
    - Pruritus
    - Vasomotor rhinitis

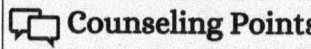 **Counseling Points**
- Counsel patients to remove their contact lens, insert the medication and then wait for 10 minutes to put reinsert.

Mechanism of Action
- Alpha-1 agonist in the conjunctiva and nasal mucosa, producing vasoconstriction.

Primary Net Benefit
- Over-the-counter agents for managing common allergy-related complaints and acute care use of specific agents for numerous indications that are extensions of their central and peripheral antihistamine effect.
- Main Labs to Monitor:
    - No routine monitoring

High-Yield Basic Pharmacology
- **Drug Interactions**
    - Imidazolines should not be used concomitantly with MAO inhibitors or ergot alkaloids as the combination increases the risk of serotonin syndrome.
- **Oral Bioavailability**
    - Orally ingested topical imidazoline may be adequately absorbed to cause signs and symptoms of systemic toxicity.
    - Imidazoline overdose is potentially fatal and characterized by acute hypertension followed by hypotension, bradycardia, altered mental status, and seizures.

High-Yield Clinical Knowledge
- **Narrow-Angle Glaucoma**
    - Do not use In patients with narrow-angle glaucoma. Use with caution in patients with cardiovascular disease, diabetes, hyperthyroidism, or infection.
    - Contains benzalkonium chloride, which may cause corneal damage and be absorbed by soft contact lenses.
- **Contact Lens Insertion**
    - Patients must be instructed to remove contact lenses before ophthalmic administration.
    - Patients should wait at least 10 minutes after administering ophthalmic antihistamines before inserting contact lenses.
- **Masking of Corneal Injury**
    - Naphazoline contains benzalkonium chloride, which may cause corneal damage and be absorbed by soft contact lenses.
- **Multiple Ophthalmic Agent Administration**
    - If the patient has more than one ophthalmic medication, they should be spaced at least five minutes.
- **Symptomatic Management**

- These agents are ineffective at treating the underlying cause of ophthalmic redness, such as allergic conjunctivitis.
- Corticosteroids are more appropriate for addressing the underlying cause but are not always indicated as allergic conjunctivitis or rhinitis may be self-limiting.
- **No More Than Three Days**
  - Imidazolines should not use for more than three days due to rebound congestion.
  - Use with caution in patients with cardiovascular disease, diabetes, hyperthyroidism, or infection.
- **Common Adverse Events**
  - Common adverse events of ophthalmic imidazolines include blurred vision, lacrimation, irritation, and hypersensitivity.

High-Yield Core Evidence
- **Naloxone Reversal of Tetrahydrozoline**
  - This was a case report describing a 36-month-old male who ingested 30 mL of an ophthalmic tetrahydrozoline 0.05% product and was brought to an emergency department 1.5 hours after the ingestion.
  - The patient was lethargic on arrival, but within 30 minutes, the patient became increasingly lethargic with decreased muscle tone and did not respond to voice commands.
  - Naloxone 0.1 mg/kg was administered, and within 30 sections, the child awoke and maintained an upright posture, but this effect was short-lived as blood pressure declined and the patient became somnolent.
  - They were admitted to the PICU and successfully discharged home without further complications.
  - (Pediatr Int. 2010;52:488–489.)

High-Yield Fast-Fact
- **Cannabinoid Interaction**
  - Cannabinoids may increase the toxicity of oxymetazoline.

HIGH-YIELD BOARD EXAM ESSENTIALS
- **CLASSIC AGENTS:** Naphazoline, oxymetazoline, tetrahydrozoline
- **DRUG CLASS:** Imidazoline
- **INDICATIONS:** Allergic conjunctivitis, allergic rhinitis
- **MECHANISM:** Alpha-1 agonist in the conjunctiva and nasal mucosa producing vasoconstriction.
- **SIDE EFFECTS:** Blurred vision, lacrimation, irritation, hypersensitivity
- **CLINICAL PEARLS:**
  - Do not use in patients with narrow-angle glaucoma.
  - Use with caution in patients with cardiovascular disease, diabetes, hyperthyroidism, or infection.

Table: Drug Class Summary

Imidazoline (Nasal/Ophthalmic) - Drug Class Review High-Yield Med Reviews			
Mechanism of Action: *Alpha-1 agonist in the conjunctiva and nasal mucosa producing vasoconstriction.*			
Class Effects: *Over-the-counter agents for managing common allergy-related complaints and acute care use of specific agents for numerous indications that are extensions of their central and peripheral antihistamine effect.*			
Generic Name	**Brand Name**	**Main Indication(s) or Uses**	**Notes**
Naphazoline	<u>With pheniramine</u> Naphcon-A, Opcon-A, Visine, Visine-A	• Allergic conjunctivitis	• **Dosing (Adult):** — Ophthalmic: 1 drop in affected eye(s) up to 4 times daily • **Dosing (Peds):** — Ophthalmic: 1 drop in affected eye(s) up to 4 times daily • **CYP450 Interactions:** None • **Renal or Hepatic Dose Adjustments:** None • **Dosage Forms:** Ophthalmic solution
Oxymetazoline	Afrin, Dristan Spray, Mucinex Nasal Spray, Neo-synephrine 12 hour spray, Vicks Sinex	• Allergic conjunctivitis • Allergic rhinitis	• **Dosing (Adult):** — Intranasal: 2 to 3 sprays into each nostril twice daily — Maximum 3 days of therapy and no more than 2 doses per 24 hours • **Dosing (Peds):** — Intranasal: 2 to 3 sprays into each nostril twice daily — Maximum 3 days of therapy and no more than 2 doses per 24 hours • **CYP450 Interactions:** None • **Renal or Hepatic Dose Adjustments:** None • **Dosage Forms:** Nasal solution
Tetrahydrozoline	Visine, Opticlear, Tyzine	• Allergic conjunctivitis • Allergic rhinitis	• **Dosing (Adult):** — Intranasal: 2 to 3 sprays into each nostril q3-4h as needed — Ophthalmic: 1 drop in affected eye(s) up to 4 times daily • **Dosing (Peds):** — Intranasal: 2 to 3 drops of 0.05% each nostril q3h as needed • **CYP450 Interactions:** None • **Renal or Hepatic Dose Adjustments:** None • **Dosage Forms:** Nasal solution, Ophthalmic solution

OPHTHALMOLOGY – MAST CELL STABILIZERS

Drug Class
- Mast Cell Stabilizer
- Agents:
  - Acute Care
    - Cromolyn
    - Lodoxamide
    - Nedocromil
    - Pemirolast

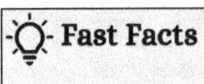

Fast Facts
- ✓ While available for use, their clinical effectiveness is limited compared to other options.

Main Indications or Uses
- Acute Care
  - Allergic conjunctivitis

Mechanism of Action
- Inhibit mast cell degranulation, preventing the release of histamine and inflammatory leukotrienes.

Primary Net Benefit
- More effective alternatives have primarily replaced ophthalmic mast cell stabilizers but may play a role in allergic conjunctivitis.
- Main Labs to Monitor:
  - No routine monitoring

High-Yield Basic Pharmacology

- Onset of Effect
  - For mast cell stabilizers to exert their maximal effect, they should be initiated one week before anticipated allergen exposure.

High-Yield Clinical Knowledge
- Symptomatic Management
  - These agents are ineffective at treating the underlying cause of ophthalmic redness, such as allergic conjunctivitis.
  - Corticosteroids are more appropriate for addressing the underlying cause but are not always indicated as allergic conjunctivitis or rhinitis may be self-limiting.
- Contact Lens Insertion
  - Patients must be instructed to remove contact lenses before ophthalmic administration.
  - Patients should wait at least 10 minutes after administering ophthalmic antihistamines before inserting contact lenses.
- Multiple Ophthalmic Agent Administration
  - If the patient has more than one ophthalmic medication, they should be spaced at least five minutes.

High-Yield Core Evidence
- Nedocromil Inferior to Ketotifen
  - This was a single-center, double-masked, contralateral, placebo, and active-controlled trial that randomized patients over the age of 10 with a history of allergic hypersensitivity responding to conjunctival allergen challenge to receive either ketotifen, nedocromil, or placebo.
  - Allergen challenges were conducted at 5 minutes post-treatment dose and 12 hours post-treatment dose.
  - Ketotifen-treated eyes experienced significantly less ocular itching than nedocromil-treated eyes and those that received placebo at both the 5-minute and 12-hour post-treatment allergen challenges.
  - Nedocromil-treated eyes showed no statistical or clinical differences from placebo at any time point.

- Although ketotifen-treated eyes showed no differences in comfort from those that received placebo, they were significantly more comfortable than nedocromil-treated eyes at 1, 2, 5, and 10 minutes after installation.
- The authors concluded that ketotifen was significantly more effective and comfortable than nedocromil at both 5 minutes and 12 hours after administration in this conjunctival allergen challenge model. (Clin Ther. 2003 Jul;25(7):1988-2005.)

High-Yield Fast-Fact
- **Alternative Properties**
    - Nedocromil is proposed to possess weak antihistamine properties.

HIGH-YIELD BOARD EXAM ESSENTIALS
- **CLASSIC AGENTS:** Cromolyn, lodoxamide, nedocromil, pemirolast
- **DRUG CLASS:** Mast cell stabilizer
- **INDICATIONS:** Allergic conjunctivitis
- **MECHANISM:** Inhibit mast cell degranulation, preventing the release of histamine and inflammatory leukotrienes.
- **SIDE EFFECTS:** Burning sensation, eye discomfort, blurry vision
- **CLINICAL PEARLS:** These agents are not effective at treating the underlying cause of ophthalmic redness, such as allergic conjunctivitis.

Table: Drug Class Summary

Mast Cell Stabilizer - Drug Class Review High-Yield Med Reviews			
Mechanism of Action: *Inhibit mast cell degranulation, preventing the release of histamine and inflammatory leukotrienes.*			
Class Effects: *More effective alternatives have primarily replaced ophthalmic mast cell stabilizers but may play a role in allergic conjunctivitis.*			
Generic Name	**Brand Name**	**Main Indication(s) or Uses**	**Notes**
Cromolyn	Intal	• Allergic conjunctivitis	• **Dosing (Adult):** — Ophthalmic: 1 to 2 drops in affected eye(s) 4 to 6 times daily • **Dosing (Peds):** — Ophthalmic: 1 to 2 drops in affected eye(s) 4 to 6 times daily • **CYP450 Interactions:** None • **Renal or Hepatic Dose Adjustments:** None • **Dosage Forms:** Ophthalmic solution
Lodoxamide	Alomide	• Allergic conjunctivitis	• **Dosing (Adult):** — Ophthalmic: 1 to 2 drops in affected eye(s) 4 times daily • **Dosing (Peds):** — Ophthalmic: 1 to 2 drops in affected eye(s) 4 times daily • **CYP450 Interactions:** None • **Renal or Hepatic Dose Adjustments:** None • **Dosage Forms:** Ophthalmic solution
Nedocromil	Alocril	• Allergic conjunctivitis	• **Dosing (Adult):** — Ophthalmic: 1 to 2 drops in affected eye(s) twice daily • **Dosing (Peds):** — Ophthalmic: 1 to 2 drops in affected eye(s) twice daily • **CYP450 Interactions:** None • **Renal or Hepatic Dose Adjustments:** None • **Dosage Forms:** Ophthalmic solution
Pemirolast	Alamast	• Allergic conjunctivitis	• **Dosing (Adult):** — Ophthalmic: 1 to 2 drops in affected eye(s) 4 times daily • **Dosing (Peds):** — Ophthalmic: 1 to 2 drops in affected eye(s) 4 times daily • **CYP450 Interactions:** None • **Renal or Hepatic Dose Adjustments:** None • **Dosage Forms:** Ophthalmic solution

OPHTHALMOLOGY – NON-STEROIDAL ANTIINFLAMMATORY DRUGS (NSAIDS)

Drug Class
- NSAIDs
- Agents:
    - Acute Care
        - Bromfenac
        - Diclofenac
        - Flurbiprofen
        - Ketorolac
        - Nepafenac

> **Warnings & Alerts**
> ✓ Use with caution or limit duration due to the risk that topical administration of ophthalmic NSAIDs, particularly in the elderly, has been associated with an increased risk of sterile corneal melts and perforations.

Main Indications or Uses
- Acute Care
    - Postoperative ocular inflammation or pain (bromfenac, diclofenac, flurbiprofen, ketorolac, nepafenac)
    - Seasonal allergic conjunctivitis (ketorolac)

Mechanism of Action
- Inhibit the conversion of arachidonic acid to prostaglandins by inhibiting COX-1 and/or COX-2 reversibly (NSAIDs).

Primary Net Benefit
- Provide local anti-inflammatory and analgesic effects and may be a therapy component after ophthalmic surgery.
- Main Labs to Monitor:
    - No routine monitoring

High-Yield Basic Pharmacology
- **Analgesic Properties**
    - Upon tissue injury and the accompanying inflammation contributing pain is caused by the release of prostaglandins by cytokines such as bradykinin.
    - Local or systemic inhibition of COX and prostaglandins by salicylates contribute to analgesia, which may be combined with other pain management strategies.

High-Yield Clinical Knowledge
- **Ocular Surface Disease**
    - The use of either topical and systemic NSAIDs, particularly in the elderly, has been associated with an increased risk of sterile corneal melts and perforations.
- **Surgical Adjunct**
    - Ophthalmic ketorolac is available in combination with phenylephrine to prevent miosis and reduce postoperative pain in patients undergoing cataract or intraocular lens replacement surgery.
- **Prostaglandin Products**
    - NSAID inhibition of cyclooxygenase decreases the production of prostaglandins, thromboxane, and prostacyclin.
        - Prostaglandin H2 typically produces prostacyclin, Prostaglandin D, E, and F, and thromboxanes.
    - Thromboxanes stimulate platelet aggregation and decrease renal blood flow.
        - Thus, inhibition of thromboxane (typically TXA2) by NSAIDs decreases platelet aggregation and may augment renal blood flow.
    - Prostaglandin inhibition may also produce vasoconstriction and bronchoconstriction.
- **Central Vs. Peripheral Prostaglandin Inhibition**
    - The anti-inflammatory properties of NSAIDs are attributed to their inhibition of peripherally located prostaglandins.
    - The analgesic properties of NSAIDs result from the inhibition of prostaglandins located in the CNS.

High-Yield Core Evidence
- **Nepafenac For Ocular Inflammation**
    - This was a multicenter, double-blind, vehicle-controlled trial that randomized patients undergoing cataract surgery with posterior chamber intraocular lens implantation to receive either nepafenac 0.1% or vehicle beginning one day before surgery and continuing on the day of surgery (day 0) for 14 days.
    - The proportion of patients randomized to nepafenac who achieved cure at day 14 (cure defined as aqueous cells score + aqueous flare score = 0) was significantly higher than patients randomized to vehicle control.
    - Furthermore, a higher percentage of patients in the nepafenac group were pain-free at all visits and had lower mean aqueous cells, flare, and cells plus flare scores at all visits.
    - There were no treatment-related ocular adverse events that occurred in either group.
    - The authors concluded that nepafenac ophthalmic suspension 0.1% was safe and effective for preventing and treating ocular inflammation and pain associated with cataract surgery. (J Cataract Refract Surg. 2007 Jan;33(1):53-8.)

High-Yield Fast-Fact
- **Adverse Events**
    - In addition to GI, renal, and cardiovascular adverse events, NSAIDs may also cause hematologic adverse events (thrombocytopenia, neutropenia, aplastic anemia), hepatic dysfunction, drug-induced asthma, and drug-induced rashes.

HIGH-YIELD BOARD EXAM ESSENTIALS
- **CLASSIC AGENTS:** Bromfenac, diclofenac, flurbiprofen, ketorolac, nepafenac
- **DRUG CLASS:** NSAIDs
- **INDICATIONS:** Postoperative ocular inflammation or pain (bromfenac, diclofenac, flurbiprofen, ketorolac, nepafenac), seasonal allergic conjunctivitis (ketorolac)
- **MECHANISM:** Inhibit the conversion of arachidonic acid to prostaglandins by inhibition of COX-1 and/or COX-2 either reversibly (NSAIDs)
- **SIDE EFFECTS:** Increased risk of sterile corneal melts and perforations
- **CLINICAL PEARLS:** The anti-inflammatory properties of NSAIDs are attributed to their inhibition of peripherally located prostaglandins. The analgesic properties of NSAIDs are a result of inhibition of prostaglandins located in the CNS.

Table: Drug Class Summary

\multicolumn{4}{c}{**Mast Cell Stabilizer - Drug Class Review**}
\multicolumn{4}{c}{High-Yield Med Reviews}
\multicolumn{4}{l}{**Mechanism of Action:** *Inhibit the conversion of arachidonic acid to prostaglandins by inhibition of COX-1 and/or COX-2 either reversibly (NSAIDs)*}
\multicolumn{4}{l}{**Class Effects:** *Provide local anti-inflammatory and analgesic effects and may be a therapy component after eye surgery.*}
Generic Name	**Brand Name**	**Main Indication(s) or Uses**	**Notes**

Bromfenac	BromSite, Prolensa	• Postoperative ocular inflammation or pain	• **Dosing (Adult):**
			  − Ophthalmic: 1 to 2 drops in affected eye(s) once to twice daily
			• **Dosing (Peds):**
			  − Not routinely used
			• **CYP450 Interactions:** None
			• **Renal or Hepatic Dose Adjustments:** None
			• **Dosage Forms:** Ophthalmic solution

Diclofenac	Voltarol Ophtha	• Postoperative ocular inflammation or pain • Ocular pain	• **Dosing (Adult):** − Ophthalmic: 1 to 2 drops in affected eye(s) 4 times daily • **Dosing (Peds):** Not routinely used • **CYP450 Interactions:** None • **Renal or Hepatic Dose Adjustments:** None • **Dosage Forms:** Ophthalmic solution
Flurbiprofen	Ocufen	• Intraoperative miosis	• **Dosing (Adult):** − Ophthalmic: 1 drop in affected eye(s) q30minutes beginning 2 hours prior to surgery • **Dosing (Peds):** Not routinely used • **CYP450 Interactions:** None • **Renal or Hepatic Dose Adjustments:** None • **Dosage Forms:** Ophthalmic solution

Ketorolac	Acular, Acuvail	• Postoperative ocular inflammation or pain
		• Seasonal allergic conjunctivitis
			• **Dosing (Adult):**
			  − Ophthalmic: 1 drop in affected eye(s) four times daily
			• **Dosing (Peds):**
			  Ophthalmic: 1 drop in affected eye(s) four times daily
			• **CYP450 Interactions:** None
			• **Renal or Hepatic Dose Adjustments:** None
			• **Dosage Forms:** Ophthalmic solution

Nepafenac	Ilevro, Nevanac	• Postoperative ocular inflammation or pain	• **Dosing (Adult):**
			  − Ophthalmic: 1 drop in affected eye(s) three times daily
			• **Dosing (Peds):**
			  − Ophthalmic: 1 drop in affected eye(s) three times daily
			• **CYP450 Interactions:** None
			• **Renal or Hepatic Dose Adjustments:** None
			• **Dosage Forms:** Ophthalmic solution

OPHTHALMOLOGY – PROSTAGLANDIN ANALOGS

Drug Class
- Prostaglandin Analogs
- Agents:
  - Acute and Chronic Care
    - Bimatoprost
    - Latanoprost
    - Latanoprostene
    - Tafluprost
    - Travoprost

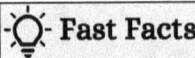

Fast Facts
- ✓ Chronic use of prostaglandin analogs can cause changes in iris pigmentation in patients with mixed-color irises and also cause prolongation of the eyelashes.

Main Indications or Uses
- Acute and Chronic Care
  - Elevated intraocular pressure (bimatoprost, latanoprost, latanoprostene, tafluprost, travoprost)
  - Hypotrichosis of the eyelashes (bimatoprost)

Mechanism of Action
- Synthetic analogs of prostaglandin F2-alpha (PGF2a) are hydrolyzed to PGF2a, which modifies ciliary muscle tension, and improves aqueous humor outflow tracts.

Primary Net Benefit
- First-line intraocular pressure (IOP) lowering agents that can often be administered once daily with sustained IOP control for up to 24-hours.
- Main Labs to Monitor:
  - Intraocular pressure (baseline, at 4-6 weeks, then every 3-4 months)
  - Ophthalmic exam

High-Yield Basic Pharmacology
- Latanoprostene
  - The prodrug of latanoprost, latanoprostene, is activated through a nitric oxide donating process, which adds to its antiglaucoma effects by further increasing aqueous humor outflow.
- Benzalkonium Chloride
  - The common preservative in many ophthalmic preparations, benzalkonium chloride, has been associated with worsening dry eyes and should be avoided, if possible.

High-Yield Clinical Knowledge
- Diurnal Effect
  - The diurnal IOP lowering effect of prostaglandin analogs allows for consistent control of IOP throughout the day, including at night when IOP is the highest during sleep.
- Iris Pigmentation
  - With long-term administration of prostaglandin analogs, iris pigmentation is likely to occur in patients with mixed-color irises.
  - The transition of eye color to brown occurs gradually over 3 to 12 months of continued use and is irreversible upon discontinuation.
  - Hyperpigmentation may also occur around the lids and lashes but is reversible with drug discontinuation.
- Hypertrichosis
  - With continued use, most prostaglandin analogs may cause hypertrichosis or lengthening of eyelashes.
  - Bimatoprost specifically carries this indication for cosmetic purposes.
- Ophthalmic Drop Administration
  - Before administering any ophthalmic product, patients should be reminded to wash their hands and remove any contact lenses.
  - Most administrations should begin with 1 drop of solution in the affected eye.

- No more than 1 drop should be administered at a time, and multiple drops should be separated by at least 1 minute since the aqueous chamber cannot hold the given volume.
- If drops and ointments are to be given, the drop should be administered first, followed by the ointment.
- **Adverse Events**
  - Rare but serious adverse events associated with prostaglandin analogs include punctate corneal erosion and conjunctival hyperemia.
- **Combination Therapy**
  - If an inadequate IOP response to an initial agent occurs, the combination with another class often leads to a less than additive further IOP reduction.
  - Furthermore, increasing the dose (i.e., number of drops) per agent rarely improves IOP lowering effect.
  - Conversion to a new IOP lowering agent is often necessary if an inadequate response occurs.
- **Acute Angle-Closure Crisis**
  - Acute angle-closure crisis is a medical emergency that requires administering one or more topical ophthalmic agents and may include systemic interventions.
  - Pilocarpine is often added to induce miosis to pull the peripheral iris away from its meshwork but may worsen angle closure and should not be used alone.
  - Oral glycerin or IV mannitol can be used with prostaglandin analogs, beta-antagonists, alpha-agonists, or carbonic anhydrase inhibitors.

High-Yield Core Evidence
- **Travoprost Study Group**
  - This was a multicenter, prospective, double-blinded trial that randomized patients with open-angle glaucoma or ocular hypertension to receive travoprost (0.0015% or 0.004%) daily, latanoprost 0.005% daily, or timolol 0.5% twice daily for 12 months.
  - Travoprost significantly improved mean IOP compared to latanoprost or timolol.
  - In a subgroup analysis of black patients, travoprost 0.004% was more effective than latanoprost and timolol in reducing IOP.
  - Travoprost was also more likely to achieve a 30% or greater IOP reduction from diurnal baseline or IOP of 17 mm Hg or less.
  - Iris pigmentation change was observed more often in patients receiving latanoprost.
  - No serious, unexpected, related adverse events were reported for any therapy.
  - The authors concluded that travoprost (0.0015% and 0.004%) is equal or superior to latanoprost and superior to timolol in lowering IOP in patients with open-angle glaucoma or ocular hypertension. (Am J Ophthalmol. 2001 Oct;132(4):472-84.)
- **Scandinavian Latanoprost Study Group**
  - This was a multicenter, double-blinded, parallel-group study that randomized patients with elevations in IOP to receive either latanoprost 0.005% once daily or timolol 0.5% twice daily for six months.
  - Patients randomized latanoprost were divided equally to a group that administered the drug in the morning for three months and then in the evening for another three months, or to latanoprost with the treatment schedule reversed.
  - The efficacy of latanoprost applied in the evening was statistically superior to latanoprost used in the morning and to timolol.
  - Latanoprost was associated with an increased incidence of conjunctival hyperemia vs. timolol.
  - Furthermore, latanoprost was associated with a significantly higher incidence of sporadic episodes of mild punctate corneal epithelial erosions.
  - Increased pigmentation of the iris was also observed in latanoprost-treated eyes.
  - The authors concluded that the effect on diurnal IOP of latanoprost applied once daily in the evening is superior to that of timolol. (Ophthalmology. 1995. 102(12):1743-1752.)

High-Yield Fast-Fact
- **Unoprostone**
  - The prostaglandin analog unoprostone was discontinued in the United States but may still be available in Canada.

Table: Drug Class Summary

\multicolumn{4}{c}{**Prostaglandin Analogs - Drug Class Review**}
\multicolumn{4}{c}{High-Yield Med Reviews}
Mechanism of Action: *Synthetic analogs of prostaglandin F2-alpha (PGF2a) are hydrolyzed to PGF2a, which modifies ciliary muscle tension, and improves aqueous humor outflow tracts.*				
Class Effects: *First-line intraocular pressure (IOP) lowering agents that can often be administered once daily with sustained IOP control for up to 24-hours.*				
Generic Name	**Brand Name**	**Main Indication(s) or Uses**	**Notes**
Bimatoprost	Latisse, Lumigan	<ul><li>Elevated intraocular pressure</li><li>Hypotrichosis of the eyelashes</li></ul>	<ul><li>**Dosing (Adult):** − Ophthalmic: 1 drop in affected eye(s) once daily − Ophthalmic: place one drop on the applicator and apply evenly along the skin of upper eyelid at the base of eyelashes at bedtime</li><li>**Dosing (Peds):** − Ophthalmic: 1 drop in affected eye(s) four times daily</li><li>**CYP450 Interactions:** None</li><li>**Renal or Hepatic Dose Adjustments:** None</li><li>**Dosage Forms:** Ophthalmic solution</li></ul>
Latanoprost	Xalatan, Xelpros	<ul><li>Elevated intraocular pressure</li></ul>	<ul><li>**Dosing (Adult):** − Ophthalmic: 1 drop in affected eye(s) once daily</li><li>**Dosing (Peds):** − Ophthalmic: 1 drop in affected eye(s) four times daily</li><li>**CYP450 Interactions:** None</li><li>**Renal or Hepatic Dose Adjustments:** None</li><li>**Dosage Forms:** Ophthalmic (emulsion, solution)</li></ul>
Latanoprostene	Vyzylta	<ul><li>Elevated intraocular pressure</li></ul>	<ul><li>**Dosing (Adult):** − Ophthalmic: 1 drop in affected eye(s) once daily</li><li>**Dosing (Peds):** − Ophthalmic: 1 drop in affected eye(s) four times daily</li><li>**CYP450 Interactions:** None</li><li>**Renal or Hepatic Dose Adjustments:** None</li><li>**Dosage Forms:** Ophthalmic solution</li></ul>
Tafluprost	Zioptan	<ul><li>Elevated intraocular pressure</li></ul>	<ul><li>**Dosing (Adult):** − Ophthalmic: 1 drop in affected eye(s) once daily</li><li>**Dosing (Peds):** − Not routinely used</li><li>**CYP450 Interactions:** None</li><li>**Renal or Hepatic Dose Adjustments:** None</li><li>**Dosage Forms:** Ophthalmic solution</li></ul>

Prostaglandin Analogs - Drug Class Review
High-Yield Med Reviews

Generic Name	Brand Name	Main Indication(s) or Uses	Notes

Travoprost	Travatan Z	- Elevated intraocular pressure	- **Dosing (Adult):**
			   – Ophthalmic: 1 drop in affected eye(s) once daily
			- **Dosing (Peds):**
			   – Ophthalmic: 1 drop in affected eye(s) four times daily
			- **CYP450 Interactions:** None
			- **Renal or Hepatic Dose Adjustments:** None
			- **Dosage Forms:** Ophthalmic solution

Unoprostone	Rescula	- Elevated intraocular pressure	- **Dosing (Adult):**
			   – Ophthalmic: 1 drop in affected eye(s) twice daily
			- **Dosing (Peds):**
			   – Not routinely used
			- **CYP450 Interactions:** None
			- **Renal or Hepatic Dose Adjustments:** None
			- **Dosage Forms:** Ophthalmic solution

HIGH-YIELD BOARD EXAM ESSENTIALS
- **CLASSIC AGENTS:** Bimatoprost, latanoprost, latanoprostene, tafluprost, travoprost
- **DRUG CLASS:** Prostaglandin analog
- **INDICATIONS:** Elevated intraocular pressure, hypotrichosis of the eyelashes
- **MECHANISM:** Synthetic analogs of PGF2a are hydrolyzed to PGF2a, which modifies ciliary muscle tension, and improves aqueous humor outflow tracts.
- **SIDE EFFECTS:** Punctate corneal erosion and conjunctival hyperemia
- **CLINICAL PEARLS:** If an inadequate IOP response to an initial agent occurs, the combination with another class often leads to a less than additive further IOP reduction. Furthermore, increasing the dose (i.e., number of drops) per agent rarely leads to a further improvement in IOP lowering effect.

2025

A COMPREHENSIVE *RAPID REVIEW*

NAPLEX

Pharmacology & Drug Classes

Otic Agents

OTIC – ANTI-INFLAMMATORIES AND CERUMENOLYTICS

Drug Class
- Anti-inflammatories and Cerumenolytics
- Agents:
    - Acute Care
        - Carbamide peroxide
        - Dexamethasone
        - Fluocinolone
        - Hydrocortisone

> **Fast Facts**
> ✓ If using carbamide peroxide to clean out ear wax, make sure to advise the patient to avoid using Q-tips to aid in the removal as this can cause compaction of the ear wax and make it harder to remove.

Main Indications or Uses
- Acute Care
    - Ear wax removal (carbamide peroxide)
    - Acute otitis externa (dexamethasone, hydrocortisone)
    - Chronic eczematous external otitis (fluocinolone)

Mechanism of Action
- Carbamide peroxide
    - Softens cerumen by its foaming action from the release of hydrogen peroxide.
- Dexamethasone, Fluocinolone, Hydrocortisone
    - Suppress polymorphonuclear leukocyte migration, and decrease capillary permeability, thereby reducing inflammation.

Primary Net Benefit
- Otic steroids provide a local anti-inflammatory effect to relieve pain from otitis externa, and carbamide may be used as a ceruminolytic but has questionable efficacy.
- Main Labs to Monitor:
    - No routine monitoring

High-Yield Basic Pharmacology
- Inflammation
    - Glucocorticoids effectively counteract inflammation by preventing extravasation and infiltration of leukocytes into the affected tissue.
    - Inflammation is also inhibited through phospholipase A2 inhibition, reducing the synthesis of arachidonic acid and reducing the release of cyclooxygenase 2 and inducible nitric oxide synthase.

High-Yield Clinical Knowledge
- Ceruminolytic Age Restriction
    - Carbamide peroxide should not be used in children younger than three years, in patients with tympanostomy tubes, or in patients with perforated tympanic membranes.
- Docusate
    - As an alternative ceruminolytic, docusate capsules can be opened, with their contents emptied into the ear to attempt to loosen impacted ear wax.
- Ear Irrigation
    - Patients who fail cerumenolytics, these patients can undergo irrigation and manual removal.
        - Irrigation should use body-temperature water that may be combined with hydrogen peroxide and administered gently to aid in removing wax.
    - Carbamide peroxide may be used as an adjunct to attempt to soften wax, facilitating removal by irrigation.
- Corticosteroids for Acute Otitis Media
    - Adding corticosteroids to antimicrobials for acute otitis media may improve pain, swelling, and redness, but the evidence is lacking to support the combination treatment definitively.

- **Adrenal suppression**
  - Although systemic corticosteroids are associated with adrenal suppression, otic preparations are rarely absorbed systemically in concentrations relevant to causing HPA suppression effects.
  - Yet, adrenal suppression is a warning in the prescribing information for otic corticosteroids.

High-Yield Core Evidence
- **Cerumenolytics**
  - This was a systematic review and meta-analysis conducted to assess the effects of ear drops to remove or aid ear wax removal in adults and children.
  - Randomized controlled trials included in this meta-analysis include those in which a cerumenolytic was compared with no treatment, water or saline, an alternative liquid treatment, or another 'cerumenolytic' in adults or children with obstructing or impacted ear wax.
  - A total of ten studies was included with a range of interventions, including oil-based treatments (triethanolamine polypeptide, almond oil, benzocaine, chlorobutanol), water-based treatments (docusate sodium, carbamide peroxide, phenazone, choline salicylate, urea peroxide, potassium carbonate), other active comparators (e.g., saline or water alone) and no treatment.
  - The proportion of ears with complete clearance of ear wax was higher in the active treatment group compared with the no treatment group after five days of treatment with a number needed to treat of 8.
  - There was no evidence to show that one active agent was superior to any other.
  - The authors concluded that there is no high-quality evidence to allow a firm conclusion to be drawn, and the ideal cerumenolytic treatment remains uncertain. (Cochrane Database of Syst Rev. 2018;(7):CD012171.)

High-Yield Fast-Fact
- **Cost and Ophthalmic Agents**
  - Otic preparations are often more expensive than the same drug in an ophthalmic preparation.
  - Pharmacists can help reduce the cost of care by recommending ophthalmic preparations for otic administration.
  - However, otic medications should never be administered ophthalmically.

HIGH-YIELD BOARD EXAM ESSENTIALS
- **CLASSIC AGENTS:** Carbamide peroxide, dexamethasone, fluocinolone, hydrocortisone
- **DRUG CLASS:** Anti-inflammatories and cerumenolytics
- **INDICATIONS:** Ear wax removal
- **MECHANISM:** Carbamide peroxide - Softens cerumen by its foaming action from the release of hydrogen peroxide. Dexamethasone, Fluocinolone, Hydrocortisone - Suppress polymorphonuclear leukocytes migration, and decrease capillary permeability, reducing inflammation.
- **SIDE EFFECTS:** Local irritation
- **CLINICAL PEARLS:** Otic steroids provide a local anti-inflammatory effect to relieve pain from otitis externa, and carbamide may be used as a ceruminolytic but has questionable efficacy.

Table: Drug Class Summary

Anti-inflammatories and Cerumenolytics - Drug Class Review High-Yield Med Reviews			
Mechanism of Action: *Carbamide peroxide - Softens cerumen by its foaming action from the release of hydrogen peroxide. Dexamethasone, Fluocinolone, Hydrocortisone - Suppress polymorphonuclear leukocytes migration, and decrease capillary permeability, reducing inflammation.*			
Class Effects: *Otic steroids provide a local anti-inflammatory effect to relieve pain from otitis externa, and carbamide may be used as a ceruminolytic but has questionable efficacy.*			
Generic Name	**Brand Name**	**Main Indication(s) or Uses**	**Notes**

Carbamide peroxide	Auro, Mollifene, Debrox	- Ear wax removal	- Dosing (Adult):
			  - Otic: 5 to 10 drops twice daily for up to 4 days
			- Dosing (Peds):
			  - Otic: 1 to 10 drops twice daily for up to 4 days
			- CYP450 Interactions: None
			- Renal or Hepatic Dose Adjustments: None
			- Dosage Forms: Otic (solution)

Dexamethasone (with ciprofloxacin)	Ciprodex	- Acute otitis externa	- Dosing (Adult):
			  - Otic: 4 drops into affected ear(s) twice daily for 7 days
			- Dosing (Peds):
			  - Otic: 4 drops into affected ear(s) twice daily for 7 days
			- CYP450 Interactions: None
			- Renal or Hepatic Dose Adjustments: None
			- Dosage Forms: Otic (suspension)

Fluocinolone	DermOtic Oil, Flac	- Chronic eczematous external otitis	- Dosing (Adult):
			  - Otic: 5 drops into affected ear(s) twice daily for 7 days
			- Dosing (Peds):
			  - Otic: 5 drops into affected ear(s) twice daily for 7 days
			- CYP450 Interactions: None
			- Renal or Hepatic Dose Adjustments: None
			- Dosage Forms: Optic (oil)

Hydrocortisone (with ciprofloxacin; neomycin/polymyxin b; acetic acid; colistin, neomycin, thonzonium)	Cipro HC, PRamox-HC, Vosol HC, Cortisporin Otic, Casporyn HC, Coly-Mycin S, Cort-Biotic, Cortane-B	- Otic infections	- Dosing (Adult):
			  - Otic: 2-5 drops into affected ear two to four times daily for 7 days
			- Dosing (Peds):
			  - Otic: 2-5 drops into affected ear two to four times daily for 7 days
			- CYP450 Interactions: None
			- Renal or Hepatic Dose Adjustments: None
			- Dosage Forms: Otic (suspension, solution)

OTIC – ANTIMICROBIALS

Drug Class
- Antimicrobials
- Agents:
  - Acute Care
    - Ciprofloxacin
    - Neomycin, colistin, hydrocortisone, thonzonium
    - Neomycin, polymyxin B, hydrocortisone
    - Ofloxacin

> **Fast Facts**
> ✓ Topical (not oral) antibiotics are preferred for the treatment of otitis externa which is also commonly known as "swimmers ear". However, topical otic antibiotics will not work for inner ear infections or "otitis media".

Main Indications or Uses
- Acute Care
  - Acute otitis externa

Mechanism of Action
- **Colistin, Polymyxin B**
  - Act as cationic detergents that interact strongly with phospholipids and disrupt bacterial cell membranes' structure, leading to bacterial cell lysis.
- **Ciprofloxacin, Neomycin, Ofloxacin**
  - In Gram-Negative bacteria, fluoroquinolones inhibit DNA gyrase, causing bacterial DNA supercoiling and inhibiting bacterial growth.
  - In Gram-Positive bacteria, fluoroquinolones inhibit topoisomerase IV, preventing the separation of interlinked DNA strands from bacterial replication.

Primary Net Benefit
- Topical antimicrobials may help resolve the infection and relieve pain from otitis externa.
- Main Labs to Monitor:
  - No routine monitoring

High-Yield Basic Pharmacology
- **Polymyxins Binding Site**
  - Gram-negative bacteria sensitivity to the polymyxins is related to the phospholipids' content in the given bacterial cell wall.
    - The polymyxins' spectrum is limited to gram-negatives as their binding site to the lipopolysaccharide of the outer membrane of gram-negative bacteria inactivating it.

High-Yield Clinical Knowledge
- **Ototoxicity**
  - Topical fluoroquinolones are not believed to cause ototoxicity when the tympanic membranes are intact.
- **Ruptured Tympanic Membranes**
  - Ototoxic topical drugs may penetrate the inner ear structures in the setting of ruptured TMs and exert their damaging effects.
  - The ototoxic drugs that are most concerning are the aminoglycosides that are thought to be vestibulotoxic (gentamicin) or cochleotoxic (amikacin, neomycin, and tobramycin), or both, acetic acid altering PH and affecting cochlear function and polymyxin B with an unknown mechanism.
  - In the setting of known or suspected TM perforation, including tympanostomy tube, non-ototoxic topical preparations are preferred.
- **Neomycin hypersensitivity**
  - Neomycin is associated with acute hypersensitivity reactions (believed to be contact dermatitis) in up to 15% of patients, including those using a topical otic dosage form.

- **Ophthalmic Preparations**
  - The difference between ophthalmic products and otic products is that ophthalmic products are sterile and buffered to a neutral pH.
  - Since otic preparations are often more expensive than the same medication and concentration as an ophthalmic preparation, clinicians may substitute an otic antibiotic for an ophthalmic product.
  - However, otic medications must never be used in the eye.

High-Yield Core Evidence
- **Acute Otitis Externa**
  - This was a meta-analysis to assess the effectiveness of interventions for acute otitis externa.
  - Randomized controlled trials included evaluated ear cleaning, topical medication, or systemic therapy to treat acute otitis externa.
  - Topical antimicrobials containing steroids were significantly more effective than placebo drops, but no clinically meaningful differences were noted in clinical cure rates between the various topical interventions reviewed.
  - However, acetic acid was significantly less effective when compared with antibiotic/steroid drops in terms of cure rate at two and three weeks.
  - The authors concluded that topical treatments alone, as distinct from systemic ones, are effective for uncomplicated acute otitis externa. Furthermore, in most cases, the choice of topical intervention does not appear to influence the therapeutic outcome significantly. (Cochrane Database of Syst Rev. 2010;(1):CD004740.)

High-Yield Fast-Fact
- **Polymyxin B and Polymyxin E**
  - Although commonly referred to as colistin, it is otherwise known as polymyxin E.
  - In the historical literature, it may be referred to as polymyxin E and is marketed either as colistimethate for intravenous administration or colistin base for topical use.
  - Polymyxin B itself is not a single agent but is a mixture of polymyxins B1 and B2.
- **Quinolone vs Fluoroquinolones**
  - This drug class can be referred to as quinolones or fluoroquinolones. However, all modern agents used in the USA are fluoroquinolones, with Nalidixic acid the only non-fluorinated quinolone, but it is no longer clinically used.

HIGH-YIELD BOARD EXAM ESSENTIALS
- **CLASSIC AGENTS:** Ciprofloxacin, neomycin/colistin/hydrocortisone/thonzonium, neomycin/polymyxin B/hydrocortisone, ofloxacin
- **DRUG CLASS:** Otic antimicrobials
- **INDICATIONS:** Acute otitis externa
- **MECHANISM:** Colistin, Polymyxin B - Act as cationic detergents that interact strongly with phospholipids and disrupt bacterial cell membranes' structure, leading to bacterial cell lysis. Ciprofloxacin, Neomycin, Ofloxacin - Inhibit DNA gyrase and topoisomerase IV, exerting a bactericidal effect on susceptible pathogens.
- **SIDE EFFECTS:** Hypersensitivity, ototoxicity
- **CLINICAL PEARLS:** Ototoxic topical drugs may penetrate the inner ear structures in the setting of ruptured TMs and exert their damaging effects.

Table: Drug Class Summary

Antimicrobials - Drug Class Review
High-Yield Med Reviews
Mechanism of Action: *Colistin, Polymyxin B* - Act as cationic detergents that interact strongly with phospholipids and disrupt bacterial cell membranes' structure, leading to bacterial cell lysis. *Ciprofloxacin, Neomycin, Ofloxacin* - Inhibit DNA gyrase and topoisomerase IV, exerting a bactericidal effect on susceptible pathogens. **Class Effects:** *Topical antimicrobials may help resolve the infection and relieve pain from otitis externa.*

Generic Name	Brand Name	Main Indication(s) or Uses	Notes

Ciprofloxacin	Cetraxal, Otiprio, Vosol	- Acute otitis externa	- **Dosing (Adult):**
			  – Otic: instill 0.2 or 0.25 mL into affected ear twice daily
			- **Dosing (Peds):**
			  – Otic: instill 0.2 or 0.25 mL into affected ear twice daily
			- **CYP450 Interactions:** None
			- **Renal or Hepatic Dose Adjustments:** None
			- **Dosage Forms:** Otic (solution, suspension)

Ofloxacin	Floxin	- Acute otitis externa	- **Dosing (Adult):**
			  – Otic: instill 0.2 or 0.25 mL into affected ear twice daily
			- **Dosing (Peds):**
			  – Otic: instill 0.2 or 0.25 mL into affected ear twice daily
			- **CYP450 Interactions:** None
			- **Renal or Hepatic Dose Adjustments:** None
			- **Dosage Forms:** Otic (solution, suspension)

Neomycin, colistin, hydrocortisone, thonzonium	Coly-Mycin, Cortisporin-TC	- Acute otitis externa	- **Dosing (Adult):**
			  – Otic: instill 5 drops into affected ear 3-4 times daily
			- **Dosing (Peds):**
			  – Otic: instill 4 drops into affected ear 3-4 times daily
			- **CYP450 Interactions:** None
			- **Renal or Hepatic Dose Adjustments:** None
			- **Dosage Forms:** Otic (suspension)

Neomycin, polymyxin B, hydrocortisone	Odan-Spor-HC	- Acute otitis externa	- **Dosing (Adult):**
			  – Otic: instill 4 drops into affected ear 3-4 times daily
			- **Dosing (Peds):**
			  – Otic: instill 3 drops into affected ear 3-4 times daily
			- **CYP450 Interactions:** None
			- **Renal or Hepatic Dose Adjustments:** None
			- **Dosage Forms:** Otic (solution, suspension)

2025

A COMPREHENSIVE *RAPID REVIEW*

NAPLEX

Pharmacology & Drug Classes

Psychiatry / Mental Health

PSYCHIATRY – ALLOSTERIC GABA-A MODULATOR

Drug Class
- Allosteric GABA-A Modulator
- Agents:
  - Acute Care
    - Brexanolone

Main Indications or Uses
- Acute Care
  - Post-partum depression

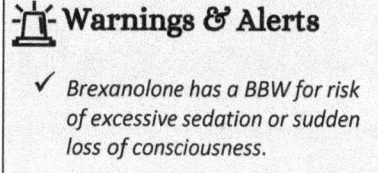

Warnings & Alerts
- Brexanolone has a BBW for risk of excessive sedation or sudden loss of consciousness.

Mechanism of Action
- Binds to the positive allosteric modulation site on the alpha subunit of GABA-A receptors, increasing receptor efficiency and potency.

Primary Net Benefit
- Single infusion management of acute post-partum depression.
- Main Labs to Monitor:
  - Continuous pulse oximetry during the administration

High-Yield Basic Pharmacology
- Endogenous Target
  - Brexanolone was designed to replace the endogenous compound allopregnanolone.
  - Allopregnanolone is a major metabolite of progesterone.

High-Yield Clinical Knowledge
- Single Indication
  - Brexanolone is only indicated for use in post-partum depression.
- Sudden Loss of Consciousness
  - As this drug is a GABA-A modulator with possible CNS depression, a black-boxed warning exists for the risk of excessive sedation or sudden loss of consciousness.
  - Time to complete recovery following a sudden loss of consciousness can range from 15 minutes to 60 minutes, during which airway and breathing support may be necessary.
- IV Administration
  - The administration of brexanolone is an IV infusion, with the single dose administered over a 60-hour continuous infusion with variable rate changes through this timeframe.
  - Brexanolone must be administered in an inpatient setting.

High-Yield Core Evidence
- Brexanolone Phase 3 Study
  - This was a single publication of two double-blind, multicenter, placebo-controlled, phase 3 trials that randomized women between the ages of 18 to 45 years old who were six months post-partum or less at screening and had post-partum depression and a qualifying 17-item Hamilton Rating Scale for Depression (HAM-D) score of at least 26 for study 1 and between 20 to 25 for study 2.
  - Patients were randomized to either brexanolone 90 mcg/kg/hr, brexanolone 60 mcg/kg/hr, or matching placebo for 60 h in study 1, or brexanolone 90 mcg/kg/hr or matching placebo for 60 h in study 2.
  - Both doses of brexanolone were associated with significantly better HAM-D scores at 60 hours than placebo in both studies.
  - The primary efficacy endpoint was the change from baseline in the 17-item HAM-D total score at 60 h, assessed in all patients who started infusion of study drug or placebo, had a valid HAM-D baseline assessment, and had at least one post-baseline HAM-D assessment.

- Although adverse events did not differ statistically between groups, patients receiving brexanolone experienced more dizziness and somnolence.
- Two patients experienced four treatment-related severe adverse events, including suicidal ideation and intentional overdose attempt during follow-up, altered state of consciousness, and syncope.
- The authors concluded that administration of brexanolone injection for post-partum depression resulted in significant and clinically meaningful reductions in HAM-D total score at 60 h compared with placebo, with rapid onset of action and durable treatment response during the study period. (Lancet. 2018 Sep 22;392(10152):1058-1070.)

High-Yield Fast-Fact
- **Post-partum Management**
    - Other antidepressants or benzodiazepines can be used alone or after brexanolone; however, specific considerations must be made for infant exposure via breast milk.

HIGH-YIELD BOARD EXAM ESSENTIALS
- **CLASSIC AGENTS:** Brexanolone
- **DRUG CLASS:** Allosteric GABA-A modulator
- **INDICATIONS:** Postpartum depression
- **MECHANISM:** Binds to the positive allosteric modulation site on the alpha subunit of GABA-A receptors, increasing receptor efficiency and potency.
- **SIDE EFFECTS:** Sudden loss of consciousness
- **CLINICAL PEARLS:** As this drug is a GABA-A modulator with possible CNS depression, a black-boxed warning exists for the risk of excessive sedation or sudden loss of consciousness.

Table: Drug Class Summary

Allosteric GABA-A Modulator - Drug Class Review			
High-Yield Med Reviews			
Mechanism of Action: *Binds to the positive allosteric modulation site on the alpha subunit of GABA-A receptors, increasing receptor efficiency and potency.*			
Class Effects: *Single infusion management of acute post-partum depression.*			
Generic Name	**Brand Name**	**Indication(s) or Uses**	**Notes**
Brexanolone	Zulresso	• Postpartum depression	• **Dosing (Adult):** — IV: 60-hour continuous infusion • **Dosing (Peds):** Not routinely used • **CYP450 Interactions:** None • **Renal or Hepatic Dose Adjustments:** — GFR < 15 mL/minute: not recommended • **Dosage Forms:** IV (solution)

PSYCHIATRY – ATYPICAL ANTIDEPRESSANTS

Drug Class
- Atypical Antidepressants
- Agents:
  - Chronic Care
    - Bupropion
    - Mirtazapine
    - Nefazodone
    - Trazodone
    - Vilazodone
    - Vortioxetine

> **Fast Facts**
> - Antidepressants carry a box warning for suicidality in adolescence to young adults.
> - Bupropion at higher doses or in an overdose can cause seizures.
> - Mirtazapine is associated with sedation and weight gain.
> - Nefazodone has a boxed warning for hepatotoxicity and thus is not used often.

Main Indications or Uses
- Chronic Care
  - Major depressive disorder
  - Aggression associated with dementia
  - Headache prophylaxis (chronic tension-type)
  - Insomnia
  - Panic disorder
  - Seasonal affective disorder (Bupropion)
  - Smoking cessation (Bupropion)

Mechanism of Action
- Bupropion
  - Norepinephrine and dopamine reuptake inhibition (NDRI)
    - Blocks norepinephrine (NE) and dopamine (D) reuptake pump causing increased neurotransmission of NE and D.
- Mirtazapine
  - Noradrenergic and specific serotonergic antidepressant (NaSSA)
  - Central alpha-2 adrenergic antagonist
    - Enhances the release of monoamines (does not block monoamine transporter) causing increased serotonergic and norepinephrine neurotransmission.
    - 5HT3 antagonism, 5HT2A antagonism, 5HT2C antagonism, and histaminic antagonism.
    - Blocks histamine receptors.
- Nefazodone and Trazodone
  - Serotonin 2A and 2C (5HT2A and 5HT2C) antagonists and reuptake inhibition (SARI)
- Vilazodone
  - Serotonin 1A partial agonist and reuptake inhibitors (SPARI)
- Vortioxetine
  - 5HT1A agonist, 5HT3 antagonist, serotonin reuptake inhibition, weak antagonism at 5HT7 and 5HT1D, and partial agonist at 5HT1B.

Primary Net Benefit
- Antidepressants as adjuncts to or as an alternative to SSRI therapy for major depressive disorder. Many agents have additional off-label indications.

High-Yield Basic Pharmacology
- Multimodal antidepressants
- Trazodone
  - In addition to its serotonin receptor effects, trazodone possesses alpha-adrenergic antagonist properties and weak antihistamine effects.
  - As a result, it is associated with CNS depression (antihistamine) and orthostatic hypotension (alpha-antagonism)

High-Yield Clinical Knowledge

- **Bupropion**
    - Numerous benefits, including treatment of depression especially with hypersomnia or fatigue, smoking cessation, cognitive slowing, and assistance with sexual dysfunction.
    - May have efficacy if SSRIs have failed (monotherapy) or produced only a partial response (adjunct therapy).
    - If used as an adjunct in bipolar depression, less likely to produce hypomania than other antidepressant agents. Though it still may occur.
    - May not be as effective for anxiety disorders as other agents.
- **Trazodone**
    - Trazodone is utilized in practice more to target sleep complaints or sexual dysfunction than depression.
- **Mirtazapine**
    - Due to its favorable adverse event profile with fewer GI complaints than other agents, mirtazapine can be added to antianxiety or antidepressant regimens, particularly its antihistamine-mediated sedative effect.
- **Vortioxetine**
    - Good evidence for use in geriatric depression with improvement in cognition along with mood.
- **Dosing and Administration**
    - Bupropion: XL is dosed once a day, SR is dosed twice daily, and immediate release is dosed 3 times daily.
    - Mirtazapine
        - Lower doses (e.g. 7.5 mg) are more likely to cause sedation than higher doses.
        - Higher doses of 45 mg to 60 mg are more likely to cause antimuscarinic effects (e.g. constipation, urinary retention)
    - Trazodone has a short half-life and is more often dosed once daily (50mg to 150 mg) at bedtime as an adjunct versus monotherapy.
        - Patients may experience carryover sedation, ataxia, and intoxicated-like feeling if dosed too aggressively, especially upon initiation.
- **Contraindications**
    - Use with monoamine oxidase inhibitors (MAOIs) within 14 days.
    - Bupropion: Active or history of seizures, eating disorders like anorexia nervosa or bulimia, with concomitant abrupt discontinuation of alcohol, benzodiazepines, or anticonvulsants.
        - XL: carries additional contraindications with things that may increase seizure likelihood: head trauma, CNS infection or tumor, stroke, etc.
- **Warnings**
    - Reports of Bupropion misuse (higher doses leading to euphoria) which increases the risk of seizure and overdose, the elderly are more likely to experience drug accumulation.
    - Caution with bupropion in those with cardiovascular disease, hepatic impairment, renal impairment, hypertension, weight loss, and cognitive impairment.
    - Trazodone: falls and fractures when used in elderly patients, cause or worsening of narrow-angle glaucoma. Use caution in epilepsy, renal impairment, hepatic impairment, and coronary artery disease.
- **Boxed Warnings**
    - Boxed warning: Increased risk of suicidality which requires close monitoring.
    - Hepatoxicity with nefazodone as rare cases of life-threatening hepatic failure have been reported.
- **Adverse Effects**
    - Drug Discontinuation Syndrome
        - Abrupt discontinuation of any atypical antidepressant can cause a sharp worsening of psychiatric symptoms, which can be worse than pre-treatment psychiatric disturbances.
        - Slow tapering is necessary to avoid this withdrawal syndrome.
    - Bupropion
        - The risk of seizure increases if chronic doses are above 450 mg/day, if a large overdose is ingested or with the immediate release formulation.
            - Seizure is a potential adverse effect of all antidepressants, but bupropion has a higher incidence associated with it.

- Additional findings from bupropion overdose include hypertension, agitation, QRS, and QT prolongation.
    - The onset of these symptoms can be delayed between 10 and 24 hours following an overdose, with seizures lasting up to 48 hours after exposure.
- The active metabolite hydroxybupropion may cause seizures by acting as a GABA antagonist and as an NMDA agonist.
- Bupropion should be avoided in those with eating disorders due to the increased risk of seizures; evidence based on past observations when bupropion immediate release was dosed at especially high levels to low body weight patients with active anorexia nervosa.
- Mirtazapine: weight gain, increased appetite, dry mouth, constipation, sedation, confusion, hypotension, flu-like symptoms (evaluate CBC as this may indicate a low WBC pr granulocyte count).
- Nefazodone is rarely used clinically as it is associated with a high risk of hepatotoxicity, which can lead to numerous physiologic effects, including jaundice, hepatitis, and hepatic necrosis.
- Trazodone is associated with CNS depression, orthostatic hypotension, QT prolongation, sedation, fatigue, headache, nausea, vomiting, blurred vision, constipation, dry mouth, and rarely priapism (if this occurs medication should be discontinued).
    - Possible mechanisms of this effect pertain to paradoxical alpha vasoconstriction in the penis, limiting blood flow.
- Vilazodone and vortioxetine: Hyponatremia, increased bleeding risk (when combined with NSAIDs, anticoagulants, antiplatelets), fractures, falls, sexual dysfunction (though the risk is lower with vilazodone and vortioxetine than with SSRIs and much less common).

- **Drug, Supplement, Food, and/or Disease Interactions**
    - Caution when combined with other CNS depressants due to the risk of additive effects.
    - Caution when combining with other antidepressants avoid combining with MAOIs.
    - Bupropion: inhibitor of CYP2D6, can increase TCA levels – avoid combination or use cautiously.
    - Mirtazapine: LFTS in those with impairment, weight, and BMI.
    - Nefazodone is a potent CYP3A4 inhibitor, contributing to numerous clinically relevant drug interactions.
    - Trazodone: metabolized by CYP3A4, may increase digoxin or phenytoin levels, and interfere with some antihypertensive agents.
    - Vilazodone: Major substrate of CYP3A4
    - Vortioxetine: Major substrate of CYP2D6
- **Monitoring**
    - Mood changes, presence of suicidality (especially in children, adolescents, or young adults), activation of mania or hypomania.
    - Weight and BMI as medications can cause weight gain (mirtazapine) or weight loss (bupropion).
    - Consider evaluating for pre-diabetes, diabetes, dyslipidemia, or consider switching to a different antidepressant if the patient gains more than 5 to 7% of their baseline weight.
    - Bupropion: Seizures, blood pressure, changes in mood, headache, insomnia, renal and liver function as dose may require adjustment. May cause a false positive urine drug screen for amphetamines (even several days after discontinuation).
    - Mirtazapine: liver function if abnormalities present or suspected, CBC for leucopenia or granulocytopenia.
    - Nefazodone: Liver function (Albumin, protein, INR, bilirubin), baseline, and periodic. Liver enzymes (AST/ALT), baseline and periodic
    - Trazodone: Sedation, orthostasis, headache, nausea, and priapism as these are common side effects that can impair patient adherence.
    - Vilazodone: High incidence of GI upset, possibly due to faster SRI activity. Taking with food may help.
- **Patient Education**
    - Medications are often titrated up slowly to start and tapered down slowly to discontinue.
        - Tapering helps avoid symptoms of withdrawal or a worsening of psychiatric symptoms.
    - Maximal therapeutic effects are not immediate and may take 4-8 weeks; however slight improvements in physical symptoms like sleep and appetite can occur within 2 to 4 weeks of treatment for some.
    - It is important to take your medication as directed every day to reach your treatment goals. If a dose is missed take it as soon as possible, but never double up on doses to catch up if a dose is missed.

- Report any side effects to your doctor or pharmacist who can help you with side effects.

High-Yield Core Evidence
- **STEP-BD**
  - This was a multicenter, double-blind, placebo-controlled study that randomized patients with bipolar depression to receive a mood stabilizer (lithium, valproate, or carbamazepine) plus an antidepressant (bupropion or paroxetine) or a mood stabilizer plus placebo to determine whether adjunctive antidepressant therapy reduces symptoms of bipolar depression without increasing the risk of mania.
  - There was no difference between groups concerning the primary outcome of the percentage of subjects in each treatment group meeting the criterion for a durable recovery.
  - However, patients randomized to a mood stabilizer plus adjunctive antidepressants experienced numerically better secondary outcomes and lower rates of the treatment-emergent effective switch.
  - The authors concluded that adjunctive, standard antidepressant medication, compared with mood stabilizers, was not associated with increased efficacy or with increased risk of a treatment-emergent effective switch.
  - N Engl J Med. 2007 Apr 26;356(17):1711-22.
- **VAST-D**
  - This was a multicenter study within the US Veterans Health Administration medical centers that randomized patients who were diagnosed with nonpsychotic major depressive disorder and were unresponsive to at least one antidepressant. Participants received either a change in their current regimen to bupropion, augmentation of their present regimen with bupropion, or augmentation with aripiprazole for 12 weeks and up to 36 weeks for longer-term follow-up.
  - The augmented treatment with aripiprazole led to a significant improvement in remission (defined as a 16-item Quick Inventory of Depressive Symptomatology-Clinician Rated score of less than five at two consecutive visits) compared to each of the other groups.
  - Aripiprazole also led to a higher likelihood of a greater than 50% reduction in QIDS-C16 score.
  - Relapse rates were similar between groups.
  - Patients randomized to bupropion experienced more anxiety, and patients randomized to aripiprazole experienced somnolence, akathisia, and weight gain.
  - The authors concluded that among a predominantly male population with major depressive disorder unresponsive to antidepressant treatment, augmentation with aripiprazole resulted in a statistically significant but only modestly increased likelihood of remission during 12 weeks of treatment compared with switching to bupropion monotherapy.
  - JAMA. 2017 Jul 11;318(2):132-145.

High-Yield Fast-Fact
- The combination of bupropion and naltrexone has demonstrated efficacy as a treatment for obesity and is currently available as a combination product for this indication

---

HIGH-YIELD BOARD EXAM ESSENTIALS
- **CLASSIC AGENTS:** Bupropion, Mirtazapine, Nefazodone, Trazodone, Vilazodone, Vortioxetine.
- **DRUG CLASS:** Atypical antidepressants.
- **INDICATIONS:** Major depressive disorder, migraine prophylaxis, panic disorder
- **MECHANISM:** Bupropion - Inhibits the reuptake of dopamine and norepinephrine, prolonging norepinephrine, and serotonergic neurotransmission. Mirtazapine - Central alpha-2 adrenergic inhibitor, causing increased serotonergic and norepinephrine neurotransmission. Nefazodone and Trazodone - Serotonin 2A and 2C (5HT2A and 5HT2C) receptor antagonists with serotonin reuptake inhibition. Vilazodone serotonin reuptake inhibition and partial 5-HT1 receptor agonism.
- **SIDE EFFECTS:** Hepatotoxicity (nefazodone), priapism (trazodone), seizures (bupropion), serotonin syndrome.
- **CLINICAL PEARLS:** Abrupt discontinuation of any atypical antidepressant can cause a sharp worsening of psychiatric symptoms, which can be worse than pre-treatment psychiatric disturbances.

Table: Drug Class Summary

Atypical Antidepressants - Drug Class Review High-Yield Med Reviews			
Mechanism of Action: ***Bupropion*** - *Inhibits the reuptake of dopamine and norepinephrine (NDRI), prolonging norepinephrine and dopaminergic neurotransmission.* ***Mirtazapine*** - *Central alpha-2 adrenergic inhibitor, causing increased serotonergic and norepinephrine neurotransmission (NaSSA).* ***Nefazodone and Trazodone*** - *Serotonin receptor 2A and 2C (5HT2A and 5HT2C) antagonists, and serotonin reuptake inhibition (SARI).* ***Vilazodone*** *serotonin partial 5-HT1 receptor agonism and serotonin reuptake inhibition (SPARI).* ***Vortioxetine*** *5HT1A agonist, 5HT3 antagonist, serotonin reuptake inhibition* **Class Effects:** Antidepressants as adjuncts or as an alternative to SSRI therapy for MDD with many additional uses.			
Generic Name	**Brand Name**	**Main Indication(s) or Uses**	**Notes**

Bupropion	Aplenzin
	Forfivo
	Wellbutrin
	Zyban
		• Major depressive disorder
		• Seasonal affective disorder
		• Smoking cessation
		• Attention deficit/ hyperactivity disorder
		• Bipolar disorder, depressive episode adjunct
		• SSRI-induced sexual dysfunction
			• **Dosing (Adult):**
			  – Oral: 100 to 450 mg daily
			• **Dosing (Peds):**
			  – Oral: 3 mg/kg/day in 2-3 divided doses
			    – Maximum 6 mg/kg/day or single dose 150 mg
			• **CYP450 Interactions:** Substrate CYP1A2, 2A6, 2B6, 2C9, 2D6, 2E1, 3A4; Inhibits CYP2D6
			• **Renal or Hepatic Dose Adjustments:**
			  – Child-Pugh class C: reduce dose by 50%
			  – CrCl < 60 mL/min: consider max of 150 mg per day.
			  – CrCl < 15 mL/min: consider alternative agent
			• **Dosage Forms:** Oral (tablet)

Mirtazapine	Remeron	• Major depressive disorder
		• Headache prophylaxis (chronic tension-type)
		• Panic disorder
			• **Dosing (Adult):**
			  – Oral: 15 to 45 mg/night
			• **Dosing (Peds):**
			  – Not routinely used
			• **CYP450 Interactions:** Minimal
			• **Renal or Hepatic Dose Adjustments:**
			  – GFR < 30 mL/minute: use an initial dose of 7.5 mg
			  – Child-Pugh class C: reduce dose by 50%
			• **Dosage Forms:** Oral (tablet)

Nefazodone	Serzone	• Major depressive disorder	• **Dosing (Adult):**
			  – Oral: 50 to 600 mg in 2 divided doses
			• **Dosing (Peds):**
			  – Not routinely used
			• **CYP450 Interactions:** Substrate CYP2D6, 3A4; Inhibits CYP3A4
			• **Renal or Hepatic Dose Adjustments:** None
			• **Dosage Forms:** Oral (tablet)

Atypical Antidepressants - Drug Class Review High-Yield Med Reviews			
Generic Name	**Brand Name**	**Main Indication(s) or Uses**	**Notes**

Trazodone	Desyrel	• Major depressive disorder
		• Aggression associated with dementia
		• Insomnia
			• **Dosing (Adult):**
			  − Oral: 25 to 400 mg/day
			• **Dosing (Peds):**
			  − Oral: 0.75 to 6.9 mg/kg/day
			    − Maximum 150 mg/dose
			• **CYP450 Interactions:** Substrate CYP2D6, 3A4
			• **Renal or Hepatic Dose Adjustments:** None
			• **Dosage Forms:** Oral (tablet)

Vilazodone	Viibryd	• Major depressive disorder	• **Dosing (Adult):**
			  − Oral: 10 mg daily x 7 days, then 20-40 mg daily (titrate every 7 days to next dose)
			• **Dosing (Peds):**
			  − Not routinely used
			• **CYP450 Interactions:** Substrate CYP2C19, 2D6, 3A4
			• **Renal or Hepatic Dose Adjustments:** None
			• **Dosage Forms:** Oral (tablet)

Vortioxetine	Trintellix	• Major depressive disorder	• **Dosing (Adult):** − Oral: 5-20 mg daily • **Dosing (Peds):** Not routinely used • **CYP450 Interactions:** CYP2D6, 2B6, 2C19, 2C8, 2C9, 2D6, 3A4 substrate • **Renal or Hepatic Dose Adjustments:** None • **Dosage Forms:** Oral (tablet)

PSYCHIATRY – MONOAMINE OXIDASE INHIBITOR

Drug Class
- Monoamine Oxidase Inhibitor
- Agents:
  - Chronic Care
    - Isocarboxazid
    - Phenelzine
    - Selegiline
    - Tranylcypromine

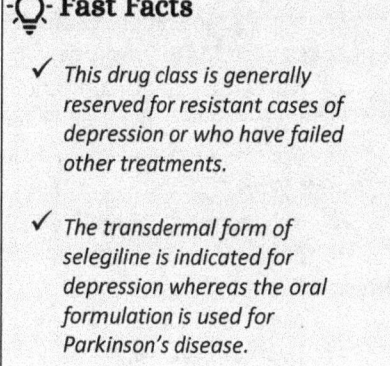

Main Indications or Uses
- Chronic Care
  - Major depressive disorder
  - Parkinson disease (only the oral form of selegiline)

Mechanism of Action
- Irreversibly bind to and inhibit monoamine oxidase-A and monoamine oxidase-B, preventing the presynaptic degradation of epinephrine, norepinephrine, dopamine, and serotonin.

Primary Net Benefit
- MAO inhibitors are reserved for refractory depression not adequately responsive to other antidepressants and when the threat of psychiatric disease outweighs the risks of MAO inhibition.
- Main Labs to Monitor:
  - Serum creatinine
  - Liver function (Albumin, protein, bilirubin, INR)
  - Blood pressure
  - Heart rate

High-Yield Basic Pharmacology
- MAO-A Vs. MAO-B
  - MAO-A normally functions to metabolize monoamines, including norepinephrine, serotonin, and dopamine, in the CNS and outside the CNS.
    - MAO-A is concentrated in the liver and intestine.
  - MAO-B selectively functions to metabolize dopamine in the CNS, primarily in the basal ganglia, but may also exist peripherally.
  - Selegiline is a selective MAO-B inhibitor, whereas isocarboxazid, phenelzine, and tranylcypromine are nonselective MAO-A and MAO-B inhibitors.
- Monoamines
  - Monoamines include not just catecholamines but also indoleamine melatonin and serotonin and naturally occurring amines such as tyramine.
- Covalent MAO Inhibition
  - Isocarboxazid, phenelzine, and tranylcypromine covalently bind to MAO and irreversibly inhibit its function, thus depleting it until new MAO can be synthesized, which can take up to 3 weeks.

High-Yield Clinical Knowledge
- Serotonin Syndrome
  - Serotonin syndrome is the combination of a rapid onset of altered mental status, autonomic instability, hyperthermia, and hyperreflexia/myoclonus.
  - MAO inhibitors are associated with the highest risk of serotonin syndrome among antidepressants.
  - Treatment of serotonin syndrome involves the management of hyperthermia through invasive or noninvasive cooling, skeletal muscle relaxation using benzodiazepines, and airway support.
    - Dantrolene and cyproheptadine have been suggested as adjuncts for managing serotonin syndrome but are of questionable patient-oriented benefit.

- **Hypertensive Crisis**
  - Although drug interactions contribute to serotonin syndrome, certain foods with high tyramine content can precipitate a similar effect, including hypertensive crisis.
    - MAO-A, located in the gut, is usually metabolized tyramine before absorption. But with MAO inhibition, tyramine becomes absorbed and can exert its vasoconstrictor effects.
- **Non-MAOI with MAOI Properties**
  - Numerous other medications possess varying degrees of MAO inhibition and, if combined, can produce hypertensive crisis and or serotonin syndrome.
  - Common examples include linezolid, procarbazine, and methylene blue.
- **St. John's Wort**
  - This common herbal cited among many adverse events and drug interactions possesses weak MAO inhibitor activity, attributed to its major components, hypericin and hyperforin.
- **Adverse Events**
  - MAO inhibitors, particularly phenelzine, are frequently associated with orthostatic or postural hypotension, weight gain, decreased libido, and anorgasmia.
  - Tranylcypromine and selegiline conversely can cause CNS stimulation and insomnia.
- **Not Just MAO Inhibition**
  - Other enzymes are inhibited by MAO inhibitors, notably including alcohol dehydrogenase.
  - Patients taking tranylcypromine should avoid alcohol due to this effect.

High-Yield Core Evidence
- **STAR-D**
  - This was a multicenter, four-tier, equipoise-stratified randomized trial in adult patients with the unipolar major depressive disorder without psychotic features who had a baseline Hamilton Depression Rating Scale score of at least 14, and patients must have sought treatment.
  - This study involved a complex randomization and patient process through the clinical trial.
  - The first step was citalopram only, and if no remission was achieved, patients were then randomly enrolled in step 2 treatment, which consisted of 7 different treatment options. Step 3 added augmentation, including lithium or triiodothyronine and nortriptyline or mirtazapine; if there was no remission, patients progressed to step 4, where tranylcypromine or venlafaxine XR plus mirtazapine were started.
  - Remission rates were higher in earlier steps, with step 1 achieving remission in 36.8% of patients, with incrementally fewer patients achieving remission in steps 2 through 4.
  - The authors concluded that lower acute remission rates and higher relapse rates during the follow-up phase are expected when more treatment steps are required. (Am J Psychiatry. 2006;163(11):1905-117.)

High-Yield Fast-Facts
- **Hydrazines**
  - Isocarboxazid and phenelzine are hydrazine compounds, similar to the hydrazine isoniazid that can cause seizures.
- **Ayahuasca**
  - Ayahuasca is a hallucinogenic drink prepared by Peruvian and other South American natives, which is a MAO inhibitor (the plan Banisteriopsis caapi) that permits dimethyltryptamine to be absorbed orally.

HIGH-YIELD BOARD EXAM ESSENTIALS
- **CLASSIC AGENTS:** Isocarboxazid, phenelzine, selegiline, tranylcypromine
- **DRUG CLASS:** MAO inhibitor
- **INDICATIONS:** Major depressive disorder, Parkinson disease
- **MECHANISM:** Irreversibly bind to, and inhibit, monoamine oxidase-A and monoamine oxidase-B, preventing the metabolism of epinephrine, norepinephrine, dopamine, and serotonin.
- **SIDE EFFECTS:** Orthostatic or postural hypotension, weight gain, decreased libido, and anorgasmia.
- **CLINICAL PEARLS:** Numerous other medications possess varying degrees of MAO inhibition, and if combined, can produce hypertensive crisis and or serotonin syndrome. Common examples include linezolid, procarbazine, and methylene blue.

Table: Drug Class Summary

Monoamine Oxidase Inhibitor - Drug Class Review **High-Yield Med Reviews**			
Mechanism of Action: *Irreversibly bind to, and inhibit monoamine oxidase-A and monoamine oxidase-B, preventing the metabolism of epinephrine, norepinephrine, dopamine, and serotonin.*			
Class Effects: *MAO inhibitors are reserved for refractory depression not adequately responsive to other antidepressants, and the risks of MAO inhibition are outweighed by the threat of psychiatric disease.*			
Generic Name	**Brand Name**	**Main Indication(s) or Uses**	**Notes**

Isocarboxazid	Marplan	- Major depressive disorder	- **Dosing (Adult):**
			    – Oral: 10 to 20 mg twice daily
			 - **Dosing (Peds):**
			    – Not routinely used
			 - **CYP450 Interactions:** None
			 - **Renal or Hepatic Dose Adjustments:** None
			 - **Dosage Forms:** Oral (tablet)

Phenelzine	Nardil	- Major depressive disorder	- **Dosing (Adult):**
			    – Oral: 15 mg TID
			       – Maximum 90 mg/day
			 - **Dosing (Peds):**
			    – Not routinely used
			 - **CYP450 Interactions:** None
			 - **Renal or Hepatic Dose Adjustments:**
			    – Child-Pugh class C: contraindicated
			 - **Dosage Forms:** Oral (tablet)

Selegiline	Emsam
	 Zelapar
		- Major depressive disorder
		 - Parkinson disease
			- **Dosing (Adult):**
			    – Oral: 1.25 to 5 mg BID
			    – Transdermal: 6 to 12 mg/24 hour patch
			 - **Dosing (Peds):**
			    – Not routinely used
			 - **CYP450 Interactions:** Substrate of CYP1A2, 2A6, 2B6, 2D6, 3A4
			 - **Renal or Hepatic Dose Adjustments:**
			    – GFR < 30 mL/minute: Use not recommended
			    – Child-Pugh Class C: Not recommended
			 - **Dosage Forms:** Oral (capsule, tablet), Transdermal patch

Tranylcypromine	Parnate	- Major depressive disorder	- **Dosing (Adult):**
			    – Oral: 10 to 60 mg/day
			 - **Dosing (Peds):**
			    – Not routinely used
			 - **CYP450 Interactions:** None
			 - **Renal or Hepatic Dose Adjustments:** None
			 - **Dosage Forms:** Oral (tablet)

PSYCHIATRY – SELECTIVE NOREPINEPHRINE / SEROTONIN REUPTAKE INHIBITOR

Drug Class
- Selective Norepinephrine/Serotonin Reuptake Inhibitor
- Agents:
    - Chronic Care
        - Desvenlafaxine
        - Duloxetine
        - Levomilnacipran
        - Milnacipran
        - Venlafaxine

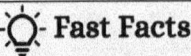

Fast Facts

✓ Venlafaxine and desvenlafaxine are classically tested on board exams to be known for causing dose-dependent increases in the blood pressure and to use with caution in patients with uncontrolled hypertension.

Main Indications or Uses
- Chronic Care
    - Anxiety
        - Duloxetine
        - Venlafaxine (including panic and social anxiety disorder)
    - Depression
        - Desvenlafaxine
        - Levomilnacipran
        - Milnacipran
        - Venlafaxine
    - Fibromyalgia
        - Duloxetine
        - Milnacipran
    - Musculoskeletal Pain
        - Duloxetine
    - Neuropathic Pain (secondary to DM)
        - Duloxetine

Mechanism of Action
- SNRI
    - Inhibits the reuptake of both norepinephrine and serotonin, prolonging norepinephrine, and serotonergic neurotransmission.

Primary Net Benefit
- Mostly used as second-line pharmacotherapy for depression and/or anxiety with improved safety compared to conventional antidepressants.
- Main Labs to Monitor:
    - No routine lab monitoring, but monitor changes in blood pressure control over time

High-Yield Basic Pharmacology
- Active Metabolites
    - The active metabolite of venlafaxine, desvenlafaxine, is commercially available as an alternative SNRI.
    - Similarly, levomilnacipran is the single-isomer of milnacipran.
- Central Beta Receptor Effects
    - Venlafaxine produces a rapid downregulation of beta-adrenergic receptors in the CNS, providing a faster relative onset of antidepressant effects than other agents.
- TCA Structure
    - Although an SNRI, duloxetine shares a tricyclic structure backbone but exhibits selective norepinephrine and serotonergic effects.

- **Non-benzodiazepine**
  - Buspirone is a non-benzodiazepine agent that acts through 5HT1A agonist activity to provide anxiolysis but lacks other common benzodiazepine properties (anticonvulsant, hypnotic, dependence, etc.)

High-Yield Clinical Knowledge
- **Overdose Risk**
  - Venlafaxine and desvenlafaxine appear to cause more morbidity and mortality after overdose than other SSRIs and other SNRIs.
  - Due to their sodium and potassium channel blocking properties, desvenlafaxine and venlafaxine may prolong the QRS and QT interval, possibly attributing to their higher overdose mortality.
- **SNRI Adverse Effects**
  - Hyperhidrosis is a common adverse event unique to SNRIs.
  - All SNRIs may also cause increases in BP, with more pronounced effects due to venlafaxine and levomilnacipran.
  - May still cause GI related adverse effects and sexual dysfunction. Most are weight neutral or promote some weight loss.
- **Drug Discontinuation Syndrome**
  - Like SSRIs, SNRIs should not be abruptly discontinued due to the risk of a sudden worsening of psychiatric symptoms, which can be worse than pre-treatment psychiatric disturbances.
    - Slow tapering is necessary to avoid this withdrawal syndrome, but agents with prolonged half-lives and active metabolites (such as fluoxetine) may have a lower likelihood due to a self-tapering effect.
- **Fibromyalgia**
  - Milnacipran is only FDA approved for treating fibromyalgia and is not routinely used to treat depression.
- **Serotonin Syndrome**
  - SNRIs carry a risk of serotonin syndrome. Risk increases when combined with other agents.
  - Serotonin syndrome is the rapid onset of altered mental status, autonomic instability, hyperthermia, and hyperreflexia/myoclonus.
  - Other antidepressants, including MAO inhibitors, are more likely to contribute to serotonin toxicity.
- **SIADH**
  - Venlafaxine and desvenlafaxine are associated with a higher risk of SIADH compared to other SNRIs and SSRIs.

High-Yield Core Evidence
- **Antidepressant Meta-Analysis**
  - This was a meta-analysis and systematic review of published and unpublished, double-blind, randomized controlled trials of antidepressant use for MDD diagnosed according to standard operationalized criteria.
  - The authors included 522 trials comprising 116,477 participants, demonstrating that all antidepressants were more effective than placebo.
  - In head-to-head studies, agomelatine, amitriptyline, escitalopram, mirtazapine, paroxetine, venlafaxine, and vortioxetine were more effective than other antidepressants.
  - Conversely, fluoxetine, fluvoxamine, reboxetine, and trazodone were the least effective drugs.
  - The fewest adverse events were reported among patients taking agomelatine, citalopram, escitalopram, fluoxetine, sertraline, and vortioxetine.
  - The authors concluded that all antidepressants were more efficacious than placebo in adults with MDD. Smaller differences between active drugs were found when placebo-controlled trials were included in the analysis, whereas there was more variability in efficacy and acceptability in head-to-head trials. (Lancet. 2018 Apr 7;391(10128):1357-1366.)

- **SNRI Systematic Review and Meta-Analysis**
  - This was a systematic review and dose-response meta-analysis of double-blind, randomized controlled trials (n=77) that examined fixed doses of five selective SSRIs in patients (n = 19,364) with MDD.
  - All SSRIs included were converted to fluoxetine equivalents, but venlafaxine and mirtazapine were not adjusted.
  - The primary outcomes were efficacy (treatment response defined as 50% or more significant reduction in depression severity), tolerability (dropouts due to adverse effects), and acceptability (dropouts for any reasons), all after a median of 8 weeks of treatment (range 4-12 weeks).
  - Fluoxetine dose equivalents between 20 mg and 80 mg demonstrated a positive dose-efficacy response, but more dropouts occurred when doses were above 40 mg of fluoxetine dose equivalents.
  - Venlafaxine doses between 75 and 150 mg were associated with a positive dose-efficacy relationship with a diminishing response with doses above 150mg daily.
  - Both venlafaxine and mirtazapine showed optimal acceptability in their lower dosing range.
  - The authors concluded that for the most used second-generation antidepressants, the lower range of the licensed dose achieves the optimal balance between efficacy, tolerability, and acceptability in the acute treatment of MDD. (Lancet Psychiatry. 2019 Jul;6(7):601-609.)

High-Yield Fast-Fact
- **Duloxetine Adverse Effects**
  - Duloxetine can cause biliary obstruction with chronic use or excessive use, leading to hyperbilirubinemia and jaundice.
  - Duloxetine can cause elevated A1c.

HIGH-YIELD BOARD EXAM ESSENTIALS
- **CLASSIC AGENTS:** Desvenlafaxine, duloxetine, levomilnacipran, milnacipran, venlafaxine
- **DRUG CLASS:** SNRI, other
- **INDICATIONS:** Fibromyalgia, generalized anxiety disorder, major depressive disorder, musculoskeletal pain, neuropathic pain, panic disorder, social anxiety disorder
- **MECHANISM:** Inhibits the reuptake of both norepinephrine and serotonin, prolonging norepinephrine, and serotonergic neurotransmission.
- **SIDE EFFECTS:** GI effects, weight neutrality or loss, increased BP, SIADH, serotonin syndrome, QRS/QT prolongation (venlafaxine)
- **CLINICAL PEARLS:** Mostly utilized as second-line after SSRIs. Effects may take 4-8 weeks. Milnacipran is indicated for fibromyalgia.

Table: Drug Class Summary

Serotonin-Norepinephrine Reuptake Inhibitors - Drug Class Review High-Yield Med Reviews			
Mechanism of Action: *Inhibits the reuptake of both norepinephrine and serotonin, prolonging norepinephrine, and serotonergic neurotransmission.*			
Class Effects: *Second-line for MDD and GAD overall, also used for various types of pain, hyperhidrosis, BP increase, weight loss; 4-8 weeks for max effect*			
Generic Name	**Brand Name**	**Main Indication(s) or Uses**	**Notes**

Desvenlafaxine	Pristiq	• Major depressive disorder	• **Dosing (Adult):** Oral: 50 to 150 mg daily
			• **Dosing (Peds):** Oral: 50 to 150 mg daily
			• **CYP450 Interactions:** CYP3A4 substrate
			• **Renal or Hepatic Dose Adjustments:**
			   – GFR 30 to 50 mL/min: Max 50 mg daily
			   – GFR < 30 mL/min: Max 25 mg daily
			   – Child-Pugh class B or C: Max 100 mg daily
			• **Dosage Forms:** Oral (tablet)

Duloxetine	Cymbalta	• Fibromyalgia
		• Generalized anxiety disorder
		• Major depressive disorder
		• Musculoskeletal pain
		• Neuropathic pain
			• **Dosing (Adult):** Oral: 20 to 120 mg daily
			• **Dosing (Peds):** Oral: 20 to 120 mg daily
			• **CYP450 Interactions:** CYP1A2, 2D6 substrate; CYP2D6 inhibitor
			• **Renal or Hepatic Dose Adjustments:**
			   – GFR < 30 mL/min Max 60 mg daily
			   – Hepatic impairment: avoid use
			• **Dosage Forms:** Oral (capsule)

Levomilnacipran	Fetzima	• Major depressive disorder	• **Dosing (Adult):** Oral: 20 to 120 mg daily
			• **Dosing (Peds):** Not routinely used
			• **CYP450 Interactions:** CYP2C19, 2C8, 2D6, 3A4, P-gp substrate
			• **Renal or Hepatic Dose Adjustments:**
			   – GFR 30 to 59 mL/min: Max 80 mg/day
			   – GFR 15 to 29 mL/min: Max 40 mg daily
			• **Dosage Forms:** Oral (capsule)

Milnacipran	Savella	• Fibromyalgia • Major depressive disorder	• **Dosing (Adult):** Oral: 50 to 100 mg BID • **Dosing (Peds):** Not routinely used • **CYP450 Interactions:** None • **Renal or Hepatic Dose Adjustments:** – GFR < 30 mL/min: Max 50 mg BID • **Dosage Forms:** Oral (tablet)

Venlafaxine	Effexor	• Generalized anxiety disorder
		• Major depressive disorder
		• Panic disorder
		• Social anxiety disorder
			• **Dosing (Adult):** Oral: 37.5 to 375 mg daily
			• **Dosing (Peds):** Oral: 12.5 to 75 mg daily
			   – Max 75 mg/day
			• **CYP450 Interactions:** CYP2C19, 2C9, 2D6, 3A4 substrate; CYP2D6 inhibitor
			• **Renal or Hepatic Dose Adjustments:**
			   – GFR < 30 mL/min: Max 150 mg/day
			• **Dosage Forms:** Oral (capsule, tablet)

PSYCHIATRY – SELECTIVE SEROTONIN REUPTAKE INHIBITORS

Drug Class
- Selective Serotonin Reuptake Inhibitors (SSRIs)
- Agents:
    - Citalopram
    - Escitalopram
    - Fluoxetine
    - Fluvoxamine
    - Paroxetine
    - Sertraline

Main Indications or Uses
- Chronic Care
    - Bipolar depression (augmentation)
    - Bulimia nervosa
    - Generalized anxiety disorder (GAD)
    - Major depressive disorder (MDD)
    - Obsessive-compulsive disorder (OCD)
    - Panic disorder
    - Post-traumatic stress disorder (PTSD)
    - Premenstrual dysphoric disorder (PMDD)
    - Social anxiety disorder
    - Treatment-resistant depression (TRD)
    - Vasomotor symptoms of menopause

> **Fast Facts**
> ✓ SSRIs have a wide variety of indications making them a very useful drug class in everyday clinical practice.
>
> ✓ Citalopram and escitalopram (s-enantiomer of citalopram) are known to have dose- or concentration-dependent effects on the QT interval more than other SSRIs.
>
> ✓ While SSRIs have a larger therapeutic index than other antidepressants, an overdose with >75 times the common daily dose could be life-threatening.
>
> ✓ Fluoxetine and paroxetine are inhibitors of CYP2D6.
>
> ✓ Paroxetine should be avoided during pregnancy due to the risk of cardiac malformations.
>
> ✓ SSRIs are widely studied and utilized in pregnancy but have been linked to rare cases of persistent pulmonary hypertension of the newborn (PPHN) and other adverse effects.

Mechanism of Action
- Selectively inhibits reuptake of serotonin by serotonin transporter, prolonging serotonergic neurotransmission.

Primary Net Benefit
- First-line pharmacotherapy for depression and many anxiety disorders as they have improved safety compared to conventional antidepressants, such as TCA and MAO inhibitors.
- Except for citalopram and escitalopram, these agents have a large therapeutic index.

High-Yield Basic Pharmacology
- Serotonin and Norepinephrine Transporters
    - SSRIs, despite their name, have weak norepinephrine and dopamine receptor-modulating effects.
    - May have effects on muscarinic, histaminic, or alpha receptors to a much lesser extent than serotonin.
    - Fluoxetine possesses serotonin and norepinephrine reuptake transporter inhibition effects, and sertraline exhibits dopamine reuptake transporter inhibition and binds at sigma 1 receptors.

High-Yield Clinical Knowledge
- First-Line Antidepressants
    - SSRIs are considered first-line agents for treating major depression and many anxiety disorders due to improved tolerability and safety, particularly after overdose, compared to conventional antidepressants (TCAs or MAOIs).
    - There is no definitive therapeutic difference between the SSRIs, but agent selection is based upon drug interactions, pharmacokinetics, pharmacogenetics, cost, and patient clinical response or adverse effects.
- Pearls
    - Citalopram: Lower max dose in elderly, hepatic impairment, or poor 2C19 metabolizers, dose dependant QT prolongation
    - Escitalopram: Lower max dose in elderly, good tolerability, s-enantiomer of citalopram, dose dependant QT prolongation.

- Fluoxetine: longest half-life (2-4 days for fluoxetine, 7-9 for metabolite), may cause activation which can be helpful in those with low energy, fatigue, or non-adherence.
- Paroxetine: most anticholinergic (drying, constipation) and histaminic (weight gain, sedation), evidence for use for vasomotor symptoms of menopause.
- Sertraline: good efficacy and tolerability, best documented cardiovascular safety, currently a preferred agent in pregnancy.
- **Dosing, Dosage Forms, and/or Administration**
  - Approximate dose equivalents: citalopram 20 mg = escitalopram 10 mg = fluoxetine 20 mg = fluvoxamine 75 mg = paroxetine 20 mg = sertraline 50 mg.
- **Treatment Effect**
  - Takes 4-8 weeks to see the full treatment effect, although some symptoms may improve faster.
  - With GAD, start with lower doses and titrate, but higher doses may be needed.
    - Therapeutic benefits may also be delayed (8-12 weeks).
- **Contraindications**
  - Use of a MAOI within 14 days.
- **Warnings**
  - Impaired cognitive performance, QT prolongation (greatest risk with citalopram and escitalopram), history of hepatic impairment, history of seizure (lowers threshold).
- **Boxed Warnings**
  - Increased risk of suicidality in pediatric to young adult patients (up to age 25).
  - Close monitoring is required in all antidepressant-treated patients for clinical worsening and for the emergence of suicidal thoughts and behaviors.
- **Adverse Effects**
  - **Acute phase side effects:** Agitation, anxiety, jitteriness, insomnia, sleep disturbances, sexual dysfunction, headache, nausea, vomiting, decreased appetite, GI distress, sweating, tremors, flushing, dizziness, drowsiness, sedation.
    - Generally, these effects go away with continued treatment so a wait-and-watch approach, supportive care, or a change in medication may be trialed.
  - **Long-term use side effects:** Weight gain, sleep disturbances, apathy, fatigue, lethargy, sexual dysfunction, diarrhea, SIADH or hyponatremia.
    - Generally switching to a more tolerable medication or adding an agent to target the symptom is done in practice to increase tolerability.
  - **Excess Serotonin Effects:** SSRIs increase serotonergic tone throughout the body, causing various effects, specifically GI distress early after initiation, but they usually resolve after one week of treatment. Excess serotonergic activity has also been associated with diminished sexual function and drive.
  - **Serotonin Syndrome:** Serotonin syndrome is the combination of a rapid onset of altered mental status, autonomic instability, hyperthermia, and hyperreflexia/myoclonus.
    - Risk increases with additional drugs that increase serotonin levels.
    - Although SSRIs have been implicated in serotonin syndrome, other antidepressants, including MAO inhibitors, are more likely to contribute to serotonin toxicity.
    - Treatment of serotonin syndrome involves the management of hyperthermia through invasive or noninvasive cooling, skeletal muscle relaxation using benzodiazepines, and airway support.
    - Dantrolene and cyproheptadine have been suggested as adjuncts for managing serotonin syndrome but are of questionable patient-oriented benefit.
  - Withdrawal
    - To avoid drug discontinuation syndrome, antidepressants should not be abruptly discontinued due to the risk of a sudden worsening of psychiatric symptoms, which can be worse than pre-treatment psychiatric disturbances.
    - "FINISH" for symptoms of discontinuation: flu-like symptoms, insomnia, nausea, imbalance, sensory disturbances, and hyperarousal.

- Slow tapering is necessary to avoid this withdrawal syndrome, but agents with prolonged half-lives and active metabolites (such as fluoxetine) may have a lower likelihood due to a self-tapering effect.
- **Antiplatelet Effect:** SSRIs increase available serotonin activity, which results in excess serotonin to inhibit platelet secretory response, platelet aggregation, and platelet plug formation and potentiate bleeding.
- **Mood changes:** Activation of mania/hypomania. Should not be used as monotherapy for bipolar depression
- **Movement Disorders:** SSRI use and its effect on serotonin and dopamine activity have been associated with the development of parkinsonism-like effects, including akathisia, dystonia, and myoclonus.
    - Although these effects are to a much lesser extent than with antipsychotic medications.
- **Dose-Dependent QT Prolongation**
    - Citalopram and escitalopram are associated with a dose-dependent increase in the QT interval.
    - To reduce Torsade de Pointes' risk, citalopram should be limited to a maximum of 20 mg/day for poor CYP2C19 metabolizers, presence of inhibitors, hepatic impairment, or those > 60 years old.
- **Sexual dysfunction** (decreased libido, inability to orgasm, erectile dysfunction, etc.)
    - More common with paroxetine and escitalopram than others
    - Can switch medication or augment with bupropion, mirtazapine, trazodone, or PDE-5i.
- **Syndrome of inappropriate antidiuretic hormone (SIADH):** SSRIs have been associated with SIADH and hyponatremia (especially in geriatric patients), which often require drug discontinuation.
- **Drug, Supplement, Food, and/or Disease Interactions**
    - Paroxetine and fluoxetine are strong inhibitors of CYP2D6 and can lead to clinically relevant drug interactions where sertraline, citalopram, and escitalopram are weak inhibitors.
    - Concomitant use of serotonergic agents.
    - Concomitant use of agents that impact coagulation/bleeding (NSAIDs, anticoagulants, antiplatelet agents)
- **Monitoring**
    - Weight, BMI.
    - Affect, behavior, mood, appetite, sleep, and suicidality.
    - Sodium levels in elderly due to risk of hyponatremia.
    - Liver function as medications require dose adjustments in declining hepatic function.
    - Renal function (citalopram, escitalopram, paroxetine) as they require renal dose adjustments.
- **Patient Education**
    - Medications should be taken as prescribed. The goal would be at least 80% adherence or more.
    - Medications should be titrated up slowly to a maximum tolerated dose & tapered slowly to discontinue
    - **Pregnancy Considerations**
        - Preconception planning is paramount in women of childbearing age.
        - SSRIs are recommended as first-line agents during pregnancy if therapy requires continuation with sertraline being most preferred.
        - Persistent pulmonary hypertension of the newborn has been reported with SSRI exposure.
        - Adverse effects in the newborn following SSRI exposure late in the third trimester may include apnea, crying, cyanosis, feeding difficulty, hyperreflexia, hypotonia, hypertonia, hypoglycemia, irritability, jitteriness, respiratory distress, required or prolonged hospitalization, seizures, temperature instability, tremor, and vomiting.
        - Paroxetine has been associated with cardiac malformations and is recommended by most data sources to be avoided.

High-Yield Core Evidence
- **SADHEART**
    - This was a multicenter, double-blind, placebo-controlled study of patients who were randomized to receive either sertraline or placebo to evaluate the safety and efficacy of sertraline on MDD in patients hospitalized for acute MI or unstable angina and free of other life-threatening medical conditions.
    - There was no difference between treatments concerning the primary safety outcome (change in LVEF).

- Furthermore, there was no difference in the secondary safety measures, including a treatment-emergent increase in ventricular premature complexes, QTc interval greater than 450 milliseconds at the endpoint, or other cardiac measures.
- However, more patients randomized to placebo experienced severe CV adverse events.
- Conversely, patients receiving sertraline had a significantly improved CGI-I score compared to placebo, but there was no significant difference in the HAM-D assessment.
- The authors concluded that sertraline is a safe and effective treatment for recurrent depression in patients with recent MI or unstable angina and without other life-threatening medical conditions.
- JAMA. 2002 Aug 14;288(6):701-9.
- **TORDIA**
  - This was a multicenter, blinded trial of adolescent patients with SSRI-resistant depression who were randomized to an alternative SSRI or venlafaxine or medication switch and cognitive-behavioral therapy.
  - There was no difference between treatment arms concerning the primary outcome of remission and relapse.
  - The likelihood of remission was much higher, and the time to remission was much faster among those who had already demonstrated clinical response by week 12.
  - The authors concluded that continued treatment for depression among treatment-resistant adolescents results in remission in approximately one-third of patients, similar to adults.
  - Am J Psychiatry. 2010 Jul;167(7):782-91.

High-Yield Fast-Facts
- **CYP2D6 and CYP2C19 Polymorphisms**
  - Most SSRIs are substrates of CYP2D6 and/or CYP2C19 and are subject to pharmacogenomic variability, leading to drug exposure changes.

HIGH-YIELD BOARD EXAM ESSENTIALS
- **CLASSIC AGENTS:** Citalopram, escitalopram, fluoxetine, paroxetine, sertraline.
- **DRUG CLASS:** SSRI
- **INDICATIONS:** Bipolar depression (adjunct), GAD, MDD, OCD, panic disorder, premenstrual dysphoric disorder, social anxiety disorder, treatment-resistant depression, vasomotor symptoms of menopause
- **MECHANISM:** Inhibits the reuptake of serotonin by the serotonin transporter, prolonging serotonergic neurotransmission.
- **SIDE EFFECTS:** Akathisia, dystonia, myoclonus, SIADH, QT prolongation (citalopram, escitalopram), sexual dysfunction (e.g., decreased libido, inability to orgasm, etc), weight gain (paroxetine)
- **CLINICAL PEARLS:**
  - Except for citalopram and escitalopram which can cause dose dependent increases in the QT interval, this drug class has a large therapeutic index.
  - The onset of clinical benefit can take up to 4-6 weeks or longer depending on the indication and titration rate.
  - Paroxetine use during pregnancy should be avoided if possible; sertraline is considered preferred.
  - Paroxetine and fluoxetine are strong inhibitors of CYP2D6 and can lead to clinically relevant drug interactions of substrates of CYP2D6.
  - Serotonin syndrome is the combination of a rapid onset of altered mental status, autonomic instability, hyperthermia, and hyperreflexia/myoclonus. Risk increases with serotonergic drugs.

Table: Drug Class Summary

Selective Serotonin Reuptake Inhibitors - Drug Class Review
High-Yield Med Reviews

Mechanism of Action: *Inhibits the reuptake of serotonin by the serotonin transporter, prolonging serotonergic neurotransmission.*

Class Effects: *First-line pharmacotherapy for MDD and others with improved safety compared to conventional antidepressants, various effects on weight or sexual dysfunction, may require 4-8 weeks to see treatment effect*

Generic Name	Brand Name	Main Indication(s) or Uses	Notes
Citalopram	Celexa	- Major depressive disorder	- **Dosing (Adult):** 　- Oral: 10-40 mg daily 　　- Max 20 mg/day for poor CYP2C19 metabolizers, presence of inhibitors, hepatic impairment, or those > 60 years - **Dosing (Peds):** 　- Oral: 5-40 mg daily - **CYP450 Interactions:** CYP2C19, 2D6, 3A4 substrate; CYP2D6 inhibitor - **Renal or Hepatic Dose Adjustments:** 　- CrCl < 20 mL/minute: use caution 　- Child-Pugh class B or C: max 20 mg/day - **Dosage Forms:** Oral (solution, tablet)
Escitalopram	Lexapro	- Generalized anxiety disorder - Major depressive disorder	- **Dosing (Adult):** 　- Oral: 5-30 mg daily - **Dosing (Peds):** 　- Oral: 2.5-30 mg daily - **CYP450 Interactions:** CYP2C19, 3A4 substrate; CYP2D6 inhibitor - **Renal or Hepatic Dose Adjustments:** 　- CrCl < 20 mL/minute: initial 5 mg 　- Child-Pugh class B or C: max 10 mg/day - **Dosage Forms:** Oral (solution, tablet)
Fluoxetine	Prozac Sarafem	- Bipolar major depression - Bulimia nervosa - Major depressive disorder - Obsessive-compulsive disorder - Panic disorder - Premenstrual dysphoric disorder - Treatment-resistant depression	- **Dosing (Adult):** 　- Oral: 10-80 mg daily - **Dosing (Peds):** 　- Oral: 0.25 mg/kg/dose or 5 mg/dose 　　- Max 20 mg/day - **CYP450 Interactions:** CYP1A2, 2B6, 2C19, 2C9, 2D6, 2E1, 3A4 substrate; CYP2C19, 2D6 inhibitor - **Renal or Hepatic Dose Adjustments:** 　- Cirrhosis or Chronic Liver Disease: decrease dose by 50% - **Dosage Forms:** Oral (capsule, solution, tablet)

Selective Serotonin Reuptake Inhibitors - Drug Class Review High-Yield Med Reviews				
Generic Name	**Brand Name**	**Main Indication(s) or Uses**	**Notes**
Fluvoxamine	Luvox	<ul><li>Bulimia nervosa</li><li>Major depressive disorder</li><li>Panic disorder</li><li>Post-traumatic stress disorder</li><li>Social anxiety disorder</li></ul>	<ul><li>**Dosing (Adult):** — Oral: 50-300 mg daily</li><li>**Dosing (Peds):** — Oral: 25-300 mg daily</li><li>**CYP450 Interactions:** CYP1A2, 2D6 substrate; CYP1A2, 2C19, 2C9, 2D6, 3A4 inhibitor</li><li>**Renal or Hepatic Dose Adjustments:** — Cirrhosis or Chronic Liver Disease: decrease dose by 50%</li><li>**Dosage Forms:** Oral (capsule, tablet)</li></ul>
Paroxetine	Paxil Paxil CR	<ul><li>Anxiety disorder</li><li>Major depressive disorder</li><li>Obsessive-compulsive disorder</li><li>Panic disorder</li><li>PTSD</li><li>Premenstrual dysphoric disorder</li><li>Social anxiety disorder</li><li>Vasomotor symptoms of menopause</li></ul>	<ul><li>**Dosing (Adult):** — Oral: 10-100 mg daily</li><li>**Dosing (Peds):** — Oral: 5-60 mg daily; Max 60 mg/day</li><li>**CYP450 Interactions:** CYP2D6 substrate; CYP2D6 inhibitor</li><li>**Renal or Hepatic Dose Adjustments:** — CrCl < 30 mL/min or Child-Pugh class C: max 40 mg/day</li><li>**Dosage Forms:** Oral (capsule, suspension, tablet)</li></ul>
Sertraline	Zoloft	<ul><li>Major depressive disorder</li><li>Obsessive-compulsive disorder</li><li>Panic disorder</li><li>Post-traumatic stress disorder</li><li>Premenstrual dysphoric disorder</li><li>Social anxiety disorder</li></ul>	<ul><li>**Dosing (Adult):** — Oral: 25-200 mg daily</li><li>**Dosing (Peds):** — Oral: 12.5-200 mg daily</li><li>**CYP450 Interactions:** CYP2B6, 2C19, 2C9, 2D6, 3A4 substrate; Inhibits CYP2D6</li><li>**Renal or Hepatic Dose Adjustments:** — Child-Pugh class A or B: reduce dose by 50%; Class C: Not recommended</li><li>**Dosage Forms:** Oral (concentrate, tablet)</li></ul>

PSYCHIATRY – TRICYCLIC ANTIDEPRESSANTS (TCA)

Drug Class
- **Tricyclic Antidepressants**
- **Agents:**
    - Chronic Care
        - Amitriptyline
        - Amoxapine
        - Clomipramine
        - Desipramine
        - Doxepin
        - Imipramine
        - Nortriptyline
        - Protriptyline
        - Trimipramine

 Fast Facts
- While TCAs are largely not used as much in clinically practice for the treatment of depression due to concerns about safety and side effects, at lower doses they are useful for treating neuropathic pain.

Main Indications or Uses
- **Chronic Care**
    - Fibromyalgia
    - Insomnia
    - Major depressive disorder
    - Migraine prophylaxis
    - Neuropathic pain
    - Obsessive-compulsive disorder
    - Panic disorder

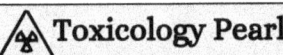 **Toxicology Pearl**
- At higher doses or concentrations, TCAs can inhibit Na+ channels in the heart and cause widening of the QRS interval. They can also inhibit Na+ channels in the CNS and eventually cause seizures.

Mechanism of Action
- Inhibit presynaptic reuptake of norepinephrine or serotonin, increasing their concentration at CNS receptors.

Primary Net Benefit
- TCAs were some of the first pharmacologic interventions for depression but are primarily reserved for resistant depression or alternative uses due to newer drug classes with improved safety.
- Main Labs to Monitor:
    - Liver enzymes and liver function (baseline and as clinically indicated)
    - Serum electrolytes (baseline and as clinically indicated)
    - ECG (baseline and as clinically indicated)
    - Blood glucose (baseline and as clinically indicated)

High-Yield Basic Pharmacology
- **Secondary or Tertiary Amine**
    - The presence or absence of a methyl group on the amine sidechain of tricyclic antidepressants classifies them as either a secondary or tertiary amine.
        - Secondary amines include amoxapine, desipramine, nortriptyline, and protriptyline.
        - Tertiary amines include amitriptyline, clomipramine, doxepin, imipramine, and trimipramine.
- **Serotonin Vs. Norepinephrine**
    - Tertiary amines are primarily inhibitors of serotonin reuptake, whereas secondary amines are more potent norepinephrine reuptake inhibitors.
- **Active Metabolites**
    - Some tertiary amines are metabolized to active compounds; for example, nortriptyline is an active metabolite of amitriptyline.

High-Yield Clinical Knowledge

- **Sodium Channel Blockade**
  - TCAs inhibit the cardiac fast sodium channels, slowing phase 0 depolarization, which manifests as QRS prolongation.
  - This QRS prolongation represents a slowing of the propagation of ventricular depolarization, leading to ventricular dysrhythmias.
  - This effect is similar to the Vaughn Williams class 1A antiarrhythmic agents.
- **Characteristic Adverse Events**
  - Compared to SSRIs, TCAs are more likely to cause antimuscarinic adverse events, sedation, orthostatic hypotension, and weight gain.
  - Antimuscarinic effects of TCAs can acutely worsen memory or cause delirium in elderly patients.
- **Sudden Cardiac Death**
  - As a result of sodium channel blockade and potential QT prolongation, TCAs may lead to sudden cardiac death.
    - An FDA warning on desipramine specifically exists regarding this increased risk of cardiac death.
- **Amoxapine**
  - Amoxapine is technically a cyclic antidepressant but is derived from the antipsychotic loxapine and acts as a norepinephrine reuptake inhibitor and dopamine antagonist.
- **Alternative Mechanisms**
  - TCAs possess numerous other mechanisms of action that more largely contribute to adverse effects or toxicity compared to efficacy.
  - TCAs possess antimuscarinic effects, peripheral alpha-1 antagonist effects, histamine-1 antagonist effects, GABA-A receptor antagonist effects, and cardiac sodium channel blockade.
- **Sodium Bicarbonate Use For Toxicity**
  - For TCA overdose or toxicity where clinically relevant ECG changes occur (QRS prolongation more significant than 100 ms), sodium bicarbonate is recommended.
  - Since TCAs are weak bases, this could hypothetically decrease their renal elimination, but sodium is needed to overcome cardiac sodium channel blockade.
  - Altering the plasma's pH to approximately 7.5 promotes the TCA movement away from the cardiac sodium channel and into the lipid membrane.
    - If patients are alkalemic or hypercarbic without appropriate ventilation, hypertonic sodium chloride can also be used as an alternative to sodium bicarbonate.

High-Yield Core Evidence

- **Mirtazapine Vs. Nortriptyline - STAR*D**
  - This was a publication describing the subgroup from the STAR*D trial in which patients had either mirtazapine or nortriptyline added to their treatment for nonpsychotic MDD.
  - Specifically, these patients had not achieved the therapeutic response following citalopram (step 1), followed by either increased citalopram or the addition of bupropion (step 2).
  - There was no significant difference between these therapies concerning the primary outcome of symptom remission based on the Hamilton Rating Scale for Depression.
  - Similarly, there was no difference in the secondary efficacy outcome of a change in QIDS-SR score (self-report of depressive symptoms) and no difference in safety events and tolerability.
  - The authors concluded that switching to a third antidepressant monotherapy regimen after two consecutive antidepressant trials resulted in low remission rates among MDD patients. (Am J Psychiatry. 2006;163(7):1161–1172.)

High-Yield Fast-Facts
- **Neurologic Toxicity**
  - TCAs may cause seizures in large exposures.
  - When the QRS is above 120 ms, the risk of seizures from TCAs is exceptionally high.
- **Drug Discontinuation Syndrome**
  - Like SSRIs and SNRIs, TCAs are associated with drug discontinuation syndrome when abruptly halted.
  - Symptoms can range from GI disturbance to psychosis and mania.

HIGH-YIELD BOARD EXAM ESSENTIALS
- **CLASSIC AGENTS:** Amitriptyline, amoxapine, clomipramine, desipramine, doxepin, imipramine, nortriptyline, protriptyline, trimipramine
- **DRUG CLASS:** TCA
- **INDICATIONS:** Fibromyalgia, major depressive disorder, migraine prophylaxis, neuropathic pain, obsessive-compulsive disorder, panic disorder
- **MECHANISM:** Inhibit presynaptic reuptake of norepinephrine or serotonin, increasing their concentration at CNS receptors.
- **SIDE EFFECTS:** Sedation, orthostatic hypotension, weight gain, QRS/QT prolongation, seizures
- **CLINICAL PEARLS:** TCAs inhibit the cardiac fast sodium channels, slowing the phase 0 depolarization, which manifests as QRS prolongation.

Table: Drug Class Summary

Tricyclic Antidepressants - Drug Class Review High-Yield Med Reviews			
Mechanism of Action: Inhibit presynaptic reuptake of norepinephrine or serotonin, increasing their concentration at CNS receptors.			
Class Effects: Mainly for resistant depression or alternative uses (neuropathic pain, migraines, and ADHD), drowsiness, weight gain, antimuscarinic effects, QT prolongation			
Generic Name	**Brand Name**	**Main Indication(s) or Uses**	**Notes**

Amitriptyline	Elavil	• Fibromyalgia
		• Major depressive disorder
		• Migraine prophylaxis
		• Neuropathic pain
			• **Dosing (Adult):**
			   – Oral: 10 to 300 mg daily
			• **Dosing (Peds):**
			   – Oral: 1 to 1.5 mg/kg/day in 3 divided doses
			   – Oral: 10 to 200 mg/day
			• **CYP450 Interactions:** CYP1A2, 2B6, 2C19, 2C9, 2D6, 3A4 substrate
			• **Renal or Hepatic Dose Adjustments:** None
			• **Dosage Forms:** Oral (tablet)

Amoxapine	Asendin	• Major depressive disorder	• **Dosing (Adult):**
			   – Oral: 25 to 600 mg/day
			     – Outpatient max 400 mg/day
			     – Inpatient max 600 mg/day
			• **Dosing (Peds):**
			   – Not routinely used
			• **CYP450 Interactions:** CYP2D6 substrate
			• **Renal or Hepatic Dose Adjustments:**
			   – Hepatic impairment: reduce dose by 50%
			• **Dosage Forms:** Oral (tablet)

Clomipramine	Anafranil	• Obsessive-compulsive disorder
		• Major depressive disorder
		• Panic disorder
			• **Dosing (Adult):**
			   – Oral: 25 to 250 mg/day
			• **Dosing (Peds):**
			   – Oral: 3 mg/kg/day or 100 mg/day, whichever is less
			• **CYP450 Interactions:** CYP1A2, 2C19, 2D6, 3A4 substrate
			• **Renal or Hepatic Dose Adjustments:**
			   – Hepatic impairment: reduce dose by 50%
			• **Dosage Forms:** Oral (capsule)

Desipramine	Norpramin	• Major depressive disorder	• **Dosing (Adult):**
			   – Oral: 25 to 300 mg/day
			• **Dosing (Peds):**
			   – Oral: 1.5 mg/kg/day divided q12h
			     – Max 3.5 mg/kg/day or 150 mg/day
			• **CYP450 Interactions:** CYP1A2, 2D6 substrate
			• **Renal or Hepatic Dose Adjustments:** None
			• **Dosage Forms:** Oral (tablet)

Tricyclic Antidepressants - Drug Class Review
High-Yield Med Reviews

Generic Name	Brand Name	Main Indication(s) or Uses	Notes

Doxepin	Silenor	- Insomnia
		- Major depressive disorder
			- **Dosing (Adult):**
			  – Oral: 3 to 50 mg/day
			- **Dosing (Peds):**
			  – Oral: 1 to 3 mg/kg/day; Max 300 mg/day
			- **CYP450 Interactions:** CYP1A2, 2C19, 2D6, 3A4 substrate
			- **Renal or Hepatic Dose Adjustments:**
			  – Hepatic impairment: reduce dose by 50%
			- **Dosage Forms:** Oral (capsule, concentrate, tablet)

Imipramine	Tofranil	- Major depressive disorder
		- Neuropathic pain
		- Panic disorder
			- **Dosing (Adult):**
			  – Oral: 25 to 300 mg/day
			- **Dosing (Peds):**
			  – Oral: 1 to 4 mg/kg/day or max 200mg/day
			- **CYP450 Interactions:** CYP1A2, 2B6, 2C19, 2D6, 3A4 substrate
			- **Renal or Hepatic Dose Adjustments:**
			  – Hepatic impairment: reduce dose by 50%
			- **Dosage Forms:** Oral (capsule, tablet)

Nortriptyline	Pamelor	- Major depressive disorder
		- Neuropathic pain
			- **Dosing (Adult):**
			  – Oral: 25 to 150 mg/day
			- **Dosing (Peds):**
			  – Oral: 0.5 to 2 mg/kg/day or 100 mg/day, whichever is less
			- **CYP450 Interactions:** CYP1A2, 2C19, 2D6, 3A4 substrate
			- **Renal or Hepatic Dose Adjustments:**
			  – Hepatic impairment: reduce dose by 50%
			- **Dosage Forms:** Oral (capsule, solution)

Protriptyline	Vivactil	- Major depressive disorder	- **Dosing (Adult):**
			  – Oral: 10 to 60 mg/day in 3-4 divided doses
			- **Dosing (Peds):**
			  – Oral: 5 to 60 mg/day in 3-4 divided doses
			- **CYP450 Interactions:** CYP2D6 substrate
			- **Renal or Hepatic Dose Adjustments:**
			  – Hepatic impairment: reduce dose by 50%
			- **Dosage Forms:** Oral (tablet)

Trimipramine	Surmontil	- Major depressive disorder	- **Dosing (Adult):**
			  – Oral: 25 to 300 mg/day
			- **Dosing (Peds):**
			  – Oral: 25 to 200 mg/day
			- **CYP450 Interactions:** CYP2C19, 2D6 substrate
			- **Renal or Hepatic Dose Adjustments:**
			  – Hepatic impairment: reduce dose by 50%
			- **Dosage Forms:** Oral (capsule)

PSYCHIATRY – ANTIPSYCHOTICS FIRST GENERATION

Drug Class
- Antipsychotics First Generation
- Agents:
  - Acute Care
    - Chlorpromazine
    - Droperidol
    - Haloperidol
    - Prochlorperazine
  - Chronic Care
    - Chlorpromazine
    - Droperidol
    - Fluphenazine
    - Haloperidol
    - Loxapine
    - Perphenazine
    - Prochlorperazine
    - Thioridazine
    - Thiothixene
    - Trifluoperazine

Main Indications or Uses
- Acute Care
  - Agitation
- Chronic Care
  - Bipolar disorder
  - Hiccups
  - Hyperactivity
  - Nausea, vomiting
  - Schizophrenia

> **Fast Facts**
> - First-generation or typical antipsychotics are more commonly associated with causing tardive dyskinesia with chronic use.
> - Haloperidol decanoate formulation is a "depot" injection that can be given every 2-4 weeks for compliance.
> - Chlorpromazine is the drug of choice for intractable hiccups.
> - Loxapine is uniquely available in an inhalation dosage form which may be helpful for compliance in those patients who smoke and feel more comfortable with that gesture.
> - Prochlorperazine (Compazine) is a common and effective antiemetic agent that can also be effective in treating acute migraine headaches in combination with other treatments.

Mechanism of Action
- Dopamine antagonist action at D2 receptors, blocking excess signaling in the mesolimbic and mesocortical pathways.

Primary Overall Net Benefit
- Useful in managing schizophrenia but offset by adverse effects leading to intolerance or permanent neurologic and psychiatric dysfunction.
- Main Labs to Monitor:
  - Strongly consider CYP2D6 testing
  - ECG

High-Yield Basic Pharmacology
- Dopamine Receptors
  - Although the principle pathophysiology of schizophrenia involves the D2 receptor pathway, other dopamine receptors (D1 through D5) have been identified.
  - The D2-like receptors include the D3 and D4 receptors, whereas the D1 receptors are closely related to the D5 receptors.
    - Dopamine receptors other than D2 do not appear to play a significant role in the current understanding of schizophrenia pathophysiology.

- **Alpha-Antagonists**
    - The first-generation antipsychotics block peripheral alpha-1 receptors to varying degrees and may cause orthostatic hypotension.
        - Chlorpromazine and fluphenazine are more likely to cause vasodilation and clinically relevant blood pressure changes than other antipsychotics, including haloperidol.
- **Muscarinic Antagonists**
    - Anticholinergic adverse events such as dry mouth, urinary retention, constipation, hypotension, and altered mental status are prevalent among the low-potency antipsychotic agents (chlorpromazine, thioridazine)

High-Yield Clinical Knowledge
- **Extrapyramidal Symptoms (EPS)**
    - EPS consists of acute dystonia, parkinsonism, akathisia, and the more severe tardive dyskinesia and neuroleptic malignant syndrome.
    - Antipsychotic agents that are more selective for the mesolimbic system are less likely to cause EPS effects.
    - High-potency antipsychotics are more likely to cause EPS but less likely to possess anticholinergic activity.
    - Conversely, low-potency antipsychotics are less likely to cause EPS but possess more anticholinergic and alpha-adrenergic antagonist activity.
- **CYP2D6**
    - Most antipsychotics are hepatically metabolized by CYP2D6, potentially leading to clinically relevant drug metabolism changes in patients with polymorphisms causing dysfunction in this oxidation pathway.
    - Numerous agents, including chlorpromazine, fluphenazine, haloperidol, loxapine, perphenazine, and thioridazine (as well as some atypical agents), are metabolized CYP2D6.
    - Among Caucasian patients, up to 25% have overexpression of CYP2D6, and 7% have functionally absent.
    - Genomic testing is suggested before starting these agents.
    - Drug interactions may also cause CYP2D6 inhibition, including commonly co-prescribed agents such as SSRI (fluoxetine, paroxetine) and bupropion.
- **Nausea and Vomiting**
    - Antipsychotics are commonly used in the acute treatment of nausea and vomiting, as dopamine receptors are present in the post-trauma area of the medulla, where the chemoreceptor trigger zone is located.
    - Other adverse effects of D2 antagonism in other areas of the brain include gynecomastia and galactorrhea (hypothalamic D2 antagonism) and parkinsonism (nigrostriatal D2 antagonism).
- **Cardiac Conduction**
    - Phenothiazine antipsychotics can cause cardiac sodium channel blockade and potassium channel blockade.
    - Although not typically relevant at standard therapeutic dosing, these effects may cause QRS and/or QT prolongation in the above therapeutic dosing or the presence of drug interactions.
        - On the one hand, the anticholinergic effects may be protective in the setting of QT prolongation, as tachycardia reduces the risk of torsade de pointes; however, it may exacerbate QRS prolongation related arrhythmias.
- **Sub-Classifications**
    - Antipsychotics are further subclassified according to their affinity for the D2 receptor, divided into low potency or high potency agents.
        - Low potency antipsychotics include chlorpromazine and thioridazine.
        - High-potency antipsychotics include fluphenazine, haloperidol, perphenazine, pimozide, and trifluoperazine.

High-Yield Core Evidence
- **CATIE**
  - This landmark multicenter, double-blind, parallel-group, controlled trial randomized patients with schizophrenia to receive olanzapine, perphenazine, quetiapine, risperidone, or ziprasidone.
  - Almost three-quarters (74%) of patients discontinued study medication before the targeted 18-month study period.
  - The time to discontinuation was significantly longer in patients receiving olanzapine compared to quetiapine or risperidone.
  - Olanzapine was associated with more discontinuation due to weight gain or metabolic effects, and perphenazine was associated with more discontinuation for extrapyramidal effects.
  - The authors concluded that among patients with schizophrenia, patients receiving olanzapine experienced a longer time to discontinuation compared with the other antipsychotic medications. Still, they experienced more significant weight gain, hyperglycemia, and hyperlipidemia. (N Engl J Med 2005; 353:1209-1223)
- **Droperidol and Nausea**
  - This was a randomized, placebo-controlled study that compared the effectiveness of droperidol 1.25 mg IV, ondansetron 8 mg IV, and saline placebo in adult emergency department patients with nausea.
  - There was no significant difference between droperidol, ondansetron, and placebo concerning the primary outcome of symptom improvement as defined by the visual analog scale rating change of -8 mm or more from baseline at 30 minutes posttreatment.
  - The authors concluded that superiority was not demonstrated for adult ED patients with nausea for droperidol or ondansetron over placebo. (Acad Emerg Med. 2019 Aug;26(8):867-877.)

High-Yield Fast-Facts
- **Hiccups**
  - Patients with intractable hiccups may benefit from using chlorpromazine 25 mg infused over 2-4 hours.
- **Droperidol Controversy**
  - Droperidol had all but disappeared from clinical practice following a black boxed warning for QT prolongation but is currently experiencing a renaissance in the treatment of nausea and vomiting.
- **ICU Delirium**
  - Haloperidol was once a mainstay in managing ICU delirium, but the therapy is mostly abandoned due to a questionable risk-benefit relationship.

HIGH-YIELD BOARD EXAM ESSENTIALS
- **CLASSIC AGENTS:** Chlorpromazine, droperidol, fluphenazine, haloperidol, loxapine, perphenazine, prochlorperazine, thioridazine, thiothixene, trifluoperazine
- **DRUG CLASS:** Antipsychotics first generation
- **INDICATIONS:** Agitation, bipolar disorder, hiccups, hyperactivity, nausea, vomiting, schizophrenia, tetanus
- **MECHANISM:** Dopamine antagonist action at D2 receptors, blocking excess signaling in the mesolimbic and mesocortical pathways.
- **SIDE EFFECTS:** Acute dystonia, parkinsonism, akathisia, QT prolongation
- **CLINICAL PEARLS:** Antipsychotics are commonly used in the acute treatment of nausea and vomiting, as dopamine receptors are present in the post trauma area of the medulla, where the chemoreceptor trigger zone is located.

Table: Drug Class Summary

Antipsychotics First Generation - Drug Class Review High-Yield Med Reviews			
Mechanism of Action: *Dopamine antagonist action at D2 receptors, blocking excess signaling in the mesolimbic and mesocortical pathways.*			
Class Effects: *Effective in managing schizophrenia but offset by adverse effects leading to intolerance or permanent neurologic and psychiatric dysfunction.*			
Generic Name	**Brand Name**	**Main Indication(s) or Uses**	**Notes**
Chlorpromazine	Thorazine	<ul><li>Agitation</li><li>Bipolar disorder</li><li>Hiccups</li><li>Hyperactivity</li><li>Nausea, vomiting</li><li>Schizophrenia</li><li>Tetanus</li></ul>	<ul><li>**Dosing (Adult):**<ul><li>Oral: 10 to 75 mg/day divided 3 to 4 times daily</li><ul><li>Up to 800 mg/day</li></ul><li>IM/IV: 25 mg q4-6h, up to 300 mg/day</li></ul></li><li>**Dosing (Peds):**<ul><li>Oral: 0.55 to 1 mg/kg/dose q6h</li><ul><li>Maximum 40 to 75 mg/day</li></ul></ul></li><li>**CYP450 Interactions:** Substrate CYP1A2, 2D6, 3A4</li><li>**Renal or Hepatic Dose Adjustments:** None</li><li>**Dosage Forms:** Oral (tablet), IV (solution)</li></ul>
Droperidol	Inapsine	<ul><li>Agitation</li><li>Nausea, vomiting</li></ul>	<ul><li>**Dosing (Adult):**<ul><li>IM/IV: 0.625 to 1.25 mg once</li></ul></li><li>**Dosing (Peds):**<ul><li>IM/IV: 0.01 to 0.015 mg/kg/dose</li><ul><li>Maximum 0.1 mg/kg/dose</li></ul></ul></li><li>**CYP450 Interactions:** None</li><li>**Renal or Hepatic Dose Adjustments:** None</li><li>**Dosage Forms:** IV (solution)</li></ul>
Fluphenazine	Prolixin	<ul><li>Psychosis</li></ul>	<ul><li>**Dosing (Adult):**<ul><li>Oral: 1 to 20 mg/day divided q6-24h</li><li>IM: 1.25 mg as needed, maximum 10 mg/day</li></ul></li><li>**Dosing (Peds):**<ul><li>Oral: 0.5 to 1 mg daily</li><ul><li>Maximum dose 24 mg/day</li></ul></ul></li><li>**CYP450 Interactions:** Substrate of CYP2D6</li><li>**Renal or Hepatic Dose Adjustments:** None</li><li>**Dosage Forms:** Oral (concentrate, elixir, tablet), IV (solution)</li></ul>

| Antipsychotics First Generation - Drug Class Review || |
| High-Yield Med Reviews || ||
Generic Name	Brand Name	Main Indication(s) or Uses	Notes
Haloperidol	Haldol	<ul><li>Agitation</li><li>Bipolar disorder</li><li>Hiccups</li><li>Hyperactivity</li><li>Nausea, vomiting</li><li>Schizophrenia</li></ul>	<ul><li>**Dosing (Adult):**<ul><li>Oral: 2 to 10 mg q6h as needed up to 30 mg/day</li><li>IM/IV: 2 to 20 mg q0.5-6h as needed</li></ul></li><li>**Dosing (Peds):**<ul><li>Oral: 0.5 to 15 mg/day or 0.05 to 0.075 mg/kg/day divided q8-12h<ul><li>Maximum 15 mg/day</li></ul></li><li>IM/IV: 0.025 to 0.1 mg/kg/dose q0.5-6h</li></ul></li><li>**CYP450 Interactions:** Substrate of CYP1A2, 2D6, 3A4</li><li>**Renal or Hepatic Dose Adjustments:** None</li><li>**Dosage Forms:** Oral (concentrate, elixir, tablet), IV (solution), IM decanoate</li></ul>
Loxapine	Adasuve	<ul><li>Agitation</li><li>Bipolar disorder</li><li>Schizophrenia</li></ul>	<ul><li>**Dosing (Adult):**<ul><li>Oral: 60 to 100 mg/day divided q6-12h<ul><li>Maximum 250 mg/day</li></ul></li><li>Inhalation: 10 mg once daily</li></ul></li><li>**Dosing (Peds):**<ul><li>Not routinely used</li></ul></li><li>**CYP450 Interactions:** Substrate of CYP1A2, 2D6, 3A4</li><li>**Renal or Hepatic Dose Adjustments:** None</li><li>**Dosage Forms:** Oral (capsule), Aerosol</li></ul>
Perphenazine	Trilafon	<ul><li>Nausea, vomiting</li><li>Schizophrenia</li></ul>	<ul><li>**Dosing (Adult):**<ul><li>Oral: 8 to 64 mg/day divided q6-12h</li></ul></li><li>**Dosing (Peds):**<ul><li>Oral: 8 to 64 mg/day divided q6-12h</li></ul></li><li>**CYP450 Interactions:** Substrate of CYP1A2, 2C9, 2C19, 2D6, 3A4</li><li>**Renal or Hepatic Dose Adjustments:** None</li><li>**Dosage Forms:** Oral (tablet)</li></ul>
Prochlorperazine	Compazine	<ul><li>Nausea, vomiting</li></ul>	<ul><li>**Dosing (Adult):**<ul><li>IM/IV/Oral: 2.5 to 10 mg q6-8h, maximum 40 mg/day</li><li>Rectal: 25 mg q12h</li></ul></li><li>**Dosing (Peds):**<ul><li>IM/IV/Oral: 0.1 to 0.15 mg/kg/dose q3-4h<ul><li>Maximum 10 mg/dose and 40 mg/day</li></ul></li></ul></li><li>**CYP450 Interactions:** None</li><li>**Renal or Hepatic Dose Adjustments:** None</li><li>**Dosage Forms:** Oral (tablet), IV (solution), Suppository</li></ul>

\multicolumn{4}{c}{**Antipsychotics First Generation - Drug Class Review**}
\multicolumn{4}{c}{High-Yield Med Reviews}
Generic Name	**Brand Name**	**Main Indication(s) or Uses**	**Notes**

Thioridazine	Mellaril	- Schizophrenia	- **Dosing (Adult):**
			   — Oral: 50 800 mg/day divided q6-12h
			- **Dosing (Peds):**
			   — Oral: 0.5 to 3 mg/kg/day divided q6-12h
			- **CYP450 Interactions:** Substrate of CYP2C19, 2D6; Inhibits CYP2D6
			- **Renal or Hepatic Dose Adjustments:** None
			- **Dosage Forms:** Oral (tablet)

Thiothixene	Navane	- Schizophrenia	- **Dosing (Adult):**
			   — Oral: 2 to 20 mg q8h, maximum 60 mg/day
			- **Dosing (Peds):**
			   — Oral: 2 to 20 mg q8h, maximum 60 mg/day
			- **CYP450 Interactions:** Substrate of CYP1A2
			- **Renal or Hepatic Dose Adjustments:** None
			- **Dosage Forms:** Oral (capsule)

Trifluoperazine	Stelazine	- Schizophrenia	- **Dosing (Adult):**
			   — Oral: 2 to 25 mg q12h, maximum 50 mg/day
			- **Dosing (Peds):**
			   — Oral: 2 to 25 mg q12h, maximum 40 mg/day
			- **CYP450 Interactions:** None
			- **Renal or Hepatic Dose Adjustments:** None
			- **Dosage Forms:** Oral (tablet)

PSYCHIATRY – ANTIPSYCHOTICS SECOND GENERATION (ATYPICAL ANTIPSYCHOTICS)

Drug Class
- Antipsychotics Second Generation (Atypical Antipsychotics)
- Agents:
  - Acute Care
    - Olanzapine
    - Ziprasidone
  - Chronic Care
    - Aripiprazole
    - Asenapine
    - Brexpiprazole
    - Cariprazine
    - Clozapine
    - Iloperidone
    - Lumateperone
    - Lurasidone
    - Olanzapine
    - Paliperidone
    - Pimavanserin
    - Quetiapine
    - Risperidone
    - Ziprasidone

Main Indications or Uses
- Acute Care
  - Agitation
    - Olanzapine
    - Ziprasidone
- Chronic Care
  - Autistic disorder irritability
  - Bipolar disorder
  - Major depressive disorder
  - Schizophrenia
  - Tourette disorder

Mechanism of Action
- Dopamine antagonist action at D2 receptors, blocking excess signaling in the mesolimbic and mesocortical pathways.

Primary Net Benefit
- Atypical antipsychotic therapy may improve safety compared to "typical" antipsychotics and aims to reduce psychiatric disease symptoms while enhancing the quality of life and daily functioning.
- Main Labs to Monitor:
  - Clozapine
    - Weekly CBC x 6 months, then q2-3months
  - ECG at baseline
  - Strongly consider CYP2D6 testing

High-Yield Basic Pharmacology
- **Serotonn Antagonists**
  - Serotonin antagonist effects at the 5HT2 (5HT2A and 5HT2C receptors) cause dopamine release and increase sympathetic outflow from the locus coeruleus.
  - Antagonism of the 5HT2 receptors improved effectiveness in treating negative schizophrenia symptoms and significantly lowered EPS incidence.
    - Higher relative 5HT2 antagonist effects with weaker D2 antagonism is associated with a lower incidence of EPS symptoms, characteristic of the second-generation or atypical antipsychotics.
  - Other serotonin receptors have been identified as targets for antipsychotics, including the 5HT1, 5HT3, and 5-HT6 receptors.

> **Fast Facts**
>
> ✓ Second generation or atypical antipsychotics not only antagonize dopamine receptors but also modulate the activity of 5-HT (serotonin) receptors. This redistribution of receptor activity causes less tardive dyskinesia and also improves not only positive symptoms of schizophrenia but also negative symptoms. As such, they are the mainstay of treatment for schizophrenia.
>
> ✓ This class of drugs comes in a number of different dosage formulations to allow for patient specific treatment. This also includes the availability of immediate release and long-acting formulations.
>
> ✓ Clozapine and olanzapine are effective agents but come at a greater costs of more side effects to include weight gain, potential increases in glucose, and dyslipidemia.

- **Partial D2 Agonists**
  - Most atypical agents are equally potent antagonists of 5HT2 and D2 receptors, except for aripiprazole and brexpiprazole, which are partial agonists of D2 receptors.
- **Alpha Antagonists**
  - Atypical agents retain the peripheral alpha-1 antagonist activity of the first-generation antipsychotics.
  - This is a relevant effect in patients receiving parenteral olanzapine, or large doses of quetiapine for agitation management, significantly increasing their risk of falls.

High-Yield Clinical Knowledge
- **Clozapine Toxicity**
  - Clozapine is restricted to patients who have failed to respond to other antipsychotics as it carries a significant risk of agranulocytosis and seizures.
  - Although only 1-2% of patients on clozapine develop agranulocytosis, this potentially fatal effect necessitates weekly CBC during the first six months of therapy.
  - Seizures are another complication of clozapine therapy as it is an antagonist of GABA-A receptors.
    - Chlorpromazine also is a similarly potent GABA antagonist but often overlooked in clinical practice.
- **Neuroleptic Malignant Syndrome**
  - NMS results from abrupt reductions in dopamine neurotransmission in the hypothalamus and striatum, leading to modifying the body's core temperature regulation and autonomic dysfunction.
  - Manifestations of NMS include "lead-pipe" rigidity, hyperthermia, and altered mental status.
  - NMS is more likely to occur during dose adjustment of D2 antagonist agents, at the start of therapy, in the presence of dopaminergic agents, or idiosyncratic.
  - High potency antipsychotics and depot formulations of antipsychotics (including atypical agents) have also been associated with NMS onset.
  - Treatment of NMS is primarily focused on reducing hyperthermia by administering benzodiazepines to facilitate muscle relaxation and possibly bromocriptine or dantrolene, which are of questionable benefit.
    - For acutely hyperthermic patients, ice baths, extravascular and/or intravascular cooling may be required.
- **Reduced EPS**
  - The atypical antipsychotics are less likely to cause EPS than first-generation agents as they are less selective for the mesolimbic system and are less likely to cause EPS effects.
  - The atypical agents are also less likely to impact prolactin concentrations, thus having a relatively lower gynecomastia risk.
- **Acute Agitation**
  - The parenteral atypical antipsychotics olanzapine and ziprasidone offer a clinical tool for managing acutely agitated patients.
  - Although these agents may have a slightly longer onset of action than haloperidol, their use is associated with marginally improved behavioral responses.
  - Ziprasidone shared similar dose-dependent QT prolongation with haloperidol and extended or high doses should prompt ECG measurement.
- **Parkinsonism**
  - Like the underlying pathophysiology of Parkinson's disease, antipsychotics may cause a blockade of nigrostriatal D2 receptors, which is the cause of the movement disorders associated with antipsychotic therapy.
- **Overdose**
  - Overdoses of antipsychotic agents are relatively common, given the underlying psychiatric disease.
  - Underlying toxicologic management principles are consistent in these patients with assessment, GI decontamination, and supportive care.
  - Patients should have serial ECGs following the QRS and QT intervals with aggressive treatment with sodium bicarbonate for QRS more significant than 100 ms and adequate replacement of serum potassium and magnesium in patients with QT prolongation.
  - The potential use of physostigmine to manage anticholinergic delirium is possible but should be guided by expert toxicologic consultation.

High-Yield Core Evidence

- **Cariprazine for Acute Schizophrenia**
  - This phase 3, multinational, double-blind, placebo- and active-controlled study randomized patients with acute exacerbation of schizophrenia to receive either placebo, cariprazine 3 mg/day, cariprazine 6 mg/day, or aripiprazole 10 mg/day for six weeks.
  - Cariprazine at both 3mg and 6 mg daily significantly improved the primary and secondary efficacy parameters of the mean change from baseline to week 6 in Positive and Negative Syndrome Scale total score and Clinical Global Impressions-Severity of Illness score compared to placebo.
  - There was no significant difference between cariprazine compared to patients who received aripiprazole.
  - Treatment-emergent adverse events were similar among groups.
  - The authors concluded that this study supports the efficacy, safety, and tolerability of cariprazine 3 and 6 mg/d in treating patients with acute exacerbation of schizophrenia. (J Clin Psychiatry. 2015 Dec;76(12):e1574-82.)
- **Brexpiprazole in acute Schizophrenia**
  - This was a multicenter, double-blind, placebo-controlled study that randomized patients with schizophrenia experiencing an acute exacerbation to brexpiprazole 0.25, 2, or 4 mg or placebo for six weeks.
  - Patients randomized to any doses of 2 or 4 mg, but not 0.25 mg of brexpiprazole significantly improved change from baseline to week 6 in Positive and Negative Syndrome Scale total score, and Clinical Global Impressions Scale severity score compared to placebo.
  - Akathisia and weight gain occurred significantly more often in patients receiving brexpiprazole and appeared in a dose-dependent fashion.
  - The authors concluded that brexpiprazole at dosages of 2 and 4 mg/day demonstrated statistically significant efficacy compared with placebo and good tolerability for patients with an acute schizophrenia exacerbation. (Am J Psychiatry. 2015 Sep 1;172(9):870-80.)

High-Yield Fast-Facts

- **Risperidone Derivative**
  - Some agents are derivative metabolites of parent compounds, such as paliperidone, which is the active metabolite of risperidone.
- **Lipid Emulsion**
  - Some overdoses of antipsychotics can be treated with intravenous lipid emulsion to partition the offending agent into the lipid rather than in the CNS or cardiac tissue.

HIGH-YIELD BOARD EXAM ESSENTIALS
- **CLASSIC AGENTS:** Aripiprazole, asenapine, brexpiprazole, cariprazine, clozapine, iloperidone, lumateperone, lurasidone, olanzapine, paliperidone, pimavanserin, quetiapine, risperidone, ziprasidone
- **DRUG CLASS:** Atypical antipsychotics
- **INDICATIONS:** Autistic disorder irritability, bipolar disorder, major depressive disorder, schizophrenia, Tourette disorder
- **MECHANISM:** Dopamine antagonist action at D2 receptors, blocking excess signaling in the mesolimbic and mesocortical pathways.
- **SIDE EFFECTS:** Parkinsonism, NMS, anticholinergic effects, agranulocytosis (clozapine)
- **CLINICAL PEARLS:** The atypical antipsychotics are less likely to cause EPS than first-generation agents as they are less selective for the mesolimbic system and are less likely to cause EPS effects.

Table: Drug Class Summary

| | Antipsychotics Second Generation (Atypical Antipsychotics) - Drug Class Review High-Yield Med Reviews |

Mechanism of Action: *Dopamine antagonist action at D2 receptors, blocking excess signaling in the mesolimbic and mesocortical pathways.*

Class Effects: *Atypical antipsychotic therapy may improve safety compared to "typical" antipsychotics and reduce psychiatric disease symptoms while enhancing the quality of life and daily functioning.*

Generic Name	Brand Name	Main Indication(s) or Uses	Notes

Aripiprazole	Abilify	• Autistic disorder irritability
		• Bipolar disorder
		• Major depressive disorder
		• Schizophrenia
		• Tourette disorder
			• **Dosing (Adult):**
			  − Oral: 2 to 30 mg daily
			  − IM: 400 mg qmonth
			• **Dosing (Peds):**
			  − Oral: 1.25 to 15 mg daily
			• **CYP450 Interactions:** Substrate of CYP2D6, 3A4
			• **Renal or Hepatic Dose Adjustments:** None
			• **Dosage Forms:** Oral (solution, tablet), IM suspension

Asenapine	Saphris	• Bipolar disorder
		• Schizophrenia
			• **Dosing (Adult):**
			  − SL: 5 to 10 mg BID
			  − Patch: 3.8 mg/24hours daily to maximum 7.6 mg/24hour
			• **Dosing (Peds):**
			  − SL: 2.5 to 10 mg BID
			• **CYP450 Interactions:** Substrate of CYP1A2, 2D6, 3A4
			• **Renal or Hepatic Dose Adjustments:**
			  − Child-Pugh class C: Use contraindicated
			• **Dosage Forms:** Oral (sublingual tablet), Transdermal patch

Brexpiprazole	Rexulti	• Major depressive disorder
		• Schizophrenia
			• **Dosing (Adult):**
			  − Oral: 0.25 to 4 mg daily
			• **Dosing (Peds):**
			  − Not routinely used
			• **CYP450 Interactions:** Substrate of CYP2D6, 3A4
			• **Renal or Hepatic Dose Adjustments:**
			  − GFR < 60 mL/minute: maximum 3 mg/day
			  − Child-Pugh class C: maximum 3 mg/day
			• **Dosage Forms:** Oral (tablet)

Cariprazine	Vraylar	• Bipolar disorder
		• Schizophrenia
			• **Dosing (Adult):**
			  − Oral: 1.5 to 12 mg daily
			• **Dosing (Peds):**
			  − Not routinely used
			• **CYP450 Interactions:** Substrate of CYP2D6, 3A4
			• **Renal or Hepatic Dose Adjustments:**
			  − GFR < 30 mL/minute: use not recommended
			  − Child-Pugh class C: use not recommended
			• **Dosage Forms:** Oral (capsule)

\multicolumn{4}{c}{**Antipsychotics Second Generation (Atypical Antipsychotics) - Drug Class Review**}
\multicolumn{4}{c}{High-Yield Med Reviews}
Generic Name	**Brand Name**	**Main Indication(s) or Uses**	**Notes**

Clozapine	Clozaril	- Schizophrenia	- **Dosing (Adult):**
			  - Oral: 6.25 to 900 mg/day
			- **Dosing (Peds):**
			  - Oral: 6.25 to 400 mg/day
			- **CYP450 Interactions:** Substrate of CYP1A2, 2D6, 3A4
			- **Renal or Hepatic Dose Adjustments:** None
			- **Dosage Forms:** Oral (suspension, tablet)

Iloperidone	Fanapt	- Schizophrenia	- **Dosing (Adult):**
			  - Oral: 1 to 12 mg BID
			- **Dosing (Peds):**
			  - Not routinely used
			- **CYP450 Interactions:** Substrate of CYP2D6, 3A4; Inhibits CYP3A4
			- **Renal or Hepatic Dose Adjustments:**
			  - Child-Pugh class C: use not recommended
			- **Dosage Forms:** Oral (tablet)

Lumateperone	Caplyta	- Schizophrenia	- **Dosing (Adult):**
			  - Oral: 42 mg daily
			- **Dosing (Peds):**
			  - Not routinely used
			- **CYP450 Interactions:** Substrate of CYP1A2, 2D6, 3A4
			- **Renal or Hepatic Dose Adjustments:**
			  - Child-Pugh class B or C: use not recommended
			- **Dosage Forms:** Oral (capsule)

Lurasidone	Latuda	- Bipolar disorder
		- Schizophrenia
			- **Dosing (Adult):**
			  - Oral: 20 to 160 mg/day
			- **Dosing (Peds):**
			  - Oral: 20 to 160 mg/day
			- **CYP450 Interactions:** Substrate and Inhibitor of CYP3A4
			- **Renal or Hepatic Dose Adjustments:**
			  - GFR < 50 mL/minute: maximum 80 mg/day
			  - Child-Pugh class B or C: use not recommended
			- **Dosage Forms:** Oral (tablet)

Antipsychotics Second Generation (Atypical Antipsychotics) - Drug Class Review
High-Yield Med Reviews

Generic Name	Brand Name	Main Indication(s) or Uses	Notes
Olanzapine	Zyprexa	<ul><li>Agitation</li><li>Bipolar disorder</li><li>Major depressive disorder</li><li>Schizophrenia</li></ul>	<ul><li>**Dosing (Adult):**<ul><li>Oral: 2.5 to 10 mg daily</li><li>IM/IV: 2.5 to 10 mg x1 followed by two additional as needed doses of 1.25 to 5 mg</li></ul></li><li>**Dosing (Peds):**<ul><li>Oral: 0.625 to 10 mg daily</li><li>IM/IV: 1.25 to 10 mg x1 followed by two additional as needed doses of 1.25 to 5 mg</li></ul></li><li>**CYP450 Interactions:** Substrate of CYP1A2, 2D6, 3A4</li><li>**Renal or Hepatic Dose Adjustments:** None</li><li>**Dosage Forms:** Oral (tablet), IV solution, IM suspension</li></ul>
Paliperidone	Invega	<ul><li>Schizophrenia</li></ul>	<ul><li>**Dosing (Adult):**<ul><li>Oral: 6 to 12 mg daily</li><li>IM: 234 mg x1 then 156 mg monthly</li><li>Extra info if needed</li></ul></li><li>**Dosing (Peds):** [same as adult]<ul><li>Extra info if needed</li><li>Extra info if needed</li></ul></li><li>**CYP450 Interactions:** Substrate of P-gp</li><li>**Renal or Hepatic Dose Adjustments:**<ul><li>GFR: 50 to 79 mL/minute: maximum 6 mg; IM 156 mg followed by 117 mg, then 78 mg qmonth</li><li>GFR: 10 to 49 mL/minute: maximum 3 mg/day; IM use not recommended</li><li>GFR < 10 mL/minute : oral not recommended</li></ul></li><li>**Dosage Forms:** Oral (tablet), IM suspension</li></ul>
Pimavanserin	Nuplazid	<ul><li>Parkinson's disease</li></ul>	<ul><li>**Dosing (Adult):**<ul><li>Oral: 34 mg daily</li></ul></li><li>**Dosing (Peds):**<ul><li>Not routinely used</li></ul></li><li>**CYP450 Interactions:** Substrate of CYP3A4</li><li>**Renal or Hepatic Dose Adjustments:** None</li><li>**Dosage Forms:** Oral (capsule, tablet)</li></ul>

| \multicolumn{4}{c}{**Antipsychotics Second Generation (Atypical Antipsychotics) - Drug Class Review**} |

Generic Name	Brand Name	Main Indication(s) or Uses	Notes

Quetiapine	Seroquel	- Bipolar disorder
		- Major depressive disorder
		- Schizophrenia
			- **Dosing (Adult):**
			  – Oral: 50 to 1,200 mg/day
			- **Dosing (Peds):**
			  – Oral: 50 to 1,200 mg/day
			    – Children 10 years or older
			- **CYP450 Interactions:** Substrate CYP2D6, 3A4
			- **Renal or Hepatic Dose Adjustments:**
			  – Hepatic impairment: slower titration
			- **Dosage Forms:** Oral (tablet)

Risperidone	Risperdal	- Autistic disorder irritability
		- Bipolar disorder
		- Major depressive disorder
		- Schizophrenia
			- **Dosing (Adult):**
			  – Oral: 0.5 to 6 mg/day
			  – IM: 25 to 50 mg q2weeks
			  – SQ: 90 to 120 mg qmonth
			- **Dosing (Peds):**
			  – Oral: 0.25 to 3 mg/day
			- **CYP450 Interactions:** Substrate CYP2D6, 3A4, P-gp
			- **Renal or Hepatic Dose Adjustments:**
			  – Renal or hepatic impairment: slower dose titration
			- **Dosage Forms:** Oral (solution, tablet), IM suspension

Ziprasidone	Geodon	- Agitation
		- Bipolar disorder
		- Schizophrenia
			- **Dosing (Adult):**
			  – IM: 10 mg q2h or 20 mg q4h, maximum 40 mg/day
			  – Oral: 20 to 120 mg BID
			- **Dosing (Peds):** [same as adult]
			  – IM: 10 mg q2h or 20 mg q4h, maximum 40 mg/day
			  – Oral: 20 to 80 mg BID
			- **CYP450 Interactions:** Substrate CYP1A2, 3A4
			- **Renal or Hepatic Dose Adjustments:** None
			- **Dosage Forms:** Oral (capsule), IM solution

PSYCHIATRY – BUSPIRONE – ANXIOLYTIC - NONBENZODIAZEPINE

Drug Class
- Anxiolytic (Non-Benzodiazepine)
- Agents:
    - Chronic Care
        - Buspirone

 Fast Facts
- ✓ While buspirone is considered a nonbenzodiazepine anxiolytic, it should not be used for the acute management of anxiety since it has a delayed onset of clinical benefit of up to 2-3 weeks.

Main Indications or Uses
- Chronic Care
    - Anxiety (prevention or maintenance)

Mechanism of Action
- Buspirone
    - Unknown, but effects are mediated mainly through 5HT1A receptors with some affinity for 5HT2 receptors and DA2 autoreceptors.

Primary Net Benefit
- Mostly used as second-line pharmacotherapy for the prevention of anxiety especially when other standard treatments have not been sufficient.
- Main Labs to Monitor:
    - No routine lab monitoring

High-Yield Basic Pharmacology
- Buspirone Drug Interactions
    - Buspirone is a substrate of CYP3A4, with potential interactions with potent inhibitors (ketoconazole, itraconazole, fluvoxamine, verapamil, etc.), and inducers (phenytoin, phenobarbital, rifampin, St. John's wort).
    - Buspirone should not be combined with MAO inhibitors, as the risk of additive serotonergic effects is high.

High-Yield Clinical Knowledge
- Onset of Clinical Effect
    - Buspirone typically takes 2 to 3 weeks for a benefit.
        - As such, it should not be used as a "PRN" treatment or for acute anxiety.
- Tolerability
    - Generally well tolerated with very rare cases of dystonic reactions from its dopamine antagonism and serotonin syndrome due to its modulation of serotonin receptor activity.
- Anxiolytics in Elderly
    - Buspirone is a reasonable option for managing anxiolysis in the elderly, as it lacks excessive sedative properties and associated risk of delirium associated with benzodiazepines.

High-Yield Fast-Fact
- Abuse Potential
    - Based on its mechanism and known history since approval in 1986, it has a very low or little abuse potential.

HIGH-YIELD BOARD EXAM ESSENTIALS
- **CLASSIC AGENTS:** Buspirone
- **DRUG CLASS:** Anxiolytic (non-benzodiazepine)
- **INDICATIONS:** Anxiety disorder (chronic prevention)
- **MECHANISM:** Unknown, but effects are mediated mainly through 5HT1A receptors with some affinity for 5HT2 receptors and DA2 autoreceptors.
- **SIDE EFFECTS:** Dizziness
- **CLINICAL PEARLS:** Delayed onset of action/benefit. Should not be used for PRN or acute treatment.

Table: Drug Class Summary

Serotonin-Norepinephrine Reuptake Inhibitors & Buspirone - Drug Class Review			
High-Yield Med Reviews			
Mechanism of Action: Unknown, but effects are mediated mainly through 5HT1A receptors with some affinity for 5HT2 receptors and DA2 autoreceptors.			
Class Effects: Prevention of anxiety with chronic use; very little side effects or abuse potential			
Generic Name	**Brand Name**	**Main Indication(s) or Uses**	**Notes**

Buspirone	Buspirone	- General anxiety	- **Dosing (Adult):**
			   – Oral: 10 to 20 mg/day divided in 2-3 doses
			   – Max 60 mg/day
			 - **Dosing (Peds):**
			   – Oral: 5 mg daily to 30 mg twice daily
			   – Max 60 mg/day
			 - **CYP450 Interactions:** Substrate CYP2D6, 3A4
			 - **Renal or Hepatic Dose Adjustments:**
			   – Severe hepatic or renal impairment: not recommended
			 - **Dosage Forms:** Oral (tablet)

PSYCHIATRY – LITHIUM

Drug Class
- Lithium
- Agents:
  - Chronic Care
    - Lithium

Main Indications or Uses
- Chronic Care
  - Bipolar disorder
  - Major depressive disorder

Mechanism of Action
- Complex pharmacology without unified agreement on its underlying mechanism.
  - Involves interaction with dopamine, norepinephrine, serotonin neurotransmission, and secondary signaling systems.

> **Fast Facts**
> ✓ Lithium is a mood stabilizer for mainly the treatment of bipolar disorder that is known to have one of the smallest or narrowest therapeutic indexes. As such, the window of therapeutic benefit is small which is why it requires drug level monitoring.

Primary Net Benefit
- This monovalent cation has been used for decades for Bipolar Disorder despite a narrow therapeutic index, chronic toxicities, and unclear mechanism of action.
- Main Labs to Monitor:
  - Renal function (baseline then q2-3 months for the first six months)
  - Basic metabolic panel (electrolytes)
  - CBC with differential
  - Thyroid function (baseline then q2-3 months for the first six months)
  - Pregnancy test
  - ECG (baseline)
  - Serum lithium levels (twice weekly, then q1-3months)
    - Therapeutic range 0.6 to 1.2 mmol/L
  - Weight

High-Yield Basic Pharmacology
- **Glycogen Synthase Kinase 3 Beta (GSK-3B)**
  - GSK-3B is a CNS kinase that plays a pivotal role in neurogenesis, neuronal function, neuronal cell survival, gene transcription, and numerous other effects.
    - GSK-3B is influenced by dopamine expression, and hyperactivity has been linked to excess dopamine in the CNS.
  - Hyperactivity and dysregulation of GSK-3B as been linked to CNS excitation, neuronal degradation, tumor growth, and Alzheimer's disease.
  - Lithium is believed to inhibit the action of GSK-3B directly and elicits behavioral responses in controlling mania.
- **Beta-Arrestins**
  - The activation of GSK-3B is regulated by the complex Akt - beta-arrestin 2 (BetaArr2) - protein phosphatase 2A (PP2A).
  - Lithium activates Akt by displacing the magnesium required to assemble the Akt-BetaArr2-PP2A complex.
  - By disrupting this Akt-BetaArr2-PP2A complex, lithium further prevents the action of GSK-3B.
- **Inositol Monophosphatases**
  - Lithium inhibits inositol monophosphatases by decreasing myoinositol concentration in the cerebral cortex, preventing secondary messengers' formation (phosphatidylinositol, diacylglycerol, phospholipase C, and inositol triphosphate).
  - Without these secondary messengers, a cascade of events to psychiatric disease is modulated, leading to lithium's observed clinical benefits on the CNS.

High-Yield Clinical Knowledge
- **Bipolar Disorder**
  - Lithium remains an essential therapy and first-line treatment for acute mania and acute bipolar depression and a core component of pharmacotherapeutic maintenance of bipolar type 1 and 2 disorders.
  - As a result of prolonged time to onset of effects and close titration to therapeutic levels, alternative agents, including modern antipsychotic agents, have been used more frequently with similar outcomes.
- **Adverse Events**
  - Lithium therapy is associated with numerous acute and chronic toxicities that may not correlate with serum levels.
  - Common adverse events early on in therapy include GI disturbances (primarily diarrhea) and mild CNS effects.
    - Diarrhea is often managed by slowing dose titration; using liquid rather than tablet or capsule products can alleviate these symptoms.
    - Hand tremors may also develop, which can respond to slower titration, lower doses, or the addition of propranolol.
  - Nephrogenic diabetes insipidus occurs in up to 50% of patients on lithium but is often reversible upon discontinuation.
  - Thyroid effects and primary hypothyroidism can occur and can be managed with supplemental thyroid hormone replacement.
- **Lithium Toxicity**
  - Acute overdoses of lithium rarely have toxic CNS concentrations and do not acutely cause neurologic dysfunction.
  - Chronic lithium toxicity is associated with intravascular volume depletion and negative water balance, worsening lithium toxicity.
    - Additionally, concomitant drugs such as ACE inhibitors or angiotensin receptor blockers (ARBs) that decrease renal blood flow or thiazide diuretics that increase lithium reabsorption can contribute to chronic lithium toxicity.
  - However, in acute-on-chronic or lithium toxicity, where serum levels are above 5 mEq/L or above 4 mEq/L in patients with renal dysfunction, hemodialysis may be required to manage altered mental status and seizures or cardiac arrhythmias.
  - Risk factors for lithium toxicity include sodium restriction, dehydration, vomiting, diarrhea, patients over the age of 50, or those with concomitant heart failure or cirrhosis.
- **Broad Neuroprotection**
  - Lithium has also been associated with neuroprotective effects owing to its downregulation of the protein p53 from modulation of the bcl-2 gene, limiting apoptosis of CNS tissue.
- **Drug-Interactions**
  - Although lithium doesn't directly impact hepatic oxidation, clinically relevant drug interactions exist.
  - ACE inhibitors/ARBs, thiazide diuretics, and NSAIDs affect lithium's renal clearance increasing lithium exposure.
  - Caffeine and theophylline conversely increase lithium renal elimination, lowering lithium exposure.
  - Numerous other clinically relevant drug interactions should prompt further review in other resources.
- **SILENT**
  - Chronic lithium therapy is associated with a syndrome of irreversible neurologic and neuropsychiatric sequelae known as the syndrome of irreversible lithium-effectuated neurotoxicity, or SILENT.
    - SILENT is a new neurologic dysfunction without prior neurologic illness and persists for at least two months after lithium cessation.
    - These effects are often attributed to other agents these patients may be taking but have occurred in patients after discontinuing these other drugs or lithium monotherapy.

High-Yield Core Evidence
- **BALANCE**
  - This was a multicenter, open-label trial of patients 16 years and older with bipolar 1 disorder that randomized patients to receive lithium, valproate, or a combination of lithium plus valproate and assess the treatment's impact in the prevention of bipolar I disorder.
  - Combination therapy with lithium and valproate was significantly better than valproate alone, but lithium monotherapy was also considerably better than valproate alone concerning the primary outcome of the initiation of a new intervention for an emergent mood episode.
  - There was no difference in the primary outcome between patients randomized to combination therapy or lithium monotherapy.
  - Serious adverse events were similar between the groups.
  - The authors concluded that long-term therapy for patients with bipolar I disorder is clinically indicated; both combination therapy with lithium plus valproate and lithium monotherapy are more likely to prevent relapse than is valproate monotherapy. This benefit seems to be irrespective of baseline severity of illness and is maintained for up to 2 years. (Lancet. 2010 Jan 30;375(9712):385-95.)
- **EMBOLDEN-I**
  - This was a multicenter, double-blinded trial that randomized patients with bipolar disorder to receive either quetiapine 300 mg/day, quetiapine 600 mg/day, lithium, or placebo to determine their respective impact on the incidence of a major depressive episode in bipolar disorder.
  - Both quetiapine doses led to a significantly improved primary outcome of the change in the Montgomery-Asberg Depression Rating Scale total score compared to lithium monotherapy and placebo.
  - There was no difference between lithium and placebo concerning this primary outcome.
  - Either dose of quetiapine was significantly better than lithium for each secondary outcome measure.
  - The authors concluded that quetiapine (300 or 600 mg/d) was more effective than a placebo to treat episodes of acute depression in bipolar disorder. Lithium did not significantly differ from placebo on the primary measures of efficacy. Both treatments were generally well tolerated. (J Clin Psychiatry. 2010 Feb;71(2):150-62.)

High-Yield Fast-Fact
- **7-Up**
  - Lithium was once found in the soda drink 7-Up, and the "7" in its name has been attributed to the atomic weight of elemental lithium.
- **Batteries**
  - Lithium is a common component of batteries, including the ones powering eclectic vehicles and cell phones.

HIGH-YIELD BOARD EXAM ESSENTIALS
- **CLASSIC AGENTS:** Lithium
- **DRUG CLASS:** Lithium
- **INDICATIONS:** Bipolar disorder, major depressive disorder
- **MECHANISM:** Complex pharmacology without unified agreement on its underlying mechanism.
- **SIDE EFFECTS:** GI disturbances (primarily diarrhea), nephrogenic DI, hypothyroidism
- **CLINICAL PEARLS:** Has a narrow therapeutic index. Although lithium does not directly impact hepatic oxidation, there are several clinically relevant drug interactions. ACE inhibitors/ARBs, thiazide diuretics, and NSAIDs affect lithium's renal clearance increasing lithium exposure.

Table: Drug Class Summary

Lithium - Drug Class Review High-Yield Med Reviews			
Mechanism of Action: *Complex pharmacology without unified agreement on its underlying mechanism.*			
Class Effects: *This monovalent cation has been used for decades for Bipolar Disorder despite a narrow therapeutic index, chronic toxicities, and unclear mechanism of action.*			
Generic Name	**Brand Name**	**Indication(s) or Uses**	**Notes**
Lithium	Lithobid	<ul><li>Bipolar disorder</li><li>Major depressive disorder</li></ul>	<ul><li>**Dosing (Adult):**<ul><li>Oral: 600 to 900 mg/day divided into 2-3 doses<ul><li>Target therapeutic levels between 0.6 and 1.2 mEq/L</li></ul></li></ul></li><li>**Dosing (Peds):**<ul><li>Oral: 8 to 40 mEq/day adjusted to target level between 0.6 to 1.2 mEq/L</li><li>Maximum 40 mg/kg/day</li></ul></li><li>**CYP450 Interactions:** None</li><li>**Renal or Hepatic Dose Adjustments:**<ul><li>GFR < 30 mL/minute: avoid use</li></ul></li><li>**Dosage Forms:** Oral (capsule, solution, tablet)</li></ul>

NEUROLOGY – OREXIN RECEPTOR ANTAGONISTS

Drug Class
- Orexin Receptor Antagonists (ORAs), Miscellaneous Hypnotics
- Agents:
  - Chronic Care
    - Daridorexant
    - Lemborexant
    - Suvorexant

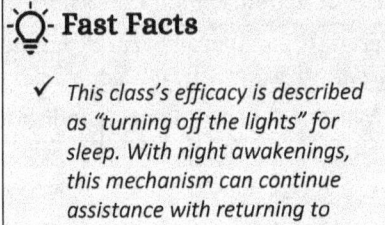

Fast Facts
✓ This class's efficacy is described as "turning off the lights" for sleep. With night awakenings, this mechanism can continue assistance with returning to sleep.

Main Indications or Uses
- Chronic Care
  - Insomnia

Mechanism of Action
- Block the binding of orexin A and B to OX1R and OX2R receptors. Orexin A and B are wake-promoting neuropeptides, so blocking their action suppresses the wake drive.

Primary Net Benefit
- Hypnotic agents are utilized to promote sleep maintenance and onset by affecting wakefulness with a more favorable safety profile than other drugs for insomnia.
  - Guidelines recommend use for sleep maintenance; prescribing information includes use for sleep onset.
- Main Labs to Monitor:
  - No routine laboratory monitoring

High-Yield Basic Pharmacology
- **Orexin Receptor Antagonism**
  - ORAs are dual receptor antagonists.
  - Orexin receptor antagonism that produces the desired sleep effects is also responsible for potential adverse effects, such as narcolepsy or cataplexy.

High-Yield Clinical Knowledge
- **Narcolepsy**
  - ORAs are contraindicated in patients with narcolepsy. Narcolepsy is associated with decreased orexin neurons and orexinergic tone, which may increase narcolepsy symptoms with ORAs.
- **CNS Depression Leading to Daytime Impairment**
  - May impair daytime wakefulness with or without clinical symptoms that can be detected by testing.
  - Daytime somnolence may require dose reductions in patients who drive to avoid driving impairment.
    - Increased risk occurs if patients do not achieve at least 7 hours of dedicated sleep time, use concomitant CNS depressants, or take higher doses.
  - Concomitant use of other CNS depressants may result in additive effects. Doses may require adjustment.
  - Avoid use with other insomnia medications and alcohol.
- **Complex Sleep Behaviors**
  - Like other hypnotics, complex sleep behaviors may include somnambulism, sleep-driving, and completing other activities while not awake. These behaviors may present at any time during therapy.
- **Worsening Depression and Suicidal Ideation**
  - Depression can worsen with ORAs. Suicidal ideations or suicide may result.
  - Intentional overdose may also be a concern from worsening depression.
- **Sleep Paralysis, Hypnagogic or Hypnopompic Hallucinations, and Cataplexy-Like Symptoms**
  - Sleep paralysis and hypnagogic or hypnopompic hallucinations may occur during sleep-wake transitions.
  - Mild cataplexy can occur and include leg weakness for up to a few minutes, especially with high doses.
- **Respiratory Disease**

- Patients with respiratory disease, including COPD and sleep apnea, should avoid or use with caution due to limited evidence in these populations.
- **Drug Abuse or Dependence**
  - ORAs are C-IV controlled substances.
  - Use cautiously in patients with a history of abuse or addiction, especially with long-term use.
  - ORAs are not associated with physical dependence.
- **Withdrawal**
  - ORAs are not associated with withdrawal symptoms.
- **Additional Adverse Effects**
  - Headache, abnormal dreams, dry mouth, GI effects, upper respiratory symptoms, tachycardia, anxiety, and pruritus have also been reported.
- **Drug Interactions**
  - ORAs are metabolized by CYP3A4 and subject to increased therapeutic effect in the presence of CYP3A4 inhibitors. Avoid strong CYP3A4 inhibitors, including some azole antifungals, macrolides, and protease inhibitors.
  - Moderate CYP3A4 inhibitors, such as non-dihydropyridine calcium channel blockers, ciprofloxacin, fluconazole, and erythromycin, should receive reduced doses.
    - Lemborexant should be avoided with moderate CYP3A4 inhibitors and limited to 5 mg with weak CYP3A4 inhibitors.
  - Avoid with strong CYP3A4 inducers.
- **Administration**
  - Administer within 30 minutes of bedtime with 7-8 hours dedicated for sleep.
  - Administration after a high-fat meal may delay T_{max} and sleep onset (1.5-2 hours).
  - If insomnia persists after 7-10 days, reevaluate therapy.
- **Special Populations**
  - Suvorexant Use
    - Women and patients with obesity demonstrate an increased risk of adverse effects with ORAs due to higher drug concentrations (5% and 15%, respectively). Increased effects may be more significant in obese women; use caution with increasing doses.
  - Geriatric patients did not demonstrate different effects than other adults. Exercise caution due to the potential for increased risk of falls.

High-Yield Core Evidence
- **Suvorexant and Lemborexant Meta-Analysis**
  - Suvorexant and lemborexant demonstrated significant and favorable outcomes for efficacy compared to placebo with a review of 8 trials.
  - Suvorexant sleep diary outcomes were significant (time to sleep onset, total sleep time, refreshed on waking, and wake after sleep onset) compared to placebo, except for number of awakenings and subjective quality of sleep at 3 months. All efficacy outcomes from rating scales and polysomnography were significantly improved with suvorexant.
  - Lemborexant efficacy measures evaluated by diaries significantly improved compared to placebo (sleep onset latency, sleep efficiency, and wake after sleep onset).
  - Safety profiles also did not differ between the drugs and placebo, except for somnolence.
    - Suvorexant demonstrated more excessive daytime sleepiness, fatigue, back pain, dry mouth, and abnormal dreams. Lemborexant demonstrated more nightmares.
  - There was no difference in hallucinations, suicidal ideations, or vehicular accidents.
  - (Front Psychiatry 13:1070522. doi: 10.3389/fpsyt.2022.1070522.)
- **Lemborexant vs Suvorexant Meta-Analysis**
  - Meta-analysis includes data from 4 trials on efficacy and safety outcomes between lemborexant, suvorexant, zolpidem ER, and placebo.
  - Outcomes compared included subjective time to sleep onset, subjective total sleep time, and subjective wake-after-sleep onset after 1 week. All active treatments performed better than placebo.

- Discontinuation rates did not differ with placebo, but lemborexant and suvorexant were associated with increased somnolence compared to placebo.
- Lemborexant 10 mg showed the largest effect size compared to placebo for all primary outcomes weighed against somnolence risk, so there may be some benefit, although associated with risk.
- (J Psychiatr Res 2020;128:68-74.)
- **Lemborexant vs. Other Insomnia Treatments Meta-Analysis**
    - Meta-analysis included 45 trials with a duration of at least 1 week. Interventions included lemborexant, suvorexant, benzodiazepines, benzodiazepine receptor agonists, trazodone, and ramelteon.
    - Lemborexant was most likely to have the best outcome for 3 out of 4 objective efficacy measures (total sleep time, latency to persistent sleep, and sleep efficiency).
    - Safety profiles were similar related to adverse effects and withdrawals.
    - Treatment effects were similar in older populations compared to adults.
    - (J Manag Care Spec Pharm 2021;27:1296-1308.)

High-Yield Fast-Facts
- Suvorexant has some evidence for use in pediatric patients ≥ 10 years old for insomnia.

HIGH-YIELD BOARD EXAM ESSENTIALS
- **CLASSIC AGENTS:** Daridorexant, lemborexant, suvorexant
- **DRUG CLASS:** Orexin receptor antagonists
- **INDICATIONS:** Insomnia
- **MECHANISM:** Block the binding of orexin A and B to OX1R and OX2R receptors. Orexin A and B are wake-promoting neuropeptides, so blocking their action suppresses wake drive.
- **SIDE EFFECTS:** Somnolence, abnormal dreams
- **CLINICAL PEARLS:** ORAs are metabolized by CYP3A4 and should be avoided with strong CYP3A4 inhibitors, including azole antifungals, macrolides, protease inhibitors, and non-dihydropyridine calcium channel blockers.

Table: Drug Class Summary

| | **Orexin Receptor Antagonists - Drug Class Review**
High-Yield Med Reviews |

Mechanism of Action: *Block orexin A and B binding to OX1R and OX2R receptors. Orexin A and B are wake-promoting neuropeptides, so blocking their action suppresses the wake drive.*			
Class Effects: Hypnotic agents utilized to promote sleep maintenance (possibly onset) by affecting wakefulness with a more favorable safety profile than other drugs for insomnia, somnolence, and abnormal dreams.			
Generic Name	**Brand Name**	**Main Indication(s) or Uses**	**Notes**

Daridorexant	Quviviq	- Insomnia	- **Dosing (Adult):**
			  - Oral: 25 to 50 mg daily within 30 min of bedtime
			- **Dosing (Peds):**
			  - Not routinely used
			- **CYP450 Interactions:** CYP3A4 substrate
			- **Renal or Hepatic Dose Adjustments:**
			  - Child-Pugh Class B: maximum 25 mg/day
			  - Child-Pugh Class C: not recommended
			- **Dosage Forms:** Oral (tablet)

Lemborexant	DayVigo	- Insomnia	- **Dosing (Adult):**
			  - Oral: 5 to 10 mg daily within 30 min of bedtime
			- **Dosing (Peds):**
			  - Not routinely used
			- **CYP450 Interactions:** CYP3A4 substrate
			- **Renal or Hepatic Dose Adjustments:**
			  - Child-Pugh Class B: maximum 5 mg/day
			  - Child-Pugh Class C: not recommended
			- **Dosage Forms:** Oral (tablet)

Suvorexant	Belsomra	- Insomnia	- **Dosing (Adult):**
			  - Oral: 10 to 20 mg daily within 30 min of bedtime
			- **Dosing (Peds):**
			  - Limited data ≥ 10 years: same as adults
			- **CYP450 Interactions:** CYP3A4 substrate
			- **Renal or Hepatic Dose Adjustments:**
			  - Child-Pugh Class C: not recommended
			- **Dosage Forms:** Oral (tablet)

NEUROLOGY – SEDATIVE HYPNOTICS – NON-BENZODIAZEPINES

Drug Class
- Non-Benzodiazepine Hypnotics
- Agents:
  - Chronic Care
    - Eszopiclone
    - Zaleplon
    - Zolpidem

Main Indications or Uses
- Chronic Care
  - Insomnia

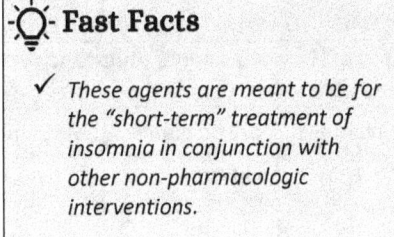

Fast Facts
- ✓ These agents are meant to be for the "short-term" treatment of insomnia in conjunction with other non-pharmacologic interventions.

Mechanism of Action
- Bind to GABA-A receptors containing the alpha-1 subunit, increasing the GABA-A channel opening frequency and potentiating GABAergic inhibition of neurotransmission.

Primary Net Benefit
- Potent hypnotic agents that, although function similarly to benzodiazepines, are less disruptive to sleep stages and lack relevant antiepileptic properties.
- Main Labs to Monitor:
  - No routine laboratory monitoring

High-Yield Basic Pharmacology
- GABA-A Receptor
  - The GABA-A receptor most commonly contains a five-subunit complex with alpha, beta, and gamma subunits.
  - The non-benzodiazepine sedative hypnotic "z-drugs" also bind to the alpha-1 subunit in a fashion similar to benzodiazepines.
- Zopiclone
  - Zopiclone is a non-benzodiazepine hypnotic not available in the United States, but its active S(+) enantiomer, eszopiclone is available.

High-Yield Clinical Knowledge
- Somnambulism
  - The Z drug compounds are frequently associated with somnambulism, otherwise known as 'sleepwalking,' a transient anterograde global amnesia.
  - Some reports have described 'sleep-eating where patients have consumed food while asleep, which has led to significant weight gain.
- Sleep Apnea
  - Although not explicitly stated in the prescribing information, z-drugs should be used with extreme caution or be avoided in patients with sleep apnea.
- Withdrawal
  - Unlike benzodiazepines, z-drug-associated withdrawal syndrome is relatively mild and not associated with significant morbidity or mortality.
    - Benzodiazepine withdrawal shares similar physiology to alcohol withdrawal with a potentially complicated course, including delirium tremens, seizures, and death.
- Overdose
  - Overdoses of z-drugs are associated with normal vital signs coma and rarely lead to clinically significant manifestations if taken alone.
  - Zopiclone has been linked to methemoglobinemia, although rare.
  - Flumazenil, a GABA-A antagonist, may reverse the hypnotic effects of z-drugs.

- **Hypnosis**
  - Eszopiclone, zaleplon, and zolpidem induce sleep without significantly affecting sleep architecture.
  - Benzodiazepines, on the other hand, will decrease the onset of sleep, increase non-REM sleep duration, reduce the time of REM sleep, and stage 4 non-REM sleep.
- **Drug Interactions**
  - Eszopiclone, zaleplon, and zopiclone are metabolized by CYP3A4 and subject to increased therapeutic effect in the presence of potent CYP3A4 inhibitors, including azole antifungals, macrolides, protease inhibitors, and non-dihydropyridine calcium channel blockers.
- **Tolerance**
  - Non-benzodiazepine hypnotic use is associated with the development of a decreased clinical effect following continuous exposure.
    - Cross-tolerance can be a feature of this effect, including other sedative-hypnotics (barbiturates), benzodiazepines, or ethanol.
  - Tolerance is thought to develop from the downregulation of GABA-A receptors as a counterregulatory response to excessive inhibition.

High-Yield Core Evidence
- **CBT Vs. Zopiclone**
  - This was a single-center, double-blind, placebo-controlled trial of elderly adult patients with chronic primary insomnia who were randomized to either cognitive-behavioral therapy (CBT), zopiclone 7.5 mg nightly, or placebo for six months.
  - The CBT-based therapy was associated with significantly improved short and long-term outcomes, including total wake time, total sleep time, sleep efficiency, and slow-wave sleep (only assessed using polysomnography), compared to either zopiclone or placebo.
  - Patients randomized to CBT experienced close to 10% improvement in sleep efficiency than patients randomized to zopiclone in whom sleep efficiency decreased.
  - The authors concluded that these results suggest that interventions based on CBT are superior to zopiclone treatment both in short- and long-term management of insomnia in older adults. (JAMA. 2006;295:2851–2858.)
- **Eszopiclone for Chronic Insomnia**
  - This was a multicenter, double-blind, placebo-controlled trial that randomized patients between the ages of 21 to 69 years with chronic insomnia and/or sleep latency to receive eszopiclone 3 mg nightly, or placebo for six months.
  - Patients randomized to eszopiclone experienced sustained and significant improvements in sleep latency, wake time after sleep onset, number of awakenings, number of nights awakened per week, total sleep time, and quality of sleep compared with placebo.
  - Eszopiclone was also associated with significant improvements in secondary endpoints, including monthly ratings of next-day function, alertness, and sense of physical well-being than with placebo.
  - There was no evidence of tolerance, and the most common adverse events were unpleasant taste and headache.
  - The authors concluded that throughout six months, eszopiclone improved all of the components of insomnia as defined by DSM-IV, including patient ratings of daytime function. (Sleep. 2003;26:793–797.)

High-Yield Fast-Facts
- **Urine Drug Screen**
  - Many clinically used urine drug screen assays use a diazepam core structure and analogs to identify the parent or metabolites of many benzodiazepines in the urine.
  - Since the Z-drugs are structurally distinct from benzodiazepines, they will not likely result positively on a typical urine drug screen.
- **Glycine Receptors**
  - Glycine receptors are similar to GABA as they're voltage-gated chloride channels, but these receptors are a Cl- inhibitory receptor in the spinal cord.
  - Strychnine and tetanus toxin are glycine receptor inhibitors.

HIGH-YIELD BOARD EXAM ESSENTIALS
- **CLASSIC AGENTS:** Eszopiclone, zaleplon, zolpidem
- **DRUG CLASS:** Non-benzodiazepine hypnotics
- **INDICATIONS:** Insomnia
- **MECHANISM:** Bind to GABA-A receptors containing the alpha-1 subunit, increasing the frequency of GABA-A channel opening and potentiating GABAergic inhibition of neurotransmission.
- **SIDE EFFECTS:** Abuse potential, daytime sleepiness, somnambulism
- **CLINICAL PEARLS:** Eszopiclone, zaleplon, and zopiclone are metabolized by CYP3A4 and subject to increased therapeutic effect in the presence of potent CYP3A4 inhibitors, including azole antifungals, macrolides, protease inhibitors, and non-dihydropyridine calcium channel blockers.

Table: Drug Class Summary

Non-Benzodiazepine Hypnotics - Drug Class Review			
High-Yield Med Reviews			
Mechanism of Action: *Bind to GABA-A receptors containing the alpha-1 subunit, increasing the frequency of GABA-A channel opening and potentiating GABAergic inhibition of neurotransmission.*			
Class Effects: *Potent hypnotic agents that, although function similarly to benzodiazepines, are less disruptive to sleep stages and lack relevant antiepileptic properties.*			
Generic Name	**Brand Name**	**Main Indication(s) or Uses**	**Notes**

Eszopiclone	Lunesta	- Insomnia	- Dosing (Adult):
			  – Oral: 1 to 3 mg immediately before bedtime
			- Dosing (Peds):
			  – Not routinely used
			- CYP450 Interactions: Substrate CYP2E1, 3A4
			- Renal or Hepatic Dose Adjustments:
			  – Child-Pugh class C: maximum 2 mg
			- Dosage Forms: Oral (tablet)

Zaleplon	Sonata	- Insomnia	- Dosing (Adult):
			  – Oral: 10 to 20 mg immediately before bedtime
			- Dosing (Peds):
			  – Not routinely used
			- CYP450 Interactions: Substrate CYP3A4
			- Renal or Hepatic Dose Adjustments:
			  – Child-Pugh class A or B: maximum 5 mg
			  – Child-Pugh class C: not recommended
			- Dosage Forms: Oral (capsule)

Zolpidem	Ambien, Edluar, Intermezzo, Zolpimist	- Insomnia	- Dosing (Adult):
			  – Oral: IR/Spray/SL: 5 to 10 mg immediately before bedtime
			  – Oral: ER: 6.25 to 12.5 mg immediately before bedtime
			- Dosing (Peds):
			  – Oral: 0.25 mg/kg before bedtime
			    – Maximum 10 mg/dose
			- CYP450 Interactions: Substrate CYP2E1, 3A4
			- Renal or Hepatic Dose Adjustments:
			  – Child-Pugh class C: maximum 2 mg
			- Dosage Forms: Oral (tablet, ER, sublingual)

PSYCHIATRY – NMDA ANTAGONIST

Drug Class
- NMDA Antagonist
- Agents:
  - Acute Care
    - Ketamine
  - Chronic Care
    - Esketamine
    - Ketamine

Main Indications or Uses
- Acute Care
  - Esketamine, Ketamine
    - Treatment-resistant depression
  - Ketamine
    - Analgesia
    - Anesthesia
    - Agitation
    - Sedation
    - Status epilepticus
- Chronic Care
  - Esketamine
    - Major depressive disorder

> **Fast Facts**
> - While ketamine has been used historically as a sedative-hypnotic as part of procedural sedation or rapid sequence intubations (RSI), it, along with esketamine, is now being use for the treatment of depression.
> - Ketamine use does not reduce the respiratory drive enough at standard doses to allow it to be used for procedures. In addition, it is generally neutral hemodynamically.
> - Ketamine can be given intranasally, IM, and IV making it clinically more useful for a number of scenarios.

Mechanism of Action
- Noncompetitive inhibition of n-methyl-d-aspartate (NMDA) receptor.

Primary Net Benefit
- Ketamine is a widely used dissociative anesthetic with many effects, including acute management of depression where its S-enantiomer, esketamine, is uniquely indicated.
- Main Labs to Monitor:
  - Blood pressure at baseline, then hourly or 1-hour post-administration.

High-Yield Basic Pharmacology
- S-Ketamine
  - Ketamine is a racemic mixture, and the s-enantiomer (esketamine) has been identified to possess the antidepressant properties of ketamine.
- Phencyclidine
  - Both esketamine and ketamine are short-acting analogs of phencyclidine, which is otherwise known by its illicit moniker, PCP.
- Active metabolites
  - Ketamine and esketamine each have active metabolites, which prolong the duration of effect with repeat or chronic use.
  - Norketamine is ⅓ as active as ketamine and is produced in a higher proportion after oral administration due to first-pass hepatic metabolism.
  - Noresketamine possesses similar characteristics to norketamine; however, data are lacking.

High-Yield Clinical Knowledge
- Antidepressant Effect
  - Esketamine or ketamine is primarily reserved for patients with depression that has not responded to conventional antidepressants.

- These agents possess advantages over continuing antidepressant treatment or further increasing doses, including rapid onset within 24 hours of administration.
- However, these antidepressant effects may not last beyond seven days.
- **Esketamine Preparation**
  - Esketamine is only available as an intranasal preparation and retains many of the pharmacokinetic characteristics of ketamine and the antidepressant effects (onset within 24 hours, duration of approximately seven days).
- **Dissociation**
  - Ketamine causes a unique dose-dependent dissociation, where the patient cannot pain, visual or auditory neurotransmission signals to the brain, but the outgoing sympathetic and parasympathetic output front the CNS is not directly affected.
  - This effect occurs at an approximate weight-based dose of 0.5 to 1 mg/kg.
  - Analgesic effects of ketamine occur lower in the dose range, approximately between 0.1 to 0.3 mg/kg.
- **Additional Actions**
  - Esketamine and ketamine each have opioid agonist properties and increase dopaminergic activity inhibition of dopamine reuptake, cholinergic effects, and voltage-sensitive calcium channel blocking effects.
- **Blood Pressure, Intracranial Pressure, Intraocular Pressure**
  - Ketamine and esketamine are thought to increase blood pressure, intracranial pressure, and intraocular pressure but do not do so in a clinically relevant manner.
    - Thus ketamine is not contraindicated specifically because of elevated blood pressure, intracranial pressure, or intraocular pressure.
- **Abuse Potential**
  - Esketamine and ketamine have high abuse potential and can lead to chronic dependence and tolerance.
  - Long-term effects of ketamine abuse can lead to neurogenic bladder or worsening underlying psychiatric disease.

High-Yield Core Evidence
- **Esketamine Vs. Placebo**
  - In this double-blind, multicenter, proof-of-concept study, patients at imminent risk of suicide patients were randomized to receive either esketamine or placebo twice weekly for four weeks, in addition to comprehensive standard-of-care treatment.
  - Patients receiving esketamine experienced a significant improvement in the primary outcome of the change in score from baseline to 4 hours after the initial dose on the Montgomery-Åsberg Depression Rating Scale.
  - This positive effect of esketamine was sustained through 24 hours but was not significantly different from the placebo at day 25.
  - However, the between-group reductions in clinician global judgment of suicide risk scores were not statistically different at any time point.
  - The authors concluded that intranasal esketamine compared with placebo, given in addition to comprehensive standard-of-care treatment, may result in significantly rapid improvement in depressive symptoms, including some measures of suicidal ideation, among depressed patients at imminent risk for suicide. (Am J Psychiatry. 2018 Jul 1;175(7):620-630.)
- **Ketamine or Etomidate for RSI in Trauma**
  - This was a four-year retrospective evaluation after a single institutional's protocol change from etomidate to ketamine as the standard induction agent for adult trauma patients undergoing rapid sequence intubation in the emergency department.
  - There was no observed difference between treatments concerning the primary outcome of in-hospital mortality (adjusted for age, vital signs, and injury severity and mechanism).
  - Furthermore, there were no statistically significant differences in secondary outcomes, including ICU-free days or ventilator-free days.
  - The authors concluded that patient-centered outcomes were similar for patients who received etomidate or ketamine. (Ann Emerg Med. 2017 Jan;69(1):24-33.e2.)

Psychiatry / Mental Health

High-Yield Fast-Fact
- **Nothing New**
  - Although recently approved for use in treatment-resistant depression, esketamine has been in use since the early 1960s.

HIGH-YIELD BOARD EXAM ESSENTIALS
- **CLASSIC AGENTS:** Esketamine, ketamine
- **DRUG CLASS:** NMDA antagonists
- **INDICATIONS:** Analgesia, anesthesia, agitation, treatment-resistant depression, sedation, status epilepticus
- **MECHANISM:** Noncompetitive inhibition of n-methyl-d-aspartate (NMDA) receptor.
- **SIDE EFFECTS:** Emergence psychosis, abuse risk
- **CLINICAL PEARLS:** Ketamine and esketamine are thought to increase blood pressure, intracranial pressure, intraocular pressure but do not do so in a clinically relevant manner.

Table: Drug Class Summary

NMDA Antagonist - Drug Class Review High-Yield Med Reviews			
Mechanism of Action: *Noncompetitive inhibition of n-methyl-d-aspartate (NMDA) receptor.*			
Class Effects: *Ketamine is a widely used dissociative anesthetic with many effects, including acute management of depression where its S-enantiomer, esketamine, is uniquely indicated.*			
Generic Name	**Brand Name**	**Indication(s) or Uses**	**Notes**

Esketamine	Spravato	- Major depressive disorder
		- Treatment-resistant depression
			- **Dosing (Adult):**
			  - Induction: IN 56 mg twice weekly or 84 mg twice weekly
			  - Maintenance: Decrease frequency to once weekly
			- **Dosing (Peds):**
			  - Not routinely used
			- **CYP450 Interactions:** text
			- **Renal or Hepatic Dose Adjustments:**
			  - Child-Pugh class C: not recommended
			- **Dosage Forms:** Nasal solution

Ketamine	Ketalar	- Analgesia
		- Anesthesia
		- Agitation
		- Treatment-resistant depression
		- Sedation
		- Status epilepticus
			- **Dosing (Adult):**
			  - IV: 0.5 to 2 mg/kg bolus
			    - IV infusion 0.05 to 2 mg/kg/hour
			  - IM/IN: 1 to 4 mg/kg
			  - Oral: 0.5 mg/kg/day, maximum 500 mg/day
			- **Dosing (Peds):**
			  - IV: 0.5 to 2 mg/kg bolus
			    - IV infusion: 0.05 to 2 mg/kg/hour
			  - IM/IN: 1 to 4 mg/kg
			  - Oral: 0.5 mg/kg/day, maximum 500 mg/day
			- **CYP450 Interactions:** Substrate of CYP2B6, 2C9, 3A4
			- **Renal or Hepatic Dose Adjustments:** None
			- **Dosage Forms:** IV (solution)

PSYCHIATRY – NOREPINEPHRINE REUPTAKE INHIBITOR

Drug Class
- Norepinephrine Reuptake Inhibitor (NRI)
- Agents:
    - Chronic Care
        - Atomoxetine
        - Viloxazine

Main Indications or Uses
- Chronic Care
    - ADHD

> **Fast Facts**
> ✓ These agents can cause worsen psychiatric conditions to include bipolar disorder.
>
> ✓ Atomoxetine has been linked to increased risk of suicidal ideations.

Mechanism of Action
- Inhibits the reuptake of norepinephrine, but the exact mechanism for benefit in ADHD is unknown.

Primary Net Benefit
- Improve symptoms and functioning of ADHD without adverse effects associated with stimulants.
- Main Labs to Monitor:
    - Liver enzymes
    - SCr, eGFR (viloxazine)

High-Yield Basic Pharmacology
- **CYP2D6 Poor Metabolizers Requiring Atomoxetine**
    - If a patient is a poor CYP2D6 metabolizer, start with 40 mg daily, then increase after a minimum of 4 weeks to 80 mg if needed. Peak concentrations demonstrated to be 5 times greater in poor metabolizers.
    - Caution with strong CYP2D6 inhibitors.
- **CYP1A2 Strong Inhibitor (Viloxazine)**
    - Viloxazine is a strong CYP1A2 inhibitor and a weak CYP2D6 and 3A4 inhibitor.
        - Avoid duloxetine melatonin, MAOIs, melatonin receptor agonists, propranolol, theophylline, and tizanidine.
    - Viloxazine is only a minor substrate of CYP2D6 and a substrate of UGT1A9 and UGT2B15.
- Viloxazine absorption may be reduced by a high-fat meal.

High-Yield Clinical Knowledge
- **Suicidal Ideations with Atomoxetine**
    - Atomoxetine has been associated with increased risk of suicidal ideations. The risk is potentially greater early during therapy.
- **Warnings**
    - Mania or hypomania may be induced in patients with bipolar disorder.
- **Adverse Effects**
    - May cause sedation or fatigue. Use caution with activities requiring alertness.
    - Increased BP and HR may occur and should be monitored.
    - GI effects are also common.
    - Atomoxetine may cause hyperhidrosis.

High-Yield Core Evidence
- **Suicide-Related Behavior or Ideation with Atomoxetine**
  - Meta-analysis of double-blind, placebo-controlled trials of atomoxetine in pediatric (n = 3883) and adult (3365) patients with ADHD.
  - Suicidal ideations were significantly more frequent with pediatric patients only.
  - No completed suicides were reported. One attempted pediatric suicide occurred.
  - Concluded that suicidal ideation was uncommon in patients, but it was reported more frequently in pediatric patients on atomoxetine versus placebo. Overall, the authors concluded there is minimal risk of suicidal ideations with pediatric patients on atomoxetine, and patients should be monitored and evaluated carefully for therapy with atomoxetine. Adults did not demonstrate greater risk of suicidal ideations with atomoxetine. (J Child Adolesc Psychopharmacol 2014;24:426-434.)

High-Yield Fast-Fact
- Atomoxetine can be discontinued without tapering.
- Atomoxetine can be used off-label for neurogenic orthostatic hypotension.
- Clonidine and guanfacine in extended-release formulations are also used in pediatric patients as nonstimulants for ADHD but have a different mechanism of action than NRIs.

HIGH-YIELD BOARD EXAM ESSENTIALS
- **CLASSIC AGENTS:** atomoxetine, viloxazine
- **DRUG CLASS:** NRI
- **INDICATIONS:** ADHD
- **MECHANISM:** Inhibits the reuptake of norepinephrine, but exact mechanism for benefit in ADHD is unknown.
- **SIDE EFFECTS:** sedation, fatigue, increased BP or HR, GI effects, hyperhidrosis (atomoxetine)
- **CLINICAL PEARLS:**
  - NRIs are nonstimulant options to manage ADHD.
  - May increase risk of mania in patients with bipolar disorder.
  - Monitor for drug interactions.
  - Atomoxetine may increase suicidal ideations, especially early in therapy.

Table: Drug Class Summary

| | Selective Norepinephrine Reuptake Inhibitor - Drug Class Review
High-Yield Med Reviews |

Selective Norepinephrine Reuptake Inhibitor - Drug Class Review			
	*Mechanism of Action:* Inhibits the reuptake of norepinephrine, but exact mechanism for benefit in ADHD is unknown.		
Class Effects: Nonstimulant drugs for ADHD,			
Generic Name	**Brand Name**	**Main Indication(s) or Uses**	**Notes**

Atomoxetine	Strattera	• ADHD	• **Dosing (Adult):**
			  – Oral: initial 40 mg daily, then increase after ≥ 3 days to 80 mg daily
			  – Max 100 mg/day
			• **Dosing (Peds):**
			  – Oral ≥ 6 years and ≤ 70 kg: initial 0.5 mg/kg/d, then increase after ≥ 3 days to 1.2 mg/kg/d
			  – Max 1.4 mg/kg/d or 100 mg whichever is less
			  – Oral ≥ 6 years and > 70 kg: same as adult
			• **CYP450 Interactions:** CYP 2D6, 2C19 substrate
			• **Renal or Hepatic Dose Adjustments:**
			  – Child-Pugh class B: dose at 50% normal dose
			  – Child-Pugh class C: dose at 25% normal dose
			• **Dosage Forms:** Oral (capsule)

Viloxazine	Qelbree	• Attention-deficit hyperactivity disorder	• **Dosing (Adult):**
			  – Oral: 200 mg daily, max 600 mg/day
			• **Dosing (Peds):**
			  – Oral: 100 mg daily, max 200 mg/day
			• **CYP450 Interactions:** CYP2D6 substrate; CYP1A2, 2D6, 3A4 inhibitor
			• **Renal or Hepatic Dose Adjustments:**
			  – GFR < 30 mL/min/1.73m^2: initial 100 mg daily, max 200 mg/day
			• **Dosage Forms:** Oral (capsule)

PSYCHIATRY – SMOKING CESSATION

Drug Class
- Smoking Cessation
- Agents:
    - Acute Care
        - Bupropion
        - Clonidine
        - Nicotine
        - Nortriptyline
        - Varenicline

> 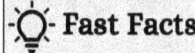 **Fast Facts**
>
> ✓ Varenicline no longer lists neuropsychiatric adverse events as a black-boxed warning, but use is still controversial.
>
> ✓ For smoking cessation, bupropion should be used for 12 weeks but may be continued for up to 1 year.

Main Indications or Uses
- Chronic Care
    - Hypertension (clonidine)
    - Major depressive disorder (bupropion, nortriptyline)
    - Neuropathic pain (nortriptyline)
    - Seasonal affective disorder (bupropion)
    - Smoking cessation (bupropion, clonidine, nicotine, nortriptyline, varenicline)

Mechanism of Action
- Bupropion
    - Inhibits the reuptake of dopamine and norepinephrine, prolonging norepinephrine and serotonergic neurotransmission
- Clonidine
    - Centrally acting alpha-2 agonist that reduces withdrawal symptoms
- Nicotine
    - Agonist of central nicotinic-cholinergic receptors, as well as at neuromuscular junctions and adrenal medulla
- Nortriptyline
    - Inhibits presynaptic reuptake of norepinephrine or serotonin, increasing their concentration in the CNS
- Varenicline
    - Partial nicotinic receptor agonist, preventing nicotinic stimulation of mesolimbic dopaminergic activity

Primary Net Benefit
- Individual or complementary interventions for smoking cessation to reduce cravings/addiction or withdrawal from nicotine
- Main Labs to Monitor:
    - Liver enzymes and liver function (baseline, and as clinically indicated)
    - Serum electrolytes (baseline, and as clinically indicated)
    - ECG (baseline, and as clinically indicated)
    - Blood glucose (baseline, and as clinically indicated)
    - Neuropsychiatric changes (varenicline)

High-Yield Basic Pharmacology
- Clonidine
    - Clonidine is a centrally acting alpha-2 agonist, thereby enhancing the activity of inhibitory neurons in the vasoregulatory regions of the CNS.
        - This ultimately leads to a *decrease* in the release of norepinephrine.
- Sodium Channel Block
    - TCAs inhibit the cardiac fast sodium channels, slowing the phase 0 depolarization, which manifests as QRS prolongation.

- This QRS prolongation represents a slowing of the propagation of ventricular depolarization, leading to ventricular dysrhythmias.
- This effect is similar to the Vaughn Williams class 1A antiarrhythmic agents.
- **Bupropion**
  - The active metabolite hydroxybupropion may cause seizures by acting as a GABA antagonist and as an NMDA agonist.

High-Yield Clinical Knowledge
- **Varenicline Neuropsychiatric Effects**
  - The prescribing information for varenicline no longer lists neuropsychiatric adverse events as a black-boxed warning, but use is still controversial.
    - This change was based on a large randomized controlled trial (EAGLES study further described below).
  - Varenicline is first-line pharmacotherapy for smoking cessation in patients with CVD.
- **Nicotine Replacement Therapy (NRT)**
  - NRT consists of numerous dosage forms of nicotine and may be added to varenicline in patients who do not adequately respond to varenicline alone.
  - Combination NRT is defined as a continuous nicotine dose (ex. nicotine patch) with the addition of as-needed nicotine for break-through cravings (gum, lozenge, or spray).
  - NRT can be used in patients with CVD and has NOT been associated with increased CVD events.
- **NRT Gum Instructions**
  - Patients who smoke more than 25 cigarettes per day should start with 4 mg gum (rather than 2 mg gum).
    - A new piece of gum should be used every 2 hours at a fixed schedule for the first 1 to 3 months.
  - Patients should be counseled to chew the gum slowly until a peppery or minty taste emerges, then the gum should be "parked" between cheek and gums to facilitate nicotine absorption through the oral mucosa.
  - While using the gum, acidic beverages (coffee, soft drinks, etc.) should be avoided since they may reduce the amount of nicotine absorbed.
- **Bupropion Combination**
  - Bupropion is an agent that is both effective for smoking cessation and may help treat certain disorders such as depression.
    - The ACC guidelines do not recommend the addition of bupropion to varenicline for smoking cessation.
    - If either agent alone is not achieving cessation, combination therapy with NRT should be used before switching agents.
  - For smoking cessation, bupropion should be used for 12 weeks but may be continued for up to 1 year.
- **Bupropion and Seizures**
  - Although bupropion has numerous benefits, including smoking cessation characteristics, minor sexual dysfunction, and less fatigue than other antidepressants, it can be more troublesome in overdose.
  - The risk of seizures increases if chronic doses are above 450 mg/day or patients ingest an overdose.
  - Additional findings from bupropion overdose include HTN, agitation, or QRS and QT prolongation.
    - The onset of these symptoms can be delayed between 10 and 24 hours following an overdose, with seizures lasting as long as 48 hours after exposure.
- **Characteristic Adverse Events of Agents**
  - Compared to SSRIs, TCAs are more likely to cause antimuscarinic adverse events, sedation, orthostatic hypotension, and weight gain.
    - Antimuscarinic effects of TCAs can acutely worsen memory or cause delirium in elderly patients.
  - Varenicline is associated with GI effects and abnormal dreams.
  - NRT Effects:
    - Patches may cause abnormal dreams. May remove before bedtime if these occur.
    - Route of administration for NRT products will determine local adverse effects associated with irritation of administration sites.

- **Sudden Cardiac Death**
  - As a result of sodium channel blockade and potential QT prolongation, TCAs may lead to sudden cardiac death.
    - An FDA warning on desipramine specifically exists regarding this increased risk of cardiac death.
- **Alternative Mechanisms**
  - TCAs possess numerous other actions that may contribute to their actions but largely contribute to adverse events and toxicity.
  - TCAs can cause antimuscarinic effects, peripheral alpha-1 antagonist properties, histamine-1 antagonist properties, cardiac sodium channel blockade, and GABA-A receptor antagonist properties.

High-Yield Core Evidence
- **EAGLES**
  - This was a multinational, double-blinded, triple-dummy, placebo- and active-controlled trial that randomized patients in two cohorts, psychiatric and non-psychiatric comorbidities, to assess neuropsychiatric safety of the smoking cessation medications varenicline and bupropion.
  - Patients aged 18 to 75 years who smoked 10 or more cigarettes/day and had an interest in quitting were randomized to receive either varenicline 1 mg twice daily, bupropion hydrochloride 150 mg twice daily, nicotine replacement therapy 21-mg/d patch with tapering, or placebo.
  - There was no significant difference between interventions concerning the primary endpoint of the incidence of a composite measure of moderate and severe neuropsychiatric adverse events, and the primary efficacy endpoint was biochemically confirmed continuous abstinence for weeks 9-12.
  - Varenicline-treated participants achieved higher abstinence rates than those on placebo, nicotine patch, and bupropion.
  - Those on bupropion and nicotine patches achieved higher abstinence rates than those on placebo.
  - The authors concluded that there was no significant increase in neuropsychiatric adverse events attributable to varenicline or bupropion relative to nicotine patches or placebo and that varenicline was more effective than placebo, nicotine patch, and bupropion in helping smokers achieve abstinence, whereas bupropion and nicotine patch was more effective than placebo. (Lancet. 2016 Jun 18;387(10037):2507-20.)
- **Cardiovascular Extension of EAGLES**
  - This was an extension of the EAGLES study expanded to include CV monitoring during and after treatment.
  - Patients aged 18 to 75 years who smoked ten or more cigarettes/day and had an interest in quitting were randomized to receive either varenicline 1 mg twice daily, bupropion hydrochloride 150 mg twice daily, nicotine replacement therapy 21-mg/d patch with tapering, or placebo.
  - Those with unstable psychiatric illness, active substance abuse, recent MI or CABG, stroke or TIA within two months, or uncontrolled HTN were excluded.
  - There was no difference between groups concerning the primary endpoint of the time to develop a major adverse CV event (CV death, nonfatal MI, or nonfatal stroke) during treatment.
  - Furthermore, no significant treatment differences were observed in time to CV events, BP, or heart rate.
  - The authors concluded there was no evidence that the use of smoking cessation pharmacotherapies increased the risk of serious CV adverse events during or after treatment. (JAMA Intern Med. 2018;178(5):622-631.)

High-Yield Fast-Facts
- **Opioid Withdrawal**
  - Clonidine has been used as an adjunct agent in the management of opioid withdrawal.
    - However, it is essential to note that despite its I2 agonist properties, clonidine predominantly acts via its central alpha-2 agonist effects and masks the sympathetic effects of opioid withdrawal.
- **Vape**
  - E-cigarettes used for "vaping" contain numerous excipients, including propylene glycol or glycerol products with a combination of nicotine, flavorings, and/or other chemicals.
  - The long-term safety of these products is unknown, and they are not recommended in smoking cessation.

HIGH-YIELD BOARD EXAM ESSENTIALS
- **CLASSIC AGENTS:** Bupropion, clonidine, nicotine, nortriptyline, varenicline
- **DRUG CLASS:** Smoking cessation agents
- **INDICATIONS:** Smoking cessation
- **MECHANISM:**
    - Nicotine - Agonist of central nicotinic-cholinergic receptors, as well as at neuromuscular junctions and adrenal medulla.
    - Varenicline - Partial nicotinic receptor agonist, preventing nicotinic stimulation of mesolimbic dopaminergic activity.
    - In general, smoking cessation agents reduce cravings/addiction or withdrawal.
- **SIDE EFFECTS:** Neuropsychiatric effects (varenicline), HTN (bupropion), hypotension (clonidine), QRS prolongation (nortriptyline)
- **CLINICAL PEARLS:** While patients with a history of depression or other neuropsychiatric illnesses may receive varenicline (although this is still controversial), bupropion is an agent that is both effective for smoking cessation and may help treat depression.

Table: Drug Class Summary

Smoking Cessation - Drug Class Review
High-Yield Med Reviews
Mechanism of Action:
Bupropion - Inhibits the reuptake of dopamine and norepinephrine, prolonging norepinephrine and serotonergic neurotransmission
Clonidine - Centrally acting alpha-2 agonist that helps with withdrawal symptoms
Nicotine - Agonist of central nicotinic-cholinergic receptors, as well as at neuromuscular junctions and adrenal medulla
Nortriptyline - Inhibit presynaptic reuptake of norepinephrine or serotonin, increasing their concentration in the CNS
Varenicline - Partial nicotinic receptor agonist, preventing nicotinic stimulation of mesolimbic dopaminergic activity
Class Effects: Individual or complementary interventions for smoking cessation to reduce cravings/addiction or withdrawal from nicotine

Generic Name	Brand Name	Main Indication(s) or Uses	Notes
Bupropion	Aplenzin Forfivo Wellbutrin Zyban	<ul><li>Major depressive disorder</li><li>Seasonal affective disorder</li><li>Smoking cessation</li></ul>	<ul><li>**Dosing (Adult):**<ul><li>Oral: 100 to 450 mg daily</li></ul></li><li>**Dosing (Peds):**<ul><li>Oral: 3 mg/kg/day in 2-3 divided doses<ul><li>Max 6 mg/kg/day or single dose 150 mg</li></ul></li></ul></li><li>**CYP450 Interactions:** CYP1A2, 2A6, 2B6, 2C9, 2D6, 2E1, 3A4 substrate; CYP2D6 inhibitor</li><li>**Renal or Hepatic Dose Adjustments:**<ul><li>Child-Pugh class C: reduce dose by 50%</li></ul></li><li>**Dosage Forms:** Oral (IR and ER tablet)</li></ul>
Clonidine	Catapres Kapvay	<ul><li>Hypertension</li><li>Smoking cessation</li></ul>	<ul><li>**Dosing (Adult):**<ul><li>Oral: Initial: 0.1 mg twice daily, > 0.6 mg/day not recommended.</li><li>TD Patch: 0.1 mg/24-hour patch once every 7 days</li></ul></li><li>**Dosing (Peds):**<ul><li>≤45 kg: Initial: 0.05 mg at bedtime</li><li>>45 kg: Initial: 0.1 mg at bedtime</li><li>Max is based on patient weight:<ul><li>27 to 40.5 kg: 0.2 mg/day</li><li>40.5 to 45 kg: 0.3 mg/day</li><li>> 45 kg: 0.4 mg/day</li></ul></li></ul></li><li>**CYP450 Interactions:** None</li><li>**Renal or Hepatic Dose Adjustments:** None</li><li>**Dosage Forms:** Topical (transdermal patch), Oral (IR and ER tablet)</li></ul>

Smoking Cessation - Drug Class Review
High-Yield Med Reviews

Generic Name	Brand Name	Main Indication(s) or Uses	Notes

Nicotine	Habitrol, NicoDerm, Nicorette, Nicotine, Nicotrol, Thrive	• Smoking cessation	• **Dosing (Adult):**
			   − Gum: chew 1 piece q1-8hours (max 24 pieces/day)
			   − Inhalation: 6 to 16 cartridges/day
			   − Lozenge: 1 lozenge q1-8hours (max 20 lozenges/day)
			   − Nasal spray: 1 to 10 doses/hour (maximum 80 sprays/day)
			   − Transdermal: 7 to 21 mg/day
			• **Dosing (Peds):**
			   − Not routinely used
			• **CYP450 Interactions:** CYP1A2, 2A6, 2B6, 2C19, 2C9, 2D6, 2E1, 3A4 substrate
			• **Renal or Hepatic Dose Adjustments:** None
			• **Dosage Forms:** Oral (gum, inhalation, lozenge), Nasal spray, Transdermal patch

Nortriptyline	Pamelor	• Major depressive disorder
		• Smoking cessation (off-label)
			• **Dosing (Adult):**
			   − Oral: 25 to 150 mg/day
			• **Dosing (Peds):**
			   − Oral: 0.5 to 2 mg/kg/day or 100 mg/day, whichever is less
			• **CYP450 Interactions:** CYP1A2, 2C19, 2D6, 3A4 substrate
			• **Renal or Hepatic Dose Adjustments:**
			   − Hepatic impairment: reduce dose by 50%
			• **Dosage Forms:** Oral (capsule, solution)

Varenicline	Chantix	• Smoking cessation	• **Dosing (Adult):**
			   − Oral: 0.5 mg daily on days 1 to 3; 0.5 mg BID days 4 to 7; 1 mg BID for at least 11 weeks
			• **Dosing (Peds):**
			   − Not routinely used
			• **CYP450 Interactions:** None
			• **Renal or Hepatic Dose Adjustments:**
			   − CrCl < 30 mL/min: max 0.5 mg BID
			   − ESRD: 0.5 mg daily
			• **Dosage Forms:** Oral (tablet)

TOXICOLOGY – SUBSTANCE ABUSE DETERRENTS

Drug Class
- Substance (Alcohol & Opioid) Abuse Deterrents
- Agents:
    - Acute Care
        - Acamprosate
        - Disulfiram
        - Naltrexone

Main Indications or Uses
- Acute & Chronic Care
    - Alcohol use disorder
    - Opioid use disorder

Mechanism of Action
- Acamprosate
    - Modulates the action of glutamate at the NMDA receptor, modulating alcohol cravings.
- Disulfiram
    - Inhibits aldehyde dehydrogenase causing an accumulation of acetaldehyde.
- Naltrexone
    - Competitive opioid receptor (including mu, kappa, and delta) antagonists.

Fast Facts

✓ The characteristic "disulfiram reaction" in the context of ethanol use consists of significant nausea with vomiting but also flushing, chest pain, tachycardia, weakness, blurred vision, and hypotension. When a patient experiences this it helps to "deter" them which is why we call them deterrents. Note: Even medications can contain alcohol. For example, lopinavir/ritonavir solution contains 42% alcohol.

Primary Net Benefit
- Acamprosate and naltrexone are well-tolerated options for alcohol use disorder and have primarily replaced disulfiram.
- Main Labs to Monitor:
    - Serum creatinine (acamprosate, naltrexone)
    - Liver function (INR/PT, albumin, protein, bilirubin) (disulfiram)

High-Yield Basic Pharmacology
- Oral Bioavailability
    - Naltrexone has a wide bioavailability range due to the first-pass metabolism of between 5 and 60%.
    - This differs from other opioid antagonists, including naloxone, minimally absorbed orally (bioavailability of approximately 2%).
- Disulfiram Like Agents
    - Numerous medications can produce a disulfiram-like effect, including NMTT cephalosporins (cefazolin, cefotetan), chlorpropamide, griseofulvin, metronidazole, nitrofurantoin, procarbazine, and first-generation sulfonylureas.
- Metal Chelating and CAD
    - Disulfiram is metabolized to diethyldithiocarbamate (DDC), available in other countries as a chelating agent for nickel or copper chelation.
    - However, DDC is further metabolized to carbon disulfide, associated with pyridoxine deficiency, seizures, atherosclerosis, and heart disease.

High-Yield Clinical Knowledge
- Naltrexone for Alcohol Abstinence
    - Naltrexone is available as an IM depot injection as adjunctive therapy in ethanol abstinence.
    - Opioid antagonism by naltrexone is proposed to inhibit central opioid-mediated ethanol craving and reduce ethanol intake and relapse incidence.
- Alcohol Withdrawal

- Naltrexone does not induce alcohol withdrawal but could precipitate opioid withdrawal in patients taking opioids.
    - However, naltrexone should not be initiated in patients suffering from acute alcohol withdrawal.
- Thorough patient history, including non-prescription/illicit drug use, must be conducted before initiation of naltrexone.
- **Disulfiram Reaction**
    - Disulfiram causes the accumulation of acetaldehyde upon consumption of ethanol, preventing the function of aldehyde dehydrogenase, but not alcohol dehydrogenase.
    - The characteristic "disulfiram reaction" consists of flushing, headache, nausea/vomiting, chest pain, tachycardia, weakness, blurred vision, and hypotension.
        - As a result, disulfiram should be avoided in patients with heart failure, arrhythmias, recent MI, or CAD risk factors.
        - Disulfiram is also associated with the abrupt onset of respiratory depression, seizures, and death.
    - This effect can persist for up to 24 hours after a given dose of disulfiram.
- **Pharmacogenomic Link**
    - The effectiveness of naltrexone appears to be related to the presence or absence of polymorphisms in the mu-opioid receptor gene, OPRM1.
    - Patients with Asn40Asp polymorphisms may experience a more pronounced response to naltrexone with a lower relapse rate.
- **Monthly Administration**
    - Naltrexone is available as a once-monthly intramuscular injection for alcohol dependence.
    - This route and dose may be more effective in reducing heavy drinking and improving abstinence.
- **CAGE and AUDIT**
    - The CAGE questionnaire or Alcohol Use Disorders Identification Test (AUDIT) tools can determine patients' alcohol abuse or dependence.
        - The AUDIT tool best quantifies alcohol misuse, whereas the CAGE questionnaire is a tool to help discuss alcohol use.

High-Yield Core Evidence
- **Acamprosate For Alcohol Dependence**
    - This was a Cochrane systematic review and meta-analysis assessing the effectiveness and tolerability of acamprosate compared to placebo and other pharmacological agents.
    - The investigators included all double-blind, randomized controlled trials that compare acamprosate's effects with placebo or active control on drinking-related outcomes.
    - Of the 24 trials included, the authors noted that acamprosate was shown to significantly reduce the risk of any drinking and significantly increase the cumulative abstinence duration compared to placebo.
    - Diarrhea was the only side effect that was more frequently reported under acamprosate than placebo, and industry-sponsored trials did not significantly differ from non-profit-funded trials.
    - The authors concluded that acamprosate appears to be an effective and safe treatment strategy for supporting continuous abstinence after detoxification in alcohol-dependent patients. (Cochrane Database Syst Rev. 2010;(9): CD004332.)
- **Opioid Antagonists for Alcohol Dependence**
    - This was a Cochrane systematic review and meta-analysis assessing the effectiveness and tolerability of opioid antagonists in alcohol dependence treatment.
    - The authors included all double-blind, randomized controlled trials which compare the effects of naltrexone or nalmefene with placebo or active control on drinking-related outcomes.
    - Naltrexone therapy was associated with a significantly reduced risk of heavy drinking, and decreased drinking days, heavy drinking days, consumed amount of alcohol, and gamma-glutamyltransferase activity, compared to placebo.
    - However, there was no effect on return to any drinking.
    - The authors concluded that naltrexone appears to be an effective and safe strategy in alcoholism treatment. (Cochrane Reviews. 2010;(12): CD001867.)

High-Yield Fast-Fact
- **Vasopressor Interaction**
  - Disulfiram inhibits dopamine beta-hydroxylase metabolism of dopamine to norepinephrine/epinephrine.
  - As a result, norepinephrine is the preferred vasopressor in patients taking disulfiram.

HIGH-YIELD BOARD EXAM ESSENTIALS
- **CLASSIC AGENTS:** Acamprosate, disulfiram, naltrexone
- **DRUG CLASS:** Alcohol abuse deterrents
- **INDICATIONS:** Alcohol use disorder, opioid use disorder (naltrexone)
- **MECHANISM:**
  - **Acamprosate** - Modulates the action of glutamate at the NMDA receptor, modulating alcohol cravings.
  - **Disulfiram** - Inhibits aldehyde dehydrogenase, causing an accumulation of acetaldehyde.
  - **Naltrexone** - Competitive opioid receptor (including mu, kappa, and delta) antagonists.
- **SIDE EFFECTS:** Disulfiram reaction (flushing, headache, nausea/vomiting, chest pain, tachycardia, weakness, blurred vision, and hypotension)
- **CLINICAL PEARLS:** Naltrexone is available as an IM depot injection as adjunctive therapy in ethanol abstinence. Opioid antagonism by naltrexone is proposed to inhibit central opioid-mediated ethanol craving, reduces ethanol intake and incidence of relapse.

Table: Drug Class Summary

Alcohol Abuse Deterrents - Drug Class Review **High-Yield Med Reviews**			
Mechanism of Action: *Acamprosate - Modulates the action of glutamate at the NMDA receptor, modulating alcohol cravings.* *Disulfiram - Inhibits aldehyde dehydrogenase, causing an accumulation of acetaldehyde.* *Naltrexone - Competitive opioid receptor (including mu, kappa, and delta) antagonists.*			
Class Effects: Acamprosate and naltrexone are well-tolerated options for alcohol use disorder and have largely replaced disulfiram.			
Generic Name	**Brand Name**	**Indication(s) or Uses**	**Notes**

Acamprosate	Campral	- Alcohol use disorder	- **Dosing (Adult):**
			    - Oral: 666 mg two to three times daily
			 - **Dosing (Peds):**
			    - Not routinely used
			 - **CYP450 Interactions:** None
			 - **Renal or Hepatic Dose Adjustments:**
			    - GFR: 30 to 50
			 - **Dosage Forms:** Oral (tablet), Suspension for intramuscular injection

Naltrexone	Vivitrol	- Alcohol use disorder
		 - Opioid use disorder
			- **Dosing (Adult):**
			    - Oral: 50 to 100 mg/day
			    - IM: 380 mg q4weeks
			 - **Dosing (Peds):**
			    - Not routinely used
			 - **CYP450 Interactions:** None
			 - **Renal or Hepatic Dose Adjustments:** None
			 - **Dosage Forms:** Oral (tablet), Suspension for intramuscular injection

Disulfiram	Antabuse	- Alcohol use disorder	- **Dosing (Adult):**
			    - Oral: 125 to 500 mg daily
			 - **Dosing (Peds):**
			    - Not routinely used
			 - **CYP450 Interactions:** None
			 - **Renal or Hepatic Dose Adjustments:** None
			 - **Dosage Forms:** Oral (tablet)

2025

A COMPREHENSIVE *RAPID REVIEW*

NAPLEX
Pharmacology & Drug Classes

Pulmonology

PULMONOLOGY – BRONCHODILATORS – ANTICHOLINERGIC – SHORT ACTING

Drug Class
- **Short-Acting Anticholinergic (Antimuscarinic) Antagonists**
- **Agents:**
  - **Acute & Chronic Care**
    - Ipratropium

Main Indications or Uses
- **Acute Care**
  - Allergic rhinitis
  - Asthma
- **Chronic Care**
  - Chronic obstructive pulmonary disease (COPD)

> 💡 **Fast Facts**
>
> ✓ Ipratropium is available in a combination therapy with albuterol which can be useful in acute asthma and COPD exacerbations where dual mechanisms for bronchodilation are needed. That product is known as DuoNeb.

Mechanism of Action
- Nonselective antimuscarinic at M1, M2, and M3 receptors which leads to reductions in cytosolic calcium concentrations with the smooth muscle cells lining the bronchioles thereby leading to smooth muscle relaxation and bronchodilation.

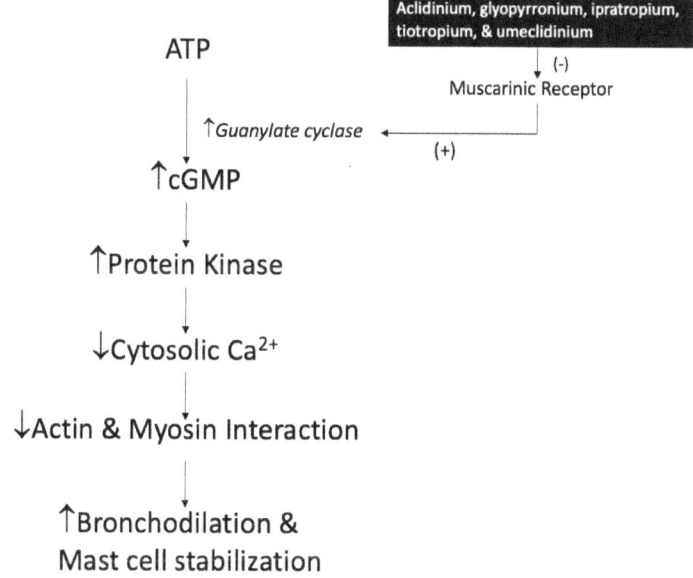

Primary Net Benefit
- Rapid-acting bronchodilator used in combination with albuterol in patients with acute severe asthma or COPD.
- Main Labs to Monitor:
  - SpO2
  - Respiratory rate
  - FEV1, Peak Flow

High-Yield Basic Pharmacology
- **Quaternary Ammonium**
  - Both tiotropium and ipratropium are quaternary ammonium structures, which prevent their absorption into the CNS across the blood-brain barrier.
  - This limits the central antimuscarinic potential of these drugs.
  - Ipratropium is poorly absorbed from the respiratory tract and further limits systemic antimuscarinic effects.

- **M2 Effect**
  - Ipratropium's inhibitory effect on M2 receptors can be counterproductive as antagonism of these receptors causes bronchoconstriction.
    - Some have argued that the paradoxical bronchoconstriction from ipratropium results from the administration of a hypotonic nebulized solution or benzalkonium chloride.
- **Onset of Action**
  - Although most prescribing and drug information describe the onset of ipratropium's effect at 30 to 60 minutes, a nebulized dose will be active within 30 seconds producing 50% maximal bronchodilation within minutes.

High-Yield Clinical Knowledge
- **Adjunctive Therapy**
  - Ipratropium is used primarily with albuterol for acute severe asthma either empirically or with an incomplete response to albuterol alone.
  - An additional 15% improvement in FEV1 can be observed when ipratropium is combined with albuterol in emergency department management of acute severe asthma.
- **Nebulized Administration**
  - Ipratropium is commonly administered via nebulization.
  - For this administration route, a tight-fitting mouthpiece is recommended to reduce the exposure of the eyes to ipratropium which may cause a local antimuscarinic effect (pupillary dilation, diminished accommodation).
    - For this reason, ipratropium should be used with caution in patients with glaucoma.
- **Maximum Frequency**
  - In patients with acute severe asthma, ipratropium should be administered at a dose of 0.5 mg q20minutes for a maximum of three doses.
    - Continued dosing beyond three doses in one hour produces no additional bronchodilatory effect but can prolong the dose-dependent duration of effect and adverse effects beyond eight hours.
- **Maximum Dose**
  - Patients who take ipratropium chronically for COPD may respond to higher doses but be administered at the same frequency (q6-8h).
    - Ipratropium can be administered as six puffs up to q6h.

High-Yield Core Evidence
- **Ipratropium Vs. Tiotropium**
  - This was a systematic review and meta-analysis to compare tiotropium's relative effects to ipratropium bromide on quality-of-life markers, exacerbations, symptoms, lung function, and serious adverse events in patients with COPD using available randomized controlled trial (RCT) data.
  - This analysis included two studies of good methodological quality of at least 12 weeks duration of participants with a mean forced expiratory volume in one second (FEV1) of 40% predicted value at baseline.
  - At three months, tiotropium, compared to ipratropium, was associated with a significantly increased FEV1, and fewer participants receiving tiotropium experienced one or more non-fatal serious adverse events.
  - Furthermore, the tiotropium group was also less likely to experience a COPD-related serious adverse event when compared to ipratropium bromide, with fewer hospital admissions and fewer patients experiencing one or more exacerbations leading to hospitalization.
  - However, there was no significant difference in mortality between the treatments.
  - The authors concluded that tiotropium treatment, compared with ipratropium bromide, was associated with improved lung function, fewer hospital admissions (including those for exacerbations of COPD), fewer exacerbations of COPD, and improved quality of life. (Cochrane Database Syst Rev. 2015 Sep 22;(9):CD009552.)

High-Yield Fast-Fact
- **Ipratropium Poor Taste**
    - Ipratropium is described as having a bitter taste that limits chronic compliance with this therapy.

HIGH-YIELD BOARD EXAM ESSENTIALS
- **CLASSIC AGENTS:** Ipratropium
- **DRUG CLASS:** SAMA
- **INDICATIONS:** Allergic rhinitis, asthma, COPD
- **MECHANISM:** Nonselective antimuscarinic at M1, M2, and M3 receptors.
- **SIDE EFFECTS:** Sinusitis, headache, UTI, dyspepsia
- **CLINICAL PEARLS:** Ipratropium is used primarily in combination with albuterol for acute severe asthma either empirically or with an incomplete response to albuterol alone. An additional 15% improvement in FEV1 can be observed when ipratropium is combined with albuterol in emergency department management of acute severe asthma.

Table: Drug Class Summary

Short-Acting Muscarinic Antagonists - Drug Class Review			
High-Yield Med Reviews			
Mechanism of Action: Nonselective antimuscarinic at M1, M2, and M3 receptors.			
Class Effects: Rapid-acting bronchodilator used in combination with albuterol in patients with acute severe asthma or COPD.			
Generic Name	**Brand Name**	**Indication(s) or Uses**	**Notes**
Ipratropium	Atrovent, Atrovent Nasal, Ipravent	<ul><li>Allergic rhinitis</li><li>Asthma</li><li>Chronic obstructive pulmonary disease</li></ul>	<ul><li>**Dosing (Adult):**<ul><li>Intranasal: two sprays in each nostril 2-4 times daily</li><li>MDI: 2 inhalations (34 mcg) 4 times daily</li><li>Nebulization: 0.5 mg q20minutes for three doses, OR 0.5 mg q6-8h</li></ul></li><li>**Dosing (Peds):**<ul><li>Intranasal: two sprays in each nostril 2-4 times daily</li><li>MDI: 1 to 2 inhalations (34 mcg) 4 times daily; Max: 12 inhalations/day</li><li>Nebulization: 0.25 to 0.5 mg q20minutes for three doses, OR 0.25 to 0.5 mg q6-8h</li></ul></li><li>**CYP450 Interactions:** None</li><li>**Renal or Hepatic Dose Adjustments:** None</li><li>**Dosage Forms:** Nasal solution, Inhalation (aerosol, solution)</li></ul>

PULMONOLOGY – BRONCHODILATORS – LONG-ACTING MUSCARINIC ANTAGONISTS

Drug Class
- Long-Acting Muscarinic Antagonists
- Agents:
    - Chronic Care
        - Aclidinium
        - Glycopyrrolate
        - Revefenacin
        - Tiotropium
        - Umeclidinium

Main Indications or Uses
- Chronic Care
    - Asthma (tiotropium only)
    - Chronic obstructive pulmonary disease

Mechanism of Action
- Selectively inhibit muscarinic receptors, M1 and M3, with slow dissociation from M3 providing a prolonged bronchodilatory effect.

Fast Facts
✓ This class of drugs have significantly helped with not only compliance when compared to ipratropium due to their longer-acting formulations but improving symptoms which help to keep COPD patients out of the hospital.

Counseling Points
✓ Counsel patients on tiotropium to NOT swallow the capsules but to insert it into the inhalation device for proper drug delivery.

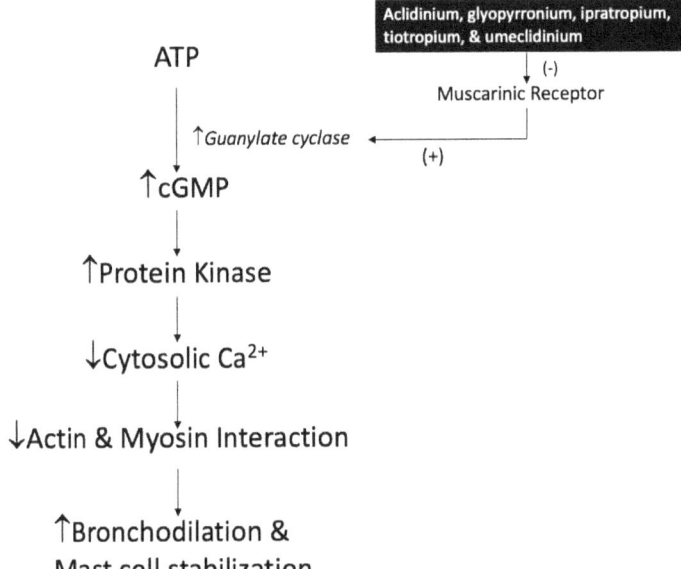

Primary Net Benefit
- LAMAs improve lung function and COPD symptoms and may reduce the risk of COPD exacerbations, but their role in asthma is reserved for severe uncontrolled asthma.
- Main Labs to Monitor:
    - SpO2
    - Respiratory rate
    - FEV1, Peak Flow

High-Yield Basic Pharmacology
- **Onset**
    - The LAMA agents glycopyrrolate and umeclidinium have rapid onsets of between 5 to 15 minutes but should not be used for acute management of COPD or asthma exacerbation.
    - Ipratropium is the preferred antimuscarinic for use with albuterol for asthma or COPD exacerbation.

- **Quaternary Ammonium**
  - LAMAs are quaternary ammonium structures that prevent their absorption into the CNS across the blood-brain barrier.
  - This limits the central antimuscarinic potential of these drugs.

High-Yield Clinical Knowledge
- **High Risk for Exacerbation**
  - In patients at high risk of COPD exacerbation, tiotropium is preferred as it has the most evidence supporting a more significant reduction in the frequency of exacerbations compared to LABA.
    - Other LAMAs may be used for this benefit; the largest amount of data supports tiotropium.
- **Long Term Benefit**
  - Evidence exists to support the long-term use of tiotropium in patients with COPD by reducing the frequency of COPD exacerbations.
  - There was also no evidence of an increased risk of cardiovascular adverse events associated with long-term use of tiotropium.
  - However, tiotropium did not have a significant impact in slowing lung function decline with long-term therapy.
- **Dosing**
  - There is no dose titration of LAMA agents, as their commercially available dosage forms are the appropriate starting dose and effective for nearly all adult patients.
- **Asthma Use**
  - LAMAs are reserved for the treatment of uncontrolled severe asthma.
    - Alternatives for uncontrolled severe asthma include high-dose inhaled corticosteroids plus LABA, LAMA plus biologic therapy, or oral corticosteroids.
  - Tiotropium decreases the frequency of severe exacerbations and reduces the need for oral corticosteroids in asthma.
- **Capsules**
  - Glycopyrrolate and tiotropium are available in capsules intended to have their contents inhaled.
  - Patients must be adequately educated to avoid ingesting these capsules, which will have no therapeutic benefit, increasing their exacerbation risk.
- **Less Pneumonia**
  - Compared to inhaled corticosteroids, LAMAs are associated with a lower risk of secondary pneumonia, with a similar reduction in exacerbation rates.

High-Yield Core Evidence
- **FLAME Trial**
  - This was a multicenter, double-blind, double-dummy, noninferiority that randomized patients with COPD and a history of at least one exacerbation during the previous year were randomly assigned to receive, by inhalation, either the indacaterol 110 mcg plus glycopyrrolate 50 mcg once daily or salmeterol 50 mcg plus fluticasone 500 mcg twice daily.
  - Indacaterol plus glycopyrrolate was met both the noninferiority to and superiority to, salmeterol plus fluticasone regarding the primary outcome of the annual COPD exacerbation rate, the yearly rate of moderate or severe exacerbations, a longer time to the first exacerbation.
  - The incidence of adverse events and deaths was similar in the two groups.
  - The incidence of pneumonia was significantly lower in the indacaterol-glycopyrrolate group compared to the salmeterol-fluticasone group.
  - The authors concluded that indacaterol-glycopyrrolate was more effective than salmeterol-fluticasone in preventing COPD exacerbations in patients with a history of exacerbation during the previous year. (N Engl J Med. 2016 Jun 9;374(23):2222-34.)

- **TALC Trial**
  - This was a multicenter, three-way, double-blind, triple-dummy crossover trial of patients with asthma.
  - Study subjects were randomized to either tiotropium plus inhaled glucocorticoid, to a doubling of the inhaled glucocorticoid dose, or the addition of salmeterol plus tiotropium.
  - Compared with doubling the dose of an inhaled glucocorticoid, tiotropium was superior in improving peak expiratory flow (PEF), evening PEF, the proportion of asthma-control days, FEV1 before bronchodilation, and daily symptoms scores.
  - Tiotropium was non-inferior to the addition of salmeterol in all assessed outcomes.
  - When added to an inhaled glucocorticoid, the authors concluded that tiotropium improved symptoms and lung function in patients with inadequately controlled asthma. Its effects appeared to be equivalent to those with the addition of salmeterol. (N Engl J Med. 2010 Oct 28;363(18):1715-26.)

High-Yield Fast-Fact
- **Glycopyrrolate Uses**
  - Glycopyrrolate has numerous other uses, including ophthalmologic indications, and parenteral uses including recovery from anesthesia and drying of mucous membranes associated with palliative care.

HIGH-YIELD BOARD EXAM ESSENTIALS
- **CLASSIC AGENTS:** Aclidinium, glycopyrrolate, revefenacin, tiotropium, umeclidinium
- **DRUG CLASS:** LAMA
- **INDICATIONS:** Asthma, COPD
- **MECHANISM:** Selectively inhibit muscarinic receptors, M1 and M3, with slow dissociation from M3 providing a prolonged bronchodilatory effect.
- **SIDE EFFECTS:** Xerostomia, secondary pneumonia, tachycardia
- **CLINICAL PEARLS:** In patients at high risk of COPD exacerbation, tiotropium is preferred as it has the most evidence supporting a more significant reduction in the frequency of exacerbations compared to LABA.

Long-Acting Muscarinic Antagonists - Drug Class Review
High-Yield Med Reviews

Mechanism of Action: *Selectively inhibit muscarinic receptors, M1 and M3, with slow dissociation from M3, providing a prolonged bronchodilatory effect.*

Class Effects: *LAMAs improve lung function and COPD symptoms and may reduce the risk of COPD exacerbations, but their role in asthma is reserved for severe uncontrolled asthma.*

Generic Name	Brand Name	Main Indication(s) or Uses	Notes
Aclidinium	Tudorza Pressair	- Chronic obstructive pulmonary disease	- **Dosing (Adult):** - Oral inhalation: 400 mcg (1 inhalation) bid - **Dosing (Peds):** Not routinely used - **CYP450 Interactions:** Substrate CYP2D6, 3A4 - **Renal or Hepatic Dose Adjustments:** None - **Dosage Forms:** Aerosol powder

Glycopyrrolate	Lonhala Magnair, Seebri Neohaler	- Chronic obstructive pulmonary disease	- **Dosing (Adult):**
			  - DPI: 1 capsule (15.6 mcg) BID
			  - Nebulization: 25 mcg BID
			- **Dosing (Peds):** Not routinely used
			- **CYP450 Interactions:** None
			- **Renal or Hepatic Dose Adjustments:** None
			- **Dosage Forms:** Inhalation (capsule, solution)

Revefenacin	Yupelri	- Chronic obstructive pulmonary disease	- **Dosing (Adult):**
			  - Nebulization: 175 mcg daily
			- **Dosing (Peds):** Not routinely used
			- **CYP450 Interactions:** Inhibits P-gp
			- **Renal or Hepatic Dose Adjustments:**
			  - Hepatic impairment: not recommended
			- **Dosage Forms:** Inhalation (solution)

Tiotropium	Spiriva	- Asthma
		- Chronic obstructive pulmonary disease
			- **Dosing (Adult):**
			  - Oral inhalation (Respimat): Two inhalations (2.5 mcg) once daily
			  - Oral inhalation (DPI): contents of 1 capsule inhaled once daily
			  - Oral inhalation (Soft-mist inhaler): Two inhalations (5 mcg) once daily
			- **Dosing (Peds):**
			  - Oral inhalation (Respimat): Two inhalations (1.25 mcg) once daily
			  - Oral inhalation (Soft-mist inhaler): Two inhalations (5 mcg) once daily
			- **CYP450 Interactions:** Substrate CYP2D6, 3A4
			- **Renal or Hepatic Dose Adjustments:** None
			- **Dosage Forms:** Inhalation (aerosol, capsule)

Umeclidinium	Incruse Ellipta	- COPD	- **Dosing (Adult):**
			  - DPI: 1 (62.5 mcg) inhalation daily
			- **Dosing (Peds):**
			  - Not routinely used
			- **CYP450 Interactions:** Substrate CYP2D6, P-gp
			- **Renal or Hepatic Dose Adjustments:** None
			- **Dosage Forms:** Inhalation aerosol

PULMONOLOGY – BRONCHODILATOR – BETA-2 AGONIST – LONG ACTING

Drug Class

- **Long-Acting Beta-2 Agonist**
- **Agents:**
    - Chronic Care
        - Arformoterol
        - Formoterol
        - Indacaterol
        - Olodaterol
        - Salmeterol
        - Vilanterol

> **Fast Facts**
>
> ✓ Formoterol is the more commonly used LABA for the treatment of exercise-induced asthma due to shorter onset of action compared to other agents.

Main Indications or Uses

- **Chronic Care**
    - Asthma
    - Chronic obstructive pulmonary disease
    - Exercise-induced bronchospasm

Mechanism of Action

- Activation of beta-2 adrenergic receptors decreases intracellular calcium entry, leading to smooth muscle relaxation.

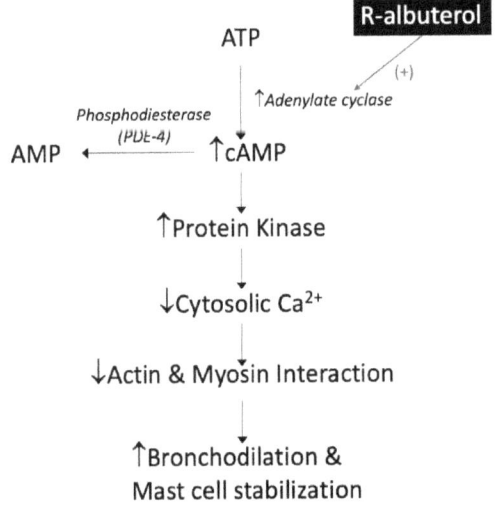

Primary Net Benefit

- Long-acting beta-2 agonists (LABA) provide selective bronchodilation, are a core component for asthma, and play a role in COPD therapy. Still, emerging evidence suggests long-acting muscarinic antagonists (LAMA) may be preferred.
- **Main Labs to Monitor:**
    - Respiratory rate
    - FEV1, Peak Flow

High-Yield Basic Pharmacology

- **Lipid-Soluble**
  - LABAs are characteristically more lipid-soluble than SABA agents, allowing penetration into the cell membrane's outer phospholipid layer, conferring a longer time of action.
- **Beta-2 Selectivity**
  - LABAs are generally more beta-2 selective than albuterol, owing to their increased time in lung tissue.
- **Dose-Response Curve**
  - The ability of beta-2 agonists to provide bronchodilation is dependent on the baseline degree of bronchoconstriction.
  - With increasing bronchoconstriction, the dose-response curve of beta-2 agonists experiences a rightward shift, with a corresponding decrease in duration of effect.
    - Patients with increasing bronchoconstriction will require higher, more frequent doses of beta-2 agonists of both short- and long-acting forms.

High-Yield Clinical Knowledge

- **LABA Role**
  - In the treatment of asthma, LABAs are preferred to inhaled corticosteroids (ICS).
  - Combinations of ICS and LABA increase asthma control, reduce the frequency of exacerbations, and do so to a more considerable degree than increasing ICS dose alone.
- **Chronic Bronchodilation**
  - LABAs must not be used for the acute management of severe asthma.
  - Although salmeterol has a rapid onset of fewer than 30 minutes, albuterol is the drug of choice as it is almost immediately effective.
- **Long Vs. Ultra-Long**
  - Formoterol and salmeterol are considered long-acting agents with a 12-hour duration of effect.
  - The ultra-long-acting beta-2 agonists include indacaterol, olodaterol, and vilanterol can be administered once daily, as their effects last 24-hours.
- **Downregulation**
  - With the long-term administration of beta-2 agonists, a decreasing number of beta-2 receptors and decreased binding affinity occurs.
    - Desensitization of beta-2 agonist effects also occurs in cardiac tissue (as well as other extrapulmonary sites), reducing systemic adverse events from chronic high dose LABA therapy.
  - The addition of systemic corticosteroids, not inhaled corticosteroids, can partially reverse this effect and prevent its occurrence.
  - The duration of bronchodilation is primarily affected, with less of a change in the peak response.
- **Transient Hypoxia**
  - Beta-2 agonists may transiently cause decreased perfusion of poorly ventilated lung units, thereby reducing arterial oxygen tension.
  - However, this effect is small and can be compensated for by administering supplemental oxygen.
- **Hypokalemia/Hyperglycemia/Hyperlactemia**
  - LABAs may produce potassium shifting intracellularly, potentially leading to conduction delays in cardiac tissue.
    - Patients with acute severe asthma or COPD exacerbations receiving SABA therapy should have their potassium closely monitored and kept above the lower limit of normal (typically above 3.5 mEq/L, but some recommend above 4.0 mEq/L.
  - High-dose LABA therapy can produce glucose and lactate elevations, as these agents augment glycolysis and cause an anaerobic metabolic shift.
  - Tachycardia is a rare effect secondary to LABAs as they rarely distribute outside of lung tissue.

High-Yield Core Evidence

- **TORCH Trial**
  - This was a multicenter, double-blind trial that randomized patients with COPD to either salmeterol 50 mcg plus fluticasone propionate 500 mcg twice daily (combination regimen) or to either placebo salmeterol alone or fluticasone propionate alone for three years.
  - There was no statistically significant difference between combination therapy and placebo concerning the hazard ratio for death.
  - The mortality rate for salmeterol alone or fluticasone propionate alone did not differ significantly from that for placebo.
  - Combination therapy did reduce the annual rate of exacerbations significantly compared to placebo and improved health status and spirometric values.
  - There was a higher risk of pneumonia among patients receiving fluticasone.
  - The authors concluded that reducing death from all causes among patients with COPD in the combination-therapy group did not reach the predetermined level of statistical significance. (N Engl J Med. 2007 Feb 22;356(8):775-89.)

- **IMPACT Trial**
  - This was a multicenter, double-blind trial of patients with COPD who were randomized to fluticasone 100 mcg plus umeclidinium 62.5 mcg plus vilanterol 25 mcg (triple therapy), fluticasone 100 mcg plus umeclidinium 62.5 mcg, or umeclidinium 62.5 mcg plus vilanterol 25 mcg.
  - Triple therapy with fluticasone, umeclidinium, and vilanterol led to a significantly lower annual rate of moderate or severe COPD exacerbations than either double therapy group and a lower rate of hospitalization to the umeclidinium, vilanterol group.
  - Patients taking fluticasone experienced a higher incidence of pneumonia compared to the umeclidinium-vilanterol group.
  - The authors concluded that triple therapy with fluticasone furoate, umeclidinium, and vilanterol resulted in a lower rate of moderate or severe COPD exacerbations than fluticasone furoate-vilanterol or umeclidinium-vilanterol in this population. (N Engl J Med. 2018 May 3;378(18):1671-1680.)

High-Yield Fast-Fact

- **Boxed Warning Removal**
  - The FDA removed the boxed warning for increased asthma-related deaths with ICS/LABA combinations as more robust evidence failed to show this relationship.

HIGH-YIELD BOARD EXAM ESSENTIALS
- **CLASSIC AGENTS:** Arformoterol, formoterol, indacaterol, olodaterol, salmeterol, vilanterol
- **DRUG CLASS:** LABA
- **INDICATIONS:** Asthma, COPD
- **MECHANISM:** Activation of beta-2 adrenergic receptors, decreasing intracellular entry of calcium, leading to smooth muscle relaxation.
- **SIDE EFFECTS:** Tachycardia, hypokalemia, hyperglycemia, hyperlactemia
- **CLINICAL PEARLS:** With long-term administration of beta-2 agonists, a decreasing number of beta-2 receptors and decreased binding affinity occurs.

Table: Drug Class Summary

Long-Acting Beta-2 Agonist - Drug Class Review			
High-Yield Med Reviews			
Mechanism of Action: *Activation of beta-2 adrenergic receptors decreases the intracellular entry of calcium, leading to smooth muscle relaxation.*			
Class Effects: *Long-acting beta-2 agonists (LABA) provide selective bronchodilation and are a core component for asthma and play a role in COPD therapy, but emerging evidence suggests long-acting muscarinic antagonists (LAMA) may be preferred.*			
Generic Name	**Brand Name**	**Main Indication(s) or Uses**	**Notes**
Arformoterol	Brovana	- Chronic obstructive pulmonary disease	- **Dosing (Adult):** - Nebulization: 15 mcg BID; Max 30 mcg/day - **Dosing (Peds):** Not routinely used - **CYP450 Interactions:** None - **Renal or Hepatic Dose Adjustments:** None - **Dosage Forms:** Nebulization solution
Formoterol	Perforomist	- Chronic obstructive pulmonary disease	- **Dosing (Adult):** - Nebulization: 20 mcg BID; Max 40 mcg/day - **Dosing (Peds):** Not routinely used - **CYP450 Interactions:** Substrate CYP2C9 - **Renal or Hepatic Dose Adjustments:** None - **Dosage Forms:** Nebulization solution
Indacaterol	Arcapta Neohaler	- Chronic obstructive pulmonary disease	- **Dosing (Adult):** - DPI: 1 capsule (75 mcg) inhaled twice daily - **Dosing (Peds):** Not routinely used - **CYP450 Interactions:** Substrate CYP2D6, 3A4, P-gp - **Renal or Hepatic Dose Adjustments:** None - **Dosage Forms:** Inhalation capsule
Olodaterol	Striverdi Respimat	- Chronic obstructive pulmonary disease	- **Dosing (Adult):** - Oral inhalation: two inhalations once daily - **Dosing (Peds):** Not routinely used - **CYP450 Interactions:** Substrate CYP2C8, 2C9, 3A4 - **Renal or Hepatic Dose Adjustments:** None - **Dosage Forms:** Inhalation (aerosol)

Salmeterol	Serevent Diskus	- Asthma
		- Chronic obstructive pulmonary disease
		- Exercise-induced bronchospasm
			- **Dosing (Adult):**
			  - DPI: 50 mcg daily
			- **Dosing (Peds):**
			  - DPI: 50 mcg daily
			- **CYP450 Interactions:** Substrate CYP3A4
			- **Renal or Hepatic Dose Adjustments:** None
			- **Dosage Forms:** Inhalation (aerosol)

Vilanterol	Only available in combinations: Breo Ellipta, Anoro Ellipta, Trelegy Ellipta	- Asthma - Chronic obstructive pulmonary disease	- **Dosing (Adult):** - Oral inhalation: 25 mcg daily - **Dosing (Peds):** Not routinely used - **CYP450 Interactions:** Substrate CYP3A4 - **Renal or Hepatic Dose Adjustments:** None - **Dosage Forms:** Inhalation (aerosol)

PULMONOLOGY – BRONCHODILATOR – BETA-2 AGONIST – SHORT ACTING

Drug Class
- Bronchodilator; Short-Acting Beta-2 Agonist (SABA)
- Agents:
  - Acute & Chronic Care
    - Albuterol
    - Levalbuterol
    - Metaproterenol
    - Racemic epinephrine
    - Terbutaline

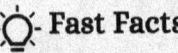 **Fast Facts**
- ✓ Levalbuterol is just the active isomer from the racemic mixture of albuterol. The is no evidence of any meaningful clinical advantage of levalbuterol over albuterol alone.

Dosing Pearl
- ✓ Terbutaline is unique in that it can be administered by subcutaneous injection and has been used in the past for tocolysis (premature labor).

Main Indications or Uses
- Acute & Chronic Care
  - Asthma
  - Chronic obstructive pulmonary disease
  - Exercise-induced bronchospasm

Mechanism of Action
- Activation of beta-2 adrenergic receptors decreases intracellular calcium entry, leading to smooth muscle relaxation.

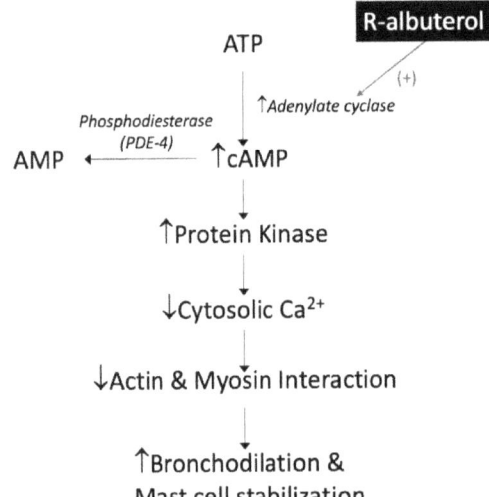

Primary Net Benefit
- Inhaled SABAs are used for the as-needed treatment of acute bronchospasm, providing a dose-dependent bronchodilatory effect. Systemic SABAs are no longer recommended due to extrapulmonary adverse events.
- Main Labs to Monitor:
  - Respiratory rate
  - FEV1, Peak Flow

High-Yield Basic Pharmacology
- **Racemic Mixture**
  - Albuterol is a racemic mixture of R-albuterol and S-albuterol.
  - R-albuterol is available separately as levalbuterol, which is metabolized more rapidly than S-albuterol, and may lack the pro-inflammatory effects that could diminish the bronchodilatory effect.

- **Racemic Epinephrine**
  - Racemic epinephrine is available as a solution for nebulization and can be used as a bronchodilator.
  - It is more commonly used to treat croup in pediatrics or for the treatment of stridor.

High-Yield Clinical Knowledge

- **Acute Bronchospasm**
  - Inhaled short-acting beta-2 agonists are the drugs of choice for acute bronchodilation and acute severe asthma management.
- **Maximum Dose**
  - Although the prescribing information of albuterol describes upper limits of recommended doses for MDI and nebulization treatments, there is no maximum clinical dose.
  - The drug information cited maximum doses should be used as surrogates for pharmacologic failure.
  - In acute bronchospasm, albuterol should be administered continuously until sufficient bronchodilatory effect is achieved or advanced airways are necessary (i.e., endotracheal intubation).
- **Hypokalemia**
  - High doses of SABAs may produce potassium shifting intracellularly, potentially leading to conduction delays in cardiac tissue.
  - Patients with acute severe asthma or COPD exacerbations receiving SABA therapy should have their potassium closely monitored and kept above the lower limit of normal (typically above 3.5 mEq/L, but some recommend above 4.0 mEq/L.
  - This effect is used proactively in the acute treatment of hyperkalemia.
- **Levalbuterol Dose**
  - Levalbuterol is commonly cited to produce less tachycardia and extrapulmonary effects than albuterol; however, this was only demonstrated when levalbuterol was administered at a dose of 0.63 mg q8h was compared to albuterol 2.5 mg and has not been able to be reproduced in other clinical studies.
- **Dose-Dependent Adverse Events**
  - High-dose SABA therapy can produce glucose and lactate elevations, as these agents augment glycolysis and cause an anaerobic metabolic shift.
    - Hyperlactemia is not necessarily harmful in all clinical situations, provided patients have sufficient oxidative capacity, hydration, and renal function.
  - Tachycardia is another common adverse event related to SABA therapy; however, it should not prevent using SABAs (albuterol) or an indication to lower the dose empirically.
- **Metaproterenol/Terbutaline**
  - Terbutaline use is limited to pediatrics, as its use in adults is accompanied by unacceptably high rates of systemic adverse events.
    - Similarly, metaproterenol is rarely used for bronchodilatory effects.

High-Yield Core Evidence

- **SMART**
  - This was a double-blind, placebo-controlled, observational study of patients over 12 years of age with asthma as judged by the study physician were eligible who were randomized to either salmeterol xinafoate or placebo added to usual asthma care.
  - After analyzing an interim analysis, the study was terminated due to findings in African Americans and difficulties in enrollment.
  - In the interim analysis, there was no difference in the primary outcome, respiratory-related deaths, or life-threatening experiences for salmeterol compared to placebo.
  - However, patients receiving salmeterol had a significant increase in respiratory-related deaths, asthma-related deaths, and in combined asthma-related deaths or life-threatening experiences.
  - A large proportion of this effect was observed in the African American subpopulation.
  - The authors concluded no significant differences between treatments. Still, there were statistically significant increases in respiratory-related and asthma-related deaths and combined asthma-related deaths or life-threatening experiences in the total population receiving salmeterol. (Chest. 2006 Jan;129(1):15-26.)

- **Novel START**
  - This was a multi-center, open-label, parallel-group, controlled trial of adult patients with mild asthma who were randomized to receive albuterol MDI for asthma, budesonide BID plus as-needed albuterol, or budesonide-formoterol as needed for asthma.
  - Patients randomized to receive budesonide-formoterol experienced a significantly lower annualized exacerbation rate than patients in the albuterol group but not in the budesonide maintenance group.
  - Severe exacerbations also occurred less frequently in the budesonide-formoterol group than in the albuterol and budesonide groups.
  - The authors concluded that budesonide-formoterol used as needed in adults with mild asthma was superior to albuterol used to prevent asthma exacerbations. (N Engl J Med. 2019 May 23;380(21):2020-2030.)

High-Yield Fast-Fact
- **NCAA Performance Enhancing**
  - Albuterol is considered a performance-enhancing drug, according to the NCAA.
  - Pharmacists should be aware that student-athletes with asthma are required to possess proof for a medical exemption so that they can continue to take albuterol and compete within the NCAA regulations.

HIGH-YIELD BOARD EXAM ESSENTIALS
- **CLASSIC AGENTS:** Albuterol, levalbuterol, metaproterenol, racemic epinephrine, terbutaline
- **DRUG CLASS:** SABA
- **INDICATIONS:** Asthma, bronchospasm, COPD
- **MECHANISM:** Activation of beta-2 adrenergic receptors, decreasing intracellular entry of calcium, leading to smooth muscle relaxation.
- **SIDE EFFECTS:** Tachycardia, tremor, hypokalemia
- **CLINICAL PEARLS:** Although the prescribing information of albuterol describes upper limits of recommended doses for MDI and nebulization treatments, there is no maximum clinical dose.

Table: Drug Class Summary

Short-Acting Beta-2 Agonist - Drug Class Review High-Yield Med Reviews			
Mechanism of Action: *Activation of beta-2 adrenergic receptors decreases intracellular calcium entry, leading to smooth muscle relaxation.*			
Class Effects: *Inhaled SABAs are used to treat acute bronchospasm as-needed treatment, providing a dose-dependent bronchodilatory effect. Systemic SABAs are no longer recommended due to extrapulmonary adverse events.*			
Generic Name	**Brand Name**	**Main Indication(s) or Uses**	**Notes**
Albuterol	ProAir, Proventil, Ventolin	<ul><li>Asthma</li><li>Bronchospasm</li><li>Chronic obstructive pulmonary disease</li></ul>	<ul><li>**Dosing (Adult):**<ul><li>MDI/DPI: 2 inhalations q4-6h as needed<ul><li>Up to 8 to 10 inhalations q20minutes for 3 doses, repeated as necessary</li></ul></li><li>Nebulization: 2.5 mg q4-6h as needed<ul><li>Up to 15 mg/hour via continuous nebulization over 1 hour</li></ul></li></ul></li><li>**Dosing (Peds):**<ul><li>MDI/DPI: 1 to 2 inhalations q4-6h as needed<ul><li>Up to 8 to 10 inhalations q20minutes for 3 doses, repeated as necessary</li></ul></li><li>Nebulization: 2.5 mg q4-6h as needed<ul><li>Up to 15 mg/hour via continuous nebulization over 1 hour</li></ul></li></ul></li><li>**CYP450 Interactions:** None</li><li>**Renal or Hepatic Dose Adjustments:** None</li><li>**Dosage Forms:** Inhalation (aerosol, nebulization solution, solution), Oral (syrup, tablet)</li></ul>
Levalbuterol	Xopenex	<ul><li>Asthma</li><li>Bronchospasm</li></ul>	<ul><li>**Dosing (Adult):**<ul><li>MDI: 2 inhalations (90 mcg) q4-6h as needed<ul><li>Up to 4 to 8 inhalations q20minutes for 3 doses, repeated as necessary</li></ul></li><li>Nebulization: 0.63 to 1.25 mg q6-8h as needed<ul><li>Up to 2.5 mg q20minutes, then 1.25 to 5 mg q1-4hours as needed</li></ul></li></ul></li><li>**Dosing (Peds):**<ul><li>MDI/DPI: 1 inhalation q4-6h as needed<ul><li>Up to 4 to 8 inhalations q20minutes for 3 doses, repeated as necessary</li></ul></li><li>Nebulization: 0.31 to 1.25 mg q4-6h as needed<ul><li>Up to 2.5 mg q20minutes, then 1.25 to 5 mg q1-4hours as needed</li></ul></li></ul></li><li>**CYP450 Interactions:** None</li><li>**Renal or Hepatic Dose Adjustments:** None</li><li>**Dosage Forms:** Inhalation (aerosol, nebulization solution)</li></ul>

Short-Acting Beta-2 Agonist - Drug Class Review
High-Yield Med Reviews

Generic Name	Brand Name	Main Indication(s) or Uses	Notes

Metaproterenol	Alupent	- Asthma	- **Dosing (Adult):**
			  - Oral: 20 mg q6-8h
			- **Dosing (Peds):**
			  - Oral: 1.3 to 2.6 mg/kg/day divided q6-8h
			    - Maximum 10 mg/dose
			- **CYP450 Interactions:** None
			- **Renal or Hepatic Dose Adjustments:** None
			- **Dosage Forms:** Oral (syrup, tablet)

Racemic epinephrine	Racepi	- Bronchospasm	- **Dosing (Adult):**
			  - MDI: 1 (0.125 mg) inhalations q4-6h as needed
			    - Up to 8 inhalations/24 hours
			  - Nebulization: 2.25% mg q4-6h as needed
			    - Up to 12 inhalations/24 hours
			- **Dosing (Peds):**
			  - MDI: 1 (0.125 mg) inhalations q4-6h as needed
			    - Up to 8 inhalations/24 hours
			  - Nebulization: 2.25% mg q4-6h as needed
			    - Up to 12 inhalations/24 hours
			- **CYP450 Interactions:** None
			- **Renal or Hepatic Dose Adjustments:** None
			- **Dosage Forms:** Inhalation (solution)

Terbutaline	Bricanyl	- Asthma/Bronchospasm
		- Extravasation management
		- Premature labor
			- **Dosing (Adult):**
			  - Oral: 2.5 to 5 mg q8h
			  - SQ: 0.25 mg/dose q20minutes for 3 doses
			  - IV: 2.5 to 5 mcg/minute, increased gradually q20-30min to maximum 25 mcg/minute
			- **Dosing (Peds):**
			  - IV infusion: 0.2 to 0.4 mcg/kg/minute, maximum 5 mcg/kg/minute
			  - Oral: 2.5 mg q8h
			  - SQ: 0.01 mg/kg/dose q20minutes x 3 doses
			- **CYP450 Interactions:** None
			- **Renal or Hepatic Dose Adjustments:** None
			- **Dosage Forms:** IV (solution), Oral (tablet)

PULMONOLOGY – CFTR MODULATOR

Drug Class
- CFTR Modulator
- Agents:
  - Chronic Care
    - Elexacaftor, tezacaftor, ivacaftor
    - Ivacaftor
    - Lumacaftor, ivacaftor
    - Tezacaftor, ivacaftor

Main Indications or Uses
- Chronic Care
  - Cystic fibrosis

Mechanism of Action
- Ivacaftor
  - Improve lung mucus viscosity and clearance by potentiating the activity of the cystic fibrosis transmembrane conductance regulator (CFTR) protein, prolonging chloride channel opening.
- Elexacaftor, lumacaftor, tezacaftor
  - Enhance the performance of mutant CFTR protein processing at the cell surface.

Primary Net Benefit
- Novel disease-modifying therapy for cystic fibrosis through targeted therapy aimed at partially restoring the function of mutated CFTR.
- Main Labs to Monitor:
  - LFT (INR/PT, albumin, protein, bilirubin) at baseline, q3months x 1 year, then annually
  - Ophthalmological exam (baseline and periodic)

High-Yield Basic Pharmacology
- Specific CFTR Targets
  - Ivacaftor functions to potentiate CFTR, but elexacaftor, lumacaftor, and tezacaftor have slightly different targets.
  - Elexacaftor, lumacaftor, and tezacaftor improve cellular processing and trafficking of normal and mutant CFTR forms, including the mutant F508del-CFTR.
- Administration
  - CFTR modulators should be taken orally with high-fat content foods to facilitate absorption.
    - Examples of high-fat foods include butter, eggs, nuts, or whole-milk dairy products.

High-Yield Clinical Knowledge
- Correctors and Potentiators
  - Combining both correctors of CFTR protein activity (elexacaftor, lumacaftor, tezacaftor) and potentiators (ivacaftor) are used in patients with Phe508del CFTR mutation.
- FEV1 Improvements
  - CFTR modulator therapy significantly improves FEV1 in patients with CF when added to background therapy.
- CFTR Locations
  - CFTR proteins are expressed not only in the lung tissue and in sweat glands and the GI tract (including intestines, pancreas, and bile duct).

- **Mutations**
  - As the cause of cystic fibrosis has been identified to be a result of mutations in the gene encoding the CFTR proteins, most have at least one copy of the Phe508del CFTR mutation.
  - Patients with homozygous mutations of the Phe508del mutation have demonstrated a clinical response to CFTR modulator therapy.

High-Yield Core Evidence
- **TRAFFIC/TRANSPORT**
  - This was a single publication of two phase 3, double-blind, placebo-controlled studies where patients with cystic fibrosis were homozygous for the Phe508del CFTR mutation were randomized to either lumacaftor 600 mg daily or 400 mg q12h in combination with either ivacaftor 250 mg q12h or placebo for 24 weeks.
  - Patients randomized to combination therapy with lumacaftor and ivacaftor experienced a significant improvement from baseline FEV1 at the study endpoint compared to placebo.
  - Additionally, the rate of pulmonary exacerbations was lower in the lumacaftor and ivacaftor combination group and the rate of hospitalization or IV antibiotics.
  - Adverse events were similar, but more patients discontinued lumacaftor and ivacaftor combination due to an adverse event compared to placebo.
  - The authors concluded that data show that lumacaftor combined with ivacaftor provided a benefit for patients with cystic fibrosis homozygous for the Phe508del CFTR mutation. (N Engl J Med. 2015 Jul 16;373(3):220-31.)
- **Elexacaftor, Tezacaftor, Ivacaftor for CF**
  - This was a phase 3, double-blind, placebo-controlled trial that randomized patients at least 12 years of age with CF and Phe508del-minimal function genotypes to receive either elexacaftor or tezacaftor ivacaftor combination therapy or placebo for 24 weeks.
  - Combination therapy significantly improved the percentage of predicted FEV1 at weeks 4 and 24 and a significantly lower incidence of pulmonary exacerbations and lower sweat chloride concentrations.
  - There were no observed serious adverse events with combination therapy compared to placebo.
  - The authors concluded that elexacaftor, tezacaftor, and ivacaftor combination therapy was efficacious in patients with cystic fibrosis with Phe508del–minimal function genotypes, in whom previous CFTR modulator regimens were ineffective. (N Engl J Med 2019; 381:1809-1819.)

High-Yield Fast-Fact
- **Sulfonamides**
  - The core structure of elexacaftor contains a sulfonamide moiety and may cause cross-sensitivity in patients with sulfonamide allergies.

HIGH-YIELD BOARD EXAM ESSENTIALS
- **CLASSIC AGENTS:** Elexacaftor, tezacaftor, ivacaftor, lumacaftor
- **DRUG CLASS:** CFTR modulator
- **INDICATIONS:** Cystic fibrosis
- **MECHANISM:** Ivacaftor - Improve lung mucus viscosity and clearance by potentiating the CFTR protein activity, prolonging chloride channel opening. Elexacaftor, lumacaftor, tezacaftor - Enhance the performance of mutant CFTR protein processing at the cell surface.
- **SIDE EFFECTS:** Hepatotoxicity, conjunctivitis, cataracts, upper respiratory tract infection
- **CLINICAL PEARLS:** As the cause of cystic fibrosis has been identified to be a result of mutations in the gene encoding the CFTR proteins, most have at least one copy of the Phe508del CFTR mutation.

Table: Drug Class Summary

CFTR Modulator - Drug Class Review High-Yield Med Reviews			
Mechanism of Action: *Ivacaftor - Improve lung mucus viscosity and clearance by potentiating the CFTR protein activity, prolonging chloride channel opening.* *Elexacaftor, lumacaftor, tezacaftor - Enhance the performance of mutant CFTR protein processing at the cell surface.* **Class Effects:** *Novel disease-modifying therapy for cystic fibrosis through targeted therapy aimed at partially restoring mutated CFTR function.*			
Generic Name	**Brand Name**	**Main Indication(s) or Uses**	**Notes**

Elexacaftor, tezacaftor, ivacaftor	Trikafta	- Cystic Fibrosis	- **Dosing (Adult):**
			   - Oral: 2 packet q12h
			- **Dosing (Peds):**
			   - Children over 12 years, use adult dose
			- **CYP450 Interactions:** Substrate CYP3A4, P-gp; Inhibits CYP3A4, P-gp
			- **Renal or Hepatic Dose Adjustments:**
			   - Child-Pugh class B: Day 1: 2 tablets in AM, Day 2: 1 tablet in AM, then alternate day 1/2
			   - Child-Pugh class C: not recommended
			- **Dosage Forms:** Oral (packet)

Ivacaftor	Kalydeco	- Cystic Fibrosis	- **Dosing (Adult):**
			   - Oral: 150 mg q12h
			- **Dosing (Peds):**
			   - Oral: 25 to 150 mg q12h
			- **CYP450 Interactions:** Substrate CYP3A4; Inhibits CYP3A4, P-gp
			- **Renal or Hepatic Dose Adjustments:**
			   - Child-Pugh class B or C: 150 mg daily
			- **Dosage Forms:** Oral (packet, tablet)

Lumacaftor, ivacaftor	Orkambi	- Cystic Fibrosis	- **Dosing (Adult):**
			   - Oral: 2 packet q12h
			- **Dosing (Peds):**
			   - Oral: 1 to 2 packet q12h
			- **CYP450 Interactions:** Substrate CYP3A4; Inhibits CYP3A4, P-gp
			- **Renal or Hepatic Dose Adjustments:**
			   - Child-Pugh class B: 2 packets in AM, 1 tablet PM
			   - Child-Pugh class C: 1 packet q12h
			- **Dosage Forms:** Oral (packet)

CFTR Modulator - Drug Class Review
High-Yield Med Reviews

Generic Name	Brand Name	Main Indication(s) or Uses	Notes
Tezacaftor, ivacaftor	Symdeko	• Cystic Fibrosis	• **Dosing (Adult):** 　− Oral: 2 packet q12h • **Dosing (Peds):** 　− Oral: 1 to 2 packet q12h • **CYP450 Interactions:** Substrate CYP3A4; Inhibits CYP3A4, P-gp • **Renal or Hepatic Dose Adjustments:** 　− Child-Pugh class B: 2 packets in AM, 1 tablet PM 　− Child-Pugh class C: 1 packet q12h • **Dosage Forms:** Oral (packet)

PULMONOLOGY – CORTICOSTEROIDS – INHALED

Drug Class
- Inhaled Corticosteroids
- Agents:
  - Acute and Chronic Care
    - Beclomethasone
    - Budesonide
    - Ciclesonide
    - Fluticasone
    - Mometasone

> **Fast Facts**
> ✓ Inhaled corticosteroids are the primary treatments for the maintenance and control of asthma but are adjuncts to those with COPD.

Main Indications or Uses
- Acute & Chronic Care
  - Asthma
  - Chronic obstructive pulmonary disease

> **Counseling Points**
> ✓ Counsel patients to rinse out their mouths after dose administration to reduce the risk of oral candidiasis or thrush.

Mechanism of Action
- Combines with intracellular glucocorticoid receptors and acts as a gene transcription factor, increasing the production of anti-inflammatory mediators, suppression of inflammatory cytokines, inflammatory cell activation/recruitment/infiltration, and decreasing vascular permeability.

Primary Net Benefit
- ICS are a core component for chronic asthma care but have a limited role in COPD. Numerous combination inhaler products improve compliance and administration of other controller agents, but patients must be educated on proper oral care to reduce the risk of oropharyngeal complications.
- Main Labs to Monitor:
  - Respiratory rate
  - FEV1, Peak Flow
  - Bone mineral density, growth (children, baseline, and periodically)
  - CBC
  - Liver enzymes (AST/ALT, alkaline phosphatase)
  - Liver function (INR/PT, albumin, protein, bilirubin)
  - Ophthalmic exam

High-Yield Basic Pharmacology
- **Corticosteroid Effects**
  - Inhaled corticosteroids increase the number of beta-2 receptors in lung tissue, thus improving SABA or LABA therapy responsiveness.
  - ICS also deduce pulmonary hypersecretion, reducing airway edema and exudation.
- **Onset of Action**
  - The bronchodilatory effects of ICS are not sufficiently rapid enough for acute management of severe asthma, where parenteral corticosteroids are more appropriate.
  - The time to maximal response for ICS therapy is approximately 4 to 8 weeks.
- **Relative Potency**
  - Many steroids are compared on their relative potency and to predict dose responses.
  - While the ICS are of differing potencies, their doses in commercially available products produce similar clinical bronchodilatory and anti-inflammatory effects.

High-Yield Clinical Knowledge
- **Asthma Vs. COPD**
  - ICS therapy is central to asthma by providing anti-inflammatory effects that improve long-term morbidity and mortality.

- However, ICS are not preferred for patients with COPD as they carry a higher risk of bacterial pneumonia and are limited to patients with severe airflow obstruction, concomitant asthma, or a history of frequent exacerbations.
- **Mouth Rinsing**
    - Patients on ICS must be educated to rinse and spit their mouths after administration to reduce the agent's oral bioavailability and reduce the risk of oral or esophageal candidiasis.
- **Systemic Steroid Effects**
    - ICS may be systemically absorbed, producing numerous adverse events similar to oral or parenteral corticosteroids.
    - These adverse events include osteoporosis, ophthalmologic complications (glaucoma, cataracts), adrenal suppression, delayed wound healing, hyperglycemia, hypertension, and psychiatric disturbances.
- **Systemic Absorption**
    - ICS are all absorbed systemically but can be rapidly metabolized via the first-pass metabolism if absorbed orally.
        - However, systemic absorption through lung tissue bypasses first-pass hepatic circulation, increasing systemic exposure to the corticosteroid.
        - Poor inhaler technique can result in enteral absorption of ICS but in the case of beclomethasone and ciclesonide, which are prodrugs, further limiting bioavailability.
- **Pediatric Growth Velocity**
    - Chronic use of ICS in pediatric patients is associated with growth suppression and occurs with low to medium dose ICS.
        - This effect is transient, and growth velocity returns to normal after 6 to 24 months of therapy and does not affect maximal growth potential.
- **Drug Interactions**
    - Protease inhibitors may significantly reduce the metabolism of inhaled corticosteroids, potentially increasing the risk of toxicity and adrenal suppression.
    - Fluticasone should not be used in patients taking protease inhibitors; however, beclomethasone is the best option as it is not a substrate of CYP3A4.

High-Yield Core Evidence
- **WISDOM**
    - This was a multicenter, double-blind, parallel-group trial of patients with a history of COPD exacerbation given tiotropium, salmeterol, and fluticasone (triple therapy) for a six-week run-in period.
    - After the run-in phase, patients were randomized to continue triple therapy or receive tiotropium salmeterol (double treatment) for 12 weeks.
    - Dual therapy with tiotropium and salmeterol was non-inferior to triple therapy (tiotropium, salmeterol, and fluticasone) from the time to the first moderate or severe COPD exacerbation (the primary outcome).
    - However, adjusted mean FEV1 was significantly higher among patients receiving triple therapy with fluticasone than dual therapy. Still, no change in dyspnea and minor changes in health status occurred in the glucocorticoid-withdrawal group.
    - The authors concluded that In patients with severe COPD receiving tiotropium plus salmeterol, the risk of moderate or severe exacerbations was similar among those who discontinued inhaled glucocorticoids and those who continued glucocorticoid therapy. (N Engl J Med. 2014 Oct 2;371(14):1285-94.)
- **Salford Lung Study**
    - This was a multicenter, controlled effectiveness trial that randomized patients with COPD to a once-daily inhaled combination of fluticasone furoate 100 mcg plus vilanterol 25 mcg or usual care.
    - Patients randomized to fluticasone plus vilanterol experienced a significantly lower moderate or severe exacerbations rate than usual care (primary outcome).
    - However, there was no difference in the rate of primary care contact (contact with a general practitioner, nurse, or other health care professional) and secondary care contact (inpatient admission, outpatient visit with a specialist, or emergency department visit), modification of the initial trial treatment for COPD, and the rate of exacerbations among patients who had had an exacerbation within three years before the trial.

- The authors concluded that for patients with COPD and a history of exacerbations, a once-daily treatment regimen of combined fluticasone furoate and vilanterol was associated with a lower rate of exacerbations than usual care without a greater risk of serious adverse events. (N Engl J Med. 2016 Sep 29;375(13):1253-60.)

High-Yield Fast-Fact
- **Dysphonia**
    - Up to 20% of patients taking ICS experience a steroid-induced myopathy of the vocal cords, producing dysphonia.
    - Proper inhaler technique and a spacer device can reduce the risk of thrush, candidiasis, and dysphonia.

HIGH-YIELD BOARD EXAM ESSENTIALS
- **CLASSIC AGENTS:** Beclomethasone, budesonide, ciclesonide, fluticasone, mometasone
- **DRUG CLASS:** Inhaled corticosteroids
- **INDICATIONS:** Asthma, COPD
- **MECHANISM:** Combines with intracellular glucocorticoid receptors and acts as a gene transcription factor, increasing the production of anti-inflammatory mediators, suppression of inflammatory cytokines, and inflammatory cell activation/recruitment/infiltration, and decreases vascular permeability.
- **SIDE EFFECTS:** Thrush, include osteoporosis, ophthalmologic complications (glaucoma, cataracts), adrenal suppression, delayed wound healing, hyperglycemia, hypertension, and psychiatric disturbances
- **CLINICAL PEARLS:** Chronic use of ICS in pediatric patients is associated with growth suppression and occurs with low to medium dose ICS.

Table: Drug Class Summary

\multicolumn{4}{c}{Inhaled Corticosteroids - Drug Class Review}
\multicolumn{4}{c}{High-Yield Med Reviews}
\multicolumn{4}{l}{**Mechanism of Action:** *Combines with intracellular glucocorticoid receptors and acts as a gene transcription factor, increasing the production of anti-inflammatory mediators, suppression of inflammatory cytokines, and inflammatory cell activation/recruitment/infiltration, and decreases vascular permeability.*}
\multicolumn{4}{l}{**Class Effects:** *ICS are a core component for chronic asthma care but limited role in COPD.*}
Generic Name	**Brand Name**	**Main Indication(s) or Uses**	**Notes**

Beclomethasone	Qvar	• Asthma
		• Chronic obstructive pulmonary disease
			• **Dosing (Adult):**
			  − Oral inhalation: 40 to 400 mcg BID
			• **Dosing (Peds):**
			  − Oral inhalation: 40 to 320 mcg BID
			• **CYP450 Interactions:** None
			• **Renal or Hepatic Dose Adjustments:** None
			• **Dosage Forms:** Aerosol powder, Inhalation solution

Budesonide	Pulmicort	• Asthma
		• Chronic obstructive pulmonary disease
			• **Dosing (Adult):**
			  − DPI: 360 to 720 mg BID
			  − Nebulization: 2 mg q6h
			• **Dosing (Peds):**
			  − Nebulization: 0.25 mg BID or 0.5 mg daily
			  − DPI: 180 to 360 mg BID
			• **CYP450 Interactions:** Substrate CYP3A4
			• **Renal or Hepatic Dose Adjustments:** None
			• **Dosage Forms:** Aerosol powder, Inhalation suspension

Ciclesonide	Alvesco	• Asthma	• **Dosing (Adult):**
			  − Oral inhalation: 80 to 320 mcg BID
			• **Dosing (Peds):**
			  − Oral inhalation: 80 to 320 mcg BID
			• **CYP450 Interactions:** Substrate CYP3A4
			• **Renal or Hepatic Dose Adjustments:** None
			• **Dosage Forms:** Inhalation aerosol solution

Fluticasone	ArmonAir, Arnuity, Flovent	• Asthma
		• COPD
			• **Dosing (Adult):**
			  − DPI (ArmonAir): 55 to 232 mcg BID
			  − DPI (Arnuity): 100 to 200 mcg daily
			  − MDI/DPI (Flovent): 100 to 1,000 mcg BID
			• **Dosing (Peds):**
			  − MDI/DPI (Flovent): 100 to 1,000 mcg BID
			• **CYP450 Interactions:** Substrate CYP3A4
			• **Renal or Hepatic Dose Adjustments:** None
			• **Dosage Forms:** Inhalation (aerosol, aerosol powder)

Mometasone	Asmanex	• Asthma	• **Dosing (Adult):**
			  − MDI: 200 to 400 mcg BID
			  − DPI: 220 to 440 mcg Daily
			• **Dosing (Peds):**
			  − MDI: 100 to 400 mcg BID
			  − DPI: 110 to 440 mcg Daily
			• **CYP450 Interactions:** Substrate CYP3A4
			• **Renal or Hepatic Dose Adjustments:** None
			• **Dosage Forms:** Inhalation aerosol

PULMONOLOGY – INHALER - COMBINATION PRODUCTS

Drug Class
- Combination Products
- Agents:
  - Chronic Care
    - Advair, AirDuo, Wixela (Salmeterol, fluticasone)
    - Anoro Ellipta (Vilanterol, umeclidinium)
    - Breo Ellipta (Vilanterol, fluticasone)
    - Bevespi (Formoterol, glycopyrrolate)
    - Breztri Aerosphere (Formoterol, budesonide, glycopyrrolate)
    - Combivent, DuoNeb (Albuterol, ipratropium)
    - Duaklir, Pressair (Aclidinium, formoterol)
    - Dulera (Formoterol, mometasone)
    - Stiolto (Tiotropium, olodaterol)
    - Symbicort (Formoterol, budesonide)
    - Trelegy Ellipta (Vilanterol, umeclidinium, fluticasone)
    - Utibron Neohaler (Indacaterol, glycopyrrolate)

Main Indications or Uses
- Chronic Care
  - COPD

Mechanism of Action
- See specific drug class Rapid Reviews

Primary Net Benefit
- Combination inhalers of bronchodilators or inhaled corticosteroids improve drug delivery to the pulmonary sites of action and enhance compliance.
- Main Labs to Monitor:
  - FEV1/FVC
  - PEF
  - Combinations with ICS
    - Bone mineral density, growth (children, baseline, and periodically)
    - CBC
    - Liver enzymes (AST/ALT, alkaline phosphatase)
    - Liver function (INR/PT, albumin, protein, bilirubin)
    - Ophthalmic exam

Table: Drug Class Summary

Combination Products - Drug Class Review High-Yield Med Reviews			
Mechanism of Action: See specific drug class Rapid Reviews.			
Class Effects: Combination inhalers of bronchodilators or inhaled corticosteroids improve drug delivery to the pulmonary sites of action and improve compliance.			
Generic Name	Brand Name	Main Indication(s) or Uses	Notes

Aclidinium, formoterol	Duaklir Pressair	- Chronic obstructive pulmonary disease	- **Dosing (Adult):**
			   - Oral Inhalation: 1 inhalation twice daily
			- **Dosing (Peds):**
			   - Not routinely used
			- **CYP450 Interactions:** Substrate CYP2C9, 2D6, 3A4
			- **Renal or Hepatic Dose Adjustments:** None
			- **Dosage Forms:** Aerosol powder

Albuterol, ipratropium	Combivent Respimat, DuoNeb	- Asthma
		- Chronic obstructive pulmonary disease
			- **Dosing (Adult):**
			   - COPD
			      - Oral Inhalation: 1 inhalation 4 times daily
			   - Asthma
			      - Oral inhalation: 8 inhalations q20minutes as needed for up to 3 hours
			      - Nebulization: 3 mL q20minutes for 3 doses or q4-6hours
			- **Dosing (Peds):**
			   - Nebulization: 1.5 to 3 mL q20minutes for 3 doses
			- **CYP450 Interactions:** None
			- **Renal or Hepatic Dose Adjustments:** None
			- **Dosage Forms:** Solution for nebulization, Solution for oral inhalation

Formoterol, Budesonide	Symbicort	- Asthma
		- Chronic obstructive pulmonary disease
			- **Dosing (Adult):**
			   - MDI: 2 inhalations once to twice daily
			- **Dosing (Peds):**
			   - MDI: 2 inhalations once to twice daily
			- **CYP450 Interactions:** None
			- **Renal or Hepatic Dose Adjustments:** None
			- **Dosage Forms:** Symbicort 160/4.5, Symbicort 80/4.5

Formoterol, Glycopyrrolate	Bevespi Aerosphere	- Chronic obstructive pulmonary disease	- **Dosing (Adult):**
			   - MDI: 2 inhalations twice daily
			- **Dosing (Peds):**
			   - Oral Inhalation
			- **CYP450 Interactions:** None
			- **Renal or Hepatic Dose Adjustments:** None
			- **Dosage Forms:** Inhalation aerosol

Combination Drugs - Drug Class Review			
High-Yield Med Reviews			
Generic Name	Brand Name	Indication(s) or Uses	Notes

Formoterol, Budesonide, Glycopyrrolate	Breztri Aerosphere	- Chronic obstructive pulmonary disease	- **Dosing (Adult):**
			  - MDI: 2 inhalations twice daily
			- **Dosing (Peds):**
			  - Oral Inhalation
			- **CYP450 Interactions:** None
			- **Renal or Hepatic Dose Adjustments:** None
			- **Dosage Forms:** [e.g., basic info]

Formoterol, Mometasone	Dulera	- Asthma
		- Chronic obstructive pulmonary disease
			- **Dosing (Adult):**
			  - MDI: 2 inhalations twice daily
			- **Dosing (Peds):**
			  - MDI: 2 inhalations twice daily
			- **CYP450 Interactions:** Substrate CYP2C9, 3A4
			- **Renal or Hepatic Dose Adjustments:** None
			- **Dosage Forms:** Dulera (50/5; 100/5; 200/5)

Indacaterol, Glycopyrrolate	Utibron Neohaler	- Chronic obstructive pulmonary disease	- **Dosing (Adult):**
			  - DPI: 1 capsule inhaled twice daily
			- **Dosing (Peds):**
			  - Not routinely used
			- **CYP450 Interactions:** Substrate CYP2D6, 3A4, P-gp
			- **Renal or Hepatic Dose Adjustments:** None
			- **Dosage Forms:** [e.g., basic info]

Salmeterol, fluticasone	Advair HFA, Advair Diskus, AirDuo, Wixela Inhub	- Asthma
		- Chronic obstructive pulmonary disease
			- **Dosing (Adult):**
			  - DPI: 1 inhalation twice daily
			  - MDI: 2 inhalations twice daily
			- **Dosing (Peds):**
			  - DPI: 1 inhalation twice daily
			  - MDI: 1 to 2 inhalations twice daily
			- **CYP450 Interactions:** Substrate CYP3A4
			- **Renal or Hepatic Dose Adjustments:** None
			- **Dosage Forms:** Advair (45/21 mcg; 115/21 mcg; 230;21 mcg), Advair Diskus (100/50; 250/50; 500/50), AirDuo (55/14; 113/14; 232/14), Wixela Inhub (100/50; 250/50; 500/50)

Tiotropium, olodaterol	Stiolto Respimat	- Chronic obstructive pulmonary disease	- **Dosing (Adult):**
			  - Oral Inhalation: two inhalations once daily
			- **Dosing (Peds):**
			  - Oral Inhalation
			- **CYP450 Interactions:** Substrate CYP2C8, 2C9, 2D6, 3A4
			- **Renal or Hepatic Dose Adjustments:** None
			- **Dosage Forms:** Stiolo Respimat 2.5 mg and 2.5 mg olodaterol

Combination Drugs - Drug Class Review High-Yield Med Reviews			
Generic Name	**Brand Name**	**Indication(s) or Uses**	**Notes**

Vilanterol, fluticasone	Breo Ellipta	- Asthma
		- Chronic obstructive pulmonary disease
			- **Dosing (Adult):**
			  – DPI: 1 inhalation once daily
			- **Dosing (Peds):**
			  – Not routinely used
			- **CYP450 Interactions:** Substrate CYP3A4
			- **Renal or Hepatic Dose Adjustments:** None
			- **Dosage Forms:** Breo Ellipta (25/100; 25/200)

Vilanterol, umeclidinium	Anoro Ellipta	- Chronic obstructive pulmonary disease	- **Dosing (Adult):**
			  – DPI: 1 inhalation daily
			- **Dosing (Peds):**
			  – Oral Inhalation
			- **CYP450 Interactions:** Substrate CYP2D6, P-gp
			- **Renal or Hepatic Dose Adjustments:** None
			- **Dosage Forms:** Anoro Ellpita (62.5/25 mcg)

Vilanterol, umeclidinium, fluticasone	Trelegy Ellipta	- Asthma
		- Chronic obstructive pulmonary disease
			- **Dosing (Adult):**
			  – DPI: 1 inhalation once daily
			- **Dosing (Peds):**
			  – Not routinely used
			- **CYP450 Interactions:** Substrate CYP2D6, 3A4, P-gp
			- **Renal or Hepatic Dose Adjustments:** None
			- **Dosage Forms:** [e.g., basic info]

PULMONOLOGY – METHYLXANTHINES

Drug Class
- Methylxanthines
- Agents:
  - Acute Care
    - Aminophylline
    - Caffeine
    - Theophylline

Main Indications or Uses
- Acute Care
  - Apnea of prematurity (caffeine)
  - Bradycardia (aminophylline)
- Chronic Care
  - Asthma (theophylline)

Mechanism of Action
- Methylxanthines nonselectively inhibit phosphodiesterases, increasing intracellular cAMP leading to smooth muscle relaxation.

> **Fast Facts**
>
> ✓ Theophylline's use in clinical practice has declined significantly over the years just is still used on occasion for asthma and/or COPD when other standard treatments have failed.
>
> ✓ Theophylline requires drug level monitoring due to toxicity, can cause tachycardia and seizures at higher doses, and is associated with drug interactions with inhibitors of CYP1A2 (e.g., ciprofloxacin).

Primary Net Benefit
- Once used as first-line agents for asthma, methylxanthines have been relegated to add-on therapy in patients who have otherwise failed alternative bronchodilators and inhaled corticosteroids.
- Main Labs to Monitor:
  - Theophylline trough (8-15 mcg/mL)
  - Liver enzymes (AST/ALT, alk phos)
  - Liver function (PT/INR, albumin, protein, bilirubin)

High-Yield Basic Pharmacology
- **Di- and Trimethylxanthine**
  - Theophylline's chemical name is 1,3-dimethylxanthine, whereas caffeine is 1,3,7-trimethylxanthine.
    - Theobromine is 3,7-dimethylxanthine.
- **Not Uric Acid**
  - The available methylxanthines are metabolized to demethylated xanthines, not uric acid (which involves xanthine oxidase).
- **Alternative Mechanisms**
  - Methylxanthines may provide bronchodilation by inhibiting adenosine's action on airway smooth muscle.
    - Adenosine has been associated with increased airway smooth muscle release of histamine.
  - Methylxanthines may also inhibit intracellular calcium influx, inhibit prostaglandins and histone deacetylation, and act as a sympathomimetic.
  - Selective phosphodiesterase 4 inhibitors have been developed, most notably roflumilast.

High-Yield Clinical Knowledge
- **Methylxanthines and Pulmonary Disease**
  - Theophylline is an effective bronchodilator that was once widely used for asthma.
  - As a result of the development of inhaled bronchodilators, the risks of theophylline due to its narrow therapeutic index outweighed any benefit compared to other available agents.
- **Apnea of Prematurity**
  - Caffeine is still routinely used in neonates to treat apnea of prematurity.
  - Administered via IV infusion, caffeine is an effective respiratory stimulant.
- **Aminophylline and Theophylline**

- Aminophylline is a water-soluble theophylline-ethylenediamine complex that is suitable for IV administration.
- These two agents are otherwise pharmacologically and kinetically similar.
- **CNS Effect**
  - All methylxanthines cross the blood-brain barrier and can exert a mild excitatory effect.
  - Caffeine is widely consumed for its cortical arousal abilities; however, the dose is larger, up to 1,000 mg, for bronchodilatory effects.
    - The potentially fatal caffeine dose is approximately 100 mg/kg, but patients can experience tachycardia and neuropsychiatric effects at much smaller doses.
- **Caffeine Citrate Vs. Sodium Benzoate**
  - Caffeine sodium benzoate should not be used in neonates as benzoate may displace bilirubin.
  - Caffeine citrate is preferred in neonatal apnea.
- **Diuresis**
  - Methylxanthines promote diuresis by increasing GFR and reducing tubular sodium reabsorption.
  - However, the diuretic effect is insufficient to allow for its use clinically as a diuretic.
- **Therapeutic Drug Monitoring**
  - Theophylline should be titrated to a target trough between 8 and 15 mcg/mL.
  - Patients consistently within the target range can be monitored once or twice yearly unless new drug interactions occur, toxicity is suspected, or the patient's disease worsens.
  - Risk factors for theophylline toxicity include elderly patients, pneumonia, heart failure, or liver dysfunction.
  - Common drug interactions include potent CYP inhibitors such as cimetidine, macrolides, fluoroquinolones, and CYP inducers, including smoking (tobacco and marijuana), phenytoin, phenobarbital, or rifampin.
- **CYP1A2**
  - The methylxanthines are metabolized by CYP1A2 and are subject to considerable pharmacokinetics in patients with CYP1A2 genetic polymorphisms.

High-Yield Core Evidence

- **Aminophylline in Bradyasystolic Arrest**
  - This was a double-blind trial that randomized adults 16 years and older presenting with asystole or pulseless electrical activity and who were unresponsive to initial treatment with epinephrine and atropine to receive either IV aminophylline 250 mg (with an additional 250 mg if necessary) or placebo.
  - There was no difference between groups regarding the primary outcome of the proportion of patients who had a return of spontaneous circulation (ROSC).
  - Significantly more patients receiving aminophylline experienced non-sinus tachyarrhythmias compared to placebo.
  - Survival to hospital admission and survival to hospital discharge was not significantly different between the groups.
  - The authors concluded that there was no evidence that aminophylline significantly increases the proportion of patients who achieve ROSC after bradyasystolic cardiac arrest. (Lancet. 2006 May 13;367(9522):1577-84.)

High-Yield Fast-Fact

- **Pentoxifylline**
  - Pentoxifylline, although used for peripheral arterial disease, is a methylxanthine. It lacks bronchodilatory effects at normal therapeutic dosing.

Table: Drug Class Summary

\multicolumn{4}{c}{**Methylxanthines - Drug Class Review**}
\multicolumn{4}{l}{**Mechanism of Action:** Methylxanthines nonselectively inhibit phosphodiesterases, increasing intracellular cAMP leading to smooth muscle relaxation.}
\multicolumn{4}{l}{**Class Effects:** Once used as first-line agents for asthma, methylxanthines have been relegated to add-on therapy in patients who have otherwise failed alternative bronchodilators and inhaled corticosteroids.}
Generic Name	**Brand Name**	**Main Indication(s) or Uses**	**Notes**

Aminophylline	Norphyl	• Asthma	• **Dosing (Adult):**
			  – IV Loading Dose: 5.7 mg/kg
			  – IV Infusion: 0.25 to 0.51 mg/kg/hour
			    – Age over 60 years: Maximum 507 mg/day
			    – Age 60 years or younger: Maximum 1,139 mg/day
			• **Dosing (Peds):**
			  – IV Loading Dose: 5.7 mg/kg
			  – IV Infusion: 0.25 to 0.51 mg/kg/hour
			• **CYP450 Interactions:** Substrate CYP1A2, 2C9, 2D6, 2E1, 3A4
			• **Renal or Hepatic Dose Adjustments:**
			  – Hepatic impairment: Maximum 507 mg/day
			• **Dosage Forms:** IV (solution)

Caffeine	NA	• Apnea of prematurity	• **Dosing (Adult):**
			  – IV: 250 to 1,000 mg caffeine base over 1 hour
			  – Oral: 100 to 200 mg q3-4h as needed
			• **Dosing (Peds):**
			  – Oral: 100 to 200 mg q3-4h as needed
			• **CYP450 Interactions:** Substrate CYP1A2, 2C9, 2D6, 2E1, 3A4; Inhibits CYP1A2
			• **Renal or Hepatic Dose Adjustments:** text
			• **Dosage Forms:** IV (solution), Oral (solution, tablet)

| Methylxanthines - Drug Class Review ||||
| High-Yield Med Reviews ||||
Generic Name	Brand Name	Main Indication(s) or Uses	Notes
Theophylline	Elixophyllin Theo-Dur	<ul><li>Bradycardia</li><li>Reversible airflow obstruction</li></ul>	<ul><li>**Dosing (Adult):**<ul><li>Oral: IR 150 to 600 mg/day divided q6-8h</li><li>Oral: ER 300 to 600 mg/day divided q12h (for 12-hour formulation) or q24h (for 24-hour formulation)</li><li>IV: 4.6 mg/kg, followed by 0.3 to 0.4 mg/kg/hour<ul><li>Age over 60 years: Maximum 400 mg/day</li><li>Age 60 years or younger: Maximum 900 mg/day</li></ul></li></ul></li><li>**Dosing (Peds):**<ul><li>IV: 4.6 mg/kg, followed by 0.3 to 0.4 mg/kg/hour</li><li>IV: 0.7 to 1.5 mg/kg/hour</li><li>Oral: IR: 12 to 20 mg/kg/day divided q4-6h<ul><li>Maximum 400 mg/day</li></ul></li><li>Oral: ER: 12 to 20 mg/kg/day divided q12-24h<ul><li>Maximum 400 mg/day</li></ul></li></ul></li><li>**CYP450 Interactions:** Substrate CYP1A2, 2E1, 3A4</li><li>**Renal or Hepatic Dose Adjustments:**<ul><li>Hepatic impairment: IV: initial dose of 0.2 mg/kg/hour; maximum 400 mg/day</li></ul></li><li>**Dosage Forms:** IV (solution), Oral (capsule, elixir, solution, tablet)</li></ul>

HIGH-YIELD BOARD EXAM ESSENTIALS
- **CLASSIC AGENTS:** Aminophylline, caffeine, theophylline
- **DRUG CLASS:** Methylxanthines
- **INDICATIONS:** Asthma, COPD
- **MECHANISM:** Methylxanthines nonselectively inhibit phosphodiesterases, increasing intracellular cAMP leading to smooth muscle relaxation.
- **SIDE EFFECTS:** Tachycardia, CNS excitation, headache, seizures, diuresis
- **CLINICAL PEARLS:** Caffeine is still routinely used in neonates for the treatment of apnea of prematurity. Administered via IV infusion, caffeine is an effective respiratory stimulant.

PULMONOLOGY – ANTI-ASTHMA – MONOCLONAL ANTIBODIES

Drug Class
- 5-Lipoxygenase Inhibitor
- Agents:
    - Chronic Care
        - Benralizumab
        - Dupilumab
        - Mepolizumab
        - Omalizumab
        - Reslizumab
        - Tezepelumab

> **Fast Facts**
> ✓ The use of these MABs in asthma comes after already implementing other appropriate treatments such as inhaled corticosteroids and bronchodilators. Thus, these are not first-line therapies and none are for acute exacerbations of asthma.

Main Indications or Uses
- Chronic Care
    - Asthma (benralizumab, dupilumab, mepolizumab, omalizumab, reslizumab, tezepelumab)
    - Chronic idiopathic urticaria (omalizumab)
    - Eosinophilic granulomatosis with polyangiitis (mepolizumab)
    - Nasal polyps (omalizumab)
    - Rhinosinusitis (dupilumab)

Mechanism of Action
- **Benralizumab**
    - IL-5 receptor antagonist, preventing eosinophilic binding to the IL-5 receptor on airway tissue.
- **Dupilumab**
    - IL-4-alpha receptor antagonist reduces IgE-mediated inflammatory response by disrupting IL-4 and IL-13 signaling pathways.
- **Mepolizumab, reslizumab**
    - Inhibit interleukin-5 (IL-5), reducing eosinophils' differentiation, recruitment, and activation of the airway.
- **Omalizumab**
    - A recombinant anti-IgE antibody, preventing IgE binding to its receptor on mast cells and basophils.

Primary Net Benefit
- Biologic therapeutics are reserved for patients with moderate to severe persistent asthma.
- Main Labs to Monitor:
    - Serum total IgE (omalizumab at baseline)
    - Blood eosinophils

High-Yield Basic Pharmacology
- **Omalizumab**
    - The action of omalizumab on inhibiting IgE from binding to its receptor on basophils and mast cells leads to a reduced release of allergen-induced inflammatory mediators.
    - Long-term therapy between 8 and 12 weeks of omalizumab decreases the expression of IgE's high-affinity receptor on airway mast cells.

High-Yield Clinical Knowledge
- **Anaphylaxis**
    - Despite a relatively low risk of anaphylaxis (less than 1%), benralizumab, mepolizumab, and reslizumab are parenterally administered in a healthcare setting prepared to respond to anaphylaxis.
    - Omalizumab carries a warning of anaphylaxis that can occur during therapy.
- **Herpes Zoster**
    - Patients 50 years or older who receive mepolizumab should receive recombinant zoster vaccination four weeks before the first dose of mepolizumab.
- **Reduced Oral Corticosteroids**

- Benralizumab, dupilumab, mepolizumab, and omalizumab have been observed to reduce the frequency of exacerbations and oral corticosteroid use in patients with severe asthma.
- **Omalizumab And Asthma Exacerbations**
    - Omalizumab may prevent asthma exacerbation in patients with frequent exacerbations by increasing the expression of type 1 interferons which improve antiviral immunity.

High-Yield Core Evidence
- **MENSA**
    - This multicenter, double-blind, double-dummy study randomized patients with recurrent asthma exacerbations and evidence of eosinophilic inflammation despite high doses of inhaled glucocorticoids one of three study groups: mepolizumab 75 mg IV, 100 mg SQ, or placebo every 4 weeks for 32 weeks.
    - Patients receiving mepolizumab experienced a significant reduction in the rate of asthma exacerbations, including exacerbations necessitating an emergency department visit or hospitalization.
    - Mepolizumab was also associated with a significant improvement from baseline FEV1 at week 32 compared to placebo.
    - The safety profile of mepolizumab was similar to that of placebo.
    - The authors concluded that mepolizumab administered intravenously or subcutaneously significantly reduced asthma exacerbations and was associated with improvements in asthma control markers. (N Engl J Med. 2014 Sep 25;371(13):1198-207.)
- **SIROCCO**
    - This was a double-blind, parallel-group, placebo-controlled phase 3 study that randomized patients between the ages of 12 to 75 years who had a physician-based diagnosis of asthma and at least two exacerbations while on high-dose ICS and LABA in the previous year.
    - Study subjects were randomized to receive either benralizumab 30 mg q4weeks or q8weeks or placebo q4weeks for 48 weeks to add to their standard therapy.
    - Both frequencies of benralizumab were associated with a significant reduction in the annual asthma exacerbation rate over 48 weeks compared to placebo.
    - Benralizumab also significantly improved prebronchodilator FEV1 in patients at week 48 compared to placebo.
    - Asthma symptoms were significantly improved in the benralizumab q8week group but not for the q4week group compared to placebo.
    - The authors concluded that benralizumab is safe and effective for patients with severe asthma and elevated eosinophils uncontrolled by high-dosage ICS plus LABA. (Lancet. 2016 Oct 29;388(10056):2115-2127.)

High-Yield Fast-Fact
- **Fraction of Exhaled Nitric Oxide**
    - FeNO can be followed as a predictor of acute asthma exacerbations and levels greater than 19.5 ppb are predictive of an exacerbation rate reduction.

HIGH-YIELD BOARD EXAM ESSENTIALS
- **CLASSIC AGENTS:** Benralizumab, dupilumab, mepolizumab, omalizumab, reslizumab
- **DRUG CLASS:** 5-Lipoxygenase Inhibitor
- **INDICATIONS:** Asthma (benralizumab, dupilumab, mepolizumab, omalizumab, reslizumab), chronic idiopathic urticaria (omalizumab), eosinophilic granulomatosis with polyangiitis (mepolizumab), nasal polyps (omalizumab), rhinosinusitis (dupilumab)
- **MECHANISM:** Benralizumab - IL-5 receptor antagonist, preventing eosinophilic binding to the IL-5 receptor on airway tissue. Dupilumab - IL-4-alpha receptor antagonist that reduces IgE mediated inflammatory response by disrupting IL-4 and IL-13 signaling pathways. Mepolizumab, reslizumab - inhibit interleukin-5 (IL-5), reducing the differentiation, recruitment, and activation of eosinophils to the airway. Omalizumab - recombinant anti-IgE antibody, preventing IgE binding to its receptor on mast cells and basophils.
- **SIDE EFFECTS:** Injection site reaction, headache
- **CLINICAL PEARLS:** Despite a relatively low risk of anaphylaxis (less than 1%), benralizumab, mepolizumab, and reslizumab are parenterally administered in a healthcare setting prepared to respond anaphylaxis. Omalizumab carries a warning of anaphylaxis that can occur at any time during therapy.

Table: Drug Class Summary

Anti-Asthma Monoclonal Antibody - Drug Class Review High-Yield Med Reviews			
Mechanism of Action: *Benralizumab* - IL-5 receptor antagonist, preventing eosinophilic binding to the IL-5 receptor on airway tissue. *Dupilumab* - IL-4-alpha receptor antagonist that reduces IgE mediated inflammatory response by disrupting IL-4 and IL-13 signaling pathways. *Mepolizumab, reslizumab* - inhibit interleukin-5 (IL-5), reducing the differentiation, recruitment, and activation of eosinophils to the airway. *Omalizumab* - recombinant anti-IgE antibody, preventing IgE binding to its receptor on mast cells and basophils.			
Class Effects: Biologic therapeutics reserved for patients with moderate to severe persistent asthma.			
Generic Name	**Brand Name**	**Main Indication(s) or Uses**	**Notes**
Benralizumab	Fasenra	• Asthma	• **Dosing (Adult):** — SQ: 30 mg q4weeks for 3 doses, then q8weeks • **Dosing (Peds):** — SQ: 30 mg q4weeks for 3 doses, then q8weeks • **CYP450 Interactions:** None • **Renal or Hepatic Dose Adjustments:** None • **Dosage Forms:** Subcutaneous auto-injector or prefilled syringe
Dupilumab	Dupixent	• Asthma • Rhinosinusitis	• **Dosing (Adult):** — SQ: 400 to 600 mg once followed by 200 to 300 mg every other week • **Dosing (Peds):** — SQ: 400 to 600 mg once followed by 200 to 300 mg every other week • **CYP450 Interactions:** None • **Renal or Hepatic Dose Adjustments:** None • **Dosage Forms:** Subcutaneous auto-injector or prefilled syringe
Mepolizumab	Nucala	• Asthma • Eosinophilic granulomatosis with polyangiitis	• **Dosing (Adult):** — SQ: 100 to 300 mg q4weeks • **Dosing (Peds):** — SQ: 40 to 300 mg q4weeks • **CYP450 Interactions:** None • **Renal or Hepatic Dose Adjustments:** None • **Dosage Forms:** Subcutaneous auto-injector or prefilled syringe

Anti-Asthma Monoclonal Antibody - Drug Class Review
High-Yield Med Reviews

Generic Name	Brand Name	Main Indication(s) or Uses	Notes

Omalizumab	Xolair	- Asthma
		- Chronic idiopathic urticaria
		- Nasal polyps
			- **Dosing (Adult):**
			  - Patient-specific dosing based on serum IgE
			    - SQ: 150 to 600 mg q4weeks
			    - SQ: 225 to 600 mg q2weeks
			- **Dosing (Peds):**
			  - Patient-specific dosing based on serum IgE
			    - SQ: 75 to 300 mg q4weeks
			    - SQ: 225 to 375 mg q2weeks
			- **CYP450 Interactions:** None
			- **Renal or Hepatic Dose Adjustments:** None
			- **Dosage Forms:** Subcutaneous auto-injector or prefilled syringe

Reslizumab	Cinqair	- Asthma	- **Dosing (Adult):**
			  - IV: 3 mg/kg q4weeks
			- **Dosing (Peds):**
			  - Not routinely used
			- **CYP450 Interactions:** None
			- **Renal or Hepatic Dose Adjustments:** None
			- **Dosage Forms:** IV (solution)

Tezepelumab	Tezspire	- Asthma	- **Dosing (Adult):**
			  - SQ: 210 mg q4weeks
			- **Dosing (Peds):** For children 12 years and older
			  - SQ: 210 mg q4weeks
			- **CYP450 Interactions:** None
			- **Renal or Hepatic Dose Adjustments:** None
			- **Dosage Forms:** IV (solution)

PULMONOLOGY – MUCOLYTICS

Drug Class
- Mucolytics
- Agents:
  - Acute & Chronic Care
    - Acetylcysteine
    - Dornase alfa
    - Hypertonic Saline
    - Mannitol

> **Fast Facts**
> ✓ Acetylcysteine has an unpleasant odor that patients complain of.
>
> ✓ Hypertonic saline may induce bronchospasm and should be preceded by a bronchodilator.

Main Indications or Uses
- Acute & Chronic Care
  - Cystic fibrosis (Dornase alfa, hypertonic saline, mannitol)
  - Mucolytic (Acetylcysteine)

Mechanism of Action
- Acetylcysteine
  - Reduces disulfide bridges that bind glycoproteins to other proteins, including albumin and IgA.
- Dornase alfa
  - Cleaves extracellular DNA, thereby decreasing the viscosity of mucus.
- Hypertonic saline, Mannitol
  - Hydrates mucous membranes and facilitates ciliary clearance of mucus.

Primary Net Benefit
- Mucolytics are a core anti-obstructive therapy for cystic fibrosis patients and should be combined with anti-inflammatory and antibiotic interventions.
- Main Labs to Monitor:
  - SpO2
  - Pulmonary function (FEV1, FVC, FEV1/FVC)

High-Yield Basic Pharmacology
- Deoxyribonuclease I
  - In response to the mucociliary dysfunction in CF pathophysiology, highly polymerized DNA is released from dead neutrophils, which leads to further mucus production and thickening.
    - This cycle of infection and mucus thickening eventually results in respiratory failure.
    - Dornase alfa works by cleaving DNA released from these neutrophils, thus reducing the secondary mucus accumulation and viscosity, ultimately preventing further airway infections and lung injury.

High-Yield Clinical Knowledge
- CF Treatment
  - Bronchodilators (including albuterol), dornase alfa, and hypertonic saline should be used in patients with cystic fibrosis who are six years of age and older.
- Dornase Alfa Cough
  - The most common complaint with dornase alfa therapy is the development of cough.
  - In small children, the PARI-BABY nebulizer facemask can aid in drug delivery but is associated with a higher incidence of cough.
    - However, dornase alfa can reduce the risk of CF exacerbations by nearly 30%, reduce mortality, and improved sustained lung function.
- NAC Effects
  - Nebulized N-acetylcysteine can be used as a mucolytic but has not been shown to reduce disease progression or prevent exacerbations in COPD patients.

- **Acetylcysteine Taste/Odor**
  - Acetylcysteine has an unpleasant odor that patients complain of if they receive nebulized treatments.
  - The taste is similar to rotten eggs and challenging to mask when administered via nebulization.
- **Hypertonic Saline**
  - The use of hypertonic saline in CF increases mucus clearance at 1 hour and 24 hours compared to baseline.
  - Hypertonic saline may induce bronchospasm and should be preceded by a bronchodilator.
- **B-HAPII**
  - The core components of treatment for CF include bronchodilators, hypertonic saline, airway clearance, Pulmozyme (dornase alfa), inhaled corticosteroids, and inhaled antibiotics.
  - Airway clearance methods include manual chest percussion, vest physiotherapy, and positive expiratory pressure ventilation.
  - Commonly used inhaled antibiotics for CF include tobramycin, aztreonam, and colistimethate.

High-Yield Core Evidence

- **NHSCF**
  - This was a double-blind, parallel-group study of patients at least six years old with stable cystic fibrosis.
  - Patients were randomized to either nebulized NaCl 7% 4 mL or NaCl 0.9% twice daily for 48 weeks.
  - There was no significant difference in the primary outcome of the rate of change in lung function during the 48 weeks of treatment.
  - However, the absolute difference in lung function between groups, favoring NaCl 7%, was significant when averaged across all post-randomization visits in the 48-week treatment period.
  - The NaCl 7% group had significantly higher FVC and FEV1 values but similar FEF25-75 values.
  - The NaCl 7% group also had significantly fewer pulmonary exacerbations and a significantly higher percentage of patients without exacerbations.
  - NaCl 7% was not associated with worsening bacterial infection or inflammation.
  - The authors concluded that NaCl 7% preceded by a bronchodilator is an inexpensive, safe, and effective additional therapy for patients with cystic fibrosis. (N Engl J Med. 2006;354(3):229–240.)
- **Pulmozyme Early Intervention Trial**
  - This was a multicenter, double-blind, placebo-controlled trial of patients with cystic fibrosis between 6 and 10 years with FVC of 85% or greater than predicted to determine whether long-term treatment with dornase alfa maintains lung function and reduces respiratory tract exacerbations.
  - Patients randomized to receive dornase alfa experienced a significant improvement in FVC, FEV1, and forced expiratory flow between 25% and 75% of vital capacity than placebo at the end of the 96-week study period.
  - Patients receiving dornase alfa had a significantly lower acute respiratory tract exacerbation risk.
  - No statistically significant difference between the groups in changes in weight-for-age percentile.
  - The authors concluded that the treatment of young patients with CF with dornase alfa maintains lung function and reduces the risk of exacerbations over 96 weeks. (J Pediatr. 2001;139(6):813–820.)

High-Yield Fast-Fact

- **Mannitol Storage**
  - Mannitol commonly crystallizes a room temperature and often requires storage in a warm location, reducing this risk of crystallization.

Table: Drug Class Summary

Mucolytics - Drug Class Review High-Yield Med Reviews			
Mechanism of Action: *Acetylcysteine - Reduces disulfide bridges that bind glycoproteins to other proteins, including albumin and IgA.* *Dornase alfa - cleaves extracellular DNA, thereby decreasing the viscosity of mucus.* *Hypertonic saline, Mannitol - Hydrates mucous membranes and facilitates ciliary clearance of mucus.*			
Class Effects: *Mucolytics are a core anti-obstructive therapy for patients with cystic fibrosis and should be combined with anti-inflammatory and antibiotic interventions.*			
Generic Name	**Brand Name**	**Main Indication(s) or Uses**	**Notes**

Acetylcysteine	Acetadote
	 Mucomyst
	 Cetylev
		- Acetaminophen overdose
		 - Mucolytic
			- **Dosing (Adult):**
			   − Oral: 140 mg/kg once (maximum 15 g) followed by 70 mg/kg (maximum 7.5g/dose) q4h for 17 doses
			   − IV: 150 mg/kg/hour for one hour (maximum 15 g), followed by 12.5 mg/kg/hour for 4 hours (maximum 5 g/dose), followed by 6.25 mg/kg/hour (maximum 10 g/dose) for 16 hours
			   − Nebulized: 6 to 10 mL (10%) or 3 to 5 mL (20%) q1-6h
			 - **Dosing (Peds):**
			   − Oral: 140 mg/kg once (maximum 15 g) followed by 70 mg/kg (maximum 7.5g/dose) q4h for 17 doses
			   − IV: 150 mg/kg/hour for one hour (maximum 15 g), followed by 12.5 mg/kg/hour for 4 hours (maximum 5 g/dose), followed by 6.25 mg/kg/hour (maximum 10 g/dose) for 16 hours
			   − Nebulized: 6 to 10 mL (10%) or 3 to 5 mL (20%) q1-6h
			 - **CYP450 Interactions:** None
			 - **Renal or Hepatic Dose Adjustments:** None
			 - **Dosage Forms:** Inhalation solution, IV (solution), Oral (Tablet)

Dornase alfa	Pulmozyme	- Cystic fibrosis	- **Dosing (Adult):**
			   − Inhalation: 2.5 mg daily
			   − Intrapleural: 5 mg twice daily
			 - **Dosing (Peds):**
			   − Inhalation: 2.5 mg daily
			   − Intrapleural: 5 mg twice daily
			 - **CYP450 Interactions:** None
			 - **Renal or Hepatic Dose Adjustments:** None
			 - **Dosage Forms:** Inhalation solution

		Mucolytics - Drug Class Review High-Yield Med Reviews	
Generic Name	**Brand Name**	**Main Indication(s) or Uses**	**Notes**
Hypertonic saline	HyperSal	• Cystic fibrosis	• **Dosing (Adult):** 　− Inhalation: NaCl 7% 4mL BID • **Dosing (Peds):** 　− Inhalation: NaCl 3% to 7% 4mL BID • **CYP450 Interactions:** None • **Renal or Hepatic Dose Adjustments:** None • **Dosage Forms:** Inhalation solution
Mannitol	Aridol Bronchitol	• Assessment of bronchial hyperresponsiveness • Cystic fibrosis	• **Dosing (Adult):** 　− Inhalation: 400 mg BID • **Dosing (Peds):** 　− Inhalation: 400 mg BID • **CYP450 Interactions:** None • **Renal or Hepatic Dose Adjustments:** None • **Dosage Forms:** Inhalation capsule, inhalation kit

HIGH-YIELD BOARD EXAM ESSENTIALS
- **CLASSIC AGENTS:** Acetylcysteine, dornase alfa, hypertonic saline, mannitol
- **DRUG CLASS:** Mucolytics
- **INDICATIONS:** Cystic fibrosis, mucolytic
- **MECHANISM:**
    - Acetylcysteine - Reduces disulfide bridges that bind glycoproteins to other proteins, including albumin and IgA.
    - Dornase alfa - cleaves extracellular DNA, thereby decreasing the viscosity of mucus.
    - Hypertonic saline, Mannitol - Hydrates mucous membranes and facilitates ciliary clearance of mucus.
- **SIDE EFFECTS:** Unpleasant odor (acetylcysteine), cough (dornase alfa)
- **CLINICAL PEARLS:** In small children, the PARI-BABY nebulizer facemask can aid in drug delivery but is associated with a higher incidence of cough. However, dornase alfa can reduce the risk of CF exacerbations by nearly 30%, reduce mortality, and improved sustained lung function.

PULMONOLOGY – PHOSPHODIESTERASE 4 INHIBITORS

Drug Class
- **Phosphodiesterase-4 Inhibitors**
- **Agents:**
    - **Chronic Care**
        - Apremilast
        - Crisaborole
        - Roflumilast

> **Fast Facts**
> ✓ Both apremilast and roflumilast are orally administered formulations which is different from most treatments in COPD.

Main Indications or Uses
- **Chronic Care**
    - Atopic dermatitis (Crisaborole)
    - Behcet disease (Apremilast)
    - Psoriasis (Apremilast)
    - Psoriatic arthritis (Apremilast)
    - COPD (Roflumilast)

Mechanism of Action
- Selective inhibition of phosphodiesterase-4 (PDE4) leads to decreased intracellular cAMP and decreased pro-inflammatory cytokines.

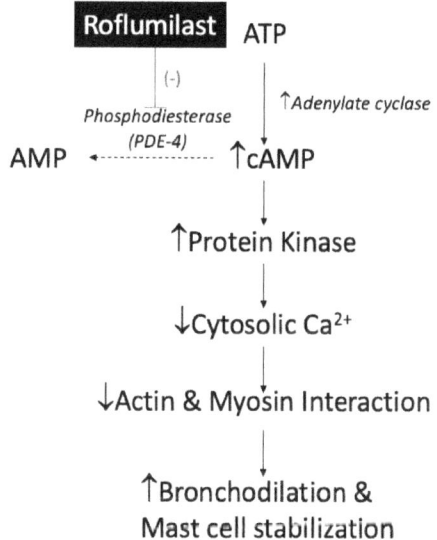

Primary Net Benefit
- Roflumilast may offer additional symptom control in select severe COPD patients on an existing therapy.
    - Roflumilast is reserved for select severe COPD patients.
    - Apremilast may be effective in patients with dermatologic conditions but carry a risk of neuropsychiatric events.
    - Crisaborole does not have a warning for neuropsychiatric effects as it is not systemically absorbed.
- Main Labs to Monitor:
    - Weight
    - Serum creatinine
    - LFT (INR/PT, albumin, bilirubin, protein)
    - Signs and symptoms of mood changes, depression, or suicidal thoughts

High-Yield Basic Pharmacology
- **Site-Specific PDE4 Inhibition**
  - Roflumilast's actions as a PDE4 inhibitor cause airway smooth muscle tissue relaxation and decrease inflammatory mediators promoting COPD disease progression.
- **Roflumilast and Methylxanthines**
  - Roflumilast similarly produces anti-inflammatory effects to methylxanthines.
  - However, methylxanthines such as theophylline produce nonselective inhibition phosphodiesterases, increasing intracellular cAMP and smooth muscle relaxation.
  - Methylxanthines should not be combined with roflumilast.

High-Yield Clinical Knowledge
- **COPD Treatment**
  - Roflumilast is reserved for severe COPD patients with chronic cough, sputum production, and a history of frequent exacerbations.
  - Roflumilast, although providing anti-inflammatory properties, does not produce meaningful bronchodilation.
- **CYP3A4 Substrates**
  - Apremilast and roflumilast are substrates of CYP3A4 and are subject to numerous drug interactions.
  - Patients taking CYP3A4 inducers (carbamazepine, phenytoin, phenobarbital, rifampin) should not begin apremilast or roflumilast as their effectiveness will be substantially diminished.
  - Potent CYP3A4 inhibitors may be combined with apremilast or roflumilast; however, increased monitoring (neuropsychiatric) should occur.
- **Roflumilast Safety**
  - Common adverse events associated with roflumilast therapy include GI events (nausea, diarrhea), decreased appetite and weight loss, and headache.
  - Neuropsychiatric events including insomnia, anxiety, new or worsening depression, and suicidal thoughts are rare but concerning effects of roflumilast.
    - Roflumilast should be avoided in patients with a history of depression or suicidality.
- **CYP1A2 and Smoking**
  - Although generally recommended to avoid and provide smoking cessation education, roflumilast AUC may be significantly lower in active smokers.
  - Cigarette smoke contains polycyclic aromatic hydrocarbons that induce CYP1A2.

High-Yield Core Evidence
- **ESTEEM 2**
  - This was a continuation to 32-weeks of a 16-week, phase 3, double-blind, placebo-controlled trial that randomized adult patients with psoriasis to receive either apremilast 30 mg twice daily or placebo.
  - At week 16, placebo patients switched to apremilast. At week 32, apremilast patients achieving at least a 50% reduction in Psoriasis Area and Severity Index (PASI) were then re-randomized to continue apremilast or receive placebo until loss of 50% of PASI improvement obtained at week 32, patients re-randomized to placebo resumed apremilast.
  - At the week 16 endpoint, significantly more apremilast patients achieved PASI 75, PASI 50, and static Physician's Global Assessment score of 0 or 1, compared to placebo.
  - Among re-randomized patients at week 32 showed now receiving apremilast showed significant improvements in quality of life and pruritus at week 16 compared with placebo.
  - The exposure-adjusted incidence of adverse events did not increase with continued apremilast treatment for up to 52 weeks.
  - The authors concluded that apremilast was influential in the treatment of moderate-to-severe plaque psoriasis over 52 weeks. (Br J Dermatol. 2015 Dec;173(6):1387-99.)

- **REACT**
  - This was a multicenter, double-blind, placebo-controlled, parallel-group, multicenter, phase 3-4 trial that randomized patients with severe COPD with severe airflow limitation, symptoms of chronic bronchitis, and at least two exacerbations in the previous year to either roflumilast 500 mcg or placebo was given orally once daily together with a fixed inhaled corticosteroid and long-acting beta-2 agonist combination.
  - There was no statistically significant difference between groups concerning the primary outcome of the rate of moderate to severe COPD exacerbations per patient per year.
  - However, using a predefined sensitivity analysis using negative binomial regression, roflumilast was associated with a significant reduction in COPD exacerbations per patient per year.
  - More patients randomized to roflumilast experienced severe adverse events, including severe COPD exacerbations, pneumonia, and deaths.
  - The authors concluded that roflumilast reduces exacerbations and hospital admissions in patients with severe COPD who are at risk of frequent and severe exacerbations despite inhaled corticosteroid and long-acting beta-2 agonist therapy, even in combination with tiotropium. (Lancet. 2015;385(9971):857-866.)

High-Yield Fast-Fact
- **Caffeine Free**
  - Many drinks and sports supplements contain labeling claiming their product is caffeine-free but have large quantities of theobromine, a similar methylxanthine (3,7-dimethylxanthine).

HIGH-YIELD BOARD EXAM ESSENTIALS
- **CLASSIC AGENTS:** Apremilast, crisaborole, roflumilast
- **DRUG CLASS:** Phosphodiesterase-4 inhibitors
- **INDICATIONS:** Atopic dermatitis (crisaborole), Behcet disease (apremilast), psoriasis (apremilast), psoriatic arthritis (apremilast), COPD (roflumilast)
- **MECHANISM:** Selective phosphodiesterase-4 (PDE4) inhibition leads to decreased intracellular cAMP and decreased pro-inflammatory cytokines.
- **SIDE EFFECTS:** GI events (nausea, diarrhea), decreased appetite, weight loss, headache, insomnia, anxiety, new or worsening depression, and suicidal thoughts
- **CLINICAL PEARLS:**
  - Roflumilast is not a first-line agent for COPD; instead is an adjunctive treatment to existing therapy. It is also orally administered which may be initially counter-intuitive for COPD.
  - Although generally recommended to avoid and provide smoking cessation education, roflumilast AUC may be significantly lower in active smokers. Cigarette smoke contains polycyclic aromatic hydrocarbons that induce CYP1A2.

Table: Drug Class Summary

\multicolumn{4}{c}{**Phosphodiesterase-4 Inhibitors - Drug Class Review**}
\multicolumn{4}{c}{High-Yield Med Reviews}
\multicolumn{4}{l}{**Mechanism of Action:** *Selective phosphodiesterase-4 (PDE4) inhibition leads to decreased intracellular cAMP and decreased pro-inflammatory cytokines.*}
\multicolumn{4}{l}{**Class Effects:** *Roflumilast is reserved for select severe COPD patients; apremilast may be effective in patients with dermatologic conditions but carry a risk of neuropsychiatric events. Crisaborole does not have a warning for neuropsychiatric effects as it is not systemically absorbed.*}
Generic Name	**Brand Name**	**Indication(s) or Uses**	**Notes**

Apremilast	Otezla	- Behcet disease
		- Psoriasis
		- Psoriatic arthritis
			- **Dosing (Adult):**
			  - Oral: 30 mg BID
			    - Titration from 10 mg once to target dose over 6 days
			- **Dosing (Peds):**
			  - Not routinely used
			- **CYP450 Interactions:** Substrate CYP3A4, P-gp
			- **Renal or Hepatic Dose Adjustments:**
			  - GFR < 30 mL/minute: slower titration and maximum 30 mg once daily
			- **Dosage Forms:** Oral (capsule)

Crisaborole	Eucrisa	- Atopic dermatitis	- **Dosing (Adult):**
			  - Topical application to the affected area BID
			- **Dosing (Peds):**
			  - Topical application to the affected area BID
			- **CYP450 Interactions:** None
			- **Renal or Hepatic Dose Adjustments:** None
			- **Dosage Forms:** Ointment

Roflumilast	Daliresp	- COPD	- **Dosing (Adult):**
			  - Oral: 250 mcg daily x 4 weeks, then 500 mcg daily
			- **Dosing (Peds):**
			  - Not routinely used
			- **CYP450 Interactions:** Substrate CYP1A2, 3A4
			- **Renal or Hepatic Dose Adjustments:**
			  - Child-Pugh class B or C: contraindicated
			- **Dosage Forms:** Oral (tablet)

PULMONOLOGY – ENDOTHELIN RECEPTOR ANTAGONIST

Drug Class
- Endothelin Receptor Antagonist
- Agents:
  - Chronic Care
    - Ambrisentan
    - Bosentan
    - Macitentan

Main Indications or Uses
- Chronic Care
  - Pulmonary arterial hypertension

Mechanism of Action
- Antagonists of endothelin-A and endothelin-B receptors prevent endothelin-induced vasoconstriction of these vessels.

> **Fast Facts**
> ✓ These agents tend to be used for WHO group 2 and 3 pulmonary hypertension.
>
> ✓ Common dose-limiting adverse events include hypotension, tachycardia, flushing, and headaches.
>
> ✓ All of these options are oral dosage formulations making them easier to take.

Primary Net Benefit
- Endothelin receptor antagonists improve exercise capacity in most patients and impact functional class and time to clinical worsening.
  - All agents require participation in prescription monitoring programs due to significant toxicities.
- Main Labs to Monitor:
  - Liver enzymes (AST/ALT) - baseline and monthly after that (bosentan)
  - Liver function (PT/INR, albumin, bilirubin, protein) - baseline and monthly after that (bosentan)
  - CBC - baseline and monthly after that (bosentan)
  - Pregnancy test

High-Yield Basic Pharmacology
- ETa Selectivity
  - Ambrisentan is highly selective for ETa, whereas bosentan is non-selective between ETa and ETb.
- Endothelin Activity
  - Endothelin has broad effects throughout the body, but concerning pulmonary arterial hypertension, it causes dose-dependent vasoconstriction in vascular beds.
  - These effects are counterbalanced by prostacyclin and nitric oxide, which are also other therapeutic targets in pulmonary hypertension.

High-Yield Clinical Knowledge
- Hepatic Injury
  - The use of bosentan is associated with an increased risk of hepatotoxicity, initially manifesting as increases in hepatic enzymes.
  - This occurs due to bile salt retention and its resulting cytotoxic action on hepatocytes due to its competition with bosentan for biliary excretion of bile salts.
  - Baseline and monthly liver enzyme and liver function tests are required during bosentan therapy.
- Teratogens
  - All endothelin receptor antagonists are teratogens and are contraindicated in pregnancy.
  - Female patients must participate in a prescription monitoring program (REMS) to receive macitentan.
  - Documentation of a negative pregnancy test is required before initiation, and compliance with two forms of contraception is necessary while taking endothelin receptor antagonists.
- Combination Therapy
  - Endothelin receptor antagonists, namely ambrisentan, can be combined with tadalafil in patients with functional classes two or three.
  - A significant reduction in clinical failure events, including death, or hospitalizations due to progressing pulmonary arterial hypertension, is observed with combination therapy.

- Other combinations recommended include riociguat and bosentan, selexipag addition to endothelin receptor antagonists, and phosphodiesterase 5 inhibitors combined with any other agents.
- **Dose-Dependent Effects**
    - The endothelin receptor antagonists all exhibit a dose-dependent effect on functional capacity, and patients should be titrated to maximum tolerable doses.
    - Common dose-limiting adverse events include hypotension, tachycardia, flushing, and headaches.
- **Drug Interactions**
    - Bosentan and macitentan are inducers of CYP2C9 and 3A4, leading to numerous drug interactions, including necessary concomitant medications for pulmonary hypertension patients, including oral contraceptives (these agents are teratogens), warfarin, cyclosporine, and glyburide.

High-Yield Core Evidence
- **SERAPHIN**
    - This was a multicenter, prospective, placebo-controlled trial that randomized patients with symptomatic pulmonary arterial hypertension to receive a placebo once daily, macitentan 3 mg once daily, or macitentan 10 mg once daily.
    - Macitentan doses of either 3 or 10 mg daily each significantly reduced the hazard ratio of the primary endpoint of the time from the initiation of treatment to the first occurrence of a composite endpoint of death, atrial septostomy, lung transplantation, initiation of treatment with intravenous or subcutaneous prostanoids, or worsening of pulmonary arterial hypertension.
    - Adverse events more frequently associated with macitentan than with placebo were headache, nasopharyngitis, and anemia.
    - The authors concluded that macitentan significantly reduced morbidity and mortality among patients with pulmonary arterial hypertension in this event-driven study.
    - (N Engl J Med. 2013;369(9):809–818.)
- **Bosentan in PAH**
    - This was a multicenter, prospective, double-blind, placebo-controlled study that randomized patients with pulmonary arterial hypertension to receive placebo or to receive bosentan 62.5 mg twice daily for four weeks followed by either of two doses of bosentan (125 or 250 mg twice daily) for a minimum of 12 weeks.
    - Patients randomized to bosentan experienced a significant improvement in the primary endpoint of the degree of change in exercise capacity compared to placebo.
    - Bosentan therapy was also associated with significant improvements in secondary endpoints, including the change in the Borg dyspnea index, the change in the World Health Organization (WHO) functional class, and the time to clinical worsening.
    - The authors concluded that bosentan is beneficial in patients with pulmonary arterial hypertension and is well tolerated at a dose of 125 mg twice daily. (N Engl J Med. 2002 Mar 21;346(12):896-903.)

High-Yield Fast-Fact
- **Heart Failure Studies**
    - Bosentan was also initially studied for heart failure; however, the REACH study was prematurely stopped due to excess toxicity and worsening heart failure.

HIGH-YIELD BOARD EXAM ESSENTIALS
- **CLASSIC AGENTS:** Ambrisentan, bosentan, macitentan
- **DRUG CLASS:** Endothelin receptor antagonist
- **INDICATIONS:** Pulmonary arterial hypertension
- **MECHANISM:** Antagonists of endothelin-A and endothelin-B receptors, preventing endothelin-induced vasoconstriction of these vessels.
- **SIDE EFFECTS:** Hypotension, tachycardia, flushing, and headaches.
- **CLINICAL PEARLS:** All endothelin receptor antagonists are teratogens and are contraindicated in pregnancy. Female patients must participate in a prescription monitoring program (REMS) to receive macitentan.

Table: Drug Class Summary

| | Endothelin Receptor Antagonist - Drug Class Review
High-Yield Med Reviews |

Mechanism of Action: *Antagonists of endothelin-A and endothelin-B receptors, preventing endothelin-induced vasoconstriction of these vessels.*

Class Effects: *Endothelin receptor antagonists improve exercise capacity in most patients and impact functional class and time to clinical worsening. All agents require participation in prescription monitoring programs due to significant toxicities.*

Generic Name	Brand Name	Main Indication(s) or Uses	Notes

Ambrisentan	Letairis	- Pulmonary arterial hypertension	- **Dosing (Adult):**
			  - Oral: 5 to 10 mg daily
			- **Dosing (Peds):**
			  - Not routinely used
			- **CYP450 Interactions:** Substrate CYP2C19, 3A4, P-gp
			- **Renal or Hepatic Dose Adjustments:**
			  - Child-Pugh class C: Not recommended
			  - AST/ALT: above 5x upper limit of normal OR 2x upper limit of normal with hepatic injury - discontinue therapy
			- **Dosage Forms:** Oral (tablet)

Bosentan	Tracleer	- Pulmonary arterial hypertension	- **Dosing (Adult):**
			  - Oral: 62.5 to 125 mg BID
			- **Dosing (Peds):**
			  - Oral: 1 mg/kg/dose twice daily
			  - Oral: 3 to 64 mg twice daily
			- **CYP450 Interactions:** Substrate CYP2C9, 3A4; Induces CYP2C9, 3A4
			- **Renal or Hepatic Dose Adjustments:**
			  - Child-Pugh class B or C: Not recommended
			  - AST/ALT: above 8x upper limit of normal OR 3x upper limit of normal with hepatic injury - discontinue therapy
			- **Dosage Forms:** Oral (tablet)

Macitentan	Opsumlt	- Pulmonary arterial hypertension	- **Dosing (Adult):**
			  - Oral: 10 mg daily
			- **Dosing (Peds):**
			  - Not routinely used
			- **CYP450 Interactions:** Substrate CYP2C9, 3A4; Induces CYP2C9, 3A4
			- **Renal or Hepatic Dose Adjustments:**
			  - AST/ALT: above 3x upper limit of normal - discontinue therapy
			  - Child-Pugh class B or C: Not recommended
			- **Dosage Forms:** Oral (tablet)

PULMONOLOGY – GUANYLATE CYCLASE STIMULATOR

Drug Class
- Guanylate Cyclase Stimulator
- Agents:
  - Chronic Care
    - Riociguat
    - Vericiguat

Main Indications or Uses
- Chronic Care
  - Pulmonary arterial hypertension
    - Riociguat only
  - Heart failure with reduced ejection fraction
    - Vericiguat only

Mechanism of Action
- Sensitizes soluble guanylate cyclase (sGC) to endogenous nitric oxide and directly stimulates sGC independent from nitric oxide.

Primary Net Benefit
- Riociguat is an alternative agent for select patients with pulmonary arterial hypertension, whereas vericiguat has been associated with reductions in heart-failure-associated hospitalizations.
- Main Labs to Monitor:
  - Pregnancy test (baseline, monthly during treatment, and one month after discontinuation)

High-Yield Basic Pharmacology
- Cigarette Smoke
  - The metabolism of riociguat and its M1 metabolite is accomplished, in part, by CYP1A1.
  - Polycyclic aromatic hydrocarbons, a component of cigarette smoke, are potent inducers of CYP1A1 and may induce the metabolism of riociguat.
  - Although patients with pulmonary arterial hypertension should not smoke, those regularly exposed to secondhand smoke may also experience induction of CYP1A1.

High-Yield Clinical Knowledge
- Pregnancy
  - Contraindicated in pregnancy as teratogenic effects have been observed.
  - To receive the drug, female patients in whom riociguat is considered must go through a REMS program.
- Adverse Events
  - Common adverse events include hypotension, dyspepsia, nausea, anemia.
  - Riociguat may also cause palpitations, headache, dysphagia, epistaxis, and abdominal distension.
- Continued Compliance
  - Strict compliance with riociguat is required, as patients who miss therapy for three or more days must restart at a lower dose due to excess risk of hypotension.
- Vericiguat In Heart Failure
  - HFrEF is associated with dysregulation of the nitric oxide-sGC-cGMP pathway, leading to impairment in diastole and microvascular dysfunction.
- Drug Interactions
  - Riociguat and vericiguat should not be combined with nitroglycerin or PDE5 inhibitors (sildenafil, tadalafil) as severe hypotension may occur.

High-Yield Core Evidence
- PATENT-1
  - This phase 3 double-blind study randomized patients with symptomatic pulmonary arterial hypertension to receive placebo or riociguat at patient-specific doses to a maximum of 2.5 mg three times daily.
  - The third group of patients received riociguat capped at 1.5 mg three times daily but were only included for exploratory and descriptive purposes.
  - Compared to placebo, patients randomized to receive riociguat experienced a significant improvement in the 6-minute walk distance at the end of week 12.
  - Riociguat was associated with significant pulmonary vascular resistance improvements, NT-proBNP levels, WHO functional class, time to clinical worsening, and Borg dyspnea score.
  - The most common serious adverse event in the placebo and 2.5 mg–maximum groups, was syncope.
  - The authors concluded that riociguat significantly improved exercise capacity and secondary efficacy endpoints in patients with pulmonary arterial hypertension. (N Engl J Med 2013;369(4):330–340.)
- VICTORIA
  - This was a phase 3, double-blind, placebo-controlled trial that randomized patients with chronic heart failure (New York Heart Association class II, III, or IV) and an ejection fraction of less than 45% to receive vericiguat at a target dose, 10 mg once daily or placebo, in addition to guideline-based medical therapy.
  - Significantly fewer patients randomized to vericiguat experienced a primary outcome event of death from cardiovascular causes or first hospitalization for heart failure compared to placebo.
  - This effect was driven by a vericiguat-associated reduction in the risk of hospitalizations for HF.
  - There was no difference in the incidence of symptomatic hypotension or syncope.
  - The authors concluded that among patients with high-risk HF, the incidence of death from CV causes or hospitalization for HF was lower among those who received vericiguat than those who received placebo. (N Engl J Med. 2013;369(4):319–329.)

High-Yield Fast-Fact
- Cinaciguat, similar to vericiguat, is being investigated for use in HFrEF, but specifically, acute decompensated heart failure.

HIGH-YIELD BOARD EXAM ESSENTIALS
- **CLASSIC AGENTS:** Riociguat, vericiguat
- **DRUG CLASS:** Guanylate cyclase stimulator
- **INDICATIONS:** HFrEF (vericiguat), pulmonary arterial hypertension (riociguat)
- **MECHANISM:** Sensitizes soluble guanylate cyclase (sGC) to endogenous nitric oxide and directly stimulates sGC independent from nitric oxide.
- **SIDE EFFECTS:** Palpitations, headache, dysphagia, epistaxis, abdominal distension, nausea/vomiting/diarrhea, and anemia
- **CLINICAL PEARLS:** Avoid use with nitroglycerin and PDE5 inhibitors due to risk of severe hypotension.

Table: Drug Class Summary

	Guanylate Cyclase Stimulator - Drug Class Review High-Yield Med Reviews
	**Mechanism of Action:** *Sensitizes soluble guanylate cyclase (sGC) to endogenous nitric oxide and directly stimulates sGC independent from nitric oxide.*
	**Class Effects:** *Used in pulmonary arterial hypertension (riociguat), used in HFrEF (vericiguat) for HF hospitalization reductions, significant hypotension, contraindicated in pregnancy and with PDE5 inhibitors.*
Generic Name	**Brand Name**	**Indication(s) or Uses**	**Notes**

Riociguat	Adempas	- Pulmonary arterial hypertension	- **Dosing (Adult):**
			  – Oral: 0.5 to 2.5 mg TID
			- **Dosing (Peds):** N/A
			- **CYP450 Interactions:** Substrate CYP2C8, 3A4, P-gp
			- **Renal or Hepatic Dose Adjustments:**
			  – GFR < 15 mL/minute: Not recommended
			  – Child-Pugh class C: Not recommended
			- **Dosage Forms:** Oral (Tablet)

Vericiguat	Verquvo	- Heart failure with reduced ejection fraction	- **Dosing (Adult):** – Oral: 2.5 to 10 mg daily - **Dosing (Peds):** N/A - **CYP450 Interactions:** Substrate P-gp - **Renal or Hepatic Dose Adjustments:** None - **Dosage Forms:** Oral (tablet)

PULMONOLOGY – SYNTHETIC PROSTACYCLIN & PROSTACYCLIN IP RECEPTOR AGONIST

Drug Class
- Synthetic Prostacyclin & Prostacyclin IP Receptor Agonist
- Agents:
  - Chronic Care
    - Epoprostenol
    - Iloprost
    - Treprostinil
    - Selexipag

Main Indications or Uses
- Chronic Care
  - Pulmonary arterial hypertension

Mechanism of Action
- Epoprostenol, Iloprost, Treprostinil
  - Prostacyclin (PGI2) synthetic analogs induce pulmonary vascular smooth muscle relaxation, vasodilation, and inhibition of platelet aggregation.
- Selexipag
  - Selective prostacyclin IP receptor agonist, increasing cAMP and relaxation of vascular smooth muscle causing pulmonary vasodilation.

> **Warnings & Alerts**
> ✓ *The synthetic PGI2, epoprostenol, has a short half-life of 3 to 5 minutes, necessitating continuous IV infusion chronically. As a result, patients must have backup supplies of medication cartridges to prevent administration gaps, leading to potentially life-threatening rebound pulmonary vasoconstriction.*

Primary Net Benefit
- Prostacyclin analogs and agonists induce pulmonary vasodilation, counteracting pulmonary arterial hypertension's physiology, but due to administration complications and toxicities, are generally reserved for WHO functional class II or higher.
- Main Labs to Monitor:
  - Liver function (INR/PT, albumin, protein, bilirubin) - selexipag
  - Blood pressure

High-Yield Basic Pharmacology
- PGI2 Physiology
  - Pulmonary arterial hypertension is a disease process of pulmonary vascular injury secondary to endothelial dysfunction, smooth muscle cell dysfunction, and pulmonary vascular matrix changes in platelet function and activation of inflammatory cascades.
  - Prostacyclin analogs and agonists directly modify this process by providing vascular vasodilation and inhibition of platelet aggregation, anti-inflammatory properties, and cytoprotective actions.
- Epoprostenol Administration
  - Epoprostenol requires continuous IV infusion, including for outpatients.
  - After initiation and dose titration in an acute care setting, patients are discharged home with a central venous catheter and pump.

High-Yield Clinical Knowledge
- Short Half-Life
  - The synthetic PGI2 epoprostenol has a short half-life of 3 to 5 minutes, necessitating continuous IV infusion, including for outpatients.
  - Patients must have backup supplies of medication cartridges to prevent administration gaps, leading to potentially life-threatening rebound pulmonary vasoconstriction.
  - Treprostinil has a longer half-life permitting subcutaneous administration, which can be limited due to injection site reactions.
    - In patients who cannot tolerate subcutaneous site reaction, IV administration of treprostinil is permissible.

- **Inhalation Administration**
  - In contrast to the other prostacyclin analogs, iloprost and treprostinil may be administered via inhalation.
  - Iloprost must be administered six to up to 9 times per day, each taking up to 10 minutes to administer, and with each administration approximately 2 hours apart over the waking hours.
  - Treprostinil is administered using three inhalations four times daily during waking hours.
    - Similar to the other prostacyclin analogs, gaps in administration can lead to acute decompensations and rebound pulmonary vasoconstriction.
- **Oral Administration**
  - Treprostinil and selexipag are orally administered prostacyclin analog or prostacyclin IP receptor agonists.
  - Treprostinil is administered two to three times daily but must be taken with food to improve absorption.
  - Selexipag is an orally administered agent that is taken twice daily.
- **Dose Titration**
  - The prostacyclin analogs and agonists must be slowly titrated to the maximum tolerable doses to achieve the therapeutic benefits.
- **Class Adverse Events**
  - Common adverse events observed with each agent include myalgias, jaw pain, nausea, diarrhea, abdominal pain, headaches, flushing, dizziness, and hypotension.
  - These effects are dose-dependent but dissipate over time with continued exposure and administration.
- **Conventional PAH Therapy**
  - The conventional therapeutic approach to managing pulmonary arterial hypertension includes oral anticoagulation, diuresis, digoxin, and supplemental oxygen therapy.
  - Calcium channel blockers may be appropriate in selected patients where a positive acute vasoreactivity test is observed.
  - Combination drug therapy targeting numerous physiologic pathways is a common approach in managing pulmonary arterial hypertension and is associated with reduced time to clinical failure and hospitalizations.

High-Yield Core Evidence
- **Oral Treprostinil**
  - This was a multicenter, double-blind, placebo-controlled trial in patients with pulmonary arterial hypertension not receiving an endothelin receptor antagonist or phosphodiesterase type-5 inhibitor background therapy to evaluate the safety and efficacy of the oral prostacyclin analog treprostinil.
  - Patients were randomized to receive either treprostinil or placebo, and the primary endpoint was the change from baseline in 6-minute walk distance at week 12.
  - Patients randomized to receive treprostinil experienced a significantly improved 6-minute walk distance at week 12 treatment compared to placebo in both the per-protocol and intent-to-treat analysis.
  - However, there were no significant changes in secondary endpoints.
  - The authors concluded that oral treprostinil improves exercise capacity in PAH patients not receiving other treatment. (Circulation. 2013;127(5):624–633.)
- **GRIPHON**
  - This was an event-driven, phase 3, double-blind, placebo-controlled trial that randomized patients with pulmonary arterial hypertension to receive placebo or selexipag in individualized doses (maximum dose, 1600 mcg twice daily).
  - Selexipag was associated with a significant improvement in the primary endpoint of the composite of death from any cause or a complication related to pulmonary arterial hypertension up to the end of the treatment period (defined for each patient as seven days after the date of the last intake of selexipag or placebo).
  - Significantly more patients in the selexipag group discontinued their assigned regimen prematurely because of adverse events.
  - The most common adverse events in the selexipag group were consistent with prostacyclin's known side effects, including headache, diarrhea, nausea, and jaw pain.

- The authors concluded that among patients with pulmonary arterial hypertension, the risk of the primary composite endpoint of death or a complication related to pulmonary arterial hypertension was significantly lower with selexipag than with placebo. (N Engl J Med. 2015;373(26):2522–2533.)

High-Yield Fast-Fact
- **Drug Development**
  - Numerous pipeline drugs are currently being investigated for the treatment of pulmonary arterial hypertension, including cromakalim (activators of Ca2+-activated and voltage-gated K+ channels and ATP-sensitive K+ channels), inhibitors of Notch signaling pathways, extracellular elastase inhibitors (elafin), and angiopoietin 1 inhibitors (trebananib).

HIGH-YIELD BOARD EXAM ESSENTIALS
- **CLASSIC AGENTS:** Epoprostenol, iloprost, treprostinil, selexipag
- **DRUG CLASS:** Synthetic prostacyclin & prostacyclin IP receptor agonist
- **INDICATIONS:** Pulmonary arterial hypertension
- **MECHANISM:** Epoprostenol, Iloprost, Treprostinil - Prostacyclin (PGI2) synthetic analogs induce pulmonary vascular smooth muscle relaxation, vasodilation, and inhibition of platelet aggregation. Selexipag - Selective prostacyclin IP receptor agonist, increasing cAMP and vascular smooth muscle relaxation causing pulmonary vasodilation.
- **SIDE EFFECTS:** Myalgias, jaw pain, nausea, diarrhea, abdominal pain, headaches, flushing, dizziness, and hypotension.
- **CLINICAL PEARLS:** In contrast to the other prostacyclin analogs, iloprost and treprostinil may be administered via inhalation. Iloprost must be administered six to up to 9 times per day, each taking up to 10 minutes to administer, and with each administration approximately 2 hours apart over the waking hours. Treprostinil is administered using three inhalations four times daily during waking hours.

Table: Drug Class Summary

Synthetic Prostacyclin & Prostacyclin IP Receptor Agonist - Drug Class Review			
High-Yield Med Reviews			
Mechanism of Action: *Epoprostenol, Iloprost, Treprostinil* - Prostacyclin (PGI2) synthetic analogs induce pulmonary vascular smooth muscle relaxation, vasodilation, and inhibition of platelet aggregation. *Selexipag* - Selective prostacyclin IP receptor agonist, increasing cAMP and vascular smooth muscle relaxation causing pulmonary vasodilation.			
Class Effects: Prostacyclin analogs and agonists induce pulmonary vasodilation, counteracting the physiology of pulmonary arterial hypertension, but due to administration complications and toxicities, they are generally reserved for WHO functional class II or higher.			
Generic Name	**Brand Name**	**Main Indication(s) or Uses**	**Notes**
Epoprostenol	Flolan, Veletri	• Pulmonary arterial hypertension	• **Dosing (Adult):** — IV: initial 2 nanogram/kg/minute, titrated by 1-2 ng/kg/minute q15minutes until dose-limiting adverse events occur — Target 25 to 40 ng/kg/minute — Inhalation: 20,000 ng/mL solution nebulized at 8mL/hour, titrating down q30min to q4h to 10,000 ng/mL, then 5,000 ng/mL, then 2,500 ng/mL • **Dosing (Peds):** — IV: initial 2 nanogram/kg/minute, titrated by 1-2 ng/kg/minute q15minutes until dose-limiting adverse events occur — Target: 25 to 40 ng/kg/minute — Continuous nebulization 20 to 50 ng/kg/minute • **CYP450 Interactions:** None • **Renal or Hepatic Dose Adjustments:** None • **Dosage Forms:** IV (solution)
Iloprost	Ventavis	• Pulmonary arterial hypertension	• **Dosing (Adult):** — Inhalation: 2.5 mcg/dose, increased to 5 mcg/dose administered 6 to 9 times daily no sooner than q2h while awake — Maximum 45 mcg/day • **Dosing (Peds):** — Inhalation: 2.5 mcg/dose, increased to 5 mcg/dose administered 6 to 9 times daily no sooner than q2h while awake — Maximum 45 mcg/day — Inhalation: 0.5 mcg/kg over 10 minutes, increased q10minutes to 2 mcg/kg • **CYP450 Interactions:** None • **Renal or Hepatic Dose Adjustments:** — Child-Pugh class B or C - Increase dosing interval to q3-4h • **Dosage Forms:** Inhalation solution

Synthetic Prostacyclin & Prostacyclin IP Receptor Agonist - Drug Class Review High-Yield Med Reviews			
Generic Name	**Brand Name**	**Main Indication(s) or Uses**	**Notes**

Treprostinil	Orenitram
	Remodulin
	Tyvaso
		• Pulmonary arterial hypertension	• **Dosing (Adult):**
			   – Inhalation: 18 mcg QID while awake, titrated by 18 mcg q1-2weeks to maximum 54 mcg/dose QID while awake
			   – Oral: 0.125 mg q8h, titrated by 0.125 mg/dose q3-4days to target 8 mg TID
			   – Oral: 0.25 mg q12h, titrated by 0.25 or 0.5 mg/dose q3-4days to target 8 mg TID
			   – IV/SQ: 1.25 nanogram/kg/minute, titrated by 1.25 nanogram/kg/minute q1week for 4 weeks, then 2.5 nanogram/kg/minute q1week to target dose of 40 to 80 ng/kg/minute
			• **Dosing (Peds):**
			   – Not routinely used
			• **CYP450 Interactions:** Substrate CYP2C8, 2C9
			• **Renal or Hepatic Dose Adjustments:**
			   – Oral dosage form only
			      – Child-Pugh class B: Avoid use
			      – Child-Pugh class C: Contraindicated
			• **Dosage Forms:** Inhalation solution, IV solution

Selexipag	Uptravi	• Pulmonary arterial hypertension	• **Dosing (Adult):**
			   – Oral: 200 to 1,600 mcg BID
			• **Dosing (Peds):**
			   – Not routinely used
			• **CYP450 Interactions:** Substrate CYP2C8, 3A4
			• **Renal or Hepatic Dose Adjustments:**
			   – Child-Pugh class B: Administer once daily
			   – Child-Pugh class C: Avoid use
			• **Dosage Forms:** Oral (tablet)

2025

A COMPREHENSIVE *RAPID REVIEW*

NAPLEX

Pharmacology & Drug Classes

Practice Exam – Drug Classes

NAPLEX PRACTICE QUESTIONS & ANSWERS – DRUG CLASS REVIEWS

PRACTICING QUESTIONS IS THE KEY TO SUCCESS!
- ✓ **FACT:** To get licensed you must pass a multiple-choice exam!
- ✓ **FACT:** Failing to practice applying concepts is a plan for failure.
- ✓ **FACT:** Buying this book gives you access to a FREE 150-question practice exam.
- ✓ **FACT:** Buying this book allows you to upgrade to our review courses at a discount!

1. Which medication has a significant drug interaction with warfarin?

    a. Amiodarone
    b. Carvedilol
    c. Pioglitazone
    d. Lamotrigine

2. Which medication would most likely cause anticholinergic adverse effects?

    a. Metformin
    b. Buspirone
    c. Atenolol
    d. Tolterodine

3. A 5-year-old patient requires amoxicillin for acute otitis media. The patient weighs 46 pounds, and a 400 mg / 5 mL suspension is available. What is the correct dosing regimen for this patient?

    a. 5 mL daily
    b. 5 mL twice daily
    c. 10.5 mL twice daily
    d. 10 mL three times daily

4. Which medication is indicated to treat infections with Pseudomonas aeruginosa?

    a. Tigecycline
    b. Azithromycin
    c. Ceftazidime
    d. Ampicillin-sulbactam

5. You are evaluating a patient has HTN, heart failure with reduced ejection fraction, COPD, type 2 diabetes, osteoporosis, and obesity. They are currently taking enalapril, metoprolol succinate, fluticasone and

vilanterol, albuterol as needed, alendronate, metformin, and liraglutide. Their blood pressure today is 145/92 mm Hg and has been elevated at home. Their glucose is well-controlled. Which medication would be best to add to their regimen if needed?

- a. Furosemide
- b. Spironolactone
- c. Dapagliflozin
- d. Amlodipine

6. Which statement is true regarding the mechanism of action for tenecteplase?
    - a. Converts fibrin-bound plasminogen to plasmin
    - b. Increase fibrin formation
    - c. Blocks factor Xa action
    - d. Inhibits the conversion of fibrinogen to fibrin

7. Which patient can safely receive the FluMist Quadrivalent vaccine?

    - a. Patient with HIV
    - b. Patient who is pregnant
    - c. Patient who is 18 months old
    - d. Patient taking tramadol

8. What adverse effect is common with HMG-CoA reductase inhibitors?

    - a. Diarrhea
    - b. Myalgias
    - c. Seizures
    - d. Tachycardia

9. Which medication is a RANKL inhibitor?

    - a. Romosozumab
    - b. Atogepant
    - c. Denosumab
    - d. Atomoxetine

10. Which medication may cause serotonin syndrome?

    - a. Succinylcholine
    - b. Gabapentin
    - c. Viloxazine
    - d. Paroxetine

11. The following drugs are known to have warnings listed in their product package inserts regarding adverse effects in patients with certain genetic polymorphisms, EXCEPT:

a. Metoprolol
b. Allopurinol
c. Carbamazepine
d. Phenytoin

12. A patient has blood cultures positive for Methicillin-resistant Staphylococcus aureus and was started on vancomycin 1 gram every 12 hours. What would be an appropriate trough concentration to continue the current dose and frequency?

    a. 8 mg/dL
    b. 12 mg/dL
    c. 18 mg/dL
    d. 28 mg/dL

13. What is the brand name of latanoprost?

    a. Lumigan
    b. Pataday
    c. Cortisporin-TC
    d. Xalatan

14. You are seeing a 42-year-old patient has a past medical history of hypertension, dyslipidemia, obesity, GERD, and allergic rhinitis. The patient is currently taking Norvasc, Lipitor, Ozempic, Protonix, and Zyrtec. Which medication was prescribed without a correct indication?

    a. Ozempic
    b. Lipitor
    c. Norvasc
    d. Protonix

15. Which of the following demonstrates the correct dosing of a new direct oral anticoagulant for stroke prevention in atrial fibrillation?

    a. Rivaroxaban 15 mg daily
    b. Edoxaban 60 mg twice daily
    c. Apixaban 5 mg twice daily
    d. Dabigatran 75 mg twice daily

16. A 52-year-old patient was discharged 1 week ago from the hospital due to an ST-segment elevation MI. Their medications include clopidogrel, lisinopril, metoprolol succinate, rosuvastatin, and nitroglycerin SL as needed, and they have no known allergies. Which medication is missing from their regimen?

a. Spironolactone
b. Aspirin
c. Enoxaparin
d. Isosorbide mononitrate

17. What should be monitored in a patient using AndroGel? Select all that apply.

    a. Hemoglobin and hematocrit
    b. Blood pressure
    c. Potassium
    d. Liver function tests

18. Which medication is recommended first-line for treatment of status epilepticus?

    a. Lorazepam
    b. Alprazolam
    c. Lamotrigine
    d. Carbamazepine

19. Which medication should be avoided in the first trimester of pregnancy?

    a. Loratadine
    b. Methimazole
    c. Nitrofurantoin
    d. Sertraline

20. Which drug has the correct dose and rate of administration for cardiogenic shock?

    a. Milrinone 1 mg/kg/minute
    b. Epinephrine 2 mg/kg/minute
    c. Dopamine 75 mcg/kg/minute
    d. Norepinephrine IV 0.5 mcg/kg/minute

ANSWERS & RATIONALE

1. A
   Amiodarone interacts with warfarin; reduce warfarin dose 30-50% with amiodarone initiation and monitor closely for further adjustment until steady state is achieved over weeks.

2. D
   Tolterodine is an anticholinergic drug used in overactive bladder treatment for its urinary retention properties associated with its anticholinergic actions. Common anticholinergic adverse effects include dry eyes, blurry vision, dry mouth, dizziness, confusion, drowsiness, hallucinations, flushing, tachycardia, or constipation.

3. C
   Convert weight to kg (46 lbs / 2.2 lbs = 20.9 kg). Dosing for acute otitis media to achieve ear penetration is 80-90 mg/kg/day (20.9 kg x 80 mg = 1672.7 mg/d). Divide into 2 doses (1672.7 mg / 2 = 836.4 mg twice

daily). Suspension is available in 400 mg / 5 mL concentration (836.4 mg / x = 400 mg / 5 mL; x = 10.5 mL twice daily). Other options would be under- or overdosing.

4. C
Ceftazidime is a third-generation cephalosporin with activity against Pseudomonas aeruginosa. Tigecycline is effective against MRSA and other gram-positive, gram-negative, and anaerobic organisms. Azithromycin is a macrolide with activity against common respiratory pathogens but not Pseudomonas. Ampicillin-sulbactam covers gram-positive, gram-negative, and anaerobic bacteria but not Pseudomonas or extended-spectrum beta-lactamases.

5. B
Spironolactone can reduce blood pressure and improve mortality in heart failure with reduced ejection fraction while improving hypertension. Patients should always be treated with medications known to reduce mortality before moving on to other treatments. Dapagliflozin would be indicated to reduce CV death and HF hospitalizations, but the patient's diabetes is controlled, and there is potential for fracture risk with SGLT2 inhibitors. Furosemide and amlodipine could be used but would not confer additional mortality benefit.

6. A
Tenecteplase converts fibrin-bound plasminogen to plasmin to break down clots in stroke and STEMI, as well as other off-label uses. A drug that increased fibrin formation would increase clotting. Factor Xa inhibitors include apixaban, edoxaban, fondaparinux, and rivaroxaban. Heparin inhibits the conversion of fibrinogen to fibrin. Out of these drugs, tenecteplase is the only one that breaks down clots.

7. D
FluMist Quadrivalent is a live vaccine that should not be given to patients who are immunocompromised or on immunosuppressant drugs, pregnant, or under 24 months old because of the increased risks of potential vaccine-induced infection. A patient taking varenicline for smoking cessation could receive FluMist Quadrivalent.

8. B
Myalgias are common adverse effects associated with statins. The other adverse effects are not commonly associated with HMG-CoA reductase inhibitors.

9. C
Denosumab is a RANKL inhibitor (osteoporosis). Atogepant is a CGRP receptor antagonist. Romosozumab is a sclerostin inhibitor. Atomoxetine is an NRI.

10. D
Paroxetine is an SSRI that may cause serotonin syndrome due to inhibiting the reuptake of serotonin. Combination with other drugs that increase serotonin further increases the risk of serotonin syndrome. The other agents do not modulate serotonin.

11. A
Genetic testing is not recommended for metoprolol. Allopurinol (HLA-B*5801) or carbamazepine (HLA-B*1502) may cause severe cutaneous adverse reactions with these alleles. Abacavir (HLA-B*5701) has a higher risk of hypersensitivity reactions with this allele. Phenytoin (HLA-B*1502 and CYP2C9*3) carries a higher risk of SJS or TEN with these genetic changes.

12. C
Vancomycin trough concentrations should be between 15-20 mg/dL. This is a surrogate marker for an AUC:MIC ratio of > 400 mg-h/L, which indicates clinical efficacy.

13. D
    Xalatan is the brand name of latanoprost.
14. A
    Ozempic does not have a correct indication based on the past medical history. Ozempic (semaglutide up to 2 mg) is indicated for type 2 diabetes. Wegovy (semaglutide 2.4 mg) is indicated for obesity.

15. C
    Apixaban 5 mg twice daily is the correct dosing for atrial fibrillation unless the patient has 2 of the following (give apixaban 2.5 mg twice daily): age ≥ 80 years, weight ≤ 60 kg, or SCr ≥ 1.5 mg/dL. Rivaroxaban is dosed at 20 mg daily for atrial fibrillation. Edoxaban is dosed at 60 mg daily and not used if CrCl > 95 mL/min. Dabigatran is dosed at 150 mg twice daily with an option to give 110 mg twice daily with an increased risk for bleeding. NOAC dosing varies based on indication, bleeding risk, renal function, age, weight, and potentially other patient-specific clinical factors.

16. B
    Aspirin and clopidogrel should be continued at least 12 months after STEMI. Spironolactone could be an option depending on the clinical scenario. Enoxaparin would be discontinued prior to discharge. Isosorbide mononitrate is used in angina and is not required.

17. A, B, D
    Monitor hemoglobin and hematocrit, blood pressure, and liver function tests with testosterone because testosterone replacement may cause polycythemia, BP elevations, and liver impairment, respectively.

18. A
    Lorazepam is recommended for status epilepticus and preferred when IV access is available. Alprazolam, lamotrigine, and carbamazepine are only available in oral dosage forms with slower onsets of action, which is inappropriate for status epilepticus.

19. B
    Methimazole is teratogenic during the 1st trimester but is preferred over propylthiouracil in the 2nd/3rd trimesters. Loratadine is used during pregnancy for allergic rhinitis. Nitrofurantoin is contraindicated between 38-42 weeks of pregnancy. Sertraline is a preferred SSRI.

20. D
    Norepinephrine 2 mcg/kg/minute is an appropriate rate of administration. The other doses and administration rates are significantly too high and would cause serious adverse effects and possibly death.

www.ingramcontent.com/pod-product-compliance
Lightning Source LLC
LaVergne TN
LVHW061931070526
838199LV00060B/3816